W9-ARY-336

FOOD SCIENCE

An Ecological Approach

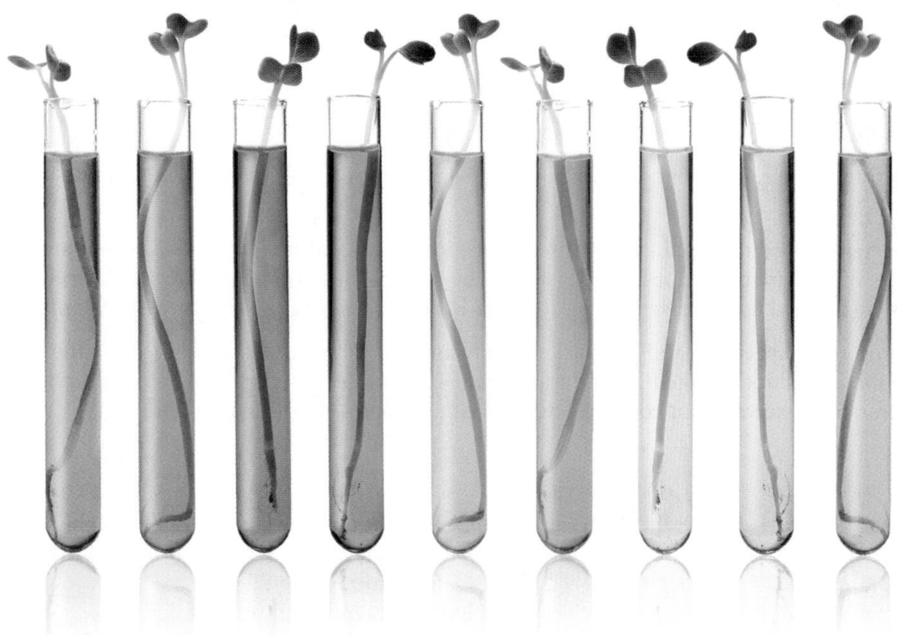

EDITED BY

SARI EDELSTEIN, PhD, RD

Department of Nutrition

Simmons College

Boston, Massachusetts

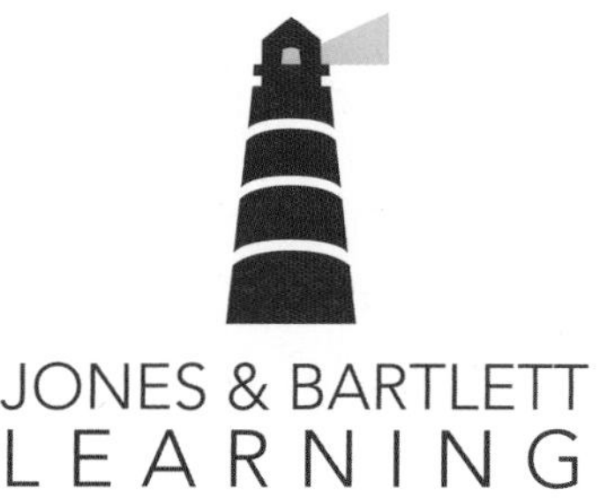

JONES & BARTLETT
LEARNING

World Headquarters
Jones & Bartlett Learning
5 Wall Street
Burlington, MA 01803
978-443-5000
info@jblearning.com
www.jblearning.com

Jones & Bartlett Learning books and products are available through most bookstores and online booksellers. To contact Jones & Bartlett Learning directly, call 800-832-0034, fax 978-443-8000, or visit our website, www.jblearning.com.

Substantial discounts on bulk quantities of Jones & Bartlett Learning publications are available to corporations, professional associations, and other qualified organizations. For details and specific discount information, contact the special sales department at Jones & Bartlett Learning via the above contact information or send an email to specialsales@jblearning.com.

Production Credits

Chief Executive Officer: Ty Field
President: James Homer
SVP, Editor-in-Chief: Michael Johnson
SVP, Chief Marketing Officer: Alison M. Pendergast
Publisher: William Brottmiller
Executive Editor: Shoshanna Goldberg
Editorial Assistant: Agnes Burt
Production Editor: Jessica Steele Newfell
Senior Marketing Manager: Jennifer Stiles
Production Services Manager: Colleen Lamy
Online Products Manager: Dawn Mahon Priest
VP, Manufacturing and Inventory Control: Therese Connell
Composition: diacriTech
Developmental Editor: Jennifer Angel
Cover and Title Page Design: Scott Moden
Rights & Photo Research Associate: Amy Rathburn
Cover, Title Page, and Front Matter Opener Image: © Nixx Photography/ShutterStock, Inc.
Printing and Binding: Courier Companies
Cover Printing: Courier Companies

To order this product, use ISBN: 978-1-4496-9477-7

Library of Congress Cataloging-in-Publication Data

Food science: an ecological approach / edited by Sari Edelstein.
p.; cm.
Includes bibliographical references and index.
ISBN 978-1-4496-0344-1 — ISBN 1-4496-0344-0
I. Edelstein, Sari.
[DNLM: 1. Food Technology. 2. Conservation of Natural Resources. 3. Dietetics. 4. Food Safety. 5. Food Supply. WA 695]
363.19'26—dc23
2012032100

6048

Printed in the United States of America
17 16 15 14 13 10 9 8 7 6 5 4 3 2 1

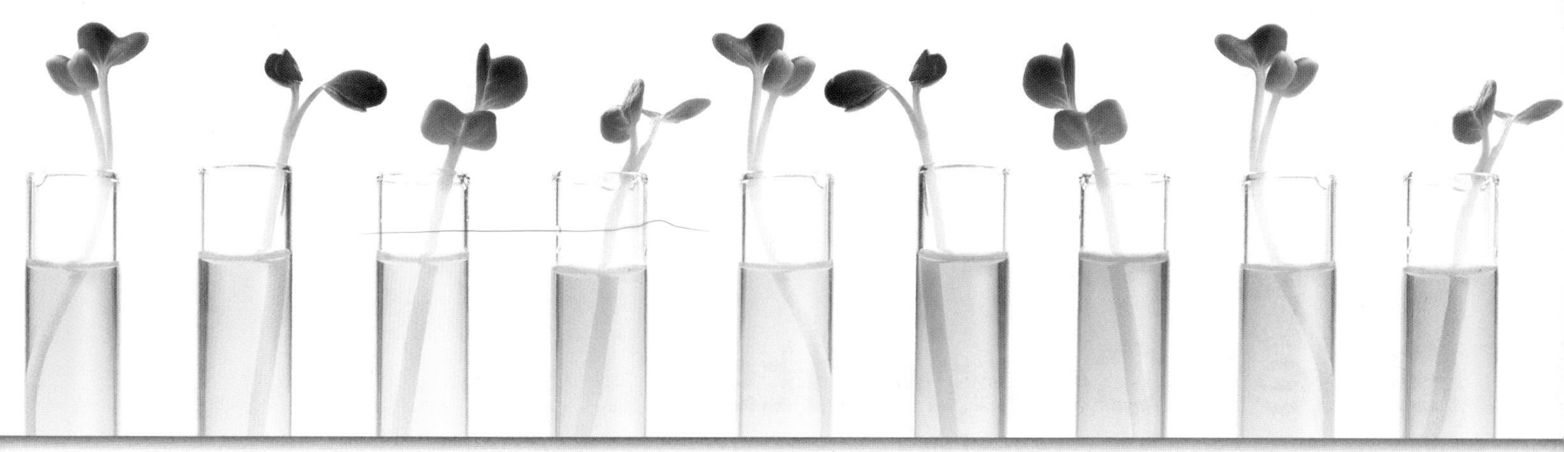

This book is dedicated to my beautiful daughters, Jodi Rachael and Staci Michelle.
No mother could be more proud of the women you have become.

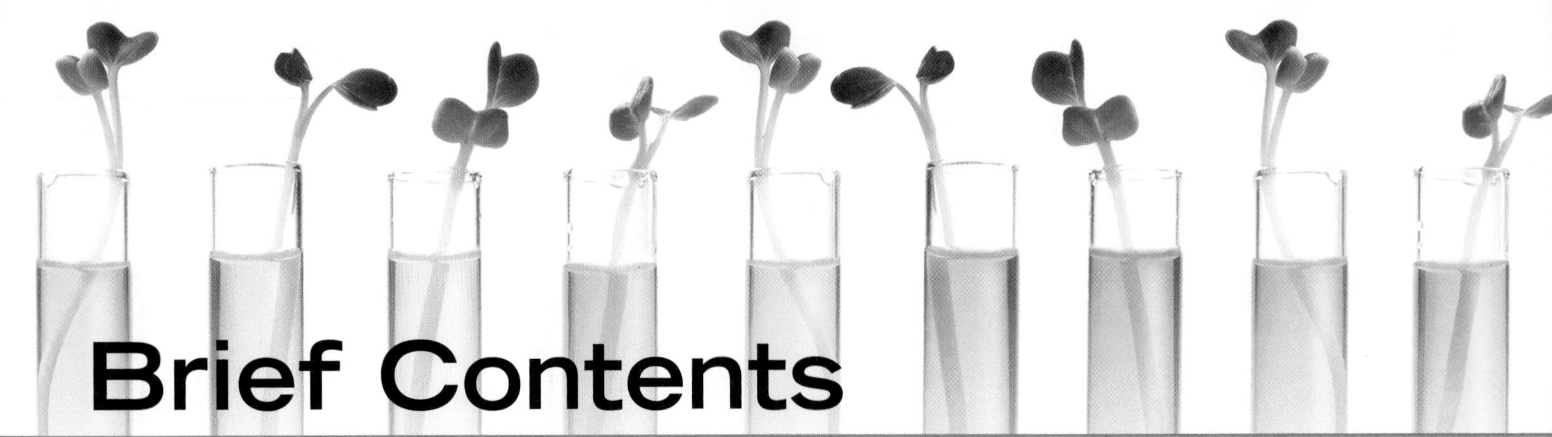

Brief Contents

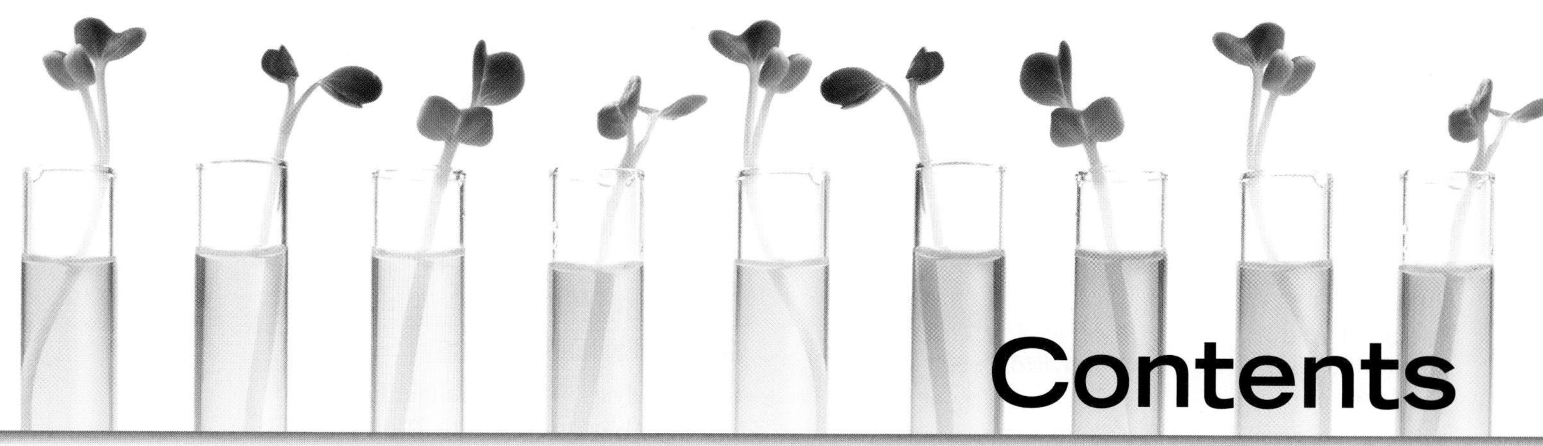

Contents

Preface

Why the Ecological Approach?

Sari Edelstein, PhD, RD

The subject of food science includes the study of plant and animal sources at the cellular level. Different species have evolved based on their environments and genetic changes over time. Ecological changes can have devastating consequences for a plant or animal species. For example, the Irish potato famine that occurred in the 1800s was the result of a virulent fungus (*Phytophthora infestans*) whose spores were spread by wind. Similarly, droughts, such as that seen in 2011 in Somalia, can have a negative effect on animal and plant life in a region. The role of food scientists in these types of scenarios is to potentially find plants that are able to survive in such changing environmental conditions.

Food scientists are being challenged to find and develop plant and animal species that are more tolerant of the Earth's changing ecology (natural or manmade) in order to provide food that is rich in nutrients (food composition and quality), cost-effective, and available to all people (food technology and delivery systems).

Let us examine some of the environmental changes (natural or manmade) that may affect the world's food supply in the future:*

- *Increases in average temperature*. An increase in the average temperature in a region can (1) lengthen the growing season in regions with a relatively cool spring and fall, (2) adversely affect crops in regions where summer heat already limits production, (3) increase soil evaporation rates, and (4) increase the chance of severe drought.
- *Changes in rainfall amounts and patterns*. Changes in rainfall can affect soil erosion rates and soil moisture, both of which are important for crop yields. In addition, it is predicted that climate change will increase the number of extreme precipitation events.
- *Increases in pollution levels*. Higher levels of ground-level ozone will limit the growth of crops. Because ozone levels in the lower atmosphere are shaped by both emissions and temperature, climate change will most likely increase atmospheric ozone concentrations.
- *Change in climatic variability and extreme events*. Increased frequency and severity of heat waves, drought, floods, and hurricanes are a potential result of climate change.

This text examines food science within the context of the modern world we live in today. Although the scientific principles remain the same, they must be viewed through a new lens, one that marries food science with present-day concerns regarding food quality, composition, and availability. Each chapter of this textbook brings to light some of these challenges facing food scientists.

This text approaches food science from an ecological perspective. The science of food remains at the very core of this book, as reflected by the concepts and principles that students are required to master. Section I of *Food Science: An Ecological Approach* presents the introductory concepts students studying food science are required to learn. Using concise language and an engaging writing style, these foundational chapters provide students with the background to understand the relationship between food science and the environment, research methods used by food scientists, and the underlying science and chemistry behind food composition.

Chapter 1, "Food Science and the Natural Environment," anchors food science within the natural environment. After reading this chapter, students will be able to conceptualize how environmental conditions affect food composition and sources. Principles such as ecosystems, crop yield, sustainable agriculture, and biodiversity are just some of the important concepts introduced in the chapter.

Chapter 2, "How Food Science Is Guided by Research," presents the traditional evidence-based research models that students will need to embrace as a part of validating food science facts. Chapter 2 also explores some of the various types of scientific studies, including analytical studies; case-control studies; case reports and case series; cohort studies; cross-sectional surveys; descriptive studies; double-blind, placebo-controlled designs; hypothesis testing; intervention

---

* Data from Parry ML, Canziani OF, Palutikof JP, van der Linden PJ, Hanson CE (eds.). *Climate Change 2007: Impacts, Adaptation, and Vulnerability. Contribution of Working Group II to the Third Assessment Report of the Intergovernmental Panel on Climate Change.* Cambridge, UK: Cambridge University Press; 2008.

studies; longitudinal surveys; observational studies; population or correlational studies; and randomized designs.

Chapter 3, "Sensory Evaluation," discusses the traditional sensory evaluation techniques food scientists use for taste tests. After reading this chapter, students will understand traditional taste panel methods, product and panelist control, sensory tests, and test scaling.

Chapter 4, "Food Composition," establishes students' foundational knowledge of the chemical structures and chemical reactions common to food. This foundational knowledge is critical to understanding the later chapters of the text. The chapter presents the chemical building blocks of foods through discussion of carbohydrates, starches, lipids, proteins, vitamins, and minerals.

Section II of *Food Science: An Ecological Approach* provides a focused discussion of the types of food and the science behind each. Using a consistent presentation, each chapter discusses each food's historical, cultural, and ecological significance; its physical and chemical properties; preparation techniques and food safety concerns; and its impact on health.

Chapter 5, "Meat and Meat Substitutes," delves into the study of meat and meat substitutes. Content coverage includes muscle structure, meat cuts, and factors affecting the composition of meat.

Chapter 6, "Poultry and Fish," explores the structure of poultry and fish as well as nutritional and environmental issues with regard to poultry and fish consumption.

Chapter 7, "Milk and Dairy Products," presents milk and dairy products. Topics include issues pertaining to the production and purchase of milk and dairy products and their uses in recipes.

Chapter 8, "Eggs and Egg Replacements," examines egg-related food science topics such as egg production, quality, and grading and the use of eggs in cooked foods.

Chapter 9, "Vegetarianism," presents information on the different types of vegetarian diets and the prevalence of vegetarianism in the United States. The chapter compares the health effects of vegetarian, vegan, and omnivorous diets.

Chapter 10, "Fruits and Vegetables," presents the classification of fruits and vegetables. It also includes a discussion of the structural parts of fruits and vegetables and the various types of pigments present in plant products. Students will learn about the health benefits of plants as a source of phytonutrients and their use as functional foods.

Chapter 11, "Grains, Cereals, Pasta, Flour, and Starch Cookery," presents the food science behind grains, cereals, pastas, and starch cookery. Students will learn about the different types of grains and cereals. The anatomy of grains and cereals and various cooking methods are also discussed. A special feature on the use of starch thickeners for use in dysphagia is also provided.

Chapter 12, "Yeast Breads, Quick Breads, and Cakes," focuses on yeast breads, quick breads, and cakes. Particular attention is paid to the mixing, kneading, rising, and baking of yeast breads. The preparation of cakes and quick breads is also discussed. Students will learn about the role of various ingredients in the preparation of doughs and batters.

Chapter 13, "Fats and Oils," discusses the role of fats and oils in food science. Among the topics discussed are saturated fats, monounsaturated fats, and fat substitutes. The effects of heat on fats and oils are explored. The effects of rancidity on foods are also presented.

Chapter 14, "Sugar and Sugar Substitutes," introduces students to the structure of sugar and sugar replacements, as well as their use in baked goods and other products. Students will become familiar with the different sources of sugar, its chemical properties, and its use in baked goods and candy making. A detailed discussion of the various sugar replacements is also provided.

Chapter 15, "Beverages," focuses on coffee, tea, and sports drinks, discussing the composition, quality, and nutritional benefits of each. Focused discussions of soda, wine, and liquors are presented individually through Special Topics features within the chapter.

Chapter 16, "Food Preservation and Packaging," presents the most current information related to food preservation and packaging. Traditional methods of food preservation are discussed, including heat treatments, freezing, drying, and irradiation. New technologies, such as high pressure treatments, pulsed light and ultrasound technology, and the use of alternative chemicals, are also presented. Different methods and materials for food packaging are also discussed.

Special Topic

Careers in Food Science

Jackeline Barreto

A food scientist, or food technologist, looks for better ways to select, preserve, process, package, and distribute food products, including the ingredients that go into them. A food scientist also must have extensive knowledge about the nature, composition, and behavior of food, such as what happens to its flavor, color, or nutritional properties when cooked or placed in storage. Biology, microbiology, chemistry, and engineering are just some of the diverse fields of study that food science draws upon to ensure safe, high-quality consumer products.[1]

Food scientists and technologists usually work at universities or food processing facilities. Their main objective is to improve food products by finding a more effective and efficient way to preserve, package, store, or deliver foods. It is the responsibility of the food scientist to analyze and determine the nutritional content of the food with respect to carbohydrates, fats, proteins, sugars, vitamins, minerals, and so on. In addition, food scientists work with government agencies and corporations to make sure that food safety, food quality, food waste, and food disposal regulations are being met.

Food scientists may be involved in discovering new food sources; analyzing a food item to determine its vitamin, fat, sugar, or protein content; or searching for substitutes for harmful or undesirable additives, such as nitrites. Other food scientists may engage in applied research, finding ways to improve the content of food or to remove harmful additives. Food scientists are also involved in exploring better ways to process, preserve, package, or store food according to industry and government regulations. Some continue to research improvements in traditional food processing techniques, such as baking, blanching, canning, drying, evaporation, and pasteurization.[2]

Because of the wealth of knowledge that food scientists must draw upon, a career in food science requires a bachelor's degree, but a master's or doctorate is often preferred. Some states require that certain food scientists have proper licensure, such as that required for soil scientists. Today, 31,000 food scientists are working in the United States, and job growth for food scientists is greater than average compared to other occupations. It can also be a well-paying career, with an average salary of $56,030 and a median income ranging from $43,600 to $81,340.[3]

References

1 U.S. Department of Agriculture. Food Science and Technology. Available at: http://www.ars.usda.gov/is/kids/scientists/foodscientist.htm. Accessed November 1, 2011.

2 Institute of Food Technology. What Is Food Science and Technology? 2011. Available at: http://www.ift.org/Knowledge-Center/Learn-About-Food-Science/What-is-Food-Science.aspx. Accessed December 6, 2011.

3 Bureau of Labor Statistics. Agricultural and Food Scientist. 2009. Available at: http://www.bls.gov/oco/ocos046.htm. Accessed December 6, 2011.

Features of This Text

Food Science: An Ecological Approach incorporates a number of engaging pedagogical features to aid in the student's understanding and retention of the material.

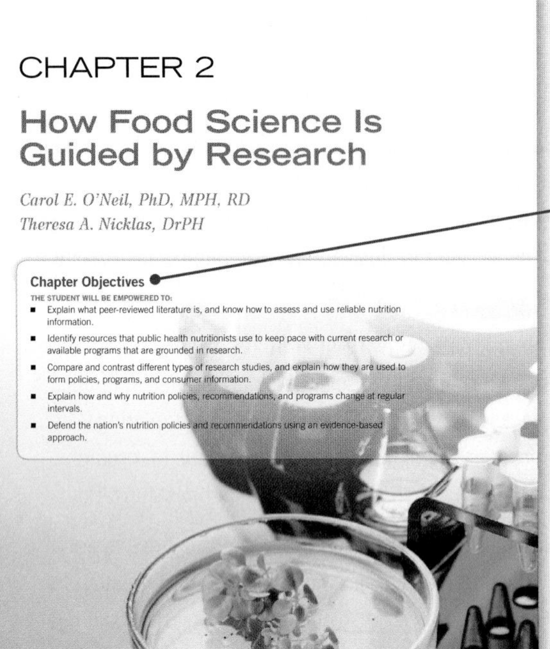
CHAPTER 2
How Food Science Is Guided by Research
Carol E. O'Neil, PhD, MPH, RD
Theresa A. Nicklas, DrPH
Chapter Objectives
THE STUDENT WILL BE EMPOWERED TO:
Explain what peer-reviewed literature is, and know how to assess and use reliable nutrition information.
Identify resources that public health nutritionists use to keep pace with current research or available programs that are grounded in research.
Compare and contrast different types of research studies, and explain how they are used to form policies, programs, and consumer information.
Explain how and why nutrition policies, recommendations, and programs change at regular intervals.
Defend the nation's nutrition policies and recommendations using an evidence-based approach.

Each chapter starts with **Chapter Objectives**, which highlight the critical points of each chapter.

shell membranes Two membranes, outer and inner, that surround the albumen (white) of an egg; they provide a protective barrier against bacterial penetration.

Salmonella Rod-shaped bacteria responsible for many foodborne illnesses.

Key Terms are defined throughout the chapter to enhance comprehension.

Chapter Review

Food science encompasses the investigation of better ways to select, preserve, process, package, and distribute food products. It includes the study of the composition of food ingredients and their manipulation during growing, production, processing, and presentation to the consumer.

Although many of the scientific principles remain the same as for traditional food science, many must be evaluated with an additional factor or concern. This factor is *ecology*, which impacts food quality, composition, and availability. Some steps to address solutions to the changing environment presented in this chapter include:

- Identifying present ecological practices and providing suggested improvements such as sustainability
- Tackling food waste and advocating the use of whole foods
- Addressing climate change and its affect on crops and providing suggestions of crop change
- Focusing on improved individual diet patterns that may be better for our environment
- Highlighting the effect of the changing environment and its impact on health
- Identifying business practices that demonstrate good nutrition with ecology in mind.

At the end of each chapter, a **Chapter Review** summarizes key ideas and helps students remember the different concepts discussed in the chapter and how the concepts interrelate.

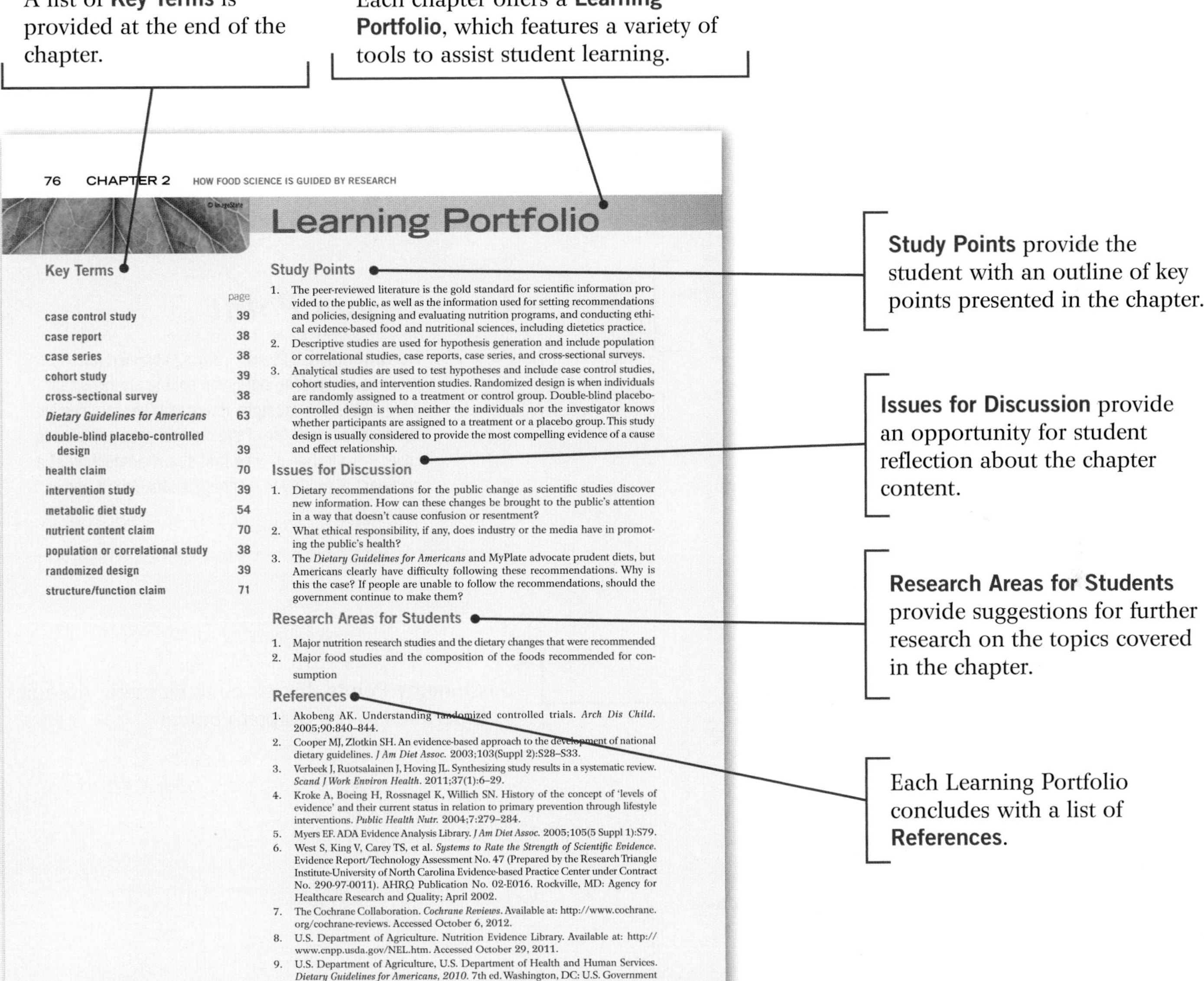

A list of **Key Terms** is provided at the end of the chapter.
Each chapter offers a **Learning Portfolio**, which features a variety of tools to assist student learning.
Study Points provide the student with an outline of key points presented in the chapter.
Issues for Discussion provide an opportunity for student reflection about the chapter content.
Research Areas for Students provide suggestions for further research on the topics covered in the chapter.
Each Learning Portfolio concludes with a list of **References.**

76 CHAPTER 2 HOW FOOD SCIENCE IS GUIDED BY RESEARCH

© ImageState

Learning Portfolio

Key Terms

	page
case control study	39
case report	38
case series	38
cohort study	39
cross-sectional survey	38
Dietary Guidelines for Americans	63
double-blind placebo-controlled design	39
health claim	70
intervention study	39
metabolic diet study	54
nutrient content claim	70
population or correlational study	38
randomized design	39
structure/function claim	71

Study Points

1. The peer-reviewed literature is the gold standard for scientific information provided to the public, as well as the information used for setting recommendations and policies, designing and evaluating nutrition programs, and conducting ethical evidence-based food and nutritional sciences, including dietetics practice.
2. Descriptive studies are used for hypothesis generation and include population or correlational studies, case reports, case series, and cross-sectional surveys.
3. Analytical studies are used to test hypotheses and include case control studies, cohort studies, and intervention studies. Randomized design is when individuals are randomly assigned to a treatment or control group. Double-blind placebo-controlled design is when neither the individuals nor the investigator knows whether participants are assigned to a treatment or a placebo group. This study design is usually considered to provide the most compelling evidence of a cause and effect relationship.

Issues for Discussion

1. Dietary recommendations for the public change as scientific studies discover new information. How can these changes be brought to the public's attention in a way that doesn't cause confusion or resentment?
2. What ethical responsibility, if any, does industry or the media have in promoting the public's health?
3. The *Dietary Guidelines for Americans* and MyPlate advocate prudent diets, but Americans clearly have difficulty following these recommendations. Why is this the case? If people are unable to follow the recommendations, should the government continue to make them?

Research Areas for Students

1. Major nutrition research studies and the dietary changes that were recommended
2. Major food studies and the composition of the foods recommended for consumption

References

1. Akobeng AK. Understanding randomized controlled trials. *Arch Dis Child.* 2005;90:840–844.
2. Cooper MJ, Zlotkin SH. An evidence-based approach to the development of national dietary guidelines. *J Am Diet Assoc.* 2003;103(Suppl 2):S28–S33.
3. Verbeek J, Ruotsalainen J, Hoving JL. Synthesizing study results in a systematic review. *Scand J Work Environ Health.* 2011;37(1):6–29.
4. Kroke A, Boeing H, Rossnagel K, Willich SN. History of the concept of 'levels of evidence' and their current status in relation to primary prevention through lifestyle interventions. *Public Health Nutr.* 2004;7:279–284.
5. Myers EF. ADA Evidence Analysis Library. *J Am Diet Assoc.* 2005;105(5 Suppl 1):S79.
6. West S, King V, Carey TS, et al. *Systems to Rate the Strength of Scientific Evidence.* Evidence Report/Technology Assessment No. 47 (Prepared by the Research Triangle Institute-University of North Carolina Evidence-based Practice Center under Contract No. 290-97-0011). AHRQ Publication No. 02-E016. Rockville, MD: Agency for Healthcare Research and Quality; April 2002.
7. The Cochrane Collaboration. *Cochrane Reviews.* Available at: http://www.cochrane.org/cochrane-reviews. Accessed October 6, 2012.
8. U.S. Department of Agriculture. Nutrition Evidence Library. Available at: http://www.cnpp.usda.gov/NEL.htm. Accessed October 29, 2011.
9. U.S. Department of Agriculture, U.S. Department of Health and Human Services. *Dietary Guidelines for Americans, 2010.* 7th ed. Washington, DC: U.S. Government

Dough Conditioners

In commercial baking, **dough conditioners** are used to improve the finished bread product, yielding better volume and softer crumb. **Crumb** refers to dry particles in the crust. Conditioners are classified by their functions on the dough:[13,19-24]

- *Oxidizing agents* adjust the acidity of dough and thereby affect the number of disulfide bonds in the gluten and gluten-forming molecules.
- *Reducing agents*, such as L-cysteine, interact with gluten to reduce elasticity.
- *Emulsifiers*, such as mono- and diglycerides, reduce the degree or rate at which bread goes stale.
- *Enzymes*, most commonly fungal amylases, are used for varying purposes, including extending product shelf life, reducing the required mix time, and improving the texture of the finished product.

Making Yeast Breads

The process of making yeast bread comprises mixing, kneading, fermenting/rising, shaping, and baking (see **Figure 12.3**).

Mixing

The most important stage of the bread making process is mixing. Mixing allows all the ingredients to be incorporated uniformly into the mixture. This promotes the development of gluten structures that trap air bubbles from the yeast, allowing the dough to rise. A number of different options are available for mixing:[13,19,20,25,26]

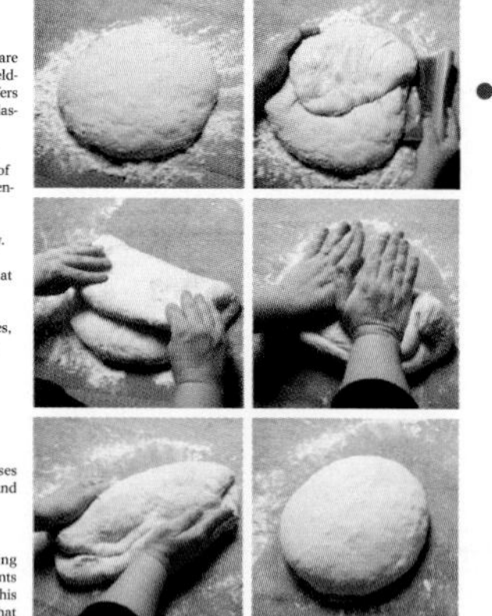

FIGURE 12.3 Making yeast bread consists of a number of steps: mixing, kneading, fermenting/rising, shaping, and baking.

A comprehensive and instructional **art package** includes color photographs and illustrations throughout this text to encourage learning with a unique visual appeal.

Green Points provide contextual suggestions for living a sustainable lifestyle.

Green Point

Commercial Bread Buying commercial bread is convenient, but home baking offers certain advantages. For example, fewer additives are needed because the shelf life of the product does not need to cover the duration of time that spans production at a commercial facility to reaching a consumer's home.

Gastronomy Point

Popcorn Popcorn has been eaten for centuries and is considered the oldest snack food. For a salt-free, low-fat treat, season plain popcorn with savory, sweet, or hot and spicy seasonings.

Gastronomy Points discuss cooking methodologies as it pertains to the chapter context.

Phytonutrient Points discuss the health benefits of food components.

Phytonutrient Point

Alpha-Linolenic Acid Alpha-linolenic acid, found in flaxseed, walnut, and canola oils, can be converted into DHA and EPA, although the efficiency of conversion is very low in the human body. Nevertheless, it is an important omega-3 fatty acid, especially in a vegetarian diet.

Innovation Point

The Internet as a Source of Information Today, for health professionals and consumers alike, a bewildering array of information is available on the Internet. Reliable sites have URLs ending in .edu or .gov. These sites often present a distillation of information from the peer-reviewed literature or other reliable sources. Using the Internet to locate information can save valuable time; however, any information found on the Internet should be approached with caution and evaluated carefully.

Innovation Points discuss developments in the field of food science.

Special Topics pays particular attention to singular points featured throughout the context of the chapter.

Special Topic 6.2

Sauces for Chicken and Fish

Maura Grimes

Sauces provide a flavorful component to chicken and fish dishes. Different ingredients result in the different tastes and textures of sauces. Cream, milk, and flour can be used to create thick sauces. Egg yolks help the sauce to emulsify, giving it a creamy texture. Vinegar provides an acidic taste and helps to tenderize fish or chicken. Butter provides a delicious fatty flavor that goes especially well with fish. Wine has a delicious flavor that enhances the overall dish. Overall, the different tastes in sauces are directly influenced by the ingredients included. The key to making a good sauce is having an understanding of the different ingredients and the effect they will have.

Roux-based sauces are white sauces that typically contain butter, flour, and milk. A basic roux is made by sautéing butter and slowly adding flour. Once the flour is dispersed, milk is slowly added to thicken the mixture into a sauce. The thickness of the sauce depends on the flour-to-milk ratio.[1,2] Different spices, such as nutmeg, can be combined with the sauce to create a variety of flavors to go with different types of dishes. Roux is typically served best with chicken and meat. One variety of roux is Mornay sauce, which has butter, flour, milk, egg yolks, gruyere cheese, and ground nutmeg. This sauce is good with chicken and fish. Another variety is supreme sauce, which is best served with chicken. It has butter, flour, chicken stock, and heavy cream. Another variety that goes well with chicken is caper sauce. This sauce has butter, flour, chicken stock, egg yolks, heavy cream, and capers. The capers add a sharp flavor to this sauce.

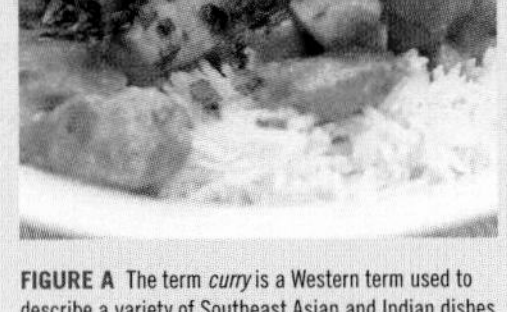

© Terry Davis/ShutterStock, Inc.

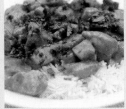

FIGURE A The term *curry* is a Western term used to describe a variety of Southeast Asian and Indian dishes that use a complex combination of spices and/or herbs and yogurt. Curry sauces can be used to complement meat, poultry, seafood, and vegetable dishes.

Yogurt-based sauces can be served with fish or chicken. Asian-Indian cultures incorporate yogurt into many of their sauces; the acidity of the yogurt helps to tenderize the meat.[1,2] The most popular yogurt-based sauce are curries, which come in many different varieties and can be served well with almost anything (see **Figure A**). Cumin, coriander, chili powder, fenugreek, cinnamon, clove, cardamom, and turmeric are all popular spices used in curries. The spices used in curries provide have many antioxidant properties.[1,2]

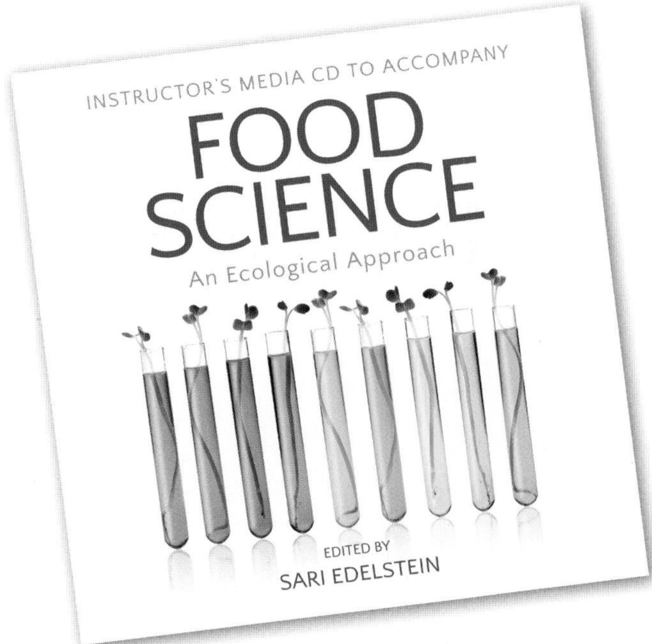

The Instructor's Media CD is a comprehensive teaching resource available to adopters of the book. It includes:

- PowerPoint Lecture Presentation Slides
- Image and Table Bank, which provides art and tables that can be imported into PowerPoint slides and tests or can be used to create transparencies

Instructor resources, including a Test Bank and Instructor's Manual, are available for download. Contact your Representative at **www.jblearning.com**.

The **companion website** for *Food Science: An Ecological Approach*, **go.jblearning.com/foodscience**, offers students and instructors an unprecedented degree of integration between their text and the online world through many useful study tools, activities, and supplementary information. Study tools include a lab manual featuring recipes correlated to chapter content with additional recipes included for cultural competency, flashcards, an interactive glossary, crossword puzzles, and practice quizzes. This interactive and informative website is accessible to students through the redeemable access code provided in every new text.

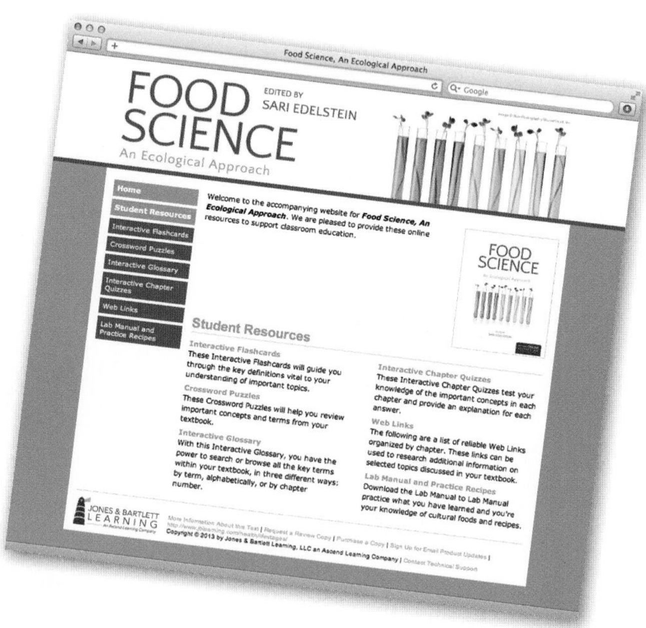

About the Editor

Sari Edelstein, PhD, RD, is an Associate Professor of Nutrition at Simmons College in Boston, Massachusetts. Dr. Edelstein's research interests are in the field of dietetics and nutrition, inclusive of systems and process management and food science. Dr. Edelstein came to Simmons College with 30 years of corporate experience, with many positions held in leadership roles. She is a prolific author, producing 10 nutrition textbooks in the last 8 years. One of her texts, *Nutrition in Public Health*, has been adopted by the American Public Health Association, which markets the book under its worldwide brand. Dr. Edelstein teaches food service systems and management, food science, and sports nutrition private practice at Simmons College. She currently works with the Boston Public Schools to form student nutrition clubs, as well as with the USDA with regard to food-insecure households.

Acknowledgments

I would like to thank all of the chapter and lab manual authors for their expertise and generous offers to participate in this cutting-edge text. Thanks also to Shoshanna Goldberg and her team at Jones & Bartlett Learning for their tireless efforts; thank you to Agnes Burt, Jessica Newfell, and Amy Rathburn for seeing this project through the production process. I also offer my appreciation to my graduate assistants, Debra Silverman, Colleen Lynch, and Melissa Przybysz, for their help. Finally, I would like to extend a warm thank you to Jennifer Angel for her countless hours providing feedback and suggestions throughout the manuscript development process.

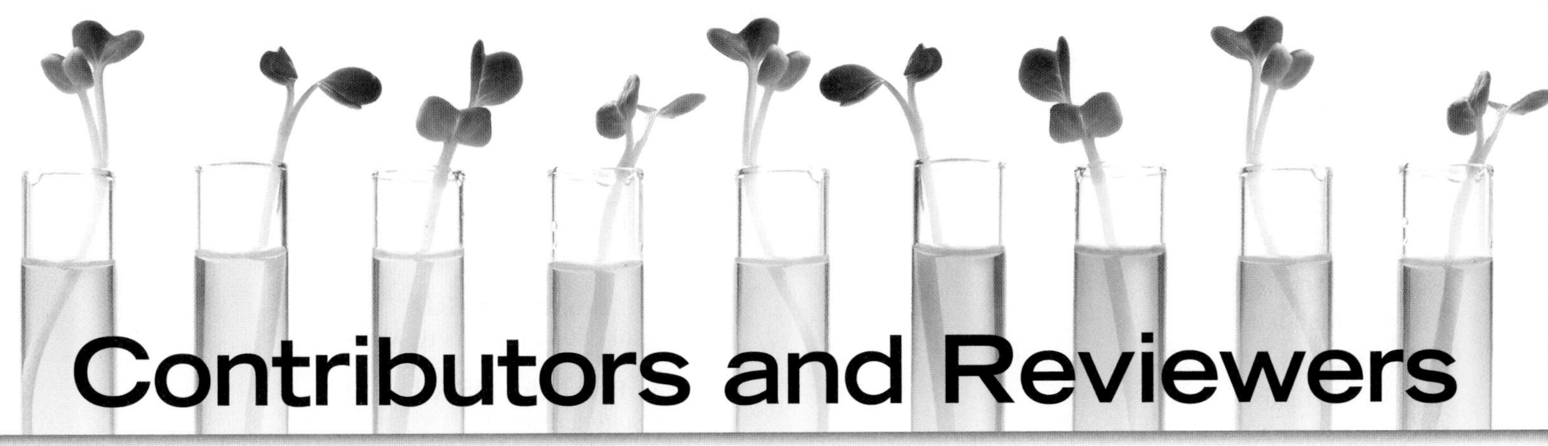

Contributors and Reviewers

Chapter Authors

Toby Amidor, MS, RD, CDN
Columbia University
FoodNetwork.com

Sung Eun Choi, PhD, RD
Queens College, CUNY

Nanna Cross, PhD, RD
Cross and Associates

Sari Edelstein, PhD, RD
Simmons College

Catherine Frederico, MS, RD, LDN
Newbury College

Bonnie Gerald, PhD, DTR
Consultant

Irana Hawkins, CAGS, MPH, RD
Simmons College

Jeannie Houchins, MA, RD
Nutrition Consultant

Debra King, MS, RD, LD
Nutrition Consultant

Zhanglin Kong, MS
Tufts University

Jennifer Lerman, RD, LDN
Massachusetts General Hospital

Mindy Beth Nelkin, MS, RD, MA
The Garden City Hotel

Carol E. O'Neil, PhD, MPH, RD
Louisiana State University

Theresa A. Nicklas, DrPH
Baylor College of Medicine

Carole Palmer, EdD, RD, LD
Tufts University

Tim Radak, DrPH, RD
Walden University

Renee Reynolds, MS, RD, LDN
Tufts University

SeAnne Safaii, PhD, RD, LD
University of Idaho

Lalitha Samuel, PhD
Lehman College

Allison Stevens, MS, RD, LD
Nutrition Consultant

Diane K. Tidwell, PhD, RD
Mississippi State University

Courtney P. Winston, MPH, RD, LD, CDE
University of Texas Health Science Center at Houston
Medical School

Contributing Section Authors from Simmons College

Lauren Adler
Bekah Angoff
Jackeline Barreto
Maria Belloso
Michelle Boutet
Lisa S. Brown
Kathryn Calcutt
Sarah Churchill
Nina Current
Danielle Flug
Sara Greeley
Maura Grimes
Kate Janisch
Emily Kaley
Brina Kelly
Erin Kunze

Zhanglin Kong
Jessica Brie Leonard
Lauren Levandowski
Colleen Lynch
Bridget Mahoney
Mary McAvoy
Jill M. Merrigan
Jacqueline Minichiello
Christina Molinski
Lauren Mudgett
Allison Mulvaney
Kimberly Owen
Michelle Palladino
Caitlin Portrie
Leslie Rathon
Andrea Roche
Veronica Salsberg
Katrina Schroeder
Debra Silverman
Isabel Smith
Jennifer Stallings
Jordan Tillery
Aisling Whelan
Christina Ypsilantis

Reviewers

Susan E. Adams, MS, RD, LDN
La Salle University

Joye M. Bond, PhD, RD
Minnesota State University, Mankato

Karen Brasfield, MS, RD, LD
Texas State University

James R. Daniel
Purdue University

Beverley Demetrius, EdD, RD, LD
Life University

Joe S. Hughes
California State University, San Bernardino

Deborah A. Hutcheon, MS, RD, LD
Bob Jones University

Carol J. Klitzke
Viterbo University

Rabia Rahman MS, RD, LD
Saint Louis University

Janelle M. Walter, PhD, RD, CFCS
Baylor University

SECTION I

Food Science Background: Food Systems in Relation to Climate Change, Research, Sensory Evaluation, and the Chemical Composition of Food

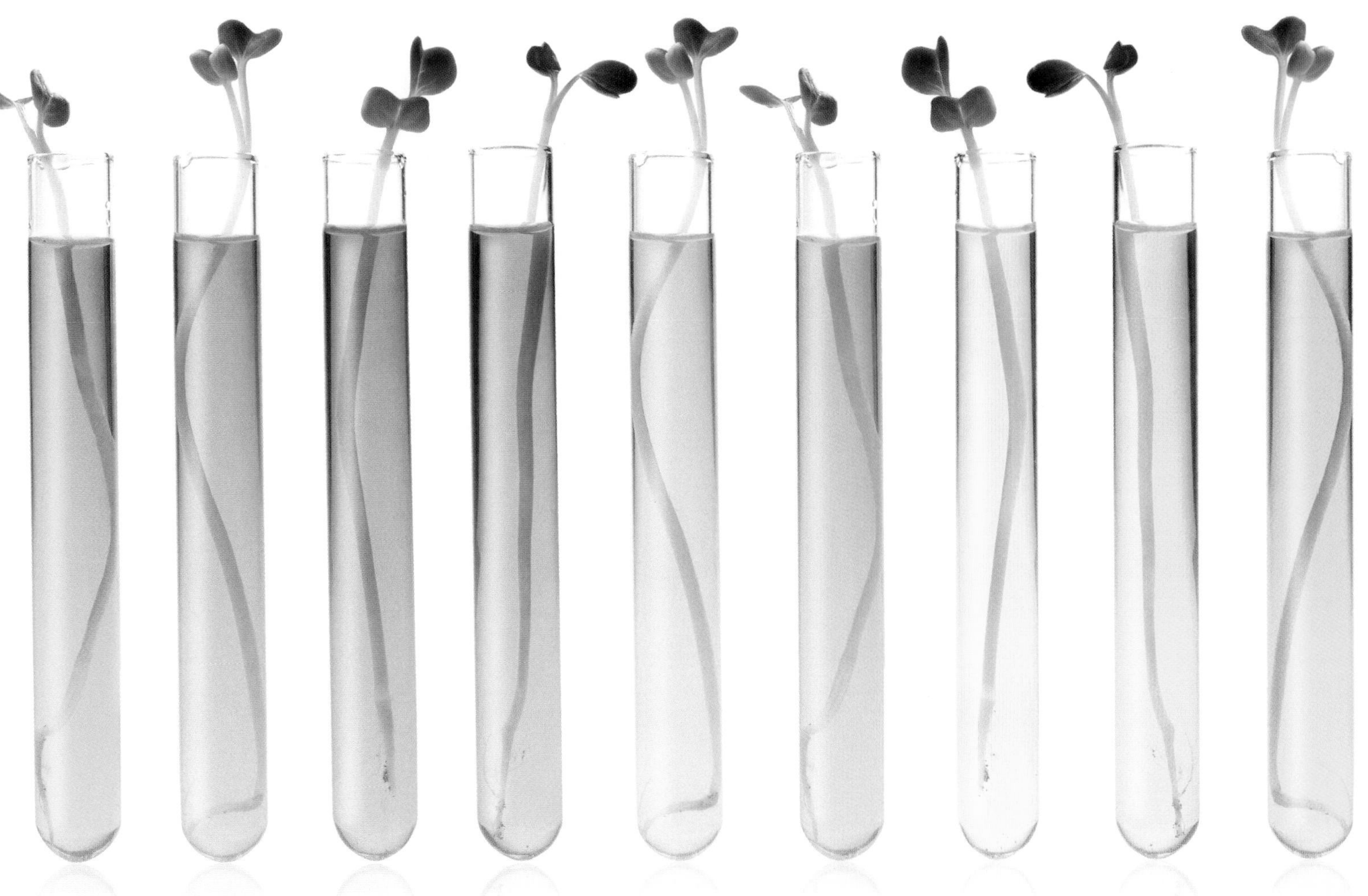

CHAPTER 1

Food Science and the Natural Environment

Irana Hawkins, CAGS, MPH, RD

Chapter Objectives

THE STUDENT WILL BE EMPOWERED TO:

- Summarize the topics encompassed by the food science discipline.
- Define *ecosystem*, *nutrition ecology*, and *ecosystem services*, and demonstrate how these terms relate to the study of food science.
- Provide examples of anthropogenic effects on the natural environment and food systems.
- Discuss current challenges to sustainably feeding the world.
- Discuss the potential impacts of climate change on food science and the potential role of dietary changes in mitigating climate change.
- Explain the concept of *nutrition transitions*, and give examples of global and national transitions currently underway.
- Give specific examples of how the principles of nutrition ecology can be applied to reduce the human impact on the natural environment.

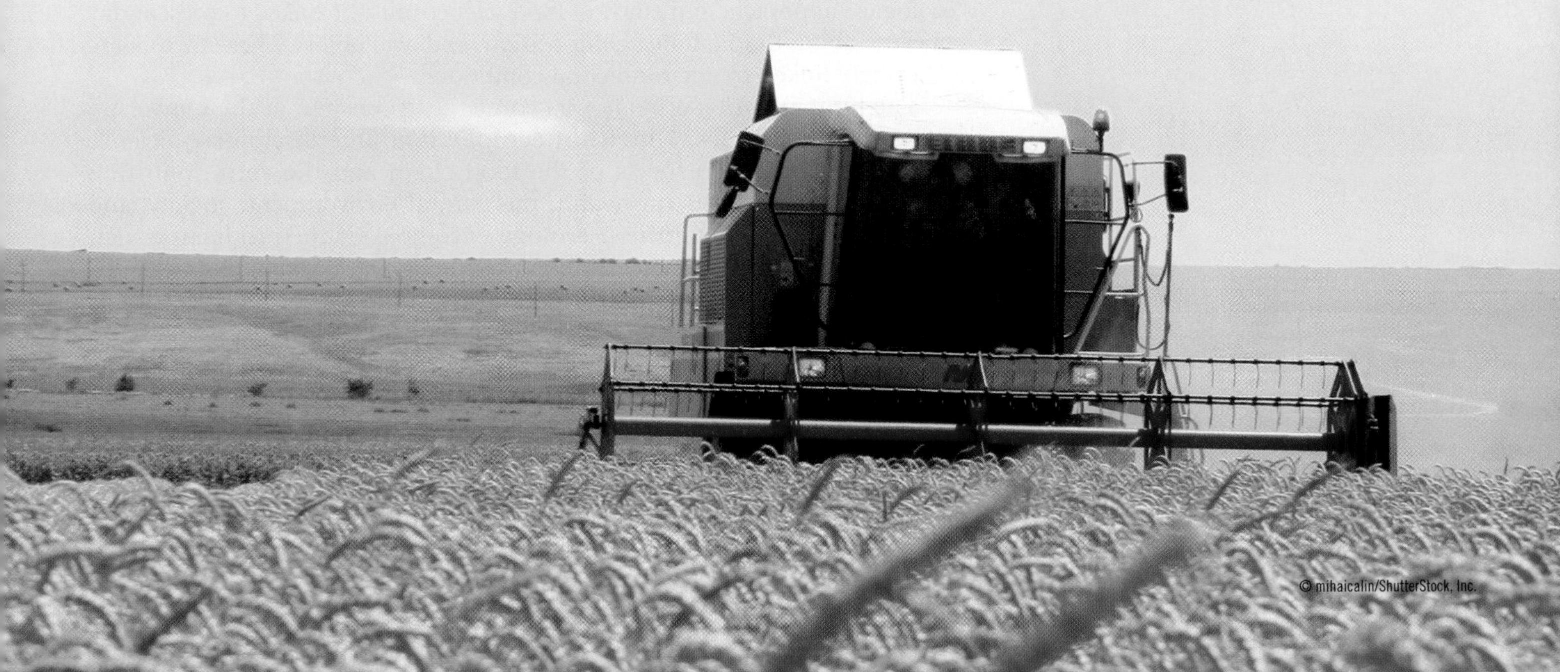

Historical, Cultural, and Ecological Significance

As one author noted, "… our relationship with food is the most intimate of all the connections we have with other beings, for we take it into our mouths and actually incorporate it into our cells."[1] Today, more than 311 million people live in the United States, and close to 7 billion people inhabit our planet.[2] The world population is expected to increase to over 9 billion people by 2044.[3] Understanding the projected impact of this population growth on the natural environment is paramount because human health is inextricably linked to the health of the natural environment.[4]

Sustaining human life requires an array of resources, the most important being food and water. Although the simple act of eating and drinking directly connects us to the natural environment at a most basic level, a burgeoning array of scientific data suggests that rapid changes in food production methods, trade, and dietary choices are affecting the living systems of the natural environment at many different levels and in ways not previously experienced. In an era of heightened environmental concern, careful consideration must be given to food- and beverage-related businesses and to agricultural and lifestyle practices.

This text explores topics on these connections among food, human health, and the natural environment. This introductory chapter broadly examines the natural environment and its relationship to food science.

food science Encompasses the investigation of better ways to select, preserve, process, package, and distribute food products.

nutrition ecology An interdisciplinary science that encompasses all aspects of the food chain and the entire nutrition system and their effects on health, the natural environment, society, and the economy.

How the Natural Environment Relates to Food Science

Food science encompasses the investigation of better ways to select, preserve, process, package, and distribute food products. As a discipline, it studies the composition of food ingredients and their manipulation during growing, production, processing, and presentation to the consumer. Therefore, a food scientist must have extensive knowledge on the nature, composition, and behavior of food, such as what happens to its flavor, color, or nutritional properties when cooked or placed in storage.

We consider food science within the context of the natural world we live in today. Although many of the scientific principles remain the same as for traditional food science, many must be viewed through a new lens. To take an "ecological approach," our study of food science must be linked to present-day concerns about food quality, composition, and availability. These factors are all strongly linked to environmental conditions.

The term *nutrition ecology* was coined 25 years ago at the University of Giessen in Germany. **Nutrition ecology** is an interdisciplinary science that encompasses all aspects of the food chain and the entire nutrition system and their effects on health, the natural environment, society, and the economy.[5] Today, nutrition ecology encompasses the production, harvesting, preservation, storage, transport, processing, packaging, trade, distribution, preparation, composition, and consumption of food as well as the disposal of waste materials.[5] Food scientists now address nutrition ecology and consider all links in the nutrition system, including the wholesomeness of foods, the sustainability of the natural environment, and food security.[6] (**Special Topic 1.1** examines food security issues in more detail.) Even today, food and nutrition professionals suggest avoiding reductionism in nutrition research and practice,[7] instead encouraging a holistic approach that considers overall dietary patterns[8] and the integrity of food systems.[9]

Special Topic 1.1

Food Insecurity in the United States

Lauren Adler

Modern food science can tell us extraordinary things about the composition of food and how it keeps us alive and nourished, but what happens when people do not have enough food to achieve a healthy diet? Although it is a more serious issue in developing countries, 17.4 million U.S. households experienced food insecurity at some point in 2010.[1]

What Is Food Insecurity?

The U.S. Department of Agriculture (USDA) defines *food security* as consistent, dependable access by all household members at all times to enough food for an active, healthy life.[1] **Food insecurity** occurs when households have difficulty at some point providing enough food for all their members due to lack of resources.

food insecurity When households have difficulty providing enough food for all their members due to lack of resources.

Food insecure households fall into two categories (see **Figure A**):

- *Low food security*: Households with low food security are able to avoid major disruptions by reducing the *kinds* of food they eat.
- *Very low food security* (formerly called *food insecurity with hunger*): Households with very low food security have one or more members of the household reduce the *amount* of food they eat; normal eating patterns are disrupted.[1]

How Is Food Insecurity Measured?

In the United States, food security status is measured using a survey called the Core Food Security Module.[2] This module consists of 18 questions (10 for households without children) and is administered by the USDA using a nationally representative sample (see **Figure B**). The following are some examples of questions in the survey:

1. "The food that we bought just didn't last and we didn't have money to get more." Was that often, sometimes, or never true for you in the last 12 months?
2. (a) In the last 12 months, did you or other adults in the household ever not eat for a whole day because there wasn't enough money for food? (Yes/No)

   (b) How often did this happen—almost every month, some months but not every month, or in only 1 or 2 months?
3. In the last 12 months, were the children ever hungry but you just couldn't afford more food? (Yes/No)

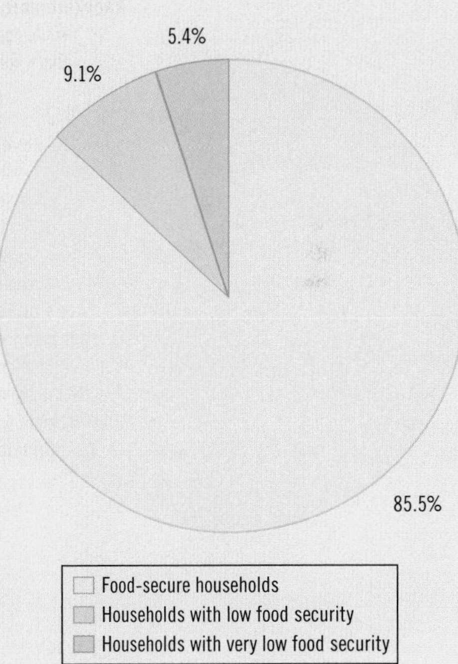

FIGURE A Food security status of U.S. households in 2010.

Note: Food insecure households include those with low food security and very low food security.

Source: Reproduced from Coleman-Jensen A, Nord M, Andrews M, Carlson S. *Household Food Security in the United States, 2010* (Figure 1). Washington, DC: U.S. Department of Agriculture, Economic Research Service; 2011. Available at: http://www.ers.usda.gov/media/121076/err125_2_.pdf.

Who Experiences Food Insecurity?

Although a variety of people experience food insecurity, food insecurity is more common in certain types of households. The highest rates of very low food security are found in:

- Households with incomes below the poverty line
- Families with children headed by single women
- African American households
- Hispanic American households
- Families with children headed by single men
- Households in principal cities of metropolitan areas[1]

A number of food assistance programs have been implemented by the U.S. government to help Americans combat food insecurity.[2] These initiatives include the Supplemental Nutrition Assistance Program (SNAP; also known as food stamps); Special Supplemental Program for Women, Infants, and Children (WIC); the National School Lunch Program, the National School Breakfast Program, and the Emergency Food Assistance Program. These programs, along with community efforts such as soup kitchens and community volunteers, help to increase food security throughout the United States.

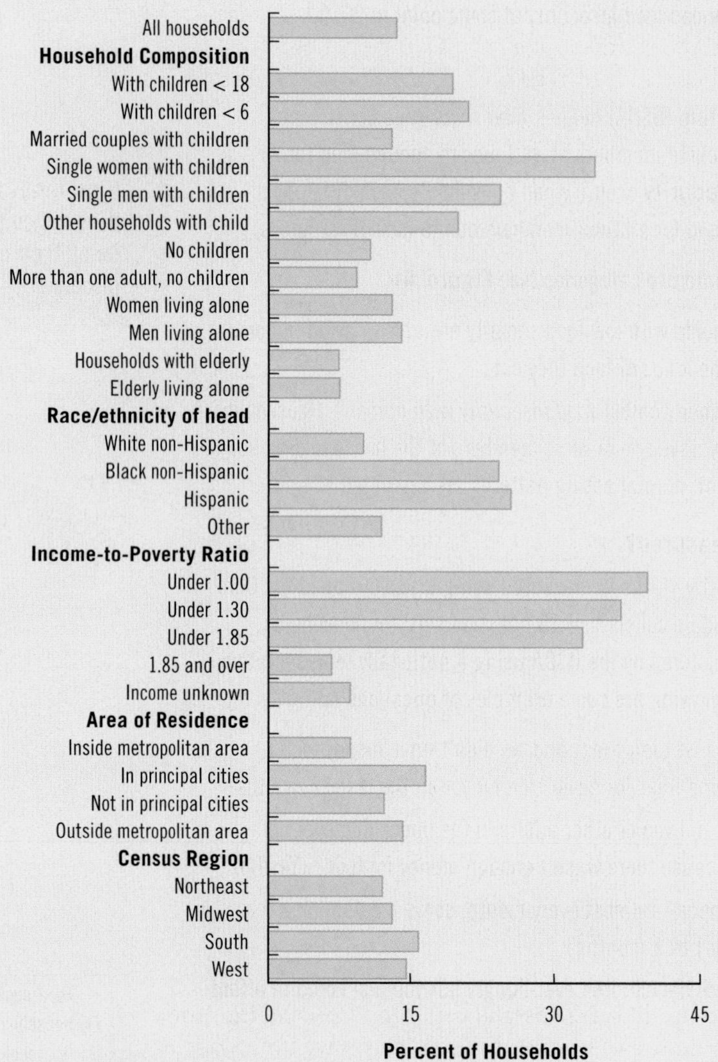

FIGURE B Percentage of U.S. households reporting indicators of food insecurity.

Source: Reproduced from Coleman-Jensen A, Nord M, Andrews M, Carlson S. *Household Food Security in the United States, 2010* (Figure 4). Washington, DC: U.S. Department of Agriculture, Economic Research Service; 2011. Available at: http://www.ers.usda.gov/media/121076/err125_2_.pdf.

References

1 Coleman-Jensen A, Nord M, Andrews M, Carlson S. *Household Food Security in the United States, 2010.* Washington, DC: U.S. Department of Agriculture, Economic Research Service; 2011.

2 Edelstein S, Gerald B, Crutchley Bushell T, Gundersen G. *Food and Nutrition at Risk in America: Food Insecurity, Biotechnology, Food Safety, and Bioterrorism.* Sudbury, MA: Jones and Bartlett Publishers; 2009.

Ecological Literacy

Our understanding of the interconnected systems that provide food and sustain the web of life is known as **ecological literacy**.[10] The following terms are important to this understanding:

- An **ecosystem** is a dynamic complex of plant, animal, and microorganism communities, as well as the nonliving environment, that interacts and functions as a unit.[11]
- **Ecosystem services** are the benefits people obtain from ecosystems, including food and water; the regulation of floods, drought, land degradation, and disease; soil formation and nutrient cycling; and cultural, recreational, spiritual, religious, and other nonmaterial benefits.[11]
- **Living systems** are the animate, interconnected components and processes of ecosystems (no matter how small or large) that continuously affect and depend on each other as well as on the integrity of the system. Living systems are characterized by interdependence, systems integrity, feedback mechanisms, biodiversity, cooperation and partnership, living cycles, optimal size, and waste equals food.[12]

ecological literacy An understanding of the interconnected systems and associated relationships that sustain the web of life.

ecosystem A dynamic complex of plant, animal, and microorganism communities, as well as the nonliving environment, that interacts and functions as a unit.

ecosystem services Benefits society obtains from ecosystems, including food and water; the regulation of floods, drought, land degradation, and disease; soil formation and nutrient cycling; and cultural, recreational, spiritual, religious, and other nonmaterial benefits.

living systems The animate, interconnected components and processes of ecosystems (no matter how small or large).

The Current Need for an Ecological Approach

Numerous scientific reports and studies have documented the degradation of the natural environment and the decline of ecosystems. The past 50 years of human activity have "altered ecosystems to an extent and degree unprecedented in human history."[13] Ecological systems are experiencing multiple severe and mutually reinforcing stresses. The root causes of ecosystem change are the increased per person consumption of ecosystem services and a growing population. Trends that will continue to disturb ecosystem functions include:[13]

- Increased demand for food, fiber, and water
- Pollution from contaminants and waste
- Eutrophication of waterways
- Global trade
- Climate change
- Overfishing, overgrazing, and overlogging
- Habitat loss and fragmentation

Another trend that may disturb the ability of ecosystems to function is the introduction of genetically modified crops and other food species into the natural world. Genetic manipulation of our food supply may have unintended consequences, as discussed in **Special Topic 1.2**.

Special Topic 1.2

Genetically Modified Organisms and Food

Jeannie Houchins, MA, RD

Genetically modified organisms (GMOs) are increasingly present in our food supply. Each country handles this technology and the end products differently. Even definitions vary slightly between the United States and the World Health Organization:

genetically modified organisms (GMOs) Organisms that have been transformed by the insertion of one or more transgenes (genes not naturally found in the organism); organisms in which the genetic material (DNA) has been altered in a way that does not occur naturally.

herbicide A type of pesticide used to kill unwanted plants. Herbicides target a specific type of plant while leaving others intact. Plants can produce natural herbicides in reaction to an encounter with an undesirable species or substance.

- According to the U.S. Department of Energy Genome Programs, **genetically modified organisms (GMOs)** are those that have been transformed by the insertion of one or more transgenes (genes not naturally found in the organism).[1]
- According to the World Health Organization (WHO), GMOs are organisms in which the genetic material (DNA) has been altered in a way that does not occur naturally.[2]

The terms *biotechnology* and *genetic modification (GM)* are commonly used interchangeably by the press; however, *biotechnology* is a more general term that refers to using organisms or their components—such as enzymes—to make products such as wine, cheese, beer, and yogurt (as well as various nonfood products).[1] *GM*, in contrast, refers to a specialized set of technologies that alter the genetic makeup of organisms.

GM technology also is called *modern biotechnology, gene technology, recombinant DNA technology*, and *genetic engineering*. With GM technology, selected individual genes can be transferred from one organism into another and also from one species to another. Such methods are used to create GM plants, which are then used to grow GM food crops. As with many scientific innovations, there are benefits and controversies associated with GMOs. These benefits and controversies are summarized in **Table A**.

According to the WHO, GM foods are developed and marketed because there is some perceived advantage either to the producer or consumer of these foods that translates into a product with a lower price or a greater benefit (in terms of durability or nutritional value), or both. Initially, GM seed developers wanted their products to be accepted by producers, so they concentrated on innovations that farmers (and the food industry more generally) would appreciate. The initial objectives for GM plants were to improve crop protection (through the introduction of resistance against plant diseases caused by insects or viruses) or to increase crop tolerance (through the use of a **herbicide**).[2]

TABLE A
Perceived Benefits and Drawbacks of Genetically Modified Organisms

Perceived Benefits	Perceived Drawbacks
Crops • Enhanced taste and quality • Reduced maturation time • Increased nutrients and yields • Better stress tolerance • Improved resistance to disease, pests, and herbicides • New products and growing techniques **Environment** • "Friendly" bioherbicides and bioinsecticides • Conservation of soil, water, and energy • Bioprocessing for forestry products • Better natural waste management • More efficient processing **Society** • Increased food security for growing populations	**Ethics** • Violation of the intrinsic value of natural organisms • Tampering with nature by mixing genes among species • Objections to consuming animal genes (and their products) in plants and vice versa **Environment and Health** • Potential environmental impacts, including unintended transfer of transgenes through cross-pollination, unknown effects on other organisms (e.g., soil microbes), and loss of biodiversity • Potential human health impacts, including allergens, transfer of antibiotic-resistance markers, unknown effects **Labeling** • Not mandatory in some countries (e.g., United States) • Mixing GM crops and non-GM ingredients in food products confounds labeling attempts **Society** • New advances may be skewed to interests of rich countries • Domination of world food production by a few companies • Increasing dependence by developing countries on industrialized nations • Biopiracy, or foreign exploitation of natural resources

Source: Modified from U.S. Department of Energy, Office of Science. Human Genome Project Information: Genetically Modified Foods and Organisms. Available at: http://www.ornl.gov/sci/techresources/Human_Genome/elsi/gmfood.shtml. Accessed August 20, 2010.

The question of whether GM foods are safe is one that the WHO takes seriously. The WHO has created parameters to assess the safety of GM foods, including the investigation of:[2]

- Direct health effects (toxicity)
- Tendencies to provoke allergic reaction (allergenicity)
- Specific components thought to have nutritional or toxic properties
- Stability of the inserted gene
- Nutritional effects associated with genetic modification
- Any unintended effects that could result from the gene insertion

Environmental risks are of particular concern with GM products. The WHO assessment process includes evaluation of a GMO's stability in the environment. The assessment considers ecological characteristics of the environment in which the introduction will take place and the potential unintended effects that may result from the insertion of the new gene.[2]

According to the WHO, GM foods currently available on the international market have passed risk assessments—they are not likely to present risks for human health. Furthermore, no effects on human health have been shown as a result of the consumption of GM foods by the general population in the countries where they have been approved. Risk assessments and postmarket monitoring are the basis for evaluating the safety of GM foods. The food regulations of every government vary; countries with provisions for GM foods usually also regulate GMOs and generally take into account health and environmental risks as well as control- and trade-related issues (such as labeling). In view of the dynamics of the debate on GM foods, legislation is likely to continue to evolve.[2]

References

1 U.S. Department of Energy, Office of Science. Human Genome Project Information: Genetically Modified Foods and Organisms. Available at: http://www.ornl.gov/sci/techresources/Human_Genome/elsi/gmfood.shtml. Accessed August 20, 2010.

2 World Health Organization. 20 Questions on Genetically Modified Foods. Available at: http://www.who.int/foodsafety/publications/biotech/20questions/en/index.html. Accessed August 15, 2010.

Human demands on the biosphere more than doubled between 1961 and 2007.[14] By assessing renewable resource utilization, it has been estimated that humans have exceeded the Earth's biocapacity by 50%.[14] **Biocapacity** represents the regenerative capacity and availability of the planet's natural resources. Even using modest projections, the calculations point to a situation defined as "ecological overshoot"[14,15]; that is, humans are using ecosystem resources faster than they can be replenished (see **Figure 1.1**).

Ecosystem health and ecosystem services are deeply affected by food production and acquisition methods, food consumption patterns, and other **anthropogenic effects**—those caused by human activities. Some suggest that the U.S. Farm Bill should mandate an environmental impact statement to decrease the ecological degradation associated with food and agricultural practices.[16] As an example, a closer examination of aquatic ecosystems—oceans, rivers, and lakes—illustrates the concern:

- Systemic overfishing of inland fresh waters has been shown to threaten **biodiversity**.[17]
- Populations of the North Atlantic basin's diadromous fish—those species that migrate between saltwater and freshwater—have suffered dramatic declines due to habitat loss, overfishing, pollution, and the negative effects of climate change, nonnative species, and aquaculture.[18]

biocapacity The regenerative capacity and the availability of the natural resources of the planet.

anthropogenic effects Those created by or caused by human activity.

biodiversity The variety of life forms that make up a community, including plants, animals, fungi, and microorganisms. In recent years, the term has come to stand for the concepts and principles of conservation.

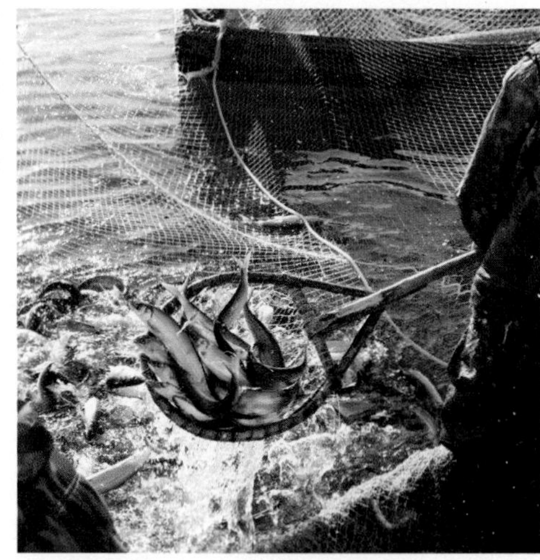

FIGURE 1.1 The health of the world's oceans is declining as a result of overfishing. Because no one country or person owns the ocean's resources, they are open to exploitation by everyone. If there are no limits on fishing, certain fish populations will collapse.

- Anthropogenic coal emissions have been implicated in levels of methyl mercury in fish that are hazardous to human consumers.[19,20]
- Organophosphorus pesticides have been found in the human body, in part due to chemicals in agricultural runoff being accumulated into the tissues of freshwater fish.[21,22]

Table 1.1 lists some of the issues studied by food scientists for each major category of food.

How This Affects the Study of Food Science

How do these issues affect the study of food science? Food scientists are now examining the impact of food production on the environment. In particular, the following food practices can decrease the impact of food production on the environment:

- Eating lower on the food chain (select more plant-based protein)
- Selectively eating local foods
- Eating organically grown foods

The federal government has developed a new product label, the Biobased label, to help consumers make smart choices when selecting environmentally friendly products. This new labeling is detailed in **Special Topic 1.3**.

TABLE 1.1
Relationship of Food Science to the Natural Environment

Food Science Category	Examples
Meat	• Effects of animal feed on meat composition • Overuse of antibiotics, leading to antibiotic resistance • Pesticide residues in animal feed and meat tissue
Fish	• Impact of overfishing on ecosystem services • Contamination of wild fish populations by aquaculture species • Antibiotics used in aquaculture showing up in the human food supply
Poultry	• Microbial contamination that affects human consumption • Overuse of antibiotics and hormones • Avian flu
Milk and dairy products	• Bovine growth hormone • Contaminants in milk and food safety • Antibiotic use
Eggs	• *Salmonella* contamination • The relationship between asthma and egg allergy in the pediatric population • Higher levels of microbial contamination in unwashed eggs
Fruits and vegetables	• Pesticide residues • Importing fruit year round, which increases the distance traveled and contributes to greenhouse gas emissions • Ability to transport food far distances may alter the picking time, which can affect flavor and nutrient content
Grains	• Pesticide use and content in grain products • Effects of grain-based animal feed on meat composition • Desertification of cropland
Fats and oils	• Effects of crop monocultures and genetically modified organisms (GMOs) • Effects of chemicals used in processing • Effects of using food crops for biofuels
Nuts	• Pesticide residues in nuts • Nut composition and food allergies • Waste practices
Sugar	• Human health implications • Destruction of native ecosystems, water contamination, and other ecosystem disturbances resulting from burning waste after harvest with certain sugar crops • The large amounts of energy involved in processing sugar

Food Science Category	Examples
Sugar replacements	• Potential health risks associated with their composition • Contamination of groundwater, manure, and sewage sludge during production
Water	• Large amounts needed to support livestock • Effect of climate change on water supplies • Groundwater contamination
Food preservation	• Nanotechnology and human health • Effects of certain food additives on human health • Food safety concerns (home canning, irradiation)
Food packaging and waste	• Leaching of food packaging chemicals into food and liquids • Excessive and unnecessary use of disposable food packaging • Expanding food composting services

Source: Adapted from Science.gov. Earth Science Applications. Available at: http://www.nasa.gov/pdf/55397main_14%20ESA.pdf. Accessed June 1, 2012.

Special Topic 1.3

USDA's Biobased Product Label

Katrina Schroeder

Today's educated consumers are constantly on the lookout for products that can help them to "do the right thing." Is a product organic? Was it sourced from sustainable material? Was it made in the United States? Were the workers treated fairly? Concern for the environment as well as worries about America's dependence on foreign materials such as oil and petroleum has led many people to ask these questions, among others, when purchasing items ranging from pet food to packaging materials.

The USDA's new BioPreferred program aims to make shopping decisions easier with its new USDA Certified Biobased Product label. Companies must apply to use the label by submitting proof to the USDA that their product is biobased.[1]

A **biobased product** is a commercial or industrial product or package made of at least 25% biological products, renewable agricultural materials (including plant, animal, and marine materials), or forestry materials. This definition was put into place by the 2002 Farm Bill and was revised in the 2008 Farm Bill to include intermediate ingredients or feedstocks as biobased products.[2] The label indicates what percentage of the product is biobased and whether it is the product itself or the packaging (or both) that is made from the renewable biological products.

biobased product A commercial or industrial product or package made of at least 25% biological products, renewable agricultural materials (including plant, animal, and marine materials), or forestry materials.

The label also indicates whether a biobased product is part of the Federal Procurement Preference Program. Preferred products will have the letters "FP" on the label in addition to the percentage. This program, which is referred to as the BioPreferred program, requires that federal agencies give preference to biobased products when making certain purchases.[3]

Products that are eligible for the new label fall into numerous categories (see http://www.catalog.biopreferred.gov for a full list of products that are currently approved to bear the label). For example, categories include toiletries, office supplies, vehicle maintenance products, industrial products, and pet supplies. Specific products that have been approved to carry the USDA Certified Biobased Product label include Pain Relief Massage Cream™ from Botanical Skin Works, Biodegradable Mechanical Pencil with Grip™ by Papermate, and Living Fresh Towels™ from Valley Forge Fabrics, Inc.

With all new initiatives come concerns about their actual effectiveness. A USDA press release dated January 19, 2011, indicated that the "growing [biobased] industry as a whole is responsible for over 100,000 jobs" and that the initiative will create green jobs and new markets for farmers. According to Agriculture Deputy Secretary Kathleen Merrigan:

> Today's consumers are increasingly interested in making educated purchasing choices for their families. This label will make those decisions easier by identifying products as biobased. These products have enormous potential to create green jobs in rural communities, add value to agricultural commodities, decrease environmental impacts, and reduce our dependence on imported oil.[1]

However, as one article on Sustainablog points out, there is no requirement that the biobased materials come from American farmers or are even American made.[4] In fact, imported products are eligible for the label as long as they adhere to the same testing standards as American products. Another issue is consumer confusion; some might think that the USDA's new label is an endorsement of sorts, and the term *biobased* can be confused with terms such as *green* and *organic*. According to the USDA's website FAQs about the label, the environmental benefits of purchasing these products are not entirely clear. On the question of whether these products are better for the environment, the USDA's answer is that:

> A USDA certified biobased label is not a guarantee or expression of environmental preferability or impact. There is an expectation that the increased use of biobased products will help reduce petroleum consumption by increasing the use of renewable resources, thus reducing the amount of new carbon released into the atmosphere, helping to better manage the carbon cycle, in turn reducing resultant adverse environmental and health impacts.[5]

At present, for a number of different reasons, consumers may be hard-pressed to find this label on any actual products. First, the USDA takes up to 601 days to approve or reject an application, a timeframe it hopes to shorten as the project picks up steam. Considering that the labeling initiative started in January 2011 and that the products must first be tested before an application can be submitted, it is not a big surprise that there are not currently a lot of labeled products on the market. Second, the cost of testing a single product to prove its biobased status and percentage is estimated by the USDA to be around $600 per product. It is possible that a company that manufactures biobased products will not see the cost benefit of paying for testing for a label that has not been proven to create more demand for a product. Currently, the USDA does not provide financial assistance for this testing; it is hoped that increased demand for testing will drive down the price over time.[5]

If the biobased product movement gains momentum, more and more products will begin to display the label. Consumers will then be able to make more educated purchases based on the product or packaging's percentage of biobased material.

References

1 U.S. Department of Agriculture. USDA Launches New Biobased Product Label to Boost Demand for Products Made from Renewable Commodities and Support Green Jobs. Available at: http://www.usda.gov/wps/portal/usda/usdahome?contentid=2011/01/0015.xml&navid=NEWS_AUSUMS&navtype=RT&parentnav=ENERGY&edeployment_action=retrievecontent. Accessed October 1, 2012.

2 U.S. Department of Agriculture. USDA BioPreferred. Biobased Products. Available at: http://www.biopreferred.gov/Biobased_Products.aspx?SMSESSION=NO. Accessed December 4, 2011.

3 U.S. Department of Agriculture. USDA BioPreferred. Federal Purchasing Requirement. Available at: http://www.biopreferred.gov/PurchasingBiobased.aspx. Accessed December 4, 2011.

4 McIntire-Strasburg J. The USDA BioPreferred Program: Consumer Empowerment ... or Confusion? Sustainablog. Available at: http://blog.sustainablog.org/2011/04/usda-biopreferred-label. Accessed December 4, 2011.

5 U.S. Department of Agriculture. USDA Biopreferred Frequently Asked Questions Available at: http://www.biopreferred.gov/FAQ.aspx. Accessed December 2, 2011.

Climate Change

The consensus among U.S. scientists and numerous intergovernmental agencies and working groups is that climate change—also called *atmospheric warming* or *global warming*—is now an extreme environmental concern.[23,24] Anthropogenic carbon dioxide emissions have been linked to irreversible, adverse changes to the global climate. These changes are projected to stress the planet's living systems.[25] The following are just some of the potential impacts of global climate change:[25]

- Rainfall patterns may be altered, adversely affecting the supply of water for humans, agriculture, and ecosystems.
- Wildfires and desertification may increase.
- Raising sea levels may flood arable land currently located near coastlines.

acidification When carbon dioxide is absorbed by oceans, it changes the chemistry of the seawater, which can impair marine life and adversely affect the oceanic food web.

Climate change also affects the chemistry of seawater in ways that may greatly affect biodiversity and ecosystem services as well as the fishing industry. If carbon dioxide emission trends continue, the ocean will continue to undergo acidification to an extent and at rates that have not occurred for tens of millions of years. **Acidification** occurs when carbon dioxide is absorbed by oceans. It changes the chemistry of seawater, which can impair marine life and ultimately adversely affect the oceanic food web. Such changes compromise the long-term viability of marine ecosystems such as coral reefs and the associated benefits they provide, including coastland protection from storm surges (see **Figure 1.2**). Coral reefs also are threatened by coastal development, pollution, exploitation, and destructive fishing practices.[26]

Recommendations for improving the health of ocean ecosystems includes limiting fossil fuel emissions and managing the resilience of marine ecosystems until they have recovered from the impacts of climate change.[26] Studies conducted in the North Pacific and the North Atlantic reveal unexpectedly large changes in deep-ocean ecosystems due to climate-driven changes.[27] Climate change affects not only oceanic surface waters and the deep sea, it also disrupts the global carbon cycle (see **Figure 1.3**), which will likely influence the ecology and biogeochemistry of the deep sea.[27]

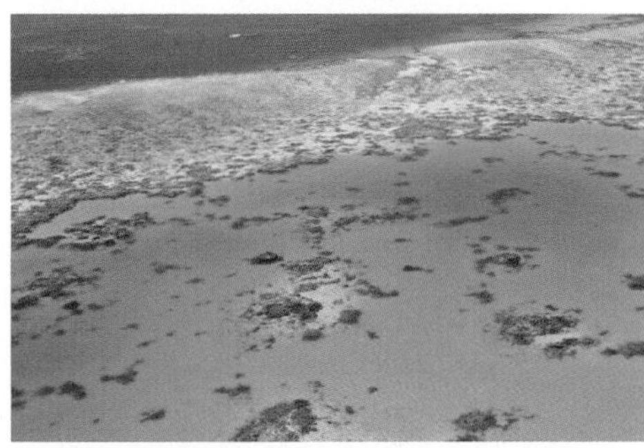

FIGURE 1.2 Climate change is one of the biggest threats to the Great Barrier Reef off the coast of Australia. Increasing ocean temperatures cause coral bleaching, whereby the coral stop producing their brightly hued pigments. It also leads to increased disease susceptibility, which negatively affects the ecology of the reef community.

Models of the effects of climate change on the United States predict that crop and livestock production will be increasingly challenged due to pests, water limitations, diseases, and weather extremes.[28] These effects are detailed in **Special Topic 1.4**. Humans will face increased health risks relating to heat stress; diseases transmitted by water, insects, and rodents; poor air quality (see **Figure 1.4**); and extreme weather events.[28] Numerous interconnected social and environmental stresses will also increase, especially when the effects of climate change are combined with pollution, population growth, the overuse of resources (see **Figure 1.5**), increased urbanization, and economic stressors.[28] However, scientific modeling indicates that decreasing anthropogenic greenhouse gas and carbon dioxide emissions immediately and into the future could reduce the amount of damage anticipated from climate change.[25]

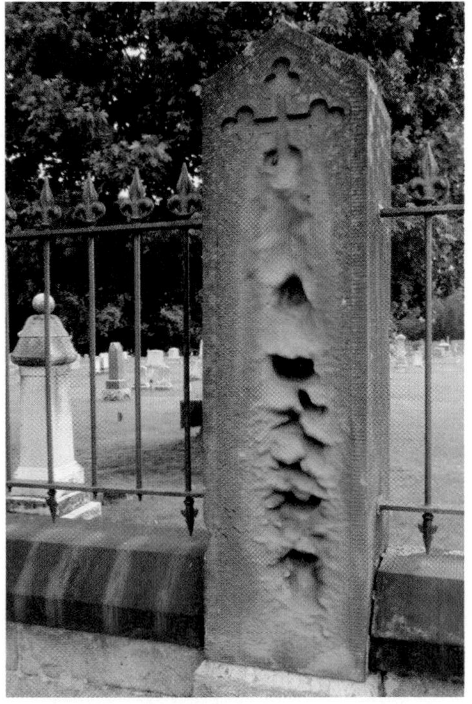

FIGURE 1.3 The global carbon cycle is the biogeochemical cycle by which carbon is exchanged among living organisms, the soil, rocks, water sources, and the atmosphere. Through the carbon cycle, carbon is recycled throughout the biosphere and all of its organisms.

Mitigating Climate Change

Intergovernmental, national, and municipal organizations are working to develop substantive policies to mitigate climate change. They are joined by the advocacy and research efforts of nongovernmental organizations, academic institutions, and nonprofit groups, including religious organizations. In particular, the United Nations (UN) Millennium Development Goals (MDGs) were developed from a compilation of priority needs of those living in the poorest countries. Climate change is predicted to most severely impact those with the fewest resources, those who in fact have contributed the least to the anthropogenic degradation of the natural environment.[29] One of the MDGs targets environmental sustainability and specifically identifies the following as notable goals:[29]

- Integrating sustainability into all levels of policies and programs
- Reversing the loss of natural resources
- Reducing biodiversity loss
- Increasing access to safe drinking water and basic sanitation
- Improving the lives of those living in slums

Special Topic 1.4

The Effects of Climate Change on the Earth's Food Supply

Lauren Levandowski

Since the beginning of the industrial era, human activity has increased the amount of carbon dioxide (CO_2) in the atmosphere, which has influenced significant changes in global weather patterns and temperatures. Large amounts of carbon dioxide and other so-called greenhouse gases emitted by human activities absorb heat, trapping it in the atmosphere and causing what is known as a **greenhouse effect**. This is a naturally occurring process, but it has been substantially increased by the amount of carbon dioxide being emitted into earth's atmosphere. In the United States, major sources of greenhouse gases include the burning of fossil fuels by power plants and automobiles, industrial and agricultural processes, and waste management practices. Electricity generation is the greatest source of these emissions in the United States, followed by transportation.[1]

greenhouse effect A naturally occurring process whereby gasses trap heat in the atmosphere. Human activities have generated more of these gases, particularly carbon dioxide, resulting in the warming of earth's atmosphere.

crop yields Also called *agricultural output*; the amount of crops harvested per unit over a given period of time; can refer to the crops as a whole as well as to an individual plant.

Climate Change and Agriculture

In general, climate change may benefit food production in many regions that have cool springs and falls by creating a warmer climate and longer growing season. However, crop production will be reduced in areas where summer temperatures already limit plant growth. Because plants use carbon dioxide in photosynthesis, higher levels of atmospheric carbon dioxide may have a positive effect on many crops, potentially increasing **crop yields**. However, studies have shown that optimizing plant growth through increased levels of carbon dioxide will not increase nutritional qualities, such as protein concentrations, in proportion to the higher crop yields.[2]

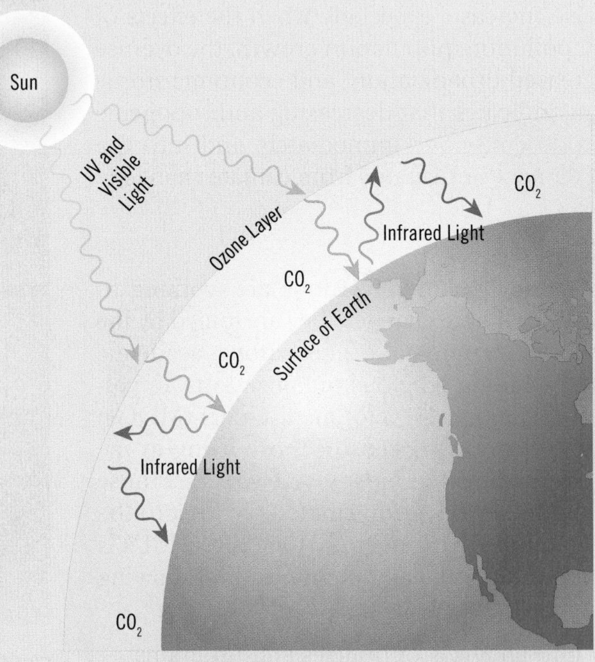

Greenhouse gases comprise only about 1% of the atmosphere, but they regulate Earth's climate by trapping heat. As the amount of atmospheric greenhouse gases increases, global temperatures increase, too.

Climate change also is likely to increase in the frequency and severity of natural disasters—such as droughts, floods, and extreme heat waves—that have devastating effects on crop production. Additionally, increased temperatures over time may change the water supply by evaporating soil moisture, making the continued production of crops in certain regions of the world unrealistic. Rising temperatures also will increase the ability of agricultural pests to survive what were traditionally harsh winters, allowing them to attack spring crops.[2] According to the Environmental Protection Agency (EPA), agriculture is very sensitive to climate variability and extreme weather patterns. An increase in frequency of heat stress, floods, and droughts negatively affects crop yields and livestock production beyond any positive impacts of climate change.[1]

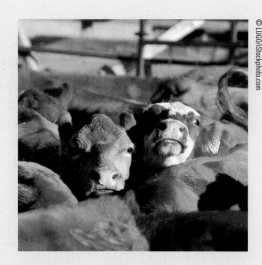

Livestock raised for human food consumption is a major source of greenhouse gasses, which includes 37% of anthropogenic methane emissions, 65% of anthropogenic nitrous oxide emissions, and 64% of anthropogenic ammonia emissions.

Lastly, rising temperatures are shrinking the amount of Arctic sea ice; currently, roughly half of the ice coverage is left, compared to measurements taken in 1979. This melting sea ice is one of the contributing causes to rising sea levels observed around the world. Some of the key concerns of rising sea levels include loss of arable land, increased risk of flooding, and increased salinity in coastal water supplies.[1]

The Future of the Food Supply

It is predicted that the greatest loss of useable cropland will likely occur in Africa and parts of South Asia; the largest gains of arable cropland will be in Russia and Central Asia. The increase in variations in global and regional weather patterns will bring a greater fluctuation in crop yields, decreasing the stability of the global food supply and overall food security. Regions currently experiencing the highest levels of undernourishment—parts of Africa and South Asia—are the same regions predicted to have the most dramatic drop in crop yields.[2]

Climate change also may increase the prevalence of food and waterborne diseases. For example, warmer temperatures may increase the risk of poisoning from toxic shellfish and reef fish. Higher temperatures in areas with traditionally temperate climates may also hinder people's ability to safely store food products. Increased flooding, especially in regions with insufficient sanitation practices, will raise the number of people at risk of waterborne diseases.

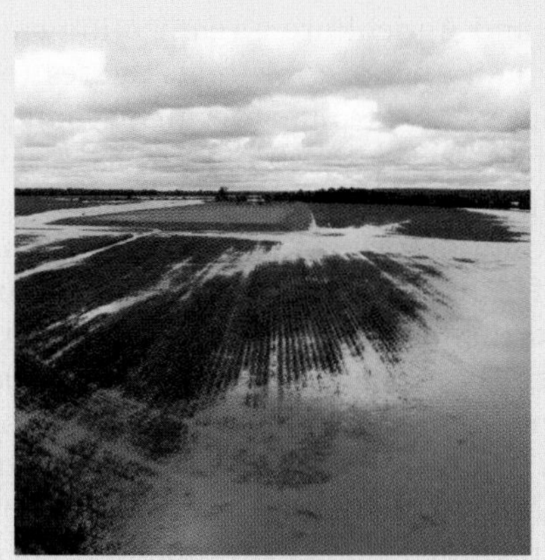

Climate change increases the risk of flooding because warmer air holds more moisture. Scientists predict that the amount of rain in the heaviest precipitation events will increase by more than 40% by 2100, increasing the risk of catastrophic floods.

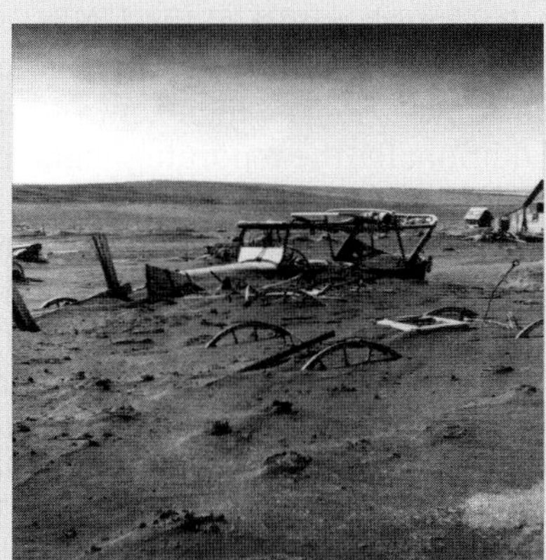

Global warming is making droughts more severe in semiarid and subhumid regions in parts of Africa, Asia, and North America.

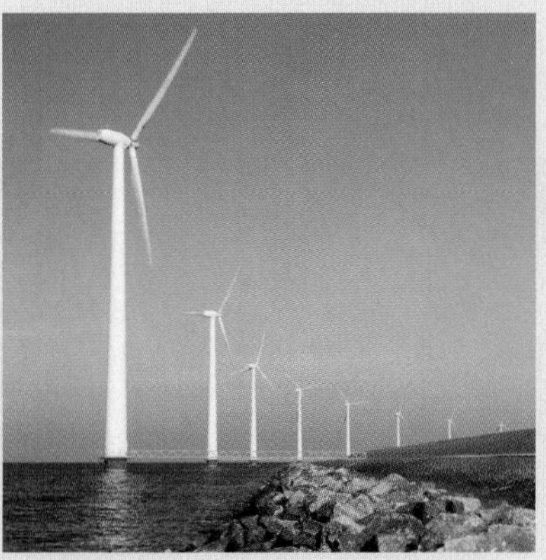

Wind power is a renewable, clean energy source that does not result in the release of greenhouse gases into the atmosphere. Development of alternative energy sources such as wind, solar, and tidal energy will decrease the release of greenhouse gases and possibly decrease the rate of climate change.

Overall, research has shown that climate change will affect food production and trade, access to food, the stability of global food supplies, and food utilization. Within much of the developing world, the adverse impacts of climate change will be felt disproportionately by the poor. Farmers in many of these regions will be unable to adapt to changing conditions.[2]

The future of the global agricultural industry lies in its ability to adapt to these changes through new technologies and sustainable, environmentally friendly agricultural practices. Adapting to changing growing seasons and altering crops to make them better suited to the changing conditions will be necessary.[1] Developing and employing clean energy sources, such as wind and solar energy, also will decrease reliance on fossil fuels and the production of greenhouse gas emissions. These steps have the potential to protect and improve the future of the food supply and the environment.

References

1 Environmental Protection Agency. Climate Change. Available at: http://www.epa.gov/climatechange. Accessed February 25, 2011.

2 Schmidhuber J, Tubiello FN. Global food security under climate change. *PNAS*. [online]. 2007;104:19703–19708. Available at: http://www.pnas.org/content/104/50/19703.full.pdf. Accessed February 25, 2011.

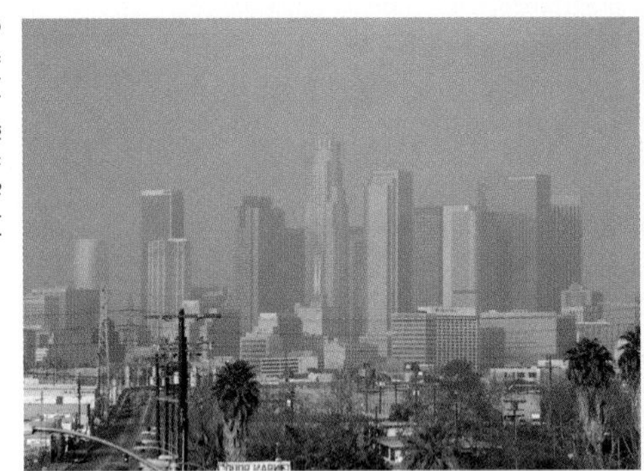

FIGURE 1.4 Los Angeles, California, is well known for its smog. Increasing global temperatures will only worsen smog in such areas, increasing the number of days per year when ozone concentrations exceed federal clean air standards, affecting the health of millions of people.

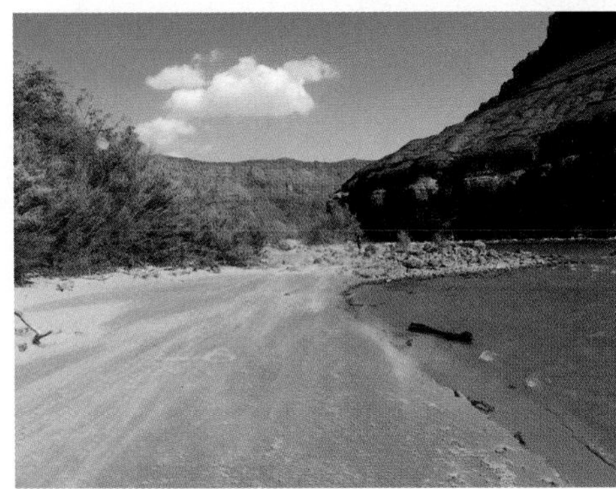

FIGURE 1.5 The Colorado River is an important source of freshwater for a number of Western states. Increased demand due coupled with rising temperatures due to global climate change increase the risk of this valuable resource drying up.

Nationally, the Centers for Disease Control and Prevention (CDC) has created a climate and health program, providing a framework for states, health departments, and communities to build capacity and anticipate problems related to climate change.[30] The National Institutes of Health (NIH) also seeks to increase research and partnership opportunities to minimize the impacts of climate change on human health.[31] *Healthy People 2020*—our nation's health goals—considers climate change to be an "emerging issue" within the purview of environmental health (see **Figure 1.6**).[32]

How This Affects the Study of Food Science

- Climate change will impact crop production.
- Partnerships and research can minimize the effects of climate change on the global food supply.

Effects of Diet on Climate Change

A landmark report of the UN's Food and Agriculture Organization stated that livestock production emits large amounts of greenhouse gases (e.g., carbon dioxide, methane, nitrous oxide) that contribute to climate change.[33] Additionally, the report highlighted other adverse effects of livestock production on the global environment, including deforestation for pastureland; water pollution due to animal waste, antibiotics, and hormones; tannery chemicals in the processing of hides; fertilizer/pesticide residue and runoff from feed crops; eroded pastures; and the loss of biodiversity.[33] Although some scientists have expressed concern about the report's calculations and suggest redefining various measures and scales, others assert that the annual worldwide greenhouse gas emissions from livestock and their byproducts have been vastly underestimated.[34,35] Many declare that approaches to public health nutrition should place climate change and environmental concern at the center of teaching, learning, advocacy, and practice.[36–38]

Vegetarianism and Plant-Based Diets

Some experts propose the adoption of a vegetarian diet as an important strategy to combat global warming/climate change (see **Figure 1.7**).[39] Numerous studies have indicated that vegetarian and plant-based diets are effective in mitigating environmental damage and minimizing resource consumption.[40–43] For example, researchers in Scotland concluded that a healthy vegetarian diet composed of locally grown organic foods, such as freshly grown vegetables available at a farmer's market (see **Figure 1.8**), could reduce Scotland's ecological footprint by nearly 40%.[44] Experimental modeling suggests that consuming plant-based diets can be an effective way to decrease greenhouse gas emissions and feasibly achieve climate stabilization goals.[45] Furthermore, plant-based diets are nutritionally sound throughout the entire lifecycle and can reduce chronic disease morbidity.[46]

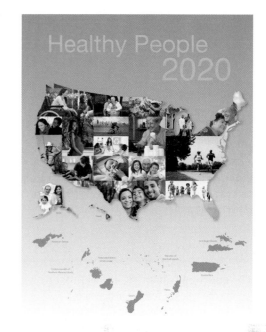

FIGURE 1.6 One of the goals of *Healthy People 2020* is to promote health for all Americans through a healthy environment.

Source: Courtesy of HealthyPeople.gov, U.S. Department of Health and Human Services.

How This Affects the Study of Food Science

- Plant-based diets can minimize resource consumption.

Effects of Food Waste on Climate Change

It has been reported that food waste in the United States has been underestimated and has increased in recent years.[47] The energy content of wasted food is important from an environmental perspective—especially considering the water and energy requirements of food production and the emissions associated with food waste.[47] The total amount of food wasted in the United States in 2007 represented more than 2030 ± 160 trillion British Thermal Units (BTUs) of embedded energy and was "more than the energy available from many popular efficiency and energy procurement strategies such as the annual production of ethanol from grains and annual petroleum available from drilling in the outer continental shelf."[48]

Domestically, food scraps represented 14.1% of the 243 million tons of solid waste generated in the United States in 2009.[49] Food scraps represent the second largest percentage of municipal solid waste after paper and paperboard products.[49] Food scraps in the 2009 study were defined as uneaten food and food preparation waste across a variety of facilities, including homes, but did

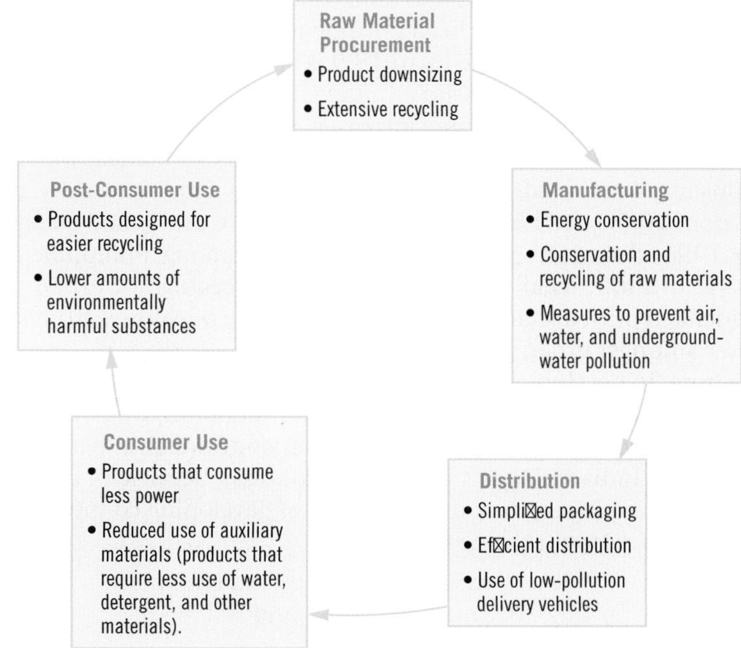

FIGURE 1.7 With the lifecycle assessment method, all the environmental impacts associated with every stage of a product's lifecycle, from beginning to end, are analyzed. The results can help consumers make informed decisions about what foods and products they choose to purchase.

Source: Adapted from Environmental Protection Agency National Risk Management Research Laboratory's Life Cycle Assessment. Available at: http://www.epa.gov/nrmrl/std/lca/lca.html.

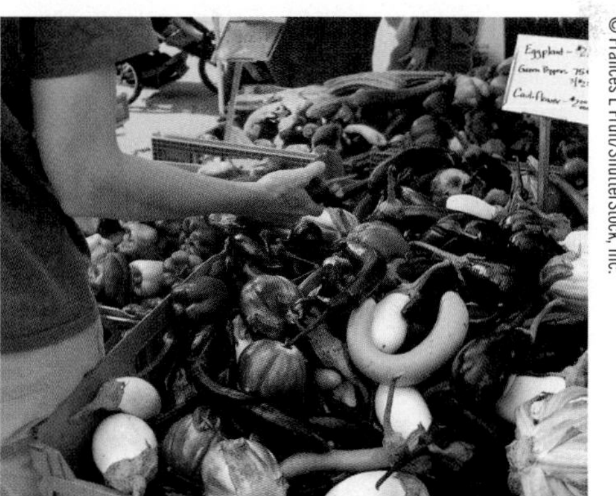

FIGURE 1.8 Buying food at the farmer's market benefits the environment in a number of ways. First, foods at the farmer's market are usually not enclosed in wasteful packaging. Second, the foods are not transported across the country by trucks that give off greenhouse gases.

not include the preconsumer waste of manufactured food products, which was classified as industrial waste.[49] The EPA has created a Food Waste Management Cost Calculator to estimate the costs of alternatives to food waste disposal.[50] Food waste diversion (keeping organic food waste out of landfills by composting or recycling) lowers greenhouse gas emissions; enriches soils and mitigates soil erosion; and improves land use.[50] Globally, there is a need for greater precision in quantitative measures of food waste.[51]

Green Point

Plant-Based Diets The adoption of plant-based diets can be an effective way to decrease greenhouse gas emissions and stabilize the climate.

How This Affects the Study of Food Science

- Composting food waste can reduce costs associated with food production and can improve soils.
- Preventing food waste has far-reaching benefits.
- Reducing food waste can save enormous amounts of energy.

Nutrition Transitions

nutrition transition The major shift in the types of foods consumed by human populations and the resultant effect upon body composition and health.

An important term in food science these days is **nutrition transition**. The term *nutrition transition* describes major shifts in the types of foods consumed by populations and their effects on general health and body composition.[52] Nutrition transitions are studied in relation to the following:[53]

- Major shifts in population growth and age structure
- The spatial distribution of populations
- The role of the food industry in determining diet structure
- Changes in women's roles
- Public concern for diet and disease prevention
- Complex interactions among epidemiological, socioeconomic, and demographic factors

Globally, a nutrition transition to foods that are energy dense and high in fats, cholesterol, and sugars has been documented.[53,54] One survey examined the dietary habits of children aged 2 to 18.9 years of age in the United States, the Philippines, China, and Russia.[55] In the United States, the percentage of calories consumed away from home increased across age groups, from 13.3% of total caloric intake in 1977 to 25.6% of total caloric intake in 1996.[55] Youth consumption of soft drinks, fruit drinks, fast food, and salty snacks doubled from 10.5% to 21.2% of total calorie intake in the United States from 1977 to 1996. Soft drink consumption doubled among Philippine youth from 1994 to 2002. In all countries, a higher percentage of urban versus rural residents reported snacking, and the percentage of calories from snacks was higher amongst urban youth.

Data from 36 developing countries shows that there are now more women with a Body Mass Index (BMI) greater than 25 (denoting overweight) than women with a BMI of less than 18.5 (denoting underweight), with the only exception being India.[56] These statistics are troubling because of the general lack of healthcare infrastructure and resources in developing countries for the treatment of diet-related chronic diseases.[57]

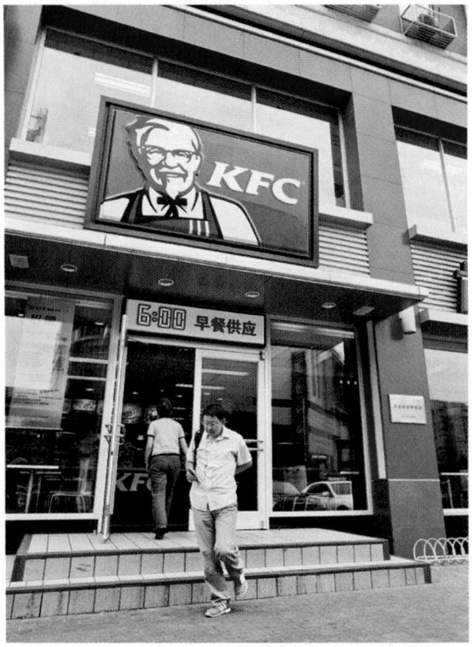

FIGURE 1.9 The increase in the number fast food outlets across the globe has made fast, cheap, and calorie-dense, but nutrient-poor, foods available to most of the world's population. It also has been associated with increasing obesity-related healthcare costs.

Globalization

Globalization has been cited in the creation of lifestyle imbalances that are linked to poor diet and limited physical activity. Specifically, globalization has resulted in the following trends across the globe:[58]

- The spread of technologies that limit energy expenditure
- Modern food processing (see **Figure 1.9**)

- Communication and distribution techniques that espouse "the Western diet"
- Global expansion of the mass media
- Disappearance of fresh food markets in the developing world

One study found that globalization afforded high-income groups the ability to use the international marketplace for monetary gain while providing low-income groups lower quality, obesity-promoting foods.[59] Globalization also has been implicated in high food prices and in reducing access of vulnerable populations to nutritious foods.[60]

Removing trade barriers has been shown to increase the amount of food entering a country, to change the types of foods being imported, and to decrease the costs of importing food, which increases competition with local food producers.[61] For example, the increased availability of animal products for import has increased animal product consumption in developing countries, while the country that produced the food often receives a subsidy for producing the products.[61] Distorted pricing mechanisms and intense promotion has also increased animal product consumption in developing countries.[62]

The consumption of animal products in China and India is likely to continue to increase over the next 30 years. It is estimated that China's meat consumption will surpass that of developed countries by 2030.[63] An increase in animal product consumption is predicted in both developed and developing countries, and most of the growth in livestock production will occur in developing countries.[63,64] Concentrated Animal Feeding Operations (CAFOs), now common in the United States, are being used as a model for meat production in the developing world.[65] This trend is likely to strain ecosystem services, particularly water resources, as discussed in **Special Topic 1.5**.

Special Topic 1.5

Sustainably Feeding the World

Jessica Brie Leonard

Any examination of the sustainability of the global food supply must first look at the **conventional agriculture** practices currently being employed to feed the world's population. These practices have become pervasive because they emphasize high production and low costs, which dovetails with health and food production policy, increasing population growth, and the realities of the ever-evolving marketplace.

The development of conventional agriculture practices stems from the post-World War II era when an emphasis was placed on drastically increasing worldwide food production. This push to increase production led to extensive use of pesticides, fertilizers, and water, in addition to the adoption of fast crop rotation and crop **monoculture**. The positive effects on yield were seen as a measure of success and the impacts of these agricultural practices on soil erosion, groundwater pollution, water overuse, and the development of chemical-resistant weeds were largely ignored or deemed an acceptable byproduct.[1]

conventional agriculture Industrialized agricultural system characterized by mechanization, crop monocultures, and the use of chemical fertilizers and pesticides. Its emphasis is on productivity and profitability.

monoculture The cultivation of a single crop year-to-year on the same land.

The push and pull between the visible and invisible effects of conventional agricultural is the cornerstone of the debate over implementation of sustainable agricultural practices. The changes to the environment that cannot be purely tasted, touched, heard, smelled, or seen create a barrier to perception, acknowledgment, and action to change the current agricultural system. Media, including the documentary *An Inconvenient Truth*, attempt to fill in the gaps of these perceptions with facts, figures, and projections of where we are headed should policy changes not be implemented. Despite a heightened sense of awareness of the problems, the actions of farmers, consumers, and industry leaders have not been drastically altered. This lack of action is tantamount to an open endorsement of these harmful practices. As one expert noted, "How we choose to know, see, and participate within the world can greatly shape how we view the world."[2]

sustainable agriculture An agricultural system that is founded in the principles of ecology; sustainable agriculture is economically viable, socially conscious, and capable of maintaining high productivity.

Many of the negative aspects of conventional agriculture that mandate a change to **sustainable agriculture** are not directly perceived by consumers. These include decreased soil fertility, reduced populations of beneficial soil microorganisms, and increases in the amount of dangerous chemicals in groundwater. What consumers do see is that conventional agriculture yields weed-free crops, pest-free fields, high yields, and product uniformity. The full costs of conventional agriculture are not apparent because they are "externalized to society at-large."[2]

The agricultural policies that have allowed for increased crop yields have now been found to be environmentally unsound and ultimately producing food lacking in nutritional quality.[3] The increased pressure set forth by policies that mandate increased crop yields at maximum profit are straining the agricultural system beyond both its physical and practical limits. The fundamental conventional agricultural practices at play here include monocultures, intense tillage, the use of petrochemical-based fertilizers, the "pesticide treadmill," environmentally unsound crop irrigation, and the unnatural selection of plant genomes.[3,4]

Whereas farming once meant the growing of crops and raising of livestock and then bringing goods to market, current practices favor monocultures where specialization has become the norm. Multiple crops and various species of livestock no longer coexist on the same farm. Conventional agriculture favors the cultivation of one crop pushed to its maximum yield because of efficiencies provided by mechanized planting and harvesting methods and fertilizer and pesticide use. Sadly, these economies of scale result in an increased need for chemical pesticides as the crop monocultures become resistant to the current pesticide preparations.[4]

Farming in a monoculture format also requires excessive tillage of the soil. The aim is to loosen the structure of the soil for better aeration, growth, irrigation, and sowing of the seed. When a singular crop is farmed and the soil is exploited through short crop rotations, the soil loosens its cover and the quality of the soil is degraded. This degradation takes many forms, including increases soil salinity, waterlogging, soil compaction, and pesticide contamination and declines in soil structure and fertility. Erosion is the most widespread form of degradation and contributes to a worldwide loss of 25,000 million tons of topsoil annually.[4] Degradation of agricultural soils, given the limited amount of arable land, makes it difficult to foresee a future for the agricultural industry.

Wasteful water practices, such as those currently used to irrigate crops, are an additional source of concern. Water is drawn from underground aquifers at rates that exceed their replenishment by natural rainfall, rivers are drained at the expense of aquaculture, and dams are built, resulting in unnatural wildlife habitats. The rate at which water is applied to crops exceeds their ability to take up the water, leaving it to evaporate or drain out of the fields. This evaporation has been shown to alter regional humidity levels and rainfall patterns.[4]

Water also serves as the thoroughfare for the petrochemical-based fertilizers and pesticides that are applied to the crops. These chemicals are washed away and enter the groundwater, entering the food chain for generations to come when the water is eventually consumed by people and animals. New chemicals are constantly entering the food chain as pesticides that once were effective become incapable of killing off the pest population and new ones must be developed and applied to take their place, only to follow the same path toward human consumption. Petrochemical-based fertilizers also are of concern because their production and pricing is dependent on the fluctuations of the global oil market.[4]

The proliferation of crop monocultures has resulted in a decline in the genetic diversity of the domesticated plants and animals. It is estimated that approximately 75% of the genetic diversity present in crop plants in 1900 has now been lost.[4] This decline in diversity has in large part been due to conventional agriculture's emphasis on short-term productivity. The development of a crop variety that has high productivity and responds to current fertilizers and pesticides supports the short-term production goal. The drawback is that the crop variety becomes vulnerable as the pest becomes resistant to the pesticide. The irony of the decline in genetic diversity is that the solution to the problem of pesticide resistance may reside in the natural plant defenses present in the plant population, though a diminishing diversity means diminishing genetic resources and thus limited possible solutions to the problem.[4]

Where Do We Start?

Sustainability is centered on "the principle that we meet the needs of the present without compromising the needs of the future."[5] This definition makes the point of addressing the future even though our ability to forecast it is very limited. The question of whether the possible remedies to the harm conventional agriculture is causing could create a new category of problems can only be addressed over time. What we can say is that the current practices are harming the environment and affecting the health of the human population.

Both simple and fundamental changes are necessary in order for the agricultural industry to discard its post-World War II mentality and focus on sustainable practices. Sustainable agriculture has three main objectives: economic profitability, environmental health, and ethical soundness. In practice, these objectives are achieved through maximizing the use of ecological processes, optimizing the use of natural resources, and restricting the use of external resources.[1,5]

The least radical strategy is to substitute, rather than overhaul, current practices. An example would be replacing toxic chemicals and mineral fertilizers with compounds that are lower-level pollutants, that leave fewer residues in the soil, and that consume fewer energy resources to produce. A substitution strategy that outlines the use of biopesticides and the farming of genetically modified plants is seen as a somewhat viable short-term strategy. The drawback is that it is not a long-term solution, due to the evolution of biocide-resistant pests and concerns over the long-term effect of growing and consuming genetically modified crops.[1] See Special Feature 1.2 on genetically modified food for a detailed explanation.

The agroecological approach is favored over a substitution approach because its goal is to apply "ecological concepts and principles to the design, development, and management of sustainable agricultural systems."[1] This approach promotes biodiversity and seeks to enhance it through cultural practices. The benefit of this approach is that it seeks to do more than substitute one problem for another. It looks to address both the agricultural and cultural components, with input from other relevant fields, such as ecology and geography.[1]

The agroecological approach acknowledges that sustainable agriculture, population growth, and societal development cannot be addressed independently of one another. Rather, they are so closely intertwined that it is difficult to separate them and create steps toward change that will positively impact them all. The best approach for shifting to sustainable agriculture lies in strategies to make better use of our existing resources, including land, water, biodiversity, and technologies. The intensity of the changes adopted is a key component of a sustainable approach to agriculture and involves using natural, social, and human capital in combination with the best practices in available technologies and ecological management. Those practices that minimize or eliminate harm to the environment are those that qualify for implementation.[6]

A shift toward a more sustainable model of agriculture does not mean that technological advances have to be ruled out; in fact, they can be part of the solution if they do not cause harm to the environment. **Table A** lists a number of resource-conserving technologies and practices that can improve an **agroecosystem**.

agroecosystem An agricultural system that includes cropland, pasture, land for livestock, and uncultivated land adjacent to a farm that supports vegetation and wildlife and the corresponding atmosphere, soil, groundwater, and drainage. A sustainable agroecosystem maintains natural resources and does not rely on artificial inputs to manage pests and disease outbreaks among the crops.

TABLE A
Practices for Building Healthy Agroecosystems

Technology/Practice	Implementation
Integrated pest management	Only use pesticides when other options fail. Use natural pests to control weeds and disease to maintain biodiversity.
Integrated nutrient management	Use crop rotation with nitrogen-fixing crops. Use natural sources of inorganic and organic sources of nutrients. Reduce runoff of nutrients from agricultural fields.
Conservation tillage	Reduce the frequency of tillage to conserve soil and avoid erosion.
Cover crops	Grow cover crops, particularly nitrogen-fixing ones, in the off-season or in conjunction with main crops to maintain healthy soil.
Agroforestry	Incorporate trees into the agricultural system.
Water harvesting in dryland areas	Improve irrigation and rainfall retention on formerly abandoned and degraded land.
Livestock reintegration into farming systems	Establish mixed crop and livestock environments to improve nutrient cycling on farms.

Although technology has a role to play, it is not a stand-alone solution. The adoption of environmentally friendly technologies can result in favorable changes, but the role that people play cannot be overlooked. It is essential to employ a holistic approach in shifting to sustainable agriculture because isolated practices will not yield a perceivable result. Education also is important. A lack of information on how to implement and manage change can be a barrier to sustainable agriculture. Therefore, the education of the farming community on sustainable agriculture practices is essential for creating a cultural foundation for future change.[6]

A survey of Iowa farmers brought to light that the shift from conventional agriculture to sustainable agriculture will be a challenge because the average farmer's planning cycle is 6 months out, at the least. The profit-driven conventional agriculture industry makes it difficult to adopt change and leaves farmers in a position where it is practically impossible for them to choose a long-term approach when faced with 1-year lease arrangements and an emphasis on short-term economic gains.[2]

Within the farming culture are additional pressures that are less likely to be validated by the greater society, including the belief that allowing weeds to be part of the biodiversity of one's crops, as they often are in sustainable agriculture practices, reflects poorly on the farmer. Manageable, incremental changes and education with regard to sustainable farming practices are key elements in fostering acceptance of sustainable agriculture in the farming community. Time and education will provide the room needed for confidence to grow and for farmers to take an active role in the innovation and evolution of new sustainable practices.[2]

Feeding and the Food System

A global strategy expands upon the agroecological approach by not only looking at the culture of agriculture but also at society as a whole and recognizing that sustainability is about more than farms. A global strategy means looking at the entire food system; that is, the relationship between farms and food consumption and at how food is marketed.[1]

Inherent in any food system and its agricultural policies is the need to feed the growing human population. Food policies cannot be focused solely on increasing the quantity of food produced; they also must address access to food, the quality of the food, and the decision of which food items to produce. A secure food supply satisfies consumers' needs without jeopardizing production processes in the short or long term. It ensures the sustainability of supplies while considering the safety of methods of production and the nutritional stability of the food produced.[3]

The relationship between food security and sustainability is addressed in the World Health Organization's (WHO) First Action Plan for Food and Nutrition Policy as follows:[3]

- The ways in and means by which food is produced and distributed respect the natural process of the earth and are thus sustainable.
- Both the production and consumption of food are grounded in and governed by social values that are just and equitable as well as moral and ethical.
- The ability to acquire food is assured.
- The food itself is nutritionally adequate and personally and culturally acceptable.
- The food is obtained in a manner that upholds human dignity.

The focus of food production and health policies shifted from increased food production and distribution in the early to mid-twentieth century to correcting nutrient deficiencies in the latter half of the twentieth century. Most recently, the focus has shifted toward considering the ecological impact of food production. This can be seen in the international resolutions in Agenda 21 that was endorsed by the UN Conference on Environment and Development that addresses the relationship between agricultural production and its environmental impact. The WHO also has begun to address concerns over the following: loss of biodiversity, desertification and ecological degradation, water and air pollution, the social and psychological effects of depleted environments, and issues of social justice and human rights and food production.[3]

agribusiness A complex system of businesses involved in the production and packaging of food. It includes farmers, both large and small operations, and the companies that provide the inputs, such as seeds, chemicals, and lines of credit, needed to produce agricultural products. This system also includes businesses involved in the processing, packaging, transportation, and marketing of food.

The current approach to food production is based in science but not environmental science. The transformation from agriculture to **agribusiness** was made possible through the genetic modification of crops and livestock; the spraying of crops and animal feed with added nutrients; and the use of chemicals to increase yields. These developments resulted in financial gains, and therefore have been widely adopted and endorsed. However, endorsement of such practices should not be mistaken as validation. The increased abundance of food and reduced food costs have increased food safety risks and damaged the environment.[1]

The Producer–Consumer Disconnect

The deficiencies that set the current food policies in motion are no longer at the forefront of nutritional concerns; thus the policies should be revised to address the current situation. A disconnect exists between society's needs and current agricultural practices. To meet the needs of the global population, the agribusiness industry must begin to address the nutrient density and the diversity of the food supply. Deterioration in the nutrient content of food has been a result of decreased biodiversity and an increase in the processing and preservation of foods with an emphasis on their visual appearance.[3]

This emphasis on product presentation has evolved simultaneously with the food industry's evolution into a player in the global marketplace. Food is moved rapidly around the world, and processing, packaging, and preserving now consume the highest percentages of each food dollar spent. Today, the farmer is left with less than 8 cents of each food dollar that is spent.[4] Farmers also face difficulties when choosing what to plant because they must ensure that a particular crop variety is commercially viable; that is, that it will be bought by a large transnational corporation.[4]

The emergence of agribusiness is a direct result of the commodification of food. This transformation of food into a global commodity has consequently influenced the tastes and behaviors of consumers. Demand is created for products with a high profit potential, such as fast foods, processed snacks, exotic fruits, and out-of-season vegetables. These foods have the highest environmental costs, and their purchase supports the least sustainable practices.[4] **Figure A** depicts food commodities with the lowest and highest environmental costs.

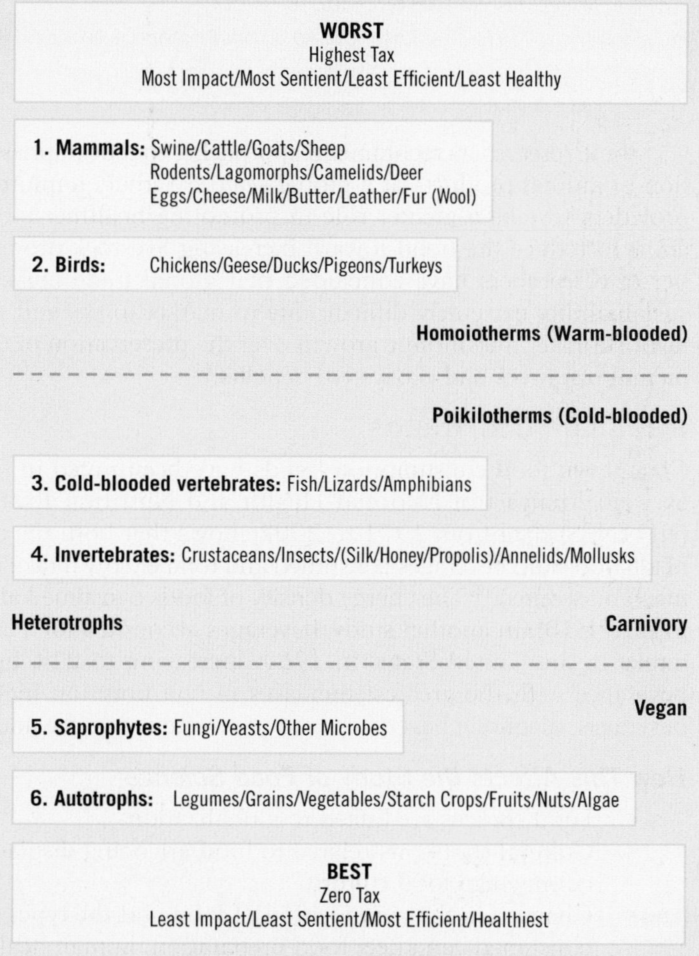

FIGURE A Different types of foods have different environmental impacts. For example, fresh produce has a much smaller environmental cost than a package of potato chips.

Source: Modified from Goodland R. Agricultural sustainability: Diet matters. *Ecological Economics.* 1997;23(3):189–200.

Community Action

A closer relationship needs to be established between consumers and farmers. Consumers should be educated on the benefits of reducing consumption of animal products and foods requiring excessive transport and processing. Farmers can be encouraged to create and protect the soil, conserve and protect water sources, manage organic wastes to avoid pollution, select plants and animals that are adapted to the local environment, encourage biodiversity, manage pests with minimal environmental impact, and limit the use of nonrenewable resources.[4,7]

Communities can support sustainable agriculture by reestablishing local farmers as the primary food source. Shorter food supply chains decreases the number of links in the food supply, creating a more cohesive food community. It also is up to the consumers and the larger community to require that food producers and manufacturers provide information—such as the food's nutritional content and origin—on the food they are purchasing. This information exchange can educate consumers on the practices their purchases are supporting and enable them to spend their food dollar more sustainably.[4]

The issues created by current conventional agricultural practices are deeply rooted in agribusiness. The adoption of more sustainable practices has the potential to have a positive impact on the environment and our food supply. It is this focus that must be adopted in order to move sustainable agricultural practices forward and allow for positive changes in our environment.

References

1 Lichtfouse E, Navarrete M, Debaeke P, et al. Agronomy for sustainable agriculture: A review. *Agron Sustain Dev.* 2005;25:1–6.
2 Carolan MS. Do you see what I see? Examining the epistemic barriers to sustainable agriculture. *Rural Sociol.* 2006;71(2):232–260.
3 World Health Organization. *Food and Health in Europe: A New Basis for Action.* WHO Regional Publications, European Series, no. 96; 2003.
4 Gliessman S. *Agroecology: The Ecology of Sustainable Food Systems.* Boca Raton, FL: CRC Press; 2007.
5 Spiertz JHJ. Nitrogen, sustainable agriculture and food security: A review. *Agron Sustain Dev.* 2010;30:13–55.
6 Pretty J. Can ecological agriculture feed nine billion people? *Monthly Review.* 2005 Nov.;61(6):16–58.
7 Horne J, McDermott M. *The Next Green Revolution: Essential Steps to a Healthy Sustainable Agriculture.* Binghamton, NY: Food Products Press, Haworth Press; 2001.

Some researchers recommend approaches that deemphasize the consumption of animal products at a global scale.[62] Others implore U.S. healthcare providers to take a greater role in promoting healthier food options in an effort to reduce the trend toward increasing livestock production.[66] A number of researchers have concluded that global trade makes environmental sustainability extremely difficult due to market forces and mechanisms that favor short-term economic growth over the preservation of essential environmental resources and ecosystem benefits.[67]

National Food Trends

Changes in food consumption trends have been noted in the United States as well. Analysis of National Health and Nutrition Examination Survey (NHANES) data from 1971 to 2002 shows that both the reported amount of all foods and beverages consumed and total energy intake increased in both men and women.[68] The energy density of foods consumed also increased (see **Figure 1.10**). In another study, beverages accounted for 12% of total caloric intake in the United States in 1965, increasing to 21% by 2002.[69] Those beverages with the greatest increases in consumption included sweetened beverages, alcoholic beverages, and unsweetened coffee and tea.

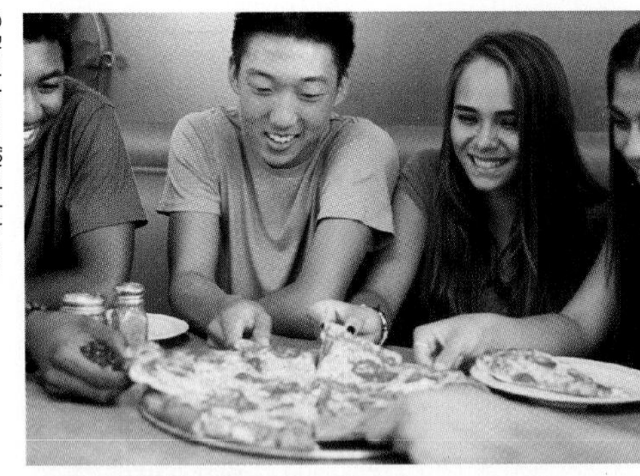

FIGURE 1.10 Today's foods are more energy dense than in the past, which can make it easy to consume too many empty calories.

How This Affects the Study of Food Science

- Food choices are linked to globalization.
- Cultural traditions related to food are being displaced by the commercial food culture.
- Changes in the composition of food and the types of foods consumed can affect food preparation, human health, and the natural environment.

Going Green with Food Science

Numerous organizations across various disciplines are working to improve or preserve the integrity of our food while simultaneously addressing the health of both humans and the natural environment:

- Health Care Without Harm is an international coalition that works to create healthcare systems that implement ecologically sound practices.[70] In its joint report with the WHO, three of seven components for a "climate-friendly healthcare facility" are food- and beverage-related: providing sustainable, locally grown foods; conserving water and avoiding bottled water; and recycling and composting.[71] Healthcare facilities are further encouraged to reduce their ecological footprint and improve patient health by limiting the amount of meat served in hospital meals and preparing their own food onsite.[71]
- The Environmental Working Group (EWG) is a nonprofit organization that uses public information to protect public health and the natural environment.[72] The EWG strives to protect vulnerable segments of the human population (i.e., children, babies, infants in the womb) from toxic contaminants, including chemicals in the food stream.[73]
- The Washington Toxics Coalition works to eliminate toxic chemicals that accumulate in the environment and in humans. It cites the ban of bisphenol A (BPA) from baby bottles, children's drink cups, and sports bottles in the state of Washington as one of its many accomplishments.[74]
- The Center for Food Safety works to curb the proliferation of harmful food production technologies and promotes sustainable agriculture.[75] Its "Cool Foods Campaign" connects food to global warming/climate change.[76]
- The Hunger and Environmental Nutrition Practice Group of the Academy of Nutrition and Dietetics envisions optimizing the nation's health by promoting access to nutritious food and clean water for a secure and sustainable food system. It aspires to: "A sustainable and resilient food system that conserves and renews natural resources, advances social justice and animal welfare, builds community wealth, and fulfills the food and nutrition needs of all eaters now and in the future."[77]
- The Center for a Livable Future is driven by the concept that diet, health, food production, the environment, population growth, and equity are all elements of a single complex system.[78]

Concern and care for the natural environment also is demonstrated by individuals within health organizations and across disciplines:[79,80]

- Some general practice physicians advocate linking patient health promotion recommendations to environmental sustainability. They do this by encouraging patients to eat more plant-based foods and fewer animal products as well as by promoting walking, biking, and using public transportation.[81]
- Some experts promote increased self-reliance for food preparation and food production, such as cooking and growing one's own food.[82,83]
- A large health benefits company in Massachusetts provides a member discount for professionally installed organic raised-bed vegetable gardens and gardening advice to make growing organic vegetables at home easier.[84]

How This Affects the Study of Food Science

- Decreasing bottled water use can help the natural environment.
- Chemicals in food packaging can accumulate in humans.
- Numerous organizations place great importance on reducing the human impact on the natural environment and improving human health via improved food and water quality.

Putting Theory into Practice

The following four narratives illustrate how specific organizations and individuals are putting the theory of nutritional ecology into practice.

The Greening of a Seattle Restaurant

The owners of Sutra, a 30-seat restaurant Sutra in Seattle, Washington, create an extraordinary culinary experience that honors community and human health while minimizing the impact on the natural environment. They achieve this through exemplary business practices. Once customers are seated for dinner, in which the entire restaurant enjoys the prix fixe menu in unison, Sutra chef Colin Patterson strikes a large bell to signal the start of the meal. When the reverberations have diminished, Patterson graciously greets his customers and extends gratitude to them for coming, to the Earth for providing the food, to those who grew and acquired the food, and to the weather pattern that created the beauty of that day.[85]

The following is an example of a dinner at Sutra:[86]

Roasted Carrot–Cauliflower–Leek Soup with an Arugula Smoked Lentil & Fennel Salad with a Green Garlic–Lime–Saffron Vinaigrette finished with Candied Sunflower Seeds

Wild Foraged Wood Sorrel Risotto–Asparagus–Shiso Roll with a Yuzu–Tomato Sauce topped with Micro Greens

Nettle–Mung Bean Spatzel with Grilled Haruka Japanese (locally grown) Turnips & Tamari–Ginger Roasted Shitake Mushrooms served with Thyme–Cashew Cream Sauce and finished with Parsnip Chips

Maple Blossom–Coconut Ice Cream (nondairy) served with a Cinnamon–Pecan Cookie and finished with a Blackberry–Port Compote

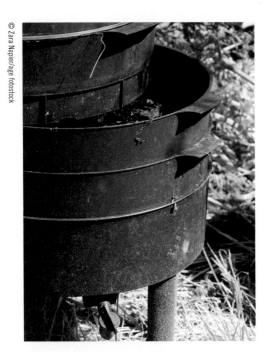

FIGURE 1.11 Vermicomposting uses worms to create a mixture of decomposing food waste, bedding materials, and vermicast. Vermicast, also known as *worm manure*, is excreted by the worms as they break down the organic matter. It is very nutrient rich and has been shown to have lower levels of contaminants than organic materials that have not been vermicomposted.

vermicomposting The use of earthworms to convert organic waste into a nutrient-rich paste that can be used to replenish the soil.

The menu itself is chic—a thick, marbled brown paper with bold italic lettering offset by a thick black border. The menu is small, 5 × 8 inches, which minimizes resource consumption compared to a multipage laminated restaurant menu. The fine print at the bottom of the menu reads: "Printed on Recycled Grocery Bags." Patterson changes the menu biweekly and never creates the same menu twice. This allows him to use his ingenuity in creating scrumptious meals that are based around produce that is currently in season. According to Patterson, "A good chef knows that you make the best food when it's fresh from the ground, and it's never going to taste any better." Although admitting that it is sometimes difficult to acquire foods locally due to unpredictable weather patterns, Patterson sources as many local foods as possible, including foraged foods.[85]

The prix fixe menu coupled with a fixed headcount conserves resources from the outset, eliminating the food waste typical of extensive restaurant menus and unpredictable customer-ordering patterns. Patterson recalls, "When I worked in other restaurants, it was very disappointing to fill three to five large garbage cans of wasted food every night." Although little food is left on customers' plates at the end of the meal, any food waste is composted on-site by way of three large vermicomposting bins (see **Figure 1.11**). **Vermicomposting** is the use of earthworms to convert organic waste into a nutrient-rich hummus that can be used to replenish the soil; the hummus is then used on a productive edible flower and herb garden located behind the restaurant. On-site composting not only facilitates nutrient recycling, but it also reduces the cost of waste disposal as well as the associated fossil fuel use and carbon output of the truck that would otherwise pick up the food scraps for commercial composting (or disposal in a landfill).[85]

Sutra does not offer take-home boxes, thus bypassing food container waste. Portion sizes are such that consumers generally eat the entire meal in the restaurant. Patterson also returns as many food service boxes as he can to food vendors for reuse.

Lastly, Patterson believes that providing healthy foods is as important as creating tasty, savory foods. He recognizes the nutritive value of many local native plant foods—for example, stinging nettle, which contains over 400 milligrams of calcium per 1 cup serving (cooked), along with 6 grams of dietary fiber. In fact, many edible plants native to the Pacific Northwest have impressive nutrient profiles; furthermore, native plants are extraordinarily beneficial to the ecosystem and ecosystem services.[85]

How This Affects the Study of Food Science

- Edible native and foraged foods can expand the palate and add valuable nutrients to the diet.
- Food waste in the restaurant setting can be minimized.
- Cooking foods shortly after they have been picked can offer superior taste.

Minimizing Food Container Waste

Lynn Foord, Director of Prerequisites for Health Professions at Massachusetts General Hospital, Institute of Health Professions, drinks a cup of coffee every day. Instead of using a disposable coffee cup made of paper and plastic components each day, Dr. Foord simply uses a reusable coffee mug (see **Figure 1.12**). She made this change when she noticed the large volume of waste the disposable cups produced. "It was when my trash can was not emptied once for a week that I literally saw the unnecessary volume of trash that I was responsible for, which moved me to reflect on my personal behaviors and propelled me to action," Dr. Foord noted. Dr. Foord also brings her lunch to work in a reusable lunch tote complete with reusable tableware, eliminating large quantities of disposable food container waste.[87]

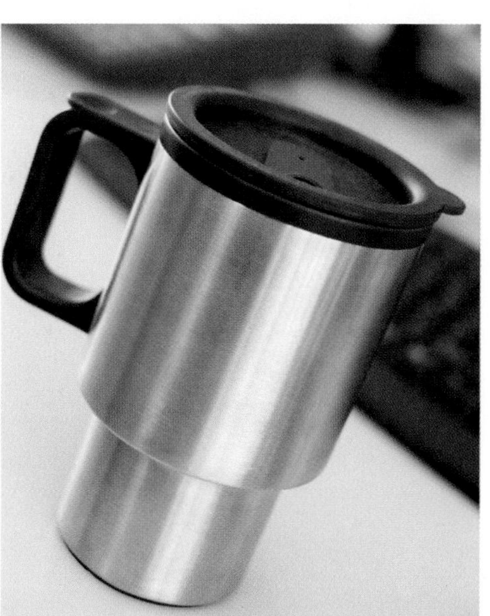

FIGURE 1.12 Making a small change, such as using reusable coffee mugs, is an easy way to reduce the amount of waste generated in an office setting.

How This Affects the Study of Food Science

- Changing personal behaviors can reduce unnecessary food container waste.
- Contemporary eating patterns have led to increased food container waste.

Using Diet and Exercise to Reduce Carbon Output

On a particularly lovely day after work, Paul Harris decided to walk to the next subway stop so he could enjoy the sunshine of the day a little longer before entering the subway. But he didn't stop there and ended up walking all the way home from work. Thereafter, Harris decided to walk those 3 miles to or from work approximately 200 days a year, using public transportation or carpooling at other times. Harris claims he only had to wake up 15 minutes earlier than usual for the 45-minute walk, and he estimates that he walked approximately 30,000 miles to and from work over 25 years.

Harris now co-chairs Climate Change Action Brookline, a citizen-led effort to reduce carbon output in the city of Brookline, Massachusetts, and helps manage the Brookline Farmers Market. By analyzing his lifestyle habits in the company of neighbors who came together to form an "Eco Team," Harris went from practicing a lifestyle associated with 26,000 pounds of carbon output

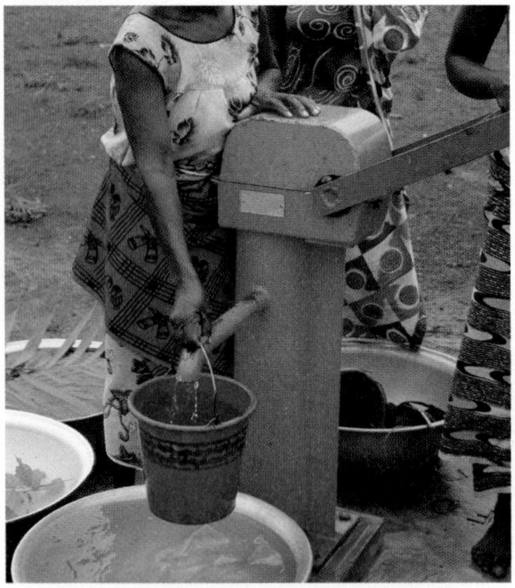

FIGURE 1.13 Purchasing safe drinking water systems for communities in the developing world is an inexpensive way to make a positive impact on the lives of those living in poverty.

per year to one associated with 16,000 pounds. His lifestyle changes included transitioning to a vegetarian diet. According to Harris, "A vegetarian diet is not as hard as I thought. I looked at it as something I can do that has multiple benefits. It's low cost and high benefit."[88]

How This Affects the Study of Food Science

- Decreasing meat consumption can reduce greenhouse gas and carbon dioxide emissions.
- Vegetarian diets are readiy accessible and can support local agricultural systems.

Closing the Loop

In an effort to save money, improve health, and eliminate paper and plastic waste, the Seattle University Engineers Without Borders (EWB) student organization has integrated nutrition ecology principles into its organizational practices. Faculty advisor Professor Phillip Thompson also realized that the money spent on their pizza-based working lunch was money that could be spent on building safe drinking water systems for communities in the developing world (see **Figure 1.13**). They acquired a full set of "gently used" porcelain tableware and decided to take full responsibility for its foodservice needs. After obtaining two slow cookers, the students and faculty now take turns preparing a slow-cooked, plant-based lunchtime meal, which has lowered the cost of feeding the entire group (15 to 30 people) to about $15 per meal. In all, the group's actions saved $170 per month, or $2,040 dollar per year. EWB used these savings to support the operation and maintenance of a safe drinking water system for a medical clinic in Haiti.[89]

How This Affects the Study of Food Science

- Returning to increased self-sufficiency for providing meals minimizes food waste and increases control over the health-related aspects of food. Simple meals can appease taste buds and the senses.

Chapter Review

Food science encompasses the investigation of better ways to select, preserve, process, package, and distribute food products. It includes the study of the composition of food ingredients and their manipulation during growing, production, processing, and presentation to the consumer.

Although many of the scientific principles remain the same as for traditional food science, many must be evaluated with an additional factor or concern. This factor is *ecology*, which impacts food quality, composition, and availability. Some steps to address solutions to the changing environment presented in this chapter include:

- Identifying present ecological practices and providing suggested improvements such as sustainability
- Tackling food waste and advocating the use of whole foods
- Addressing climate change and its affect on crops and providing suggestions of crop change
- Focusing on improved individual diet patterns that may be better for our environment
- Highlighting the effect of the changing environment and its impact on health
- Identifying business practices that demonstrate good nutrition with ecology in mind.

Learning Portfolio

Study Points

1. Restructuring our relationship with the natural environment to enact the principles of sustainability is one of the greatest challenges of our day.
2. In an era of heightened environmental concern, careful consideration must be given to lifestyle behaviors, agricultural practices, and food processing and distribution.
3. Ecological systems are experiencing multiple severe and mutually reinforcing stresses, the root causes of which are increased per person consumption of ecosystem services and a growing human population.
4. The following trends will continue to disturb ecosystems: increased demand for food, fiber, and water; ecosystem contaminants and waste; eutrophication of waterways; global trade; climate change; overfishing, vergrazing, and overlogging; and habitat loss and fragmentation.
5. Removal of trade barriers increases the amount of food that enters a country, results in the importation of new foods, and makes it more difficult for local food producers to compete in the marketplace.
6. Some scientists and healthcare and public health professionals are encouraging people to reduce their consumption of animal products in an effort to improve overall dietary patterns and benefit the environment.
7. The energy density of food has increased in recent years; snacking, soda consumption, and overall food intake also have increased.
8. Organizations and numerous people are working across a variety of disciplines and venues to improve the integrity of food systems and to promote healthy lifestyle behaviors that reduce the human impact on the living systems of the natural environment.
9. Many edible plants native have impressive nutrient profiles and are extraordinarily beneficial to ecosystems and ecosystem services.

Issues for Discussion

1. Discuss current trends that will continue to disturb ecosystem functions into the future, including increased global demand for food and water.
2. Discuss potential solutions for the following problems that threaten the global food and water supply:
   a. Ecosystem contaminants and waste
   b. Eutrophication
   c. Global trade
   d. Climate change
   e. Overfishing
   f. Overgrazing
   g. Overlogging
   h. Habitat loss and fragmentation

Research Ideas for Students

1. The multifaceted relationship between food production and the living systems of the natural environment
2. The connections among nutrition ecology, ecosystems, ecosystem services, and the concept of an ecological footprint
3. A historical timeline of anthropogenic effects on the living systems of the natural environment
4. The relationship between diet and climate change and the potential role of diet in mitigating climate change
5. Reducing the impact on the living systems of the natural environment via nutrition ecology

Key Terms

	page
acidification	13
agribusiness	22
agroecosystem	21
anthropogenic effects	9
biobased product	11
biocapacity	9
biodiversity	9
conventional agriculture	19
crop yields	14
ecological literacy	7
ecosystem	7
ecosystem services	7
food insecurity	5
food science	4
genetically modified organisms (GMOs)	8
greenhouse effect	14
herbicide	8
living systems	7
monoculture	19
nutrition ecology	4
nutrition transition	18
sustainable agriculture	20
vermicomposting	26

References

1. Suzuki DT. *The Sacred Balance: Rediscovering our Place in Nature.*Amherst, NY: Prometheus Books; 2002.
2. U.S. Census Bureau. U.S. & World Population Clocks. Updated 2011. Available at: http://www.census.gov/main/www/popclock.html. Accessed May 23, 2011.
3. U.S. Census Bureau, Population Division. International Data Base, World Population: 1950–2050. Updated 2011. Available at: http://www.census.gov/ipc/www/idb/worldpopgraph.php. Accessed May 23, 2011.
4. Chivian E, McCally M, Hu H, Haines A (eds.). *Critical Condition: Human Health and the Environment.* Cambridge, MA: The MIT Press; 1993.
5. Leitzmann C. Nutrition ecology: The contribution of vegetarian diets. *Am J Clin Nutr.* 2003;8(suppl):657S–659S.
6. Lietzmann C. Nutrition ecology: Origin and definition. *Forum Nutr.* 2003;56:220–221.
7. Hoffman I. Transcending reductionism in nutrition research. *Am J Clin Nutr.* 2003;78(suppl):514S–516S.
8. Messina M, Lampe JW, Birt DF. Reductionism and the narrowing nutrition perspective: Time for reevaluation and emphasis on food synergy. *J Am Diet Assoc.* 2001;101(12): 1416–1419.
9. Tagtow A, Harmon A. Healthy Land, Healthy Food, & Healthy Eaters. October 2008. Available at: http://www.iatp.org/documents/healthy-land-healthy-food-healthy-eaters. Accessed June 18, 2012.
10. Capra F. The new facts of life: Connecting the dots on food, health, and the environment. *Public Library Quarterly.* 2009;28: 242–248.
11. Millennium Ecosystem Assessment Responses Working Group. MA conceptual framework. In: *Ecosystems and Human Well-Being: Policy Responses*, vol. 3. Washington, DC: Island Press; 2005: 1–25.
12. Sweeney LB. Remembering what we already know: Using our systems intelligence to meet 21st century challenges. Prepared lecture materials for the Organizational Systems Renewal Graduate Program, April 2009, Seattle, Washington.
13. Hassan R, Scholes R, Ash N (eds.). *Ecosystems and Human Well-Being: Current State and Trends. Findings of the Condition and Trends Working Group.* Washington, DC: Island Press; 2005: no. 1.
14. World Wild Fund for Nature. *Living Planet Report 2010: Biodiversity, Biocapacity and Development.* 2010. Available at: http://wwf.panda.org/about_our_earth/all_publications/living_planet_report/living_planet_report_timeline/2010_lpr2. Accessed June 17, 2012.
15. Wackernagel M, Schulz NB, Deumling D, et al. Tracking the ecological overshoot of the human economy. *Proc Natl Acad Sci USA.* 2002;99(14):9266–9271.
16. La Seur CL, Abelkop AD. Forty years after NEPA's enactment, it is time for a comprehensive Farm Bill environmental impact statement. *Harvard Law & Policy Review.* 2010;4:201–227.
17. Allan JD, Abell R, Hogan Z, et al. Overfishing of inland waters. *BioScience.* 2005;55(12):1041–1051.
18. Limburg KE, Waldman JR. Dramatic declines in North Atlantic diadromous fishes. *BioScience.* 2009;59(11):955–965.
19. Driscoll CT, Han Y, Chen CY, et al. Mercury contamination in forest and freshwater ecosystems in the Northeastern United States. *BioScience.* 2007;57(1):17–28.
20. Mergler D, Anderson HA, Chan, et al. Methylmercury exposure and health effects in humans: A worldwide concern. *Ambio.* 2007;36(1):3–11.
21. Hayes T, Haston K, Tsui M, et al. Herbicides: Feminization of male frogs in the wild. *Nature.* 2002;419(6910): 895–896.
22. Hayes TB, Case P, Chu S, et al. Pesticide mixtures, endocrine disruption, and amphibian declines: Are we underestimating the impact? *Environ Health Perspect.* 2006;1141(suppl 1): 40–50.
23. Rosenberg S, Vedlitz A, Cowman DF, Zahran S. Climate change: A profile of US climate scientists' perspectives. *Climate Change.* 2010;101:311–329.
24. Barker TI, Bashmakov L, Bernstein JE, et al. Technical Summary. In: *Climate Change 2007: Mitigation. Contribution of Working Group III to the Fourth Assessment Report of the Intergovernmental Panel on Climate Change.* Metz B, Davidson OR, Bosch PR, Dave R, Meyer LA (eds.). New York: Cambridge University Press; 2007: 26–93.
25. Solomon S, Plattner G, Knutti R, Friedlingstein P. Irreversible climate change due to carbon dioxide emissions. *Proc Natl Acad Sci USA.* 2009;106(6):1704–1709.
26. McLeod E, Salm RV, Anthony K, et al. The Honolulu Declaration on Ocean Acidification and Reef Management. The Nature Conservancy, U.S.A., and IUCN, Gland, Switzerland; 2008. Available at: http://icriforum.org/icri-documents/associated-publications/honolulu-declaration-ocean-acidification-and-reef-management. Accessed June 12, 2012.
27. Smith KL, Ruhl HA, Bett BJ, et al. Climate, carbon cycling, and deep-ocean ecosystems. *Proc Natl Acad Sci.* 2009; 106(46):19211–19218.
28. Karl TR, Melillo JM, Peterson TC (eds.). *Global Climate Change Impacts in the United States.* New York: Cambridge University Press; 2009.
29. United Nations. *The Millennium Development Goals Report 2010.*2010. Available at: http://www.un.org/millenniumgoals/pdf/MDG%20Report%202010%20En%20r15%20-low%20res%2020100615%20-.pdf. Accessed June 12, 2012.
30. Centers for Disease Control and Prevention. Climate and Health Program. Updated 2011. Available at: http://www.cdc.gov/climateandhealth/about.htm. Accessed October 2, 2012.
31. Rosenthal JP, Jessup CM. Global climate change and health: Developing a research agenda for the NIH. *Trans Am Clin Climatol Assoc.* 2009;120:129–141.
32. U.S. Department of Health and Human Services. *Healthy People 2020* Topics and Objectives: Environmental Health. Available at: http://www.healthypeople.gov/2020/topicsobjectives2020/overview.aspx?topicid=12. Updated 2011. Accessed June 15, 2011.
33. Food and Agriculture Organization of the United Nations. Livestock's Long Shadow: Environmental Issues and Options. 2006. Available at: http://www.fao.org/docrep/010/a0701e/a0701e00.HTM. Accessed June 12, 2012.
34. Pitesky ME, Stackhouse KR, Mitloehner FM. Clearing the air: Livestock's contribution to climate change. *Adv Agron.* 2009;103:1–40.

35. Goodland R, Anhang J. Livestock and climate change: What if the key actors in climate change are ... cows, pigs, and chickens? *World Watch*. 2009 Nov/Dec:10–19.
36. Yngve A, Margetts B, Tseng M, et al. Climate change: Time to redefine our profession [editorial]. *Public Health Nutr.* 2010;13(3):301–302.
37. Tapsell LC. Food and nutrition issues for the future [editorial]. *Nutr & Diet*. 2010;67(1):2–3.
38. Holdsworth M. Sustainability should be integral to nutrition and dietetics [editorial]. *J Hum Nutr Diet.* 2010;23(5):467–468.
39. Mohr N. A New Global Warming Strategy: How Environmentalists Are Overlooking Vegetarianism as the Most Effective Tool Against Climate Change in Our Lifetimes. An EarthSave International Report. 2005. Available at: http://www.earthsave.org/globalwarming.htm. Accessed June 12, 2012.
40. Baroni L, Cenci L, Tettamanti M, Berati M. Evaluating the environmental impact of various dietary patterns combined with different food production systems. *Eur J Clin Nutr*. 2007;61:279–286.
41. Carlsson-Kanyama A, Gonzalez AD. Potential contributions of food consumption patterns to climate change. *Am J Clin Nutr.* 2009;89(5):1704S–1709S.
42. Eshel G, Martin PA. Diet, energy, and global warming. *Earth Interactions*. 2006;10:1–17.
43. Marlow HJ, Hayes WK, Soret S, et al. Diet and the environment: Does what you eat matter? *Am J Clin Nutr*. 2009;89(5): 1699S–1703S.
44. Frey S, Barrett J. The Footprint of Scotland's Diet: The Environmental Burden of What We Eat. A Report for Scotland's Global Footprint Project. Stockholm Environment Institute. 2006. Available at: http://assets.wwf.org.uk/downloads/the_footprint_of_scotlands_diet.pdf. Accessed June 12, 2012.
45. Stehfast E, Bouwman L, vanVuuren DP, et al. Climate benefits of changing diet. *Climate Change*. 2009;95:83–102.
46. Craig WJ, Mangels AR. Position of the American Dietetic Association: Vegetarian diets. *J Am Diet Assoc.* 2009;109(7): 1266–1282.
47. Hall KD, Guo J, Dore M, Chow CC. The progressive increase of food waste in America and its environmental impact. *PLoS One.* 2009;4(11):e7940.
48. Cuellar AD, Webber ME. Wasted food, wasted energy: The embedded energy in food waste in the United States. *Environ Sci Technol.* 2010;44:6464–6469.
49. Environmental Protection Agency. Municipal Solid Waste in the United States: 2009 Facts and Figures. EPA530-R-10-012. 2010. Available at: http://www.epa.gov/osw/nonhaz/municipal/pubs/msw2009rpt.pdf. Accessed June 12, 2012.
50. Environmental Protection Agency. Food Waste Management Cost Calculator. Version 1.0:1-13. 2009. Available at: http://www.epa.gov/epawaste/conserve/materials/organics/food/tools/index.htm.
51. Parfitt J, Barthel M, Macnaughton S. Food waste within food supply chains: Quantification and potential for change to 2050. *Philos Trans R Soc Lond B Biol Sci.* 2010;365(1554): 3065–3081.
52. Popkin BM. Nutrition in transition: The changing global nutrition challenge. *Asia Pac J Clin Nutr.* 2001;10(suppl):S13–S18.
53. Popkin BM. Nutritional patterns and transitions. *Pop Dev Rev*. 1993;19(1):138–157.
54. Zhai F, Wang H, Du S, et al. Prospective study on nutrition transition in China. *Nutr Rev.* 2009;67(suppl 1):S56–S61.
55. Adair LS, Popkin BM. Are child eating patterns being transformed globally? *Obes Res.* 2005;13(7):1281–1299.
56. Mendez MA, Monteiro CA, Popkin BM. Overweight exceeds underweight among women in most developing countries. *Am J Clin Nutr.* 2005;81(3):714–721.
57. Kennedy E. The global nutrition agenda: 2008 and beyond. *Brown J World Aff.* 2008;15(1):121–134.
58. Popkin BM. Global nutrition dynamics: The world is shifting rapidly toward a diet linked with noncommunicable diseases. *Am J Clin Nutr.* 2006;84(2):289–298.
59. Hawkes C. Uneven dietary development: Linking the policies and processes of globalization with the nutrition transition, obesity and diet-related chronic diseases. *Global Health*. 2006 Mar 28;2:4.
60. Brinkman H, dePee S, Sanogo I, et al. High food prices and the global financial crisis have reduced access to nutritious food and worsened nutritional status and health. *J Nutr.* 2010;140(suppl):153S–161S.
61. Throw AM. Trade liberalisation and the nutrition transition: Mapping the pathways for public health nutritionists. *Public Health Nutr*. 2009;12(11):2150–2158.
62. Popkin BM, Du S. Dynamics of the nutrition transition toward the animal foods sector in China and its implications: A worried perspective. *J Nutr*. 2003;133:3898S–3906S.
63. Schmidhuber J, Prakash S. The nutrition transition to 2030: Why developing countries are likely to bear the major burden. *Acta Agriculturae Scand Section C.* 2005;2:150–166.
64. Rosegrant MW, Leach N, Gerpacio RV. Alternative futures for world cereal and meat consumption. *Proc Nutr Soc.* 1999;58: 219–234.
65. Pew Commission on Industrial Farm Animal Production. Putting Meat on the Table: Industrial Farm Animal Production in America. A Report of the Pew Commission on Industrial Farm Animal Production. 2008. Available at: http://www.pewtrusts.org/uploadedFiles/wwwpewtrustsorg/Reports/Industrial_Agriculture/PCIFAP_FINAL.pdf. Accessed June 12, 2012.
66. Akhtar AZ, Greger M, Ferdowsian H, Frank E. Health professionals' roles in animal agriculture, climate change, and human health. *Am J Prev Med.* 2009;36(2):182–187.
67. Ulhoi JP, Ulhoi BP. Beyond climate focus and disciplinary myopia: The roles and responsibilities of hospitals and healthcare professionals. *Int J Environ Res Public Health.* 2009;6(3):1204–1214.
68. Kant AK, Graubard BI. Secular trends in patterns of self-reported food consumption of adult Americans: NHANES 1971–1975 to NHANES 1999–2002. *Am J Clin Nutr.* 2006;84:1215–1223.
69. Duffey KJ, Popkin BM. Shifts in patterns and consumption of beverages between 1965 and 2002. *Obesity (Silver Spring)*. 2007;15(11):2739–2747.
70. Health Care Without Harm. Health Care Without Harm: What We Do. Available at: http://www.noharm.org/all_regions/about. Accessed June 15, 2011.
71. World Health Organization and Health Care Without Harm. *Healthy Hospitals-Healthy Planet-Healthy People: Addressing*

Climate Change in Health Care Settings. 2009. Available at: http://www.who.int/globalchange/publications/healthcare_settings/en/index.html. Accessed June 12, 2012.
72. Environmental Working Group. About the Environmental Working Group. Available at: http://www.ewg.org/about. Accessed June 15, 2011.
73. Environmental Working Group. Historical EWG Accomplishments. Available at: http://www.ewg.org/historicalaccomplishments#food. Accessed June 15, 2011.
74. Washington Toxics Coalition. Washington Toxics Coalition Mission Statement. Available at: http://watoxics.org/about. Accessed June 15, 2011.
75. Center for Food Safety. About Us. Available at: http://truefoodnow.org/about. Accessed June 15, 2011.
76. Center for Food Safety. Cool Foods Campaign. Available at: http://www.coolfoodscampaign.org. Accessed June 15, 2011.
77. Hunger and Environmental Nutrition Practice Group of the American Dietetic Association. Who We Are. Available at: http://www.hendpg.org/hen.cfm?page=who-we-are. Accessed June 15, 2011.
78. Johns Hopkins University Center for a Livable Future. Key Interconnections. Available at: http://www.jhsph.edu/research/centers-and-institutes/johns-hopkins-center-for-a-livable-future/about/key_interconnections. Accessed October 2, 2012.
79. Truckner RT. Health care provider beliefs concerning the adverse health effects of environmental and ecosystem degradation. *Wilderness Environ Med.* 2009;20:199–211.
80. Edelstein S, Chiu D, Weber L. Reported use of eco-friendly products by nutrition professionals. *Top Clin Nutr.* 2010; 25(3):272–279.
81. Horton G, Magin P. Healthy patients, healthy planet: Green recommendations for GP health promotion. *Aust Fam Physician.* 2007;36(12):1006–1008.
82. Begley A, Gallegos D. Should cooking be a dietetic competency? *Nutr Diet.* 2010;67(1):41–46.
83. Lombard KA, Forster-Cox S, Smeal D, ONeill MK. Diabetes on the Navajo nation: What role can gardening and agriculture extension play to reduce it? *Rural Remote Health.* 2006;6(4):1–16.
84. Harvard Pilgrim Health Care. Harvard Pilgrim Health Care: Green City Growers. Available at: https://www.harvardpilgrim.org/portal/page?_pageid=213,290236&_dad=portal&_schema=PORTAL. Accessed June 28, 2011.
85. Patterson C. Personal communication. April 23, 2011.
86. Patterson C. Sutra Vegetarian Restaurant Menu. April 23, 2011.
87. Foord L. Personal communication. April 23, 2011.
88. Harris P. Personal communication. April 23, 2011.
89. Thompson P. Personal communication. April 23, 2011.

CHAPTER 2

How Food Science Is Guided by Research

Carol E. O'Neil, PhD, MPH, RD

Theresa A. Nicklas, DrPH

Chapter Objectives

THE STUDENT WILL BE EMPOWERED TO:

- Explain what peer-reviewed literature is, and know how to assess and use reliable nutrition information.
- Identify resources that public health nutritionists use to keep pace with current research or available programs that are grounded in research.
- Compare and contrast different types of research studies, and explain how they are used to form policies, programs, and consumer information.
- Explain how and why nutrition policies, recommendations, and programs change at regular intervals.
- Defend the nation's nutrition policies and recommendations using an evidence-based approach.

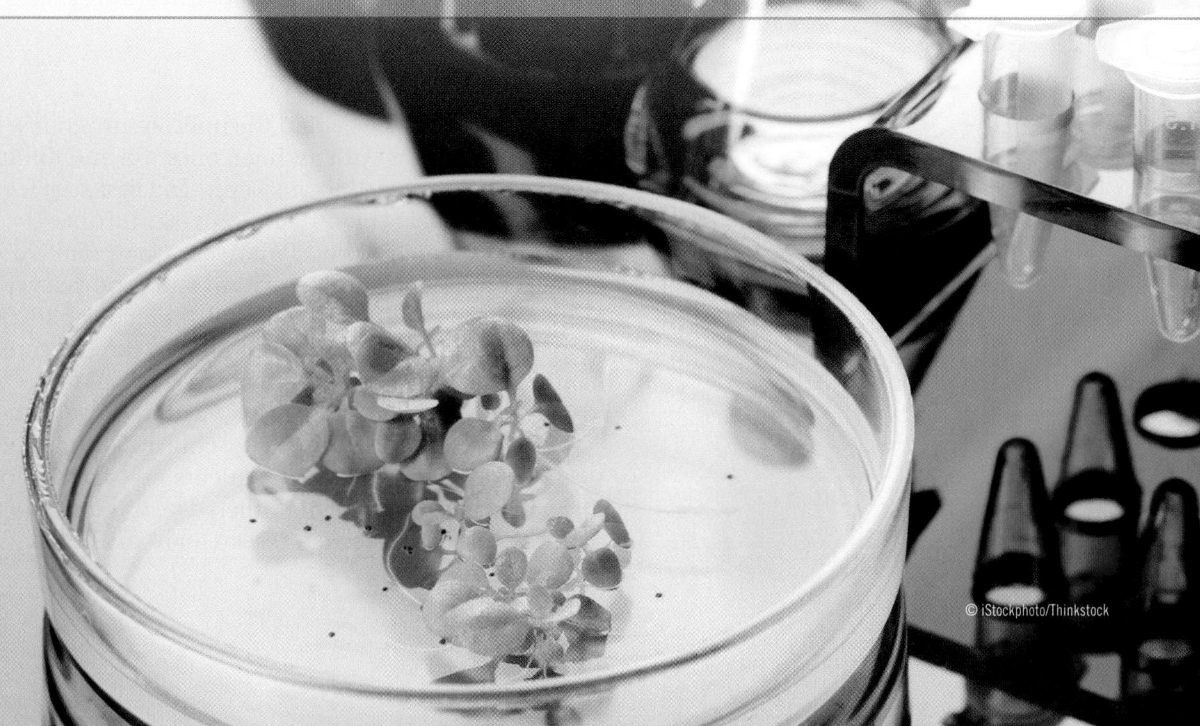

Food Science and Research

Food science and nutrition are complementary fields that examine all aspects of food, diet, health, and disease. Nutrition researchers have determined that a poor diet can lead to deficiency diseases, such as rickets or scurvy, or to chronic conditions and diseases, such as obesity, cardiovascular disease (CVD), type 2 diabetes, osteoporosis, and cancer. Diets associated with these diseases are high in saturated fatty acids, trans fats, sugar, and sodium or low in essential nutrients, such as dietary fiber, calcium, vitamin D, and potassium. Although nutritionists recommend specific amounts of foods and nutrients to optimize health, food scientists apply these recommendations to develop products that can provide optimal amounts of these nutrients. These symbiotic fields share a common literature, research methods, and study designs. This chapter explains how to evaluate the literature in either field and discusses how this research is used to formulate policy.

How to Interpret Research: An Evidence-Based Approach

Peer-reviewed literature is the gold standard for scientific information that is provided to the public. It also provides the information used in developing recommendations and policies, designing and evaluating nutrition programs, and conducting ethical evidence-based food and nutritional studies. The peer-reviewed literature consists of scholarly works and usually represents the most recent original research in a field. Prior to publication, the manuscript describing the study is reviewed, or refereed, by academic and professional peers. Review criteria typically include the significance of the work (i.e., whether it made an important and original contribution to the literature), the methodology (i.e., the data were gathered and analyzed appropriately for the discipline), and whether the results were interpreted correctly.

Navigating the Peer-Reviewed Literature

The peer-reviewed literature can be difficult to understand, especially by those inexperienced in the food science field. The literature can be contradictory because similar studies can produce different results. The use of different study designs, populations, and methods, including statistical analyses, contributes to the confusion.

Asking a Question

Assessing the science behind the policies, programs, practices, and consumer information begins with asking a question and finding, reading, and evaluating the articles needed to answer it. The first step is to locate the appropriate literature. This can be a daunting task; fortunately, databases are available that make it much easier. PubMed is the premiere database for articles on medical topics, including nutrition and food science. This database includes more than 21 million citations for biomedical articles from MEDLINE and numerous life science journals. PubMed can be searched by key word, author name, article title, or journal name. Many citations in PubMed include links to full-text articles from PubMed Central or publisher websites.

University libraries often subscribe to journals or provide resources, such as EBSCO Host, that allow students and faculty to obtain full-text articles that might not be available otherwise. Other important databases for food science or nutrition-related research are described in **Table 2.1**.

TABLE 2.1
Important Databases for the Food and Nutrition Sciences

Database	Online Location	Description
AGRICOLA	http://agricola.nal.usda.gov	Provides citations in agriculture and related fields.
AGRIS (International System for Agricultural Science and Technology)	http://www.ntis.gov/products/agris.aspx	The international information system for the agricultural sciences and technology.
Behavioral Risk Factor Surveillance System: Survey Data	http://www.cdc.gov/brfss	Includes eight databases on specific illnesses or aspects of chronic disease prevention and health promotion; designed to help public health professionals and educators locate program information.
CARIS	http://cris.nifa.usda.gov	Contains information about current agricultural research projects being carried out by or on behalf of developing countries.
The Cochrane Library	http://www.thecochranelibrary.com/view/0/index.html	Contains reliable evidence from Cochrane and other systematic reviews, clinical trials, and more.
Directory of Open Access Journals	http://www.doaj.org	This database increases the visibility and ease of use of open access journals, promoting their use and impact.
Embase	http://www.embase.com	The most comprehensive source for answers on biomedical questions.
ERIC (Education Resources Information Center)	http://www.eric.ed.gov	Includes information on research on educational research and resources; early childhood education, junior colleges and higher education; reading and communications skills; languages and linguistics; education management; counseling and personnel services; library and information science; information resources.
Food Safety Research Database	http://fsrio.nal.usda.gov/nal_web/fsrio/advsearch.php	Provides information on publicly funded, and to the extent possible, privately funded food safety research initiatives to prevent unintended duplication of food safety research and to assist the executive and legislative branches of the government and private research entities to assess food safety research needs and priorities.
FSTA (Food Science and Technology Abstracts)	http://www.foodsciencecentral.com	The largest collection of food science, food technology, and food-related human nutrition abstracts. Contains over 580,000 records, with approximately 2,000 new records added every month. Includes journal articles (~80%) plus patents, theses, standards, legislation, books, reviews, and conference proceedings.
Health Source: Nursing/Academic Edition	http://www.lib.utexas.edu/indexes/titles.php?id=176	Offers access to nearly 600 scholarly full-text journals, including approximately 450 peer-reviewed journals focusing on many medical disciplines. Also featured are abstracts and indexing for nearly 850 journals.
ISTP (Index to Scientific & Technical Proceedings)	http://www.library.dmu.ac.uk/Resources/Databases/index.php?page=164&id=31	Indexes the published literature of the most significant conferences, symposia, seminars, colloquia, workshops, and conventions in a wide range of disciplines in science and technology over the last 5 years.
LILACS (Latin American and Caribbean Health Sciences Literature)	http://bases.bireme.br/cgi-bin/wxislind.exe/iah/online/?IsisScript=iah/iah.xis&base=LILACS&lang=i&form=F	Bibliographic control and dissemination of health scientific-technique literature from Latin American and Caribbean countries, which is often absent from other the international databases.
MEDLINE	http://www.nlm.nih.gov/bsd/pmresources.html	MEDLINE, which is sponsored by the National Library of Medicine, contains citations and abstracts to international biomedical literature from over 3,700 journals on topics such as primary research, clinical practice, administration, policy issues, and healthcare services.

(*continues*)

TABLE 2.1
Important Databases for the Food and Nutrition Sciences (*continued*)

Database	Online Location	Description
Merck Index Online	http://library.dialog.com/bluesheets/html/bl0304.html	An encyclopedia of chemicals, drugs, and biologicals that contains more than 10,000 monographs, 32 supplemental tables, and 450 organic name reactions. Nearly 4,000 of the entries cover drugs and pharmaceuticals, 2,000 describe common organic chemicals and laboratory reagents, another 2,000 cover naturally occurring substances and plants, 1,000 focus on the elements and on inorganic chemicals, and approximately 1,000 pertain to compounds of agricultural significance.
Nursing and Allied Health Source	http://www.proquest.com/en-US/catalogs/databases/detail/pq_nursingahs.shtml	Provides users with reliable healthcare information related to nursing, allied health, alternative and complementary medicine, and related topics.
PubMed	http://www.ncbi.nlm.nih.gov/pubmed	PubMed comprises more than 21 million citations for biomedical literature from MEDLINE, life science journals, and online books. Citations may include links to full-text content from PubMed Central and publisher websites.
Science Citation Index	http://www.thomsonscientific.com/cgi-bin/jrnlst/jloptions.cgi?PC=K	This database covers the journal literature of the sciences.
Science Direct	http://www.sciencedirect.com	An information source for scientific, technical, and medical research. It offers access to more than 1,100 journals in 16 fields of science, including the social sciences.
Scopus	http://www.scopus.com/home.url	The largest abstract and citation database of the peer-reviewed literature.
Web of Science	http://thomsonreuters.com/products_services/science/science_products/a-z/web_of_science	Index of more than 5,800 major journals across 164 scientific disciplines.

Conducting a Search

After formulating a question and determining the appropriate database to use, the next stage is to select the descriptors and conduct the search. The descriptors and the search limits depend on the question being asked. For example, if the question is "What is the effect of 100% fruit juice consumption on weight in children?" your descriptors could be "fruit juice" OR "fruit" AND "weight" OR "BMI" AND "children" OR "adolescents." The search might be easier if the search limits were "All Children," in which case the last two descriptors could be eliminated. Scanning the abstracts that appear following an initial search will allow you to determine which articles are appropriate for answering your question.

Accessing and Assessing the Articles

The next step is to obtain and read the full-text articles, either by downloading them or visiting the library. This is not a casual reading to prepare a summary, but a critical evaluation of the published study. **Table 2.2** shows the steps to take when reviewing a peer-reviewed article.

TABLE 2.2
How to Assess an Article from the Peer-Reviewed Literature

Section of the Article	How to Assess
Title	1. Did the title reflect what was actually done in the study? The purpose, the populations used, the findings, and conclusions can be reflected in the title. A positive statement about the contents, rather than a title that is a question, is preferred.
Abstract	1. Did the abstract clearly outline all aspects of the manuscript? a. The purpose of the study b. The methods c. The results d. The conclusions 2. Was enough information provided to understand what was done and what was found?
Introduction	1. Did the authors provide enough background information to understand why the study was done? 2. Did the authors provide enough background information to let you know what others have done on this topic and where there might be gaps in the literature?* 3. Were important studies omitted from the introduction? This might suggest bias. 4. Did the authors clearly state the purpose of the study? A hypothesis or research question should have been stated. Not all study designs are appropriate for testing hypotheses; for example, cross-sectional studies generate hypotheses.
Material and Methods	1. Was the type of study clearly defined? 2. Did the experimental design allow the research question or hypothesis to be tested? 3. If appropriate, was a control group included? Was it comparable to the test group? 4. Was the population appropriate for the study? 5. Was the population suitable to generalize the results? 6. Was the population well defined? a. Adequate sample size for appropriate statistical power. b. Gender, age, race/ethnicity, income, etc. c. Inclusion/exclusion criteria for the study. d. If the study population was a subset of a larger population, was it clear how the study population differed from the larger population? This could indicate bias. e. Was a convenience sample used, or were the participants randomized? 7. Were there ethical concerns if human subjects or vertebrate animals were used? Was there a clear statement that the research was approved by the appropriate committee? 8. Were the methods presented in enough detail so the research could be repeated (or built upon) by another research team? 9. Were the methods used reliable and valid? 10. Statistical methods: a. Were they appropriate? b. Were outcome variables clearly defined? c. Did the authors control for potential confounding variables? d. Was a statistical probability level clearly stated? 11. Was it clearly stated how the data will be presented in the results [e.g., data are presented as mean + standard error (SE)]? Were all terms defined?
Results	This section should present study results only. No methodology should be presented and, unless it is a combined Results and Discussion section, there should be no interpretation of the information. 1. Were results organized in a logical sequence? Did the results follow the same order as the methods? 2. Were demographics presented? 3. Were the graphics appropriate? a. Were the graphics needed? Should more/less be included? b. Was the information clearly presented in labeled tables and figures? Can the tables and figures stand alone? 4. From a biological standpoint, were the data reasonable?

(*continues*)

TABLE 2.2
How to Assess an Article from the Peer-Reviewed Literature (*continued*)

Section of the Article	How to Assess
Discussion	1. Were the study objectives met? 2. Did the authors adequately interpret their results? 3. Did the authors discuss their results and compare them with the current literature? 4. Was the discussion related directly to the results, or was it overly speculative? 5. If nonstandard methods were used, were they adequately discussed? 6. Were limitations of the study clearly stated? 7. Were conclusions drawn? Were they supported by the results?
References	1. Were the references cited appropriate? Were they accurate? Were they timely? 2. Were enough references presented so a cogent whole was presented in the manuscript?
Acknowledgments	1. Were the funding sources clearly identified? 2. Were there real or apparent conflicts of interest that could suggest bias?

* This is difficult for those unfamiliar with the literature, but it becomes easier with practice and familiarity with the topic.

Identifying the Study Design

A critical consideration when reviewing an article is the study design—the type of experimental design that was used to produce the test results—and whether it was relevant to the disease, condition, or program being examined.

Descriptive Studies

Descriptive studies can be used to generate hypotheses. Descriptive studies can focus on populations or on individuals. The following are the most common types of descriptive studies:

- A **population or correlational study** uses data from entire populations to compare event (such as disease) frequencies with an exposure in different groups during the same time period or in the same group at different points in time. These studies look at whole populations rather than individuals, thus it is impossible to link an individual exposure with the occurrence of disease in that individual.
- A **case report** is a detailed report regarding a single patient. Case reports can be suggestive, but it often is difficult to exclude alternative explanations for a particular condition. These studies are usually used to study rare diseases.
- **Case series** are compiled from multiple case reports describing the same conditions. Routine surveillance programs can often be used to compile case series.
- A **cross-sectional survey** looks at individuals with respect to both exposure and disease at a point in time. Because both exposure and disease are assessed at the same time, it can be difficult to determine whether the exposure predated the disease.

Analytical Studies

Analytical studies can be used to test specific hypotheses. They include both observational studies and intervention studies. Observational studies are popular in the food and nutrition literature and include case control studies and cohort studies. A **case control study** is a case series of individuals who have the disease of interest and a group of similar individuals who do not have the disease/exposure. Comparisons are made between the two groups. A **cohort study**, such as the Nurses' Health Study, classifies participants on the presence or absence of exposure and follows them over time to assess disease development. In a *retrospective cohort study*, the disease of interest has

population or correlational study Study that uses data from entire populations to compare event (such as disease) frequencies with an exposure in different groups during the same time period or in the same group at different times. Because these studies look at whole populations rather than individuals, it is impossible to link an individual exposure with the occurrence of disease in that individual—a major limitation of this type of study.

case report Detailed reports of a condition or disease in a single individual. Case reports can be suggestive, but it often is difficult to exclude alternative explanations for a condition/disease. These studies are usually used to study rare diseases.

case series Compiled from multiple case reports describing the same conditions. Routine surveillance programs can often be used to compile a case series.

cross-sectional survey Examines individuals with respect to both exposure and disease at a specific point in time. Because exposure and disease are assessed at the same time, it can be difficult to determine whether the exposure predated the disease.

already occurred at the time the study begins; in a *prospective cohort study*, the disease has not yet occurred at that time.

An **intervention study** is a type of prospective cohort study where the exposure is controlled by the investigator. These studies can be considered therapeutic (secondary prevention) or preventative. DASH and DASH Sodium (discussed later in this chapter) were intervention studies. Intervention studies often use a **randomized design.** With a randomized design, individuals are randomly assigned to a treatment or control group. With a **double-blind placebo-controlled design**, neither the individuals nor the investigator know whether participants are assigned to the treatment or placebo group. This study design is usually considered to provide the most compelling evidence of a cause-and-effect relationship; however, this design is susceptible to bias. Some study designs are more powerful than others in providing evidence on a topic. This has given rise to the concept of a "hierarchy of evidence" with regards to the effectiveness of interventions, treatments, practice protocols, or policies.[1] From bottom (least convincing) to top (best evidence), the hierarchy is generally presented as: expert opinion, case reports, case series, case-control studies; cross-sectional surveys; prospective or retrospective cohort studies; randomized clinical trials (RCTs); and, finally, systematic reviews of multiple RCTs. Keep in mind; however, that this hierarchy assumes that all studies were well designed and executed. A poor RCT may not provide the same level of evidence as a very well-designed cross-sectional survey.

Evaluating Statistics

Most peer-reviewed publications in the food and nutrition literature include an array of statistics in the results and conclusion. A review of the quantitative measure statistics used can provide useful information about the value of the study and its generalizability to the larger population. **Table 2.3** provides a brief overview of some statistical terms that are often found in the literature.

TABLE 2.3
How to Evaluate Statistics

Statistic	How to Evaluate
Sample size	The number of units (e.g., people, animals) used in the study. Although there is no magic number for the correct number of "units" in a study, the sample size should be determined by the variability in the data. The more variable the data, the larger the sample size needed to establish statistical significance.
Effect size	The salience of the treatment relative to the noise in measurement. Thought should be given as to whether the effect is only statistically significant or if it also is biologically or clinically significant.
Alpha (α) level	The probability level, or the odds, that the observed result is due to chance. There is no specific alpha level that should be used, but many studies use 0.05, which means that there is only a 5% chance of making a type I error, or rejecting a true null hypothesis.
Power	The probability that the statistical test will reject a false null hypothesis, or not make a type II error. As power increases, the chance of making a type II error decreases. The probability of a type II error is referred to as beta (β), and power is equal to $1 - \beta$. Power analyses should be done before (a priori) the data is collected, but it can be done afterward (post hoc). There are no formal standards for power; however, many scientists use 0.80 as the standard.

case control study A case series on individuals who have the disease of interest and a group of similar individuals who do not have the disease. Exposure comparisons can be made.

cohort study Participants are classified based on the presence or absence of exposure and then followed over time to assess disease development. In a *retrospective cohort study*, the disease of interest has already occurred at the time the study begins; in a *prospective cohort study*, the disease has not yet occurred.

intervention study A type of prospective cohort study where the exposure is controlled by the investigator. These studies can be considered therapeutic (secondary prevention) or preventative. Dietary Approaches to Stop Hypertension (DASH) was an intervention study.

randomized design A study design whereby individuals are randomly assigned to a treatment or control group.

double-blind placebo-controlled design A design whereby neither the participants nor the investigator knows who has been assigned to a treatment or a placebo group. This study design is usually considered to provide the most compelling evidence of a cause-and-effect relationship.

Assessing a Body of Literature

A single peer-reviewed article, or even several, is not sufficient for making ethical evidence-based practice decisions, setting public health goals, or designing nutrition programs for health professionals and the public. To accomplish any of these goals, the strength of a body of scientific studies must be assessed, usually by conducting a systematic review or a meta-analysis.[2–5] A meta-analysis combines the results of several studies.

Various agencies, including the Agency for Healthcare Research and Quality (AHRQ), Cochrane Reviews, the U.S. Department of Agriculture's Nutrition Evidence Library (NEL), and the Academy of Nutrition and Dietetics' Evidence Analysis Library (EAL) have developed methods for developing evidence reports and technology assessments to assist public- and private-sector organizations.[5–8] The EAL process was recognized by the Joint Commission (the accreditation agency for healthcare organizations) as being exemplary in bringing the best research to practice. In addition, it has been adapted by the FDA to assess the type of qualified health claims that can be put on food labels. Each of these agencies has its own criteria for assessing a research question and a body of literature; however, they are generally similar. The following domains are generally assessed:

- The *quality* of the studies, including the extent to which bias was minimized (see **Table 2.4**)
- The *consistency* of the findings across studies
- The *quantity* of the studies, including the magnitude of effect, the number of studies conducted, and the sample size and statistical power of the study
- The *impact* of the studies, including the importance of the outcomes and the magnitude of the effect
- The *generalizability* of the findings to the larger population

Different agencies have different grading scales to assess a given body of evidence. The EAL and the USDA's NEL have five categories of evidence: strong, moderate, limited, expert opinion only, and grade not assignable. How the domains evaluated, the study design, and the evidence category come together in the USDA's NEL is shown in **Table 2.5**.

TABLE 2.4
Potential Sources of Research Bias*†

Source of Bias	Description
Funding sources	• Government/foundation funding is not as susceptible to bias as industry funding. However, government agencies direct the funding, and thus unconventional ideas, no matter how valid, are unlikely to be funded. • Industry funding often is perceived as being biased toward the product. Although this has been reported in food and nutrition research, additional systematic reviews and meta-analyses are needed to determine the extent of the problem. • Industries may require investigators to test hypotheses that are consistent with their own financial interests. • Industry sponsors may delay publication of results that are unfavorable to their products.

Source of Bias	Description
Investigator bias	• Conflicts of interest may occur when a financial or personal consideration compromises or appears to compromise the integrity of the study in any way. Conflicts of interest may include, but are not limited to, funding sources, selection of study participants, hiring of personnel, purchase of equipment, choice of analyses, and interpretation of the data. • Investigators may interpret the study results in ways that favor the funding agencies. • Investigators writing scientific reviews that are funded by industry may under- or overrepresent specific viewpoints.
Study population bias	• Noncoverage errors result from sampling in a way that excludes some individuals as a result of the way the population was selected. Study inclusion and exclusion criteria should be clearly stated and adhered to. • Volunteers may be more interested in or knowledgeable about the topic; this may skew results of interviews or focus group discussions. • Volunteers also may be more compliant; lack of compliance can confound treatment efficacy. • Nonrespondent bias, which is similar to that seen with volunteers, can bias survey results. • Preconception bias may occur unless the study is blinded or is double blind. • Test subjects may be treated differently from controls. A double-blind study can ameliorate this problem, but in some types of studies (e.g., weight-loss trials) groups often can be identified by treatment effect. • Nonsystematic withdrawal bias may occur if subjects withdraw or are withdrawn from treatment or control groups at different rates. Participants in a placebo or no-treatment group are more likely to drop out of a study than those receiving treatment.
Measurement or reporting bias	• Recall or memory bias can be a problem if outcomes being measured require that subjects recall past events. This is a problem with most diet assessment studies. • Reporting errors commonly occur in diet assessment studies; factors contributing to these include: recency of consuming the foods, weight of the respondent, types of food consumed, failure to understand portion size, and the skill of the interviewer. • Procedural bias can occur when time pressure is applied to participants; for example, not allowing ample time to fill out a questionnaire.
Interviewer bias	• Can occur if the interviewer gives subtle cues to the respondent; double-blind studies can help to prevent this, but it's not always possible to use this design.
Contamination bias	• Can occur when investigators have a preconceived idea of the study's effects.
Statistical bias	• Choice of statistical tests or probability levels to favor a given hypothesis. • Choice of covariates or confounding factors favor a given hypothesis.
Confirmation bias	• The evidence may be evaluated in ways that support the investigators' prior beliefs.
Rescue bias	• Discounting of data by finding selective faults in the experiment.
Auxiliary hypothesis bias	• Introduction of ad hoc modifications that imply that an unanticipated finding would have been different if the study design had been different.
Mechanism bias	• Scientists are less skeptical when the underlying data is credible. • Studies showing positive results are more likely to be published than those showing negative or neutral results. • Positive results within a given study are more likely to be published than negative or neutral results. • Data may be suppressed or remain unpublished because the findings are perceived to challenge the interests of the funding agency or because they fail to support the researcher's ideological opinions.

* Bias should not be confused with scientific misconduct.

† For a fuller description of these and other types of investigator bias, see Kaptchuk TJ. Effect of interpretive bias on research evidence. *BMJ.* 2003;326(7404): 1453–1455. Full disclosure of all potential sources of bias should be disclosed in the manuscript. This is usually done in a section called "Study Limitations." Funding sources and potential conflicts of interest of all authors should also be disclosed. This is sometimes done in a section called "Funding Sources" and sometimes as part of the acknowledgments.

TABLE 2.5
The Grading Chart Used by the USDA's National Evidence Library to Evaluate the Strength of the Body of Evidence Supporting Conclusion Statements

Element	Strong	Moderate	Limited	Expert Opinion Only	Grade Not Assignable
Quality					
• Scientific rigor and validity • Study design and execution	Studies of strong design Free from design flaws, bias, and execution problems	Studies of strong design with minor methodological concerns OR only studies of weaker study design for question	Studies of weak design for answering the question OR inconclusive findings due to design flaws, bias, or execution problems	No studies available Conclusion based on usual practice, expert consensus, clinical experience, opinion, or extrapolation from basic research	No evidence that pertains to question being addressed
Consistency					
• Consistency of findings across studies	Findings generally consistent in direction and size of effect or degree of association, and statistical significance with minor very exceptions	Inconsistency among results of studies with strong design OR consistency with minor exceptions across studies of weaker design	Unexplained inconsistency among results from different studies OR a single study unconfirmed by other studies	Conclusion supported solely by statements of informed nutrition or medical commentators	N/A
Quantity					
• Number of studies • Number of study participants	One large study with a diverse population or several good quality studies Large number of subjects studied Studies with negative results have sufficiently large sample size for adequate statistical power	Several studies by independent investigators Doubts about adequacy of sample size to avoid Type I and Type II error	Limited number of studies Low number of subjects studied and/or inadequate sample size within studies	Unsubstantiated by published research studies	Relevant studies have not been done
Impact					
• Importance of studied outcomes • Magnitude of effect	Studied outcome relates directly to the question Size of effect is clinically meaningful Significant (statistical) difference is large	Some doubt about the statistical or clinical significance of the effect	Studied outcome is an intermediate outcome or surrogate for the true outcome of interest OR size of effect is small or lacks statistical and/or clinical significance	Objective data unavailable	Indicates area for future research
Generalizability					
• Generalizability to population of interest	Studied population, intervention and outcomes are free from serious doubts about generalizability	Minor doubts about generalizability	Serious doubts about generalizability due to narrow or different study population, intervention, or outcomes studied	Generalizability limited to scope of experience	N/A

Source: Reproduced from U.S. Department of Agriculture. 2010 DGAC Conclusion Grading Chart. Nutrition Evidence Library. Available at: http://www.nutritionevidencelibrary.com/topic.cfm?cat=3210. Accessed June 5, 2012.

For example, the 2010 Dietary Guidelines Advisory Committee used the USDA's NEL to support a variety of broad topics when developing the *Dietary Guidelines for Americans, 2010*.[9] These broad topics included alcohol, carbohydrates, energy balance and weight management, fatty acids and cholesterol, food safety and technology, nutrient adequacy, protein, sodium, potassium, and water. Individual questions were posed under each of these categories. For example, under *food safety and technology*, one subtopic was *washing produce*. Under this subtopic, two questions were posed:

- What techniques for washing fresh produce are associated with favorable food safety outcomes?
- To what extent do U.S. consumers follow techniques for washing fresh produce that are associated with favorable food safety outcomes?

Innovation Point

The Internet as a Source of Information Today, for health professionals and consumers alike, a bewildering array of information is available on the Internet. Reliable sites have URLs ending in .edu or .gov. These sites often present a distillation of information from the peer-reviewed literature or other reliable sources. Using the Internet to locate information can save valuable time; however, any information found on the Internet should be approached with caution and evaluated carefully.

Qualitative Studies

Data for qualitative studies is collected through observations, surveys, or interviews. Surveys and surveillance studies are designed to describe the general characteristics of a disease, such as cardiovascular disease (CVD) or type 2 diabetes, especially in relation to person, place, and time. Indices of "person" include age; sex; race/ethnicity; marital status; occupation; income; and lifestyle variables, including diet, physical activity, and smoking status. Surveys are a type of cross-sectional study in which variables are measured at a single point in time. Interviews can be with individuals or focus groups, which involve a group of respondents assembled to answer questions on a given topic. In nutrition or food science research, either can be used to determine knowledge, attitude, or behaviors of consumers or other target groups.

Some qualitative studies can be exploratory. Because of their inherent design limitations, such studies are used to generate, rather than to test, hypotheses. Qualitative studies also may be components of larger studies. The data generated from these studies is used to validate instruments or to determine the focus of nutrition education programs, possibly through a focus group discussion.

The collection of nutrition- and health-related information from a population is critical for designing and evaluating policies and programs that improve health status and decrease risk factors. To be useful, information must be collected in a timely manner and presented to scientists, policymakers, and the public in a readily understandable form. Without monitoring, decisions may be made using insufficient information or incorrect assumptions. Nutrition monitoring can be conducted using several methods within the broad categories of screening, assessment, and surveillance.

Nutrition Screening

Nutrition screening is a systematic approach that can be used to quickly identify nutrition problems or individuals at nutritional risk who are in need of further assessment or who require intervention. Two widely used screening instruments are the Nutrition Screening Initiative's DETERMINE questionnaire and the mini-nutritional assessment, which is used in screening populations of older adults.[10] Many other screening tools are available to nutrition professionals, including those designed to determine malnutrition, diabetes risk, and food security.[11–13]

Nutrition Assessment

Nutrition assessment involves measurement of indicators of dietary status using such methods as 24-hour diet recalls, food frequency questionnaires (FFQ), and food diaries. Other methods used to determine intake include direct observation, weighed plate waste, and food records with or without the weighing of foods. Newer dietary assessment methods include using digital photography or mobile phones to keep food records.[14–19]

24-Hour Diet Recalls

With 24-hour diet recalls, study participants are asked to list all the foods they have eaten in the past 24 hours. The strengths of 24-hour diet recalls are that they provide detailed information about the types and amounts of food consumed on a given day, have a low response burden, and are cost-effective.[20,21] However, because they are memory dependent, respondents may under- or over-report consumption. A single 24-hour diet recall should not be used to assess diets of individuals. Collection of group data from 24-hour diet recalls with mean reporting, for example as performed by the National Health and Nutrition Examination Survey (NHANES), is an appropriate use of 24-hour diet recalls. However, it has long been recognized that 24-hour diet recalls may not reflect usual intake.[22–24]

In 2003, in an effort to improve the accuracy of 24-hour diet recalls, staff members of NHANES began to use two 24-hour diet recalls to collect participant information. The National Cancer Institute and the Center for Nutrition Policy and Promotion then developed a statistical method to calculate usual intake using both recalls.[25–28] The standard for assessing intake is multiple 24-hour dietary recalls using the multiple-pass method. Because intake may differ on weekends, it is important to include both weekday and weekend days in the recalls.[29–31]

Innovation Point

Digital Tracking When using dietary assessment methods that incorporate the use digital photography or smartphones to keep food records, it is imperative that the staff, study participants, or clients are trained appropriately to take consistent photographs.

Questionnaires

With the food frequency questionnaire (FFQ), study participants are asked to record their food consumption in categories such as number of food items, food groups, and portion sizes—all of which are indicators of nutrient intake.[32,33] An advantage of FFQs is that they can be self-administered; thus, they are suitable for large epidemiologic studies. A disadvantage is that FFQs often underestimate intake of total energy; however, energy adjustments can be used to reduce the effects of measurement error.[34–37] A wide variety of FFQs are in use, but some have not been validated against 24-hour recalls or direct observation. The effectiveness of FFQs depends on the range of food options presented. Meta-analyses have found that FFQs with longer food lists (200 items) have higher correlation coefficients than FFQs with shorter food lists (100 items) for most nutrients.[38] It is important to include appropriate ethnic foods that may be consumed by the population of interest when designing an FFQ.

Surveillance

In 1968, the World Health Assembly described *surveillance* as "the systematic collection and use of epidemiologic information for planning, implementation, and assessment of disease control."[39] In contrast to surveys, surveillance is continuous, and the data collected can be used to provide a framework for public health policies and a rationale for intervention. Surveillance also provides a way to monitor the effectiveness of specific interventions. They can "complete the loop"; that is, surveillance studies can be used to determine nutritional problems or nutritional needs and then following the intervention they can be used to evaluate whether the problems remain or if the intervention was effective.

Ensuring Accuracy

Accurate measurements are critical when determining a population's food intake. Intake of food groups can be determined using conventional instruments such as the SuperTracker system.[40,41] Nutrient intake can be assessed using the Nutrient Data Laboratory of the Agricultural Research Service, the Food and Nutrient Database for Dietary Studies, and commercial diet analysis programs.[42,43] Whenever possible, dietary intake should be confirmed using appropriate biomarkers, such as serum folate or vitamin C levels.[44,45] Intake of nutrients or food groups can be compared with recommended values for specific populations, and, in turn, with the prevalence or incidence of chronic disease.

Government Monitoring Programs

Most governments track the health and nutrition status of their population. For example, the U.S. government has tracked information on food consumption and the food supply for more than 100 years, starting with the USDA's Food Supply Series in 1909. The first USDA Household Food Consumption Survey (known as the Nationwide Food Consumption Survey after 1965) was started in the 1930s. In 1960, The National Health Examination Survey was initiated. However, the survey did not include provide information on nutrition and its link with diet, thus federal officials could not provide information on diet and disease or undernutrition to Congress. The first comprehensive nutrition survey in the United States was the Ten-State Nutrition Survey, which was conducted between 1968 and 1970 in California, Kentucky, Louisiana, Massachusetts, Michigan, New York, South Carolina, Texas, Washington, and West Virginia. The National Health and Nutrition Examination Survey (NHANES) I and II and the Pediatric Nutrition Surveillance Systems were initiated in the 1970s.

National Nutrition Monitoring and Related Research Program

In 1990, the National Nutrition Monitoring and Related Research Program (NNMRRP) established a comprehensive, coordinated program for nutrition monitoring and related research to improve the health and nutrition assessment of the U.S. population. The NNMRRP required the establishment of:

- A program to coordinate federal nutrition monitoring efforts and to assist states and local governments in participating in a nutrition monitoring network
- An interagency board to develop and implement the program
- A nine-member advisory council to provide scientific and technical advice and to evaluate program effectiveness
- Dietary guidelines to be issued every 5 years, and any dietary guidance issued by the federal government for the general public must be reviewed by the secretaries of Agriculture and Health and Human Services

The NNMRRP encompasses more than 50 surveillance activities that monitor and assess health and nutritional status in the United States. Monitoring efforts are divided into five overarching areas: nutrition and related health measurements; food and nutrient consumption; knowledge, attitude, and behavior assessments; food composition and nutrient databases; and food supply determinants. Important monitoring programs are summarized in **Table 2.6**. Most of the datasets generated by this program are available to the public. Some are restricted, due to confidentially or disclosure rules. The data can be accessed by researchers through application to the Research Data Center (RDC) in the National Center for Health Statistics headquarters in Hyattsville, Maryland. Proposals are reviewed by the RDC staff.

TABLE 2.6
National Nutrition-Related Health Assessments*

Survey Name	Date	Target	Data Collected	Department/Agency
Nutritional and Related Health Measurements				
NHANES†	1999–present	Civilian, noninstitutionalized persons 2 months or older; oversampling of adolescents, African Americans, Mexican Americans, and adults older than age 60	Survey elements are similar to NHANES III and NHIS**; this is a continuous monitoring system	NCHS, CDC (HHS)
NHANES III	1988–1994	Civilian, noninstitutionalized persons 2 months or older; oversampling of adolescents, non-Hispanic blacks, Mexican Americans, children younger than 6 years and adults older than 60	Demographics, dietary intake (e.g., 24-hour recall, food frequency), biochemical analysis of blood and urine, physical examination, anthropometry, blood pressure, bone densitometry, diet and health behaviors, health conditions	NCHS, CDC (HHS)
NHANES III Supplemental Nutrition Survey of Older Persons	1988–1994	Representative U.S. elderly population	Demographics, dietary intake (e.g., 24-hour recall, food frequency), biochemical analysis of blood and urine, physical examination, anthropometry, blood pressure, bone densitometry, diet and health behaviors, health conditions	NCHS, NIH/NIA
HHANES	1982–1984	Civilian, noninstitutionalized Mexican Americans in five southwestern states, Cuban Americans in Dade County, Florida, and Puerto Ricans in New York, New Jersey, and Connecticut, aged 6 months to 74 years	Demographics, dietary intake (24-hour recall and food frequency), biochemical analysis of blood and urine, physical exam, anthropometry, blood pressure, diet and health behaviors, health conditions	NCHS (HHS)
NHANES II	1976–1980	Civilian, noninstitutionalized persons aged 6 months to 74 years	Demographics, dietary intake, biochemical analysis of blood and urine, physical exam, anthropometry	NCHS (HHS)
NHANES I	1971–1974	Civilian, noninstitutionalized population of the conterminous states aged 1 to 74 years	Demographics, dietary information, biochemical analysis of blood and urine, physical exam, anthropometry	NCHS (HHS)
PedNSS	1973, continuous	Low-income, high-risk children, birth to 17 years, emphasis on birth to 5 years	Demographics, anthropometry, birth weight, hematology	NCCDPHP, CDC (HHS)
PNSS	1973, continuous	Convenience sample of low-income, high-risk pregnant women	Demographics, pregravid weight and maternal weight gain, anemia, behavioral risk factors, birth weight, and formula-feeding data	NCCDPHP, CDC (HHS)

Survey Name	Date	Target	Data Collected	Department/Agency
Food and Nutrient Consumption				
CSFII**	1994–1996 1989–1991 1985–1986	Individuals of all ages with oversampling in low-income households	One- and three-day food intakes, times of eating events, sources of food eaten away from home	ARS, HNIS
TDS	1961, annual	Specific age and gender groups	Determines levels of nutrients and contaminants in the food supply; analyses are performed on foods that are "table-ready"	FDA (HHS)
Consumer Expenditure Survey	1980, continuous	Noninstitutionalized population and a portion of the institutionalized population in the United States	Demographics, food stamp use, average annual food expenditures	U.S. Bureau of Labor Statistics
NFCS	1977–1978, 1987	Households in the conterminous states—all income and low income	Households: quantity (pounds), dollar value, and nutritive value of food eaten Individuals: food intake, times of eating events, and sources of foods eaten away from home	HNIS (USDA) ARS (USDA)
SNDA II	1998	Public schools in the 48 contiguous states and the District of Columbia that participate in the National School Lunch Program	School and food service characteristics, nutrients by food group and relationship to the RDA and DGA by meals, source of meals, and nutrient content of USDA meals	FNS/USDA
WIC Feeding Practices Study	1994–1995	Pre- and postnatal women and their children who participate in WIC	Demographics, rates of breast and formula feeding, factors associated with breastfeeding	FNS/USDA
5 a Day for Better Health Baseline Survey	1991	Adults 18 years and older	Demographics; fruit and vegetable intake; and knowledge, attitudes, and practices regarding intake	NCI (HHS)
Knowledge, Attitude, and Behavior Assessments				
YRBBS‡	Biennial	Civilian, noninstitutionalized adolescents aged 12 to 18 years	Demographics; diet and weight; drug, alcohol and tobacco use; seat belt and bicycle helmet use; behaviors that contribute to violence; suicidal tendencies	CDC (HHS)/ NCCDPHP
BRFSS§	1984, continuous	Adults 18 years and older in households with telephones located in participating states	Demographics, questions that assess risk factors associated with leading causes of death, alcohol and tobacco use, weight, seat belt and helmet use, use of preventative medical care	CDC (HHS)/ NCCDPHP
DHKS	1994–1996	Adults 20 years and older who participated in CSFII 1994–1996	Demographics, self-perceptions of relative intake, awareness of diet and health relationships, food-label use, perceived importance of following diet and health recommendations, beliefs about food safety, and knowledge of sources of nutrients; data can be linked with intake through CSFII data	ARS/USDA

(*continues*)

TABLE 2.6
National Nutrition-Related Health Assessments* (*continued*)

Survey Name	Date	Target	Data Collected	Department/Agency
Infant Feeding Practices Survey	1993–1994	New mothers and healthy infants to 1 year of age	Demographics, prior infant feeding practices, baby's social situation, characteristics associated with breast feeding, development of allergies	FDA
Consumer Food Handling Practices	1992–1993, 1998	Civilian, noninstitutionalized adults older than 18 years with telephones	Demographics, prevalence of unsafe food handling practices, knowledge of food safety principles, use of sources of information about safe food handling, incidence of foodborne illnesses	FDA
Food Composition and Nutrient Databases				
National Nutrient Data Bank	—	—	This is the repository for information on approximately 7,100 foods and up to 80 components. Essentially all food composition databases are derived from this databank.	ARS (USDA)
Food Label and Package Survey	1977–96, biennially	All brands of processed foods regulated by the FDA	Prevalence of nutrition labeling, declaration of select nutrients, prevalence of label claims and other descriptors	FDA (HHS)
Food Supply Determinations				
AC Nielsen SCANTRACK	1985, monthly	~3,000 U.S. supermarkets	Sales and physical volume of specific market items, selling price, percent of stores selling the product	ERS/USDA
U.S. Food and Nutrient Supply Series	1909, annually	U.S. population	ERS = Amount of food commodities that disappear into the food distribution system; CNPP = nutrient levels of food supply; results are totaled for each nutrient and converted to per day basis	ERS/CNPP/USDA

Abbreviations: ARS, Agricultural Research Service; BRFSS, Behavioral Risk Factor Surveillance System; CDC, Centers for Disease Control and Prevention; CNPP, Center for Nutrition Policy and Promotion; CSFII, Continuing Survey of Food Intakes by Individuals; DHKS, Diet and Health Knowledge Survey; ERS, Economic Research Service; FDA, Food and Drug Administration; HHANES, Hispanic Health and Nutrition Examination Survey; HHS, Health and Human Services; HNIS, Human Nutrition Information Service; NFCS, Nationwide Food Consumption Survey; NCCDPHP, National Center for Chronic Disease Prevention and Health Promotion; NCHS, National Center for Health Statistics; NCI, National Cancer Institute; NHANES, National Health and Nutrition Examination Survey; NHIS, National Health Interview Survey; NIA, National Institute on Aging; NIH, National Institutes of Health; PedNSS, Pediatric Nutrition Surveillance System; PNSS, Pregnancy Nutrition Surveillance System; SNDA, School Nutrition Dietary Assessment Study; TDS, Total Diet Study; USDA, United States Department of Agriculture; WIC, Women, Infants, and Children; YRBSS, Youth Risk Behavioral Surveillance System.

* A complete guide to nutrition monitoring in the United States can be found at: http://www.cdc.gov/nchs/data/misc/nutri98.pdf.

† The complete survey content of NHANES 1999–2004 can be found at http://www.cdc.gov/nchs/data/nhanes/dxa/dxa_techdoc.pdf.

** CSFII and NHANES have now been combined into a single survey.

‡ The YRBSS report for 2004 can be found at http://www.cdc.gov/mmwr/PDF/rr/rr5312.pdf. MMWR summary reports are available through the CDC website.

§ Full information on the Behavioral Risk Factor Surveillance System is available at http://www.cdc.gov/brfss/#about_BRFSS.

National Health and Nutrition Examination Survey

The National Health and Nutrition Examination Survey (NHANES) is a program of studies designed to assess the health and nutritional status of the U.S. population (see **Table 2.7**). The survey combines health interviews and physical examinations with dietary information (see **Table 2.8**).

TABLE 2.7
Goals of NHANES

- Estimate the number and percent of persons in the U.S. population, and designated subgroups, with selected diseases and risk factors.
- Monitor trends in the prevalence, awareness, treatment, and control of selected diseases.
- Monitor trends in risk behaviors and environmental exposures.
- Analyze risk factors for selected diseases.
- Study the relationship among diet, nutrition, and health.
- Explore emerging public health issues and new technologies.
- Establish a national probability sample of genetic material for future genetic research.
- Establish and maintain a national probability sample of baseline information on health and nutritional status.

Source: Data from Centers for Disease Control and Prevention. *Nutrition Monitoring in the United States*. Available at: http://www.cdc.gov/nchs/data/misc/nutri98.pdf. Accessed June 5, 2012.

TABLE 2.8
Data Gathered by the NHANES

Measurement Category	Information Gathered
Health measurements by participant age and gender	• Physical exam (all ages) • Blood pressure (8 years and older) • Bone density (8 years and older) • Condition of teeth (5 years and older) • Vision test (12 years and older) • Hearing test (12 to 19 years and 70 years and older) • Height, weight, and other body measures (all ages) • Ophthalmology exam for eye diseases (40 years and older) • Breathing tests (6 to 79 years)
Lab tests on urine (6 years and older)	• Kidney function tests (6 years and older) • Sexually transmitted infections (STIs) • Chlamydia and gonorrhea (14 to 39 years) • Exposure to environmental chemicals (selected persons 6 years and older) • Pregnancy test (females 12 years and older and girls 8 to 11 years who have periods)
Lab tests on blood (1 year and older)	• Anemia (all ages) • Total and HDL cholesterol (6 years and older) • Glucose measures (12 years and older) • Infectious diseases (2 years and older) • Kidney function tests (12 years and older) • Lead (1 year and older) • Cadmium (1 year and older) • Mercury (1 year and older) • Liver function (12 years and older) • Nutrition status (1 year and older) • Thyroid function test (12 years and older) • Prostate specific antigen (PSA; males 40 years and older) • Sexually transmitted infections (STIs) • Genital herpes (14 to 49 years) • Human immunodeficiency virus (HIV) (18 to 49 years) • Human papillomavirus (HPV) antibody (14 to 59 years) • Exposure to environmental chemicals (selected persons 6 years and older)
Lab tests on water	• Environmental chemicals (12 years and older in half of households)
Other lab tests	• Vaginal swabs (self-administered; females 14 to 59 years) • Human papillomavirus (HPV; ages 14 to 59 years)

(*continues*)

TABLE 2.8
Data Gathered by the NHANES (*continued*)

Measurement Category	Information Gathered
Private health interviews	• Health status (ages 12 and older) • Questions about drug and alcohol use (no drug testing will be done; 12 years and older) • Reproductive health (females 12 years and older) • Questions about sexual experience (14 to 69 years) • Tobacco use (12 years and older)
Anthropometry measurements from the mobile examination center	• Body mass index (BMI); for children 2 to 19 years of age, BMI z-score also is determined • Waist circumference • Skinfold measurements and body fat measures through DXA
Dietary information from the mobile examination center	• Two 24-hour dietary recalls; parents or guardians report for children 0 to 5 years of age; children 6 to 11 years are assisted by an adult; children older than 12 years of age self-report • Food frequency questionnaire (some years)
After the visit to the mobile examination center	• Participants asked about the foods they eat will receive a phone call 3 to 10 days after their exam for a similar interview (all ages); participants, or an adult for participants ages 1 to 15 years old, are asked about their food-shopping habits • Persons who test positive for hepatitis C will be asked to participate in a brief telephone interview 6 months after the exam; parents will respond for children

Source: Data from Centers for Disease Control and Prevention. Nutrition Monitoring in the United States. Available at: http://www.cdc.gov/nchs/data/misc/nutri98.pdf. Accessed June 5, 2012.

Beginning in 1999, the NHANES became a continuous surveillance program, with data released to the public biannually. The NHANES does not use a random sample; however, a complex, multistage, probability sampling design is used to select participants representative of the civilian, noninstitutionalized U.S. population. Data collection by the NHANES occurs at three levels: a brief household screener interview, an in-depth household survey interview, and a medical examination. Because detailed interviews and clinical, laboratory, and radiological examinations are conducted, the response burden to participants is significant. The interviews and medical examinations take place in a mobile examination center.

In 2002, the Department of Health and Human Services (DHHS) and the USDA integrated NHANES and the Continuing Survey of Food Intakes by Individuals (CSFII), the two major diet and health surveys, into a continuous data collection system. Thus, diet and nutrition information can now be linked directly to health status information. The data can be accessed from the NHANES website. The integrated dietary component of the NHANES, titled *What We Eat in America*, provides nutrient intake breakdowns by age, gender, race/ethnicity, and income, as well as by meal.[46] The NHANES website also features data briefs, research articles, and links to the NHANES dietary tutorial, which can be used to gain a more in-depth understanding of the data, including how it is collected and how it can be used.

It is difficult to quantify the tremendous impact that NHANES and related programs have had on health policy and health research in the United States.[47] One way is to look at the number of publications generated using NHANES data. For instance, a PubMed search on the term "NHANES" in December 2012 produced 19,251 publications on diverse topics, including self-reported physical activity/sedentary behavior in pregnant women; cardiovascular risk factors; prevalence and treatment of mental disorders in U.S. children as a correlate of television viewing and computer use; body mass index in children and adolescents; and the association of consumption of 100% fruit juice and nutrient intake in children. NHANES has also provided valuable information on ethnic and racial differences in dietary intake; the clustering of cardiovascular risk factors based on socioeconomic status; and variations in hypertension rates by geographic region.[48–52]

Findings from NHANES studies have been used to generate hypotheses that can be tested through randomized clinical trials. Hypotheses are carefully constructed statements generated from inferences. Three methods of hypothesis formation about the etiology of disease are derived from inductive reasoning:

- *Method of difference:* If the frequency of a condition is markedly different in two sets of circumstances, the condition may be caused by a factor that differs between them.
- *Method of agreement:* The observation that a single factor is common to a number of circumstances in which the disease occurs with high frequency.
- *Method of concomitant variation:* Refers to circumstances in which the frequency of a factor varies in proportion to the frequency of disease. This is particularly useful in generating hypotheses from correlational data.

When assessing studies using NHANES data, it is important to understand the strengths and limitations of the NHANES dataset. The following are the strengths of NHANES data:

- The data is collected from a representative sample of the U.S. population; data from all ages and ethnicities is available.
- The sample size is large and can be increased further by combining datasets.
- Since 2003, two 24-hour recalls have been collected and, from these, usual intake can be calculated.
- A wide array of demographic and lifestyle variables and biomarkers of disease are available, which can be used as either covariates or outcome variables in statistical analyses.
- The data and support documentation are publicly available.

The limitations of NHANES data are as follows:

- Because information on exposure and disease are collected at the same time, it is not possible to determine if the exposure preceded or resulted in the disease. Thus, causal inferences cannot be drawn. This is one of the most important limitations.
- It is impossible to control for all potential confounders.
- Even with the ability to calculate usual intake, the dietary data ultimately are reliant on a method that is memory dependent.

Epidemiologic Studies

In addition to data collected by the National Center for Health Statistics, a number of long-term, primarily government-funded, epidemiologic studies on adults and children/adolescents have provided critical information that has been used to guide the nation's health policies and federal programs. The Bogalusa Heart Study (BHS), the Framingham Heart Study, and the Coronary Artery Risk Development in Young Adults (CARDIA) are leading examples. Other important epidemiologic studies in the United States that have contributed to our knowledge of risk reduction and disease prevention are the Nurses' Health Study (170,000 female registered nurses between the ages of 30 and 55 years at the beginning of the study), the Nurses' Health Study II (established in 1989, 117,000 female nurses between the ages of 25 and 42 years); and the all-male Health Professional Follow-up Study (initiated in 1986 with 2-year scheduled follow-ups). This latter study was designed to complement the Nurses' Health Study, relating nutritional factors to the incidence of serious illnesses, such as cancer, heart disease, and other vascular diseases, in 51,529 male health professionals. Another important epidemiologic study is the Iowa Women's Health Study, a cohort of 41,837 postmenopausal women who have been followed since 1985. Combined, these studies have generated more than 2,000 publications and have helped shape medical care, risk reduction programs, health promotion, and public policy.

The Bogalusa Heart Study

The Bogalusa Heart Study (BHS) was designed initially to examine the early development of coronary heart disease and essential hypertension in a biracial (African American–Caucasian) pediatric population.[53–55] The BHS population consists of approximately 5,000 individuals who have been studied at various growth phases and have been followed for as long as 15 years. The mixed epidemiologic design of the study has included cross-sectional and longitudinal surveys to provide information on several questions, including:

- What is the distribution and prevalence of CVD risk factors in a defined pediatric population, and how are abnormal serum lipid levels, blood pressure, and other risk factors defined in children?
- Do cardiovascular risk factors track and change over time?
- What is the interrelationship among these risk factors?
- What is the interaction of genetics and the environment?

Data from the BHS has contributed significantly to our knowledge and understanding of CVD risk factors in children, as well as the history of CVD in early life. For example, data on children, adolescents, and young adults from birth to 31 years has provided information to develop a framework for desirable cholesterol levels in children and has led investigators to recommend screening of cardiovascular risk factors for *all* children, not only those with a parental history of heart disease or dyslipidemia (high blood lipids), beginning at elementary school age. Data also suggest that risk factors for CVD "track"; that is, they remain in a rank relative to peers over time. For example, children with elevated serum total cholesterol or low-density lipoprotein (LDL) cholesterol levels are likely to have dyslipidemia in adulthood.

The BHS data has been used to characterize and to identify trends in children's diets for more than 30 years.[56] The American Academy of Pediatrics used BHS data in formulating its recommendation that the *Dietary Guidelines for Americans, 2010* apply to all healthy children ages 2 years and older. The Academy of Nutrition and Dietetics' used BHD data in its position paper on dietary guidance for healthy children 2 to 11 years of age.[57]

One of the major accomplishments of the BHS did not come from epidemiologic data *per se* but rather from autopsy studies of participants, usually those killed in accidents.[58] BHS data confirmed and extended earlier studies that showed that fatty streaks in the aorta were evident in the first decade of life and that the extensiveness of these lesions was highly associated with serum total cholesterol and LDL cholesterol levels.[59]

The Framingham Heart Study

The Framingham Heart Study has been described as "one of the most impressive medical works in the twentieth century."[60] The Framingham Study has provided critical information on the causes, complications, and management of atherosclerosis. Initiated under the auspices of the National Heart Institute (now the National Heart Lung and Blood Institute; NHLBI) in 1948, 1,980 men and 2,421 women were enrolled in a 3-year observational study in Framingham, Massachusetts. At the time, this study design was quite a novel idea. The first report, published in 1961, identified high blood pressure, smoking, and high cholesterol as major factors in heart disease, and it conceptualized them as risk factors. Continued study of the population has provided health professionals with multifactorial risk profiles for cardiovascular disease, which have assisted in identifying individuals at high risk, as well as providing the basis for preventative measures. During its more than 50-year history, the Framingham Heart Study has introduced the concept of biological, environmental, and behavioral risk factors; identified major risk factors associated with heart disease, stroke, and other diseases; revolutionized preventive medicine; and changed how the medical community and general population regard disease pathogenesis. The National Cholesterol Education Program (NCEP) used the Framingham risk scoring system to determine the 10-year risk of coronary heart disease in adults.[61] The Framingham Heart Study also has supplied valuable information to the Seventh Report of the Joint National Committee on the Prevention, Detection, Evaluation, and Treatment of High Blood Pressure.[62]

In 1971, the Framingham Heart Offspring Study was implemented. It included 5,124 men and women ages 5 to 70 years who were offspring and spouses of the offspring of the original Framingham cohort. The objectives of this study were to study the incidence and prevalence of CVD and its risk factors, trends in CVD incidence and its risk factors over time, and family patterns of CVD and risk factors. The Offspring Study provided the opportunity to evaluate a second generation of participants, assess new or emerging risk factors and outcomes, and provide a resource for future genetic analyses.[63]

Data Quality

The quality of data from surveys and epidemiologic studies depends on the training of personnel and adherence to rigid protocols. It also depends on the validity and reliability of the test instruments used, as well as on the subjects' responses. Instruments may need to be modified for specific populations. For example, in the BHS, the 24-hour diet recall method had to be adapted for use in children.[64] To improve the reliability and validity of the 24-hour diet recall, quality controls included:

- The use of a standardized protocol that specified exact techniques for interviewing, recording, and calculating results
- Standardized, graduated food models to quantify foods and beverages consumed
- A product identification notebook for commonly forgotten snacks, foods, and beverages
- School lunch assessment to identify all school lunch recipes, preparation methods, and average portion sizes of menu items reflected in each 24-hour diet recall
- Follow-up telephone calls to parents to obtain information on brand names, recipes, and preparation methods of meals served at home
- Research of products in the field to obtain updated information on ingredients, preparation, and weights (primarily of snack foods and fast foods)[65]

- Participation of all interviewers in rigorous training sessions and pilot studies before the field surveys to minimize interviewer effects
- Collection of one 24-hour diet recall per study participant
- Collection of duplicate recalls from a 10% random subsample to assess interviewer variability[66]

Clinical Trials

Clinical trials are commonly used to assess diet or dietary interventions or to determine the efficacy of drugs or other pharmacologic agents.

Metabolic Diet Studies

metabolic diet study Randomized control trial conducted in a clinical research center where study participants are randomized into test or control groups and fed an experimental diet or a "regular" diet, respectively.

A **metabolic diet study** is a randomized control trial conducted in a clinical research center where study participants are randomized into test or control groups and fed an experimental diet or a "regular" diet, respectively. Different designs are available for metabolic diet studies; the one that provides the most valid results is the double-blind, placebo-controlled study.[67] In these studies, neither the investigator nor the participant knows whether the test or control diet is offered. Because it is difficult and expensive to do these studies, they are usually short in duration and have a small sample size; compliance and dropout rates are problems.

DASH

A classic example of a double-blind, placebo-controlled metabolic diet study is the Dietary Approaches to Stop Hypertension (DASH) trials.[67,68] The DASH investigators examined data from epidemiologic studies, other clinical trials, and studies using experimental animals that showed that consumption of nutrients, notably low levels of sodium and high levels of potassium and calcium, lowered blood pressure. To test the impact of diet on blood pressure, the initial DASH study was conducted at four academic medical centers and included 459 adult participants. Inclusion criteria were untreated systolic blood pressure of less than 160 mm Hg and diastolic blood pressure of 80–95 mm Hg. For 3 weeks, participants ate a control diet. They were then randomized to 8 weeks of one of three diets: a control diet; a diet rich in fruits and vegetables; or a combination diet rich in fruits, vegetables, and low-fat dairy foods and low in saturated fatty acids, total fat, and cholesterol. Salt intake and weight were held constant; each diet contained the same number of calories (all food was prepared in a metabolic kitchen where calories were carefully measured). The combination diet, or "DASH diet," was shown to quickly (within 2 weeks) and substantially lower blood pressure.

DASH Sodium

In DASH Sodium, a subsequent study, 412 participants were assigned to a control diet or a DASH diet. Within the assigned diet, participants ate meals with high (3,450 mg/2,100 kcals), intermediate (2,300 mg/2,100 kcals), or low (1,150 mg/2,100 kcals) levels of sodium for 30 consecutive days each, in random order. Reduction of sodium intake to levels below the current recommendation of the DASH diet substantially lowered blood pressure, with the most significant effect seen with the lowest sodium concentration. The DASH diet has been widely embraced for the treatment of hypertension. Nutrition education materials on this diet plan are readily available.[69]

The PREMIER study

As elegant and persuasive as the DASH studies were, one drawback to this kind of study design is that participants receive all foods during the course of the study; thus, it is unclear how compliant people will be after the study.[67] The PREMIER study demonstrated that free-living individuals (individuals not in a clinical setting with prescribed diets) were able to make the lifestyle changes associated with decreased blood pressure.[70]

Pharmacologic Intervention Studies

When clinical trials of diet involve pharmacologic intervention, they carry a risk that is not usually seen with metabolic diet studies. The classical example of this was seen in the Alpha-Tocopherol, Beta-Carotene Cancer Prevention Study (ATBC Study)[71] and the Beta-Carotene and Retinol Efficacy Trial (CARET).[72] Based on epidemiologic data that showed a relationship between dietary intake of fruits and vegetables or, specifically, of beta-carotene, and reduced risk of developing lung cancer, especially in smokers, the ATBC and CARET studies used high-dose beta-carotene in major cancer chemopreventive trials.[73–76] Investigators expected to see reductions in lung cancer by as much as 49% in some high-risk groups.[72] In actuality, beta-carotene increased the risk of lung cancer, forcing the CARET study to be stopped early.[77] These studies clearly point to the necessity of additional research and have important public health implications.[78]

Animal Studies

Animal studies are important in nutrition research for many reasons. For one, variables can be easier to control in animals than in humans. Laboratory animals that are genetically identical and exposed to the same environmental conditions can be fed carefully prepared diets with different combinations of nutrients. Second, invasive treatments—such as ovariectomies to mimic the physiologic state of postmenopausal women—can be performed on animals.[79] Third, because the lifespan of most laboratory animals is short, the effects of dietary manipulation can be followed over several generations. Finally, animals can be sacrificed at the end of the experiment and the effect of the treatment can be examined closely at the organ, tissue, or cellular level.

Animal studies can explore molecular mechanisms behind a given observation in humans. For example, ferrets were used to determine that high doses of beta-carotene caused keratinized squamous metaplasia in the lung tissues, which was exacerbated by exposure to cigarette smoke.[80] This explains the paradoxical relationship between beta-carotene and smoking seen in the ATBC and CARET trials discussed earlier. It also points out another use of animal studies; that is, the metabolism of natural products should be investigated using animal models *before* beginning human intervention trials, particularly if nutrient doses exceed recommended levels.[81]

Rats, mice, rabbits, guinea pigs, dogs, sheep, and monkeys are the animals most commonly used in nutrition research. The species selected for a given experiment should be one whose metabolism is the most similar to human metabolism for a particular nutrient. The importance of this criterion is illustrated in the classic studies of vitamin C metabolism. A review of the literature will show that only guinea pigs are used for vitamin C research. This makes sense because guinea pigs are the only laboratory animal that, like humans, has an obligatory requirement for this nutrient.

Many of the elements that make animal studies so appealing in nutrition research also are drawbacks. For example, interactions between genetics and the environment are easy to study in animals, but the results are difficult to translate to humans because, with the exception of monozygotic twins, humans are not genetically identical. Thus, no matter how carefully a human experiment is controlled, responses to dietary manipulations may be different due to individual genetic backgrounds.

Using Nutrition Research to Inform Policy and Improve Public Health

The main reasons for conducting nutrition research are to establish public health goals, to determine policy or enact laws, to generate consumer messages, and to improve public health practice. Public health goals for the nation are set forth in *Healthy People 2020*.[82] The nutrition policy for the nation is the *Dietary Guidelines for Americans* with the accompanying consumer education component, MyPlate.[9,83]

Numerous programs and organizations rely on research to help shape recommendations and program policy. For example, the Institute of Medicine relies on research to develop Dietary Reference Intakes (DRIs).[84] The Food and Drug Administration uses research for its Food Labels program,[85] and the USDA Food and Nutrition Service relies on research when formulating guidelines for its Supplemental Nutrition Assistance Program (SNAP), school lunch programs, and the Supplemental Nutrition for Women, Infants, and Children (WIC) program.[87–89] The National Institutes of Health not only generates research, but also uses published studies when forming recommendations, including those for the NCEP and the National High Blood Pressure Education Program (NHBPEP).[61,90] Finally, programs geared for consumers, such as the CDC's Fruits and Veggies More Matters, are based on research.[91]

Healthy People 2020

Individual health is closely linked to community health—the health of the community and environment in which individuals live, work, and play. Community health, in turn, is profoundly affected by the collective beliefs, attitudes, and behaviors of everyone who lives in that community. *Healthy People*, published by the Department of Health and Human Services, is the comprehensive health promotion and disease prevention agenda for the nation. The Healthy People program grew out of health initiatives pursued over the last 25 years. In 1979, *Healthy People: The Surgeon General's Report on Health Promotion and Disease Prevention* provided nutrition goals for reducing premature deaths and preserving independence for older adults. In 1980, *Promoting Health/Preventing Disease: Objectives for the Nation* targeted 226 health objectives for the nation to achieve over the next 10-year period.[92,93] These were followed by *Healthy People 2000*, *Healthy People 2010*, and the current *Healthy People 2020* goals.[82]

The overarching goals presented in *Healthy People 2020* are for Americans to:

- Attain high-quality, longer lives free of preventable disease, disability, injury, and premature death.
- Achieve health equity, eliminate disparities, and improve the health of all groups.
- Create social and physical environments that promote good health for all.

- Promote quality of life, healthy development, and healthy behaviors across all life stages.

Over the course of Healthy People 2020, four foundation health measures will be used to monitor progress toward promoting health, preventing disease and disability, eliminating disparities, and improving quality of life:[94]

1. *General health status* includes life expectancy, healthy life expectancy, and chronic disease prevention.
2. *Health-related quality of life and well-being* includes measures of physical, mental, and social health-related quality of life.
3. *Determinants of health* include biology, genetics, individual behavior, access to health services, and the environment in which people are born, live, learn, play, work, and age.
4. *Health disparities* include measures of disparities and inequality based on race/ethnicity, gender, physical and mental ability, and geography.

Healthy People 2020 has 42 topic areas. Each topic area includes evidence-based interventions and resources from the U.S. Preventive Services Task Force Clinical Preventive Services, the Guide to Community Preventive Services, and the Quick Guide to Healthy Living Information for Consumers (see http://www.healthfinder.gov).[95–97] The topic areas likely to be of most interest to nutrition or food science students are Food Safety and Nutrition and Weight Status; other important nutrition-related topic areas are those on chronic diseases, including cancer, chronic kidney disease, diabetes, and heart disease and stroke. Many states also have developed their own Healthy People plans. Development of state-specific plans enables states to prioritize health problems, address needs of specific racial or ethnic groups, and develop solutions that are economically feasible for state budgets.

The National Center for Health Statistics is responsible for coordinating efforts to monitor the country's progress toward meeting the Healthy People objectives. Data is gathered from more than 190 different data sources from more than seven federal government agencies, including Health and Human Services; the Departments of Commerce, Education, Justice, Labor, and Transportation; and the Environmental Protection Agency. Data also is obtained from voluntary and private nongovernmental organizations. As appropriate, data for the objectives is provided for subgroups defined by relevant dimensions (e.g., sociodemographic subgroups of the population, health status, or geographic classifications) through DATA 2010, an interactive database system, and the CDC Wonder System.[98] Quarterly reports are available to the public.

The NHLBI's 2010 Cardiovascular Gateway demonstrates how one agency linked goals from *Healthy People 2010*, the *Dietary Guidelines for Americans, 2010*, and the NCEP to provide information and ideas to the public and health professionals. *Improving Health/Changing Lives: Communities Taking Action* describes effective community health campaigns—the Healthy Heart Project in rural West Virginia and Helping Educators Attack Cardiovascular Risk Factors Together—that were funded by the NHLBI and that used Healthy People goals to reduce heart disease and cardiovascular risk factors. To support the Healthy People initiative, the NHLBI also provides nutrition education material and sponsors conferences, meetings, exhibits, and distance-learning opportunities.[99]

The objectives in *Healthy People 2020* related to nutrition and weight status are presented in **Table 2.9**. The data sources used to generate the objectives are included in *Healthy People 2020*; oftentimes NHANES data was used. Several objectives were retained or modified slightly from *Healthy*

TABLE 2.9
***Healthy People 2020* Objectives Related to Nutrition and Weight Status**

Healthier Food Access	
NWS-1	Increase the number of states with nutrition standards for foods and beverages provided to preschool-aged children in child care.
NWS-2	Increase the proportion of schools that offer nutritious foods and beverages outside of school meals: • NWS-2.1: Increase the proportion of schools that do not sell or offer calorically sweetened beverages for students. • NWS-2.2: Increase the proportion of school districts that require schools to make fruits or vegetables available whenever other food is offered or sold.
NWS-3	Increase the number of states that have state-level policies that incentivize food retail outlets to provide foods that are encouraged by the *Dietary Guidelines for Americans.*
NWS-4	(Developmental) Increase the proportion of Americans who have access to a food retail outlet that sells a variety of foods that are encouraged by the *Dietary Guidelines for Americans.*
Health Care and Worksite Settings	
NWS-5	Increase the proportion of primary care physicians who regularly assess body mass index (BMI) in their patients. • NWS-5.1: Increase the proportion of primary care physicians who regularly assess body mass index (BMI) in their adult patients. • NWS-5.2: Increase the proportion of primary care physicians who regularly assess body mass index (BMI) for age and sex in their child or adolescent patients.
NWS-6	Increase the proportion of physician office visits that include counseling or education related to nutrition or weight. • NWS-6.1: Increase the proportion of physician office visits made by patients with a diagnosis of cardiovascular disease, diabetes, or hyperlipidemia that include counseling or education related to diet and nutrition. • NWS-6.2: Increase the proportion of physician office visits made by adult patients who are obese that include counseling or education related to weight reduction, nutrition, or physical activity. • NWS-6.3: Increase the proportion of physician visits made by all child or adult patients that include counseling about nutrition or diet.
NWS-7	(Developmental) Increase the proportion of worksites that offer nutrition or weight management classes or counseling.
Weight Status	
NWS-8	Increase the proportion of adults who are at a healthy weight.
NWS-9	Reduce the proportion of adults who are obese.
NWS-10	Reduce the proportion of children and adolescents who are considered obese. • NWS-10.1: Children aged 2 to 5 years. • NWS-10.2: Children aged 6 to 11 years. • NWS-10.3: Adolescents aged 12 to 19 years. • NWS-10.4: Children and adolescents aged 2 to 19 years.
NWS-11	(Developmental) Prevent inappropriate weight gain in youth and adults. • NWS-10.1: Children aged 2 to 5 years. • NWS-10.2: Children aged 6 to 11 years. • NWS-10.3: Adolescents aged 12 to 19 years. • NWS-10.4: Children and adolescents aged 2 to 19 years. • NWS-10.5: Adults 20 years and older.
Food Insecurity	
NWS-12	Eliminate very low food security among children.
NWS-13	Reduce household food insecurity and in doing so reduce hunger.

Food and Nutrient Consumption	
NWS-14	Increase the contribution of fruits to the diets of the population aged 2 years and older.
NWS-15	Increase the contribution of total vegetables to the diets of the population aged 2 years and older. • NWS-15.1: Increase the contribution of total vegetables to the diets of the population aged 2 years and older. • NWS-15.2: Increase the contribution of dark green vegetables, orange vegetables, and legumes to the diets of the population aged 2 years and older.
NWS-16	Increase the contribution of whole grains to the diets of the population aged 2 years and older.
NWS-17	Reduce consumption of calories from solid fats and added sugars in the population aged 2 years and older. • NWS-17.1: Reduce consumption of calories from solid fats. • NWS-17.2: Reduce consumption of calories from added sugars. • NWS-17.3: Reduce consumption of calories from solid fats and added sugars.
NWS-18	Reduce consumption of saturated fat in the population aged 2 years and older.
NWS-19	Reduce consumption of sodium in the population aged 2 years and older.
NWS-20	Increase consumption of calcium in the population aged 2 years and older.
Iron Deficiency	
NWS-21	Reduce iron deficiency among young children and females of childbearing age. • NWS-21.1: Children aged 1 to 2 years. • NWS-21.2: Children aged 3 to 4 years. • NWS-21.3: Females aged 12 to 49 years.
NWS-22	Reduce iron deficiency among pregnant females.

Source: Reproduced from U.S. Department of Health and Human Services. Office of Disease Prevention and Health Promotion. *Healthy People 2020.* Washington, DC. Available at: http://healthypeople.gov/2020/topicsobjectives2020/objectiveslist.aspx?topicId=29. Accessed June 5, 2012.

People 2010, either because they remain important or were not met in *Healthy People 2010*.[100,101] For example, the goals for objectives related to weight were not met, as shown in **Figure 2.1**. When public comments were examined, many people asked the question, "What is a healthy weight?" Without this basic knowledge, it is unlikely that the public can ever meet the *Healthy People* goals. This is the reasoning for including objectives in *Healthy People 2020* related to education and counseling on weight and overweight.

Nutrient Requirements

The first Recommended Daily Allowances (RDAs) were published in 1941 as a "guide for advising on nutrition problems in connection with national defense."[102] The first edition included recommendations for only nine nutrients: protein, thiamine, riboflavin, niacin, ascorbic acid, vitamins A and D, calcium, and iron. In the seventh edition (1968), additional nutrients were included: folate; vitamins B_6, B_{12}, and E; phosphorous; magnesium; and iodine. The last edition of the RDAs (1989) added vitamin K, zinc, and selenium. The RDAs are applicable to *groups* of healthy people, such as those in the military or receiving school lunch programs, rather than *individuals*. The RDAs are, however, often used to assess the adequacy of an individual's diet.

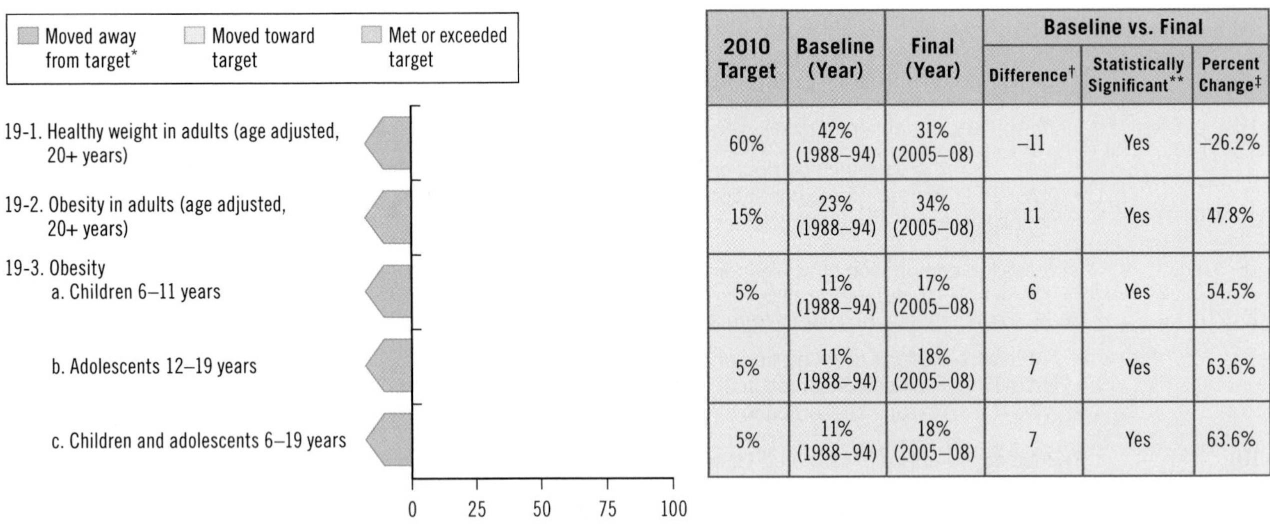

2010 Target	Baseline (Year)	Final (Year)	Baseline vs. Final		
			Difference†	Statistically Significant**	Percent Change‡
60%	42% (1988–94)	31% (2005–08)	–11	Yes	–26.2%
15%	23% (1988–94)	34% (2005–08)	11	Yes	47.8%
5%	11% (1988–94)	17% (2005–08)	6	Yes	54.5%
5%	11% (1988–94)	18% (2005–08)	7	Yes	63.6%
5%	11% (1988–94)	18% (2005–08)	7	Yes	63.6%

FIGURE 2.1 Summary of progress toward attainment of objectives related to weight in adults and children in *Healthy People 2010*. Note that the failure to meet these goals has resulted in the carryover of these goals to *Healthy People 2020*.

Notes:

* Movement away from target is not quantified using the percent of targeted change achieved.

† Difference = Final Value – Baseline Value

Differences between percentages are measured in percentage points.

** When estimates of variability are available, the statistical significance of the difference between the final value and the baseline value is assessed at the 0.05 level.

‡ $\frac{\text{Final value} - \text{Baseline Value}}{\text{Baseline Value}} \times 100$

§ $\frac{\text{Final value} - \text{Baseline Value}}{\textit{Healthy People } 2010 - \text{Target Baseline Value}} \times 100$

Source: Reproduced from Centers for Disease Control and Prevention. *Healthy People Data 2010.* Figure 19-1. Progress Toward Target Attainment for Focus Area 19: Nutrition and Overweight. Available at: http://www.cdc.gov/nchs/data/hpdata2010/hp2010_final_review_focus_area_19.pdf. Accessed June 8, 2012.

In 1993, the question of whether the RDAs should be changed was posed by the Institute of Medicine's Food and Nutrition Board. A number of reasons were offered in support for changing the RDAs. Specifically, sufficient new scientific information had accumulated to substantiate reassessment of the recommendations. For example, sufficient data for efficacy and safety and upper tolerable limits was now available. Also, the RDAs were focused on preventing deficiency diseases. New RDAs were needed to take into account the reduction of diet-related chronic diseases. Finally, components of food not meeting the traditional concept of a nutrient, such as phytochemicals, were not included in the RDAs. If adequate data existed for these important chemicals, then reference intakes should be established.

Dietary Reference Intakes

Between 1994 and 2004, the Food and Nutrition Board extended and replaced the former RDAs. Similarly, the Canadian government revised its Recommended Nutrient Intakes (RNIs). Dietary Reference Intakes (DRIs) take into account age, gender, and life stage (e.g., pregnant, breastfeeding). They cover more than 40 nutrient substances and are available online.[84] The reference values for heights and weights of adults and children used in the DRIs are from NHANES III.

Conceptually, the DRIs are the same as the RDAs, in that their formulation relies on the best scientific evidence available at the time of issuance, that they are designed for healthy individuals over time, and that they can vary depending on life cycle stage or gender.[103] The DRIs differ from the original RDAs in that they incorporate the concepts of disease prevention, upper levels of intake and potential toxicity, and nontraditional nutrients. The latter establishes a precedent; as scientists learn more about how phytochemicals, herbals, and botanicals affect health, these, too, can be incorporated into the recommendations.

Where scientific evidence is available, the DRIs include at least four nutrient-based reference values:

- The estimated average requirement (EAR) is the median intake estimated to meet the requirements of half of healthy individuals. It is based on specific criteria of adequacy and careful review of the scientific evidence. Not all nutrients have an EAR because there may not be an acceptable scientific basis upon which to define one.
- The Recommended Daily Allowance (RDA) is calculated from the EAR, where the RDA = EAR + 2 standard deviations (SD) of the requirement. The RDA is the average daily dietary intake level sufficient to meet the nutrient requirement of approximately 98% of individuals.
- If there is no EAR for a nutrient, there can be no RDA. If this is the case, an adequate intake (AI) for the nutrient is provided. AI values are calculated by experts and are intended to meet or exceed the needs of a healthy population. The AI can be used as a guide for intake, but it cannot be used for all the applications for which the EAR can. If an AI is used instead of an EAR or RDA, it indicates that additional research is required for that nutrient. The assumption is that when this research is completed and evaluated, the AI can be replaced by an EAR and RDA.
- The tolerable upper limit (UL) is the highest level of continued daily nutrient intake that is unlikely to pose an adverse health effect. It is important to note that the word "tolerable" was chosen to avoid implying a possible beneficial effect.

The Institute of Medicine has published DRIs and related information for electrolytes and water; energy, carbohydrate, fiber, fat, fatty acids, cholesterol, protein, and amino acids; vitamin A, vitamin K, arsenic, boron, chromium, copper, iodine, iron, manganese, molybdenum, nickel, silicon, vanadium, and zinc; dietary antioxidants and other related compounds; folate and other B vitamins; and calcium, phosphorus, magnesium, vitamin D, and fluoride.[104–108]

How the DRIs Are Used

The DRIs are used for individual diet planning, dietary guidance, institutional food planning, military food and meal planning, planning for food assistance programs, food labeling and fortification programs, the development of new or modified food products, and food safety. In planning menus/diets for individuals or groups, it is important to meet the RDA or AI without exceeding the UL. The Institute of Medicine has incorporated the DRIs and other data into a series of reports, including *School Meals: Building Blocks for Healthy Children*; *Local Government Actions to Prevent Childhood Obesity*; *The Public Effects of Food Deserts (Workshop Summary)*; *Nutrition Standards and Meal Requirements for National School Lunch and Breakfast Programs: Phase I. Proposed Approach for Recommending Revisions*; and *The Use of Dietary Supplements by Military Personnel*.[109–113] Summaries of the development of the DRIs as well as the uses of the DRIs in dietary assessment and menu planning can be found in the literature.[114–117]

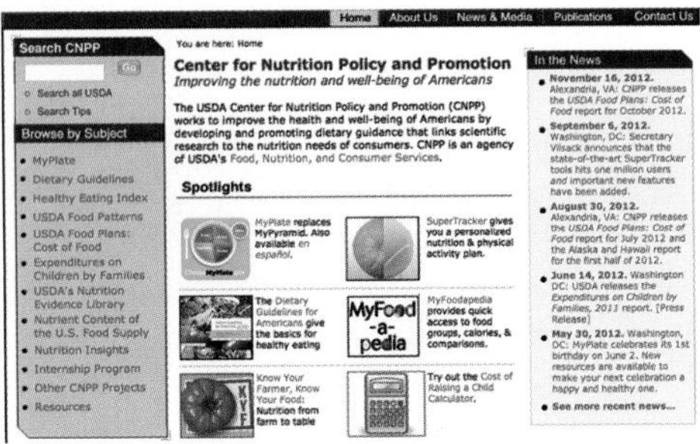

FIGURE 2.2 The Center for Nutrition Policy and Promotion plays an important role in developing and promoting dietary guidance that links scientific research to the nutrition needs of consumers. It seeks to advance and promote food and nutrition guidance for all Americans, with the goal of improving the nation's health.

Source: U.S. Department of Agriculture. Center for Nutrition Policy and Promotion. Available at: http://www.cnpp.usda.gov. Accessed August 17, 2012.

The Center for Nutrition Policy and Promotion

The Center for Nutrition Policy and Promotion (CNPP) was created in December 1994; it is one of the two offices of the USDA's Food, Nutrition, and Consumer Services. The other office is the Food and Nutrition Service (FNS). The CNPP's mission is "to improve the health of Americans by developing and promoting dietary guidance that links scientific research to the nutrition needs of consumers."[118] The CNPP carries out its mission to improve the health of Americans by: (1) advancing and promoting food and nutrition guidance for all Americans; (2) assessing diet quality; and (3) advancing consumer, nutrition, and food economic knowledge. **Table 2.10** shows the three major divisions of the CNPP. Major projects administered by CNPP are shown in **Figure 2.2**.

TABLE 2.10
The Main Divisions of the Center for Nutrition Policy and Promotion

The Evidence Analysis Library Division
Providing the latest evidence-based science to inform nutrition policy programs that support nutrition guidance provided to all Americans. To meet its goal, this division: • Leads a wide range of scientific review projects that inform and support federal nutrition policy programs and guidance, as well as serve as the basis for nutrition promotion and education. • Provides professional leadership to the nation's nutrition researchers, educators, and health professionals in the development and application of systematic evidence analysis to public health nutrition. • Makes accessible to the public systematic, evidence-based reviews. • Evaluates systematically scientific research to support the development and implementation of the *Dietary Guidelines* and on making nutrition education and social marketing, and health communication methods more effective.
The Nutrition Guidance and Analysis Division
Providing national leadership, technical expertise, and cooperation for development of the legislatively mandated Dietary Guidelines for Americans. To meet its goal, this division: • Works closely with federal partners to promote national nutrition policy. • Coordinates and shares efforts related to the Federal Advisory Committee Act, thus ensuring that federal dietary guidance is consistent with the *Dietary Guidelines for Americans* and is supported across federal departments. • Provides professional leadership in promoting national food and dietary guidance by translating science-based guidance into research-based patterns for food intake and message strategies that consumers will use to make informed decisions and positively change behavior. • Conducts policy research on food consumption patterns, nutrients in the U.S. food supply, and consumer expenditures on children to inform national and state policy.
The Nutrition Marketing and Communication Division
Designing, leading, and implementing a wide range of nutrition education, marketing, communications, and promotion projects. To meet its goal, this division: • Helps consumers, on a national scale, adopt behaviors for making wise food choices and being physically active. • Plans and coordinates marketing and communications research involving consumers, health professionals, and nutrition educators. • Develops, leads, and manages public and private partnerships to help multiply the reach of tested, actionable nutrition and health messages. • Provides customer support to consumers and professionals. • Creates and manages the CNPP and USDA's MyPlate.gov websites. • Represents CNPP in a multitude of professional conferences and meetings.

Source: Reproduced from the Center for Nutrition Policy and Promotion. USDA. Available at: http://www.cnpp.usda.gov/AboutUs.htm. Accessed June 5, 2012.

The *Dietary Guidelines for Americans*

The ***Dietary Guidelines for Americans*** provides nutrition, dietary, and food safety recommendations that are designed to promote health and reduce the risk of chronic disease for healthy Americans ages 2 years and older. The *Dietary Guidelines for Americans* is the foundation of federal nutrition policies, nutrition education programs, and information activities. The *Dietary Guidelines for Americans* makes it possible for all federal programs to provide consistent and evidence-based information. By law (PL 101-445), the *Dietary Guidelines for Americans* is developed and published jointly by the HHS and USDA every 5 years. The seventh edition (2010) was released on January 31, 2011 (earlier editions were published in 1980, 1985, 1990, 1995, 2000, and 2005). The *Dietary Guidelines for Americans, 2010,* will remain in effect until the 2015 edition is released. Changes in the *Dietary Guidelines for Americans* for each 5-year time period must reflect current scientific and medical knowledge available at the time of publication.[119] Earlier in this chapter, it was noted that the 2010 Dietary Guidelines for Americans Advisory Committee uses an evidence-based approach with information from the NEL to formulate the guidelines. Two important documents demonstrate the necessity of relying on evidence-based science: the 1988 *Surgeon General's Report on Nutrition and Health* and the 1989 National Research Council's report, *Diet and Health: Implications for Reducing Chronic Disease Risk*.[120,121]

Dietary Guidelines for Americans Nutrition, dietary, and food safety recommendations that are designed to promote health and reduce the risk of chronic disease for healthy Americans ages 2 years and older. The *Dietary Guidelines for Americans* are the foundation of federal nutrition policies, nutrition education programs, and information activities.

Importance of the *Guidelines*

The *Dietary Guidelines for Americans* dictates federal nutrition policies, which directly affect:

- Nearly 32.6 million Americans receiving benefits from SNAP
- Approximately 31 million children participating in USDA Child Nutrition Programs
- Approximately 9.1 million people receiving WIC benefits
- More than 3 million adults older than 60 years of age through the Elderly Nutrition Program

The *Dietary Guidelines for Americans* also affects information policy, as evidenced in MyPlate, food labels, and federal nutrition education programs, such as SNAP's education program. These pivotal uses of the *Dietary Guidelines for Americans* ensure that the nutrition information advocated by the government is consistent. The *Dietary Guidelines for Americans* also provides the foundation for nutrition recommendations and programs offered by nongovernmental agencies and nonprofits, such as the American Heart Association and the American Cancer Society.

The specific guidelines are usually presented as succinct statements of nutrition recommendations for the public.[9] As shown in **Figure 2.3**, the *Dietary Guidelines for Americans, 2010,* advises, as part of its *Let's Eat for the Health of It* campaign, the following central messages: build a healthy plate; cut back on foods high in solid fats, added sugars, and salt; eat the right amount of calories for you; be physically active your way; and use food labels to make better choices.

The recommendations of the *Dietary Guidelinesfor Americans, 2010*, were similar to those of the 2005 edition in that they quantified physical activity recommendations and food serving recommendations in terms of household measures. Further, the 2010 edition also discusses specific food groups, such as grains, and nutrients, such as potassium, and includes a recommendation for trans fats.

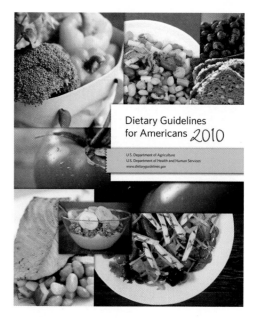

FIGURE 2.3 The overarching goal of the *Dietary Guidelines for Americans, 2010*, is to help Americans make better food choices to improve their long-term health.

Source: Reproduced from U.S. Department of Agriculture and U.S. Department of Health and Human Services. Dietary Guidelines for Americans, 2010. 7th ed. Washington, DC: US Government Printing Office; December 2010.

The policy document, an executive summary, selected messages, slide presentations, consumer brochures, and a message calendar are all available on *Dietary Guidelines* website (http://www.cnpp.usda.gov/dietaryguidelines.htm). Additional resources continue to be developed, so check the website frequently for updates.

Food Group Plans

In the United States, the federal government has promoted food group plans based on current scientific knowledge to provide dietary guidance for almost 100 years. The USDA published its first recommendations in 1916. Between 1916 and the 1940s, different food group plans published by various agencies had between 5 and 16 separate food groups. In 1943, as part of the wartime effort, the USDA published the *National Wartime Nutrition Guide*, which included the Basic Seven food guide. This guide was used until 1955, when the Department of Nutrition at the Harvard School of Public Health recommended collapsing the groups to four. This format was accepted by the USDA in 1956; in 1979, a fifth group—fats, sweets, and alcohol—was added. These plans all had one thing in common: They were designed to meet nutrient requirements and to prevent nutritional deficiencies.[122]

Food Guide Pyramid

With the recognition of the relationship between diet and chronic disease risk, a food guidance system was needed that included recommendations for preventing the excesses or poor food choices associated with chronic disease.[123] These efforts culminated with the Food Guide Pyramid, which was released in 1992.[122,124] Like the *Dietary Guidelines for Americans*, it emphasized overall health, was based on scientific research, addressed the total diet, and was built on successful elements of previous food plans.[125] The food patterns of the original Food Guide Pyramid were designed to help Americans make food choices that would allow them to meet federal nutrition standards, but moderate their intake of energy (calories), total and saturated fatty acids, sugar, and salt. Food patterns were assessed by comparing them to the 1980 RDAs and the 1980 *Dietary Guidelines*.[123] Later, they were assessed to the 1989 RDAs and the 1985 and 1990 *Dietary Guidelines*.[124] The Food Guide Pyramid supported the 2000 *Dietary Guidelines*; however, it was more specific and allowed consumers to understand food choices more fully.

Consumer testing prior to its original release showed that a pyramid was the most effective graphic; the shape helped to convey key dietary concepts of variety, proportionality, and moderation.[126] The Food Guide Pyramid's foundation was grains and cereals. Fruits and vegetables constituted the next tier; these were followed by milk and dairy products and meat and meat alternatives. Fats, oil, and sweets constituted the tip of the pyramid.

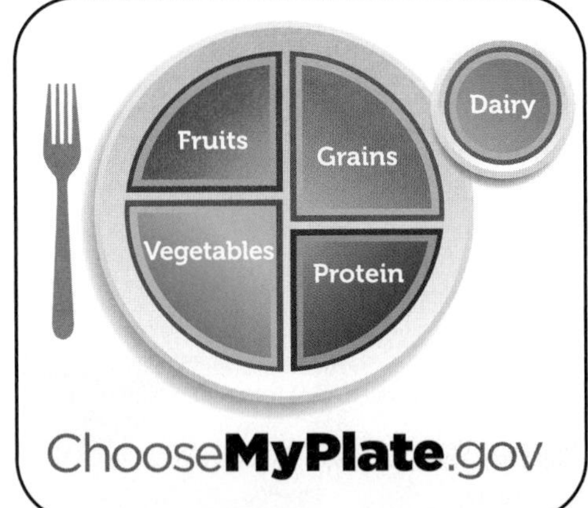

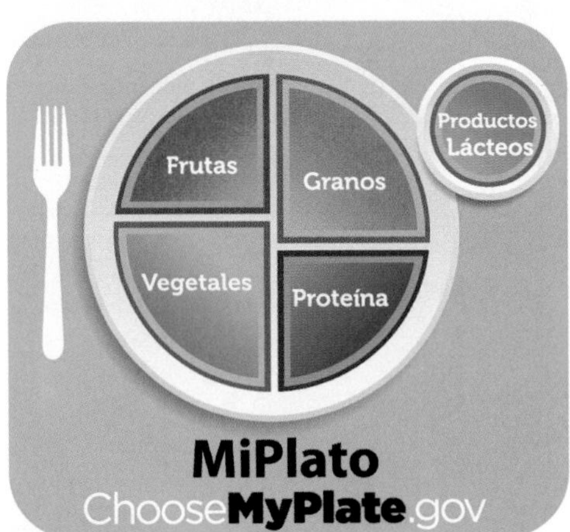

FIGURE 2.4 MyPlate, with its informative dinner plate graphic, is part of a communication initiative based on the *Dietary Guidelines for Americans, 2010* to help consumers make better food choices. It shows the five food groups using a familiar mealtime visual, a place setting.

Source: Courtesy of the U.S. Department of Agriculture.

MyPlate

In 2011, MyPlate was introduced. It is based on the *Dietary Guidelines for Americans, 2010*.[83] The MyPlate icon (see **Figure 2.4**) corresponds to seven consumer messages of the *Dietary Guidelinesfor Americans, 2010* (see **Table 2.11**). MyPlate was designed to serve as a visual reminder for healthy eating. Consumer focus-group testing determined that this visual—a dinner plate—was a familiar mealtime symbol. "My" emphasizes the personalized approach initiated by MyPlate. Serving sizes are based on common household measures and provide the basis for serving size recommendations for the *Dietary Guidelines for Americans*.[122]

TABLE 2.11
Selected Messages for Consumers from the *Dietary Guidelines for Americans, 2010*

Balancing calories	Enjoy your food, but eat less. Avoid oversized portions.
Foods to increase	Make half of your plate fruits and vegetables. Make at least half of your grains whole grains. Switch to fat-free or low-fat (1%) milk.
Foods to reduce	Compare sodium in foods like soup, bread, and frozen meals—and choose the foods with lower numbers. Drink water instead of sugary drinks.

Source: Data from the U.S. Department of Agriculture, Center for Nutrition Policy and Promotion. Dietary Guidelines for Americans, 2010. Washington, DC.

Healthy Eating Index

The Healthy Eating Index (HEI) was developed to provide a single summary method of assessing adherence to dietary recommendations. It was originally developed in 1995 using 1989–1990 data from the Continuing Survey of Food Intakes by Individuals (CSFII); it was later updated using 1994–1996 data and 1999–2000 NHANES data to assess and monitor the dietary status and dietary changes of Americans.[127–129] The 2005 revision of the *Dietary Guidelines* required a new HEI (i.e., HEI-2005) to accommodate the changes in recommendations for whole grains, vegetables, whole fruits, saturated fatty acids, and discretionary calories. The HEI-2005 measures diet quality in terms of conformity with MyPlate. The HEI-2005 uses a density approach and is expressed as a percent of calories, or "per 1,000 calories," as shown in **Table 2.12**.[83,130–132]

The HEI-2005 has been used in several ways. The CNPP used the HEI-2005 to examine the quality of diets of children and adolescents aged 2 to 17 years and found that their diets needed improvement. Overall, children and adolescents need to increase their consumption of whole fruits, whole grains, dark green and orange vegetables, and legumes. Also, calories from solid fats and added sugars should be reduced. Others have looked at whether the HEI-2005 score can be associated with improved endpoints for chronic diseases.[133] Researchers found that adherence to the *Dietary Guidelines* was associated with only a small reduction in major chronic disease risk in a population of over 100,000 American adults. (However, a limitation of this study was that few people adhered to the *Dietary Guidelines*.[133])

The Food Label

The Nutrition Labeling and Education Act (NLEA) of 1990 (PublicLaw 101-535) amended the Federal Food, Drug, and Cosmetic Act to provide, among other things, that certain nutrients and food components be included on the product's label. The regulatory authority for the food label rests with the FDA and the Federal Trade Commission (FTC). The Secretary of Health and Human Services (and by delegation, the FDA) can add or delete nutrients included in the food label or other package labeling if this action is necessary to assist consumers in maintaining healthy dietary practices. In response to these provisions, in the *Federal Register* of November 27, 1991, the FDA published a proposed rule: "Food Labeling; Reference Daily Intakes and

TABLE 2.12
Healthy Eating Index—2005: Components and Standards for Scoring*

Component	Maximum Points	Standard for Maximum Score	Standard for Minimum Score of Zero
Total fruit (includes 100% juice)	5	≥ 0.8 cup equiv. per 1,000 kcal	No fruit
Whole fruit (not juice)	5	≥ 0.4 cup equiv. per 1,000 kcal	No whole fruit
Total vegetables	5	≥ 1.1 cup equiv. per 1,000 kcal	No vegetables
Dark green and orange vegetables or legumes†	5	≥ 0.4 cup equiv. per 1,000 kcal	No dark green or orange vegetables or legumes
Total grains	5	≥ 3.0 oz equiv. per 1,000 kcal	No grains
Whole grains	5	≥ 1.5 oz equiv. per 1,000 kcal	No whole grains
Milk**	10	≥ 1.3 cup equiv. per 1,000 kcal	No milk
Meat and beans	10	≥ 2.5 oz equiv. per 1,000 kcal	No meat or beans
Oils‡	10	≥ 12 grams per 1,000 kcal	No oil
Saturated fat	10	≤ 7% of energy§	≥ 15% of energy
Sodium	10	≤ 0.7 gram per 1,000 kcal§	≥ 2.0 grams per 1,000 kcal
Calories from solid fats, alcoholic beverages, and added sugars (SoFAAS)	20	≤ 20% of energy	≥ 50% of energy

* Intakes between the minimum and maximum levels are scored proportionately, except for saturated fat and sodium (see §).
† Legumes counted as vegetables only after Meat and Beans standard is met.
** Includes all milk products, such as fluid milk, yogurt, and cheese, and soy beverages.
‡ Includes nonhydrogenated vegetable oils and oils in fish, nuts, and seeds.
§ Saturated Fat and Sodium get a score of 8 for the intake levels that reflect the 2005 Dietary Guidelines, < 10% of calories from saturated fat and 1.1 grams of sodium/1,000 kcal, respectively.
Source: Reproduced from U.S. Department of Agriculture, Center for Nutrition Policy and Promotion. Healthy Eating Index—2005. Available at: http://www.cnpp.usda.gov/Publications/HEI/healthyeatingindex2005factsheet.pdf. Accessed June 25, 2012.

Daily Reference Values; Mandatory Status of Nutrition Labeling and Nutrient Content Revision." The proposed rule required that food nutrition labels list certain nutrients and the amount of those nutrients in a serving of the food. A history of the FDA and details about an important piece of recent legislation, the Food Safety Modernization Act, are provided in **Special Topic 2.1** and **Special Topic 2.2**, respectively.

Placement of information on the label, the type size, the manufacturer's name and contact information, and other information related to content also is mandated. Special requirements apply to foods sold in small packages. Further, the USDA regulates poultry in accordance with the Poultry Products Inspection Act and meat under the Federal Meat Inspection Act.

Percent Daily Values (%DV) are one of the key elements on the food label. These are the daily dietary intake standards used for nutrition labeling. The first daily intake standards, referred to as the U.S. Recommended Daily Allowances, for the nutrition label were established in 1973 and were based on the RDAs.[134,135]

Having an understanding of food labels, including how to use of labels to make careful food selections, can help people reduce their risk of chronic disease. In addition, individuals with certain diseases can use food labels to understand how a particular food fits into a total food plan. Information on how to read a food label as well as additional consumer information is available online.[136]

Special Topic 2.1

Major Food Policy Timeline of the Food and Drug Administration

Kate Janisch

The Food and Drug Administration (FDA) is responsible for the safety and regulation of food (other than meat and poultry), drugs used on humans and animals, therapeutic agents of biological origin (such as vaccines), medical devices, cosmetics, animal feed, and radiation-emitting products. The FDA has undergone many changes in its scope of responsibility as well as where it resides in the federal government. The following is a brief outline of the FDA's history and its food policies:[1]

- **1862**: The FDA was established with a single chemist in the Division of Chemistry of the Department of Agriculture.
- **1867**: The FDA investigated misbranded and adulterated agricultural commodities, the primary reason for which it was created.
- **1883**: Harvey Washington Wiley was named the FDA's chief chemist. He campaigned for Congress to draft a law to regulate food and drug products.
- **1906**: The Food and Drug Act (also known as the Wiley Act) was signed by President Roosevelt on June 30, 1906. Prior to the act, states set their own domestic regulations with regard to food and drug commodities. The Wiley Act set uniform standards for all states. It prohibited the addition of any ingredients that would substitute for the food, conceal damage, pose a health hazard, or constitute a filthy or decomposed substance. In addition, the food or drug label could not be false or misleading in any way, and the presence and amount of 11 dangerous ingredients, including alcohol, heroin, and cocaine, had to be listed. Separate laws were established to set standards for specific foods, such as apples and butter, as well as canned foods.
- **1907**: The Board of Food and Drug Inspection was created to enforce laws.
- **1908**: The Referee Board of Consulting Scientific Experts was formed to advise the FDA on safety issues associated with food additives. This was brought about largely due to Wiley's extremist beliefs about food additives and a more conservative view from the Secretary of Agriculture, James Wilson.
- **1912**: Wiley resigned, and the agency turned its focus to drug regulation.
- **1927**: The agency was renamed the Food, Drug, and Insecticide Administration, and nonregulatory research aspects of the agency were moved elsewhere.

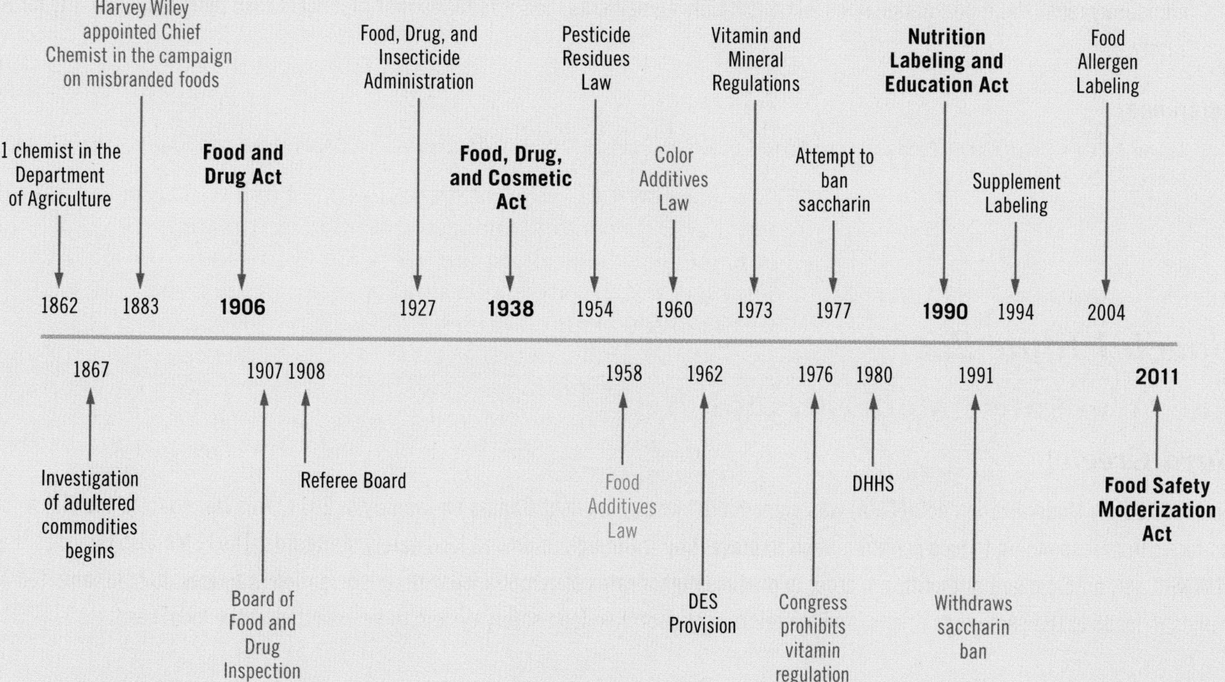

This timeline shows a brief history of the FDA and the food policies it has implemented.

- **1938**: The Food, Drug, and Cosmetic Act replaced the 1906 Food and Drug Act. This bill had floated around Congress for 5 years until disaster occurred. An untested medicinal product killed over 100 people, many of whom were children. The bill sought to cover the gaps that the first bill left open. New policies addressed food packaging and labeling and food quality. The new bill set recipe standards for many foods (e.g., if a food varied, it had to be labeled as "imitation"), established the right for the federal government to conduct factory inspections, and set forth standards for product advertising. The new bill also stated that cosmetics and medical devices were under the agency's purview, as was the premarket approval of drugs. (The Federal Trade Commission kept the rights to regulate drug advertising.)
- **1940**: The FDA moved into the new Federal Security Agency.
- **1954**: The Delaney Law specified allowable pesticide residues on foods.
- **1958**: The Delaney Law specified limits on chemical additives and banned carcinogenic additives.
- **1960**: The Delaney Law specified regulations for color additives.
- **1962**: The DES (Diethylstilbestrol) Proviso modified the Delaney Clause regarding carcinogenic additives; this proviso allowed the use of possible carcinogens to promote growth in animals as long as residues of the product did not remain in edible tissues.
- **1973**: The FDA issued regulations for vitamins, minerals, and enriched products, along with their health claims.
- **1976**: Congress prohibited the FDA from controlling the potency of supplements, but permitted its regulation of enriched foods.
- **1977**: The FDA tried banning saccharin as a sweetener because of its possible carcinogenic effects; Congress denied the ban and required a label on the package instead.
- **1980**: The FDA moved into the Department of Health and Human Services, where it remains today.
- **1990**: The Nutrition Labeling and Education Act required a standard set of nutrients on food labels, as we see it today.
- **1991**: The FDA formally withdrew its saccharin ban statement, and Congress removed its requirement of a statement on packages.
- **1994**: Supplements are allowed to be sold as long as they have a label stating "not evaluated by the FDA."
- **2004**: The Food Allergen Labeling and Consumer Protection Act passed, requiring all food products to emphasize any of the top eight food allergens unless they are in the common form (such as a bag of peanuts).
- **2011**: The Food Safety Modernization Act was passed on January 4, 2011. The goal of this act is to reduce the risks of foodborne illnesses by shifting the focus of federal regulators from responding to contamination to preventing it. The act incorporates mandatory recalls and international inspections/safety agreements, and it requires that producers take more responsibility for food safety.

Reference

1 Swann J. FDA's Origin. 2009. Food and Drug Administration. Available at: http://www.fda.gov/AboutFDA/WhatWeDo/History/Origin/ucm124403.htm. Accessed December 7, 2011.

Special Topic 2.2

The Food Safety Modernization Act

Sara Greeley

The Food Safety Modernization Act (FSMA) was signed into law by President Obama on January 4, 2011. This law enables the FDA to shift its focus from responding to food contamination to preventing it through improved food safety standards. The FSMA also provides the FDA with new enforcement authorities in order to produce higher rates of compliance with its prevention practices, to hold imported and domestic foods to the same regulations, and to create a collaborative food safety system to be executed at the local level.[1]

According to the Centers for Disease Control and Prevention (CDC), approximately 48 million people (1 in 6 Americans) get sick, 128,000 are hospitalized, and 3,000 die each year due to foodborne illnesses.[2] The aim of FSMA is to eliminate this public health burden with the implementation of a five-step process—prevention, inspection and compliance, response, imports, and enhanced partnerships—within 18 months to 2 years of enactment.

The prevention process mandates that a preventive plan to pinpoint hazards that could affect food safety be developed by every U.S. food facility. The plan must include monitoring strategies, documentation requirements, and specific action plans in case of a hazard. The prevention plan also establishes minimum standards for safe production of produce, and it regulates against intentional contamination of food.[3]

The inspection and compliance component of the FMSA tasks the FDA with overseeing mandated inspections of increasing frequency of both domestic and foreign facilities and accessing facility records. For example, all high-risk domestic facilities must be inspected within 5 years of the FMSA's enactment and no less than every 3 years thereafter.[3] Food testing will be carried out by accredited laboratories.

The FMSA provides the FDA with new tools for the response process. These new tools include mandatory recalls, flexible standards for detaining products that are in violation of standards, facility registration suspensions, enhanced tracking abilities for domestic and imported foods, and additional record-keeping requirements for high-risk foods.[1] A designated fee or suspension by the FDA may be applied to companies that require a recall.[4]

The import process grants the FDA jurisdiction to better confirm that imported products meet U.S. standards. The new import rules include improved importer accountability, third-party certification that the foreign food facilities comply with U.S. standards, certification for high-risk foods, and the right to refuse entry of foreign products that do not comply with FSMA standards.

Lastly, the enhanced partnership process builds a collaborative regulation system with other foreign and domestic agencies, which enforces the legislation and recognizes that all food safety agencies need to work together in an integrated way to achieve the highest standards of food safety.[1]

According to the FDA, this legislation is a necessity in the fight against foodborne illness. The risks of foodborne illnesses have intensified in recent years due to globalization—15 percent of the U.S. food supply is imported. This legislation also is needed because our food supply is more high tech and complex, there are more food marketplaces now, and new food hazard issues are being uncovered. In addition, the growing global population increases the number of foodborne illness cases.[5]

Many groundbreaking advances have occurred since the passage of the FMSA. In April 2011, the FDA issued updated guidelines to the seafood industry, created a more consumer-friendly recall search engine on the FDA website, and submitted its first annual report on food facilities, food imports, and FDA foreign offices to Congress. In July 2011, the FDA, the USDA, and the National Institute of Food and Agriculture entered into an agreement to collaborate on a grant program for food safety training; the FDA issued an antismuggling strategy in coordination with the Department of Homeland Security; and draft dietary guidelines for the dietary supplement industry were submitted to Congress. In August 2011, the FDA implemented a fee schedule for facilities that fail to comply with recall orders. In September 2011, the FDA created an emergency response system for food testing labs in the event of a biological, chemical, or radiological contamination event.[1]

References

1 U.S. Food and Drug Administration. Background on FDA Food Safety Modernization Act (FSMA). Available at: http://www.fda.gov/Food/FoodSafety/FSMA/ucm239907.htm. Accessed December 7, 2011.

2 Food Safety Modernization Act: Putting the Focus on Prevention. Available at: http://www.foodsafety.gov/news/fsma.html. Accessed December 7, 2011.

3 Food Safety Act: 18 Changes to Food Safety the Law Will Bring. *Huffington Post.* Available at: http://www.huffingtonpost.com/2010/12/23/food-safety-bill_n_800236.html#s213429&title=Fees_For_Reinspection. Accessed December 7, 2011.

4 Compromise Bill Grants FDA 50 Million Boost to Implement FSMA. Food Navigator-U.S.A. Available at: http://www.foodnavigator-usa.com/Regulation/Compromise-bill-grants-FDA-50m-boost-to-implement-FSMA. Accessed December 7, 2011.

Exemptions

Under the NLEA, the following foods are exempt from food-labeling laws:

- Food served for immediate consumption (e.g., served in hospital cafeterias and airplanes)
- Food sold by food service vendors (e.g., mall cookie counters, sidewalk vendors, vending machines)
- Ready-to-eat food that is not for immediate consumption but is prepared primarily on site (e.g., bakery, deli)
- Food shipped in bulk, as long as it is not for sale in that form to consumer
- Medical foods, such as those used to address the nutritional needs of patients with certain diseases
- Plain coffee and tea and some spices
- Foods lacking in significant amounts of nutrients

A voluntary point-of-purchase nutrition information program (21 CFR 101.42 through 101.45) is available for stores that sell raw fruit, vegetables, and fish. The FDA has created downloadable posters that stores can print and display that show the 20 most frequently consumed items in these categories.

Health Claims

As mandated by the NLEA of 1990, the FDA issued food labeling rules for health claims. These rules were updated in 2008. Manufacturers of conventional foods and dietary supplements can make four types of claims with regards to their products.[137]

Nutrient Content Claims

A **nutrient content claim** is are fairly straightforward, for example, a package label that claims, "Contains 100 calories." Food manufacturers also can state that a particular food is a "good source" of a nutrient when it contains 10–19% of the RDI or that a food is a "high" source of a nutrient when it contains at least 20% of the RDI.

Disclosure statements also are required to call the consumer's attention to one or more nutrients in a food that may increase the risk of a disease or health-related condition that is diet related. A disclosure statement is required when a nutrient in a food exceeds certain levels. For example, if a low-fat food is high in sodium, this must be noted on the label.

nutrient content claim Statement that a food company can place on a product label that reflects the product's nutrient content. For example, a package label may state that the product "Contains 100 calories." Companies also can state that a particular food is a "good source" of a nutrient or that a food is a "high" source of a nutrient.

health claim Claim on a food label that states there is a relationship between a substance or nutrient in the food product and a disease or health-related condition. Such claims must be reviewed and approved by the FDA.

Health Claims

Food manufacturers can place a **health claim** on foods and dietary supplements once they have been reviewed and authorized by FDA. Food manufacturers must meet stringent requirements before a claim can be placed on a label. In addition, any food product with a health claim must meet a number of specific criteria.[138] The FDA has provided industry guidance on the evidence-based review system that it uses to evaluate the publicly available scientific evidence for significant scientific agreement (SSA) health claims or qualified health claims on the relationship between a substance and a disease or health-related condition.[138] **Table 2.13** describes the health claims allowed on food labels.[139]

Qualified Health Claims

The FDA has determined that consumers benefit from having more information about diet and health on food labels.[140] Thus, the FDA has established interim procedures whereby *qualified health claims* (QHCs) can be made for conventional foods and dietary supplements. The courts have ruled that the

TABLE 2.13
Health Claims Allowed on Food Labels

Health Claims Subject to Enforcement Discretion	Qualified Health Claims Subject to Enforcement Discretion
• Calcium and osteoporosis and calcium, vitamin D, and osteoporosis • Dietary lipids and cancer • Saturated fat, trans fat, and cholesterol and the risk of coronary heart disease • Dietary noncariogenic carbohydrate sweeteners and dental caries • Fiber-containing grain products, fruits, and vegetables and cancer • Folic acid and neural tube defects • Fruits and vegetables and cancer • Fruits, vegetables, and grain products that contain fiber, particularly soluble fiber, and the risk of coronary heart disease • Sodium and hypertension • Soluble fiber from certain foods and risk of coronary heart disease • Soy protein and risk of coronary heart disease • Stanols/sterols and risk of coronary heart disease	Qualified claims about cancer risk: • Tomatoes and/or tomato sauce and prostate, ovarian, gastric, and pancreatic cancers • Calcium and colon/rectal cancer and calcium and recurrent colon/rectal polyps • Green tea and cancer • Selenium and cancer • Antioxidant vitamins and cancer Qualified claims about cardiovascular disease risk: • Nuts and heart disease • Walnuts and heart disease • Omega-3 fatty acids and coronary heart disease • B vitamins and vascular disease • Monounsaturated fatty acids from olive oil and coronary heart disease • Unsaturated fatty acids from canola oil and coronary heart disease • Corn oil and heart disease Qualified claims about cognitive function: • Phosphatidylserine and cognitive dysfunction and dementia Qualified claims about diabetes: • Chromium picolinate and diabetes Qualified claims about hypertension: • Calcium and hypertension, pregnancy-induced hypertension, and preeclampsia Qualified claims about neural tube defects: • 0.8 mg folic acid and neural tube birth defects

Sources: Data from Food and Drug Administration. Health Claims Meeting Significant Scientific Agreement (SSA). Available at: http://www.fda.gov/Food/LabelingNutrition/LabelClaims/HealthClaimsMeetingSignificantScientificAgreementSSA/default.htm. Accessed June 20, 2012; and Food and Drug Administration. Summary of Qualified Health Claims Subject to Enforcement Discretion. Available at: http://www.fda.gov/Food/LabelingNutrition/LabelClaims/QualifiedHealthClaims/ucm073992.htm. Accessed June 20, 2012.

FDA must allow for health claims based on less scientific evidence, rather than just on the standard of SSA, as long as the claims do not mislead the consumers. The FDA began considering QHCs under its interim procedures on September 1, 2003. Refer to Table 2.13 for a list of permitted QHCs.[141]

Structure/Function Claims

A **structure/function claim** differs from health claims in that it describes the role of a substance intended to maintain a structure in or function of the human body. Structure/function claims do not require preapproval by the FDA. Products with structure/function claims must include the following disclaimer: "This statement has not been evaluated by the Food and Drug Administration. This product is not intended to diagnose, treat, cure, or prevent any disease." Examples of structure/function claims are: "Calcium builds strong bones" and "Antioxidants maintain cell integrity."

structure/function claim Claim on a food package that describes the role of a substance in the food in maintaining a structure in or function of the human body. Such claims do not require preapproval by the FDA.

Allergens

Food label requirements continue to change to meet current scientific research and public demand. For example, the Food Allergen Labeling and Consumer

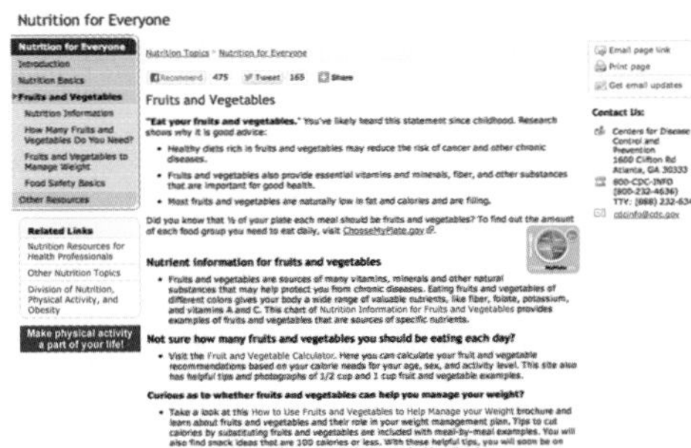

FIGURE 2.5 The Fruits & Veggies More Matters program is an excellent example of how government agencies and private groups can use evidence-based science to promote public health goals.

Source: Reproduced from Centers for Disease Control and Prevention. Nutrition for Everyone: Fruits and Vegetables. Available at: http://www.fruitsandveggiesmatter.gov. Accessed August 17, 2012.

Protection Act of 2004 (Public Law 108-282, Title II) mandated that as of January 1, 2006, foods containing or potentially containing any of the eight most common food allergens include the food name on the label in plain English; for example, "This product contains eggs." These eight foods—milk, eggs, fish, crustacean shellfish, tree nuts, peanuts, wheat, and soybeans—account for 90% of allergic reactions to food in children and adults. The FDA also provides guidance for industry from a standpoint of allergens and potential allergens in the food.

Bringing Nutrition Recommendations to the Public

A number of programs based on scientific data have been designed to improve the health of Americans. The CDC's Fruits & Veggies More Matters (see **Figure 2.5**) serves as a model program.[91] The CDC works with a number of partners with this program, including the National Cancer Institute, the CNPP, the American Cancer Society, the FDA, and the National Council of Fruit and Vegetable Nutrition Coordinators.[142] These high-profile partnerships reinforce the importance of this health message.

Like MyPlate, the Fruits & Veggies More Matters program is targeted at both health professionals and consumers. For health professionals, the program's website provides surveillance data on fruit and vegetable intake, research-to-practice information, the research behind the program, and state indicator reports.

Surveillance data are from the Behavioral Risk Factor Surveillance System, the world's largest, ongoing telephone health survey system, which has tracked health conditions and risk behaviors in the United States annually since 1984.[143] Data also are collected from the Youth Risk Behavior Surveillance System, which monitors priority health-risk behaviors and the prevalence of obesity and asthma among youth and young adults.[144] These surveillance systems clearly show that individuals are not consuming the recommended amounts of fruit and vegetables daily. For example, in 2009, the last year for which compiled survey data are available, only 22.3% of students had eaten fruits and vegetables five or more times per day during the 7 days before the survey.[145] This finding has been supported repeatedly in the literature, demonstrating the need to increase consumption across all age and ethnic groups. An array of resources, including presentation materials and consumer brochures, are available on this site that health professionals can use to help individuals make better food choices.

The program is backed by scientific research. For example, the relationship between increased consumption of fruits and vegetables and the reduced the risk of some types of cancer is one of the best established tenets of nutritional epidemiology.[73–75,146–159] Note, however, that studies supporting this finding are not consistent for all types of cancer.[147,160,161] Some studies have shown that consuming fruit, but not vegetables, reduces the risk of some types of cancer, whereas others have shown that the effect is linked with vegetable intake only.[149,150] Other studies have shown no association or only a weak one.

Intake of fruits and vegetables also has been reported to reduce the risk of other diseases, notably hypertension.[162] The importance of including fruit and vegetables in the diet is underscored by their prominent recommendations in *Healthy People 2020*, the *Dietary Guidelines for Americans, 2010*, and MyPlate. Every major health organization recommends a diet rich in fruits and vegetables for the prevention of chronic disease. Therapeutic diet regimens, including the DASH Diet and the NCEP's Adult Treatment Plan III diet, also recommend diets rich in fruit and vegetables.[61,68,69,163]

Is Fruits & Veggies More Matters effective in helping Americans to increase their intake of fruits and vegetables? At this time it is unclear whether the program has been effective. The program is relatively new and is an extension of the 5 a Day marketing campaign. Some studies showed that the 5 a Day program was successful, whereas others did not.[164–168] Some studies suggest that it is important to consider characteristics of the specific target population, including barriers to consumption and stages of change, to deliver positive messages.[169–171] Despite the success of some intervention studies, a recent report suggests that there has been no change in consumption of fruit and vegetables in U.S. adults from 1994 to 2005.[172] This clearly indicates that more work needs to be done to encourage individuals to consume fruits and vegetables and to provide them with the resources to do so.

People often complain that nutrition recommendations are conflicting and confusing. However, overall, they are actually remarkably similar across agencies, as detailed in **Table 2.14**. They are similar because this is what the science behind the programs dictates. The challenge for all nutrition professionals is to critically evaluate the scientific evidence before it is translated into public health practice. Nutrition professionals need to use this information to design, execute, and evaluate programs and policies and bring positive recommendations to the public in a unified way to ensure that consumers are getting the best possible information available that will enable them to

TABLE 2.14
Weight, Diet, and Physical Activity Recommendations for Health Promotion and Disease Prevention**

Factor	***Dietary Guidelines for Americans, 2010*** **and MyPlate**	**ATP III**	**DASH† for Hypertension**	**AHA**	**NCI**
Weight	Maintain in a healthy range; lose weight if needed	Maintain desirable weight/lose weight if needed	Maintain a healthy weight	Use up as many calories as you take in	Avoid obesity
Grains	6 ounce equivalents with half whole grains	≥ 6 servings	6–8 servings	6–8 servings with half as whole grains	
Fruit	2 cups	2–4 servings	2 to 2½ cups	4–5 servings	Women: 7 servings Men/teenage boys: 9 servings
Vegetables	2½ cups	3–5 servings	2 to 2½ cups	4–5 servings	
Dairy	3 cups low fat or fat free	2–3 servings low fat or fat free	2 to 3 cups low-fat or fat free	2–3 servings low-fat or fat free	
Meat/alternates	5½ ounce equivalents lean, low-fat, or fat free	< 5 ounces	≤ 6 ounces	< 6 ounces low fat; eat fish at least twice a week	
Fat (total)	20–35% energy	25–35% energy	DASH had 27% of energy from fat; no other recommendations		
Saturated fat	< 10% energy	< 7% energy			
Trans fat		≤ 20% of energy			
Monounsaturated fat		≤ 10% of energy		< 7% of energy < 1% of energy	

(continues)

TABLE 2.14
Weight, Diet, and Physical Activity Recommendations for Health Promotion and Disease Prevention (*continued*)**

Factor	*Dietary Guidelines for Americans, 2010* and MyPlate	ATP III	DASH† for Hypertension	AHA	NCI
Nuts, seeds, legumes	Legumes: 3 cups/ week	Encouraged but no specific recommendation	4–5 servings/week	4–5 servings/week	
Cholesterol	< 300 mg	< 200 mg	150 mg	< 300 mg	
Sodium	< 2,300 mg**	< 2,400 mg	< 2,300 mg, then lower to 1,500 mg	< 2,300 mg	Minimize salt-cured, salt-pickled, or smoked foods
Fiber	14 g/1,000 kcals	20–30 g	30 g	25 g	20–30 g with upper limit of 35 g
Added sugar	No recommendation	No recommendation	~2 teaspoons	Women: 100 kcals Men: 150 kcals	
Alcohol	Men: ≤ 2 drinks per day, if at all Women: ≤ 1 drinks per day, if at all	Men: ≤ 2 drinks per day, if at all Women: ≤ 1 drinks per day, if at all	Men: ≤ 2 drinks per day, if at all Women: ≤ 1 drinks per day, if at all	Men: ≤ 2 drinks per day, if at all Women: ≤ 1 drinks per day, if at all	Men ≤ 2 drinks per day, if at all Women ≤ 1 drinks per day, if at all
Physical activity	30 minutes most days of the week	Follow Surgeon General's recommendations	30 minutes of brisk exercise on most days for persons with hypertension	30 to 60 minutes on most days of the week at 50–80% capacity	Moderate intensity at least 30 minutes a day for most days

Abbreviations: ATP III = Third Report of the Expert Panel on Detection, Evaluation, and Treatment of High Blood Cholesterol in Adults; DASH = Dietary Approaches to Stop Hypertension; AHA = American Heart Association; NCI = National Cancer Institute.

* The *Dietary Guidelines for Americans* and American Heart Association amounts presented are for a 2,000 kcal reference diet. Unless otherwise stated, recommendations are per day. The Centers for Disease Control and Prevention recommends that individuals follow either MyPlate or the DASH diet.

† The Seventh Report of the Joint National Committee on the Prevention, Detection, Evaluation, and Treatment of High Blood Pressure recommends that people follow a DASH diet plan to help reduce blood pressure

** Individuals with hypertension, blacks, and older Americans should limit intake to 1,500 mg/day.

Source: Data from U.S. Department of Agriculture and U.S. Department of Health and Human Services. *Dietary Guidelines for Americans, 2010.* 7th ed. Washington, DC: U.S. Government Printing Office; 2010. Available at: http://health.gov/dietaryguidelines/dga2010/DietaryGuidelines2010.pdf. Accessed June 5, 2012.

make positive lifestyle changes. **Figure 2.6** shows the interrelationship among research, legislation, policies and programs, and the people affected.

Chapter Review

There often are complaints that nutrition recommendations are conflicting and confusing—however, they are actually remarkably similar across governmental agencies. Why? Because this is what the science behind the programs dictates. The challenge for all nutritionist professionals is to evaluate critically the scientific evidence before it is translated into public health practice. Nutrition professionals need to use this information to design, execute, and evaluate programs and policies and bring positive recommendations to the public in a unified way to assure that consumers are getting the best possible information available that allows them to make positive life style changes. This chapter reviewed the science behind public health policies, programs, nutrition education materials, and legislation.

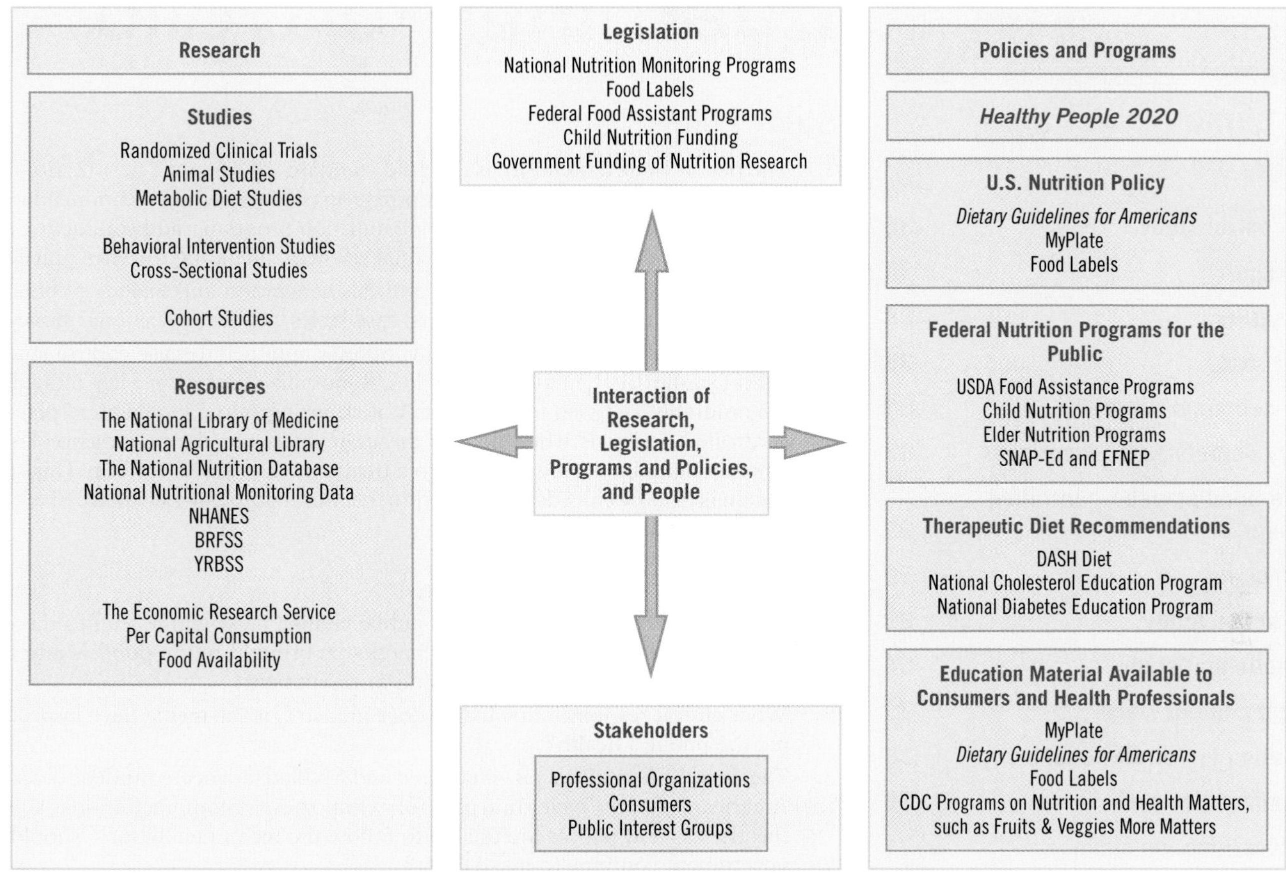

FIGURE 2.6 The relationships among nutrition research, legislation, stakeholders, and nutrition programs and policies.

Abbreviations: NHANES, National Health and Examination Survey; BRFSS, Behavioral Risk Factor Surveillance System; YRBSS, Youth Risk Behavior Surveillance System; HEI, Healthy Eating Index; CNPP, Center for Nutrition Policy and Promotion; SNAP, Supplemental Nutrition Assistance Program; EFNEP, Expanded Food and Nutrition Education Program; DASH, Dietary Approaches to Stop Hypertension; CDC, Centers for Disease Control and Prevention.

Source: Data from U.S. Department of Health & Human Services, Secretary's Advisory Committee on National Health Promotion & Disease Prevention Objectives for 2020. Available at: http://www.healthypeople.gov/hp2020/advisory.

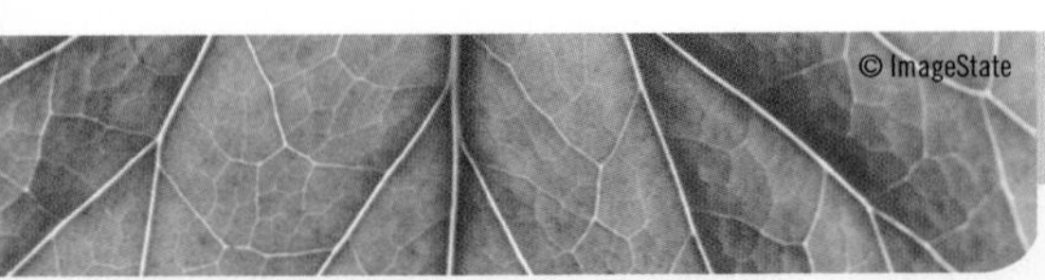

Learning Portfolio

Key Terms

	page
case control study	39
case report	38
case series	38
cohort study	39
cross-sectional survey	38
Dietary Guidelines for Americans	63
double-blind placebo-controlled design	39
health claim	70
intervention study	39
metabolic diet study	54
nutrient content claim	70
population or correlational study	38
randomized design	39
structure/function claim	71

Study Points

1. The peer-reviewed literature is the gold standard for scientific information provided to the public, as well as the information used for setting recommendations and policies, designing and evaluating nutrition programs, and conducting ethical evidence-based food and nutritional sciences, including dietetics practice.
2. Descriptive studies are used for hypothesis generation and include population or correlational studies, case reports, case series, and cross-sectional surveys.
3. Analytical studies are used to test hypotheses and include case control studies, cohort studies, and intervention studies. Randomized design is when individuals are randomly assigned to a treatment or control group. Double-blind placebo-controlled design is when neither the individuals nor the investigator knows whether participants are assigned to a treatment or a placebo group. This study design is usually considered to provide the most compelling evidence of a cause and effect relationship.

Issues for Discussion

1. Dietary recommendations for the public change as scientific studies discover new information. How can these changes be brought to the public's attention in a way that doesn't cause confusion or resentment?
2. What ethical responsibility, if any, does industry or the media have in promoting the public's health?
3. The *Dietary Guidelines for Americans* and MyPlate advocate prudent diets, but Americans clearly have difficulty following these recommendations. Why is this the case? If people are unable to follow the recommendations, should the government continue to make them?

Research Areas for Students

1. Major nutrition research studies and the dietary changes that were recommended
2. Major food studies and the composition of the foods recommended for consumption

References

1. Akobeng AK. Understanding randomized controlled trials. *Arch Dis Child.* 2005;90:840–844.
2. Cooper MJ, Zlotkin SH. An evidence-based approach to the development of national dietary guidelines. *J Am Diet Assoc.* 2003;103(Suppl 2):S28–S33.
3. Verbeek J, Ruotsalainen J, Hoving JL. Synthesizing study results in a systematic review. *Scand J Work Environ Health*. 2011;37(1):6–29.
4. Kroke A, Boeing H, Rossnagel K, Willich SN. History of the concept of 'levels of evidence' and their current status in relation to primary prevention through lifestyle interventions. *Public Health Nutr.* 2004;7:279–284.
5. Myers EF. ADA Evidence Analysis Library. *J Am Diet Assoc.* 2005;105(5 Suppl 1):S79.
6. West S, King V, Carey TS, et al. *Systems to Rate the Strength of Scientific Evidence.* Evidence Report/Technology Assessment No. 47 (Prepared by the Research Triangle Institute-University of North Carolina Evidence-based Practice Center under Contract No. 290-97-0011). AHRQ Publication No. 02-E016. Rockville, MD: Agency for Healthcare Research and Quality; April 2002.
7. The Cochrane Collaboration. *Cochrane Reviews*. Available at: http://www.cochrane.org/cochrane-reviews. Accessed October 6, 2012.
8. U.S. Department of Agriculture. Nutrition Evidence Library. Available at: http://www.cnpp.usda.gov/NEL.htm. Accessed October 29, 2011.
9. U.S. Department of Agriculture, U.S. Department of Health and Human Services. *Dietary Guidelines for Americans, 2010.* 7th ed. Washington, DC: U.S. Government

Printing Office; 2010. Available at: http://www.cnpp.usda.gov/DietaryGuidelines.htm. Accessed October 29, 2011.

10. Texas Department of Aging and Disability Services. DETERMINE Your Nutritional Health Screening Initiative. Available at: http://www.dads.state.tx.us/providers/AAA/Forms/standardized/NRA.pdf. Accessed October 29, 2011.
11. Isenring EA, Bauer JD, Banks M, Gaskill D. The Malnutrition Screening Tool is a useful tool for identifying malnutrition risk in residential aged care. *J Hum Nutr Diet.* 2009;22(6):545–550.
12. Bang H, Edwards AM, Bomback AS, et al. Development and validation of a patient self-assessment score for diabetes risk. *Ann Intern Med.* 2009;151(11):775–783.
13. U.S. Department of Agriculture, Economic Research Service. Food Security in the United States. Available at: http://www.ers.usda.gov/Briefing/FoodSecurity/surveytools.htm#household. Accessed October 29, 2011.
14. Jonnalagadda SS, Mitchell DC, Smiciklas-Wright H, et al. Accuracy of energy intake estimated by a multiple pass, 24-hour dietary recall technique. *J Amer Diet Assoc.* 2000;100:303–308.
15. Subar AF, Crafts J, Zimmerman TP, et al. Assessment of the accuracy of portion size reports using computer-based food photographs aids in the development of an automated self-administered 24-hour recall. *J Am Diet Assoc.* 2010;110:55–64.
16. Martin CK, Newton RL Jr, Anton SD, et al. Measurement of children's food intake with digital photography and the effects of second servings upon food intake. *Eat Behav.* 2007;8:148–156.
17. Martin CK, Han H, Coulon SM, et al. A novel method to remotely measure food intake of free-living individuals in real time: The remote food photography method. *Br J Nutr.* 2009;101:446–456.
18. Williamson DA, Allen HR, Martin PD, et al. Comparison of digital photography to weighed and visual estimation of portion sizes. *J Am Diet Assoc.* 2003;103:1139–1145.
19. Six BL, Schap TRE, Zhu FM, et al. Evidence-based development of a mobile telephone food record. *J Am Diet Assoc.* 2010;110:74–79.
20. Dodd KW, Guenther PM, Freedman LS, et al. Statistical methods for estimating usual intake of nutrients and foods: A review of the theory. *J Am Diet Assoc.* 2006;106:1640–1650.
21. Johnson RK, Driscoll P, Goran MI. Comparison of multiple-pass 24-hour recall estimates of energy intake with total energy expenditure determined by the doubly labeled water method in young children. *J Am Diet Assoc.* 1996;96:1140–1144.
22. Hennekens CH, Buring J. *Epidemiology in Medicine.* Baltimore, MD: Lippincott Williams & Wilkins; 1987.
23. Garn SM, Larkin FA, Cole PE. The real problem with 1-day diet records. *Am J Clin Nutr.* 1978;31:1114–1116.
24. Hegsted DM. Problems in the use and interpretation of the Recommended Dietary Allowances. *Ecol Food Nutr.* 1972;1:255–265.
25. Subar AF, Dodd KW, Guenther PM, et al. The food propensity questionnaire: concept, development, and validation for use as a covariate in a model to estimate usual food intake. *J Am Diet Assoc.* 2006;106(10):1556–1563.
26. Tooze JA, Midthune D, Dodd KW, et al. A new statistical method for estimating the usual intake of episodically consumed foods with application to their distribution. *J Am Diet Assoc.* 2006;106(10):1575–1587.
27. Dodd KW, Guenther PM, Freedman LS, et al. Statistical methods for estimating usual intake of nutrients and foods: A review of the theory. *J Am Diet Assoc.* 2006;106(10):1640–1650.
28. National Cancer Institute. Usual Dietary Intakes: The NCI method. Available at: http://riskfactor.cancer.gov/diet/usualintakes/method.html. Accessed October 29, 2011.
29. Bliss RM. Researchers produce innovation in dietary recall. *Agric Res.* 2004;52(6):10–12.
30. Raper N, Perloff B, Ingwersen L, et al. An overview of USDA's Dietary Intake Data System. *J Food Compos Anal.* 2004;17(3–4):545–555.
31. McBride J. Was it a slab, a slice, or a sliver? High-tech innovations take survey to new level. *Agric Res.* 2001;49(3):4–7.
32. Jain M, McLaughlin J. Validity of nutrient estimates by food frequency questionnaires based either on exact frequencies or categories. *Ann Epidemiol.* 2000;10:354–360.
33. Kuskowska-Wolk A, Holte S, Ohlander EM, et al. Effects of different designs and extension of a food frequency questionnaire on response rate, completeness of data and food frequency responses. *Int J Epidemiol.* 1992;21:1144–1150.
34. Kroke A, Klipstein-Grobusch K, Voss S, et al. Validation of a self-administered food-frequency questionnaire administered in the European Prospective Investigation into Cancer and Nutrition (EPIC) Study: Comparison of energy, protein, and macronutrient intakes estimated with the doubly labeled water, urinary nitrogen, and repeated 24-h dietary recall methods. *Am J Clin Nutr.* 1999;70:439–447.
35. Andersen LF, Tomten H, Haggarty P, et al. Validation of energy intake estimated from a food frequency questionnaire: A doubly labeled water study. *Eur J Clin Nutr.* 2003;57:279–284.
36. Day NE, Ferrari P. Some methodological issues in nutritional epidemiology. In: Riboli E, Lambert R (eds.). *Nutrition and Lifestyle: Opportunities for Cancer Prevention.* IARC Scientific Publication No. 156, 2002, pp. 5–10.
37. Willett WC. Dietary diaries versus food frequency questionnaires: A case of undigestible data. *Int J Epidemiol.* 2001;30:317–319.
38. Molag ML, de Vries JH, Ocké MC, et al. Design characteristics of food frequency questionnaires in relation to their validity. *Am J Epidemiol.* 2007;166:1468–1478.
39. World Health Organization. Report of the technical discussions at the twenty-first World Health Assembly on "national and global surveillance of communicable diseases." A2.1. 18-5-1968. Geneva, Switzerland.
40. U.S. Department of Agriculture. MyPlate Tracker. Available at: http://www.MyPlatetracker.gov. Accessed October 29, 2011.
41. U.S. Department of Agriculture. MyPlate Equivalents Database. Available at: http://www.ars.usda.gov/Services/docs.htm?docid=17558. Accessed October 29, 2011.
42. U.S. Department of Agriculture. National Nutrient Database for Standard Reference. Nutrient Database Laboratory. Available at: http://www.nal.usda.gov/fnic/foodcomp/search. Accessed October 29, 2011.

43. U.S. Department of Agriculture. Food And Nutrient Database for Dietary Studies. Available at: http://www.ars.usda.gov/Services/docs.htm?docid=12089. Accessed October 29, 2011.
44. Bingham SA. Biomarkers in nutritional epidemiology. *Public Health Nutr.* 2002;5:821–827.
45. Kaaks RJ. Biochemical markers as additional measurements in studies of the accuracy of dietary questionnaire measurements: Conceptual issues. *Am J Clin Nutr.* 1997;65(4 Suppl): 1232S–1239S.
46. U.S. Department of Agriculture. What We Eat in America. Available at: http://www.ars.usda.gov/Services/docs.htm?docid=15044. Accessed October 29, 2011.
47. Woteki CE. Integrated NHANES: uses in national policy. *J Nutr.* 2003;133:582S–584S.
48. Arab L, Carriquiry A, Steck-Scott S, Gaudet MM. Ethnic differences in the nutrient intake adequacy of premenopausal US women: Results from the Third National Health Examination Survey. *J Am Diet Assoc.* 2003;103:1008–1014.
49. Ford ES, Ballew C. Dietary folate intake in US adults: Findings from the third National Health and Nutrition Examination Survey. *Ethn Dis.* 1998;8:299–305.
50. Looker AC, Loria CM, Carroll MD, et al. Calcium intakes of Mexican Americans, Cubans, Puerto Ricans, non-Hispanic whites, and non-Hispanic blacks in the United States. *J Am Diet Assoc.* 1993;93:1274–1279.
51. Sharma S, Malarcher AM, Giles WH, Myers G. Racial, ethnic and socioeconomic disparities in the clustering of cardiovascular disease risk factors. *Ethn Dis.* 2004;14:43–48.
52. Hicks LS, Fairchild DG, Cook EF, Ayanian JZ. Association of region of residence and immigrant status with hypertension, renal failure, cardiovascular disease, and stroke, among African-American participants in the third National Health and Nutrition Examination Survey (NHANES III). *Ethn Dis.* 2003;13:316–323.
53. Berenson GS (ed.). *Causation of Cardiovascular Risk Factors in Childhood: Perspectives on Cardiovascular Risk in Early Life.* New York: Raven Press; 1986.
54. Berenson GS, McMahan CA, Voors AW, et al. *Cardiovascular Risk Factors in Children: The Early Natural History of Atherosclerosis and Essential Hypertension.* New York: Oxford University Press; 1980.
55. Berenson GS, Wattigney WA, Bao W, et al. Rationale to study the early natural history of heart disease: The Bogalusa Heart Study. *Am J Med Sci.* 1995;310(suppl 1):S22–S28.
56. Nicklas TA, Demory-Luce D, Yang SJ, et al. Children's food consumption patterns have changed over two decades (1973–1994): The Bogalusa heart study. *J Am Diet Assoc.* 2004;104:1127–1140.
57. Nicklas TA, Hayes D. Position of the American Dietetic Association: Nutrition guidance for healthy children ages 2 to 11 years. *J Am Diet Assoc.* 2008;108(6):1038–1044, 1046–1047.
58. Berenson GS, Wattigney WA, Tracy RE, et al. Atherosclerosis of the aorta and coronary arteries and cardiovascular risk factors in persons aged 6 to 30 years and studied at necropsy (The Bogalusa Heart Study). *Am J Cardiol.* 1992;70:851–858.
59. Strong JP, McGill HC Jr. The natural history of coronary atherosclerosis. *Am J Pathol.* 1962;40:37–49.
60. Metha NV, Khan AI. Cardiology's 10 greatest discoveries of the 20th century. *Tex Heart Inst J.* 2002;29:164–171.
61. National Institutes of Health; National Heart, Lung, and Blood Institute. Third Report of the Expert Panel on Detection, Evaluation, and Treatment of High Blood Cholesterol in Adults (Adult Treatment Panel III). Final Report, 2002. Available at: http://www.nhlbi.nih.gov/guidelines/cholesterol/atp3full.pdf. Accessed October 29, 2011.
62. The Seventh Report of the Joint National Committee on Prevention, Detection, Evaluation, and Treatment of High Blood Pressure (JNC 7). Available at: http://www.nhlbi.nih.gov/guidelines/hypertension. Accessed October 29, 2011.
63. Framingham Heart Study. Offspring Cohort. Available at: http://www.framinghamheartstudy.org/participants/offspring.html. Accessed October 29, 2011.
64. Farris RP, Nicklas TA. Characterizing children's eating behavior. In: Suskind RM, Suskind LL (eds.). *Textbook of Pediatric Nutrition.* New York: Raven Press; 1993, pp. 505–516.
65. Nicklas TA, Forcier JE, Webber LS, Berenson GS. School lunch assessment as part of a 24-hour dietary recall for children. *J Am Diet Assoc.* 1991;91:711–713.
66. Frank GC, Hollatz AT, Webber LS, Berenson GS. Effect of interviewer recording practices on nutrient intake: Bogalusa Heart Study. *J Am Diet Assoc.* 1984;84:1432–1436.
67. Most MM, Ershow AG, Clevidence BA. An overview of methodologies, proficiencies, and training resources for controlled feeding studies. *J Am Diet Assoc.* 2003;103:729–735.
68. Appel LJ, Moore TJ, Obarzanek E, et al. A clinical trial of the effects of dietary patterns on blood pressure. DASH Collaborative Research Group. *N Engl J Med.* 1997;336:1117–1124.
69. Sacks FM, Svetkey LP, Vollmer WM, et al. Effects on blood pressure of reduced dietary sodium and the Dietary Approaches to Stop Hypertension (DASH) diet. DASH-Sodium Collaborative Research Group. *N Engl J Med.* 2001;344:3–10.
70. Funk KL, Elmer PJ, Stevens VJ, et al. PREMIER: A trial of lifestyle interventions for blood pressure control: intervention design and rationale. *Health Promot Pract.* 2008;9(3):271–280.
71. Albanes D, Heinonen OP, Taylor PR, et al. Alpha-tocopherol and beta-carotene supplements and lung cancer incidence in the alpha-tocopherol, beta-carotene cancer prevention study: Effects of base-line characteristics and study compliance. *J Natl Cancer Inst.* 1996;88:1560–1570.
72. Omenn GS, Goodman G, Thornquist M, et al. The beta-carotene and retinol efficacy trial (CARET) for chemoprevention of lung cancer in high risk populations: Smokers and asbestos-exposed workers. *Cancer Res.* 1994;54(7 suppl):2038S—2043S.
73. Block G, Patterson B, Subar A. Fruit, vegetables, and cancer prevention: A review of the epidemiological evidence. *Nutr Cancer.* 1992;18:1–29.
74. Steinmetz KA, Potter JD. Vegetables, fruit, and cancer. Epidemiology. *Cancer Causes Control.* 1991;2:325–57.
75. Le Marchand L, Hankin JH, Kolonel LN, et al. Intake of specific carotenoids and lung cancer risk. *Cancer Epidemiol Biomarkers Prev.* 1993;2:183–87.
76. Steinmetz KA, Potter JD, Folsom AR. Vegetables, fruit, and lung cancer in the Iowa Women's Health Study. *Cancer Res.* 1993;53:536–543.
77. Smigel K. Beta carotene fails to prevent cancer in two major studies: CARET intervention stopped. *J Natl Cancer Inst.* 1996;88:145.

78. Pryor WA, Stahl W, Rock CL. Beta carotene: From biochemistry to clinical trials. *Nutr Rev*. 2000;58(2 Pt 1):39–53.
79. Roy HJ, Keenan MJ, Zablah-Pimentel E, et al. Adult female rats defend "appropriate" energy intake after adaptation to dietary energy. *Obes Res*. 2003;11:1214–1222.
80. Wolf G. The effect of low and high doses of beta-carotene and exposure to cigarette smoke on the lungs of ferrets. *Nutr Rev*. 2002;60:88–90.
81. Russell RM. The enigma of beta-carotene in carcinogenesis: What can be learned from animal studies. *J Nutr*. 2004;134:262S–268S.
82. U.S. Department of Health and Human Services. Office of Disease Prevention and Health Promotion. *Healthy People 2020*. Washington, DC: U.S. Government Printing Office; 2010. Available at: http://www.healthypeople.gov/2020/default.aspx. Accessed October 29, 2011.
83. U.S. Department of Agriculture. MyPlate. Available at: http://www.cnpp.usda.gov/MyPlate.htm. Accessed October 29, 2011.
84. Institute of Medicine, Food and Nutrition Board. Dietary Reference Intakes (DRIs): Estimated Average Requirements. Available at: http://www.iom.edu/Activities/Nutrition/SummaryDRIs/~/media/Files/Activity%20Files/Nutrition/DRIs/5_Summary%20Table%20Tables%201-4.pdf. Accessed October 29, 2011.
85. U.S. Department of Health and Human Services, U.S. Food and Drug Administration. Labeling and Nutrition. Available at: http://www.fda.gov/food/labelingnutrition/default.htm. Accessed October 29, 2011.
86. U.S. Department of Agriculture. Food Plans. Available at: http://www.cnpp.usda.gov/USDAFoodPlansCostofFood.htm. Accessed October 29, 2011.
87. U.S. Department of Agriculture. Supplemental Nutrition Assistance Program. Available at: http://www.fns.usda.gov/snap. Accessed October 29, 2011.
88. U.S. Department of Agriculture. Child Nutrition Programs. Available at: http://www.fns.usda.gov/cnd. Accessed October 29, 2011.
89. U.S. Department of Agriculture. Women, Infants, and Children. Available at: http://www.fns.usda.gov/wic. Accessed October 29, 2011.
90. National Institutes of Health. National Heart, Lung, and Blood Institute. National High Blood Pressure Education Program. Available at: http://www.nhlbi.nih.gov/about/nhbpep/nhbp_pd.htm. Accessed October 29, 2011.
91. Centers for Disease Control and Prevention. Fruits & Veggies Matter More. Available at: http://www.fruitsandveggiesmatter.gov. Accessed October 29, 2011.
92. U.S. Department of Health and Human Services. *Healthy People: The Surgeon General's Report on Health Promotion and Disease Prevention*. Washington, DC: Government Printing Office; 1979.
93. Perspectives in disease prevention and health promotion implementing the 1990 prevention objectives: Summary of CDC's seminar. *MMWR*. 1983;32:21–24.
94. Healthy People 2020. Foundation Health Measures. Available at: http://healthypeople.gov/2020/about/tracking.aspx. Accessed October 29, 2011.
95. U.S. Preventive Services Task Force (USPSTF) Clinical Preventive Services. Available at: http://www.uspreventiveservicestaskforce.org/index.html. Accessed October 29, 2011.
96. Guide to Community Preventive Services. Available at: http://www.thecommunityguide.org/index.html. Accessed October 29, 2011.
97. Quick Guide to Healthy Living Information for Consumers. Available at: http://healthfinder.gov/prevention. Accessed October 29, 2011.
98. Centers for Disease Control and Prevention. CDC Wonder. DATA 2010. Available at: http://wonder.cdc.gov/data2010. Accessed October 29, 2011.
99. National Institutes of Health. National Heart, Lung, and Blood Institute's HP 2010 Cardiovascular Gateway. Available at: http://hp2010.nhlbihin.net/cvd_frameset.htm. Accessed October 29, 2011.
100. Healthy People 2010 Archive File. Available at: http://www.healthypeople.gov/2010. Accessed October 29, 2011.
101. Healthy People 2010 Final Review. Available at: http://www.cdc.gov/nchs/healthy_people/hp2010/hp2010_final_review.htm. Accessed October 29, 2011.
102. U.S. Department of Agriculture, Food and Nutrition Board. *Recommended Dietary Allowances*. 10th ed. Washington, DC: National Academies Press; 1989.
103. Food and Nutritional Information Center. National Agricultural Library. Dietary Reference Intakes. Available at: http://fnic.nal.usda.gov/nal_display/index.php?info_center=4&tax_level=3&tax_subject=256&topic_id=1342&level3_id=5141. Accessed October 29, 2011.
104. Institute of Medicine, Food and Nutrition Board. *Dietary Reference Intakes for Water, Potassium, Sodium, Chloride, and Sulfate*. Washington, DC: National Academies Press; 2005.
105. Institute of Medicine, Food and Nutrition Board. *Dietary Reference Intakes for Energy, Carbohydrate, Fiber, Fat, Fatty Acids, Cholesterol, Protein, and Amino Acids (Macronutrients)*. Washington, DC: National Academies Press; 2005.
106. Institute of Medicine, Food and Nutrition Board. *Dietary Reference Intakes: Proposed Definition and Plan for Review of Dietary Antioxidants and Related Compounds*. Washington, DC: National Academies Press; 1998.
107. Institute of Medicine, Food and Nutrition Board. *Dietary Reference Intakes for Thiamin, Riboflavin, Niacin, Vitamin B_6, Folate, Vitamin B_{12}, Pantothenic Acid, Biotin, and Choline*. Washington, DC: National Academies Press; 1998.
108. Institute of Medicine, Food and Nutrition Board. *Dietary Reference Intakes for Calcium, Phosphorus, Magnesium, Vitamin D, and Fluoride*. Washington, DC: National Academies Press; 1997.
109. Institute of Medicine, Food and Nutrition Board. *School Meals: Building Blocks for Healthy Children*. Washington, DC: National Academies Press; 2009.
110. Institute of Medicine, Food and Nutrition Board. Local Government Actions to Prevent Childhood Obesity. 2009. Available at: http://iom.edu/Reports/2009/Local-Government-Actions-to-Prevent-Childhood-Obesity.aspx. Accessed October 29, 2011.
111. Institute of Medicine, Food and Nutrition Board. *The Public Health Effects of Food Deserts*. Washington, DC: National Academies Press; 2009.
112. Institute of Medicine, Food and Nutrition Board. *Nutrition Standards and Meal Requirements for National School Lunch*

and Breakfast Programs: Phase I. Proposed Approach for Recommending Revisions. Washington, DC: National Academies Press; 2008.

113. Institute of Medicine, Food and Nutrition Board. *The Use of Dietary Supplements by Military Personnel.* Washington, DC: National Academies Press; 2008.
114. Yates AA. Process and development of dietary reference intakes: Basis, need, and application of recommended dietary allowances. *Nutr Rev*. 1998;56(4 Pt 2):S5–S9.
115. Murphy SP, Poos MI. Dietary Reference Intakes: Summary of applications in dietary assessment. *Public Health Nutr*. 2002;5:843–849.
116. Murphy SP, Barr SI, Poos MI. Using the new dietary reference intakes to assess diets: A map to the maze. *Nutr Rev*. 2002;60:267–275.
117. Barr SI, Murphy SP, Agurs-Collins TD, Poos MI. Planning diets for individuals using the dietary reference intakes. *Nutr Rev*. 2003;61:352–360.
118. U.S. Department of Agriculture. Center for Nutrition Policy and Promotion. Available at: http://www.cnpp.usda.gov. Accessed October 29, 2011.
119. Dwyer JT. Nutrition guidelines and education of the public. *J Nutr*. 2001;131(11 Suppl):3074S–3077S.
120. U.S. Department of Health and Human Services, Public Health Service. The Surgeon General's report on nutrition and health. DHHS (PHS) Publication No. 88-50215, 1988.
121. National Academy of Sciences, National Research Council, Food and Nutrition Board. *Diet and Health: Implications for Reducing Chronic Disease Risk*. Washington, DC: National Academies Press; 1989.
122. Welsh S, Davis C, Shaw A. A brief history of food guides in the United States. *Nutrition Today*. 1992;November/December:6–11.
123. Cronin FJ, Shaw AM, Krebs-Smith SM, et al. Developing a food guidance system to implement the dietary guidelines. *J Nutr Ed.* 1987;19:281–232.
124. Welsh S, Davis C, Shaw A. *USDA's Food Guide: Background and Development.* Washington, DC: U.S. Department of Agriculture, Human Nutrition Information Service; 1993. Misc. Publication 1514.
125. Davis CA, Britten P, Myers EF. Past, present, and future of the food guide pyramid. *J Am Diet Assoc*. 2001;101: 881–885.
126. Goldberg JP, Belury MA, Elam P, et al. The obesity crisis: Don't blame it on the pyramid. *J Am Diet Assoc.* 2004;104: 1141–1147.
127. Kennedy ET, Ohls J, Carlson S, Fleming K. The Healthy Eating Index: Design and applications. *J Am Diet Assoc*. 1995;95: 1103–1108.
128. Bowman SA, Lino M, Gerrior SA, Basiotis PP. *The Healthy Eating Index: 1994–96.* U.S. Department of Agriculture, Center for Nutrition Policy and Promotion. Washington, DC: CNPP-5; 1998.
129. Basiotis PP, Carlson A, Gerrior SA, et al. *The Healthy Eating Index: 1999–2000.* U.S. Department of Agriculture, Center for Nutrition Policy and Promotion. Washington, DC: CNPP-12; 2002.
130. Guenther PM, Krebs-Smith SM, Reedy J, et al. USDA Center for Nutrition Policy and Promotion Fact Sheet No. 1, 2008. Available at: http://www.cnpp.usda.gov/Publications/HEI/healthyeatingindex2005factsheet.pdf. Accessed October 29, 2011.
131. Guenther PM, Reedy J, Krebs-Smith SM, et al. Development and evaluation of the Healthy Eating Index—2005: Technical report. Center for Nutrition Policy and Promotion, U.S. Department of Agriculture; 2007. Available at: http://www.cnpp.usda.gov/Publications/HEI/HEI-2005/HEI-2005TechnicalReport.pdf. Accessed June 25, 2012.
132. Guenther PM, Reedy J, Krebs-Smith SM. Development of the Healthy Eating Index—2005. *J Am Diet Assoc*. 2008;108: 1896–1901.
133. Willett WC, McCullough ML. Dietary pattern analysis for the evaluation of dietary guidelines. *Asia Pac J Clin Nutr*. 2008;17(Suppl 1):75–78.
134. Pennington JA, Hubbard VS. Derivation of daily values used for nutrition labeling. *J Am Diet Assoc*. 1997;97(12):1407–1412.
135. Origin and framework of the development of dietary reference intakes. *Nutr Rev*. 1997;55(9):332–334.
136. U.S. Food and Drug Administration. Consumer Information on the Food Label. Available at: http://www.fda.gov/food/labelingnutrition/consumerinformation/ucm078889.htm. Accessed October 29, 2011.
137. U.S. Food and Drug Administration. Food Label Claims. Available at: http://www.fda.gov/Food/GuidanceComplianceRegulatoryInformation/GuidanceDocuments/FoodLabelingNutrition/FoodLabelingGuide/ucm064908.htm. Accessed October 29, 2011.
138. U.S. Food and Drug Administration. Guidance for Industry: Evidence-Based Review System for the Scientific Evaluation of Health Claims—Final. January 2009. Available at: http://www.fda.gov/Food/GuidanceComplianceRegulatoryInformation/GuidanceDocuments/FoodLabelingNutrition/ucm073332.htm. Accessed October 29, 2011.
139. U.S. Food and Drug Administration. List of Health Claims from the Federal Food and Drug Administration. Available at: http://www.fda.gov/Food/LabelingNutrition/LabelClaims/HealthClaimsMeetingSignificantScientificAgreementSSA/default.htm. Accessed October 29, 2011.
140. U.S. Food and Drug Administration. Consumer Health Information for Better Nutrition Initiative. Available at: http://www.fda.gov/Food/LabelingNutrition/LabelClaims/QualifiedHealthClaims/QualifiedHealthClaimsPetitions/ucm096010.htm. Accessed October 29, 2011.
141. U.S. Food and Drug Administration. List of Qualified Health Claims from the Federal Food and Drug Administration. Available at: http://www.fda.gov/Food/LabelingNutrition/LabelClaims/QualifiedHealthClaims/ucm073992.htm. Accessed October 29, 2011.
142. Association of State and Territorial Public Health Nutrition Directors. Fruit and Vegetable Nutrition Council. Available at: http://www.astphnd.org/chapter_contents.php3?sid=fbf4ae&chapter_id=5&member_id=. Accessed October 29, 2011.
143. Centers for Disease Control and Prevention. Behavioral Risk Factor Surveillance System. Available at: http://www.cdc.gov/brfss. Accessed October 29, 2011.

144. Centers for Disease Control and Prevention. YRBSS: Youth Risk Behavior Surveillance System. Available at: http://www.cdc.gov/healthyyouth/yrbs. Accessed October 29, 2011.

145. Centers for Disease Control and Prevention. 2009 National Youth Risk Behavior Survey Overview. Available at: http://www.cdc.gov/healthyyouth/yrbs/pdf/us_overview_yrbs.pdf. Accessed October 29, 2011.

146. Key TJ, Schatzkin A, Willett WC, et al. Diet, nutrition, and the prevention of cancer. *Public Health Nutr.* 2004;7:187–200.

147. Chainani-Wu N. Diet and oral, pharyngeal, and esophageal cancer. *Nutr Cancer*. 2002;44:104–126.

148. Steinmetz KA, Potter JD. Vegetables, fruit, and cancer prevention: A review. *J Am DietAssoc.* 1996;96:1027–1039.

149. Riboli E, Norat T. Epidemiologic evidence of the protective effect of fruit and vegetables on cancer risk. *Am J Clin Nutr*. 2003;78(3 Suppl):559S–569S.

150. Kampman E, Arts IC, Hollman PC. Plant foods versus compounds in carcinogenesis; Observational versus experimental human studies. *Int J Vitam Nutr Res.* 2003;73:70–78.

151. Temple NJ, Gladwin KK. Fruit, vegetables, and the prevention of cancer: Research challenges. *Nutrition.* 2003;19: 467–470.

152. Smith-Warner SA, Spiegelman D, Yaun SS, et al. Intake of fruits and vegetables and risk of breast cancer: A pooled analysis of cohort studies. *JAMA.* 2001;285:769–776.

153. Kim DJ, Holowaty EJ. Brief, validated survey instruments for the measurement of fruit and vegetable intakes in adults: A review. *Prev Med.* 2003;36:440–447.

154. Ziegler RG. Vegetables, fruits, and carotenoids and the risk of cancer. *Am J Clin Nutr.* 1991;53(1 Suppl):251S–259S.

155. Duthie GG, Gardner PT, Kyle JA. Plant polyphenols: Are they the new magic bullet. *ProcNutr Soc.* 2003;62:599–603.

156. La Vecchia C, Altieri A, Tavani A. Vegetables, fruit, antioxidants and cancer: A review of Italian studies. *Eur J Nutr*. 2001;40: 261–267.

157. Reddy L, Odhav B, Bhoola KD. Natural products for cancer prevention: A global perspective. *Pharmacol Ther.* 2003;99:1–13.

158. Van Duyn MA, Pivonka E. Overview of the health benefits of fruit and vegetable consumption for the dietetics professional: Selected literature. *J Am Diet Assoc.* 2000;100:1511–1521.

159. van't Veer P, Jansen MC, Klerk M, Kok FJ. Fruits and vegetables in the prevention of cancer and cardiovascular disease. *Public Health Nutr.* 2000;3:103–107.

160. Bazzano LA, Serdula MK, Liu S. Dietary intake of fruits and vegetables and risk of cardiovascular disease. *Curr Atheroscler Rep.* 2003;5:492–499.

161. Hu FB. Plant-based foods and prevention of cardiovascular disease: An overview. *Am J Clin Nutr.* 2003;78(3 Suppl): 544S–551S.

162. Dauchet L, Amouyel P, Dallongeville J. Fruits, vegetables and coronary heart disease. *Nat Rev Cardiol.* 2009;6(9): 599–608.

163. National Heart Lung and Blood Institute. Your Guide to Lowering Your Blood Pressure with DASH. Available at: http://www.nhlbi.nih.gov/health/public/heart/hbp/dash/new_dash.pdf. Accessed October 29, 2011.

164. Anderson JV, Bybee DI, Brown RM, et al. 5 a Day fruit and vegetable intervention improves consumption in a low income population. *J Am Diet Assoc.* 2001;101:195–222.

165. Havas S, Anliker J, Damron D, et al. Final results of the Maryland WIC 5-A-Day Promotion Program. *Am J Public Health.* 1998;88:1161–1167.

166. Sorensen G, Stoddard A, Peterson K, et al. Increasing fruit and vegetable consumption through worksites and families in the Treatwell 5-a-day study. *Am J Public Health.* 1999;89: 54–60.

167. Beresford SA, Thompson B, Feng Z, et al. Seattle 5 a Day worksite program to increase fruit and vegetable consumption. *Prev Med.* 200132:230–238.

168. Stables GJ, Subar AF, Patterson BH, et al. Changes in vegetable and fruit consumption and awareness among US adults: Results of the 1991 and 1997 5 A Day for Better Health Program surveys. *J Am Diet Assoc.* 2002;102:809–817.

169. Havas S, Treiman K, Langenberg P, et al. Factors associated with fruit and vegetable consumption among women participating in WIC. *J Am Diet Assoc.* 1998;98:1141-1148.

170. Langenberg P, Ballesteros M, Feldman R, et al. Psychosocial factors and intervention-associated changes in those factors as correlates of change in fruit and vegetable consumption in the Maryland WIC 5 A Day Promotion Program. *Ann Behav Med.* 2000;22:307–315.

171. Campbell MK, Reynolds KD, Havas S, et al. Stages of change for increasing fruit and vegetable consumption among adults and young adults participating in the national 5-a-Day for Better Health community studies. *Health Educ Behav*. 1999;26: 513–534.

172. Blanck HM, Gillespie C, Kimmons JE, et al. Trends in fruit and vegetable consumption among U.S. men and women, 1994–2005. *Prev Chronic Dis.* 2008;5(2):A35.

CHAPTER 3

Sensory Evaluation

Sung Eun Choi, PhD, RD

Chapter Objectives

THE STUDENT WILL BE EMPOWERED TO:

- Identify the sensory characteristics of food.
- Discuss the factors affecting the outcomes of sensory evaluation.
- Demonstrate an understanding of the process for sensory evaluation tests.
- Formulate an effective sensory evaluation strategy by selecting appropriate test design, panelists, and instruments.
- Discuss how to analyze and interpret the sensory data and recognize specific methodological advances related to sensory evaluation.

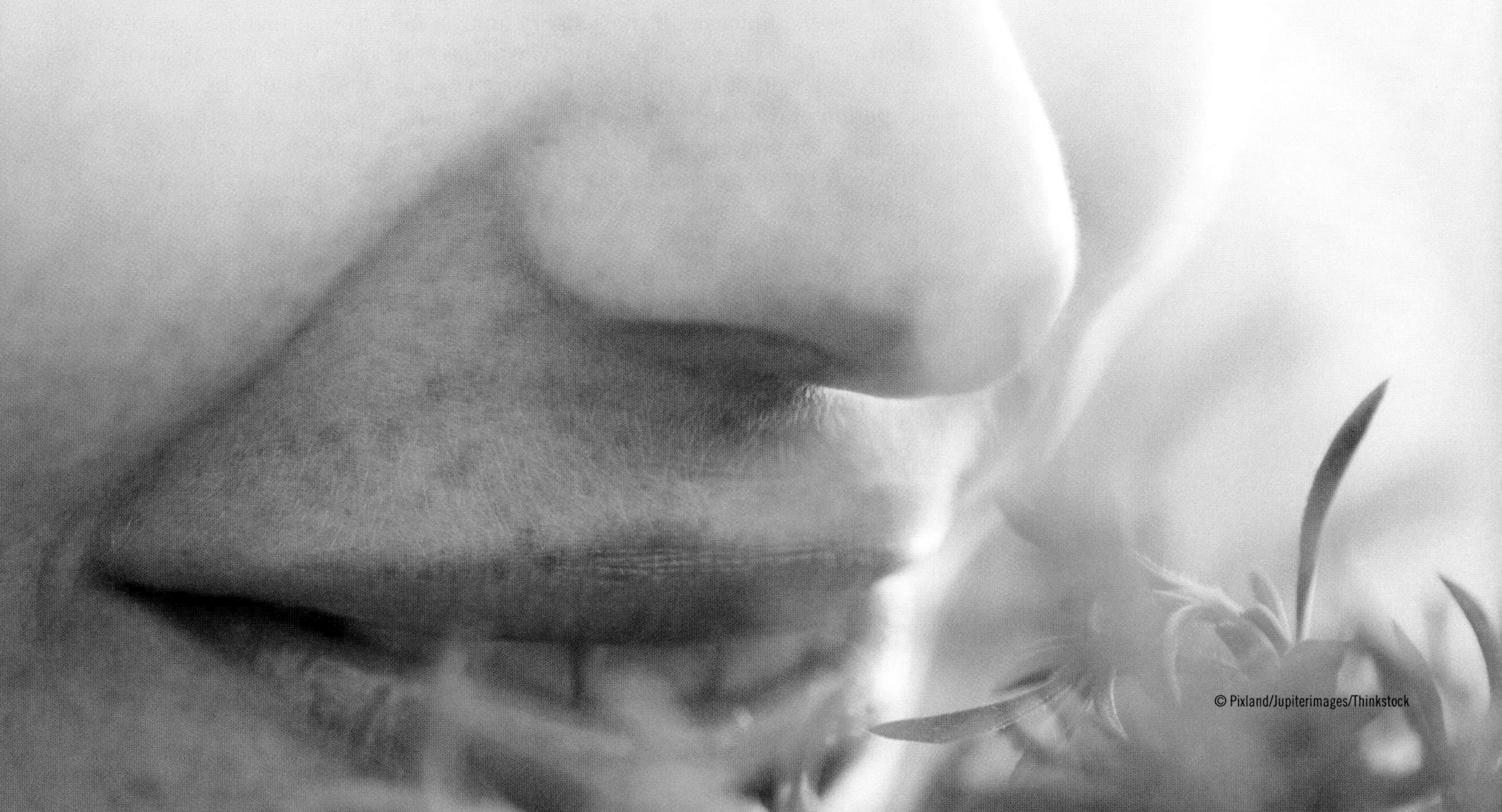

Introduction

Determining how food products affect consumers' senses is one of the most important goals of the food industry. It also is a primary concern for nutritionists and dietitians who develop healthier recipes. Because our five senses act as the gatekeeper of our bodies, the benefits of healthy food will be reaped only if our senses accept it. Therefore, consumer reaction, as perceived by the five senses, is considered a vital measure of food development. Because no apparatus can substitute for the senses in evaluating food, humans are used as test subjects. Such studies are becoming more prevalent, despite the potential biases of humans and the costs involved.

sensory evaluation The scientific measurement method of food quality based on sensory characteristics as perceived by the five senses.

Sensory evaluation is a scientific method that evokes, measures, analyzes, and interprets responses to products, as perceived through the senses of sight, smell, touch, taste, and sound.[1] This widely accepted definition is used by sensory evaluation committees within various professional organizations, including the Institute of Food Technologists and the American Society for Testing and Materials.[2] Like other scientific methods of taking measurements, sensory evaluation is concerned with precision, accuracy, and sensitivity and with avoiding false-positive results.[3] Reliable sensory evaluation is based on the skill of the sensory analyst in optimizing four factors: definition of the problem, test design, instrumentation, and interpretation of the results:[4,5]

- *Definition of the problem:* The item to be measured must be defined precisely.
- *Test design:* Not only must the design take into account unknown sources of bias, but it also must minimize the amount of testing required to produce the desired accuracy of the results.
- *Instrumentation:* The panelists must be selected and trained to give a reproducible result.
- *Interpretation of the results:* The analyst should select appropriate statistics based on the correct statistical assumptions and draw only those conclusions that are supported by the data.

The benefits of well-performed sensory evaluation can be realized in many ways; however, if the sensory analyst fails to optimize one of the four factors, much time and money is wasted. For effective sensory evaluation, the analyst should duly recognize the purpose of the study, select the appropriate experimental design, use panelists who fit the purpose, choose the proper method for preparing and presenting the samples, and analyze the data correctly. A sensory researcher should always consider whether the method is appropriately implemented and whether errors have been introduced at any stage of the experiment.

In this chapter, the principles of sensory evaluation will be introduced. Examples will be provided to demonstrate the use of sensory evaluation techniques and the application of the results toward developing and modifying food recipes.

The Human Senses

The characteristics of food are perceived by the five senses: sight, smell, taste, sound, and touch.

Sight

The eyes perceive the initial quality of food, receiving such information as color, size, shape, texture, consistency, and opacity. Light entering the lens of the eye is focused on the retina, where the rods and cones convert it to neural impulses that travel to the brain via the optic nerve.[5] Perception by the visual system of light of wavelengths 400–500 nanometers (nm; blue), 500–600 nm (green and yellow), and 600–800 nm (red) is commonly expressed in terms of the hue, value, and chroma of the Munsell color system.[5]

Color may accurately indicate ripeness, strength of dilution, and the degree to which the food has been heated. Color is used to evaluate a food's desirability and acceptability. Greenish bananas, burnt meat, and dark brown avocado send visual signals that can change a person's choices. Color often triggers certain expectations in the mind; for example, the creamy color of vanilla ice cream evokes an expectation of richness.

But, color can be deceiving. The quality of food can be masked by changes in color. For instance, if yellow coloring is added to a food without actual fat having been added, the quality of low-fat products can be improved. Color changes alone can increase a food's acceptability considerably.

Even small visual details such as adjacent or background colors and the relative sizes of areas of contrasting color can affect a consumer's perception. Parameters of size and shape, such as width, length, thickness, particle size, geometric shape, and distribution of pieces, also provide information on food quality. The dullness, shininess, smoothness, or roughness of a surface and the clarity of liquids evoke preconceptions about the food. See **Special Topic 3.1** for more information on some of the latest trends chefs use to create dishes that delight the senses.

Special Topic 3.1

Molecular Gastronomy

Sarah Churchill

The concept of molecular gastronomy was founded by Hervé This, editor at *Pour la Science*, and Nicholas Kurti, a low-temperature physicist. They coined the term **molecular gastronomy** to encompass all the physical and chemical changes that occur during food production and cooking. In an effort to identify the methods for creating the best flavor and texture, they compared existing recipes with old proverbs and old wives' tales.[1] In 1992, they established the first international Workshop on Molecular and Physical Gastronomy.[2] The workshop still takes place today; however, the field of molecular gastronomy has moved from the scientific realm into the media limelight, becoming a cultural phenomenon.

molecular gastronomy Form of modern gourmet cooking that seeks to identify all the physical and chemical changes that occur during food production and cooking to create the best flavor and texture.

Today, popular culture uses the term *molecular gastronomy* to refer to the way modern chefs innovate with ingredients and techniques to bring excitement to the dining experience. The practice of molecular gastronomy also has been referred to as *culinary constructivism*, *experimental cuisine*, *molecular cooking*, *modernist cuisine*, *culinary deconstructivism*, and *progressive cuisine*. For example, the modern chefs Ferran Adriá of el Bulli, Heston Blumenthal of The Fat Duck, and Grant Achatz of Alinea are attempting to understand the chemical and physical nature of cooking as well as the best ingredients and techniques to improve upon traditional methods. They accomplish these goals through the deconstruction of certain recipes, the transformation of the physical states of foods (i.e., gases, liquids, solids), and the use of different equipment and ingredients to change cooking methods.[3]

Such chefs do not necessarily ascribe their innovations to molecular gastronomy, however. Adriá and Blumenthal say they go beyond the mere scientific exploration promoted by This and Kurtis. They also dispute the claim that the cuisine they are creating is pure novelty. They explain that they view food with a certain openness and embrace new ingredients and cooking methods without forsaking tradition. They affirm that their methods help them realize the full potential of each ingredient by questioning traditions about the best way to cook a food and finding the best way to maintain flavor. The result is a unique cuisine that gives consumers a chance to engage and confuse all of their senses.[4]

What innovations are used to create this bold new cuisine? Modern chefs use centrifuges, syringes, freeze dryers, blast chillers, and carbon dioxide dispensers. Canapés can be created from centrifuged frozen peas to create a buttery spread. A syringe can even be used to inject a small amount of unexpected flavor. Sometimes molecular gastronomy turns a traditional dish on its head. For example, instead of pasta with grated cheese, how would you like cheese with grated pasta? Parmesan noodles can now be made from boiling the cheese, pressing out the water, and passing it through a pastry bag; the cheese noodles can be topped with grated freeze-dried pasta.[5]

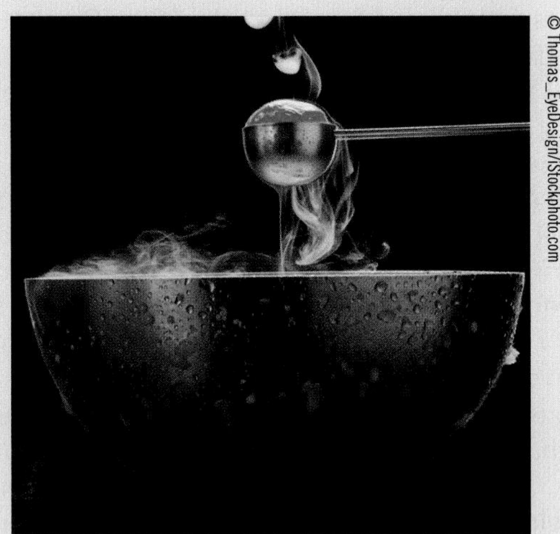

The kitchen of a chef cooking using molecular gastronomy techniques may look more similar to a high-end chemistry or physics laboratory than the kitchen of the local greasy spoon. A fusion of chemistry and cooking, molecular gastronomy seeks to transform common cooking ingredients into novel forms through the use of new technologies and techniques.

New ingredients at the modern chef's disposal include xantham gum, alginate, calcium salts, soy lecithin, agar-agar, and liquid nitrogen. These ingredients are becoming as prevalent in the modern chef's pantry as spices. They can be used to make gels, foams, and spheres without adding unwanted flavor.[6] Liquid nitrogen can be used to freeze something immediately and even make it shatter. Soy lecithin is crucial in making foams because it helps emulsify and hold ingredients together. Spheres resemble the texture and appearance of caviar but can be made using any liquid.

With the help of new technology and new ingredients, these chefs are able to create unique, artistic dishes. Chefs want to amaze consumers, and they really have. Whatever this cuisine should be called, it has become very popular. Of the 50 best restaurants in the world, the top 3 are associated with molecular gastronomy. Diners are becoming more experimental in their choices, even bravely trying tobacco- or crab-flavored ice cream. Innovation in cuisine is always progressing. With increased knowledge and technology, we'll just have to wait to see what comes next!

References

1 Molecular gastronomy: Food science raises the culinary bar. *Env Nutri.* 2010;33(9):7.

2 Blanck JF. Molecular gastronomy: Overview of a controversial food science discipline. *J Agr Food Inf.* 2007;8(3):77–85.

3 Lanchester J. Incredible edibles: The mad genius of "modernist cuisine." *The New Yorker.* 2011 March:87, 64.

4 Adria F, Blumenthal H, Keller T, McGee H. Statement on the 'new cookery.' *The Observer.* 2006. Available at: http://www.guardian.co.uk/uk/2006/dec/10/foodanddrink.obsfoodmonthly. Accessed June 28, 2012.

5 Adler J. Extreme cuisine. *Smithsonian.* 2011;42:60–66.

6 Ehrenberg R. What's cooking? *Science News.* 2008;173(13):202–203.

olfactory Relating to the sense of smell.

Smell

Our sense of smell, or **olfactory** sense, also contributes to our evaluation of food quality. The volatility of odors is related to temperature. Because only volatile molecules, in the form of gas, carry odor, it is easier to smell hot foods than cold ones. For example, hot tea is much easier to detect than iced tea, and the odor of a baked item is more intense than that of ice cream.

Lighter molecules that can become volatile are detected by the olfactory epithelium in the nasal cavity through one of two pathways: (1) directly through the nose or (2) after entering the mouth and flowing retro-nasally, or toward the back of the throat and up into the nasal cavity.[6] If you drink a carbonated beverage and laugh unexpectedly, you may experience the tingling of bubbles in the nose, showing how the mouth and nose are connected and how molecules can reach the olfactory epithelium by either route.

The gradual decrease in the ability to distinguish between odors over time is called **adaptation**. Adaptation occurs to prevent sensory overload. Dairy farmers who are exposed daily to the smell of manure will gradually become unaware of it, whereas visitors to the farm may be taken aback by the smell. Human subjects have varying sensitivities to odors, depending on hunger, satiety, mood, concentration, presence or absence of respiratory infections, and gender (e.g., women who are menstruating or are pregnant may perceive odors differently).[7] Because different people perceive a given odorant differently, identifying a new odor from a food product requires as large a panel as possible to get valid results.

adaptation The gradual decrease in the ability to distinguish between odors over time.

gustatory Relating to the sense of taste.

taste buds The small parts of gustatory and supportive cells; usually found on the upper surface of the tongue.

papillae Rough bulges or protuberances in the surface of the tongue, some of which contain taste buds.

Taste

Taste, or the perception of **gustatory** input, is the most influential factor in a person's selection of a particular food. For a substance to be tasted, it should be dissolved in water, oil, or saliva. Taste is perceived by the **taste buds** (see **Figure 3.1**), which are primarily on the surface of the tongue, by the mucosa of the palate, and in areas of the throat.

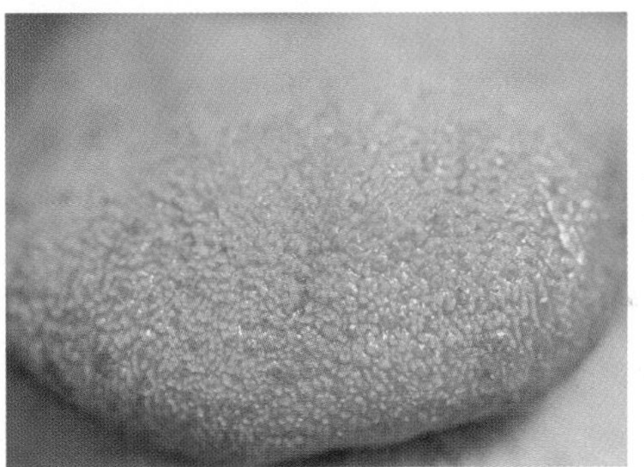

© F.C.G./ShutterStock, Inc.

FIGURE 3.1 On the tongue, the majority of the taste buds sit on raised protrusions of the tongue surface called papillae. On average, the human tongue has 2,000–8,000 taste buds.

In the middle of each taste bud lies a pore, where saliva collects. When food enters the mouth, bits of it are dissolved in the saliva pools and come into contact with cilia, small hairlike projections, from the gustatory cells.[6] The gustatory cells signal to the brain through cranial nerves. The brain, in turn, translates the nervous electrical impulses into sensations that people recognize as "taste."[6]

Taste buds are found in the **papillae** of the tongue. Two types of papillae contain taste buds. The mushroom-like fungiform papillae on the sides and tip of the tongue generally contain taste buds, and the circumvallate papillae (elevated, large papillae in the form of a "V" toward the back of the tongue) always contain taste buds.[8] As people get older, the original 9,000 to 10,000 taste buds begin to decrease in number, so that people older than age 45 often seek more spices, salt, and sugar in their food.[6]

Genetic Variation

Individual variation in taste likely has a genetic component. Studies have demonstrated a link between the ability to taste bitter thiourea compounds and a newly discovered taste receptor gene, *TAS2R38*.[9] Thus, the ability to taste these bitter compounds—phenylthiocarbamide (PTC) or the safer, chemically related compound 6-n-propylthiouracil (PROP)—may be used as a phenotypic marker for genetic differences in perceptions of taste.[10–12] In the United States, the frequency of nontasters is estimated to be 20% to 25% of the population.[13] The frequency varies by gender and race.[13,14]

One factor that may explain variation in taste and the perception of physical sensations is the anatomy of the anterior portion of the tongue. For example, PROP tasters have the most fungiform papillae (FP).[13,15–17] **Special Topic 3.2** provides more information on how genetic variations may influence how we perceive food.

Beyond genetics, variation in taste perception also depends on how perceptible sweet, fatty, and bitter components are in foods and beverages. It also depends on the value a consumer places on other factors, such as health and convenience.[18,19]

Special Topic 3.2

Nutrigenomics

Jill M. Merrigan

nutrigenomics Study of how food affects our genes and the way our bodies respond to nutrients.

Nutrigenomics studies the naturally occurring compounds in the foods and how they affect our bodies based our individual genetic differences.[1] "There is good evidence that nutrition has significant influences on the expression of genes, and, likewise, genetic variation can have a significant effect on food intake, metabolic response to food, individual nutrient requirements, food safety, and the efficacy of disease-protective dietary factors," explains nutrigenomic researcher L. R. Ferguson.[2]

The existence of a particular gene or mutation in many cases indicates a predisposition to a particular disease. Once genetic predisposition has been established, determining whether the disease will progress can be investigated by examining the relationship between the human genome and environmental and behavioral factors. The study of nutrigenomics looks at the expression of the genome with regard to nutrition. According to researcher M. Nathaniel Mead, "although genes are critical for determining function, nutrition modifies the extent to which different genes are expressed, and thereby modulates whether individuals attain the potential established by their genetic background."[3] Today, scientists are exploring nutrigenomics to determine how nutrients may be able protect the genome from damage.

Through the study of nutrigenomics, it may become possible to develop dietary interventions based on an understanding of an individual's nutritional requirements, nutritional status, and genotype. Studying how foods affects individual genes and genotypes will make it possible to design "personalized nutrition" plants that may prevent and cure chronic disease.

Studies have been completed on humans, animals, and cell cultures that reveal that macronutrients (fatty acids and proteins), micronutrients (vitamins), and naturally occurring phytochemicals (such as flavonoids, carotenoids, coumarins, and phytosterols) regulate gene expression in various ways. Micronutrients and bioreactive chemicals in foods are involved in metabolic reactions that determine hormonal balances and immune competence, as well as detoxification processes. Additionally some biochemicals found in foods, such as genistein and resveratrol, act as transcription factors, and therefore alter gene expression. Signal transduction pathways and chromatin structures are altered by other biochemicals, such as choline, and therefore indirectly affect gene expression.[3]

One example of nutrigenomics is folate and the gene for MTHFR (methylenetetrahydrofolate reductase). MTHFR has a role in supplying methionine. Methionine plays a central role in certain metabolic pathways, including those involved in the production of neurotransmitters and in the regulation of gene expression. Folate is required for MTHFR to function efficiently. MTHFR has a common polymorphism that leads to two forms of protein: the reference version (C), which functions normally, and the thermal-labile version (T), which has reduced activity. When individuals have two copies of the reference sequence gene (CC), they have normal folate metabolism. However, individuals who have two copies of the reduced version (TT) and low dietary folate accumulate homocysteine and have less methionine. This combination puts them at an increased risk for vascular disease and premature cognitive decline. By making these connections, individuals with the unstable (TT) genes can take folic acid supplements or increase their folate from food sources to metabolize excess homocysteine and restore their methionine levels to normal.[1]

Additional studies have determined that there are nine key nutrients that may have an influence on genomic integrity in a handful of ways. Six of these nutrients—folate, vitamin B_{12}, niacin, vitamin E, retinol, and calcium—are associated with a reduction in DNA damage. The other three—riboflavin, panthenic acid, and biotin—are associated with an increase in DNA damage similar to that seen upon occupational exposure to genotoxic and carcinogenic chemicals. This suggests that nutritional deficiency or excess can lead to DNA damage as damaging as that seen with exposure to environmental toxins. Other nutrigenomic studies have shown that many antioxidant nutrients and phytochemicals enhance DNA repair and reduce oxidative DNA damage.[3]

Recent research indicates that nutrigenomics may have the potential to prevent, mitigate, and treat chronic diseases and certain cancers by making small but highly useful changes to an individual's diet. In the future, scientists, doctors, and dieticians may be able to move forward to be able to identify a patient's DNA profile for a specific disease and ultimately be able to shape a diet that will reduce their chances of developing that disease. Nutrigenomics may be the answer to the obesity epidemic and improve the way individuals age with better bone and brain health; it may also decrease the risk of developing certain cancers.

References

1 Astley SB. An introduction to nutrigenomics developments and trends. *Genes Nutri.* 2007;2(1):11–13.

2 Ferguson LR. Nutrigenomics: Integrating genomic approaches into nutrition research. *Mol Diagn Ther.* 2006;10(2):101–108.

3 Mead MN. Nutrigenomics: The genome–food interface. *Env Health Persp.* 2007;115(12):A582–A589.

Basic Components of Taste

For many years, four basic tastes were recognized: sweet, salty, sour, and bitter. A fifth, umami, was added more recently. These tastes can be characterized as follows:

- *Sweet:* Substances that produce sweet taste include sugars, glycols, alcohols, aldehydes, and alternative sweeteners.[20]
- *Salty:* The salty taste comes from ionized salts, such as the ions in sodium chloride (NaCl) or other salts found naturally in some foods.
- *Sour:* The sour taste comes from the acids found in food. It is related to the concentration of hydrogen ions (H^+) that are found in the natural acids of fruits, vinegar, and certain vegetables.
- *Bitter:* Bitterness is imparted by compounds such as caffeine (tea, coffee), theobromine (chocolate), and phenolic compounds (grapefruit).[6] Many bitter substances are alkaloids that often are found in poisonous plants.
- *Umami:* This is a most recently defined component of taste, which was identified from a study of seaweed broth.[8] **Umami** is a Japanese word meaning "delicious"—it is evoked by glutamate compounds, which are commonly found in meats, mushrooms, soy sauce, fish sauce, and cheese. Some taste experts do not recognize umami as a taste at this time.

Flavor

Whereas taste relies on the sensation produced through the stimulation of the taste buds, flavor is a broader concept. **Flavor** is the combined senses of taste, aroma, and mouthfeel. **Mouthfeel** encompasses textural and chemical sensations such as astringency, spice heat, cooling, and metallic flavor.

Among the flavor components, aroma is especially important; it provides approximately 75% of the impression of flavor.[21] To get an idea of how the ability to smell affects the perception of flavor, pinch your nose and begin to eat a certain flavor of jellybean. Then, as you are chewing, unpinch your nose: You will clearly sense the difference between when the nose is pinched and unpinched. Suppose you are eating a buttered popcorn–flavored jellybean. While pinching your nose, you can only perceive sweetness, but as soon as you unpinch your nose you can recognize the buttered popcorn flavor. As another example, consider when you have a cold with a badly stuffed-up nose. Everything tastes different. (This is why pinching people's nostrils shut is helpful in mitigating the flavor of an unpleasant medicine.)

Gastronomy Point

Monosodium Glutamate Monosodium glutamate, better known by its abbreviation MSG, is one substance that contributes to the perception of umami.

umami Taste category based on glutamate compounds, which are commonly found in meats, mushrooms, soy sauce, fish sauce, and cheese.

flavor The combined sense of taste, odor, and mouthfeel.

mouthfeel The way that a particular type of food feels in the mouth.

Innovation Point

A New Taste? Research is underway for a sixth taste component relating to our perception of fats. Genetic variation in "fat taste" may help explain our food choices and dietary habits, which, in turn, could influence our nutritional and health status.

Sound

Sound is another sense used in evaluating food quality. Sounds such as sizzling, crunching, popping, bubbling, squeaking, dripping, exploding, and crackling can communicate much about a food. Most of these sounds are affected by water content; thus, their characteristics indicate a food's freshness and ripeness.[6]

Sound is detected as vibrations in the local medium, usually air. The vibrations are transmitted via the small bones in the middle ear to create hydraulic motion in the fluid of the inner ear, the cochlea. The cochlea is a spiral canal covered in cilia that, when agitated, sends neural impulses to the brain.[5]

Touch

texture The sensory manifestation of the structure or inner makeup of products in terms of their feel as measured by tactile nerves on the surface of the skin of the hands, lips, or tongue.

descriptive panel A panel commonly used to determine differences between food samples. The descriptive panelist is experienced in the type of food being tested and receives extensive training prior to the testing.

consumer panel A panel selected from the public according to the demographics necessary to taste test a product.

The sense of touch delivers impressions of a food's texture to us through oral sensations or the skin. Texture is a very complex perception: The first input is visual; second comes touch, either directly through the fingers or indirectly via eating utensils; the third is the feeling in the mouth (mouthfeel), as detected by the teeth and tactile nerve cells on the tongue and palate. **Texture** is the sensory manifestation of the structure or inner makeup of products in terms of their reactions to stress, which are measured as mechanical properties (such as hardness/firmness, adhesiveness, cohesiveness, gumminess, springiness/resilience, and viscosity) by the kinesthetic sense in the muscles of the hands, fingers, tongue, jaw, or lips.[5] Texture also includes tactile feel properties, which are measured as geometric properties (i.e., grainy, gritty, crystalline, flaky) or moisture properties (i.e., wetness, oiliness, moistness, dryness) by the tactile nerves in the surface of the skin of the hands, lips, or tongue.[5] The greater surface sensitivity of the lips, tongue, face, and hands makes easy detection of small differences in particle size and thermal and chemical properties possible among food products.

Variables Controlled During Sensory Evaluation

During sensory evaluation, panelists are typically seated at tables, cubicles, or booths, and the food is presented in a uniform fashion. To obtain valid, reproducible results during a sensory evaluation, the environment in which the sensory panel evaluates foods or beverages should be carefully controlled, as should variables pertaining to the panelists. This section discusses the many variables that should be considered when designing a sensory evaluation test.

Panel Management

Two general types of panels are used in sensory evaluation. A **descriptive panel** is commonly used to determine differences between food samples. The descriptive panelist is experienced in the type of food being tested and receives extensive training prior to the testing. A **consumer panel** is selected from the public according to the demographics necessary to taste test a product.

Panel Selection

When assembling a panel, it is preferred to use an equal number of men and women. The age distribution of the panel should also be considered because it may affect test results.[6] The sensory analyst must recruit the people who can make a reliable commitment of time and who also know what is expected of them during the test. General taste panels usually consist of people who meet the following criteria:

- They are in good health and free of illness related to sensory properties, such as chronic colds, food allergies, or diabetes.
- They are nonsmokers (smoking can dull olfactory and gustatory sensations).

- They are not color blind.
- They have no strong likes or dislikes for the food to be tested.

Panelist Preparation

The level of training for descriptive panels and consumer panels is quite different, given the differences in purpose of the evaluations in which they participate.

Descriptive Panels

Because the investment in a descriptive panel is large in terms of time and human resources, it is wise to conduct an exhaustive screening process rather than train unqualified panelists.[2] If the ability to detect subtle differences is essential, the sensory analyst may need to screen the sensory acuity of potential panelists on key properties of the product(s) that will be tested.

Descriptive panels can be selected through a series of tests that may include a set of prescreening questionnaires, a set of acuity tests, a set of ranking/rating tests, and a personal interview. However, it is not necessary to have only the most highly discriminating panelists because the average panelists will improve markedly with training and some people may be very discriminating in general but just have one or two problem areas.[2]

The amount of training required is determined by the task and the level of sensory sensitivity desired. For most descriptive panels, expensive and in-depth training is necessary.[2] During the training, the trainer must make sure the panelists realize that sensory testing work is difficult and requires attention and concentration. If team spirit can be developed by the panelists during the training sessions, this will smooth the way for the main evaluation and facilitate panelist performance. The performance of trained panelists used over long periods of time may fluctuate because of a loss of focus and a lack of motivation during the evaluation sessions.

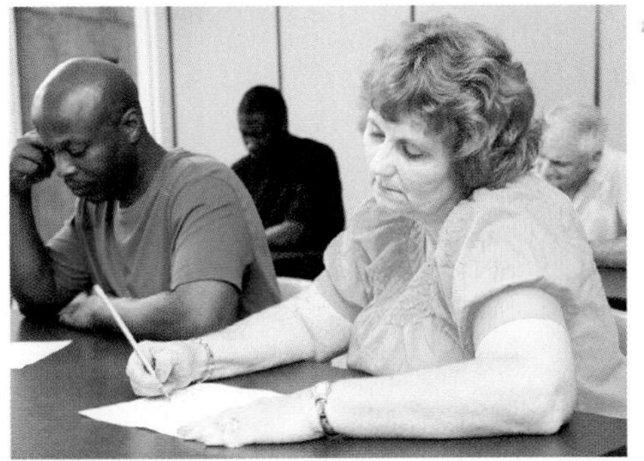

FIGURE 3.2 Manufacturers, scientists, food technologists, and marketers can use consumer panels to gain a clear perception of what ordinary consumers may experience when tasting a particular food item.

Consumer Panels

In contrast to descriptive panels, consumer panels typically require a larger number of panelists and may range from 200 to 500 people (see **Figure 3.2**). Consumer panelists can be screened on a test criteria; for example, demographics or potential use of product. The questions asked of consumer panels should be answerable by untrained panelists.

Other Considerations

Other considerations also should be taken into account to optimize panelist performance during a sensory evaluation:

- It is wise to schedule the evaluation of certain product types at the time of day when that product is normally used or consumed.[5] For example, breakfast cereals would be better tested in the morning. In contrast, it would not be recommended to test highly flavored or alcoholic products in the early morning.
- Midmornings or midafternoons (such as 11 AM or 3 PM) are considered the best times for testing because at these times people are not usually overly hungry or full.[6]
- Panelists should not ingest any other food for at least 1 hour before testing and should not chew gum immediately before testing.[6]
- The instructions provided to the panelists should be very clear and concise. It is frequently desirable to give the instructions on how to perform the sensory evaluation verbally, before the panelists enter the booth area, and then also in written form on the score sheet.[2]
- Incentives usually are given as a token of appreciation to motivate people to participate voluntarily.[2] Common incentives include snacks or small gifts.

Environmental Controls

Physical and chemical factors present at the location of the sensory evaluation must be carefully controlled so that any possible extraneous effects of the surroundings on the test results are minimized and each panelist experiences the food in the same environment.

Temperature, Humidity, and Air Circulation

The ambient temperature should be comfortable, and the surroundings should be quiet and odor-free. The temperature and relative humidity for the sensory evaluation area should be 72–75°F (22–24°C) and 45–55%, respectively.[5] The use of replaceable active carbon filters in the ventilation system ducts is recommended. A slight positive pressure should be maintained in the booth areas to prevent odor contamination.[5] The sensory scientist should check if any unnecessary odors are detected in sensory testing areas.

Color and Lighting

The color and lighting in the sensory lab should be planned to permit adequate viewing of samples while minimizing distractions.[22,23] The walls of the sensory evaluation area should be off-white; the absence of hues of any color will prevent unwanted effects on food appearance.[5] Illumination in the booths should be uniform, shadow-free, and at least 300–500 lx at the table surface.[2] An ideal lighting system is controllable with a dimmer switch to a maximum of 700–800 lx, the common illumination intensity in offices.[2] Incandescent lights can control both the light intensity and the light color, but they generate heat, which will require cooling. Fluorescent lights generate less heat and allow for choice of whiteness; for example, cool white, warm white, or simulated north daylight.[5] Colored lights are used to mask visual differences among samples, calling for the subject to determine by flavor or texture only. A choice of low-intensity red, green, and/or blue lights using colored bulbs or special filters is a common feature of sensory booths.[5]

Product Controls

Variables pertaining to the product samples themselves must also be controlled.

Sample Preparation

Food samples must be of the same size (usually enough for two bites or sips) and from the same portion of the food (e.g., middle versus outside). The sensory analyst should determine and control the amount of product to be used in all the tests, including the amount of each added ingredient, the preparation process, and **holding time**, which is defined as the minimum and maximum time after preparation that a product can be used for a sensory test. For instance, suppose the test sample is a pumpkin muffin. The sensory analyst needs to decide the size of the muffin, exactly how the muffins will be baked, the appropriate holding time, and at which temperature and on what plate the sample will be served.

holding time The minimum and maximum time after preparation that a product can be used for a sensory test.

The sensory analyst should be very careful to standardize all serving procedures and sample preparation techniques except the variable under evaluation. If the appearance of the sample is not the variable under evaluation, then the samples should appear identical. Samples should be blind-labeled with random three-digit codes, and the sample order should be randomized to avoid bias due to order of presentation. A reasonable number of samples, say two to four, should be tested at a time to avoid taste fatigue.

Sample Temperature

Samples must be presented at the same temperature, which must be specified in the test protocol. For example, ice cream should be tempered at 5–9°F (–15°C to –13°C) for at least 12 hours before serving because scooping is not easy if the ice cream is colder.[2]

Presentation

Samples should be presented in containers or on plates that are the same size, shape, and color. White or clear containers are usually chosen so as not to influence panelists' perceptions of the food's color. The sensory analyst should choose the container that is most convenient. However, the choice of container should not negatively affect the flavor characteristics of the food product.

Carriers

Carriers refer to materials that form a base or vehicle for the food being tested but may more broadly be considered as any other food that accompanies the one being tested so they are ingested, too.[2] Examples include spaghetti sauce on a spaghetti noodle, cream fillings in pastries, butter on bread, chips with salsa, and carrots with ranch dips. A carrier can mask or disguise differences or minimize the panelist's abilities to perceive the difference due to the addition of other flavors and modifications to texture and mouthfeel characteristics. However, for a product that is rarely consumed alone and almost always involves a carrier, the artificial situation where the carrier is not provided may affect test results, especially in consumer testing.[2] Therefore, whether a carrier is used should be carefully determined.

Palate Cleansers

Room temperature water or plain bread is made available for panelists to eat between samples to prevent carryover tastes. A rest period of at least 30 seconds is scheduled between samples. Paper towels or napkins are provided, and, because swallowing the food or beverage influences the taste of subsequent samples, small containers into which samples may be spit are provided.

One study that evaluated the effects of a range of palate cleansers (i.e., chocolate, pectin solution, table water crackers, warm water, water, whole milk) on foods representing various tastes and mouthfeels concluded that table water crackers were the only palate cleanser effective across all representative foods.[24] These foods included jelly beans (sweet), coffee (bitter), smoked sausage (fatty), tea (astringent), spicy tortilla chip (pungent), mint (cooling), and applesauce (nonlingering).

Measurement Theory

Measurement Hierarchy

Four levels of measurement are commonly used in sensory evaluation: nominal, ordinal, interval, and ratio.[25] It is important to recognize that there is a hierarchy in the level of measurement. At lower levels of measurement, assumptions tend to be less restrictive and data analyses tend to be less sensitive. At each level up the hierarchy, the current level includes all of the qualities of the one below it and adds something new. In general, it is desirable to have a higher level of measurement (such as interval or ratio) rather than a lower one (such as nominal or ordinal).[26]

Nominal

With nominal measurement, the numbers simply identify unique attributes; they are not ordered. For example, gender may be coded by assigning a "1" to males and a "2" to females. With nominal data, common descriptive statistics such as range, mean, or standard deviation are not appropriate. Instead, frequency counts, number of categories, or mode can be used to get some idea of the distribution of nominal data.

Ordinal

With ordinal measurement, the attributes can be ordered, but the difference between levels is not equal. It is not normally distributed and often is skewed. For example, cakes can be ordered by rank for perceived overall sweetness. The interval between values is not interpretable for ordinal measurement. In this case, the rank number can tell us where the cake falls in order of sweetness; however, we cannot draw conclusions about the differences among the products.

Interval

With interval measurement, there are ordered levels, and the difference between levels is equal. However, there is no true zero. For example, when we measure the oven temperature in degrees Fahrenheit, the distance from 100°F to 200°F is the same as the distance from 300°F to 400°F. Because the interval between the values is interpretable, it makes sense to calculate the average of the interval variable. However, in interval scaling, ratios do not make sense: 200°F is not twice as hot as 100°F, although the value is twice as large.

Ratio

With ratio measurement, there are ordered levels in which the difference between levels is equal, and there is a true zero. For example, weight is a ratio measurement. We can say that 200 pounds of sugar weighs twice as much as 100 pounds of sugar, and zero pounds of sugar means that there is no sugar.

Common Scales Used in Testing

Category Scales

Category scaling may be the oldest method of scaling; it involves the choice of discrete response alternatives to signify increasing sensation intensity in terms of degrees of liking and/or preference. The most popular category scale used in sensory testing is the **hedonic scale**, which measures the extent of like or dislike for the sensory characteristics of food. Examples of category scales are shown in **Figure 3.3**. Due to their simplicity, category scales are well suited for consumer panels. In addition, they offer some advantages in data coding and tabulation (for speed and accuracy) because they are easier to tabulate than line markings or the more variable magnitude estimates, described below.

hedonic scale A scale with which judges indicate the extent of their like or dislike for the sensory characteristics of food.

Line Scales

Line scales may also be referred to as graphic ratings or visual analog scales. Examples of line scales are shown in **Figure 3.4**. With line scales, the test participant's response is recorded as the distance of the mark from one end of the scale, usually whatever end is considered "lower." Line scaling differs from category scaling in the sense that the person's choices seem more continuous and less limited. Stone et al. recommended the use of line scaling for Quantitative Descriptive Analysis (QDA), then a relatively new approach to specifying the intensities of all the important sensory attributes.[27]

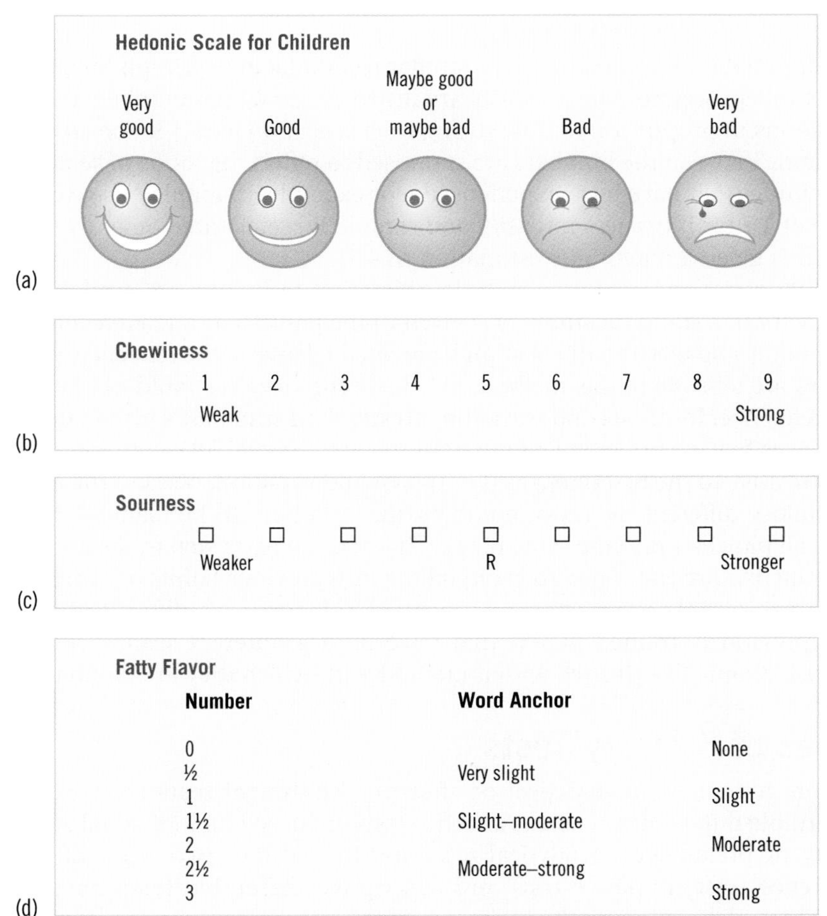

FIGURE 3.3 Examples of category scales. (a) Hedonic scale for children. (b) Chewiness. (c) Sourness. (d) Fatty flavor.

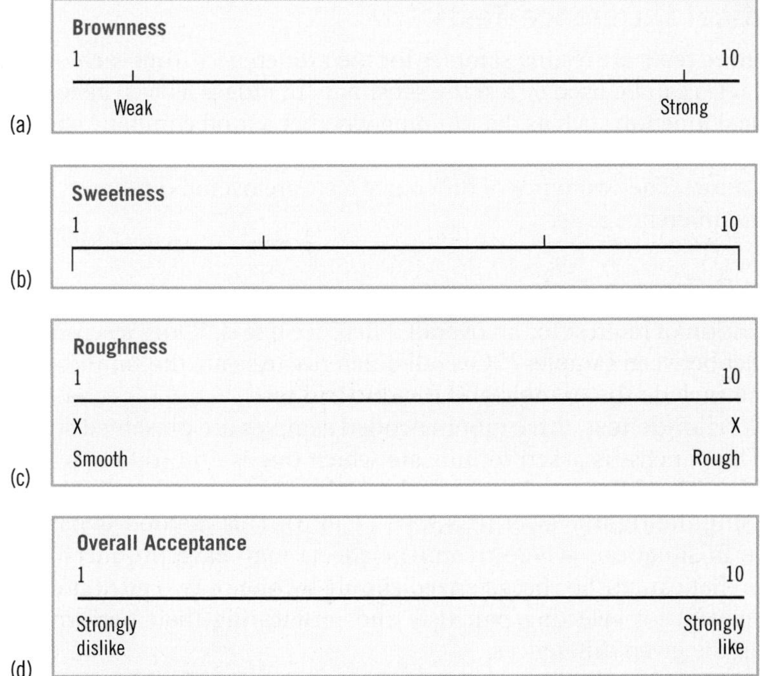

FIGURE 3.4 Examples of line scales. (a) Brownness. (b) Sweetness. (c) Roughness. (d) Overall acceptance.

Magnitude Estimation Scales

Magnitude estimation scaling is a popular technique in psychophysical studies. In this procedure, the panelists are instructed to assign numbers to their sensations in proportion to how strong each sensation feels.[2] In the analysis, the ratios between the numbers are supposed to reflect the ratios of sensation magnitudes that have been experienced. For example, if sample A is given the value of 15 for bitterness intensity and sample B seems three times as bitter, then B is given a magnitude estimation of 45.

Two variations of the magnitude estimation technique are available. In one method, a standard stimulus is given to the panelist as a reference with a fixed value, and all subsequent stimuli are rated relative to the reference. Values of zero are allowed in this method, but the rating of zero should not be used as a reference. In the second variation, no standard stimulus is given, and the panelist is free to choose any number for the first sample. All samples are then rated relative to the first intensity. For the second variation, because the panelists choose different ranges of numbers, the data have to be manipulated to bring all panelists into the same range. This adds an extra step to the analysis.

Panelists are cautioned to avoid falling into previous habits of using only category scales that they are used to using.[2] This may be a difficult problem with previously trained panels that have used a different scaling method because people like to stick with a method with which they are familiar.

analytical tests Sensory tests used to detect discernible differences.

affective tests Sensory tests used to determine differences in acceptability or preference between products.

difference tests Sensory tests designed to detect discernible differences.

triangle test A difference test in which three samples are presented simultaneously (two of which are the same), and the judge is asked to identify the odd sample.

Types of Sensory Tests

Sensory tests may be analytical or affective. **Analytical tests** are based on discernible differences, whereas affective tests are based on individual acceptability or preferences. Analytical tests are divided into two types of tests: difference (discriminative test) and descriptive. **Affective tests** have two categories, depending on the main task of the test: acceptance or preference. The primary task of an acceptance test is "rating," whereas the primary task of a preference task is "choice."[5]

Analytical Difference Tests

Difference tests are testing samples for their differences from each other. Difference tests can be used to test the sensitivity of judges as well as to perform a practical function such as determining whether a food company should buy an inexpensive ingredient to replace a more expensive one in formulating a food product. The two types of difference tests are overall difference tests and attribute difference tests.

Overall Difference Tests

The question of interest for an overall difference test is, "Does a sensory difference exist between samples?" Overall difference tests are the simplest sensory tests and include the triangle and the duo-trio test.

In a **triangle test**, three number-coded samples are presented simultaneously. The panelist is asked to indicate which one is odd (different from the other two). The difference in this method of presentation reduces the chance of guessing the right answer to 33.3% (1 in 3). This method is particularly effective in situations where treatment effects may have produced product changes that cannot be characterized simply by one or two attributes. It also can be useful for selecting panelists and monitoring their performance to discriminate given differences.

In a triangle test, six possible serving orders (AAB, ABA, BAA, BBA, BAB, ABB) are counterbalanced across all panelists. It should be conducted with 20 to 40 participants who have been screened for their sensory acuity to common product differences and who are familiar with the test procedure.

If differences are large and easy to identify, as few as 12 panelists may be employed.[5] The following is an example application of the triangle test:

- *Situation:* A food service management director wishes to confirm whether there is a significant sensory difference between a canned product and a paper carton product before changing the product. She is considering changing the chicken broth product from cans to cartons because of the clients' desires for "greener" packaging.
- *Test objective:* The objective is to determine if the change of product packaging causes an overall difference in sensory reactions to the chicken broth.
- *Test design:* The test design is shown in **Table 3.1**. There are 48 panelists with no replication.
- *Score sheet:* An example score sheet is shown in **Figure 3.5**.
- *Results and analysis:* The actual number of panelists who correctly identified the odd sample from the triangle test is counted. Out of 48 panelists, 25 correctly chose the odd sample. When a statistical test is applied, it is determined that the panelists could detect a difference between samples.
- *Conclusion*: A significant overall difference was found between the canned product and paper carton product.

Please taste the samples from left to right. Two samples are the same, and one is different. Circle the number of the sample that is different.

Sample code ______ ______ ______

Thank you!

FIGURE 3.5 Example of a triangle score sheet.

For detailed statistics regarding this example, see the Appendix at the end of this chapter.

The **duo-trio test** is another test of overall difference. In this test, the reference sample is presented first; it is followed by two other samples, one of which is the same as the reference. The panelists are requested to identify which of the latter two samples is the same as or different from the reference. With the duo-trio test, there is a 50% chance of being right by chance alone. The following example shows an application of the duo-trio test:

duo-trio test A difference test in which three samples are presented at the same time. A reference is designated, and the judge is asked to select the one most similar to the reference.

- *Situation:* A catering manager is faced with two very similar fluid egg products. Product A has been used for years; product B is a new product offered at a cheaper price. He wants to confirm whether there is an overall difference in perception between the two products.
- *Test objective:* The test objective is to determine whether the source of the fluid egg causes any overall difference in sensory perception of the scrambled egg.

TABLE 3.1
Triangle Test Design

Sample Identification	**Codes in Sets with Two As**	**Codes in Sets with Two Bs**
A: Canned product	624, 738	325*
B: Paper carton product	199*	801, 514
Panelist Number	**Serving Pattern**	**Codes in Order**
1, 7, 13, 19, 25, 31, 37, 43	AAB	624, 738, 199*
2, 8, 14, 20, 26, 32, 38, 44	ABA	624, 199*, 738
3, 9, 15, 21, 27, 33, 39, 45	BAA	199*, 624, 738
4, 10, 16, 22, 28, 34, 40, 46	BBA	801, 514, 325*
5, 11, 17, 23, 29, 35, 41, 47	BAB	801, 325*, 514
6, 12, 18, 24, 30, 36, 42, 48	ABB	325*, 801, 514

* Odd sample/correct answer.

- *Test design:* The test is conducted with 40 subjects who regularly eat eggs. Each of the two samples is used as the reference in half (20) of the evaluations. Scrambled eggs are made using the same method and equipment. The only variable that changes is the fluid egg product. Samples are presented without any condiment and at the same temperature.
- *Score sheet:* An example score sheet is shown in **Figure 3.6**.
- *Results and analysis:* Thirteen out of 40 panelists correctly matched the sample to the reference. Therefore, the panelists could not detect a difference between samples.
- *Conclusion:* The manager can conclude that there is no significant overall difference between the two fluid egg products.

Please taste the samples from left to right. The left sample is a reference. Circle the number of the sample that matches the reference. If no difference is apparent between the two unknown samples, you must guess.

Reference _______
Sample code _______
Sample code _______

Thank you!

FIGURE 3.6 Example of a duo-trio score sheet.

For detailed statistics regarding this example, see the Appendix at the end of this chapter.

Attribute Difference Tests

Attribute difference taste tests focus on a single sensory attribute such as sweetness or moistness. Attribute tests often are administered to evaluate qualitative differences in taste, color, and texture.

The **paired comparison test** is a test of difference in which a specific characteristic is designated. The subject is asked to test the two samples presented to identify the sample with the greater amount of the characteristic being measured. With this type of test, the subject has a 50% chance of being right by chance alone. The following example shows an application of the paired comparison test:

paired comparison test A difference test in which two samples are presented, and the judge is asked to select the one that has more of a particular characteristic.

ranking test A difference or preference test in which more than two samples are presented and all samples are compared by ranking them from lowest to highest for the intensity of a specific characteristic.

- *Situation:* A cookie manufacturer receives reports from the market that her cookie (cookie A) is deemed insufficiently sweet, so a test cookie (cookie B) is made using more sweetener. She wants to produce a cookie that is perceptibly sweeter, but not excessively so.
- *Test objective:* The test objective is to compare cookie A with cookie B to determine whether a small but significant increase in sweetness has been attained.
- *Test design:* A paired comparison test is chosen because the characteristic of interest is only sweetness, nothing else. The sensory analyst codes the cookies "796" and "308" and offers them to a panel of 30 subjects with proven ability to detect small changes in sweetness. The panelists are not asked, "Is 308 sweeter than 796?" but rather, "Which cookie is sweeter?" so as to eliminate the potential for bias.
- *Score sheet:* An example score sheet is shown in **Figure 3.7**.
- *Results and analysis:* Significantly more panelists (22) identified test cookie B as being sweeter.
- *Conclusion:* There is a significant sweetness difference between cookies A and B. The test cookie was successful.

There are two samples in each of the two paired comparison sets for you to evaluate. Taste each of the coded samples in the sequence presented from left to right. Please write down the code of the sweeter sample.

Sample code _______ Sample code _______

Which sample is sweeter? _______

Thank you!

FIGURE 3.7 Example of a paired comparison score sheet.

For detailed statistics regarding this example, see the Appendix at the end of this chapter.

The **ranking test** is valuable when several samples need to be evaluated for a single characteristic. Ranking test procedures have the advantage of simplicity in instructions to panelists, ease of data handling, and minimal assumptions about the level of measurement because the data are ordinal.

Although ranking tests are most often applied to hedonic data, they also are applicable to questions of sensory intensities. The following example shows an application of the ranking test:

- *Situation:* A sandwich maker wishes to compare the saltiness among different types of cheese to select a cheese for a new sandwich menu.
- *Test objective:* The test objective is to determine whether there is a significant difference in saltiness among three types of cheese (mozzarella, cheddar, and provolone).
- *Test design:* The ranking test is suitable because it is simple to carry out and does not require much training. The three samples are tested with a panel of 28 students. The panelists receive the samples (coded with three-digit numbers) in balanced, random order.
- *Score sheet:* An example score sheet is shown in **Figure 3.8**.
- *Results and analysis:* When compared to the minimum critical differences, no significant differences are found among the samples because all of the differences are less than 18.
- *Conclusion:* There is no significant difference in saltiness among the three types of cheese.

For detailed statistics regarding this example, see the Appendix at the end of this chapter.

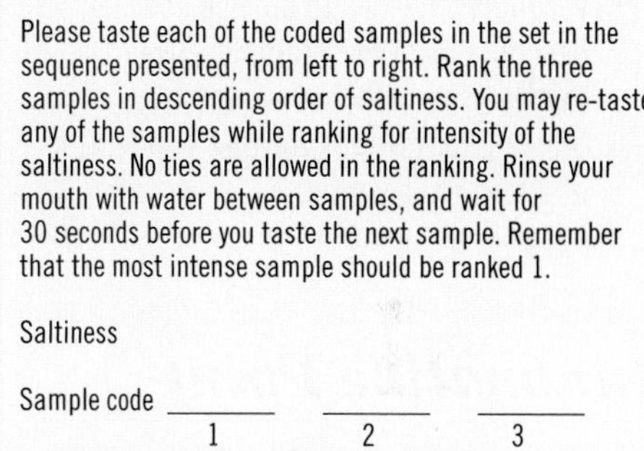
Please taste each of the coded samples in the set in the sequence presented, from left to right. Rank the three samples in descending order of saltiness. You may re-taste any of the samples while ranking for intensity of the saltiness. No ties are allowed in the ranking. Rinse your mouth with water between samples, and wait for 30 seconds before you taste the next sample. Remember that the most intense sample should be ranked 1.

Saltiness

Sample code ______ ______ ______
1 2 3

Thank you!

FIGURE 3.8 Example of a ranking score sheet.

The **rating difference test** among multiple samples is used when a rating scale is applied. The following example shows an application of the rating difference test:

rating difference test Test to differentiate among multiple samples that uses a rating scale. Products are ranked using a rating scale to assess for differences between samples.

- *Situation:* A baker is producing a new low-fat pound cake prepared by replacing butter with applesauce. He is making four samples with four levels of applesauce substitution (0%, 33%, 66%, and 100%). He discovers that moistness is the sensory characteristic that shows the most noticeable difference among samples; thus, it is the variable most likely to affect product acceptability.
- *Test objective:* The test objective is to compare the moistness of four pound cakes in order to determine which product has no significant difference in moistness from the control product and has the lowest fat content.
- *Test design:* A completely randomized design is used, in which all samples are compared together using a rating scale. Twelve subjects evaluate the moistness for four samples on scale of 1 to 9.
- *Score sheet:* An example score sheet is shown in **Figure 3.9**.
- *Results and analysis:* There are significant differences in moistness between 100% applesauce pound cake and the other three products (control with butter and no applesauce, and 33% applesauce, and 66% applesauce).
- *Conclusion:* The 66% applesauce pound cake should be chosen because it is the product with the lowest fat content that shows no significant difference from the control in moistness.

For detailed statistics regarding this example, see the Appendix at the end of this chapter.

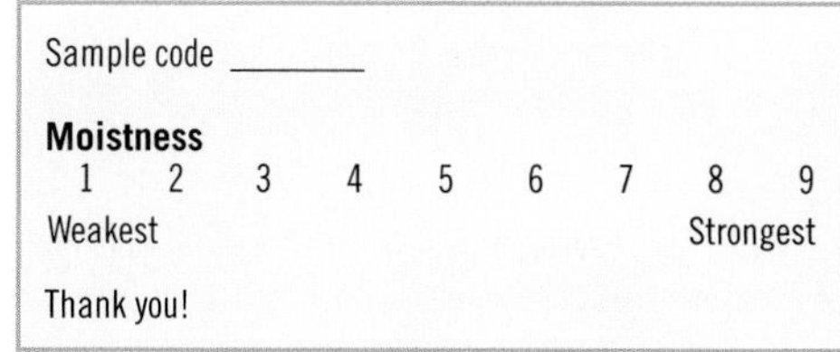
Sample code ______

Moistness
1 2 3 4 5 6 7 8 9
Weakest Strongest

Thank you!

FIGURE 3.9 Example of a rating difference score sheet.

Analytical Descriptive Tests

The descriptive sensory test is the most comprehensive and informative test used in sensory evaluation. The question for the descriptive test is, "How do products differ in specific sensory characteristics?" **Descriptive tests** enable researchers to characterize their products through selective, critical scoring of specific attributes of each product. The descriptive techniques are frequently used for developing new products and for quality assurance. The information from these methods can be especially valuable for dealing with sensory problems that consumers may detect.

descriptive tests Sensory tests designed to provide information on the specific sensory characteristics of food samples and to quantify the sensory differences.

profiling A group of highly trained panelists work together to develop the vocabulary needed to provide specific descriptions of food samples; used to detail the specific flavors (flavor profiling) or textures (texture profiling) of a food or beverage.

Descriptive tests require a well-trained panel and tend to be expensive. Descriptive tests should never be used with consumers because consistent and reproducible data are an essential part of descriptive tests.[2] Descriptive testing is usually conducted by using a scorecard containing precise word descriptions that structure the form of the responses. Each of the characteristics of a sample to be evaluated is described over a range, and the panelist selects the specific description matching the sample for each item on the scorecard. The responsibility for selecting the appropriate vocabulary to elicit an accurate picture of the samples rests with the researcher who has developed the scorecard; a well-constructed scorecard will give the desired information.[2]

Innovative Point

Approaches to Descriptive Tests The four major approaches of descriptive tests are flavor profile, quantitative descriptive analysis, texture profile, and sensory spectrum.

Profiling is another approach to descriptive testing. To conduct **profiling**, a group of highly trained panelists work together to develop the vocabulary needed to provide specific descriptions of food samples. This technique is used to detail the specific flavors (flavor profiling) or textures (texture profiling) of a food or beverage.

Flavor Profile Analysis®

Flavor Profile Analysis (FPA) is based on the concept that flavor consists of identifiable taste, odor, and chemical-feel factors as well as an underlying complex of sensory impressions that are not separately identifiable.[28] Scientists at Arthur D. Little developed this technique in the late 1940s and early 1950s, and the name and the technique were trademarked to Arthur D. Little and Co.[2] The method is a qualitative descriptive test that involves formal procedures for describing and assessing the aroma, flavor, and aftertaste of a product in a reproducible manner. FPA is a consensus technique.[2] The vocabulary used to describe the sample and the sample evaluation itself are achieved by panel members who work together to come to an agreement.

Quantitative Descriptive Analysis®

Quantitative Descriptive Analysis (QDA) was developed during the 1970s to correct some of the perceived problems associated with FPA.[1,27] Unlike FPA data, QDA data are not generated through consensus discussion, and panel leaders are not active participants. Unstructured line scales are used to describe the intensity of rated sensory attributes. Stone et al.[27] chose the linear graphic scale, a line that extends beyond fixed verbal endpoints, based, in part, on earlier studies.[29]

In QDA, 10 to 12 panelists begin their training by generating a consensus vocabulary.[27] They are exposed to many possible variations of the product to facilitate the acquisition of an accurate concept, and the panel leader acts only as a facilitator by directing discussion and supplying materials such as references and other samples required by the panel.[2] The actual product evaluations are performed by each panelist individually, usually in an isolation booth.

Texture Profile Analysis®

Texture profile analysis (TPA) was developed by scientists working for General Foods during the 1960s and was subsequently modified by several sensory specialists.[30–35] The TPA uses a standardized terminology to describe textural characteristics by both their physical and sensory aspects.[2] Definitions and listing order of the terms are determined through consensus by the TPA panelists. The reference scales anchor both the range and the concept for each term.[35] The full range of a specific parameter by reference products helps panelists confirm the intensity increments within each scale. The use of the same reference frame is the key to a successful TPA. Sample preparation, presentation, and evaluation should be strictly controlled. Panelists should also be trained to bite, chew, and swallow in a standardized way.

Sensory Spectrum®

Gail Civille, who became a TPA expert at General Foods, subsequently created the Sensory Spectrum (SS) technique.[2] This technique is an expansion on descriptive analysis techniques. The unique characteristic of the SS technique is that panelists do not generate a panel-specific vocabulary to describe sensory attributes of products, but rather use a standardized word list (lexicon).[36] The terminology used to describe a particular product is chosen *a priori* and remains the same for all products within a category over time.[2] Because panelists are trained to use the scales in an identical manner, use of the SS technique should allow data from experiments that include only one sample to be compared against data from different samples used in other studies.

Panelist training for the SS technique is much more extensive than that for QDA, and the panel leader has a more directive role than in QDA.[2] Similar to the TPA, panelists are provided lexicons that are used to describe perceived sensations associated with the samples. The panelists use a numerical intensity scale—usually a 15-point scale—and they are supplied with reference standards.

Affective Tests

For a food product to be successful in the marketplace, consumers must prefer it over other products. Therefore, consumer panels often are used to indicate preference of one sample over another. The panelist rates his or her preference for one of the samples on a specific quality on the score sheet. Hedonic rating scales can be used to measure the degree of pleasure experienced with each sample. Sometimes, the frequency that a panelist might desire to eat the sample is measured as a way to determine the acceptability of the various samples.

Acceptance Tests

Acceptance tests involve rating the difference in acceptance between two samples. The following example shows an application of a rating acceptance test:

- *Situation:* A restaurant manager wishes to compare acceptance between two types of chocolate candies (products A and B). She wants to give the more-liked chocolate product as a customer appreciation present at the end of a meal.
- *Test objective:* The test objective is to determine which chocolate product is more liked.
- *Test design:* 20 panelists are asked to evaluate acceptance for the two chocolate products using 5-point hedonic scales. Two samples (coded with random three-digit numbers) are presented simultaneously at the same temperature. Half of the panelists test product A first; the other half test product B first.
- *Score sheet:* An example score sheet is shown in **Figure 3.10**.

Please taste each sample, and indicate how well you like it.

318 (A)			442 (B)		
______	Like very much	(5)	______	Like very much	(5)
______	Like moderately	(4)	______	Like moderately	(4)
______	Neutral	(3)	______	Neutral	(3)
______	Dislike moderately	(2)	______	Dislike moderately	(2)
______	Dislike very much	(1)	______	Dislike very much	(1)

Thank you!

FIGURE 3.10 Example of a 5-point acceptance score sheet.

- *Results and data analysis:* Product A has a higher acceptance rate than product B. The calculated *t*-value for the difference values exceeds the reference *t*-value and is statistically significant.
- *Conclusion:* Product A is selected as a consumer appreciation present because product A is significantly more acceptable than product B.

For detailed statistics regarding this example, see the Appendix at the end of this chapter.

Sometimes, rating acceptance tests involve more than two samples. The following is an example application of a rating acceptance test that uses multiple samples:

- *Situation:* A dietitian is developing gluten-free chocolate chip cookies prepared by replacing all-purpose flour with brown rice and chickpea flours.
- *Test objective:* The test objective is to determine whether the gluten-free chocolate chip cookies (100% brown rice flour, 50% brown rice/50% chickpea flour, and 100% chickpea flour) are sufficiently acceptable against 100% all-purpose flour cookies.
- *Test design:* A completely randomized design that compares all samples together using a rating scale is used. One hundred subjects evaluate the overall acceptability of four samples on a 9-point hedonic scale.
- *Score sheet:* An example score sheet is shown in **Figure 3.11**.
- *Results and analysis:* The 100% chickpea flour cookie product has a significantly higher acceptance rate than other gluten-free cookies (50% brown rice/50% chickpea flour cookies and 100% brown rice flour cookie products); however, there is no significant difference among the control (all-purpose flour) and 100% chickpea flour cookies.
- *Conclusion:* The 100% chickpea flour cookies are acceptable gluten-free alternatives to the conventional all-purpose flour cookie.

Taste each sample, and indicate how well you like it.

Sample code _______

☐ Like extremely
☐ Like very much
☐ Like moderately
☐ Like slightly
☐ Neither like nor dislike
☐ Dislike slightly
☐ Dislike moderately
☐ Dislike very much
☐ Dislike extremely

Thank you!

FIGURE 3.11 Example of a 9-point verbal hedonic scale sensory sheet.

For detailed statistics regarding this example, see the Appendix at the end of this chapter.

Preference Tests

The question of interest for the preference test is, "Which sample do you prefer?" The following example shows an application of a paired preference test:

- *Situation:* A caterer wants to know determine which brand of soft drink she should use. She wants to compare the preferences for two prospective products.
- *Test objective:* The test objective is to determine which soft drink product is preferred over the other product.
- *Test design:* One hundred subjects who are soft-drink drinkers are invited to a central location where the company caters. Two products (A and B) coded with three-digit random numbers are presented simultaneously at the same temperature. Half the participants receive the soft drinks in the order A–B, and the other half receive them in the order of B–A. The serving temperature and serving time after opening the containers are carefully controlled. (Both are particularly important variables to control for carbonated beverages.)
- *Score sheet:* An example score sheet is shown in **Figure 3.12**.

Taste the sample on the left first and the sample on the right second. Which one do you prefer? Please choose one.

337 ☐ 198 ☐

Thank you!

FIGURE 3.12 Example of paired preference score sheet.

- *Results and analysis:* The number (66) that chose sample A is larger than the critical value (61) at a level of statistical significance.
- *Conclusion:* There is a significant preference difference between soft drink products. The analyst recommends that the caterer serve soft drink product A.

For detailed statistics regarding this example, see the Appendix at the end of this chapter.

The final example in this chapter details the application of a ranking preference test:

- *Situation:* A school dietitian wishes to compare preferences for three different varieties of apples.
- *Test objective:* The test objective is to determine whether there is a significant difference in preference among three types of apples (products A, B, and C).
- *Test design:* The three samples are ranked by 100 panelists. Each panelist receives three samples coded with three-digit numbers and served in balanced, random order.
- *Score sheet:* An example score sheet is shown in **Figure 3.13**.
- *Results and analysis:* When compared to the minimum critical differences at $\alpha = 0.05$ (34), product B is preferred over products A and C. There is no significant preference difference between products A and C.
- *Conclusion:* It is recommended that the school serve apple B, which is preferred over apples A and C.

For detailed statistics regarding this example, see the Appendix at the end of this chapter.

Please taste each of the coded samples in the set in the sequence presented from left to right. Rank the three samples in descending order of preference. You may re-taste any of the samples while ranking for the preference. No ties are allowed in the ranking. Remember that the most preferred sample should be ranked 1.

Sample code ______ ______ ______
1 2 3

Thank you!

FIGURE 3.13 Example of a preference ranking score sheet.

Chapter Review

Sensory evaluation is a scientific testing method for accurate measurement of human responses as perceived by the five senses. Sensory evaluation is a vital part of food development because it is the essential means of determining how consumers will react to a food. Reliable sensory evaluation can be performed by optimizing four steps: definition of the problem, test design, instrumentation, and interpretation. People evaluate a particular food primarily based on how it looks, smells, tastes, sounds, and feels. The food attributes that are typically perceived through the human senses are appearance, odor, taste, flavor, consistency, and texture.

The environment in which the sensory test is conducted should be carefully controlled, and samples must be prepared and presented in a uniform fashion so as not to influence panelists' perception of the food's quality. Panelists who are well suited to the purpose of the sensory test should be selected and trained appropriately.

The two types of sensory tests are analytical and affective. Analytical tests are based on discernible differences, whereas affective tests are based on individual acceptability or preferences. Analytical tests are divided into two types of tests: difference tests (discriminative tests) and descriptive tests. Depending on the main task of the test, affective tests are either acceptance tests or preference tests. The primary task of acceptance tests is to rate the degree of liking, whereas with preference tests the goal is to identify the item that is more liked.

© ImageState

Learning Portfolio

Key Terms

	page
adaptation	87
affective tests	96
analytical tests	96
consumer panel	90
descriptive panel	90
descriptive tests	100
difference tests	96
duo-trio test	97
flavor	89
gustatory	87
hedonic scale	94
holding time	92
molecular gastronomy	85
mouthfeel	89
nutrigenomics	88
olfactory	86
paired comparison test	98
papillae	87
profiling	100
rating difference test	99
ranking test	98
sensory evaluation	84
taste buds	87
texture	90
triangle test	96
umami	89

Study Points

1. Sensory evaluation is a scientific testing method for accurate measurement of human responses as perceived by the five senses.
2. The food attributes that are typically perceived through the five senses are appearance, odor, taste, flavor, consistency, and texture.
3. The environment in which the sensory test is conducted, as well as sample preparation and presentation, should be carefully controlled so as not to bias the results of the test. Panelists who are well suited to the purpose of the sensory test should be selected and trained appropriately.
4. The two types of sensory tests are analytical and affective. Analytical tests are based on discernible differences, whereas affective tests are based on acceptability or preferences.
5. Analytical tests include difference tests (discriminative tests) and descriptive tests. The two types of difference tests are overall difference tests and attribute difference tests.
6. The triangle test is an overall difference test. In the triangle test, three samples are presented simultaneously; two samples are alike and one is different. Panelists are asked to indicate the odd sample. The chance of obtaining a correct answer by guessing is 33.3% (1 in 3) in the triangle test.
7. The duo-trio test is an overall difference test. In the duo-trio test, the reference sample is presented first; it is then followed by two other samples, one of which is the same as the reference. The judge is asked to identify which of the last two samples is same as or different from the reference. There is a 50% chance of being right by simply guessing in a duo-trio test.
8. The paired comparison test is an attribute difference test in which a specific characteristic is designated. The subject is asked to test the two samples presented to identify the sample with the greater amount of the characteristic being measured. The subject has a 50% chance of being right by chance alone.
9. Descriptive sensory tests are the most comprehensive and informative tools used in sensory evaluation. Descriptive tests require a well-trained panel and should never be used with consumers because consistent and reproducible data are an essential part of descriptive tests. Examples of descriptive tests include the Flavor Profile Analysis (FPA), Quantitative Descriptive Analysis (QDA), Texture Profile Analysis (TPA), and the Sensory Spectrum (SS) technique.
10. Affective tests include acceptance tests and preference tests. The primary task of acceptance testing is to rate the degree of liking, whereas the preference task seeks to identify the product that is liked more.

Issues for Discussion

1. Are sensory preferences due to genetic or environmental causes?
2. Should the food industry provide foods with preferred tastes that may be sugar and salt based or try to provide healthier foods, knowing that the taste sensations may not be what most consumers prefer? Is there an ethical choice?

Research Ideas for Students

1. Taste preferences of different ethnic groups and possible reasons for such differences
2. Taste preferences of cancer patients

References

1. Stone H, Sidel JL. *Sensory Evaluation Practices.* 3rd ed. San Diego, CA: Academic Press; 2004.
2. Lawless HT, Heymann H. *Sensory Evaluation of Food: Principles and Practices.* 2nd ed. New York: Springer; 2010.

3. Meiselman HL. Critical evaluation of sensory techniques. *Food Qual Pref.* 1993;4:33–40.
4. Pfenninger HB. Methods of quality control in brewing. *Schweizer Brauerei-Rundschau.* 1979;90:121.
5. Meilgaard MC, Civille GV, Carr BT. *Sensory Evaluation Techniques.* 4th ed. Boca Raton, FL: CRC Press; 2007.
6. Brown A. *Understanding Food: Principles and Preparation.* 3rd ed. Belmont, CA: Thompson-Wadsworth; 2008.
7. Maruniak JA. The sense of smell. In: Piggott JR (ed.). *Sensory Analysis of Foods.* 2nd ed. London: Elsevier; 1988.
8. McWilliams M. *Foods: Experimental Perspectives.* 6th ed. Upper Saddle River, NJ: Pearson/Prentice-Hall; 2008.
9. Kim UK, Jorgenson E, Coon H, et al. Positional cloning of the human quantitative trait locus underlying taste sensitivity to phenylthiocarbamide. *Science.* 2003;299(5610):1221–1225.
10. Blakeslee AF. Genetic of sensory thresholds: taste for phenylthiocarbamide. *ProcNatlAcadSci USA.* 1932:120–130.
11. Fox AL. The relationship between chemical constitution and taste. *Proc Natl Acad Sci USA.* 1932:115–120.
12. Lawless HT. A comparison of different methods for assessing sensitivity to the taste of phenylthiocarbamide PTC. *Chem Senses.* 1980;5:247–256.
13. Bartoshuk LM, Duffy VB, Miller IJ. PTC/PROP tasting: anatomy, psychophysics, and sex effects. *Physiol Behav.* 1994;56(6): 1165–1171.
14. Guo SW, Reed DR. The genetics of phenylthiocarbamide perception. *Ann Hum Biol.* 2001;28(2):111–142.
15. Tepper B, Nurse R. Fat perception is related to PROP taster status. *Physiol Behav.* 1997;61(6):949–954.
16. Reedy F Jr, Bartoshuk LM, Miller I, et al. Relationship among papillae, taste pores, and 6-n-propylthiouracil (PROP) suprathreshold taste sensitivity. [abstract]. *Chem Senses.* 1996;21:616.
17. Hosako NY, Lucchina LA, Synder DJ, et al. Number of fungiform papillae in non-tasters, medium tasters and supertasters of PROP (6-n-propylthiouracil). [abstract]. *Chem Senses.* 1996;21:616.
18. Duffy VB, Bartoshuk LM. Food acceptance and genetic variation in taste. *J Am DietAssoc.* 2000;100:647–655.
19. Duffy VB, Peterson JM, Dinehart ME, Bartoshuk LM. Genetic and environmental variation in taste. *Top Clin Nutr.* 2003;18(4): 209–220.
20. Godshall MA. How carbohydrates influence food flavor. *Food Tech.* 1997;51(1):62–67.
21. De Roos KB. How lipids influence food flavor. *Food Tech.* 1997;51(5):60–62.
22. Amerine MA, Pangborn RM, Roessler EB. *Principles of Sensory Evaluation of Food.* New York: Academic Press; 1965.
23. International Organization for Standardization (ISO). Sensory analysis-general guidance for the design of test rooms. In: International Standard ISO 8589. Geneva, Switzerland: International Organization for Standardization; 1998.
24. Lucak CL, Delwiche JF. Efficacy of various palate cleansers with representative foods. *Chemosensory Perception.* 2009;2:32–39.
25. Stevens SS. Mathematics, measurement and psychophysics. In: Stevens SS (ed.). *Handbook of Experimental Psychology.* New York: Wiley; 1951: 1–49.
26. Trochim WM. *Research Methods: The Concise Knowledge Base.* Cincinnati, OH: Atomic Dog Pub; 2005.
27. Stone H, Sidel J, Oliver S, et al. Sensory evaluation by quantitative descriptive analysis. *Food Tech.* 1974;28:24–29, 32, 34.
28. Hootman RC (ed.). *Manual on Descriptive Test for Sensory Evaluation.* ASTM Manual Series MNL 13. Philadelphia, PA: American Society for Testing and Materials; 1992.
29. Anderson NH. Functional measurement and psychological judgment. *Psych Rev.* 1970;153–170.
30. Brandt MA, Skinner EZ, Coleman JA. The texture profile method. *J Food Sci.* 1963;28:404–409.
31. Civille GV, Liska IH. Modifications and applications to foods of the general foods sensory texture profile technique. *J Texture Studies.* 1975;6:19–31.
32. Szczesniak AS. Texture measurements. *Food Tech.* 1966;20: 1292–1298.
33. Szczesniak AS. General foods texture profile revisited—Ten years perspective. *J Texture Studies.* 1975; 6:5–17.
34. Szczesniak AS. Classifications of textural characteristics. *J Food Sci.* 1963;28:385–389.
35. Szczesniak AS, Brandt MA, Friedman HH. Development of standard rating scales for mechanical parameters of texture and correlation between the objective and the sensory methods of texture evaluation. *J Food Sci.* 1963;28:397–403.
36. Civille GV, Lyon B. *ASTM Lexicon Vocabulary for Descriptive Analysis.* Philadelphia, PA: American Society for Testing and Materials; 1996.

Appendix

Sensory Evaluation

Data Analysis for the Triangle Test

Step 1: Refer to the reference minimum number of correct responses for the triangle test.[1]

- *Application*: Because the number of panelists (trials) in this example is 48, the minimum number of correct responses corresponding to the probability level of 0.05 is 22.[1]

Step 2: Count the number of panelists who correctly identified the odd sample.

- *Application*: Out of 48 panelists, 25 correctly chose the odd sample.

Step 3: If the value (step 2) is same or larger than the reference value (step 1), we can say that the panelists could detect a significant difference between the samples at a probability of 5%.

- *Application*: The value (25) from step 2 is larger than the reference value. Therefore, the panelists could detect a difference between samples.

Data Analysis for the Duo-Trio Test

Step 1: Refer to the critical number of correct responses in the duo-trio test.[1]

- *Application*: Because the number of panelists (trials) in this example is 40, the critical number of correct responses corresponding to the probability level of 0.05 is 26.[1]

Step 2: Count the number of panelists who correctly matched the sample to the reference.

- *Application*: Out of 40 panelists, 13 correctly matched the sample to the reference.

Step 3: If the value (step 2) is the same or larger than the table value (step 1), we can say that the panelists could detect a significant difference between the samples at a probability of 5%.

- *Application*: The value (13) from step 2 is smaller than the reference value. Therefore, the panelists could not detect a difference between samples.

Data Analysis for the Paired Comparison Test

Step 1: Refer to the reference minimum number of correct judgments for the paired comparison test.[1]

- *Application*: In our case, the number of trials is 28 and the probability level is 0.05. The reference value is 19.[1]

Step 2: Count the number of panelists who chose sample A or B, respectively.

- *Application*: Six panelists chose sample 796 (cookie A, the original) as the sweeter sample and 22 panelists chose sample 308 (cookie B, the new one).

Step 3: If the value (step 2) is the same or larger than the reference value (step 1), we can say that the sample that was chosen more often is significantly different (sweeter) than the other sample.

- *Application*: The value (22) from step 2 is larger than the table value (19). Therefore, the panelists could detect a difference in sweetness between samples.

Data Analysis for the Ranking Test

The ranking data can be analyzed either by using the Basker's tables[2] or those by Newell and MacFarlane.[3] This analysis used a reworked table[1] from Newell and MacFarlane's.[3] **Table A** shows how the results are organized. The ranks are summed, and the differences between sums are compared to the critical values in the table. From the table in the reference, the corresponding number of samples on the horizontal axis (in our example, 3 samples) and the number of panelists from the vertical axis (in our example, 28 panelists) are selected. The number where the two points cross will be the critical values for the difference. In our case, the critical value is 18. If the difference of sum of their rank between each pair of samples is greater than the critical value, it is considered that the samples are significantly different in saltiness.

TABLE A
Results of the Ranking Test for the Saltiness of Three Types of Cheeses

Panelist No.	*A* (183, Mozzarella)	*B* (479, Cheddar)	*C* (862, Provolone)
1	3	2	1
2	3	2	1
3	2	3	1
4	2	1	3
5	1	2	3
6	3	1	2
7	3	2	1
8	2	1	3
9	2	1	3
10	2	3	1
11	2	1	3
12	2	1	3
13	2	1	3
14	1	3	2
15	2	1	3
16	2	1	3
17	3	2	1
18	3	2	1
19	2	1	3
20	2	3	1
21	3	1	2

(*continues*)

TABLE A
Results of the Ranking Test for the Saltiness of Three Types of Cheeses (*continued*)

Panelist No.	*A* (183, Mozzarella)	*B* (479, Cheddar)	*C* (862, Provolone)
22	1	2	3
23	1	2	3
24	3	1	2
25	1	2	3
26	3	1	2
27	3	1	2
28	3	2	1
Column sum	62	46	60
Differences	*A* vs. *B* = 16	*B* vs. *C* = 14	*A* vs. *C* = 2

Data Analysis for the Rating Difference Test

The data is evaluated by one-way analysis of variance (ANOVA). There are 4 treatments and 12 observations per treatment (see **Table B**). Because the *F*-value (26.65) is very significant ($P < 0.0001$) (see **Table C**), there are significant differences between treatments.

TABLE B
Results of the Rating Test for the Moistness of Four Types of Pound Cake

Panelist No.	Treatment			
	0% Applesauce (Control)	33% Applesauce	66% Applesauce	100% Applesauce
1	9	8	8	5
2	8	8	7	6
3	9	7	7	4
4	6	5	5	3
5	7	8	6	5
6	8	9	8	5
7	9	7	7	5
8	9	8	8	4
9	8	7	8	4
10	7	8	7	5
11	7	6	6	5
12	7	8	8	4

TABLE C
Completely Randomized Design One-Way Analysis of Variance of Results in Table B

Source of Variation	Sum of Squares	Degree of Freedom	Mean Square	*F*-value	*P*-value
Treatments	77.06	3	25.69	26.65	< 0.0001
Error	42.42	44	0.96		
Total	119.48	47			

To determine which samples are significantly different, perform a Tukey Honestly Significant Difference (HSD) multiple comparison test. The results are as follows:

Control, 0% applesauce	7.83b
33% applesauce	7.42b
66% applesauce	7.08b
100% applesauce	4.58a

Data Analysis for the Affective Test: Chocolate Candies

The result of the acceptance test for two types of chocolate candies and the *t*-value calculation are shown in **Table D**. In this case, the critical *t*-value (degree of freedom = 19) from the Student's *t*-distribution table at $\alpha = 0.05$ is 2.093 (a student's *t*-distribution table can be found in most statistics books or online [see http://www.itl.nist.gov/div898/handbook/eda/section3/eda3672.htm]). Because the calculated *t*-value (2.62) is larger than the reference *t*-value, a significant acceptance difference exists between the samples.

TABLE D
Results of the Acceptance Test for Two Types of Chocolate Candies

Panelist	Original (*A*)	Modified (*B*)	Difference ($A - B = D$)	D^2
1	4	4	0	0
2	5	3	2	4
3	3	3	0	0
4	4	2	2	4
5	4	3	1	1
6	4	3	1	1
7	3	4	−1	1
8	4	4	0	0
9	5	3	2	4
10	4	4	0	0
11	3	3	0	0
12	5	4	1	1
13	4	2	2	4
14	3	3	0	0
15	4	4	0	0
16	5	4	1	1
17	4	5	−1	1
18	5	4	1	1
19	3	3	0	0
20	5	5	0	0
Sum	81	70	11	23

Sum of $D = 11$, Mean of $D = 0.55$, Sum of $D^2 = \sum D^2 = 23$

$$\sqrt{\frac{\sum D^2 - (\sum D)^2/N}{N - 1}}$$

Standard deviation (SD) of $D =$

$$\sqrt{\frac{23 - (121/20)}{20 - 1}} = \sqrt{\frac{23 - 6.05}{19}} = \sqrt{\frac{16.95}{19}} = \sqrt{0.892} = 0.94$$

Standard error (SE) of $D =$ SD of $D/\sqrt{N} = 0.94/\sqrt{20} = 0.94/4.47 = 0.21$

$t =$ Mean of D/SE of $D = 0.55/0.21 = 2.62$

Data Analysis for the Affective Test: Cookie Formulations

The result of one-way analysis of variance for the overall acceptance of gluten-free cookies is shown in **Table E**.

TABLE E
Completely Randomized Design One-Way Analysis of Variance for the Overall Acceptance of Gluten-Free Cookies

Source of Variation	Sum of Squares	Degree of Freedom	Mean Square	*F*-value	π-value
Treatments	968.84	3	322.95	439.23	< 0.0001
Error	291.16	396	0.74		
Total	1260.00	399			

Because the *F*-value is statistically significant, there are significant differences among treatments. Therefore, the Tukey Honestly Significant Difference (HSD) Post-hoc test was performed. The results of the Tukey HSD test are as follows:

Control, 100% all-purpose flour cookies	7.87c
100% brown rice flour cookies	4.21a
50% brown rice/50% chickpea flour cookies	6.57b
100% chickpea flour cookies	8.15c

Data Analysis from the Paired Preference Test

Step 1: Refer to the reference minimum number of agreeing judgments for the paired preference test.[2]

- *Application:* In our case, the number of trials is 100, and the probability level is 0.05. The critical reference value is 61.[1]

Step 2: Count the number of subjects who chose sample *A* or *B*, respectively.

- *Application*: 66 subjects chose sample 337 (soft drink *A*) as the preferred sample and 34 panelists chose sample 108 (soft drink *B*).

Step 3: If the value (step 2) is same or larger than the critical value (step 1), we can say the sample that was chosen more is significantly preferred over the other sample.

Data Analysis for Ranking Preference Test

Ranks are added, and the differences between the sums are compared to the critical reference value.[1] Similar to the data analysis for the difference ranking test, select the corresponding number of samples on the horizontal axis and then select the number of panelists from the vertical axis in the reference table.[1] Find the number where the two points cross. In this example, because 100 panelists ranked three products, the critical value is 34.[1] If the difference of the rank sum between each pair of samples is greater than the critical value, then the samples are significantly different in preference. Because the rank scale used was 1 = preferred most and 3 = preferred least, the smallest rank sum means that that the product is the most preferred.

In **Table F**, because the differences of rank sum between product *B* and the other products (*A* and *B*, *B* and *C*) are larger than the critical value (34), product *B* is significantly preferred over the other products.

TABLE F
Results of the Ranking Preference Test for Three Varieties of Apples

	908 (*A*)	144 (*B*)	862 (*C*)
Rank sum	216b	164a	220b
Differences	*A* vs. *B* = 52	*B* vs. *C* = 56	*A* vs. *C* = 4

References

1. Lawless HT, Heymann H. *Sensory Evaluation of Food: Principles and Practices.* 2nd ed. New York: Springer; 2010: 563, 565, 566.
2. Basker D. Critical values of differences among rank sums for multiple comparisons. *Food Tech.* 1988 July:88–89.
3. Newell GJ, MacFarlane JD. Expanded tables for multiple comparison procedures in the analysis of ranked data. *J Food Sci.* 1987;52:1721–1725.

CHAPTER 4

Food Composition

Lalitha Samuel, PhD

Chapter Objectives

THE STUDENT WILL BE EMPOWERED TO:

- Explain the structure, properties, and functions of water in foods.
- Classify carbohydrates, and explain their functions in foods.
- Briefly discuss starch gelatinization, and identify factors that influence the quality of starch pastes and gels.
- Explain the structure of triglycerides, and identify saturated and unsaturated fatty acids, omega-3 and omega-6 fatty acids, and cis and trans double bonds.
- Explain the role of triglycerides in food processing.
- Discuss the hierarchy of protein organization with regard to its role in food processing.
- Differentiate between enzymatic and nonenzymatic browning.
- Explain the stability of vitamins and minerals in processed foods.

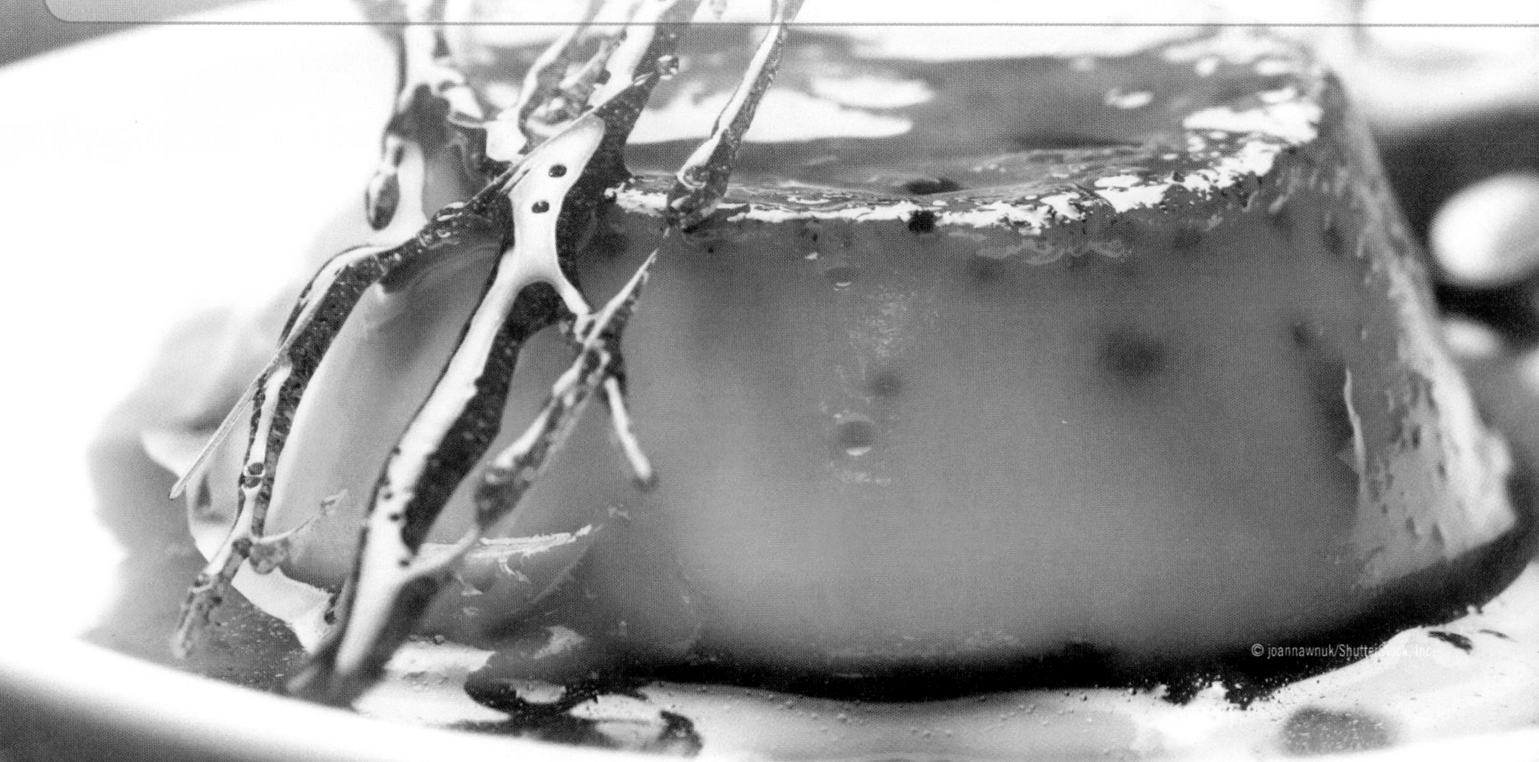

Food Composition

Throughout the history of humankind, food has been consumed for its nutritive value. The nutritive value of a food is derived from its composition. Although the energy content of foods is largely derived from carbohydrates, fats, and proteins, the vitamins and minerals present in foods are critical to the optimal functioning of the energy-yielding pathways in our bodies. Food composition is critical not only because of its nutritive value, but also because of its physical, chemical, and biological properties. For example, the water content of foods plays a vital role in their sensory properties and shelf life. This chapter discusses water, carbohydrates, lipids, proteins, vitamins, and minerals from a functional perspective, including their role in the nutritive, sensory, preservative, and processing aspects of foods.

Researchers also have identified the role of certain foods in disease prevention. In the last decade, plant foods have taken a new role as vehicles of disease prevention due to their myriad phytonutrients, as discussed in **Special Topic 4.1**. **Special Topic 4.2** discusses the regulation of health claims surrounding phytonutrients.

Special Topic 4.1

Phytonutrients and Functional Foods

Lalitha Samuel, PhD

phytonutrients Non-nutritive chemicals derived from plants that may play a role in disease prevention and human health. Also known as *phytochemicals*.

Simply put, **phytonutrients** (or *phytochemicals*) are non-nutritive chemicals derived from plants. Unlike carbohydrates, fats, proteins, vitamins, and minerals, phytonutrients are not essential for life; however, they can promote good health. They are found in vegetables and fruits, whole grains, herbs, teas, and spices. A summary of some of various phytochemicals and their food sources is provided in **Table A**.

TABLE A
Phytochemicals Found in Different Plant-Based Foods

Phytonutrient	Food Sources
Anthocyanidins	Berries, cherries, red grapes
Beta-carotene	Carrots, various fruits
Caffeic acid, ferulic acid	Apples, pears, citrus fruits, some vegetables
Diallyl sulfide, allyl methyl trisulfide	Garlic, onions, leeks, scallions
Dithiolthiones	Cruciferous vegetables such as broccoli, cabbage, bok choy, collard greens
Flavanols (catechins, epicatechins, procyanidins)	Tea, cocoa, chocolate, apples, grapes
Flavanones	Citrus fruits
Flavonols	Onions, apples, tea, broccoli
Lutein, zeaxanthin	Kale, collard greens, spinach, corn, citrus fruits
Lycopene	Tomatoes, processed tomato products
Proanthocyanidins	Cranberries, cocoa, apples, strawberries, grapes, wine, peanuts, cinnamon
Sulforaphane	Cauliflower, broccoli, Brussels sprouts, cabbage, kale, horseradish

Source: Adapted from Newell-McGloughlin M. Impact of biotechnology on food supply and quality. In: Damodaran S, Parkin KL, Fennema, OL, eds. *Food Chemistry.* Boca Raton, FL. CRC Press; 2008:1076–1077.

Phytonutrients include carotenoids, flavonoids, isothiocyanates, phenolic compounds, phytosterols, phytoestrogen, and sulfides (thiols). They may positively influence health through a number of different mechanisms:

- By quenching free radicals and protecting against oxidation, carotenoids, flavonoids, isothiocyanates, and phenols may help prevent cardiovascular diseases, cancer, and neurodegenerative diseases such as Alzheimer's disease.[1–3] The protective effects of fruits, vegetables, and whole grains against these diseases has been attributed to the antioxidants found in these foods.
- Carotenoids such as lutein and zeaxanthin have been associated with a lower incidence of age-related macular degeneration.[4]
- Flavonoids have been researched widely for their protective effect against cancers, mostly through their modulation of cell-signaling pathways; inhibition of cancer cell proliferation, tumor invasion, and angiogenesis; and anti-inflammatory effects.[5–9] Flavonoids from cranberries have been researched extensively for their ability to prevent *Helicobacter pylori*–induced stomach ulcers and cancers.[10,11]

The effect of processing on the phytochemical content of foods has been a hot topic for research. Here are some of the findings:

- The phytochemicals in red apples are strong antioxidants, but processing of apples decreases the amount of phenols present in the juice. The phenolic compounds are retained in the pomace (the squashed fruit that remains after pressing). The pomace can then be used as a value-added ingredient with potent antioxidant activity.[1]
- The flavonoid content of tea is minimally affected by processing.[12]
- Lycopene, a heat-stable carotenoid in tomatoes, becomes concentrated when processed into sauces and pastes.[13,14]
- Fermented soybean seeds do not have as many isoflavones or saponins compared to unfermented seeds.[15,16]
- The bulk of the phytochemicals in cereal grains is localized in the bran and germ layers; processed cereals and flours can lose up to 99% of their phytochemical content.

Although myriad phytochemicals have been isolated from foods, their ability to prevent disease appears to be maximized when they are consumed in whole foods rather than in extracts. Within the intact fruit or vegetable, phytochemicals offer protection against free radicals, insect infestation, and ultraviolet rays from the sun. The weight of evidence in favor of the health-promoting and disease-preventing effects of whole fruits and vegetables has been the driving force for the introduction of the "5 a Day" program by the Centers for Disease Control and Prevention (CDC).

A **functional food** is one that provides a health benefit beyond basic nutrition. Foods containing phytochemicals are all functional foods. Functional foods can fall into any of the following categories:

functional food Food or food component that offers health benefits beyond basic nutrition.

- Whole foods with naturally high concentrations of phytonutrients (e.g., carrots and oatmeal)
- Whole foods that have enhanced levels of selected bioactive compounds through the following methods:
  - Genetic engineering (e.g., tomatoes that have been genetically altered to have a higher lycopene content)
  - Traditional breeding (e.g., oats bred through artificial selection to have higher amounts of beta-glucans)
  - Specialized livestock feeding (e.g., incorporating flaxseed into chicken feed to produce eggs with higher amounts of omega-3 fatty acids)
- Purified extracts of bioactive compounds (e.g., garlic capsules, fish oil capsules, soy isoflavone extracts)
- Processed foods with added bioactive components (e.g., orange juice fortified with calcium and vegetable-based spreads with added phytosterols and omega-3 fatty acids)

The Academy of Nutrition and Dietetics states that regular consumption of functional foods has potential beneficial health effects.[17] However, despite the high sales success of functional foods, caution is needed because research pertaining to the safety limits for most phytochemicals is still its infancy. The optimal levels for consumption of different phytochemicals have yet to be established. Some animal studies indicate that high concentrations isothiocyanates may induce cancer, whereas lower concentrations have been shown to be protective against the development of cancer.[18] Similarly, soy phytoestrogens have been found to be a double-edged sword. The bioactive compound in soy phytoestrogens, genistein, has been shown to increase bone mineral density and act as an antioxidant and to also stimulate some types of tumorigenic activity.[18,19]

References

1 Boyer JJ, Liu RH. Apple phytochemicals and their health benefits. *Nutr J.* 2004;3:5.

2 Singh RP, Sharad S, Kapur S. Free radicals and oxidative stress in neurodegenerative diseases: Relevance of dietary antioxidants. *J Ind Acad Clin Med.* 2004;5(3):218–225.

3 Spector A. Review: Oxidative stress and disease. *J Ocol Pharmacol Ther.* 2000;16(2):193–201.

4 Stahl W. Macular carotenoids: Lutein and zeaxanthin. *Dev Ophthalmol.* 2005;38:70–88.

5 Ramos S. Effects of dietary flavonoids on apoptotic pathways related to cancer chemoprevention. *J Nutr Biochem.* 2007;18(7):427–442.

6 Bagli E, Stefaniotou M, Morbidelli L, et al. Luteolin inhibits vascular endothelial growth factor-induced angiogenesis: Inhibition of endothelial cell survival and proliferation by targeting phosphatidylinositol 3'-kinase activity. *Cancer Res.* 2004;64(21):7936–7946.

7 Kim MH. Flavonoids inhibit VEGF/bFGF-induced angiogenesis in vitro by inhibiting the matrix-degrading proteases. *J Cell Biochem.* 2003;89(3):529–538.

8 O'Leary KA, de Pascual-Tereasa S, Needs PW, et al. Effect of flavonoids and vitamin E on cyclooxygenase-2 (COX-2) transcription. *Mutat Res.* 2004;551(1–2):245–254.

9 Williams RJ, Spencer JP, Rice-Evans C. Flavonoids: Antioxidants or signaling molecules? *Free Radic Biol Med.* 2004;36(7):838–849.

10 Burger O, Ofek I, Tabak M. A high molecular mass constituent of cranberry juice inhibits *Helicobacter pylori* adhesion to human gastric mucus. *FEMS Immunol Med Microbiol.* 2000;29:295–301.

11 Shmuely H, Yahav J, Samra Z, et al. Effect of cranberry juice on eradication of *Helicobacter pylori* in patients treated with antibiotics and a proton pump inhibitor. *Mol Nutr Food Res.* 2007;51(6):746–751.

12 Balentine DA, Paetau-Robinson I. Tea as a source of dietary antioxidants with a potential role in prevention of chronic diseases. In: Mazza G, Oomah BD (eds.). *Herbs, Botanicals, & Teas.* Lancaster, PA: Technomic Publishing; 2000: 265–287.

13 Agarwal A, Shen H, Agarwal S, Rao AV. Lycopene content of tomato products: Its stability, bioavailability and in vivo antioxidant properties. *J Medicinal Food.* 2001;4(1):9–15.

14 Dewanto V, Wu X, Adom KK, Liu RH. Thermal processing enhances the nutritional value of tomatoes by increasing total antioxidant activity. *J Agric Food Chem.* 2002;50(10):3010–3014.

15 Coward L, Barnes NC, Setchell KDR, Barnes S. Genistein, daidzein, and their beta-glycoside conjugates: Antitumor isoflavones in soybean foods from American and Asian diets. *J Agric Food Chem.* 1993;41(11):1961–1967.

16 Fenwick DE, Oakenfull D. Saponin content of soya beans and some commercial soya bean products. *J Sci Food Agric.*1981;32:273–278.

17 Academy of Nutrition and Dietetics. Position of the American Dietetic Association: Functional foods. *J Am Diet Assoc.* 2009;109(4):735–746.

18 Hasler CM. Functional foods: Their role in disease prevention and health promotion. *Food Tech.* 1998;52(2):57–62.

19 Rao CV, Wang CX, Simi B, et al. Enhancement of experimental colon cancer by genistein. *Cancer Res.* 1997;57:3717–3722.

Special Topic 4.2

Government Regulation of Phytonutrient Health Claims

Allison Mulvaney

Food shoppers today are bombarded with thousands of food products from which to choose. Many of these products come with advertisements and nutritional claims designed to grab our attention and influence our purchasing. As the relationship between food and chronic disease becomes more evident, more food and beverage manufacturers are promoting their products as having health benefits. How are we to interpret all these claims? The regulation of health claims involving nutrients and phytochemicals is controlled by the U.S. government. These health claims often reach beyond nutrition, entering the world of government policy and litigation.

The Food and Drug Administration (FDA) is a federal agency that oversees multiple aspects of the food, beverage, and supplement industry. One of the FDA's responsibilities is to assess the validity of nutrient and health claims made by manufacturers on product packaging. Manufacturers are governed by the food-labeling guide produced by the FDA in Title 21 of the Code of Federal Regulations.[1] Title 21 provides the guidelines that are used to authorize and regulate food claims. The FDA distinguishes between three different types of food claims: nutrient content claims, health claims, and structure/function claims.

Nutrient content claims are focused on the amount or level of a specific nutrient in a food.[1] Nutrient content claims are usually characterized by descriptive words such as *high* or *good source*. For example, the phrase *high in fiber* is a nutrient content claim. The use of nutrient content claims is governed by strict guidelines defining the descriptive terms used. Its use is usually based on the established % Daily Value (%DV) and the Reference Amount Customarily Consumed (RACC).[2] For instance, for a food nutrient content claim to state that a food is high in or an excellent source of a nutrient, it must contain at least 20% or more of the %DV per RACC. A good source only needs to contain 10–19% of the %DV per RACC, and a food that is labeled as fortified or enriched must have a minimum of 10% of the %DV per RACC.

Nutrient content claim guidelines also dictate the use of terms such as *free*, *low*, and *reduced*. These have separate requirements for total calories, total fat, saturated fat, cholesterol, sodium, and sugar. For nutrients that do not have a set %DV, such as omega-3 fatty acids, manufacturers may advertise the specific amount of the nutrient that the product contains; for example, "contains 4 grams of omega-3 fatty acids."[2]

The regulations are not without their flaws. For example, manufacturers are allowed to advertise products as having no trans fats if there is less than 0.50 grams of trans fat per serving.[2] By decreasing the serving size, a manufacturer can offer a product that contains trans fats but advertise it as having none. For instance, suppose a consumer buys a box of cookies in which the serving size is one cookie. If each cookie contains 0.45 grams of trans fat, then it qualifies as being free of trans fat according to the FDA guidelines. Unfortunately, after the consumer eats five cookies, he or she has just consumed 2.25 grams of trans fat from a container that advertises that it has no trans fat. By reading the ingredients list, consumers can look for discrepancies. In the trans fat example, a consumer who notes that partially or fully hydrogenated oil is listed in the ingredients would be alerted that the product does actually contain trans fats.

Health claims directly relate the food substance to its effect on a specific disease or health condition.[2] This means that the claim must relate to some type of illness, such as the prevention of cancer or heart disease. Prior to any health claim being permitted for use, the FDA will conduct a review of the available scientific literature to confirm its validity. The FDA recognizes that diseases such as cancer can have many different forms affecting different areas of the body and that they can be caused by different factors. Therefore, claims must be specific to the exact health conditions they are asserting to benefit so that the FDA can tailor its research review to substantiate the particular claim. For example, a cereal manufacturer may state that "soluble fiber, as part of a diet low in saturated fat and cholesterol, may reduce the risk of heart disease." Because the FDA has previously approved health claims regarding soluble fiber and heart disease, the manufacturer may use the claim. Examples of other health claims that have been approved by the FDA are the relationship between calcium and osteoporosis, sodium and hypertension, and folate and neural tube defects.[2]

Qualified health claims have been permitted by the FDA since 2003 for use on foods and supplements as part of the Consumer Health Information for Better Nutrition Initiative.[2] Qualified health claims have not been held to the same scientific standards as authorized health claims, but they are permitted to provide consumers more information about the foods they are purchasing. The basis behind allowing qualified health claims on products is that the more information consumers have available, the more informed choices they can make.

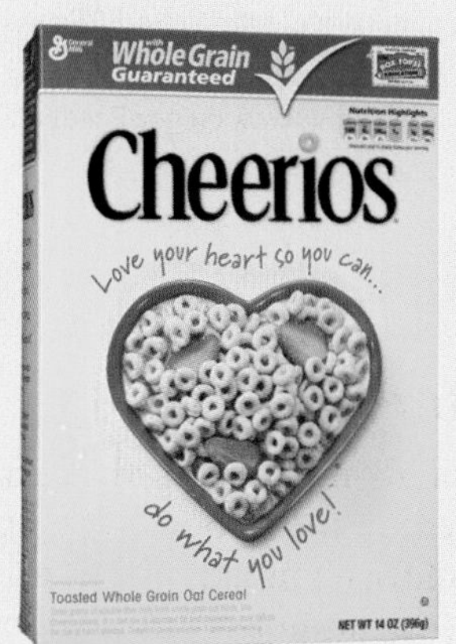

© smartstock/iStockphoto.com

According to Title 21, food manufacturers cannot make unsubstantiated health claims on product packages. But even when the health claim is backed up by research, manufacturers must be careful in how they make their claim. For example, in May 2009 the FDA issued a letter to General Mills about its claims that Cheerios can lower cholesterol by 4% percent in less than 2 months. The FDA said that this claim was similar to a drug claim.

Qualified health claims that have been approved include claims on the relationship between green tea and cancer, eicosapentaenoic acid (EPA) and docosahexaenoic acid (DHA) omega-3 fatty acids and coronary heart disease, and walnuts and heart disease.[2] Although there is some scientific research to support these claims, it is not as conclusive as the research supporting an authorized health claim.

For a manufacturer to use a qualified health claim on a product, it must first petition the FDA for approval. When a qualified nutrient claim is petitioned to the FDA, the FDA will perform a literature review and then rule on the claim. The timeline for a petition is as follows: within 15 days of submission the FDA will acknowledge the petition for a qualified health claim. The FDA will then file the petition within 45 days of being received and assign it a docket number. After the petition is assigned a docket number it becomes available for public comment via the Federal Dockets Management System website. At this time, the public can access the docket and submit commentary during a 60-day open period. Lastly, the FDA will take into account all scientific evidence available regarding the qualified health claim, as well as the public commentary, and formulate a decision on the petition. If a decision is not reached within 270 days of the initial receipt, the qualified health claim is automatically passed.[2]

Many qualified health claims are made with regard to phytonutrients. When such a health claim is made, it needs to identify the specific phytonutrient as well as the food products that contain the nutrient.[1] In 2005, manufacturers petitioned the FDA to allow claims stating that lycopene in tomatoes and tomato-based products had an effect on certain types of cancers. The FDA did not find significant scientific evidence to support the claim as an authorized health claim, although the FDA does allow it as a qualified health claim.[2] As technology advances and research continues on phytonutrients, health claims will continue to be a critical topic in terms of affecting both public health and revenue for food and beverage producers.

Structure/function claims are the least regulated type of claim. These claims are often found on a food package or supplement bottle with the intent of explaining how the product affects structures and/or functions of the human body.[2] Structure/function claims are required by law to include a disclaimer, such as "This statement has not been evaluated by the Food and Drug Administration. This product is not intended to diagnose, treat, cure, or prevent any disease."[2] This disclaimer stems from the Dietary Supplement Health and Education Act of 1994 which seeks to distinguish between supplements and drugs because a drug is specifically intended to treat and cure disease.[2]

Structure/function claims are broader than nutrient content claims and health claims, and they do not mention any relationship between the food product and a specific disease. For example, "builds strong bones" or "slows aging" are structure/function claims. In addition to the required disclaimer, a structure/function claim must be truthful and not misleading.

The FDA requires that any manufacturer who prints a structure/function claim on a product submit a copy of the claim to the FDA within 30 days of manufacturing. Unfortunately, this means that the general public is the first to view these claims, not the FDA, culminating in a largely unregulated supplement market.[2]

References

1 U.S. Department of Health and Human Services, U.S. Food and Drug Administration. *Code of Federal Regulations.* 21 CFR101.9–101.14. Revised April 2010. Available at http://www.accessdata.fda.gov/scripts/cdrh/cfdocs/cfcfr/CFRSearch.cfm?CFRPart=101. Accessed February 28, 2011.

2 U.S. Department of Health and Human Services, U.S. Food and Drug Administration. *Guidance for Industry: A Food Labeling Guide.* September 1994; revised April 2008; revised October 2009. Available at: http://www.fda.gov/FoodLabelingGuide. Accessed February 28, 2011.

Water

Although not always thought about as such, water is the most abundant nutrient in most foods. The fluid component in intra- and extracellular fluids is comprised mostly of water. The moisture content of foods can range from zero (e.g., as in lard and oil) to over 90% (e.g., as in cucumbers and tomatoes) (see **Figure 4.1**). For a particular food item, processing can significantly alter moisture content. For example, raw grapes are about 81% water; grape drinks have about 88% water; and raisins have only about 15%.

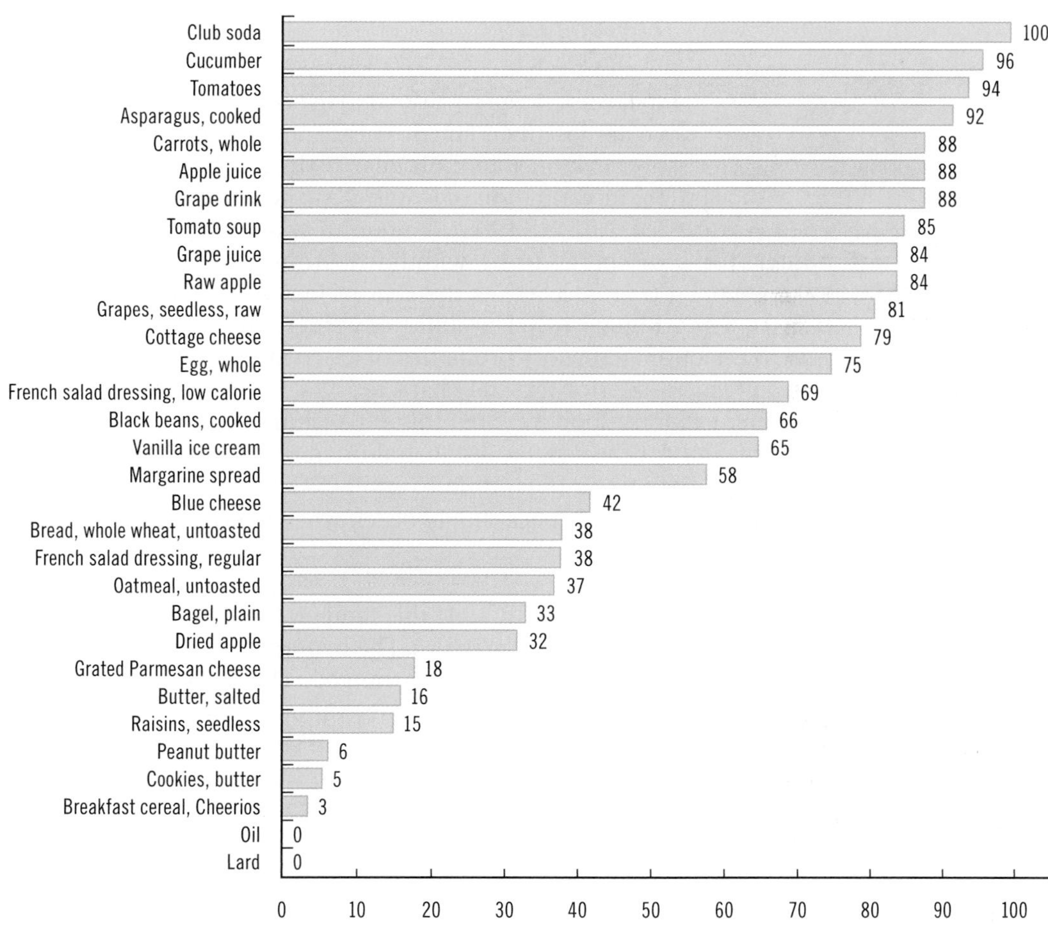

FIGURE 4.1 As shown in this graph, the moisture content of food ranges widely.

Source: Data from Gebhardt SE, Thomas RG. Nutritive value of foods. U.S. Department of Agriculture, Agricultural Research Service. *Home and Garden Bulletin.* 2002;72. Available at: http://www.ars.usda.gov/SP2UserFiles/Place/12354500/Data/hg72/hg72_2002.pdf. Accessed January 3, 2011.

Physical and Chemical Properties of Water

Water is a compound; each water molecule consists of two atoms of hydrogen covalently bonded with one oxygen atom. The H–O–H bonding angle is almost 105 degrees, giving the molecule a polar structure, as shown in **Figure 4.2A**. Although the molecule is polar, it is neutral in charge. Electrostatic attractions between the partially negative oxygen atom of one water molecule and the partially positive hydrogen atoms of a neighboring water molecule result in the formation of hydrogen bonds (see **Figure 4.2B**).

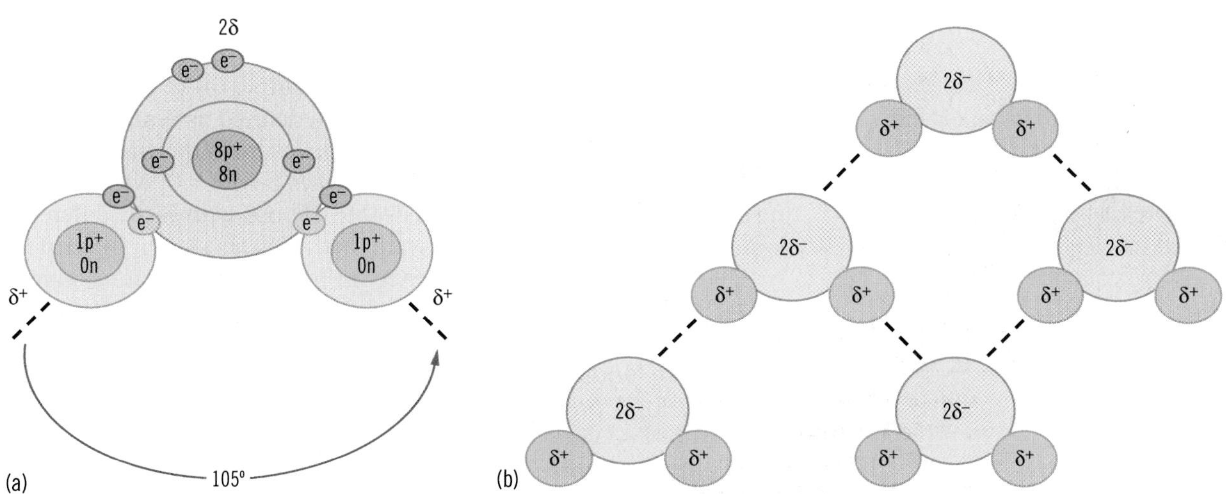

FIGURE 4.2 (a) Water is a polar and yet neutral compound, with an H–O–H bond angle of 105°. (b) Hydrogen bonds arise as a result of weak interactions between the slightly positively charged hydrogen atom of one water molecule with the slightly electronegative oxygen of another water molecule.

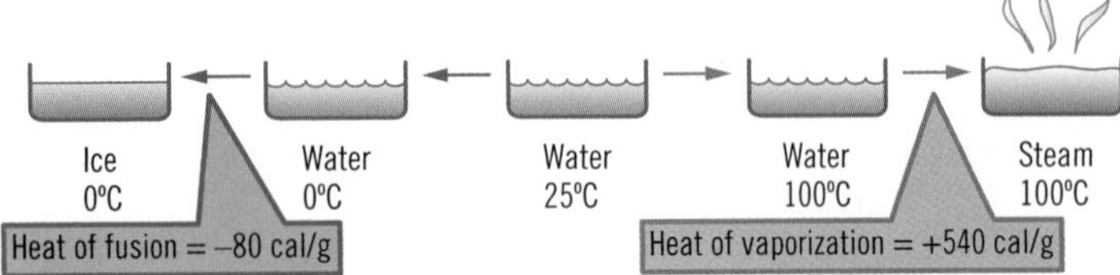

FIGURE 4.3 Water changes phase depending on the temperature and energy transfer. At 32°F (0°C), 80 calories must be lost to convert 1 gram of water into ice. At the other end of the temperature scale, at 212°F (100°C) 540 calories of energy is required to convert 1 gram of water into steam.

Freezing Point

At atmospheric pressure, water freezes at 32°F (0°C). As the temperature is lowered to the freezing point, water molecules lose their kinetic energy, move closer to each other, and exhibit intermolecular hydrogen bonding, resulting in the formation of a crystalline network that we know as ice. At 32°F (0°C), 1 gram of water requires 80 calories of energy to be withdrawn from it to convert into ice. This is called as the *heat of fusion* or *solidification* (see **Figure 4.3**). The ability of water to freeze into fine crystals is critical to the optimal sensory properties of ice cream. Conversely, large ice crystals can lead to inferior textural characteristics in frozen fruits and vegetables. Water expands upon freezing; this expansion of the crystalline structure is responsible for the cellular disintegration in frozen produce. Similarly, containers filled with water often rupture upon freezing due to the expansive nature of ice. Sufficient headspace should be left when freezing aqueous foods.

Boiling Point

Pure water boils at 212°F (100°C). At this temperature, the vapor pressure of water equals the atmospheric pressure. The hydrogen bonds between and among the water molecules become rearranged. The molecules can then escape from the surface, changing into water vapor, or steam. The amount of energy required to change 1 gram of water into steam is called the *heat of vaporization* and is equal to 540 calories. It is this high energy that accounts for the faster cooking time of steam as compared to liquid water.

The atmospheric pressure is lower at higher altitudes. Thus, water molecules encounter less resistance to transition to the gaseous phase, which reduces the boiling point. This is why cooking by boiling takes a longer time in mountainous regions or areas at high elevation. The decrease in boiling point at higher altitudes can be simulated by using a partial vacuum in commercial food applications involving heat-labile food components, such as flavors.

At normal atmospheric pressures near sea level, temperatures during boiling do not exceed 212°F (100°C). The use of pressure cookers, however, allows boiling to occur at higher temperatures and food to be cooked for shorter periods of time. Because they take less time, such high-temperature heat treatments preserve the nutritive and sensory qualities of foods and also conserve energy. Pressure cooking is normally used for cooking rice, legumes, and meat cuts with high amounts of connective tissue.

Water Activity

water activity (a_w) The ratio of the vapor pressure of a food sample (p) to the vapor pressure of pure water (p_0) at the same temperature. In thermodynamic terms, it is a measure of the energy status of water in a system.

The ratio of the vapor pressure of a food sample (p) to the vapor pressure of pure water (p_0) at the same temperature is defined as **water activity (a_w)**. In thermodynamic terms, water activity is a measure of the energy status of water in a system. Water activity of foods is always below 1.0, with most foods having a water activity level that exceeds 0.90. Foods with vastly different moisture contents may have comparable water activities, as shown in **Table 4.1**.

The importance of water activity in foods arises from its significant role in food spoilage. Fresh foods, such as meat, vegetables, milk, and some fruits, have a water activity in the range of 0.95 to 1.0. Such high water activity makes these foods very susceptible to microbial spoilage.

Many food preservation methods focus on lowering the water activity levels in foods. Very few microbes survive at a water activity of less than 0.80, and all microbial growth ceases at water activity of less than 0.5. Food preservation methods that reduce water activity include dehydration (e.g., raisins), freezing (e.g., frozen meats), salting (e.g., hams, pickles), and the addition of sugars (e.g., jams, jellies).

TABLE 4.1
Water Activity of Some Common Foods

Type of Product	Water Activity (a_w)
Fresh meat and fish	0.99
Bread	0.95
Aged cheddar	0.85
Jams and jellies	0.80
Plum pudding	0.80
Dried fruit	0.60
Biscuits	0.30
Milk powder	0.20
Instant coffee	0.20

Source: Reproduced from Water Activity in Food. Pathogen Modeling Program (PMP) Online, Division of Food Science and Technology Fact Sheet. Available at: http://pmp.arserrc.gov/PMPOnline/References/WaterActivity.aspx. Accessed March 3, 2011.

Water Hardness

Water may be classified as soft or hard, depending on the mineral salts present. Hard water contains salts such as bicarbonates and/or sulfates of calcium and magnesium. When hard water is boiled, some of these salts are precipitated. Water containing bicarbonates is termed *temporarily hard water* because the bicarbonate salts precipitate out after boiling, often depositing as "scum" on the walls of a frequently used vessel. When preparing tannin-containing beverages such as iced tea, these precipitates can cause an undesirable cloudiness to the drink. In contrast, *permanently hard water* contains calcium and magnesium sulfates, which cannot be precipitated by boiling.

Water hardness has a detrimental effect on its cleansing ability as well as its ability to soften legumes. The mineral salts interact with chemicals present in legumes and inhibit the softening process. Hard water can be demineralized through the use of ion-exchange resins, but the resulting soft water will have higher than normal amounts of sodium and other anions.

Functions of Water in Foods

The unique physical and chemical properties of water allow it to play many useful roles in foods and cooking.

Water as Medium for Heat Transfer

Both in its liquid and gaseous form, water is the most commonly used medium for heat transfer. This is because of its superior ability to absorb heat. Water has a specific heat of 1.0; this means that the energy equivalent to 1 calorie is required to raise the temperature of 1 gram of water through 1 degree Celsius (this is the specific heat of water) at normal atmospheric pressure. The relatively high specific heat of water allows it to buffer changes in food temperature. This property of water is useful in moist-cooking methods of food preparation such as boiling, braising, simmering, and steaming.

Water as a Solvent

The perception of food flavors and tastes is attributed to the dissolution of flavor molecules in saliva. Electrolytes such as sodium chloride can dissolve in water, owing to its polarity, whereas molecules such as glucose dissolve due

solution When solute molecules completely dissolve in a solvent without precipitating out.

saturated solution Solution that has the maximum amount of solute that can be dissolved in the solvent.

dispersion Formed when substances called colloids are too large to dissolve in a solvent. Instead, they remain in the solvent as an unstable dispersion. Dispersions are further classified as suspensions or emulsions.

suspension A type of dispersion where the large colloidal molecules remain suspended in the media and are visibly distinct, such as when starch is suspended in cold water.

emulsion A type of dispersion where the colloidal particles disperse completely within the medium (the second phase). Milk, mayonnaise, and gravies are examples of emulsions.

hydrolysis Chemical reaction where a water molecule is used to split a compound into simpler molecules.

to the formation of hydrogen bonds. Water also is the dispersing medium in many food mixtures—milk, soups, gravies, cake batters, and salad dressings all contain numerous macromolecules dispersed in water.

Based on their molecular size, different solutes may combine with water to form solutions and dispersions. A **solution** is formed when solute molecules completely dissolve in the solvent without precipitating out. At concentrations normally used during food preparation, both sugar and salt form solutions with water. This property is very useful in allowing water-soluble ingredients to be incorporated into food; however, it also results in the loss of vital water-soluble nutrients (such as B vitamins) during washing or by cooking methods that discard the cooking water. A **saturated solution** contains the maximum amount of solute that can be dissolved in the solvent. When a saturated solution is heated, the dissolving capacity of the solvent increases and more solute can be added. The excess solute precipitates out during cooling, as exemplified when making candy.

A **dispersion** is formed when certain substances called *colloids* are too large (i.e., they have a high molecular weight) to dissolve in a solvent. Instead, they remain in the solvent as an unstable dispersion. Dispersions are further classified as suspensions or emulsions. In a **suspension**, the large colloidal molecules remain suspended in the media and are visibly distinct, such as when starch is suspended in cold water. In an **emulsion**, the colloidal particles disperse completely within the medium (the second phase). Milk, mayonnaise, and gravies are examples of emulsions. The stability of emulsions may be decreased (and its sensory qualities compromised) by heating, mechanical forces, and freezing.

Water as a Reactant

Almost all food processing methods include a chemical reaction involving water. Ionization and hydrolysis reactions are the most commonly encountered reactions involving water in foods.

Ionization Reactions

Solutes such as salts dissolve in water and ionize into electrolytes. These electrolytes participate in weak ionic interactions with other ingredients, and they influence the freezing and boiling points of water. For example, the addition of sugar or salt will depress the freezing point. This is why ice cream mixes take a long time to freeze, and sometimes adequate freezing is possible only in commercial freezers.

Hydrolysis Reactions

In **hydrolysis**, water breaks the chemical bonds of a molecule, splitting it into two smaller molecules. Some commonly encountered hydrolysis reactions in food preparation include the hydrolysis of sucrose into glucose and fructose, a common reaction in candy making, and the hydrolysis of triglycerides into glycerol and the component fatty acids, which is a cause of rancidity in certain high-fat foods (mainly dairy products and meats).

pH

pH is a measure of the degree of acidity or alkalinity of a solution. Hydrogen ions (H^+) are characteristic of acids, whereas hydroxyl ions (OH^-) characterize bases (alkalis). The pH scale ranges from 1 through 14, with 7 characterizing a neutral pH. A pH below 7 is characterized as acidic, whereas a pH greater than 7 is alkaline. **Table 4.2** lists the pH of some common foods.

TABLE 4.2
pH Values of Some Common Foods

Food	pH
Fruits and Vegetables	
Lemon	2.2
Strawberries	3.4
Tomatoes	4.2
Bananas	4.6
Carrots	4.9–5.2
Kale, cooked	6.4–6.8
Beans	5.7–6.2
Olives	3.6–3.8
Bakery Snacks	
Bread	5.3–5.8
Biscuits	7.1–7.3
Angel food cake	5.2–5.6
Chocolate	7.2–7.6
Egg Products	
Egg whites	7.0–9.0
Egg yolks	6.4
Whole eggs	7.1–7.9
Dairy Products	
Milk	6.3–8.5
Acidophilus milk	4
Camembert cheese	7.4
Roquefort cheese	5.5–5.9
Butter	6.1–6.4
Buttermilk	4.5
Fish Products	
Most fresh fish	6.6–6.8
Tuna	5.2–6.1
White fish	5.5
Crabs	7.0
Meat and Poultry Products	
Beef, ground	5.1–6.2
Beef, ripened	5.8
Beef, unripened	7.0
Pork	5.3–6.9
Chicken	6.5–6.7
Others	
Vinegar	2.9
Sauerkraut	3.4–3.6
Orange marmalade	3
Jams and jellies	3.1–3.5
Sugar	5.0–6.0

Source: Reproduced from Food and Drug Administration. pH Values of Various Foods. Available at: http://www.fda.gov/Food/FoodSafety/FoodborneIllness/FoodborneIllnessFoodbornePathogensNaturalToxins/BadBugBook/ucm122561.htm. Accessed January 3, 2011.

carbohydrates One of the four major classes of nutrients. With an energy value of 4 calories per gram, these compounds are one of the most basic nutrients in foods.

glycogen The primary carbohydrate in animal muscle; it is converted to lactic acid after slaughter.

Carbohydrates

Chemically, **carbohydrates** refer to the polyhydroxy aldehydes and ketones found in foods. With an energy value of 4 calories, these compounds are one of the most basic nutrients in foods. They are indispensable in foods by virtue of their role as sweeteners; thickening, bulking, and gelling agents; and as contributors of flavors and pigments uniquely present in thermally processed foods.

Sugars are the basic units of carbohydrates. Based on the number of sugar entities linked together, carbohydrates are classified as follows:

- *Monosaccharides*—single sugar molecules
- *Disaccharides*—two sugar molecules
- *Oligosaccharides*—short chains of sugar molecules
- *Polysaccharides*—long chains of numerous (thousands) of sugar molecules

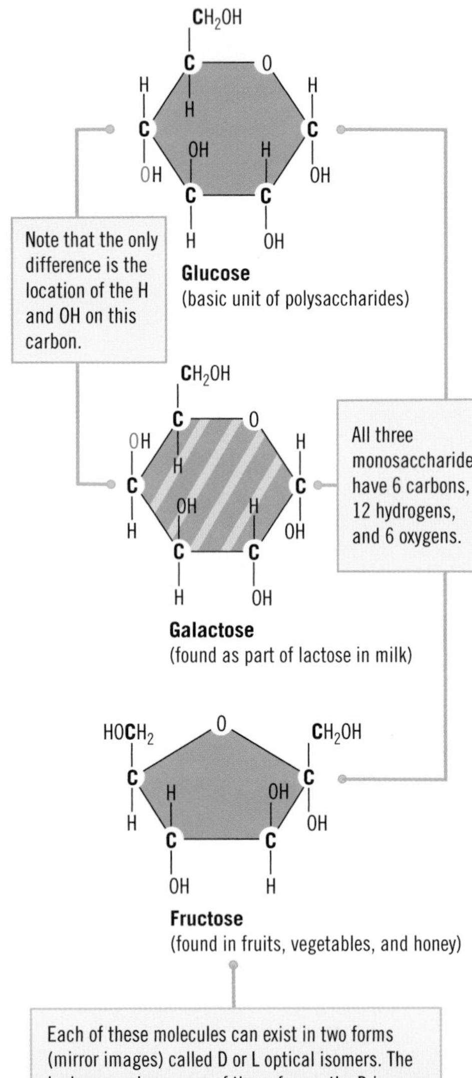
Note that the only difference is the location of the H and OH on this carbon.
Glucose
(basic unit of polysaccharides)
All three monosaccharides have 6 carbons, 12 hydrogens, and 6 oxygens.
Galactose
(found as part of lactose in milk)
Fructose
(found in fruits, vegetables, and honey)
Each of these molecules can exist in two forms (mirror images) called D or L optical isomers. The body can only use one of these forms, the D isomer.

FIGURE 4.4 Because glucose and galactose share similar six-sided hexagonal structures, they can be difficult to tell apart, but fructose's five-sided pentagon stands out.

Food Sources of Carbohydrates

Plants are the primary source of carbohydrates in the human diet. Plant carbohydrates include starches, sugars, polysaccharides, and fibers derived from the seeds, roots, stems, and fruits of the plant. Animal products are not a significant source of carbohydrates in the human diet. The primary carbohydrate in animal muscle is **glycogen**, which is converted to lactic acid after slaughter.

Common plant sources of carbohydrates include the following:

- Cereals such as rice, corn, and wheat (seeds)
- Legumes such as lentils and beans (seeds)
- Vegetables such as carrots (roots) and sweet potatoes (root tubers)
- Vegetables such as potatoes (stem tubers) and celery and sugarcane (stems)
- Fruits
- Dairy products (the sole source of lactose, commonly called *milk sugar*)

Monosaccharides

Monosaccharides are the simplest sugars found in nature. These carbohydrate molecules cannot be broken down into simpler molecules by hydrolysis. Depending on the number of carbon atoms in the molecule, simple sugars are further classified as *trioses*, those having three carbon atoms; *tetroses*, those having four carbon atoms (rarely found); *pentoses*, those having five carbon atoms; and *hexoses*, those having six carbon atoms. Trioses are not found natively in foods but are metabolic intermediates of respiration. Pentoses and hexoses are found in varying forms and proportions in foods; they contribute to the unique sensory characteristics of certain foods when subjected to thermal processing.

Hexoses are the most common monosaccharides found in foods. Fructose, glucose, and galactose are hexose sugars (see **Figure 4.4**). Although all three sugars have the same empirical formula of $C_6H_{12}O_6$, they differ in their solubility, sweetness, and extent of browning reactions. These differences arise due to the different positions of the chemical groups present in these sugars. As shown in **Table 4.3**, glucose is an aldo sugar, with an aldehyde group (–CHO) at the terminal carbon position. Fructose is a keto sugar, with a ketone group (–CO) at the carbon molecule adjacent to the terminal carbon.

TABLE 4.3
Monosaccharides, Disaccharides, and Polysaccharides Commonly Found in Foods

	Molecular Structure
Glucose	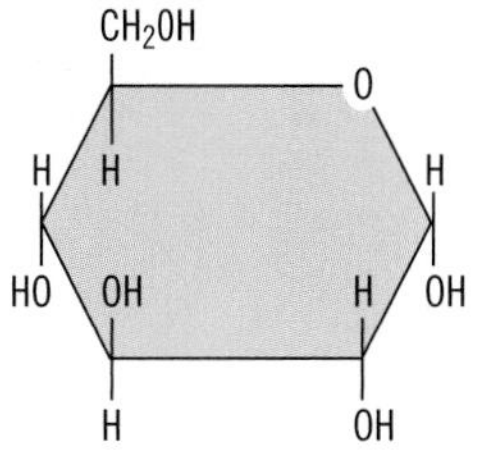 CH_2OH, O, H, H, H, HO, OH, H, OH, H, OH
Fructose	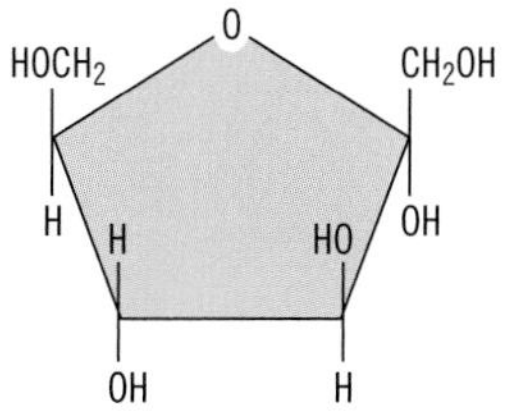 $HOCH_2$, O, CH_2OH, H, H, HO, OH, OH, H
Galactose	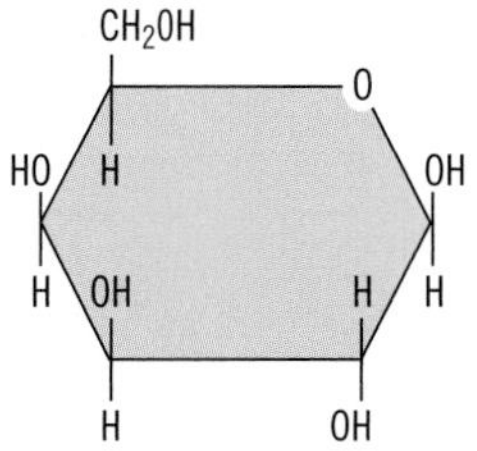 CH_2OH, O, HO, H, OH, H, OH, H, H, H, OH
Ribose	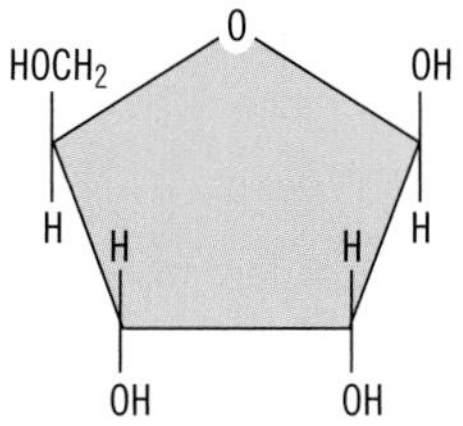 $HOCH_2$, O, OH, H, H, H, H, OH, OH
Arabinose	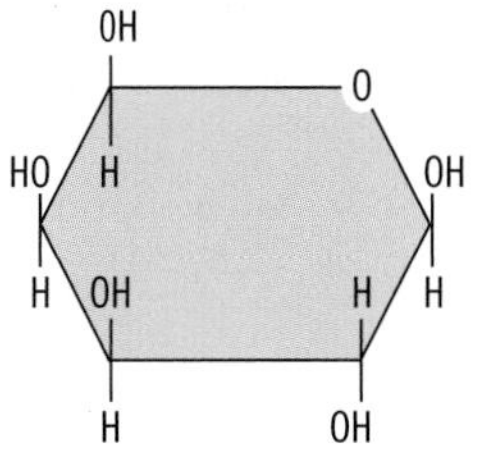 OH, O, HO, H, OH, H, OH, H, H, H, OH
Lactose	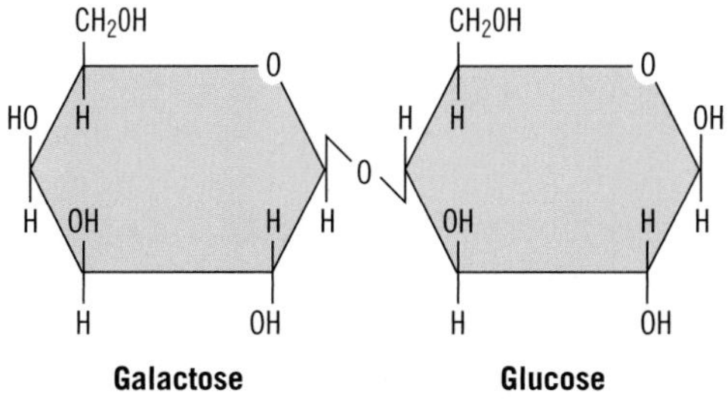 CH_2OH, O, HO, H, H, OH, H, H, H, OH, **Galactose** — O — CH_2OH, O, H, H, OH, OH, H, H, H, OH, **Glucose**

(*continues*)

TABLE 4.3
Monosaccharides, Disaccharides, and Polysaccharides Commonly Found in Foods (*continued*)

	Molecular Structure
Sucrose	**Glucose** **Fructose**
Maltose	**Glucose** **Glucose**
Raffinose	**Galactose** **Sucrose**
Stachyose	**Galactose** **Galactose** **Sucrose**

Amylose	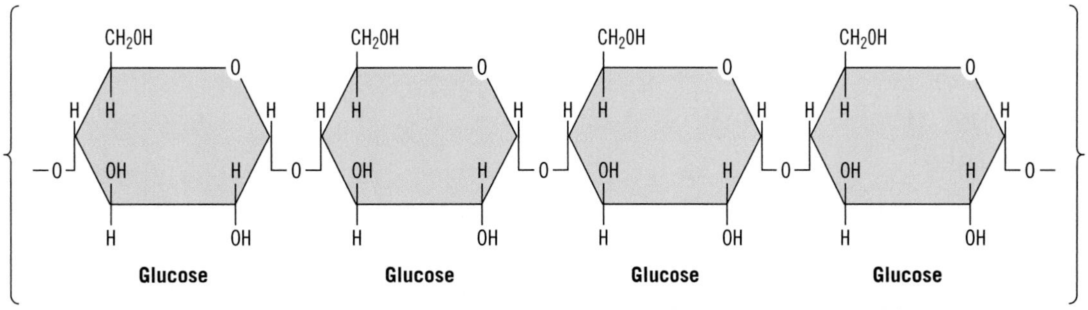 Glucose Glucose Glucose Glucose
Amylopectin	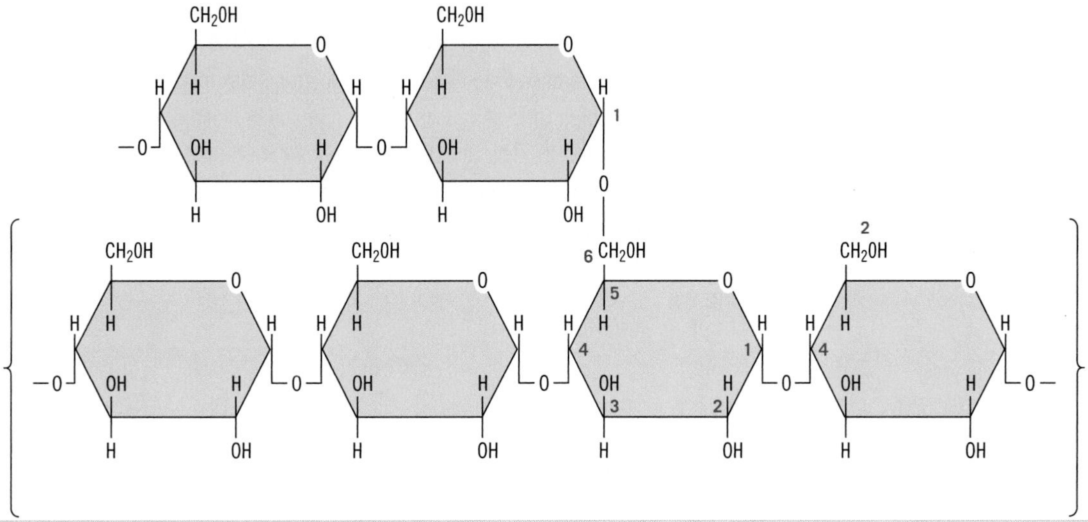
Glycogen	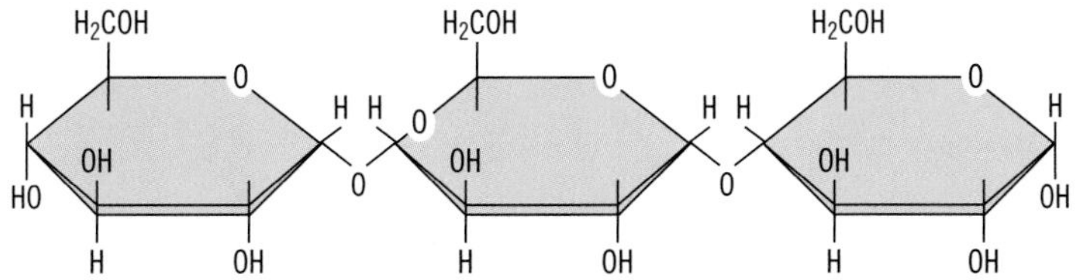
Cellulose	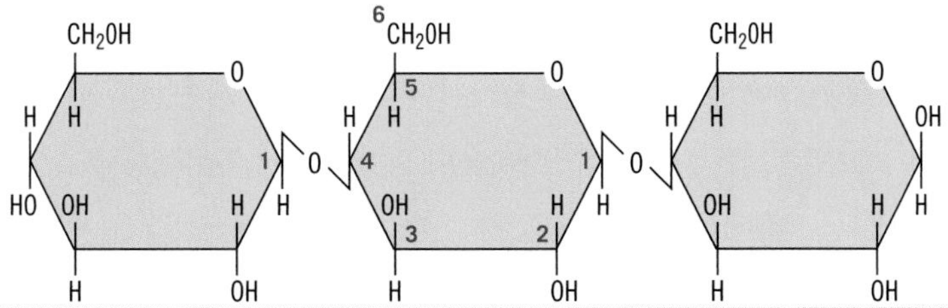

Glucose

Glucose is the most common monosaccharide found in foods. It is a building block for the disaccharide lactose, which is found in dairy products, and for the polysaccharides starch, cellulose, and glycogen. It is found in small amounts in its free form in fruits, some plant juices, and honey. Glucose is the major component of corn syrup, which is used extensively in the food industry as a sweetener, a **humectant** (i.e., helps products retain water), a bulking agent, an inhibitor of crystallization, a component of certain browning reactions, and a source of fermentable carbohydrates. Commercially, corn syrup is produced by chemical hydrolysis of cornstarch. Glucose is also the sugar that circulates in the bloodstream (measured as "blood sugar"). High amounts of circulating glucose in the bloodstream is a clinical manifestation of diabetes. The measurement of the effect carbohydrates have on blood glucose levels is discussed in **Special Topic 4.3**.

humectant A food component used to retain moisture in the matrix.

Special Topic 4.3

Glycemic Index of Food

Erin Kunze

glycemic index (GI) A ranking system that quantifies the effect that food carbohydrates have on blood glucose levels.

After a meal is ingested, the digestible carbohydrates are broken down by the body and converted into glucose for use. How fast the carbohydrate is converted to glucose in the body varies for different foods.[1] The **glycemic index (GI)** is a ranking system that quantifies the effect that food carbohydrates have on blood glucose levels. Foods are assigned a number between 1 and 100 (see **Table A**). Glucose is used as the reference value and has a glycemic index of 100. High GI foods fall in the range of 70–100, and low GI foods fall in the range of 0–55. A high GI food causes a fast increase in blood glucose levels, whereas a low GI food causes a slow and extended increase in blood glucose levels.[1] The GI value of a food is determined by the increase in blood glucose levels following consumption of 50 grams of the food over a 2-hour period. The rise in blood glucose caused by the sample food is compared to the rise in blood glucose caused by 50 grams of the reference food, glucose, over a 2-hour period.[2]

TABLE A
GI Values of Various Foods

Food	Glycemic Index Value
Fruits	
Grapefruit	25
Cherries	22
Banana	52
Apple	38
Orange	42
Vegetables	
Kale	32
Carrot	16
Broccoli	32
Winter squash	75
Onion	32
Breads	
White bread	73
Whole wheat bread	71
Sour dough	54
Rye bread	58
Bagel	72
Dairy	
Whole milk	27
Skim milk	32
Low-fat plain yogurt	36
Swiss cheese	27
Butter	50
Meat/Chicken/Fish	
Steak (beef)	0
Pork chop	0

Fried chicken breast	95
Steamed lobster	50
Cod	50
Snacks	
Potato chips	54
Cashews	22
Peanut butter	14
Pretzels	83
Granola bar	61
Starches	
Potato	72
White rice	64
Brown rice	55
Corn	53
Spaghetti	42
Desserts	
Apple pie	59
Gum drops	78
Sugar cookie	55
Cheese cake	50
Fruit leather	99

Note: For a full list, refer to http://riskfactor.cancer.gov/tools/glycemic.

Source: Data from National Cancer Institute. Glycemic Index Values Database. Available at: http://riskfactor.cancer.gov/tools/glycemic. Accessed December 3, 2011.

The glycemic index is a measure of how fast 50 grams of a certain food will raise blood glucose levels; however, a normal serving size does not always contain 50 grams of carbohydrates. A more practical and useful concept is **glycemic load**, which takes into account the quality as well as the quantity of carbohydrates by considering serving sizes of carbohydrate-containing foods.[3] Glycemic load is calculated by taking the glycemic index of a food, multiplying it by the grams of carbohydrates in the serving, and dividing by 100.[1] As with the glycemic index, the higher the glycemic load, the faster blood glucose levels will rise after consumption.

glycemic load Calculated by taking the glycemic index of a food, multiplying it by the grams of carbohydrates in the serving, and dividing by 100. Takes into account the quality as well as the quantity of carbohydrates by considering serving sizes of carbohydrate-containing foods.

Other factors also can affect a food's GI value. The glycemic index of carbohydrates is lower when they are eaten with protein and fat. Also, the particle size of a food affects the glycemic index. The smaller the particle size, the higher the GI value. Fiber slows the absorption of food within the gastrointestinal tract, therefore lowering the GI value. Acidic foods also slow gastric emptying, and thus they have lower GI values. Lastly, highly processed foods have higher GI values than their unprocessed equivalents.[4]

Because GI values measure how quickly particular carbohydrates raise blood glucose levels, they are also a reliable indicator of how quickly insulin is released in the body. A high GI food causes a surge in blood glucose, and as insulin is released blood glucose is brought down very quickly. A low GI food, in contrast, causes a gradual increase in blood glucose, and therefore a slow insulin release response (blood glucose levels neither peak nor drop too quickly). Knowing the GI values of foods is helpful in the management of type 2 diabetes. By knowing and choosing low GI foods, people with diabetes can help manage their blood glucose levels, preventing them from reaching levels either too high or too low.[5] Athletes also may benefit from knowing the GI or glycemic load of certain foods; for example, they may choose high glycemic foods for quick energy when training.[4]

Current research shows mixed evidence for an association between the consumption of high GI foods and the risk of type 2 diabetes. The evidence also is mixed for an association between high GI foods and cardiovascular disease. In addition, research has not found a relationship between high GI foods and obesity, and there is a negative epidemiological association between high GI foods and cancer.[2]

References

1 Searching for a good carbohydrate. Available at: http://www.ars.usda.gov/News/docs.htm?docid=9236. Accessed December 3, 2011.

2 Report of the DGAC on the *Dietary Guidelines for Americans, 2010.* Part D, Section 5: Carbohydrates. Available at: http://www.cnpp.usda.gov/Publications/DietaryGuidelines/2010/DGAC/Report/D-5-Carbohydrates.pdf. Accessed December 3, 2011.

3 Gropper SS, Smith JL. *Advanced Nutrition and Human Metabolism.* 5th ed. Belmont, CA: Wadsworth; 2009.

4 Glycemic index. Available at: http://web.mit.edu/athletics/sportsmedicine/wcrglycemicindex.html. Assessed December 3, 2011.

5 Whitney E, Rolfes SR. *Understanding Nutrition.* 12th ed. Belmont, CA: Wadsworth; 2008.

Fructose

Commonly referred to as *fruit sugar*, fructose is considered to be the sweetest monosaccharide.[1] It is most commonly found in its free form in honey and in ripening fruits. In processed foods, fructose is commonly found in bakery products, candy, and soft drinks and in the high fructose corn syrup (HFCS) that is often added to these products. In its free form, fructose is rarely used in foods due to its high solubility and hygroscopicity (i.e., propensity to absorb moisture). The high solubility results in significant lowering of the freezing point, which is undesirable in frozen desserts such as ice cream, because it results in faster melting. Excessive stickiness in bakery items is often attributed to the use of high amounts of moisture absorbed by a hygroscopic sweetener such as fructose.

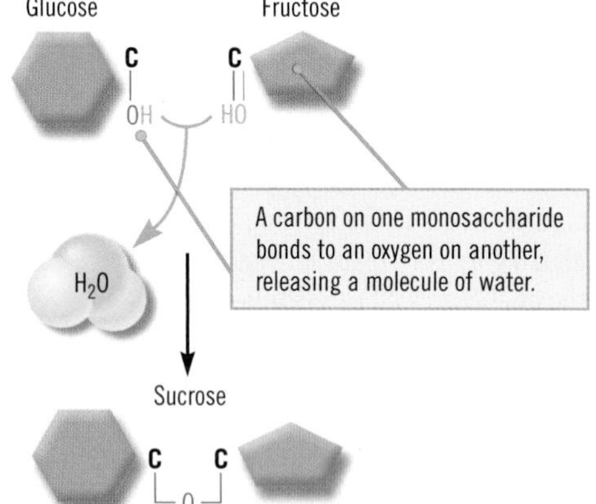

FIGURE 4.5 The formation of a glycosidic bond between two monosaccharides results in the elimination of a water molecule.

cryoprotectant A molecule that protects biological tissue against structural damage (due to ice formation) during freezing and thawing.

Galactose

Galactose is found predominantly in milk as a component of lactose. It is also found in certain oligosaccharides, along with glucose and fructose.

Disaccharides

Disaccharides are formed as a result of the condensation of two monosaccharides. In a condensation reaction, the formation of a glycosidic bond between two sugars eliminates a molecule of water, as indicated in **Figure 4.5**. Sucrose, lactose, and maltose are the most common disaccharides found in foods.

Sucrose

Often referred to as *table sugar*, sucrose is the most common disaccharide found in its free form. It is a nonreducing sugar formed by the condensation reaction between glucose and fructose. Commercially, sucrose is extracted from sugarcane and sugar beets. Because sucrose is extremely hydrophilic (i.e., water loving) and water soluble, highly concentrated sugar syrups are often used as preservatives. Highly concentrated sugar solutions depress the freezing point of water, functioning as a **cryoprotectant**; that is, an agent that gives protection against freezing. As the freezable water in a sugar solution crystallizes into ice, the concentration of sugar in the unfrozen matrix increases. This increases the viscosity of the solution and restricts the mobility of the molecules. The remaining water molecules cannot be frozen, thereby preventing the loss of structure and texture that is often attributed to dehydration in frozen foods. In the presence of the enzyme sucrase or invertase, sucrose can be hydrolyzed into equal amounts of glucose and fructose. The mixture is called *invert sugar* and is used to control crystallization of sugar during the manufacture of crystalline candies.

Lactose

Commonly called *milk sugar*, lactose is composed of the monosaccharides glucose and galactose. It is found naturally only in dairy products. Undigested lactose is implicated as the cause for lactose intolerance in some individuals.

Maltose

Maltose is composed of two molecules of glucose. It is only found in plants and in corn syrup as a result of the partial hydrolysis of starch. Commercially, maltose is produced by enzymatic hydrolysis of starch by beta-amylase and by malting of grains, most commonly barley. It is commonly referred to as *malt sugar*.

Oligosaccharides

Oligosaccharides are short-chain carbohydrates comprising 3 to 10 monosaccharide units linked by glycosidic bonds. Raffinose (a trisaccharide) and stachyose (a tetrasaccharide) are found in legumes. The human digestive system lacks the enzymes required for their digestion; instead, these sugars are fermented by intestinal microflora in the colon, resulting in gas formation.

Innovation Point

Beano Commercially available enzymes such as Beano may be taken orally to alleviate the discomfort of gas caused by the fermentation of certain oligosaccharides. Beano contains the enzyme alpha-galactosidase, which is derived from selected strains of the food-grade fungus *Aspergillus niger*. It must be consumed before eating the offending foods to act as a digestive aid.

Polysaccharides

Polysaccharides are complex carbohydrates composed of numerous monosaccharides linked by glycosidic bonds in a linear or branched manner. Common polysaccharides found in foods include starch, dextrin, cellulose, and plant gums. Homo-polysaccharides consist of the same type of monosaccharide. These include linear glucose polymers such as cellulose and starch amylose, as well as branched glucose polymers such as starch amylopectin. Hetero-polysaccharides such as guar and locust bean gum have two or more different monosaccharides. The number of monosaccharides present in a polysaccharide is referred to as its *degree of polymerization* (DP). The DP for starch amylose is around 1,000; 7,000 to 15,000 for cellulose; and can exceed 60,000 for starch amylopectin.

Unlike low-molecular-weight carbohydrates, which can depress the freezing point or increase the boiling point of water, polysaccharides do not significantly affect these properties of water (largely due to their low concentration). However, polysaccharides can protect the quality of frozen foods. Upon freezing a polysaccharide solution, a two-phase system of solid ice (crystalline water) and liquid (a mixture of about 70% polysaccharide and 30% nonfreezable water) is formed. Similar to highly concentrated sucrose solutions, the nonfreezable water is a highly concentrated matrix; the extremely high viscosity of this solution restricts the mobility of the water molecules.[2]

Polysaccharides are used in foods as thickening and/or gelling agents. They can be added at very low concentrations (0.25–0.50%) to increase viscosity or cause gelation of a liquid food matrix. Gels are formed when water is entrapped within an extensive three-dimensional network of polymer chains. Examples of gels include jams, jellies, gum drops, and dessert gels.

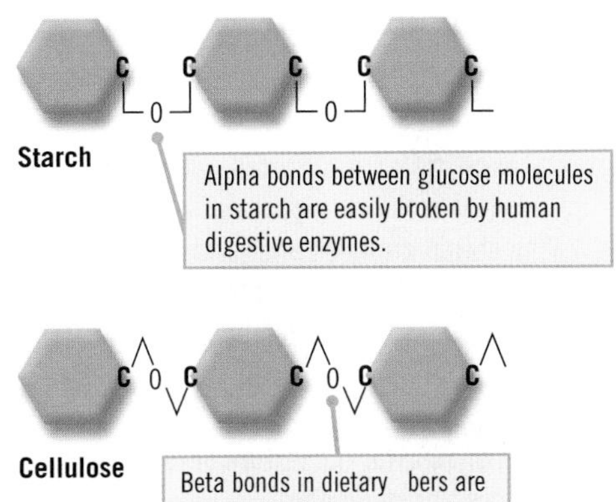

FIGURE 4.6 Glycosidic bonds in starch and cellulose. Alpha-glycosidic bonds are easily digested, but the human digestive system lacks the enzymes to cleave the beta-glycosidic bonds in cellulose, making it indigestible and of no calorific value.

Cellulose

Cellulose is a high-molecular-weight, linear, water-insoluble homo-polymer of glucose linked by beta-glycosidic linkages, as shown in **Figure 4.6**. It is classified as dietary fiber and is discussed further in the section on dietary fiber.

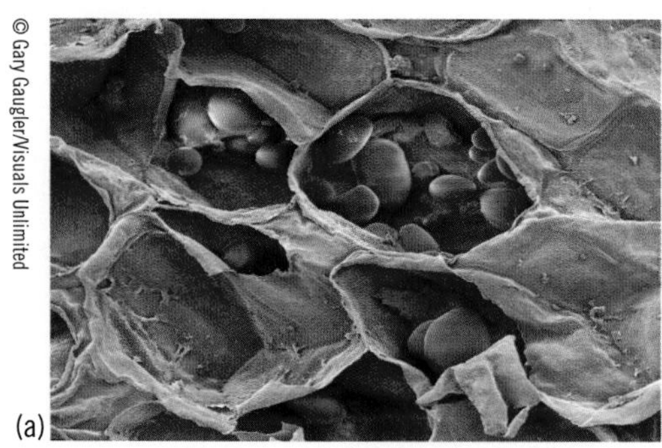
(a)

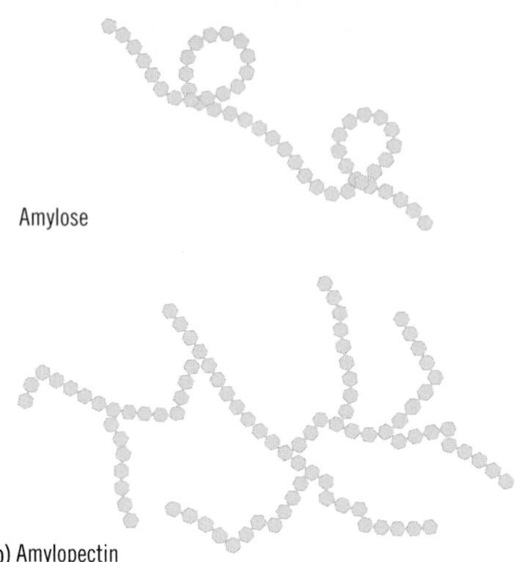

FIGURE 4.7 (a) A scanning electron microscopic image of starch granules within potato tuber cells. (b) The starch within these granules is composed of the linear fraction, amylase, and the branched fraction, amylopectin.

starch gelatinization The loss of molecular organization within starch granules characterized by irreversible swelling and loss of birefringence.

starch gelation Process whereby amylose molecules leach out of the starch granules and form intermolecular hydrogen bonds. The result is a three-dimensional network of amylose molecules with entrapped water and starch granules. Responsible for the texture of many sauces and puddings.

Starch

Starch is the predominant form of stored energy in plants and is approximately 70–80% of the calories in the human diet. Predominant sources of starch in the human diet are cereal grains, tubers, and roots. Starch is found in plants as aggregate structures called *granules*. Starch granules vary in size and shape. Tuber starches tend to have larger granules than cereal starches. Starch granules have two polymers, a linear glucose homo-polymer called *amylose* and a branched glucose homo-polymer called *amylopectin* (see **Figure 4.7**). In both polymers, glucose molecules are linked by alpha-glycosidic linkages. The branch points in amylopectin are also characterized by alpha-glycosidic linkages, as shown in Table 4.3.

Gelatinization (Pasting)

Undamaged starch granules are insoluble in water. At room temperature, starch granules swell slightly because they absorb water. Because they return to their original size when dried, this process is called *reversible absorption*. In contrast, when a starch–water mixture is heated, the starch granules lose their molecular organization. This loss of molecular organization within the granules is called **starch gelatinization** and is characterized by irreversible swelling and loss of birefringence (the transmission of light unequally in different directions of the starch granule as well as increased viscosity of the starch-water solution).

During gelatinization (also called pasting), amylose leaches from the granules, and the starch granules disintegrate. These changes in the starch granule organization increase the viscosity of the starch–water mixture, resulting in a thick paste. Gelatinization is characterized by the peak viscosity attained by the mixture, which occurs over a temperature range rather than at a specific temperature. Starch gelatinization is responsible for the textural changes associated with cooked rice, pasta, and potatoes. When this mixture is held at high temperatures, the swollen starch granules degrade and the contents are released into the surrounding water. The viscosity of the mixture decreases, resulting in pasting.

Gelation

The amylose molecules that leach out of the starch granules during gelatinization are highly mobile. As the temperature of the mixture decreases, the amylose molecules lose energy, become less mobile, and form intermolecular hydrogen bonds (junction zones). The result is a three-dimensional network of amylose molecules with entrapped water and starch granules. This phenomenon is called **starch gelation** and is responsible for the texture of many sauces and puddings.

Factors Affecting Pastes and Gels

The friable, cooked texture often attributed to starchy foods is the result of the interplay among many factors, such as the amount of available water for hydration of starch granules, the temperature and duration of cooking, shear, and the presence of ingredients such as sugar, acid, fat, and protein.

Water

Sufficient amounts of water must be present when cooking rice and pasta. The amount of water added must account for losses by evaporation and yet be enough to accommodate a threefold volume increase due to water absorption by the starch granules.

Temperature

Starch gelatinization generally takes place over a temperature range of 140–158°F (60–70°C) within which the starch–water mixture begins to thicken. Tubers such as potatoes have larger starch granules; they can absorb much more water than the smaller granules in cereals such as those found in rice and corn. Tuber starches such as potatoes and root starches such as tapioca have lower gelatinization temperatures than cereal starches. Thus, starchy tubers and roots cook faster than cereals.

Duration of Cooking

Continued application of heat beyond gelatinization temperatures results in degradation of the starch granules. Both amylose and amylopectin leach out into the water. The mixture of amylose, amylopectin, and granule remnants in the water results in an undesirable pasty texture. This phenomenon of pasting is exemplified by the gumminess associated with overcooked rice, pasta, and potatoes.

Shear

Vigorous stirring during and after gelatinization can break down the starch granules, resulting in a pasty product with a decreased viscosity. For optimal texture, the starch–water mixture should be stirred only during the initial stages of cooking to ensure homogeneous distribution of the granules. This is especially important when flavors are added to puddings and sauces.

Acidity

Under acidic conditions, specifically at a pH below 4, hydrolysis of amylose chains occurs. The hydrolytic end products, being of lower molecular weight, are more mobile; they therefore reduce the viscosity of the starch paste. Starch pastes or gels that have lemon juices or other acidic components as part of the product formulation (e.g., pie fillings, salad dressings) are very susceptible to the "thinning" ability of the acid component. Such thinning may be prevented by adding the acidic ingredient after gelatinization has occurred or by using a chemically modified starch that is acid resistant (e.g., a cross-linked starch).

Sugar

It is still unclear how sugars delay gelatinization. It has been hypothesized that sugars, being hygroscopic, compete with starch for the water available for gelatinization, and thus reduce the water activity (a_w) of the mixture. The gelatinization temperature is thereby increased, and onset of gelatinization is delayed. The type of sugar influences the temperature required for onset of gelatinization. Ranked in ascending order of their effectiveness in increasing gelatinization temperatures, they are fructose, glucose, maltose, and sucrose.[3,4]

Rate of Cooling

Both rapid and slow cooling can result in "weeping" of the starch gel, which is more formally called **syneresis**. If a starch paste is cooled rapidly, the amylose chains will not have sufficient time to form the interchain bonds that are necessary for the formation of the three-dimensional gel structure. Very slow rates of cooling may facilitate excessive alignment of the amylose chains, expelling the liquid portion. This also can happen during freezing of starch gels or with severe temperature cycling.

syneresis "Weeping" of a starch gel due to rapid heating or cooling.

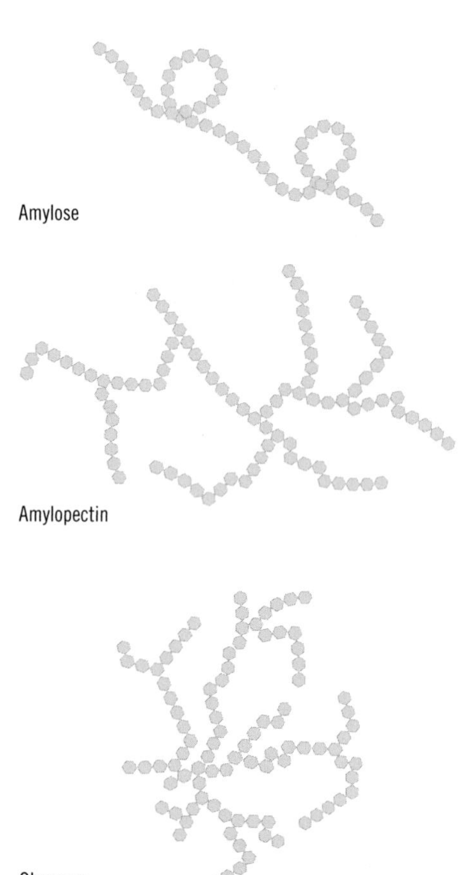

FIGURE 4.8 Amylose, amylopectin, and glycogen are glucose polymers. They differ in the extent of branching. Amylose is a linear polymer, amylopectin exhibits some branching, and glycogen exhibits extensive branching, making it bulky.

Amylose–Amylopectin Ratios

Amylose molecules are linear chains that can orient to form the intermolecular bonds necessary for successful gel formation. Amylopectin molecules, in contrast, are highly branched, bulky molecules that do not exhibit much propensity for gel formation (see **Figure 4.8**). Rather, these branched molecules contribute to the increased viscosity (thickness) of the starch paste.

The proportion of amylose and amylopectin in different plant sources accounts for the unique behavior of different plant-based foods. Most starches contain about 25% amylose and 75% amylopectin. Regular corn starch has almost 25–30% amylose and is capable of forming a very strong gel. Waxy corn starches, in contrast, are composed almost entirely of amylopectin. Thus they form a very thick paste when heated with water and do not gel.

Starch Dextrinization

When flour is dry roasted, the starches present react with water and are split into shorter chains called *dextrins*. These short-chain molecules are sweeter and more mobile in paste; they do not have the gelling ability of the native starch molecule. The result of this dextrinization process explains the slightly sweeter taste of toasted bread.

Undigestible Starches

Starch that cannot be enzymatically digested by humans is called **resistant starch (RS)**. There are four categories of resistant starch:

- *RS1:* Starches present in plant cell walls that are inaccessible to alpha-amylase activity. Whole grains and partially milled grains are good sources of RS1.
- *RS2:* Ungelatinized granules of starch commonly found in uncooked potatoes and unripe bananas.
- *RS3:* Retrograded starches formed by heating and cooling starch pastes. Extruded starchy foods, such as corn starch and sorghum flour, are good sources of RS3.
- *RS4:* Starches that are chemically modified to make them indigestible, including starch esters and cross-bonded starches. The more refined a food, the less resistant starch that is present. The less resistant starch present, the more sugars that are released during digestion. Thus, such foods have been implicated for disorders associated with hyperglycemia.[5]

Unrefined, whole grains have higher amounts of resistant starch than their refined counterparts. **Table 4.4** summarizes the amount of resistant starches present in some selected foods.

Dietary Fiber

Fiber is the indigestible polysaccharide found in plant cells. It is a component of plant cell walls and the intercellular cementing material. Carbohydrates and lignin that are intrinsic to a plant's structure but that are indigestible by human digestive enzymes are called **dietary fiber**. Dietary fiber has an important role in ensuring proper gastrointestinal function (as roughage or bulking agents) and for preventing diseases and conditions such as hypercholesterolemia, diverticulitis, constipation, and colon cancer.[6,7] Recent research also suggests that dietary fiber may play a critical role in strengthening immunity as well as in reducing obesity-related inflammatory responses.[8] Plant sources of dietary fiber include cellulose, hemicelluloses, lignin, inulin, pectins, and plant gums.

resistant starch (RS) Starch that cannot be enzymatically digested by humans.

dietary fiber Carbohydrates and lignin that are intrinsic to a plant's structure but that are indigestible by human digestive enzymes.

TABLE 4.4
Resistant Starches in Selected Foods

Product	Percent of Resistant Starch
Long-grain white and brown rice	1.7
Pudding, canned	0.2
Whole wheat breads	1.9–2.8
Refined grain products	0.2–1.1
Skinned potatoes	0.5
Legumes	3.4–3.5

Source: Data from the U.S. Department of Agriculture. What Is Resistant Starch? Available at: http://www.ars.usda.gov/SP2UserFiles/Place/36070500/InfoDianehasuploaded/Meera'sPresentations/MKweon-IDF-2009.pdf. Accessed July 8, 2012.

Indigestible carbohydrates that have been isolated, extracted, or manufactured and that have been clinically proven to have a physiological benefit are called **functional fiber.**[9] Functional fiber may be soluble or insoluble, depending on its solubility in hot water. *Soluble fiber* (such as pectin) is readily soluble in water; it changes into a gel in the digestive tract, thus delaying gastric emptying and decreasing glucose absorption. Dried beans, oat bran, fruits, and vegetables are good sources of soluble fiber. *Insoluble fiber* (such as cellulose and lignin) does not dissolve in hot water. These fibers speed up intestinal transit time and increase fecal bulk. Insoluble fiber is predominantly found in whole grains and vegetables.

functional fiber Indigestible carbohydrates that have been isolated, extracted, or manufactured and that have been clinically proven to have a physiological benefit.

cellulose A homo-polysaccharide of glucose that is indigestible by human enzymes. Cellulose is the predominant component of plant cell walls and, being indigestible, has no caloric contribution.

Cellulose

Like starch, **cellulose** is a homo-polysaccharide of glucose. However, unlike starch, cellulose is a linear polysaccharide with beta-glycosidic bonds that are indigestible by human enzymes, as was shown in Figure 4.6. Cellulose is the predominant component of plant cell walls and, being indigestible, has no caloric contribution. Powdered cellulose often is added to reduced-fat and reduced-sugar bakery goods to provide noncaloric bulk, moistness, and dietary fiber.

Hemicellulose

Hemicellulose is a combination of hetero-polysaccharides, including glucose, xylose, mannose, galactose, arabinose, and glucuronic acid. Hemicellulose is predominantly found in the outer cell wall layers of legumes and other vegetables and in the bran layer of many cereal grains. Some recipes that include legumes involve the addition of baking soda. This decreases the pH of the food, which causes the hemicelluloses to disintegrate, speeding up the cooking process. However, note that the addition of baking soda destroys some of the B vitamins and thus is not recommended.

Lignin

Lignin is a polymer chain of phenolic alcohols. In plant tissue, lignin acts as protective glue that cross-links cellulose and hemicelluloses. As plants age, lignin concentrations increase. Lignin gives vegetables such as celery and carrots their tough, stringy texture.

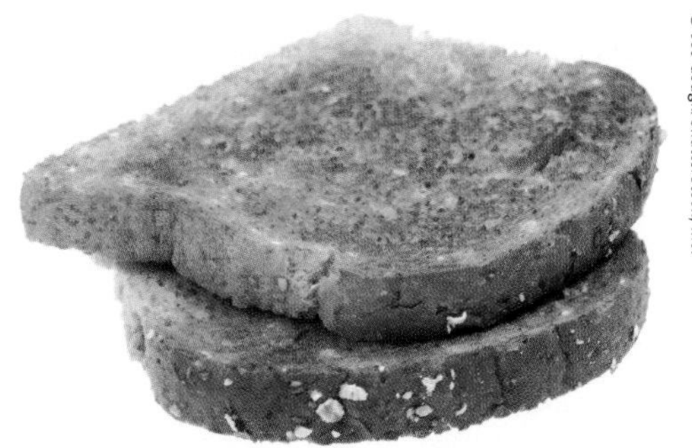

Inulin

Primarily extracted from chicory and Jerusalem artichoke, inulin also occurs as a storage carbohydrate in onions, garlic, asparagus, and bananas. It is found

Innovation Point

Microcrystalline Cellulose and Carboxymethyl Cellulose Purified wood pulp cellulose can be hydrolyzed to yield microcrystalline cellulose (MCC), which is often used as a flavor carrier, as an anticaking agent in shredded cheese, and as a fat and oil replacement in salad dressings and frozen desserts. Another cellulose derivative is carboxymethyl cellulose (CMC), which is obtained by treating purified wood pulp cellulose with sodium hydroxide and chloroacetic acid. CMC is used extensively as a food gum.

together with fructo-oligosaccharides. The human digestive system is not able to digest inulin. It often is added to food formulations as a prebiotic. Being a soluble fiber, it also is used to impart a creamy texture to reduced-fat frozen desserts such as low-fat ice cream.

Pectins

Pectins are polymers of galacturonic acid linked by alpha-glycosidic linkages. They are most commonly found as the intercellular cementing material in fruits and vegetables. Pectic substances include protopectin, pectin, and pectic acid, which are found in unripe, ripe, and overripe fruits, respectively.

In the presence of acids (pH ~3.2) and sugars (~65%) or in the presence of calcium ions, one form of pectin (low methoxyl pectin) has the unique property of being able to form a spreadable gel. Commercially, this property is used in the manufacture of fruit jellies, marmalades, and jams. Cranberries have high amounts of pectin, which is why it is so easy to make cranberry sauce. For gel formation, it is necessary that fruits be at their optimal ripeness; protopectin (found in unripe fruits) and pectic acid (found in overripe fruit) both lack the ability to form gels in the presence of acids and sugar.

Plant Gums

Plant gums are a broad class of polysaccharides obtained from seaweeds and from the bark exudates of certain trees and shrubs. Plant gums are also obtained from seeds, bacteria, and commercial chemical synthesis. They do not contain glucose; rather, galactose is a significant component. Some commonly used plant gums include locust bean gums, xanthan, carrageenans, and algins. Being hydrophilic, they can be used to increase the viscosity and mouthfeel of a wide range of reduced- and low-fat products such as ice creams, salad dressings, and meat analogs. **Table 4.5** summarizes the uses of various plant gums and other polysaccharides in food processing.

TABLE 4.5
Applications of Various Polysaccharides Used in Food Processing

Food Source Stabilizer	Polysaccharide
Anti-syneresis	Algin, karaya gum, xanthan gum, carboxymethyl cellulose
Emulsions in condensed and chocolate milks	Carrageenan, carboxymethyl cellulose, pectin
Gelation of jelly candies, jelly beans, glaze, icing	Pectin, algin, carrageenan, modified starches
Ice cream (against the formation of ice crystals, melting, and separation)	Carboxymethyl cellulose, algin, xanthan gum, modified starches, locust bean gum
Sediment prevention in fruit juices, thickening and gelation of fruit pulp	Pectin, algin
Thickening and gelation in puddings	Pectin, algin, xanthan gum, modified starches, locust bean gum
Water binding in processed meats (corned beef, sausages), jellies made from meat, fish and vegetable products	Agar, karaya gum, locust bean gum, algin, carrageenan

Source: Data from U.S. Food and Drug Administration. Listing of Food Additive Status List. Available at: http://www.fda.gov/Food/FoodIngredientsPackaging/FoodAdditives/FoodAdditiveListings/ucm091048.htm. Accessed March 11, 2011.

Summary of Roles of Carbohydrates in Food Processing

Carbohydrates play many roles in food processing. For example, sugars (monosaccharides and disaccharides) are predominantly used as sweeteners. In small amounts, they can also be used to reduce the perception of acidity and saltiness in foods. Sugars also contribute bulk, volume, and texture to baked goods, such as cakes and cookies. In fermented products such as bread, sugars act as the substrate for yeast metabolism. Sugars also may be used for their preservative effect because they reduce water activity. Starches contribute to food texture principally by undergoing gelatinization, which is significantly affected by the amount of sugars and acids present. Vegetable gums are used as stabilizers and texture modifiers in reduced-fat products.

Lipids

Lipids are organic compounds that are soluble in organic solvents. Like carbohydrates, lipids are composed of carbon, hydrogen, and oxygen; however, lipids have higher proportions of hydrogen and less of oxygen. Depending on their physical state at ambient temperature, lipids are fats (solids) or oils (liquids). When comparing naturally occurring lipids, those derived from animal sources are fats, whereas plant-derived lipids are oils. Coconut oil (plant-derived but solid at room temperature) and fish oils (animal-derived but liquid at room temperature) are exceptions.

From a nutrition standpoint, of all the components of food fats have the highest caloric density (9 calories per gram) and contribute the most to satiety after a meal. From a sensory viewpoint, lipids are critical to the unique mouthfeel and flavor that they attribute to foods. Lipids also have the unique ability to be heated to temperatures higher than the boiling point of water. Thus, lipids can be used for heat transfer during food preparation without burning the food. Lipids enable sautéing, deep-fat frying, and pan-frying, resulting in the formation of unique textures (such as crispy crusts) and flavors.

Edible lipids are categorized into three major groups: triglycerides, phospholipids, and sterols. Triglycerides constitute about 95% of the lipids found in foods. These include fats and oils.

lipids Organic compounds that are soluble in organic solvents. Like carbohydrates, lipids are composed of carbon, hydrogen, and oxygen; however, lipids have higher proportions of hydrogen and less of oxygen.

glycerol A three-carbon compound with three alcohol (hydroxyl) groups, each of which is esterified with a fatty acid.

Food Sources of Lipids

A significant portion of lipids in the American diet comes from vegetable oils, margarine, butter, and lard, which is commonly used for cooking and food processing. High amounts of fats are present in meats, poultry, and dairy products. Common plant sources of lipids include coconut, avocado, nuts, oilseeds (i.e., rape, peanut, cotton, or any seed from which oil can be extracted), and olives.

Lipid Chemistry

Lipids are formed by esterification reactions between a glycerol molecule and three molecules of fatty acids; the result is a triglyceride (lipid), as shown in **Figure 4.9**. All three fatty acids involved in the reaction may be identical, or they may be distinct. The properties of triglycerides are dependent on the structure of the fatty acids present therein.

Glycerol

The backbone of any triglyceride molecule is **glycerol**—a three-carbon compound with three alcohol (hydroxyl) groups, each of which is esterified with a fatty acid.

fatty acid Aliphatic chains with a carboxylic acid (–COOH) functional group.

Aliphatic chains with a carboxylic acid (–COOH) functional group make up the **fatty acid** component of a triglyceride, as shown in **Figure 4.10**. Although approximately 40 fatty acids are found in nature, only 2 are essential in the human diet. These are linoleic acid, which has 18 carbons with two double bonds, and alpha-linolenic acid, which has 18 carbons with three double bonds. Fatty acids differ from one another based on:

- *Chain length.* Most naturally occurring fatty acids in foods have an even number of carbon atoms, with a chain length ranging from 2 to 20 carbon atoms. Fatty acids with an odd number carbons or branched chains are found in microorganisms and dairy fat. With just two carbons, acetic acid is the shortest fatty acid. Butyric acid is a four-carbon fatty acid commonly found in milk and dairy products. Palm kernel oils are a good source of medium-chain fatty acids such as caproic (6 carbons), caprylic (8 carbons), and lauric (12 carbons) acids. Long-chain fatty acids include palmitic acid (16 carbons) and oleic acid (18 carbons) and their unsaturated forms, as shown in **Figure 4.11**.

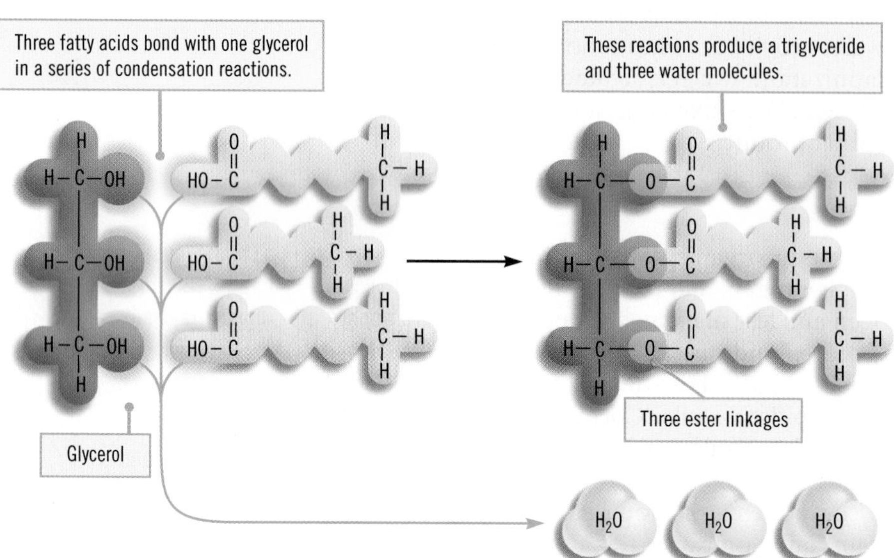

FIGURE 4.9 Triglycerides are formed by the esterification of glycerol with three fatty acids.

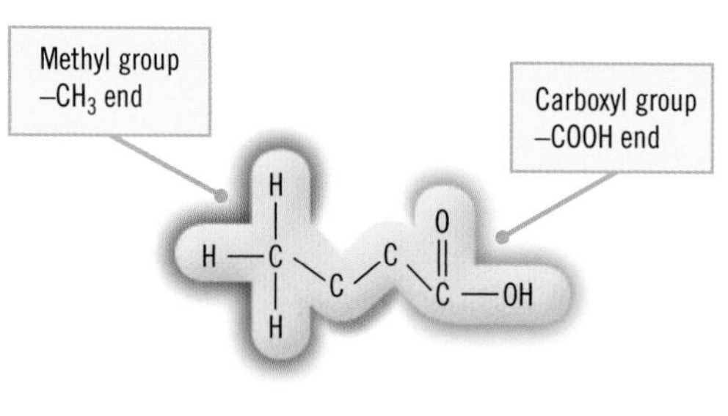

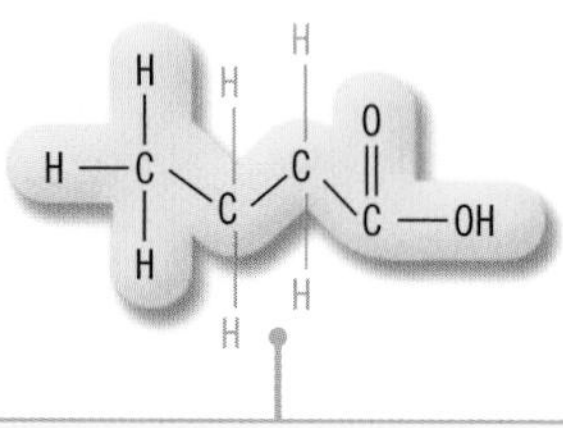

For simplicity, in most instances, the hydrogens are omitted from all but the end carbons.

FIGURE 4.10 The basic structure of a fatty acid is a carbon chain with a methyl end ($-CH_3$) and a carboxylic end (–COOH).

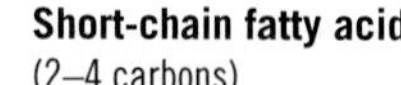

Short-chain fatty acid
(2–4 carbons)

Butyric C4:0

Medium-chain fatty acid
(6–10 carbons)

Caprylic C8:0

Long-chain fatty acid
(12 or more carbons)

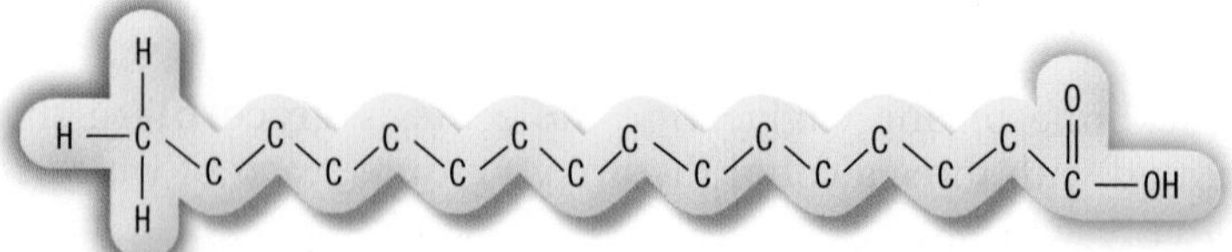

Palmitic C16:0

FIGURE 4.11 Fatty acids range from having 2 to 20 carbons in their chain.

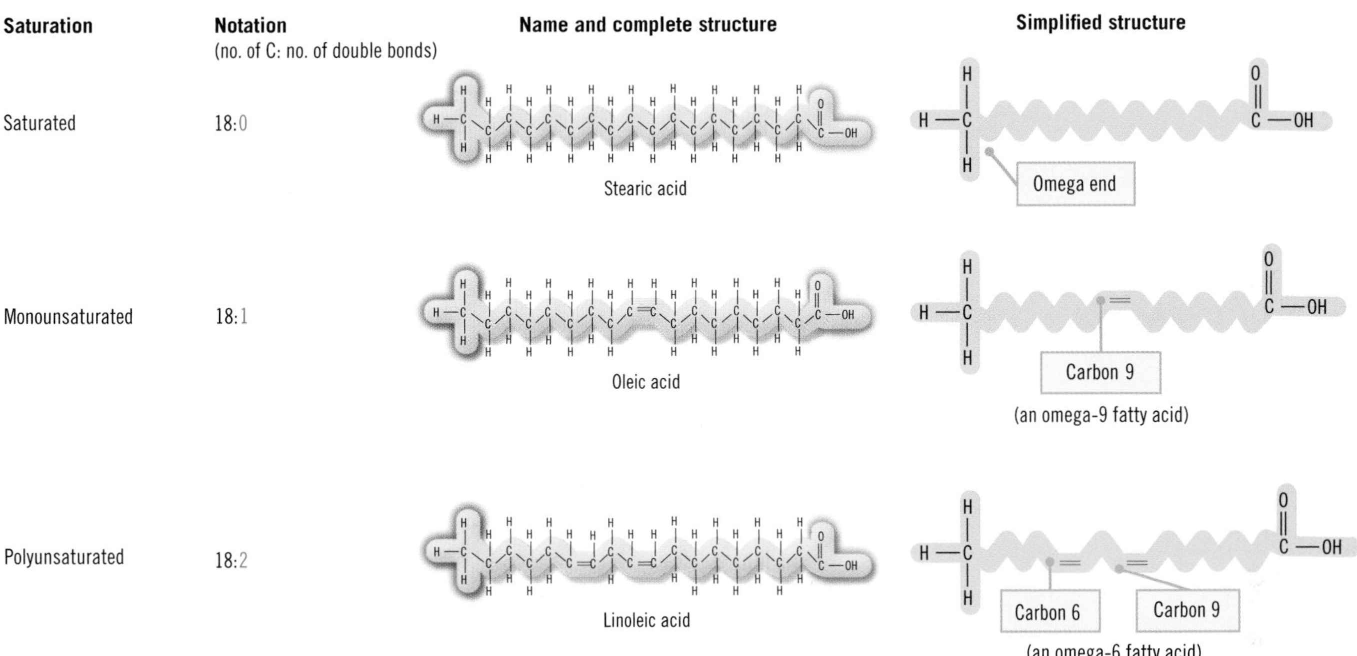

FIGURE 4.12 Fatty acids may be saturated, monounsaturated, or polyunsaturated.

- *Degree of saturation.* Fatty acids that do not have any double bonds between the individual carbon atoms are called *saturated fatty acids*. In these fatty acids, all of the carbon atoms (apart from the carboxylic functional group) are bonded to as many hydrogen atoms as possible (i.e., they are "saturated"). The presence of a carbon–carbon double bond in the chain renders the fatty acid unsaturated. As shown in **Figure 4.12**, at the point of unsaturation one hydrogen atom from each of the two adjacent carbon atoms is missing. A *monounsaturated* fatty acid has a single double bond; a *polyunsaturated* fatty acid has two or more double bonds.
- *Type of double bond.* Double bonds can exist in a cis or trans configuration in three-dimensional space. A cis configuration arises when the hydrogen atoms attached to the carbon atoms are on the same side of the double bond. When the hydrogen atoms on adjacent carbon atoms are on opposite sides of the double bond, a trans configuration occurs, as illustrated in **Figure 4.13**.

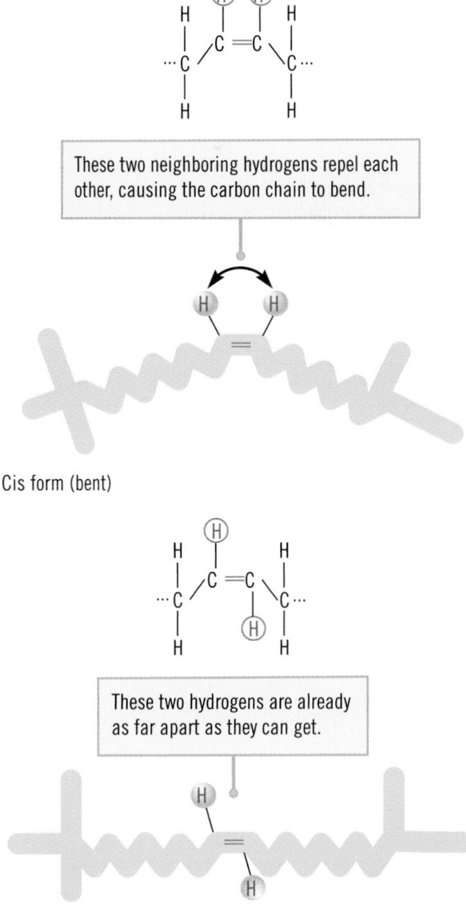

FIGURE 4.13 Double bonds may be in the cis or trans forms. A cis double bond results in significant bending of the fatty acid molecule.

Melting Points

The properties of triglycerides are influenced by the carbon chain length, the degree of unsaturation, and the cis/trans configuration of their fatty acid chains. Long-chain fatty acids have a higher melting point than their short-chain counterparts, as depicted in **Figure 4.14** and **Table 4.6**. Saturated fatty acids, being linear, tend to pack tightly, and therefore also have a higher melting point. For this reason, triglycerides such as animal fats, which are composed predominantly of long-chain fatty acids and/or saturated fatty acids, are more likely to be in a solid state at room temperature as compared to their short-chain and/or unsaturated counterparts (see **Figure 4.15**).

Conversely, vegetable oils containing high amounts of mono- and polyunsaturated fatty acids are liquid at room temperature. Unsaturation bends the fatty acid molecule at the position of the double bond, which means the molecules cannot pack tightly, and less energy is required to melt them. Consequently, they have lower melting points and tend to be liquid at room

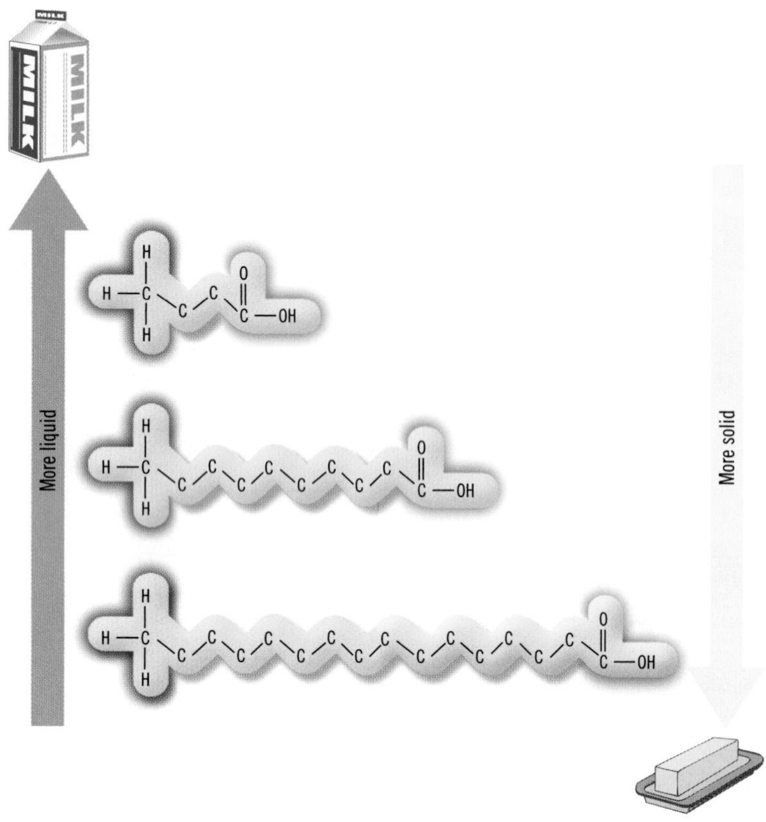

FIGURE 4.14 Fatty acids become more solid at room temperature with increasing chain length.

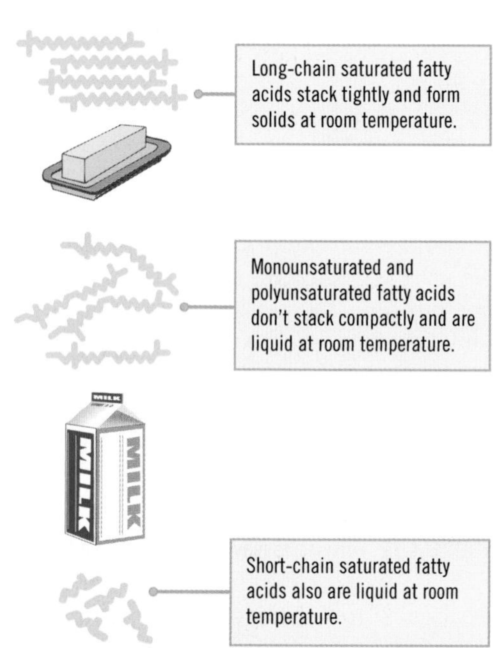

Long-chain saturated fatty acids stack tightly and form solids at room temperature.
Monounsaturated and polyunsaturated fatty acids don't stack compactly and are liquid at room temperature.
Short-chain saturated fatty acids also are liquid at room temperature.

FIGURE 4.15 Short-chain saturated fatty acids and unsaturated fatty acids cannot pack tightly and therefore tend to be liquid at room temperature.

TABLE 4.6
Effect of the Degree of Unsaturation on the Melting Point of Fatty Acids

Fatty Acid	Chemical Formula	Melting Point	Source
Lauric acid	$CH_3(CH_2)_{10}COOH$	113°F (45°C)	Cinnamon, coconut and palm oils
Myristic acid	$CH_3(CH_2)_{12}COOH$	131°F (55°C)	Nutmeg, coconut and palm oils
Palmitic	$CH_3(CH_2)_{14}COOH$	145°F (63°C)	Palm oil, sunflower oil
Stearic acid	$CH_3(CH_2)_{16}CO_2H$	156°F (69°C)	Beef tallow, pork lard
Oleic acid	$CH_3(CH_2)_7CH{=}CH(CH_2)_7COOH$ (*cis*)	57°F (14°C)	Olive oil, canola oil, avocado
Elaidic acid	$CH_3(CH_2)_7CH{=}CH(CH_2)_7COOH$ (*trans*)	111°F (44°C)	Partially hydrogenated vegetable oil
Linoleic acid	$CH_3(CH_2)_4CH{=}CHCH_2CH{=}CH(CH_2)_7COOH$	23°F (–5°C)	Safflower oil, sunflower oil, corn oil, rice bran oil
Linolenic	$CH_3CH_2CH{=}CHCH_2CH{=}CHCH_2CH{=}CH(CH_2)_7COOH$	12°F (–11°C)	Chia seeds, flax, soybean

temperature. Melting point decreases further with increasing levels of unsaturation. For example, stearic acid, oleic acid, and linolenic acid are all fatty acids with 18 carbons, but only stearic acid solidifies upon refrigeration. This difference in physical state can be explained by the effect of the degree of saturation/unsaturation.

The presence of a trans double bond in an unsaturated fatty acid also increases its melting point. For example, oleic acid and elaidic acid are 18-carbon fatty acids with a single double bond at the ninth carbon. The cis double bond of oleic acid makes the carbon chain slightly angular. Thus, its melting point is 57°F (14°C), and it is liquid at room temperature. In contrast, the presence of a trans double bond in elaidic acid gives the fatty acid an almost linear configuration, similar to saturated fatty acids. This raises the melting point to around 111°F (44°C), and it is thus solid at room temperature.

Hydrogenation

Historically, commercial baking applications used lard and tallow, both of which are solids at room temperature. In the early 20th century, it was discovered that unsaturated vegetable oils could be made solid at room temperature through a process called hydrogenation. **Hydrogenation** is the addition of hydrogen atoms to an unsaturated fatty acid, causing the double bonds (unsaturated) to become single bonds (saturated). Hydrogenation turns vegetable oil into shortening.

Complete hydrogenation results in all double bonds being converted into single bonds—an unsaturated fatty acid becomes saturated. Such a modification "hardens" the shortening, giving it a very hard texture that is unsuitable for baking. In contrast, with *partial hydrogenation* some of the cis double bonds are saturated and some of the double bonds are reconfigured from the cis form into the trans form. The result is a *partially hydrogenated fat,* or *trans fat.* The melting point of the fatty acids is increased but not to the same extent as with complete hydrogenation. This reconfiguration results in the shortening having a texture that is conducive to baking.

Because trans fats are an economical alternative to animal fats, their production increased steadily through the last century until research in the 1990s began to link trans fats to coronary heart disease. To comply with the FDA's requirements for zero trans fat labeling, manufacturers have reformulated shortenings, mostly by mixing completely hydrogenated vegetable oils with unsaturated oils.

hydrogenation The addition of hydrogen atoms to an unsaturated fatty acid, causing the double bonds (unsaturated) to become single bonds (saturated).

omega-3 fatty acids Polyunsaturated fatty acids that have their first double bond on the third carbon from the methyl end of the fatty acid chain. They are essential to the human diet and include docosahexaenoic acid (DHA), eicosapentaenoic acid (EPA), and alpha-linolenic acid (ALA).

omega-6 fatty acids Polyunsaturated fatty acids that have the first double bond on the sixth carbon atom from the methyl end. These essential PUFAs, when consumed in moderate amounts, help regulate metabolism, stimulate growth of skin and hair, and maintain bone health. Dietary sources include palm, soybean, rapeseed, and sunflower oils.

Omega-3 and Omega-6 Fatty Acids

Omega-3 and omega-6 fatty acids are essential in the human diet. Because the body cannot make them, they need to be taken in through food. **Omega-3 fatty acids** are polyunsaturated fatty acids (PUFAs), so named because they have their first double bond on the *third* carbon from the methyl end of the fatty acid chain (see **Figure 4.16**). (The methyl end carbon is called the *omega* carbon.) They include docosahexaenoic acid (DHA) and eicosapentaenoic acid (EPA) obtained from fish oil and alpha-linolenic acid (ALA) obtained from walnuts and vegetable oils (e.g., soybean, flaxseed, canola). Omega-3 fatty acids are concentrated in the brain and may be particularly critical to cognitive development. Research also suggests their role in reducing inflammation, possibly preventing the onset of heart diseases and arthritis.[10]

Omega-6 fatty acids such as linoleic acid are so named because they have the first double bond on the *sixth* carbon atom from the methyl end (see **Figure 4.17**). These essential PUFAs, when consumed in moderate amounts, help regulate metabolism, stimulate growth of skin and hair, and maintain bone health. Dietary sources include palm, soybean, rapeseed, and sunflower oils.

By current estimates, the average western diet has somewhere around a 16:1 ratio of omega-6 to omega-3 essential fatty acids. Excessive intakes of

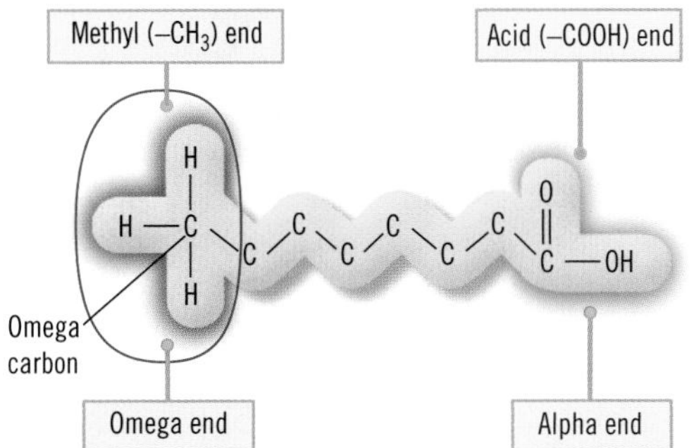

FIGURE 4.16 Fatty acid nomenclature. The carbons are identified by their locations in the chain. Although some disciplines count from the alpha carbon, nutritionists count from the omega carbon.

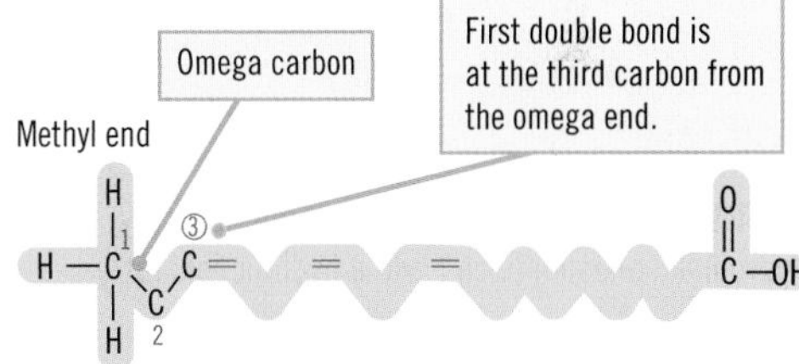

Alpha-linolenic (an omega-3 fatty acid)

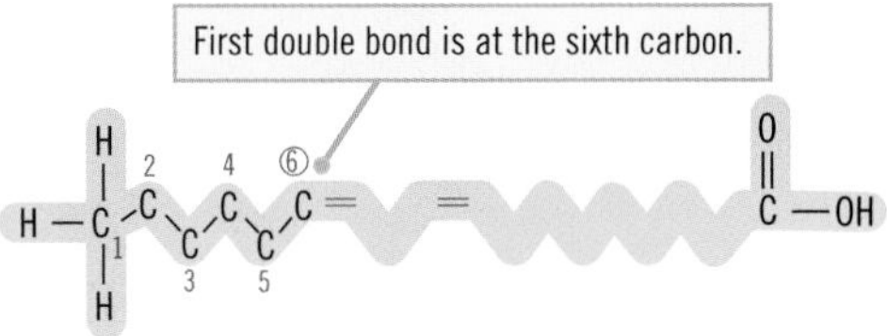

Linoleic (an omega-6 fatty acid)

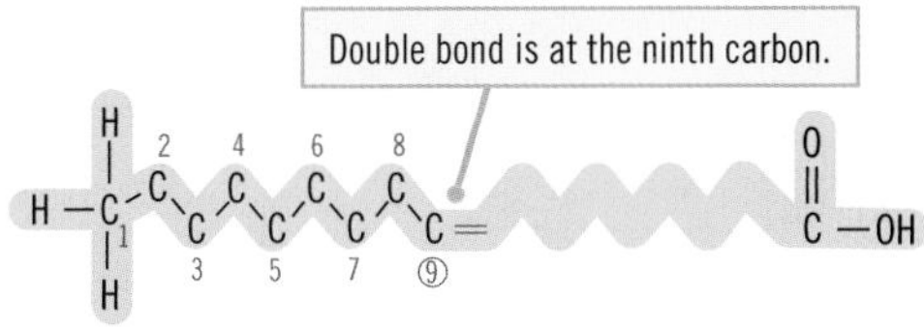

Oleic (an omega-9 fatty acid)

FIGURE 4.17 Fatty acids may be classified as omega–3, –6, or –9 fatty acids based on the position of the first double bond (from the methyl end).

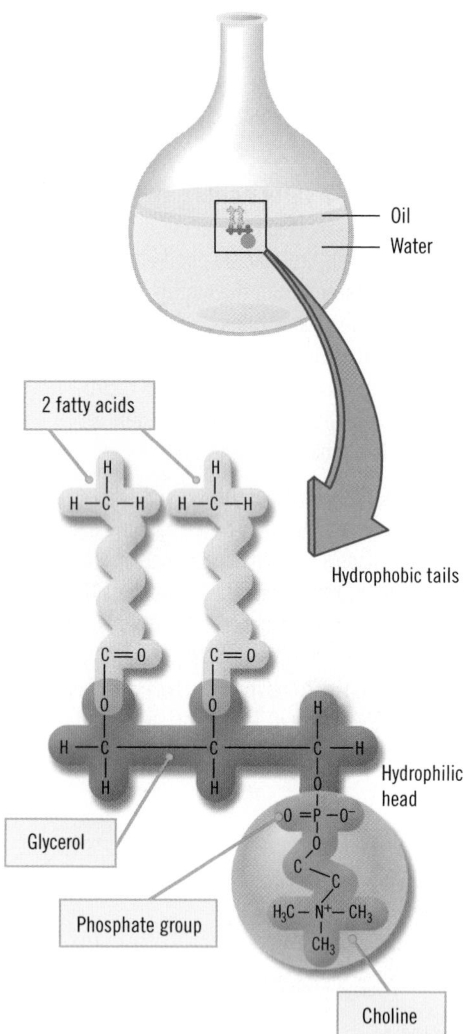

FIGURE 4.18 Phospholipids are characterized by ahydrophilic phosphate end and a hydrophobic fatty acid end.

omega-6 fatty acids have been implicated in promoting the pathogenesis of cardiovascular disease, cancer, and inflammatory and autoimmune diseases, whereas increased levels of omega-3 fatty acids (a low omega-6 to omega-3 ratio) exert suppressive effects.[10] Recent recommendations to decrease the ratio of omega-6 to omega-3 have triggered the incorporation of alpha-linolenic acid, DHA, and EPA into foods and dietary supplements.

Phospholipids

When one of the fatty acids in a triglyceride is replaced by a phosphate group, the resulting diglyceride is called a **phospholipid** (see **Figure 4.18**). This substitution drastically changes the molecule's solubility. The phosphate end is now water soluble (hydrophilic), whereas the fatty acid components are fat soluble (lipophilic). The presence of both hydrophilic and lipophilic ends in the same molecule gives phospholipids the unique ability to create emulsions (i.e., they are emulsifiers). Phospholipids are most commonly used in ice creams, sauces, pourable dressings, mayonnaise, and bakery and dairy products to prevent the separation of their water and oil components. The hydrophilic (phosphate) end of the emulsifier is attracted to the water components in the food, whereas the hydrophobic or lipophilic (fatty acid) end attracts the oil components. The ability of the phospholipids to form a "bridge" between the water and oil molecules prevents the destabilization of these food products, as illustrated in **Figure 4.19**. Lecithin, derived from egg yolk and soybean (as a byproduct of soybean oil refining), is the phospholipid most commonly used as an emulsifier by the food industry.

Sterols

Sterols are lipophilic hydrocarbons with multiple ring structures (see **Figure 4.20**). Most sterols do not contain fatty acids. In foods, sterols are found as cholesterol in animal products and as phytosterols in plant foods. High amounts of cholesterol are found in organ meats (e.g., brain, liver), egg yolk, and in the butterfat portion of dairy products. Phytosterols have a chemical structure similar to cholesterol but are absorbed in the body to a lesser extent. In fact, phytosterols are gaining popularity due to their possible role in lowering intestinal absorption of cholesterol and their potential role in protecting against cancer.

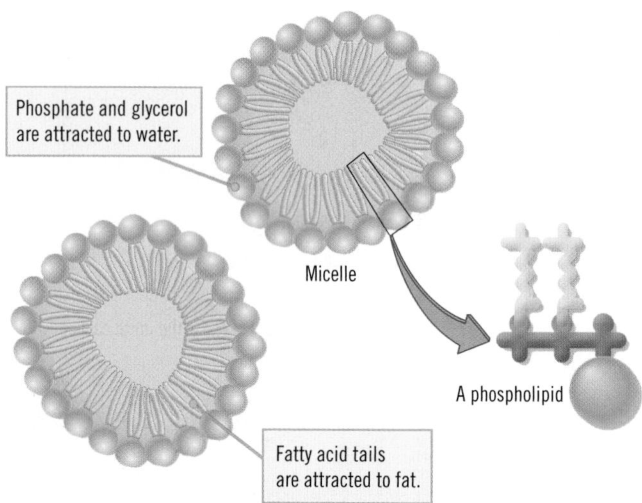

FIGURE 4.19 The amphiphilic nature of phospholipids is the principle behind their use as emulsifiers.

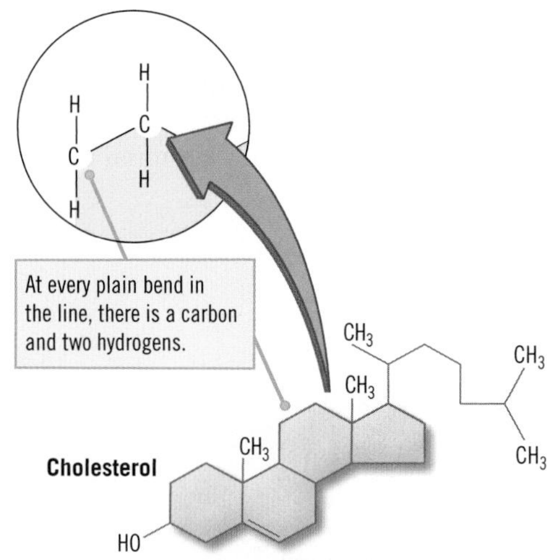

FIGURE 4.20 Structure of cholesterol, a sterol found in animal products.

Proteins

Proteins are complex polymers of amino acids. **Amino acids** are organic molecules containing carbon, hydrogen, oxygen, and nitrogen. Twenty-two amino acids are found in nature. The basic structure of amino acids involves an alpha-carbon atom linked to an amino (NH_2) group, a carboxylic group (COOH), a hydrogen atom, and a side group denoted by the letter *R*. The chemical structure of the side group distinguishes the amino acids from each other in terms of their physical and chemical properties. **Figure 4.21** shows the basic structure of a generic amino acid, plus several specific examples. Glycine is the simplest amino acid, the R group being a single hydrogen atom.

phospholipid The resulting diglyceride when one of the fatty acids in a triglyceride is replaced by a phosphate group.

proteins Complex polymers of amino acids.

amino acids Organic molecules containing carbon, hydrogen, oxygen, and nitrogen. Twenty-two amino acids are found in nature. The basic structure of amino acids involves an alpha-carbon atom linked to an amino (NH_2) group, a carboxylic group (COOH), a hydrogen atom, and a side group denoted by the letter R.

peptide bond Covalent bond between the nitrogen of one amino acid with the carbon of the carboxylic group of the adjacent amino acid. Also known as an *amide bond*.

primary structure Linear arrangement of amino acids in a protein chain.

secondary structure Foldings or coilings within a protein structure that are stabilized by hydrogen bonding.

tertiary structure Final three dimensional structure of protein that involves numerous noncovalent interactions between amino acids.

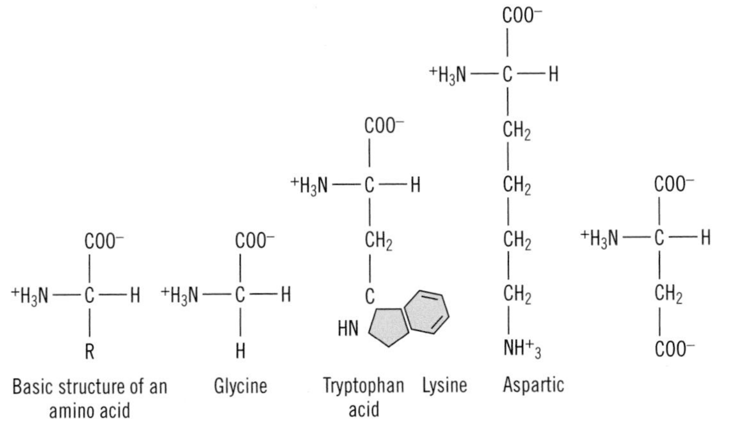

Protein Organization

Although most proteins contain all 22 amino acids, they differ in chain length, amino acid sequence, and inter- and intrachain bonds. The amino acids comprising a protein are linked to each other by peptide bonds. A **peptide bond** (also called an *amide bond*) is a covalent bond between the nitrogen of one amino acid with the carbon of the carboxylic group of the adjacent amino acid, as shown in **Figure 4.22**. Peptide bonds result in a backbone chain with alternating nitrogen and carbon atoms (–N–C–N–C–N–C–). The side group, hydrogen, and oxygen portions of the functional groups extend outward from this backbone chain.

Primary Structure

The **primary structure** of a protein is the most basic level of its organization. It is the amino acids comprising it in order.

Secondary Structure

Intramolecular hydrogen bonding between the nitrogen and carbonyl (–C=O) groups of neighboring amino acids results in the bending of the primary structure into a helical or pleated structure called the **secondary structure**.

Tertiary Structure

The helical secondary structure can be further folded into various configurations by the formation of hydrogen bonds, salt bridges, and hydrophobic interactions between the different side groups that extend from the backbone chain. This convoluted structure is called the **tertiary structure**, and it is the final level of protein organization in most proteins.

FIGURE 4.21 Structure of an amino acid. All amino acids have a similar generic structure: a central carbon attached to an amino group (NH_2), a carboxylic group (COOH), hydrogen (H) and a variable side chain (R). The side group gives each amino acid its unique identity.

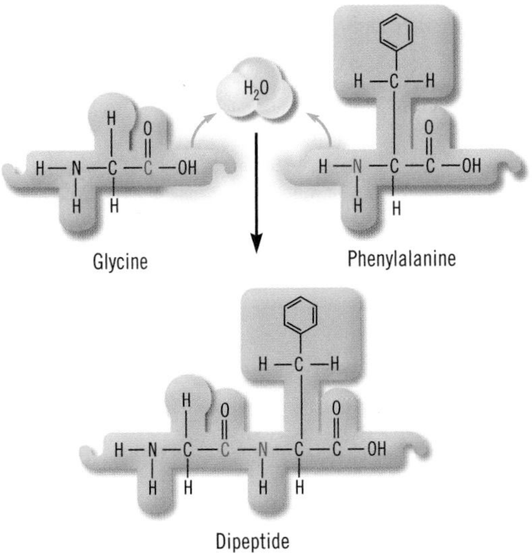

FIGURE 4.22 Amino acids are linked together by peptide bonds.

quaternary structure How multiple peptide chains are aggregated together by hydrogen bonds, disulfide linkages, and salt bridges into a final specific protein shape.

complete proteins Proteins containing all essential amino acids. Examples include meat and dairy proteins and soybeans.

incomplete proteins Proteins that lack one or more essential amino acid. Most plant proteins are incomplete proteins.

Quaternary Structure

Some proteins, such as hemoglobin, gelatin, insulin, and chlorophyll, exhibit a quaternary level of organization. **Quaternary structure** defines how multiple peptide chains are aggregated together by hydrogen bonds, disulfide linkages, and salt bridges into a final specific shape. The various levels in the hierarchy of protein organization are shown in **Figure 4.23**.

Dietary Sources of Proteins

Animal sources of protein include eggs, dairy (yogurt, milk, and cheese), fish, meat, and poultry. With the exception of gelatin, animal proteins are **complete proteins**, meaning that they supply all essential amino acids. Plant sources of proteins include legumes (e.g., beans, lentils) and cereal grains. These are **incomplete proteins**, with the exception of soybean, quinoa, and amaranth.

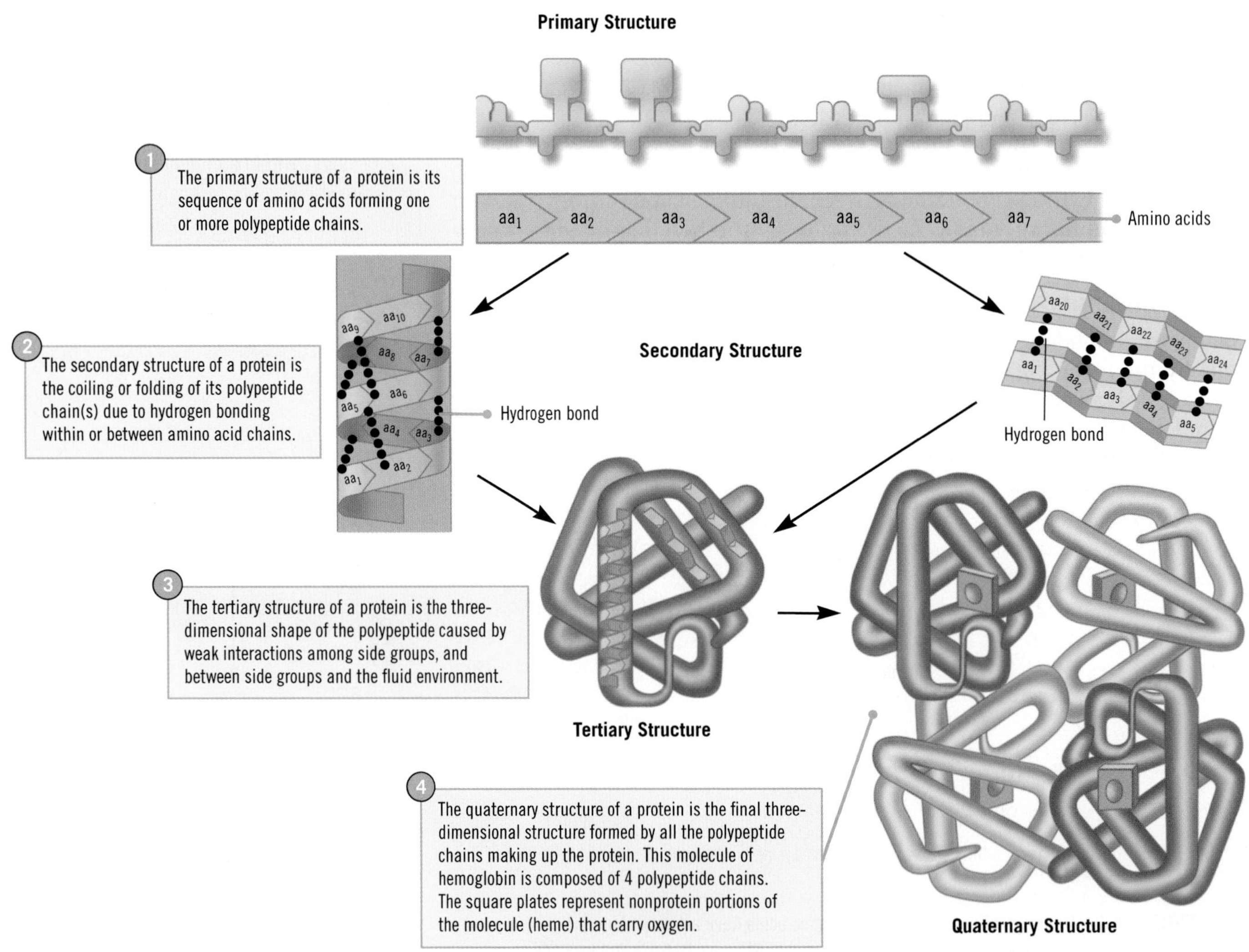

Primary Structure
1
The primary structure of a protein is its sequence of amino acids forming one or more polypeptide chains.
aa1 aa2 aa3 aa4 aa5 aa6 aa7
Amino acids
2
The secondary structure of a protein is the coiling or folding of its polypeptide chain(s) due to hydrogen bonding within or between amino acid chains.
Hydrogen bond
Secondary Structure
Hydrogen bond
3
The tertiary structure of a protein is the three-dimensional shape of the polypeptide caused by weak interactions among side groups, and between side groups and the fluid environment.
Tertiary Structure
4
The quaternary structure of a protein is the final three-dimensional structure formed by all the polypeptide chains making up the protein. This molecule of hemoglobin is composed of 4 polypeptide chains. The square plates represent nonprotein portions of the molecule (heme) that carry oxygen.
Quaternary Structure

FIGURE 4.23 Proteins can be described by their primary, secondary, tertiary, or quaternary structure.

Protein complementation—mixing multiple sources of plant proteins to consume all essential amino acids—is recommended for individuals who solely depend on plants as their dietary source of protein.

protein complementation Combining two or more different protein sources to have a better amino acid balance than when consuming either protein alone.

food foam Two-phase system where air is dispersed in a continuous liquid or solid phase.

Functional Properties of Proteins

During food processing and cooking, proteins are involved in a wide range of reactions that are responsible for the varied texture and color of processed and cooked foods.

Protein Hydration

Water modifies the physicochemical properties of proteins by binding to several groups in the amino acid residues of a protein molecule. The hydration (or water-binding) capacity of a protein is related to its amino acid composition: Proteins with a greater number of charged amino acid residues have greater hydration capacities than those with predominantly nonpolar residues. The hydration capacity of proteins is also influenced by pH, salt concentration, and temperature. Proteins are least hydrated at their isoelectric pH (the pH at which proteins have zero net charge); hydration capacities increase at low salt concentrations and decrease with increasing temperature. Many food applications, such as solubility, dispersibility, viscosity, gelation, and foaming, depend on these protein–water interactions.[11] In food applications, the water-holding capacity of proteins (e.g., the amount of free water released from meat after grinding) is more critical than water-binding capacity (e.g., the amount of bound water left in the meat after grinding). The ability of proteins to entrap water within its three dimensional network is associated with the juiciness and texture of comminuted meat products, sausages, and gelled fish products.

Gelatin, the most commonly used gelling agent in food preparation, is obtained from the hydrolysis of collagen (connective tissue in meat products). When dissolved in water, gelatin forms a viscous matrix, which upon cooling forms a gel. Gelatin is widely used as a thickener in sauces, jams, and yogurt; as a fat replacer in reduced-fat products to mimic the creamy mouthfeel of their full-fat counterparts; and in a myriad of food products, including gelatin desserts, marshmallows, and gummy candy.

Protein-Surface Properties

Proteins are amphiphilic molecules. Thus, in emulsion-type products, they will spontaneously migrate to the oil–water interface and have a stabilizing effect. Proteins are important as emulsifiers in several natural and processed foods, including milk, egg yolks, salad dressings, frozen desserts, sausages, and cakes. The stabilizing effect of proteins is exemplified during milk homogenization. In raw milk, a lipoprotein membrane stabilizes the fat globules. During homogenization, the lipoprotein membrane is replaced by a stronger protein film (comprising casein and whey proteins). Homogenization thus renders the milk fat globule smaller and more stable against creaming.

A **food foam** is a two-phase system where air is dispersed in a continuous liquid or solid phase. Whipped cream, meringues, cakes, soufflés, bread, and mousses are examples of foams. Proteins are the most important surface-active ingredient in maintaining foam stability. Whipping, bubbling, or shaking a protein solution results in the formation of a thin film at the gas–liquid interface, entrapping large numbers of gas bubbles. This is particularly evident when beating egg whites; the ovalbumin, conalbumin, and lysozyme proteins present contribute to the foaming properties of egg whites. Foam formation and stability is influenced by temperature and the presence of lipids, acids, salts, and sugars in the food matrix.

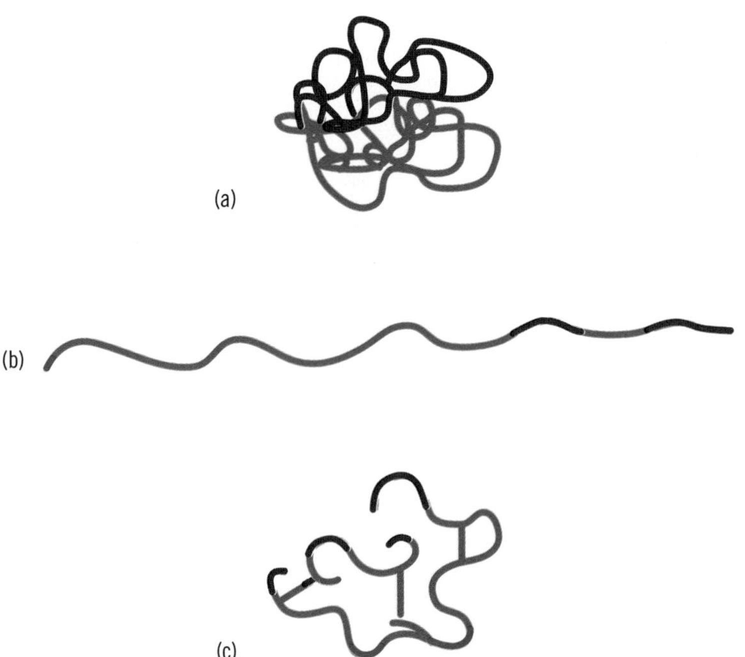

FIGURE 4.24 Denaturation, which can be achieved by the application of heat or acid, is required for protein coagulation. When an egg is cooked, the ovalbumin in the egg white becomes denatured, causing the egg white to coagulate into a white solid. (a) Native protein, tightly coiled. (b) Denatured protein, unfolding of the protein chain. (c) Coagulated protein, denatured protein binds together.

Flavor Binding

Proteins themselves are odorless compounds, but they can bind to flavor molecules and undermine the sensory attributes of oil products. For example, aldehydes and ketones generated during oxidation of unsaturated fatty acids often bind to oilseed proteins, imparting characteristic off-flavors. However, some proteins are used to enhance the flavors of processed foods. For example, simulated meat flavors are added to the plant proteins in meat analogs, enhancing the sensory acceptability of such products.[11]

Denaturation and Coagulation

Protein denaturation refers to the disruption of bonds that make up the tertiary and secondary structure of proteins. During protein denaturation, the weak (nonbonded) intra- and intermolecular secondary linkages are lost, unraveling the secondary structure. (Peptide linkages are not affected, leaving the primary structure intact.) Protein denaturation can occur through the addition of heat, alcohol, acids, salts, enzymes, and mechanical shear. Denatured proteins can congeal and separate out, a phenomenon called **protein coagulation** (protein gel formation), as shown in **Figure 4.24**. These irreversible changes in protein structure are seen when egg whites stiffen upon beating or harden upon heating. Cheese production also takes advantage of protein coagulation. Adding lactic acid and the enzyme rennin to milk denatures the milk proteins, which are then coagulated and separated for ripening and/or salting.

protein denaturation The disruption of bonds that make up the tertiary and secondary structure of proteins. Can occur through the addition of heat, alcohol, acids, salts, enzymes, and mechanical shear.

protein coagulation Congealing and separating out of denatured proteins.

enzymes Biocatalysts that speed up the rate of biochemical reactions, without getting destroyed themselves. Not all proteins are enzymes, but all enzymes are proteins. Each enzyme catalyzes a specific type of reaction.

Proteins as Enzymes

Enzymes are biocatalysts that speed up the rate of biochemical reactions, without getting destroyed themselves. Not all proteins are enzymes, but all enzymes are proteins. Each enzyme catalyzes a specific type of reaction. **Figure 4.25** summarizes the mechanism of enzymatic activity for sucrose hydrolysis. The reactant, in this case sucrose, binds to the active site of the enzyme sucrase. The enzyme–reactant complex is reconfigured, lowering the activation energy for the hydrolysis reaction. Sucrose is then cleaved into glucose and fructose. The newly formed products (glucose and fructose) are released from the enzyme's active site, which is now free to accept more reactant molecules.

Factors Affecting Enzyme Activity

Enzymes, being proteins, are very susceptible to denaturation and loss of function. Each enzyme has a specific pH and temperature for optimal activity. The optimal condition for most enzymes is a neutral pH (around 7) and a temperature range of 95 to 104°F. At extremes of pH and temperature, enzymes become denatured and no longer effective as biocatalysts. pH and temperature during food processing are controlled based on whether the application requires the enzymes to be active or inactive. For example, the enzyme invertase is added to fondant to catalyze the liquefaction of a candy center (as in chocolate-covered cherries). To maintain enzyme activity, invertase must be added to the candy mixture only after the molten mixture has cooled down.

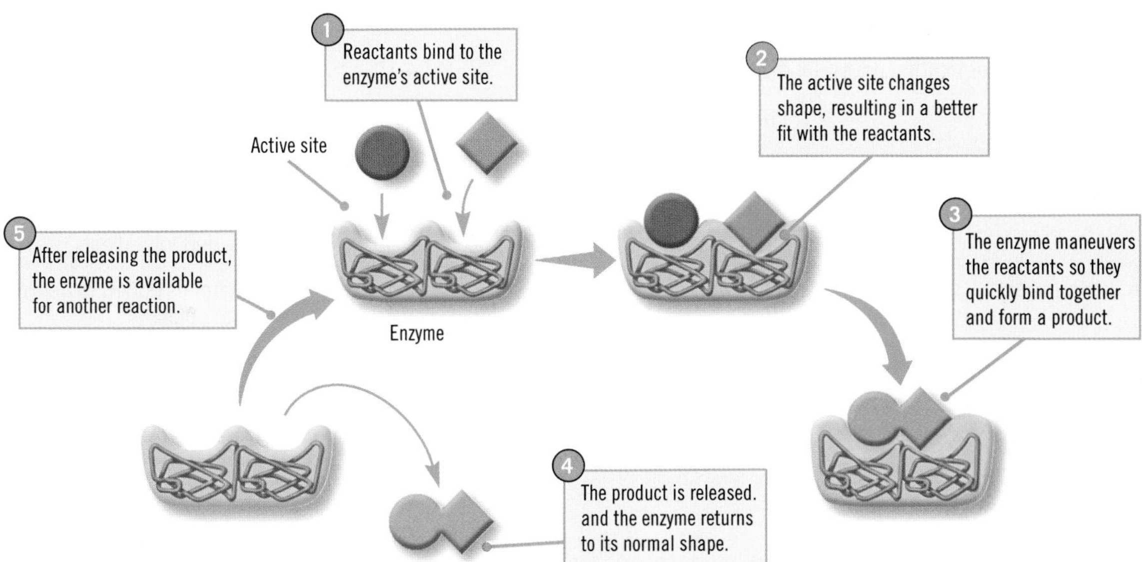
Reactants bind to the enzyme's active site.
The active site changes shape, resulting in a better fit with the reactants.
Active site
After releasing the product, the enzyme is available for another reaction.
The enzyme maneuvers the reactants so they quickly bind together and form a product.
Enzyme
The product is released. and the enzyme returns to its normal shape.

FIGURE 4.25 The hydrolysis of sucrose is speeded by the presence of the enzyme sucrase.

Other applications require enzyme inactivation to preserve or improve food quality. Examples include blanching potatoes to inactivate the polyphenol oxidase enzyme responsible for oxidative browning. Fresh pineapples should not be added to a gelatin salad. The enzyme bromelain from pineapple can hydrolyze the gelatin, resulting in loss of gel structure.

Gastronomy Point

Raw Fruits Raw fruits such as pineapple and papaya contain proteolytic enzymes (bromelain and papain, respectively) that can hydrolyze gelatin and reduce its gelling ability. These fruits can be incorporated into a gelatin salad only in their cooked (or canned) forms.

Applications of Enzymes

Enzymes are used in a variety of different types of food preparations:

- *Using lactase to make lactose-free milk.* Lactase hydrolyzes the lactose into glucose and galactose, which renders the milk suitable for individuals with lactose intolerance.
- *Heating custard mixtures and pie fillings containing egg yolk and starch denatures the enzyme amylase in egg yolks.* During storage, residual amylase activity in the custard can degrade starch amylose into smaller molecules. The high mobility of these small molecules reduces the viscosity and or/gel strength of the custard.
- *Encouraging (or inhibiting) browning.* In a process called **enzymatic browning**, the enzyme polyphenol oxidase (PPO) catalyzes the oxidation of phenols into brown-colored melanins, which are formed in the production of black tea, cocoa, and red wine. However, PPO must be inhibited to prevent the undesirable browning of potato chips; fruit salads containing apples, pears, and bananas; and guacamole. Enzymatic browning can be prevented by blocking the availability of oxygen for the reaction, inhibiting PPO activity, or by inactivating the enzyme. Some commonly used methods to inhibit enzymatic browning are summarized in **Table 4.7**. Another type of undesirable enzymatic browning occurs in mushrooms, when the enzyme tyrosinase catalyzes the oxidation of the amino acid tyrosine into brown-colored melanin compounds. Although melanins are not harmful for consumption, they are responsible for the inferior sensory qualities of some fresh and frozen produce.

enzymatic browning Process whereby the enzyme polyphenol oxidase (PPO) catalyzes the oxidation of phenols into brown-colored melanins.

TABLE 4.7
Commonly Used Methods to Inhibit Enzymatic Browning in Foods

Method	Principle Involved	Examples
Addition of acidulants (e.g., citric acid, ascorbic acid)	Reduces the pH to below the optimal levels for PPO activity	• Homemade fruit platters containing apples often are sprinkled with lemon juice. • Guacamole recipes often have lemon juice as an added ingredient.
Addition of reducing agents	Removal of oxygen	• Sulfite often is added to dehydrated fruits and vegetables.
Blanching	High temperature treatment inactivates PPO	• Potatoes are blanched immediately after slicing and prior to freezing.
Refrigeration and freezing	At temperature < 44.6°F (7°C), PPO activity is inhibited, although enzyme is not inactivated	• Refrigerated and frozen storage of produce.

- *Adding pectinases to fruit juices (pectin hydrolysis) to clarify juice.* Pectinases also are used to increase juice yield, especially from grapes.
- *Producing high fructose corn syrup from cornstarch.* High fructose corn syrup (HFCS) is produced from cornstarch using a sequence of enzymes: alpha-amylase, glucoamylase, and glucose isomerase. HFCS is used in a wide range of processed foods.
- *Using glucose oxidase to reduce sugar content.* Glucose oxidase is added to dried egg whites, potatoes, and flour to reduce sugar content and minimize browning reactions.
- *Adding rennin to milk to make cultured milk products.* The enzyme rennin acts on the milk protein casein, causing milk to curdle. The curd can then be processed into unripened cheese (e.g., cottage) or ripened cheese (e.g., Swiss, cheddar). Microbial cultures added during the ripening process produce enzymes (proteases, peptidases, lipases) bring about the strong flavors unique to ripened cheese.
- *Using alkaline phosphatase and peroxidase to optimize heat treatments used during milk pasteurization.* Both of these enzymes are found in milk. Alkaline phosphatase is denatured at a temperature exceeding that required to kill *Mycobacterium tuberculosis* (a pathogen present in raw milk that causes tuberculosis). The presence of this enzyme is therefore an indicator of inadequate heat treatment. Peroxidase is denatured at 176°F (80°C); its absence is indicative of excessive heat treatment. Excessive heating negatively affects milk's nutritive and sensory properties.[12]

Innovation Point

Enzymes Traditionally, the food industry has used enzymes in solution form. Unfortunately, this practice allows the enzymes to be used only once, which may be cost-prohibitive for some products. Innovations have allowed enzymes to be immobilized by various methods, including cross-linking them to inert carrier molecules. Immobilized enzyme systems allow repetitive use of a single batch of enzyme, improve the enzyme's heat stability, and result in enzyme-free end products.

nonenzymatic browning The most common type of browning in processed foods. These reactions occur at elevated temperatures and include the caramelization of sugars and Maillard reactions between amino acids and sugars.

carmelization A series of reactions involving dehydration, isomerization, and polymerization, resulting in the formation of polymeric caramels (caramel colloids). Caramels are responsible for the dark brown colors of certain foods.

Nonenzymatic Browning

In addition to enzymatic browning, foods may also be browned in nonenzymatic reactions. **Nonenzymatic browning** is the most common type of browning in processed foods. These reactions occur at elevated temperatures and include the caramelization of sugars and Maillard reactions between amino acids and sugars.

Caramelization

Carmelization occurs when foods containing high amounts of sugars are dry-heated. **Carmelization** involves a series of reactions involving dehydration, isomerization, and polymerization, resulting in the formation of polymeric caramels (caramel colloids). These caramels are responsible for the dark brown colors of certain foods. In addition, flavor compounds such as diacetyl (buttery flavor) and hydroxymethyl furfural are also formed through carmelization. Caramelization contributes to the desirable brown colors in caramel syrup (such as in flan), roasted coffee, carbonated colas, and beer.

Maillard Reactions

The series of nonenzymatic reactions between reducing sugars and amino acids at high temperatures that result in browning are called **Maillard reactions**. The reactions usually take place at temperatures greater than 194°F (90°C); however, some food products exhibit Maillard browning at room temperature, albeit very slowly (such as browning of milk powders during prolonged storage at room temperature). These reactions are critical to many forms of food preparation, especially baking and frying, and are partially responsible for the brown color and flavor in cakes, cookies, breads, sweetened condensed milk, roasted and browned meats, chocolate, and coffee, to name a few. Although the color and flavor changes due to Maillard reactions are generally appreciated by consumers, they do reduce the nutritive value slightly because some of the food item's sugars and amino acids are lost during the reactions.

Maillard reactions Series of nonenzymatic reactions between reducing sugars and amino acids at high temperatures that result in browning.

vitamins Organic, nutritionally essential compounds that are mostly heat labile. They are classified as water soluble or fat soluble.

Health Concerns About Acrylamide

Maillard reactions also can result in carcinogenic end products. One such end product is acrylamide, formed by the Maillard reactions between the amino acid asparagine and reducing sugars (e.g., glucose, fructose, lactose) when starchy foods are heated beyond 356°F (180°C), especially during baking and frying. The most common processed foods with elevated acrylamide levels include potato chips, French fries, cereals, crackers, and bread. Based on evidence from experiments with animals, acrylamide is reasonably anticipated to be a human carcinogen.[13]

Research towards reducing acrylamide levels has been wide ranging. Farming practices to reduce nitrogen content of the soil and increase sulfide content have been shown to reduce acrylamide levels.[13] Genetically engineered potatoes with lower levels of reducing sugars and/or asparagine may decrease the amount of reactants available for Maillard reactions.[14] The enzyme asparaginase also has been used successfully to reduce asparagine in foods, thereby reducing acrylamide levels in the cooked products.[15] The simplest solution may lie in alternative cooking methods. Because acrylamide levels increase with prolonged exposure to high temperatures, it is recommended that boiling and steaming be used, instead of baking and frying, and that overcooking be avoided.

Phytonutrient Point

Alpha-Linolenic Acid Alpha-linolenic acid, found in flaxseed, walnut, and canola oils, can be converted into DHA and EPA, although the efficiency of conversion is very low in the human body. Nevertheless, it is an important omega-3 fatty acid, especially in a vegetarian diet.

Innovation Point

Benecol Benecol spread, launched in 1995, was the first functional food containing phytosterols. Owing to their cholesterol-lowering effect, phytosterols have now been incorporated into bakery products, beverages, mayonnaise, salad dressings, and yogurt-based drinks.

Vitamins and Minerals

Both vitamins and minerals are quantitatively minor constituents of foods. They are noncaloric, but they are vital for proper metabolism and other physiological functions. **Vitamins** are organic, nutritionally essential compounds that are mostly heat labile. They are classified as water-soluble (B complex and vitamin C) or fat-soluble (A, D, E and K) vitamins. Vitamin C is found naturally only in plants; Vitamin B_{12} is found naturally in animal foods, yeast, and fermented plant products such as tempeh and tofu. Vitamins A, C, and E and the mineral iron are added during the processing of some foods. Vitamins A, C, and E act as scavengers of free radicals. Free radicals can drastically alter the sensory and nutritive values of food products (especially high-fat products). **Table 4.8** shows the changes in the nutrient composition of food during processing, cooking, and storage.

TABLE 4.8
Effect of Processing (and Cooking) and Storage Conditions on Nutrient Composition of Foods

Nutrient	Significant Food Sources	Effect of Processing and Storage Conditions
Carbohydrates	Cereal grains (rice, wheat, corn), whole and processed products Vegetables such as potatoes and tapioca, lactose from milk and dairy products	Sugars undergo Maillard reactions with proteins at high temperatures. Starches dextrinize under dry heat and gelatinize under most heat.
Proteins	Animal proteins (meat, poultry, fish, milk, egg), plant proteins (legumes, beans, lentils)	React with sugars at high temperatures (Maillard reactions). Denature and coagulate at high temperatures.
Fats	Butter, margarine, vegetable oils	Oxidative and hydrolytic rancidity when exposed to air and water, respectively. The reactions are accelerated by exposure to light.
Vitamin A (Carotenoids)	Sweet potato, carrot, pumpkin, beef liver, cheese, milk	Heat labile, oxidize when exposed to heat and light.
Vitamin B_1 (Thiamin)	Breakfast cereals (whole grain), enriched rice, enriched pasta, pork, salmon, legumes (soybeans, chickpeas, kidney beans)	Heat labile, leach out in cooking water. Destroyed under alkaline conditions and exposure to sulfating agents.
Vitamin B_2 (Riboflavin)	Breakfast cereals (whole grain), beef liver, yogurt, cheese, milk, spinach, legumes (soybeans, chickpeas, kidney beans), pork, salmon, lamb	Destroyed by exposure to light. Highly stable under acidic conditions, rapidly destroyed under alkaline pH. Negligible loss from dehydrated foods during storage at ambient temperatures.
Vitamin B_3 (Niacin)	Breakfast cereals (whole grain), beef liver, chicken, tuna, barley, rice	Stable to heat and light. Leach into the cooking water.
Folate	Breakfast cereals (whole grain), legumes and lentils, broccoli, spinach, collards	High retention during processing and storage of fortified foods. High losses during home cooking through leaching out into aqueous cooking media.
Vitamin B_6 (Pyridoxine)	Breakfast cereals (whole grain), bananas, potato and sweet potato, broccoli, chicken, pork, tuna	Susceptible to light-induced degradation and loss through leaching out into aqueous cooking media.
Vitamin B_{12}	Breakfast cereals (whole grain), beef liver, salmon, beef, cheese, yogurt	Stable to most commonly used methods of food processing and storage. Some loss during prolonged heating at neutral pH.
Biotin	Egg yolk, cheese, cauliflower	Stable to heat, light, and oxygen. Extremes of pH can cause degradation.
Vitamin C (Ascorbic acid)	Red pepper, strawberries, Brussels sprouts, broccoli, pineapple, kiwi fruit, tomatoes	High loss through leaching from freshly cut/bruised fruits and vegetables. Leached into aqueous cooking media. Loss during cooking and storage is largely dependent on food composition and exposure to metal ions and oxygen.
Vitamin D	Salmon, sardines, milk	Oxidative losses during exposure to light.
Vitamin E	Breakfast cereals, sunflowers seeds and oil, almonds, peanuts, spinach, canola oil	Fairly stable under anaerobic conditions, rapid degradation in the presence of oxygen and free radicals.

enrichment Adding back of nutrients after processing of a food. The Flour Enrichment Act of 1972 mandated the addition of thiamin, riboflavin, niacin, and iron to flour.

Enrichment and Fortification

Food processing often results in the loss of certain nutrients. These nutrients may be added back to the processed foods by the process of **enrichment**. The Flour Enrichment Act of 1972 mandated the addition of thiamin, riboflavin, niacin, and iron to flour. Rice also can be enriched, but riboflavin is excluded from the vitamin mixture used for enrichment of white rice because it imparts a yellowish coating on the rice.

Foods also may be used as carriers to deliver certain nutrients as a means to prevent specific nutrient deficiencies in the population, a process called as **fortification**. Fortification renders the food a good or superior source of the added nutrients. Examples include fortification of salt with iodine, milk with vitamins A and D, and orange juice with calcium.

fortification Addition of certain nutrients to a food as a means to prevent specific nutrient deficiencies in the population.

The stability of the added nutrients under the rigors of processing conditions must be considered during enrichment and fortification. For example, the naturally occurring form of folic acid, tetrahydrofolic acid, is highly susceptible to oxidation, whereas the synthetic form is very stable. Therefore, the synthetic form is used for fortification of breakfast cereals, pasta, breads, and other cereal products.

Losses of Vitamins During Food Production

Most growing, harvesting, handling, storage, and processing techniques are adapted to minimize nutrient loss. However, vitamin losses are inevitable as part of the postharvest food processing chain. A number of factors are responsible for these losses.

Inherent Variation

The vitamin content of fruits and vegetable varies based on the climate in which they were grown, the particular cultivar, and the stage of maturity. For example, in tomatoes the highest concentration of ascorbic acid is attained before full maturity, and folic acid concentrations decrease during ripening. Variations in agricultural practices, such as fertilizer use and the irrigation regimen, also are likely have an impact on the rate of synthesis and degradation of vitamins in plants.[16]

Handling

Loss in vitamin content can occur during postharvest handling and distribution of produce, postslaughter handling and distribution of meat products, and storage and distribution of milk products. For example, milk products are excellent sources of riboflavin. However, riboflavin is light sensitive, so milk products must be packaged in opaque containers. Loss of cellular compartmentation in fruits and vegetables during postharvest activities can release oxidative and hydrolytic enzymes, which can decrease the concentration and/or bioavailability of vitamins. The extent of enzymatic activity depends on the severity of the postharvest handling methods. Because plant produce is metabolically active after harvest, mishandling of produce through prolonged exposure to ambient temperatures can cause significant loss in vitamin content.

Food Processing

Pretreatment of fruits and vegetables, such as trimming, peeling, and cutting, results in the loss of some water-soluble vitamins. The extent of loss is greater under alkaline pH; therefore, it is not advisable to use baking soda to facilitate peeling, to brighten colors, or to speed up cooking time for legumes. Folates are easily lost into the cooking water, although the overall loss varies among different vegetables and is a function of the chemical environment (such as pH and the presence of enzymes or oxidants).[17] Vitamin and mineral retention is maximized by minimizing leaching and chemical changes, such as oxidation and interaction with other food constituents.

In cereal grains, major losses of vitamins occur during the refining process. Because many vitamins are concentrated in the bran and germ layers, removal of these layers during the refining process drastically reduces the vitamin content of refined cereals.[18] Although enrichment of refined cereal products with riboflavin, niacin, thiamin, iron, and calcium can improve their nutritive value, the impetus has been towards increased consumption of whole grains.

Innovation Point

Golden Rice Project Under the auspices of the Golden Rice Project, Swiss scientists Ingo Potrykus and Peter Beyer were successful in transferring the genes for beta-carotene synthesis from daffodils into the genome of a temperate strain of rice. In its current form, Golden Rice contains 35 micrograms of beta-carotene per gram of rice, which converts to vitamin A in the human diet. It is hoped that Golden Rice will alleviate vitamin A deficiencies in many parts of the developing world where rice is a part of the staple diet.

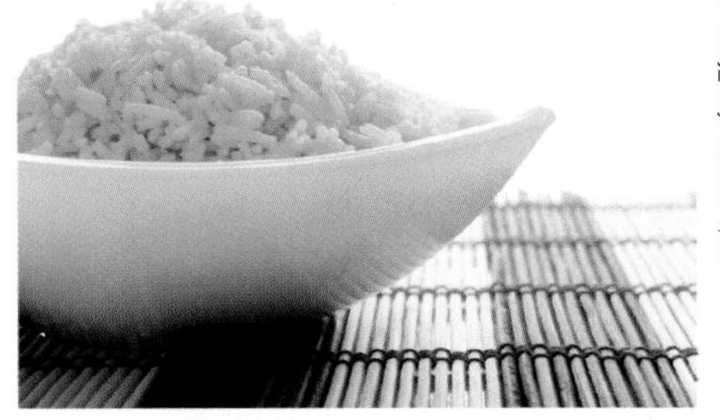

Blanching of fruits and vegetables, especially before freezing and canning, inactivates enzymes that could potentially have a detrimental effect on vitamin content. Sulfites are added as an antimicrobial agent to wines and as an inhibitor of enzymatic browning in dried fruits. (Added sulfites must be indicated on the label.) These compounds have a protective effect on ascorbic acid, but a detrimental effect on thiamin and pyridoxine. Acidic environments stabilize ascorbic acid and thiamin, whereas alkalizing compounds reduce the stability of ascorbic acid, thiamin, pantothenic acid, and folate.[18]

An exception to the effect of food processing on the bioavailability of vitamins is that of biotin from egg yolk. The protein avidin present in egg whites binds to biotin and prevents its absorption from raw eggs. Heat processing destroys avidin, allowing biotin to be readily absorbed from cooked eggs.

Minerals

mineral An element other than carbon, hydrogen, oxygen, and nitrogen that is present in food. Minerals is heat stable and are classified as major or trace, depending on their concentrations in plants and animals.

The term **mineral** in food and nutrition usually refers to an element other than carbon, hydrogen, oxygen, and nitrogen that is present in food. Minerals are heat stable and are classified as major or trace, depending on their concentrations in plants and animals. Major minerals include calcium, phosphorus, magnesium, sodium, potassium, and chloride. Trace minerals include iron, iodine, zinc, selenium, chromium, copper, and fluorine.[19] Although trace minerals are present in minute amounts, they play very important roles in the diet, and modern analytical methods are extremely sensitive to accurately measure them in foods.

Even though they are present in relatively low concentrations, by virtue of their interactions with other food components minerals have tremendous impact on the physical and chemical properties of foods.[19] Salt (sodium chloride) is the only mineral that is consumed in its native form by humans. It is most often added as a food preservative. Dairy products are a major source of calcium, whereas meats are good sources of iron and zinc. The food sources and functional roles of various minerals are detailed in **Table 4.9**.

Chapter Review

Foods are complex systems; their nutritional value and behavior under normal handling conditions are dependent on their composition. The high water activity of most fresh produce, meat, fish, and milk makes these food systems very susceptible to spoilage due to microbial and chemical reactions. Many food preservation methods, such as dehydration, freezing, and the addition of high amounts of salt or sugar, aim to reduce the water activity levels in the target food systems.

Carbohydrates are the primary source of calories in the human diet. In food processing, they are important as sweeteners, bulking agents, and texture modifiers (through starch gelatinization). They also are the reactants in caramelization and Maillard reactions. Lipids are the most energy dense nutrient and contribute to a food's mouthfeel, texture, and flavor. Fats are lipids that are in a solid state at room temperature, whereas oils are liquids at room temperature. The liquid state of oils is attributed to the presence of double bonds in the constituent fatty acids, which lowers their melting points. In foods, fats are used to shorten gluten fibers during baking, oils are used as media for heat transfer, and phospholipids are used as emulsifiers. Proteins are complex polymers of amino acids. Heat-coagulated egg proteins in soufflés and custards, acid- or enzyme-coagulated milk proteins in cheese, enzymes such as pectinases used for minimizing cloudiness in fruit juices, and the use of the enzyme rennin for cheese making are just some of the most commonly

TABLE 4.9
Functional Roles of Minerals in Foods

Mineral	Significant Food Sources	Functions in Foods (Processed)
Aluminum	Food additives	Sodium aluminum sulfate (SAS) is used as a leavening agent. Aluminum lake pigment is used as a food colorant. SAS also is used as leavening agent (baking), emulsifier (processed cheese), and buffering agent (flour mixes).
Bromine	Citrus-flavored soft drinks	Brominated vegetable oil is used as an emulsifier in citrus-flavored soft drinks.
Copper	Organ meats, seafood, nuts	Catalyst for lipid peroxidation, ascorbic acid oxidation, and nonenzymatic oxidative browning. Also acts as a texture stabilizer in egg-white foams.
Iodine	Iodized salt, seafood	Potassium iodate is used as a dough improver to improve the baking quality of flour.
Iron	Fortified cereals, legumes, meat	Catalyst for lipid peroxidation. Color modifier in meat, as a component of myoglobin. Reacts with sulfide ions to impart black discoloration (iron sulfide) to canned products.
Magnesium	Whole grains, nuts, legumes, green leafy vegetables	Color modifier in green vegetables; removal of magnesium ions during canning causes discoloration of green vegetables.
Nickel	Plant foods	Catalyst for hydrogenation of vegetable oils.
Phosphates	Present in most foods, widely used as additive	Phosphoric acid is used as an acidulant in soft drinks. Calcium pyrophosphate is used as a fast-acting leavening agent. Sodium tripolyphosphate is used to aid moisture retention in comminuted meats (e.g., hot dogs, sausage). Phosphates are used as emulsifiers in processed meats and processed cheeses.
Potassium	Fruits and vegetables, meats	Potassium chloride is used as a salt substitute. Potassium acid tartarate is used as a leavening agent.
Sodium	Sodium chloride (salt), monosodium glutamate (MSG), food additives, milk, breakfast cereals, most processed snack foods	Sodium chloride is used as a flavor modifier and preservative. Sodium bicarbonate and sodium aluminum phosphate are used as leavening agents.
Sulfur	Food additives	Sulfites and sulfur dioxide are used as inhibitors of nonenzymatic and enzymatic browning reactions (especially dried fruits). Antimicrobial agent in wines.
Zinc	Meats, fortified foods, nuts	Zinc oxide is used in the lining of cans to prevent the formation of black-colored iron sulfide during the canning process.

Source: Adapted from Miller DD. Minerals. In: Damodaran S, Parkin KL, Fennema, OL, eds. *Food Chemistry.* Boca Raton, FL. CRC Press; 2008:561.

encountered food applications of proteins. The sensory acceptance of foods often relies on the chemical interactions involving carbohydrates, proteins, and their derivatives. Both vitamins and minerals are found in varying amounts in different foods. However, while vitamin content is diminished during food processing, the mineral content is generally unaffected. A thorough knowledge of the composition of foods and the various interactions is an invaluable tool to understand the sensory, nutritional, and shelf-life changes in foods during processing and storage.

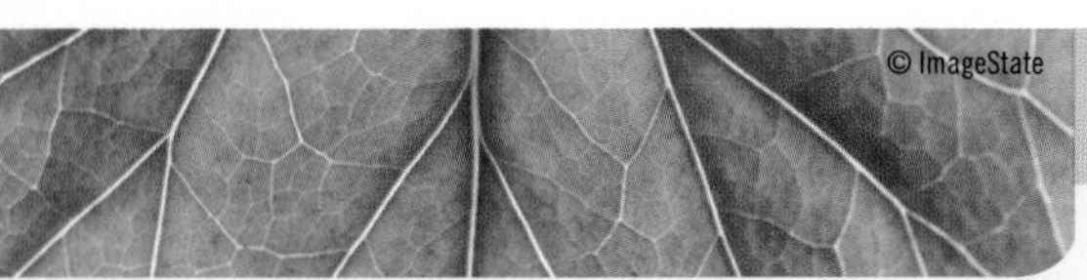

Learning Portfolio

Key Terms

	page
amino acids	143
carbohydrates	124
carmelization	148
cellulose	135
complete proteins	144
cryoprotectant	130
dietary fiber	134
dispersion	122
emulsion	122
enrichment	150
enzymatic browning	147
enzymes	146
fatty acid	138
food foam	145
fortification	151
functional fiber	135
functional food	115
glycemic index (GI)	128
glycemic load	129
glycerol	137
glycogen	124
humectant	127
hydrogenation	141
hydrolysis	122
incomplete proteins	144
lipids	137
Maillard reactions	149
mineral	152
nonenzymatic browning	148
omega-3 fatty acids	141
omega-6 fatty acids	141
peptide bond	143
phospholipid	143
phytonutrients	114
primary structure	143

Study Points

1. In most foods, water is the largest component. It has the ability to dissolve many molecules, including sugar, salt, and flavor molecules. The water activity of foods is the most significant influence on a food's shelf life. Water activity represents the energy level of water in a food system, and the shelf life of many foods may be increased by reducing the water activity. The boiling and freezing points of water solutions are influenced by the number of solute molecules present in a solution.
2. Monosaccharides, such as glucose, are the simplest carbohydrates. Monosaccharides may be linked together by glycosidic bonds to form disaccharides (e.g., maltose) or polysaccharides (e.g., amylose).
3. Indigestible carbohydrates often are classified as fiber. The human digestive tract lacks the enzymes to hydrolyze the glycosidic bonds in these polysaccharides. They often are used in reduced- and low-fat foods because they can contribute to a creamy mouth feel by absorbing large amounts of water.
4. Fats are lipids that exist in the solid state at ambient temperatures. Lipids that exist in the liquid state at ambient temperatures are called oils. Phospholipids and sterols are other common lipids found in foods.
5. The physical state of triglycerides is influenced by the length of the fatty acid chain, the absence or presence of double bonds, and the configuration (cis or trans) of the double bond in the fatty acids comprising triglycerides. Melting point decreases as the number of double bonds increases. Consequently, triglycerides comprising fatty acids with more than two double bonds (PUFAs) generally exist as oils.
6. When one of the fatty acids in a triglyceride is replaced by a phosphate group, the resulting compound is called a phospholipid. The hydrophilic phosphate group and the hydrophobic fatty acid ends enable these compounds to function as emulsifiers.
7. Proteins are long chains of amino acids linked together by peptide bonds. The primary structure of proteins may be further arranged into secondary, tertiary, and quaternary structures by bending of the primary chain, interactions within the side groups of a chain, and interactions between different peptide chains, respectively.
8. Proteins may be denatured by heat, changes in pH, mechanical shearing, and addition of salts and alcohol. During denaturation, the weak intra- and intermolecular secondary (noncovalent) linkages are lost, exposing the primary structure. Denaturation can result in loss of enzymatic activity, a property that is used to minimize enzymatic browning in potatoes and apples.
9. When foods high in carbohydrates and protein content are exposed to high temperatures, they often become brown in color. These nonenzymatic browning reactions may be further categorized as caramelization and Maillard reactions. Caramelization occurs when sugars are subjected to temperatures above their melting points. Maillard reactions are a series of high temperature interactions between carbohydrates and proteins that produce the golden brown color of cakes and cookies after baking.
10. Vitamins and minerals comprise minor constituents of foods. Whereas many vitamins are heat labile, minerals cannot be destroyed by the cooking process. Vitamins and minerals are often added to foods through the processes of fortification and enrichment.

Issues for Discussion

1. How does the carbohydrate composition of a banana change during ripening? Discuss these changes in relation to taste and glycemic control when consuming ripe bananas.
2. Protein denaturation is inevitable during food processing. Identify examples where denaturation is desirable in food products. Identify examples of food applications where it must be avoided or minimized.

3. Enzymatic browning often causes inferior sensory acceptance of bananas, apples, and mushrooms. Discuss food applications where enzymatic browning may be a desirable trait.

Research Ideas for Students

1. How packaged breakfast cereal remains crisp but the fruits (e.g., raisins, strawberries, blueberries) in the package stay moist
2. The negative health effects of acrylamide in foods

References

1. Chinachoti P. Carbohydrates: Functionality in foods. *American J Clin Nutr.* 1995;61(suppl.):922S.
2. BeMiller JN, Huber KC. Carbohydrates. In: Damodaran S, Parkin KL, Fennema OL (eds.). *Food Chemistry.* Boca Raton, FL: CRC Press; 2008: 83–154.
3. Johnson JM, Davis EA, Gordon J. Interactions of starch and sugar water measured by electron spin resonance and differential scanning calorimetry. *Cereal Chem.* 1990;67(3):286–291.
4. Ahmad FB, Williams PA. Effect of sugars on the thermal and rheological properties of sago starch. *Biopolymers.* 1999;50:401–412 (1999).
5. Hendrich S. Battling obesity with resistant starch. *Food technology.* 2010;64(3):23–29.
6. Gropper SS, Smith JL, Groff JL. *Advanced Nutrition and Human Metabolism*. Belmont, CA: Wadsworth Cengage Learning; 2009.
7. Marcason W. What is the latest research regarding the avoidance of nuts, seeds, corn and popcorn in diverticular disease? *J Am Diet Assoc.* 2008;108(11):1956.
8. Sherry CL, Kim SS, Dilger RN, et al. Sickness behavior induced by endotoxin can be mitigated by the dietary soluble fiber, pectin, through up-regulation of IL-4 and Th2 polarization. *Brain Behav Immunity.* 2010;24(4):631–640.
9. Food and Nutrition Board. *Dietary Reference Intakes for Energy, Carbohydrate, Fiber, Fat, Protein and Amino Acids.* Washington, DC: National Academies Press; 2002.
10. Simopoulos AP. The importance of the ratio of omega-6/omega-3 essential fatty acids. *Biomed Pharmacother.* 2002;56(8):365–379.
11. Damodaran S. Proteins. In: Damodaran S, Parkin KL, Fennema OL (eds.). *Food Chemistry.* Boca Raton, FL: CRC Press; 2008: 217–330.
12. Early R. *Technology of Milk Products.* 2nd ed. New York: Springer-Verlag; 1997.
13. Scientific Committee on Food 2002. Opinion of the scientific committee on food on new findings regarding the presence of acrylamide in food. Available at: http://ec.europa.eu/food/fs/sc/scf/out131_en.pdf. Accessed January 3, 2011.
14. Rommens CM, Ye J, Richael C, Swords K. Improving potato storage and processing characteristics through all-native DNA transformation. *J Agri Food Chem.* 2006;54(26):9882–9887.
15. Pedreschi F, Kaack K, Granby K. The effect of asparaginase on acrylamide formation in french fries. *Food Chem.* 2008;109(2):386–392.
16. Malewski W, Markakis P. A research note: Ascorbic acid content of developing tomato fruit. *J Food Sci.* 1971;36(3):537.
17. McKillop DJ, Pentieva K, Daly D, et al. The effect of different cooking methods on folate retention in various foods that are amongst the major contributors to folate intake in the UK diet. *British J Nutr.* 2002;88:681–688.
18. Gregory JF Jr. Vitamins. In: Damodaran S, Parkin KL, Fennema OL (eds.). *Food Chemistry.* Boca Raton, FL: CRC Press; 2008: 439–522.
19. Miller DD. Minerals. In: Damodaran S, Parkin KL, Fennema OL (eds.). *Food Chemistry.* Boca Raton, FL: CRC Press; 2008: 523–570.

protein complementation	145
protein denaturation	146
protein coagulation	146
proteins	143
quaternary structure	144
resistant starch (RS)	134
secondary structure	143
saturated solution	122
solution	122
starch gelatinization	132
starch gelation	132
suspension	122
syneresis	133
tertiary structure	143
vitamins	149
water activity (a_w)	120

SECTION II

Categorized Food and Beverage Groupings, Vegetarianism, Food Preservation, and Packaging

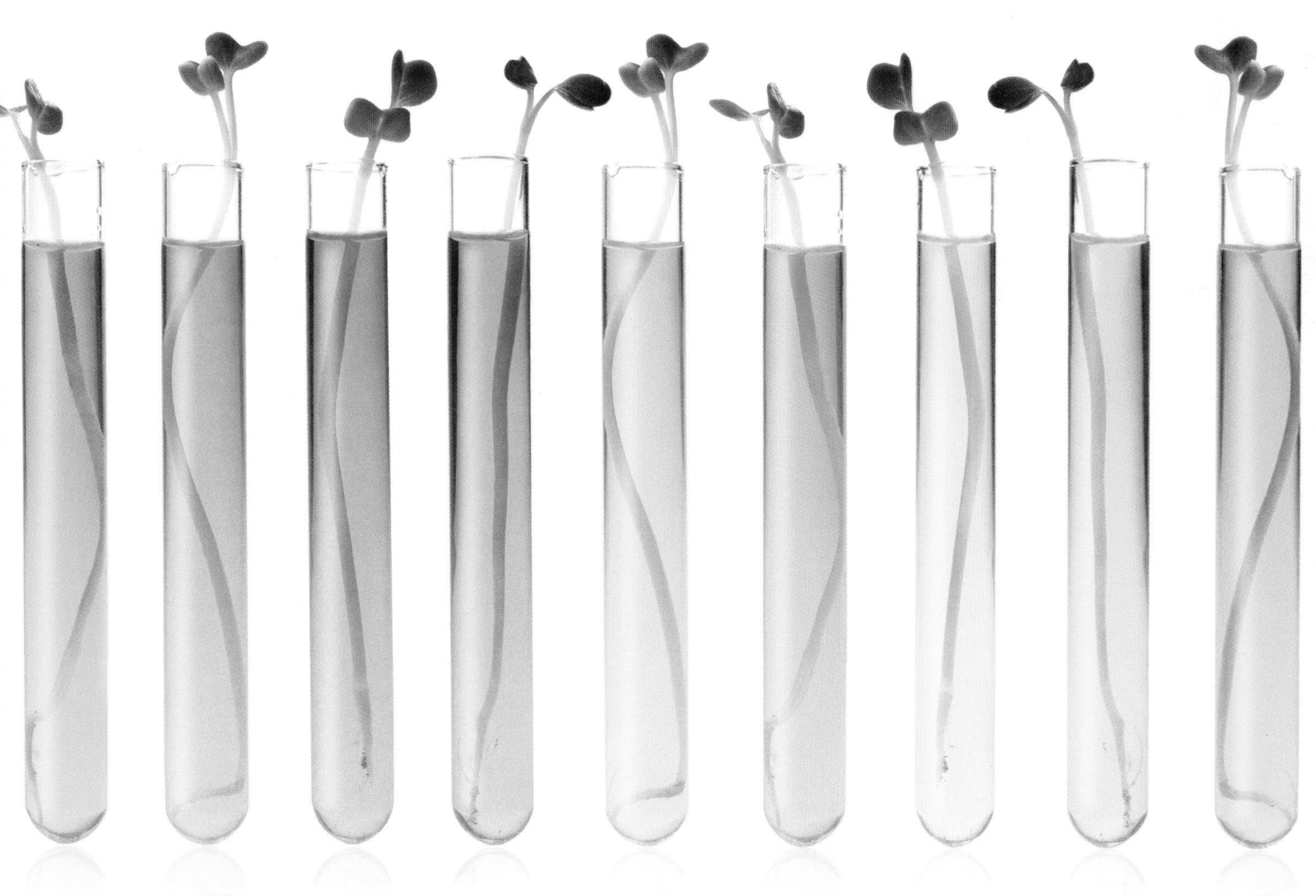

CHAPTER 5

Meat and Meat Substitutes

Courtney P. Winston, MPH, RD, LD, CDE

Chapter Objectives

THE STUDENT WILL BE EMPOWERED TO:

- Define the animal origins and cultural histories of various types of red meat.
- Describe properties of meat, such as its structural components, marbling, and pigmentation.
- Explain the changes meats undergo during aging, preserving, and other processing methods.
- Define various cuts of meats.
- Compare and contrast commonly used dry heat and moist heat cooking methods.
- Explain the nutritional contribution of meat to the human diet.
- Discuss the impact that the meat industry has on the environment and ways in which this impact might be reduced.
- List steps consumers of meat should take to prevent foodborne illness.
- Summarize the meat inspection and meat-grading procedures followed in the United States.

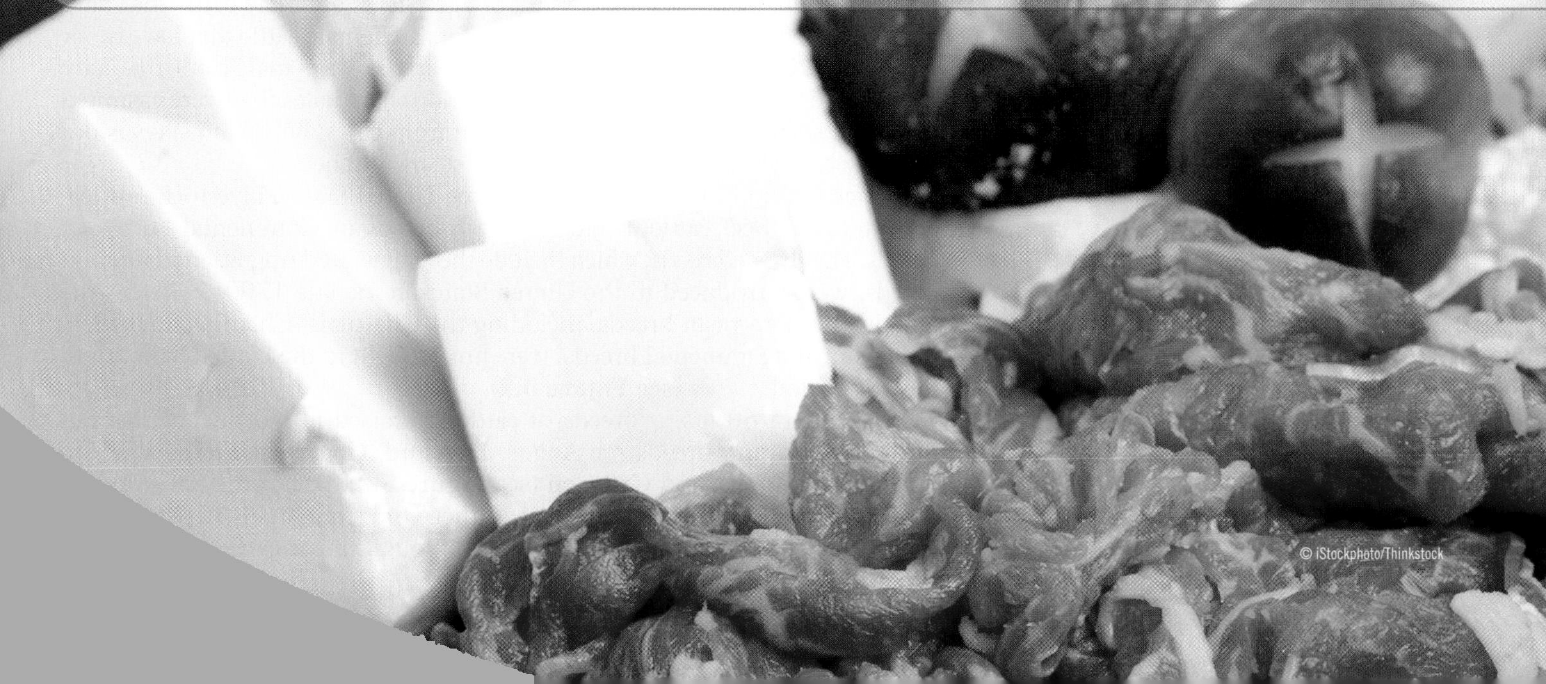

Historical, Cultural, and Ecological Significance

Livestock serves multiple purposes in supporting the biological and ecological well-being of our planet. Among their many purposes, domesticated cattle, swine, and sheep play a large role in the food chain by providing food for human beings. Their muscle, organs, and fat are marketed to consumers as protein-rich, nutrient-dense meats, contributing significantly to the diets of those who consume them. Animals also provide humans with nutritional by-products such as milk and blood, which in some cultures are considered a central part of the diet. In addition, suppliers market other portions of the animals, such as their hides, wool, bones, and blood, to consumers. Leather, a durable material crafted from cowhide, is one example of an expensive animal by-product marketed to the clothing and furniture industries. Compared to the cost of raising plants, the cost of raising animals for food is extremely high; therefore, those who raise animals try hard to sell all parts of the animal in order to improve profitability.

Gastronomy Point

Chinese Pork Archeologists have found recipes from over 2,000 years ago that demonstrate that the Chinese raised domesticated swine (pork) for human consumption.

Animals have long served as food sources for human beings. In the Stone Age, humans consumed the meat of wild boar. However, because of the large size and difficult temperament of wild animals, the process of hunting and slaughtering was very challenging. Domestication of animals made meat production much easier. Animals, beginning with sheep, were first domesticated for food around 9000 B.C. in the Fertile Crescent of the Middle East. About 2,000 years later, humans began domesticating other animals, including pigs (immature hogs) and cattle. These newly domesticated breeds were raised to be much smaller and more docile than their ancestors, and some even had alternative purposes. For example, domesticated cattle became popular for their strength and power shortly after the invention of the plow. The popularity of these domesticated animals quickly spread to other countries and continents.

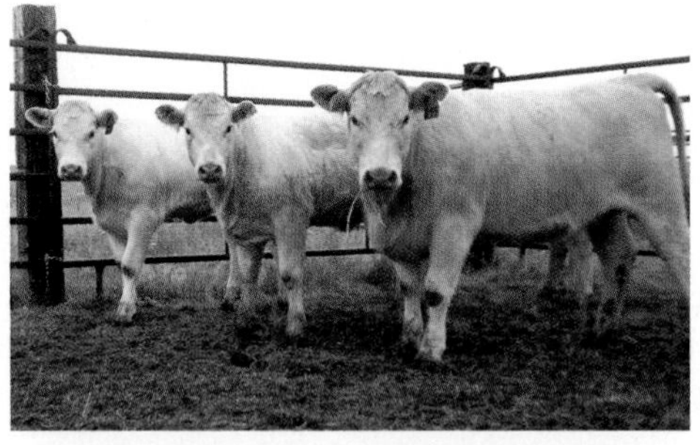

FIGURE 5.1 Charolais cattle were developed in Charolais, France. It is a large-muscled breed, with bulls weighing up to 1,100 pounds.

Courtesy of the USDA, Farm Service Agency. Photo by Darcy Vial.

Many of the animals domesticated for food purposes are not indigenous to North America. Cattle and sheep were brought to the Western Hemisphere by Columbus and the Spaniards in 1493. Hernando De Soto brought the first domesticated hogs to the New World in 1525. As these animals were bred and raised over the following centuries, large ranches and farms emerged in areas known today as Mexico, Texas, and Florida.

Beef

Beef primarily comes from the muscle tissue of full-grown steers and heifers brought to market at around 2 years of age. Steers are male cattle that have been castrated before sexual maturity; heifers are female cattle that have never reproduced. Beef can also come from the meat of cows (female cattle that have reproduced), bulls (noncastrated males), and stags (males that were castrated following sexual maturity); however, meat from cows, bulls, and stags is not typically as high in quality as meat from steers and heifers.

Over 100 million beef cattle roam the United States. Livestock producers categorize beef cattle as either British breeds or Continental European breeds. The British breeds, which include the Angus, Red Angus, and Hereford breeds, were introduced to the United States in the late 1700s, whereas the Continental European breeds, including the Charolais, Chianina, Gelbvieh, Limousin, and Simmental breeds, were not brought to the United States until the 1960s and 1970s (see **Figure 5.1**).

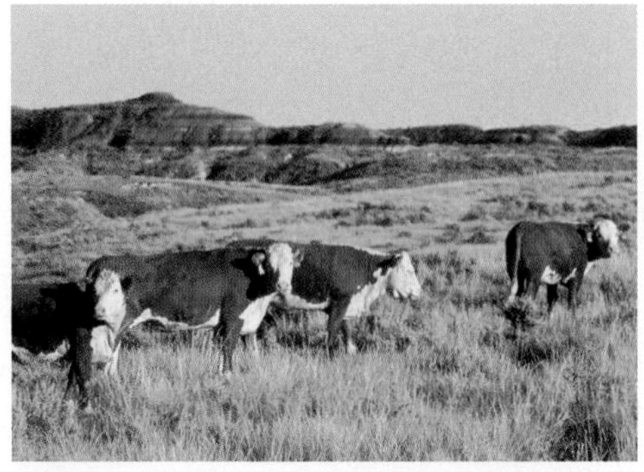

FIGURE 5.2 Even though the breed was not introduced into the United States until the 1960s, today Charolais cattle are a common breed used by beef producers in the United States.

Courtesy of the USDA Agricultural Research Service. Photo by Keith Weller.

More than 60 major breeds of cattle are raised in North America, but the most common breeds are Angus, Hereford, Charolais, Limousin, Simmental, Red Angus, and Gelbvieh (see **Figure 5.2**). Beef cattle have varying degrees of fatness and palatability, and these traits are highly dependent on the breed type. Regardless of the breed, though, most cattle weigh about

1,000 pounds and can provide roughly half their weight in edible meat at the time of slaughter.

The raising of beef cattle starts with young calves that are milk-fed immediately after birth. Calves are typically weaned onto either a grass- or grain-based diet at around 6 to 8 weeks of age. Beef cattle are typically grass fed, or pasture raised, immediately after weaning; dairy cattle usually transition straight to a grain-based diet. Beef cattle require large ranges and primarily consume forage until they are transported to a feedlot. In the feedlot, producers feed them a grain-based diet until slaughtering (see **Figure 5.3**). The diet that is given to cattle and other meat-producing animals in the final months leading up to their slaughter is called the **finishing diet**.

A small percentage of beef cattle are allowed to roam free and consume forage until slaughter. Some people ague this form of feeding is more natural and humane and has a lighter environmental impact than feedlot finishing. However, due to limited space for grazing, most cattle farms in the United States cannot accommodate the large amount of land necessary for exclusively grass-fed cattle. In addition, the grain-based diet that is provided in the final 4 to 6 months of life helps to increase the cattle's overall body weight and, in turn, profitability.

Most cattle are routinely injected with vaccines, antibiotics, and hormones soon after birth and prior to being brought to market. All cattle, including cattle that will be marketed as organic or natural and that do not receive any hormones or antibiotics, are vaccinated early in life to protect against liver abscesses and respiratory and clostridial diseases. Later on, most cattle receive antibiotics rich in ionophores—fat-soluble molecules that decrease bloating and reduce the risk of acidosis. Bloating and acidosis are two feeding problems commonly seen in cattle, and these problems can significantly decrease both feed efficiency and weight gain in beef cattle. Hormones are also commonly administered to cattle in order to promote the absorption and metabolism of nutrients and to enhance weight gain. A study from Australia found that implantation of **hormonal growth promotants (HGPs)** resulted in slaughter weights 4% and 7% greater than slaughter weights of cattle that did not receive HGPs.[1]

Veal

Veal is the meat that originates from a young calf raised to age 16 to 18 weeks. Most veal found on the market is produced from male calves because, unlike females, male cattle do not produce milk and cannot be used as dairy cows. In the United States, most veal is raised in Wisconsin, Indiana, Michigan, Ohio, New York, and Pennsylvania. Note that these are also the states where many dairy cows are raised.

Because calves used for veal are taken to market at an early age, these animals primarily consume milk-based diets or milk replacers. Milk replacers come in three formulas: a starter, a grower, and a finisher. The starter formula is higher in protein than the finisher feed, but both feeds contain about 18% of calories from fat. Veal is lighter in color than beef because milk replacers are low in iron, which lowers the iron content of the meat and lightens the color of the final product. Ideally, veal will gain 2.5 pounds per day until they reach 375 to 475 pounds; at this weight, the veal can be brought to market.

The conditions under which calves are raised have received much scrutiny in recent years; however, the American Veterinary Medical Association has worked closely with the industry to develop guidelines for the production and humane care of these animals. Although the calves are separated from their mothers within 24 hours after birth, they do receive their mothers' colostrum

Gastronomy Point

Kobe Beef The Tajimi-ushi breed of Wagyu cattle is well-known because it is from this breed that Kobe beef, a delicate beef known for its desirable flavor and tenderness, is produced.

finishing diet The diet fed to livestock animals immediately prior to slaughter.

hormonal growth promotants (HGPs) Hormones administered to livestock to promote weight gain prior to slaughter.

Green Point

Natural Cattle Natural cattle are not administered antibiotics or hormones at any time after birth or before slaughter, but they are still vaccinated to prevent liver abscesses and respiratory and clostridial diseases.

Innovation Point

CLA in Milk Increasing the amount of conjugated linoleic acid (CLA) in the milk replacer can increase the amount of CLA in the veal after slaughter. This makes the final veal product higher in this essential fatty acid, which has been associated with health-protective effects.

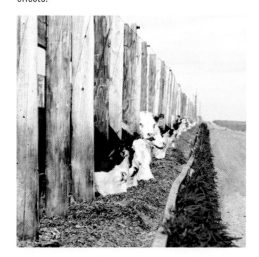

FIGURE 5.3 Meat producers can minimize preslaughter fasting stress in cattle by feeding the animals regularly. This practice helps to maintain the normal balance of rumen microbes and suppress bacteria such as the dangerous *E. coli* 0157:H7.

to protect them against disease. Once calves are separated from their mothers, they are placed in individual stalls where they have adequate room to stand up, lie down, and groom themselves. They are separated from other calves by a small partition that allows them to partially see each other. The benefit of separating these young animals is that it limits the spread of disease and it keeps them from being stressed by other animals. The stalls are normally controlled at 60–70°F (15.5–21.1°C) for the first 2 weeks after birth and then the temperature is lowered to 55°F (12.7°C).

The per capita consumption of veal is high in the United States, Uruguay, Argentina, Australia, Brazil, and New Zealand. Veal was first described in ancient Roman recipes, and by the Middle Ages, references to veal were seen in many dishes in France and England. In some cultures, veal is considered a delicacy because of its tenderness and its light coloration. Countries with large populations of Hindus, such as India, have a low per capita consumption of these beef and veal products. This is primarily because Hindus consider cattle to be sacred and thus prohibit their consumption.

Lamb

Although the typical American only eats about 0.8 pounds of lamb annually, this meat originates from one of the oldest domesticated meat species. Lamb is a common main entrée in the Middle East and is widely consumed in Arab countries, North Africa, central Asia, and northern India. In the Middle East and Asia, lamb often is served along with spiced rice or rice pilaf. In northern Africa, it is commonly served alongside couscous (a wheat product).

The palatability and characteristics of sheep meat are highly dependent on the age of the sheep. Meat from young sheep—lamb—is commonly marketed from animals between 4 and 12 months of age. The biological point at which a sheep can no longer be marketed as a lamb is when the animal gets its first pair of permanent teeth, which usually occurs around 1 year of age. Meat from older sheep, also known as mutton, hog, or hogget, remains suitable for human consumption; however, mutton tends to be tougher and to have a much stronger, and often less desirable, flavor than lamb.

Gastronomy Point

Suckling Lambs In some European and Middle Eastern countries, suckling lambs, or lambs that have only been fed their mother's milk, are marketed and sold as a delicacy.

Young lambs are usually weaned from their mothers to diets of hay and fortified feed. Some lambs can be fed special diets to produce unique flavors, such as those in France that graze in salt marshes to produce saltier meat. Immediately prior to slaughtering, most lamb will be transferred to a feedlot and transitioned to a nutrient-dense finishing feed. While in the feedlot, lambs may be given growth-promoting hormones through tags on the lambs' ears. Lambs who receive such hormones require a 40-day holding period prior to slaughter. Similarly, antibiotics may also be administered to lambs, and like the waiting period for hormones, there is also an FDA-determined holding period between the time of antibiotic administration and the time of slaughter. This holding period ensures that residues from the antibiotic have had sufficient time to exit the animal and that the residues are not consumed by humans.

At the time they are brought to market, most lambs weigh around 120 pounds and provide 60 to 72 pounds (inclusive of bone) of retail cuts. Lamb fat, which also can be harvested from the carcass, is not traditionally consumed in western cultures, but it is frequently used in the manufacture of tallow candles.

Pork

In early 2009, the U.S. Department of Agriculture Economic Research Service estimated that there were 67 million hogs and pigs in the United States.[2] Sixty-two percent of these animals were located in the Corn Belt (Iowa, Indiana,

Illinois, and parts of Ohio, Missouri, Nebraska, Kansas, and Minnesota), and 15% were in North Carolina. The United States is the largest exporter of pork and pork products in the world, producing more than 22.1 billion pounds of pork in 2010. Per capita pork consumption is highest in countries such as Denmark, Spain, Germany, and Hong Kong.

Pork is the meat that comes from hogs, the modern-day, domesticated version of the wild boar. Hogs were first domesticated for food consumption in the Middle East shortly after the domestication of sheep. The ancient Greeks and Romans were known to have cherished suckling pigs, or young hogs that had not been weaned from their mothers, as a fine dining delicacy. Romans also enjoyed cured pork products, such as ham.

Hogs are not indigenous to North America; they were introduced by Spanish explorers in the 16th century. Pork quickly gained in popularity, and, in part because of its long shelf-life when preserved, it became one of the most popular meats in the American diet. Today, a variety of hog breeds are raised around world, but in the United States popular breeds include the Yorkshire, Duroc, and Poland China.

Pork can originate from pigs or hogs of different sexes. Animals up to 4 months of age are considered to be pigs; animals older than 4 months are considered to be hogs. Among females, gilts are young females that have not given birth, and sows are females that have either been pregnant or have previously given birth. Among males, barrows are males that have been castrated prior to sexual maturity, staffs are males that have been castrated after sexual maturity, and boars are males that have never been castrated. Hogs reach sexual maturity around 6 to 8 months of age, and it is typically between 6 and 12 months of age that they are brought to market.

Pigs and hogs are typically raised on commercial hog feeds that are composed of proteins from soybean meal, fish meal, milk, and meat by-products. These feeds are also high in carbohydrates, which primarily come from corn. Vitamin B_{12} and other supplements may also be added to the feed to help promote growth and weight gain. Over the years, hogs have been bred to be leaner and less fatty than their ancestors, and much of this is because of the decreased market demand for pork lard.

Green Point

Stomachs As opposed to cattle, pigs and hogs only have one stomach and, as a result, do not produce as much in digestive gas emissions. Pork production constitutes less than 1% of U.S. greenhouse gas emissions.

At the time of slaughter, most hogs weigh 175 to 240 pounds. Although it does tend to take smaller birth weight pigs longer to reach market weight, the quality and palatability of pork is not affected by the animal's birth weight.[3] Smaller, younger hogs are used to produce fresh pork, which is tender and has a mild flavor. Older, larger animals are used for cured meats, such as bacon and ham. Overall, approximately one-third of pork meat is marketed as fresh pork, or "porkers," and the rest is marketed to consumers in cured forms, such as sausage, luncheon meats, and ham. The by-products of the hog are also retained and marketed, reducing the amount of leftover waste. For example, manufacturers will often purchase pork skin and use it in the production of gelatin.

After slaughter, the hog carcass is "dressed," and all edible organs are inspected by a trained veterinarian. The carcass is then dissected into its major cuts (i.e., hams, loins, bellies, back fat, shoulder) prior to being shipped to meat distributors.

Pork is commonly consumed in countries around the world. In areas such as China, Southeast Asia, and Polynesia, pork is considered a staple meat. In contrast, Japan is not a large consumer of pork products, but it does import a substantial amount of pork from the United States. Because Judaism and Islam discourage the consumption of pork as being unclean, countries with large Jewish and Muslim populations do not have a large per capita consumption of pork products.

Special Topic 5.1

H1N1, or "Swine Flu"

Zhanglin Kong, MS

H1N1 influenza (swine flu) was a global pandemic that first caused illness in Mexico and the United States in 2009. In April 2009, 59 deaths were caused by H1N1 in Mexico City alone. On June 11, 2009, the World Health Organization (WHO) raised the worldwide pandemic alert level to Phase 6 to signal a global pandemic of this novel influenza A strain.[1] This action was a reflection of the spread of the new viral strain and its potential for harm, rather than the actual number of deaths, which were far fewer than those caused by regular seasonal flu.

H1N1 influenza was initially named "swine flu" to indicate a swine origin. However, transmission of the virus from pigs to humans is not common and does not always lead to human influenza, often resulting only in the production of antibodies in the blood. Although the genes of the H1N1 virus are a combination of genes most closely related to North American swine-lineage H1N1 and Eurasian swine-lineage H1N1 influenza viruses, investigations of initial human cases did not identify exposures to pigs. It became apparent that this new virus was circulating among humans and not among U.S. pig herds, which means that H1N1 flu is not a foodborne disease and is not caused by eating pork or pork products.[2]

The symptoms of H1N1 flu are very similar to a regular flu—fever, cough, sore throat, runny or stuffy nose, body ache, headache, chills, fatigue, and sometimes vomiting or diarrhea. The H1N1 virus is spread mainly through the coughs and sneezes of infected people.[3]

Vaccine and Antiviral Treatment

In the United States, the Centers for Disease Control and Prevention (CDC) and local animal and human health officials work closely on epidemiological investigations, vaccine development, communications, and other responses.[1] Vaccination offers protection from the H1N1 flu. Producing the vaccine involves a number of complicated steps:[2]

- Obtain a high yield of virus by growing it in chicken eggs.
- Purify the virus particles to make vaccine.
- Distribute the vaccine to targeted individuals via hospitals and clinics.

Target individuals for initial focus when a vaccine supply is limited are (1) people who are most likely to develop illness or spread infection and (2) people who account for the majority of severe illnesses and deaths. For the H1N1 vaccine, pregnant women, children, young adults younger than age 24, adults with certain chronic health conditions or compromised immune systems, and healthcare and emergency medical services personnel are prioritized to receive the vaccine. Infected people are suggested to avoid close contact with others, especially those who might easily get the flu.[3]

The majority of individuals infected with the H1N1 virus recover without complications and without treatment or with only supportive therapy. Antiviral treatment is recommended by the CDC for patients with influenza who require hospitalization or who are at risk for severe disease or complications. The treatment benefit is greatest if antivirals are started early, usually within 2 days of the onset of symptoms.[3]

During the summer season, many students and families travel internationally. In the 2009 H1N1 pandemic, it was recommended that travelers get the H1N1 vaccine at least 2 weeks before the start of their trip to reduce their of getting sick. Many international airports across the globe use a health-screening form and a body temperature detector to identify possible H1N1–infected travelers.[3]

Lessons from the H1N1 Pandemic

The first pandemic that emerged in the twenty-first century has taught us much. Some of the most important lessons follow:[4–7]

- The current methods of vaccine production in this country are not efficient enough for an adequate response to a pandemic. This is not only because very little vaccine-manufacturing capacity is left in the pharmaceutical industry but also because there is a lack of official channels for pandemic-level vaccine distribution.

- Information sharing in the future must be more effective. The distrust caused by the perception that officials overreacted to the H1N1 pandemic needs to be overcome. Cultural diversity and the timeliness, coordination, and consistency of message delivery should be considered.
- Social media reports should be given close attention because they tend to interpret data to extremes.

References

1 Centers for Disease Control and Prevention. 2009 H1N1 Flu. Updated August 11, 2010. Available at: http://www.cdc.gov/h1n1flu.
2 Flu.gov. H1N1 (Swine Flu). Available at: http://www.flu.gov/individualfamily/about/h1n1/index.html.
3 Infectious Diseases Society of America. Information on Influenza: Seasonal and Novel A: H1N1. Available at: http://www.idsociety.org/Content.aspx?id=14220#H1N1.
4 Leung GM, Nicoll A. (2010). Reflections on pandemic (H1N1) 2009 and the international response. *PLoS Medicine* 7(10):e1000346. doi:10.1371/journal.pmed.1000346.
5 National Institute of Allergy and Infectious Diseases. H1N1 (Swine) Flu. Updated September 30, 2009. Available at: http://www.niaid.nih.gov/topics/flu/h1n1/Pages/Default.aspx.
6 Walsh B. One Year Later: 5 Lessons from the H1N1 Pandemic. (April 27, 2010). Available at: http://www.time.com/time/health/article/0,8599,1985009-3,00.html.
7 World Health Organization. Pandemic (H1N1) 2009. Available at: http://www.who.int/csr/disease/swineflu/en/index.html.

Physical and Chemical Properties

Structure of Meats

Cuts of meat from cattle, lamb, and pork have similar components. The main component of meat, and what most people desire when they consume meat, is the actual muscle tissue. Muscle tissue is roughly 75% water, 18% protein, 4–10% fat (depending on the animal and the cut), and minimal carbohydrate. In addition to the muscle tissue, meat cuts include bone, including bone marrow; connective tissue; and fat.

Muscle

Because most consumers select their meat based on the cut's muscle tissue, it is important to understand how muscle tissue is constructed. Most of the muscle tissue is actually water. When heated, the size of the meat will shrink in size; partially due to the evaporation of the water from the muscle tissue. Shrinkage is also the result of actions of the muscle proteins.

Muscle proteins range from large to a small. Muscle tissue, in general, is composed of individual muscle cells, or muscle fibers. As shown in **Figure 5.4**, each muscle cell is surrounded by a membrane, called the *sarcolemma*, and contains a fluidlike center, called the *sarcoplasm*.

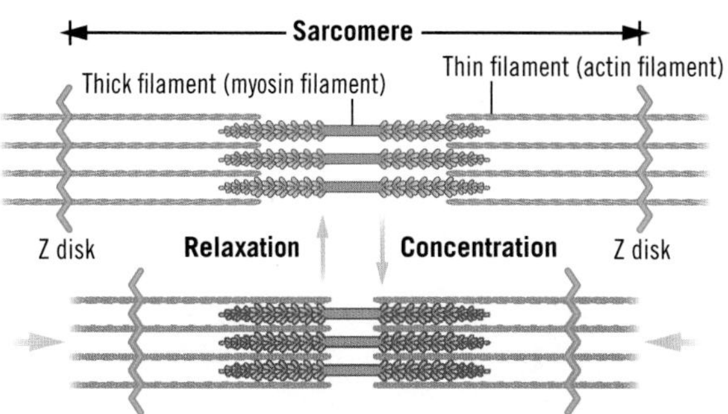

FIGURE 5.4 Muscle fibers are the basic cellular units of living muscle and of meat. Each muscle fiber consists of rod-shaped myofibrils. Myofibrils and connective tissue are the main structural components of muscle.

Inside the muscle cell are the muscle myofibrils; each muscle cell can contain 2,000 or more muscle myofibrils. The muscle myofibrils play an important role in determining the taste of the muscle tissue because small muscle myofibrils give the muscle a smooth, delicate mouthfeel.

Within the muscle myofibrils are regions called *sarcomeres*, which house the two main muscle proteins, myosin and actin. **Myosin** is the thick filament found in muscle tissue; **actin** is the thinner filament. During muscle contraction, adenosine triphosphate (ATP) and calcium cause myosin and actin to come together and form cross-bridges. The resulting, shortened state is called actomyosin; the sarcomere will remain in this shortened state until it becomes relaxed again.

myosin Thick filament in muscle fibrils that binds with actin in muscle contraction and relaxation.

actin Thin filament in muscle fibrils that binds with myosin in muscle contraction and relaxation.

Bone

Another component of meat is bone. The presence of bones in meat is especially useful when determining the cut of meat and where the meat originated. The size of bones can also help determine the age of the animal at slaughter and can be an indicator of meat tenderness. Both yellow and red bone marrows also contribute to the flavor of meat. For this reason, chefs often choose to cook bone-in meats instead of boneless cuts. Bones and their bone marrow are also commonly used in the making of broths and stocks to add flavor. When purchasing meat cuts with bones, the price per unit weight is typically lower than the price per unit weight of boneless cuts. Because bones are not consumed and can sometimes weigh more than the muscle that is consumed, the price difference between bone-in and bone-out cuts needs to be considered when purchasing meats.

Connective Tissue

Meats also are composed of connective tissues, which hold the meat together. The amount of connective tissue found in meats will have a significant impact on the tenderness of the meat. High quantities of connective tissue cause most meats to become tough and less tender.

collagen Connective tissue found in meats that will break down and form gelatin under moist heat.

elastin Connective tissue found in meats that must be physically removed or trimmed prior to consumption of the meat product.

marbling Fat interspersed throughout muscle tissue.

Connective tissues are visible to the naked eye as a white, tough substance. One of the more abundant connective tissues found in meat is **collagen**, a substance found within and around muscle tissue. When exposed to warm, moist heat, collagen will turn into a gel (gelatin). Collagen has the amino acids proline, hydroxyproline, and glycine. Collagen prevents the stretching of muscle and becomes more tightly cross-linked as the animal ages. Reticulin is a small connective tissue fiber made of collagen that surrounds and protects muscle cells.

Elastin is another, less abundant type of connective tissue found in meats. As its name implies, elastin is more elastic and flexible than collagen. Physiologically, elastin allows muscle and other organs in the body to return to their original shape after stimulation and contraction; however, the presence of elastin contributes to toughness of meat and often makes the meat less palatable.

Fat

Adipose tissue, or fat, is another component of meat that must be considered during purchasing and preparation. Fat can comprise 4–10% of meat, depending on the animal and the cut of meat. Fat covers the muscle tissue and can also be located within the muscle tissue. Fat that covers the muscle tissue is desirable because it helps the meat to retain moisture. Intramuscular fat contributes to the **marbling** of the meat; highly marbled meat tends to be juicy and has a more palatable flavor than its leaner counterparts (see **Figure 5.5**).[4]

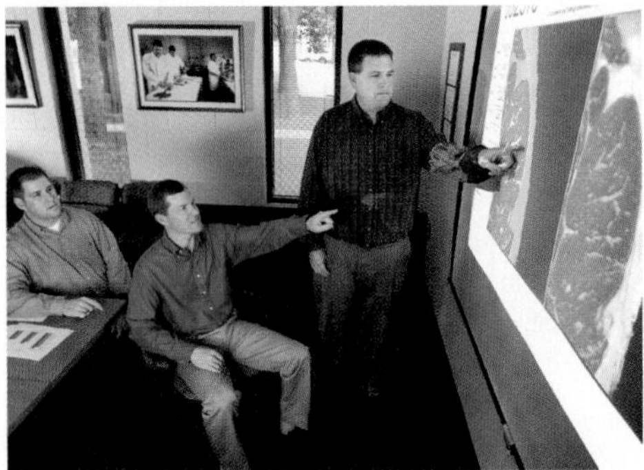

FIGURE 5.5 Food technologists analyze the intramuscular fat, or marbling, of beef slices. It usually appears as a series of small white flecks in the cut of meat. Marbling helps meat retain moisture during cooking and contributes to mouthfeel.

Courtesy of the USDA Agricultural Research Service. Photo by Stephen Ausmus.

The amount of fat found on cuts of meat varies widely. Older animals tend to have less fat, and therefore do not produce meat as juicy and tender as that from younger animals. The nutritional composition of the animal's diet can also affect the fat content of the meat. Beef fat is often extremely soft due to the high concentration of polyunsaturated fatty acids found in beef finishing feed. Animals with high-calorie finishing diets tend to have more fat and usually produce more tender meats. Interestingly, the carotenoid content of finishing diets will also affect the color of fat in the meat product. Animal feed containing high amounts of carotenoids will cause the fat to turn yellow; animals fed carotenoid-deficient diets will usually have fat that is white.

Meat cuts from lean animals are extremely tough and difficult to chew. Likewise, cuts of meat from muscles that are involved in regular exercise, such as the leg muscles, are also tougher than muscles that perform little or no exercise and that contain higher amounts of fat. Genetic mutations can also affect the tenderness of meat. In beef, an addition in the myostatin gene decreases the fat content of the meat, which results in a less desirable flavor of the final meat product (see **Figure 5.6**).[5]

Pigments

Meats contain pigments that give the cut a unique coloration. The main pigments in beef, lamb, and pork come from the proteins hemoglobin and **myoglobin**. Hemoglobin has a higher molecular weight than myoglobin. Despite having a smaller molecular weight, myoglobin is important because it contributes to the redness of meat. Myoglobin is found in higher quantities in beef and lamb than is found in poultry and fish, and this is the reason why beef and lamb are considered red meat and poultry and fish are considered white meats.

The pigments found in meat contain both iron and heme. Iron is particularly important because when this element changes its chemical state by binding to oxygen the color of the meat is immediately affected. By itself, myoglobin contains an iron molecule in the ferrous state (Fe^{++}); meat containing this state of iron exhibit a purplish-red color. When meat is cut and exposed to oxygen, myoglobin and oxygen form a compound known as **oxymyoglobin**, and the meat then exhibits a bright red color. Excessive exposure to oxygen causes water to bond with iron, causing the iron to turn into its ferric state (Fe^{+++}). When this happens, the oxymyoglobin turns into **metmyoglobin**, and the meat exhibits a brownish-red color. Although this brownish-red color does not indicate the meat is old or spoiled, it is usually undesirable to the consumer. For this reason, food manufacturers take caution when packaging meats and use techniques such as vacuum packing to reduce the raw meat's exposure to oxygen.

The pigmentation of meat can be affected by other factors besides oxygen exposure. Muscles that are frequently exercised have a higher oxygen demand and a resulting cherry-red color. The species of animal and the animal's age also affect the color of the meat. Beef has a darker color than veal because it is slaughtered at an older age and contains more myoglobin. The addition of preservatives, particularly sodium nitrite, also can affect the color of meat. In preservation, sodium nitrite converts to nitric oxide and binds with myoglobin to form **nitric oxide myoglobin**. Nitric oxide myoglobin is the bright red color often seen in uncooked processed meats, such as sausage, and it causes the preserved meat to turn pink when heated or cooked.

Slaughtering and Aging

The conditions under which an animal is slaughtered will significantly impact the quality of the meat. Animals should be slaughtered under conditions that are humane and not stressful to the animal. Ideally, the animal will be brought to market at a time when its muscles are loaded with glycogen and when the animal has not recently been exercised or excited. After slaughter, the animal is no longer taking in oxygen, thus aerobic respiration will cease. As a result, the animal's glycogen stores will gradually convert to pyruvate and eventually to **lactic acid**. The buildup of lactic acid proceeds slowly as the animal carcass begins to enter a state known as rigor mortis. During rigor mortis, which occurs approximately 6 to 24 hours after slaughter, the presence of lactic acid lowers the pH of the meat to a desirable level of 5.4 to 5.8. Maintaining this low pH allows the meat to bind water and retain moisture, and these desirable conditions will prevent carcass meat from becoming dry.

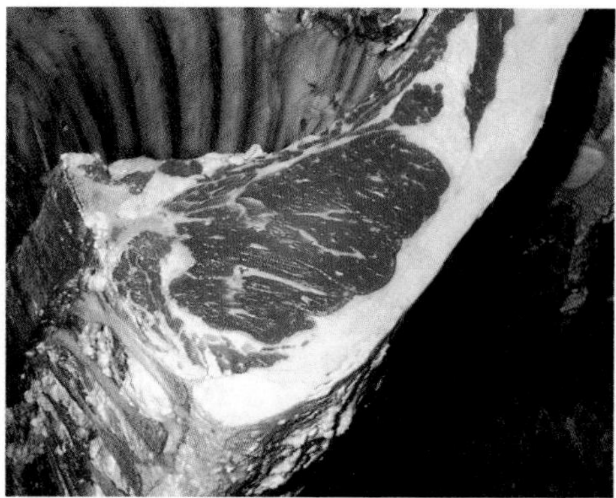

(a)

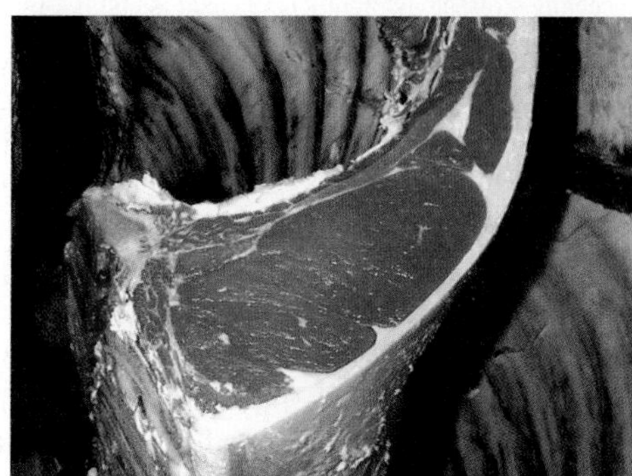

(b)

FIGURE 5.6 (a) Beef with no copies of the inactive myostatin gene. This meat has more marbling than meat from cattle with the myostatin gene. (b) Beef with two copies of the inactive myostatin gene. This meat is leaner and has less marbling than meat from cattle with fewer or no copies of the myostatin gene.

myoglobin Primary pigment found in meats.

oxymyoglobin Compound formed when the myoglobin pigment comes into contact with oxygen, causing the meat to become bright red.

metmyoglobin Compound formed when myoglobin is exposed excessively to oxygen and the iron converts to the ferric state, causing the meat to become brownish-red.

nitric oxide myoglobin Pigment found in cured meats that causes the meat to turn pink.

lactic acid Biological compound that builds up in animal carcasses after slaughter, reducing the pH of the meat.

Live export of animals to the slaughterhouse may induce stress in animals, causing them to exhaust their glycogen prior to slaughter. Thus, soon after death, lactic acid will build quickly, and the pH will drop prior to the onset of rigor mortis. As a result, the pH during rigor mortis will exceed 5.8, and the meat may develop an undesirable sticky texture and brownish-purple color. To avoid this, some producers do not transport their cattle to a slaughterhouse but instead slaughter their livestock in areas close to where the cattle are already being held.

As the animal carcass passes through rigor mortis, it is common for the meat to be hung from a beam. This hanging allows the meat fibers to be stretched, which promotes a more tender end product. Likewise, many carcasses are also aged after rigor mortis. Aging can be done by leaving the carcass hanging in a temperature and humidity-controlled environment (dry aging) or by vacuum packing the carcass in its own juices (wet aging). Some cuts of beef, such as the short loin, may have decreased yields and increased cutting times as a result of dry versus wet aging; however, the palatability of the end product remains similar.[6] Both dry and wet aging processes promote tenderness and flavor development, and these processes can be ongoing for up to 4 weeks postslaughter.

Green Point

Transportation for Slaughter Some livestock producers do not transport their animals prior to slaughter. This keeps the animal from becoming stressed. An additional benefit is that it reduces greenhouse gas emissions resulting from the transportation process.

Tenderizing Meats

Prior to cooking, tenderizing agents can be added to meats to help further break down connective tissue and make the final product less tough. The two most common chemical tenderizing agents used are papain and bromelain. Both of these enzymes originate from plant sources; papain comes from the papaya fruit, whereas bromelain comes from pineapple. These enzymes act by breaking down collagen to produce a more tender texture. It is important to remember that, like all other proteins, these enzymes become denatured and inactive when heated to extreme temperatures; however, they are mostly inactive at room temperature. Papain is most active at temperatures around 151°F (66°C).[7] Bromelain becomes active at 104°F (40°C) and is deactivated around 149°F (65°C). Regardless of which enzyme is used, the meat should be poked with a sharp fork or spear (Jaccard meat tenderizer) prior to tenderizing so that the enzymes can reach the inner portions of the meat cut. Otherwise, the outer portions of the meat will be tender, and the inner portions will remain tough.

Mechanical tenderization is another means by which meat can be tenderized. Mechanical tenderization may occur while the entire meat carcass remains intact, or it may occur once the meat has been cut into pieces. A commercial meat tenderizer is a large piece of equipment with blades and needles that cuts through excessive connective tissue. Other pieces of commercial equipment may cube the meat into smaller pieces with shorter segments of connective tissue. Meat carcasses and smaller cuts can also be pounded with a meat mallet to further break down remaining connective tissue. As a final step, carving meat against the grain (the muscle fibers) also will help to disrupt any remaining chunks of connective tissue.

Heating Meats

The addition of heat to meat will cause numerous changes, particularly to meat proteins. The shape, composition, and length of proteins determine characteristics such as flavor, juiciness, and tenderness of the meats. As meat is heated, the proteins, or muscle fibers, become denatured and decrease in length. This process causes a reduction in the water-binding capacity of the protein, thereby limiting the amount of liquid that the fibers will be able to

TABLE 5.1
Cooking Temperatures for Various Degrees of Doneness in Beef Steak

Degree of Doneness	Temperature
Rare*	< 145°F (< 63°C)
Medium rare*	145°F (63°C)
Medium	160°F (71°C)
Well done	170°F (77°C)

*Consuming rare meats is not generally recommended due to the risk of bacterial contamination and foodborne illness.

Source: Data from Texas Beef Council. Cooking School: Meat Doneness. Available at: http://www.txbeef.org/cooking_school/meat_doneness. Accessed July 25, 2012.

bind. The addition of heat will also dehydrate the myosin, thus ridding the meat of water already retained and making the final product less juicy than its original uncooked state. Heat will also cause the denatured proteins to cross-link and coagulate, giving the meat a tough and less tender texture. Meats can be cooked to a wide range of temperatures or doneness; varying degrees of doneness are provided in **Table 5.1**.

Connective tissues, such as collagen, will also begin to break down when exposed to heat. Exposure to moist heat will allow the hydrogen bonds in collagen to break, forming gelatin. This conversion of collagen to gelatin is essential when tenderizing tough meats such as beef pot roast. If the gelatin is allowed to seep into the meat drippings, these drippings can be chilled, and the resulting gel can be seen by the naked eye. Tough cuts of meat are ideally prepared using a slow, moist heat so collagen can be converted to gelatin without overheating and toughening the meat's protein. The other connective tissue found in meats, elastin, is not altered by heating, thus meats with elastin will remain tough throughout heating, and the elastin must be physically removed before consumption.

Altering the pH of the meat can cause changes in meat texture during cooking. For this reason, meats may be soaked in acidic marinades for several hours before cooking. The acid in the marinade will tenderize the meat as well as impart unique flavors that will be retained throughout cooking.

Freezing Meats

Freezing meats and meat products enables the consumer to keep the food for a longer period of time than when simply keeping the foods in the refrigerator. **Table 5.2** shows the estimated amount of time that a meat can be kept in the frozen state.

When freezing a meat, quick, low-temperature freezing is imperative. Because water freezes at a different temperature than the meat, water can separate from the protein, and once the water does begin to freeze (usually around 28–29°F [−2.2 to −1.7°C), it forms large crystals that break apart the surrounding tissues and result in a low-quality end product.

The freezing of meats also can result in drip losses when the product is eventually thawed. Again, if water is allowed to separate from the other proteins in the meat it will be lost when the meat is thawed, resulting in a less juicy final product. The freezing of meats may impact their overall tenderness once thawed and prepared; however, investigation into this issue has not always produced consistent results.[8–11]

TABLE 5.2
Cold Storage Estimated Expiration Dates for Beef, Veal, Lamb, and Pork

Meat	Shelf Life at 40°F (4°C)*	Shelf Life at 0°F (–18°C)
Ground meats Stew meat Organ and miscellaneous meats (tongue, liver, heart, kidney)	1–2 days	3–4 months
Chops Roasts Steaks	3–5 days	4–12 months
Prestuffed chops	1 day	Not recommended
Leftover and reheated meats, casseroles	3–4 days	2–3 months
Corned beef, in pouch with pickling juices	5–7 days	Drained, 1 month
Bacon	7 days	1 month

*ServSafe recommends 41°F (4.4°C).

Source: Reproduced from U.S. Department of Agriculture, Food Safety and Inspection Service. Keep Food Safe! Food Safety Basics. Available at: http://www.fsis.usda.gov/factsheets/Keep_Food_Safe_Food_Safety_Basics/index.asp. Accessed January 3, 2011.

For large-scale facilities where meat carcasses are stored frozen, specific conditions should be met. Freezer temperatures should be kept around –5°F, and air velocities should be maintained at 500–1,000 feet per minute.[12] These conditions will bring the temperature of meat down quick enough to prevent formation of ice crystals, and it also will limit the growth of bacteria in the product.

Preserved and Processed Meats

curing Preservation technique used in making meat products such as sausage and frankfurters.

Agriculturalists and food scientists have mastered the art of processing meats to produce products with various flavors and textures desirable to the consumer. Ham, corned beef, pastrami, bacon, and hot dogs are all commonly consumed meats that undergo extensive processing. **Curing** is one of the most common techniques used in meat preservation. Curing includes processes such as salting, smoking, and drying.

When curing a meat, several agents, such as sodium chloride (salt), sodium nitrite, sucrose (common table sugar), and ascorbates, are usually dissolved in water to form brine, which is the curing solution:

- Sodium chloride imparts a distinct flavor on the final product, and it also reduces the amount of free water available. By reducing the food's water content, bacterial growth is also limited, thus preserving the food. It should be noted that salts used in curing may contain trace amounts of copper or other metals, and this can speed up oxidative rancidity in the final product. For this reason, cured meats need to be handled carefully and stored properly.
- Sodium nitrite functions as an antioxidant to prevent oxidative rancidity. It can also protect against botulism, a foodborne illness, by preventing the growth of *Clostridium botulinum*, a spore-producing bacterium. It is important to note, however, that

excessive nitrite can be toxic, thus the USDA Food Safety and Inspection Service (FSIS) regulates the amount of nitrite that may be added to a product.
- Sucrose is added during curing to reduce the salty flavor imparted by sodium chloride. If added in appropriate amounts, sucrose also can cause a desirable brown coloration on the final cured product.
- Ascorbates, another group of preservatives, are reducing agents; they reduce nitrites to nitric oxide. After reduction, nitric oxide will combine with the metmyoglobin pigments and produce the pink color (nitrosyl hemochrome) commonly associated with cured meats.

The conditions under which a meat is cured depend on the size of the meat cut and the temperature under which it is cured. Large meat cuts, such as hams, need to be cured for an extended period of time because it takes a while for the brine to penetrate the thick cut of meat. Temperature also affects curing. All curing should take place at temperatures below 40°F (4.4°C) to minimize bacterial growth; however, if the temperature is too far below 40°F (4.4°C), the desired chemical reactions can be slowed or completely halted unless additional chemicals are added. In general, a piece of meat cured in brine should take about 3 1/2 to 4 days per pound to undergo the curing process if the temperature is held at 36–40°F (2.2–4.4°C). The speed of this process can be increased dramatically if the brine is injected directly into the meat; in this case, the amount of time required to finish curing a ham may be decreased to as little as 24 hours. To cure bacon, brine is injected directly into the pork belly; within a few minutes, the curing process is finished.

After the meat product has been subjected to the curing agents, the product may be smoked in a commercial smoke box or smokehouse. Wood logs and sawdust from trees such as oak and hickory are commonly used when smoking hams because the phenols and carbonyls produced by smoking impart a distinct and desirable flavor on the final product. The process of smoking must raise the internal temperature of the product enough to destroy *Trichinella spiralis*, a parasite commonly found in hogs. Hams that have been cured and smoked are considered to be precooked hams; although they are "cooked," the consumer should still reheat these hams to at least 140°F (60°C) prior to consumption.

Gastronomy Point

Salami Salami, a cured meat, has been commonly consumed in southern European cultures for centuries due to its shelf stability.

Sausage is another commonly consumed processed meat product. The meat used to make fresh sausage originates from low-grade cattle and hogs, and by U.S. government regulation sausage cannot have a fat content greater than 50%. When making fresh sausage, the meat is ground and combined with other herbs and seasonings, such as salt, pepper, and sage. The ground product is then stuffed into a natural or synthetic casing. Natural casings are usually made from the lining of sheep intestines, whereas synthetic casings may be made from food-grade plastics. After being stuffed, fresh sausage should be prepared and stored at around 32°F (0°C) to limit bacterial growth and prevent oxidative rancidity.

Frankfurters, commonly known as hot dogs, are another type of sausage consumed widely in the United States and throughout the world. This processed meat is typically made from beef and pork, although due to consumer demand some frankfurters are now made from poultry and soy products. Like fresh sausage, frankfurters are typically combined with other seasoning agents, such as pepper, mustard, and garlic, to give the final product a desirable flavor. Unlike fresh sausage, though, frankfurters are cured and smoked before being packaged and sold. The curing process involves the addition of nitrites and ascorbates, a process similar to that seen in the preparation of ham. Fat and other emulsifiers also may be added before the meat slurry is pumped into its casing and smoked in chamber. Once packaged, the final product is kept at about 32°F (0°C). Unless frozen, the product will eventually spoil and become slimy or turn green. The green color seen on some expired frankfurters or bologna is the result of a chemical reaction between hydrogen peroxide produced by bacteria and the pigment nitrosohemochrome found in the meat.

Because of the public interest in lowering the fat content of meats and meat products, many processed meats are now made with leaner meat and have bulking agents added to the meat slurry instead of fat. These bulking agents may be protein-containing ingredients, such as whey concentrates, or carbohydrate-based ingredients, such as fiber, gums, and modified starches.[13]

Meat Alternatives

textured soy protein (TSP) A protein-rich meat alternative made from defatted soy flour or soybeans.

meat extenders Protein substances added to meat; sometimes used synonymously with "meat fillers," which are usually carbohydrate substances.

Due to personal preference, health issues, and food and environmental concerns, many people have turned to using meat alternatives. Soy-based alternatives, particularly **textured soy protein (TSP)**, which is also known as *textured vegetable protein* (TVP), is commonly marketed to consumers who avoid eating animal-based products. When making TSP, soy flour or soybeans are defatted and their proteins isolated.[14] The protein-rich concentrate produced by this process is then dehydrated, and the final product is shelf stable for nearly 12 months when stored in an airtight container.

Nutritionally, TSP is an excellent meat alterative due to its high protein content. By weight, TSP is at least 50% protein; furthermore, the proteins found in TSP are complete because they contain all of the amino acids not able to be synthesized in the human body. When producing foods with TSP, processing must proceed carefully and under controlled conditions. Otherwise, products containing large amounts of TSP may develop an undesirable "beany" flavor. The development of this flavor and its accompanying odor results from the oxidation of unsaturated fatty acids in the TSP.[15] Because the development of these characteristics will make the final food product unpalatable, food scientists may limit the amount of TSP they add to meat substitutes and meat analogs, and they may also experiment with the cooking techniques used to prepare products made with TSP. For example, one study found that the majority of consumers enjoyed chicken- or shrimp-flavored TSP products when they were fried, whereas less than one-third of the consumers liked the same products when they were baked.[16]

In food science, TSP also can be used as a **meat extender**. Because of its high protein and relatively low fat content, TSP usually has a more favorable nutrition profile than high-fat, high-cholesterol meats. Some processed meat products, therefore, may have their fat content lowered by substituting meat with TSP. In addition, TSP often is cheaper than meat so food manufacturers also can incorporate TSP into meat products as a means to lower the final product's overall cost.

Phytonutrient Point

Isoflavones TSPs contain isoflavones, phytonutrients that are associated with prevention of some types of cancer.

Green Point

Meat Alternatives Because TSP comes from plants, the energy required for its manufacture and production is much lower than that required for the maintenance, slaughter, and processing of animals. Thus, meat alternatives often are considered to be more environmentally friendly than meat.

Food Selection and Menu Planning

Meats are often the centerpiece of a meal, around which other foods and beverages are paired. As such, meat should be selected carefully well in advance of the designated meal time, and an appropriate preparation and cooking plan should then be followed. The method by which the meat is cooked is highly dependent on the cut of the meat, thus an understanding of the composition of various cuts of meat is imperative.

Cuts of Meats

Wholesale and retail cuts of meats vary widely in their fat, muscle, and connective tissue content. As a result, consumers must consider the overall composition of the meat when selecting the appropriate cut. In general, cuts from muscles that receive regular exercise will be leaner and tougher than those from areas on the animal that do not receive exercise.

Beef

In the United States, butchers divide cattle carcasses into two symmetric pieces and then cut each piece in half. The front half, known as the forequarter, includes the chuck, rib, short plate, brisket, and fore shank. Common cuts such as stew beef, ribeye roll steak, rib roast, and beef brisket all originate from forequarter cuts. The back half of the carcass, known as the hindquarter, includes the short loin, tenderloin, flank, and round cuts. Many of the popular steaks, such as flank steak, top sirloin butt steak, tenderloin steak, and filet mignon, originate from the hindquarter region (see **Figure 5.7**).

Veal

Because of the animal's small size, veal has many fewer cuts than beef or pork. The main primal cuts, or the first cuts from the whole carcass, include leg (round), sirloin, loin, rib, shoulder, foreshank, and breast. Because veal is slaughtered at a young age compared to other animals, most veal roasts contain a high amount of fat and are therefore extremely tender (see **Figure 5.8**).

Lamb

Lamb has four primal cuts: shoulder, rack, loin, and leg. These are then broken down into several retail cuts typically seen in the grocery stores, including the neck, foreshank, breast/brisket, and flank. Most cuts of lamb are fairly tender and do not require the same amount of tenderization as corresponding cuts of pork and beef (see **Figure 5.9**).

Pork

The American primal cuts of pork include shoulder blade, arm shoulder, loin, leg, and side. The loin is popular because the pork loin chop and roast originate from this area, as does the pork loin tenderloin and Canadian bacon. Spare ribs and bacon originate from the side primal cut, which is sometimes referred to as the "belly" of the hog. Although any region of the animal can be cured, the leg region of the hog is typically used to produce cured ham (see **Figure 5.10**).

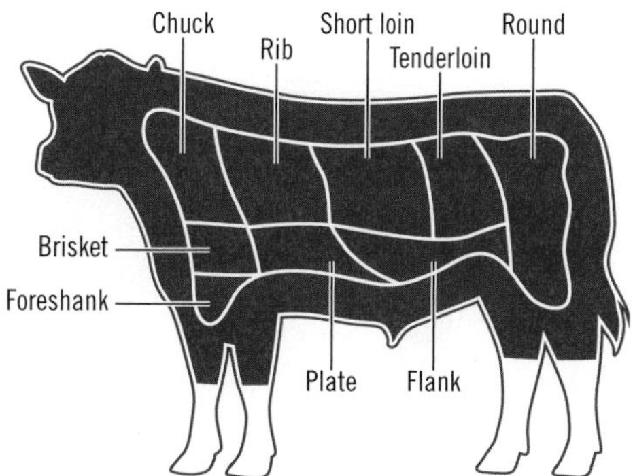

FIGURE 5.7 Standard cuts of cattle.

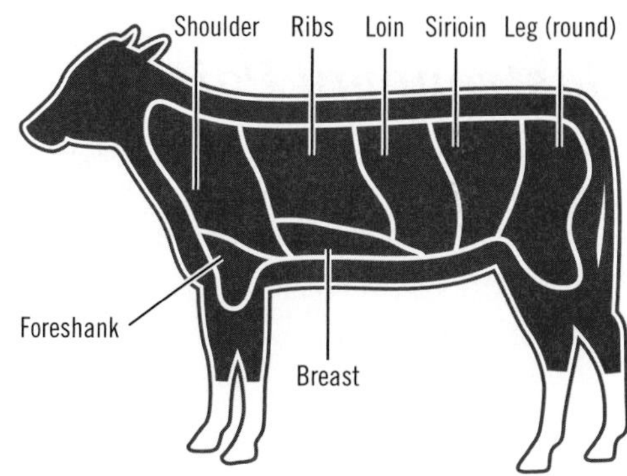

FIGURE 5.8 Standard cuts of veal.

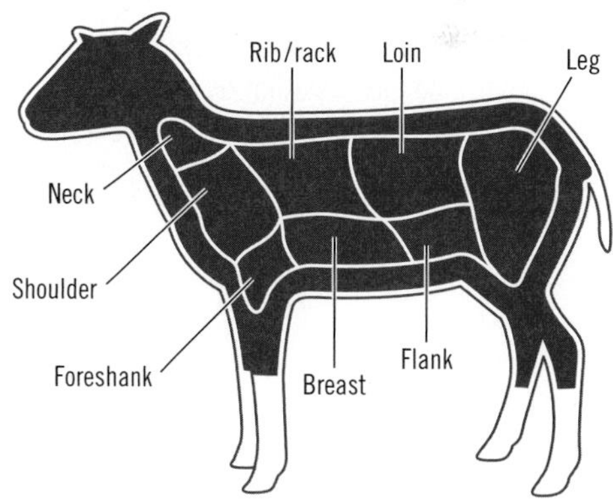

FIGURE 5.9 Cuts of lamb.

Choosing Healthy Cuts

Many consumers are interested in reducing their intake of saturated fat and are therefore choosing lean and low-fat cuts of meat. Among trimmed beef cuts, a 3-ounce serving of flank steak, T-bone steak, or sirloin steak all meet government guidelines for lean meat. Top round roast and steak and 95% fat-free ground beef also meet these guidelines. The leanest cuts of veal include the sirloin, rib chop, loin chop, and leg cutlet. With only 2.98 grams of fat per 3-ounce serving, pork tenderloins are also considered a health-conscious choice of meat.

Creating Well-Rounded Meals with Meats

It is important to balance a meal with additional side items that complement the flavor, temperature, and texture of the meat. For example, when meat is served warm, it is appropriate to balance it with a chilled salad, such as a fruit

Gastronomy Point

Yin and Yang In ancient Chinese culture, meals were created based on the yin and yang principles of balance. Meats, which were typically considered yin, were combined with yang foods, such as barley, bean curd, and broccoli.

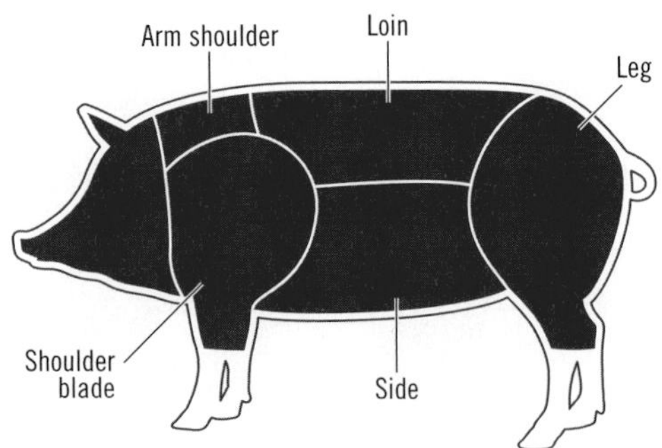

FIGURE 5.10 Cuts of pork.

or vegetable salad. Tender cuts of meat may also be complemented by the crunchy texture of a raw salad. Stew meats are traditionally served in a stew along with cooked vegetables, such as potatoes, carrots, and celery.

In some cultures, it is customary to serve wine with meat-based meals; typically, red meats are expected to be served with a room-temperature red wine. A fruity pinot noir may be used to complement the intense flavor of lamb, or a peppery-flavored shiraz may be paired with a pepper steak. In the end, however, the flavors of wine vary widely, as do personal tastes. The final decision on wine pairing should always rest with the consumer and his or her palate.

Gastronomy Point

Wine and Meat The tannins in the wine, which when isolated cause a bitter taste, bind with the proteins in the meat, causing the wine's flavor to soften.

Basic Meat Preparation Techniques

Heating and Cooking Methods

The methods used to cook meat depend on the characteristics of the meat. Well-marbled and juicy cuts of meat are best prepared using dry heat methods, whereas lean and less juicy cuts of meat are better prepared using moist heat methods. The type and amount of heat applied ultimately affect the physical changes in the meat and the outcome of the final product. The length of time heat is applied also impacts the safety of the food being consumed.

Before meats are cooked, they are typically prepared by removing the outer layers of fat and connective tissue as well as excess water found on the surface of the meat. Although the fat and connective tissue serve to protect the meat while it is raw, they can contribute to poor flavor and texture if left on during cooking. Water on the surface of meat should be removed prior to cooking in order to minimize the loss of color and nutrients during the heating process.

dry heat cooking methods Meat preparation methods that do not include the addition of liquid, such as broiling, grilling, frying, and roasting.

Dry Heat Methods

Cuts of meat that contain intramuscular fat and moisture are best prepared using **dry heat cooking methods** such as broiling, grilling, frying, and roasting. These techniques use minimal amounts of water-based liquids and rely on the composition of the meat to promote a desirable flavor and texture. As with any cooking method, the application of heat will cause the proteins in meat to become denatured and move closer to each other. As these strands of proteins coalesce, water is expelled from the product, causing shrinkage. In dry heat methods, the water released from the meat will drain away, causing the meat to contain less moisture and to be less juicy. Thus, dry heat methods are typically used on highly marbled pieces of meat that maintain their palatability because of their high fat content.

Broiling

Broiling involves the application of intense, direct, high heat for a short period of time. Broiling is usually done in an oven heated to a temperature of 375–500°F (190.6–260°C); broiling is never done at a temperature less than 350°F (176.6°C). Pieces of meat sliced up to 3 inches thick are placed on a broiling pan specially designed for this cooking technique. A basic broiling pan contains openings that allow the grease and drippings to drain away from the heat source, minimizing the potential for smoke and fire. Meats are cooked with one side facing the heat source for 6 to 14 minutes and then turned over with tongs so that the other side can be exposed for an additional, but shorter, amount of time. The longer the meat is exposed to heat, the more well done the meat will be.

Green Point

Appliances To conserve energy and to reduce your carbon footprint when cooking, you should only use large appliances when preparing large quantities of food. When cooking a small amount of food, it is more energy-efficient to use smaller appliances (e.g., toaster oven, small grill).

Thick cuts should be placed on racks located in a lower position in the oven. For example, a steak that is 3 inches thick should be placed on a rack that is in the lowest position and farthest away from the oven's heat source.

In contrast, a 1-inch thick steak should be placed on a rack that is close to the heat source and is only one or two positions away from the top. The goal of broiling is to heat the center of the meat to the desired doneness while also producing adequate browning on the outside of the meat. These characteristics can be achieved through correct positioning of the broiling pan in the oven and careful monitoring of cooking time.

Pan-broiling

Pan-broiling is similar to broiling in that it involves the application of high heat to a piece of meat. However, pan-broiling is carried out on the stovetop range using a flat grill, griddle, or heavy pan. Cuts of meats that are prepared via pan-broiling should be no thicker than ½ inch in order to reach the desired browning and internal texture. Ground beef patties and thinly sliced steaks and lamb chops are commonly prepared using this technique. During the cooking process, drippings, grease, and accumulating liquid should be removed to prevent splattering and to avoid frying the meat in the fluid.

Grilling

Grilling is another dry heat method similar to broiling. In grilling, however, heat is applied below the meat as opposed to above it. When grilling, meats should be less than 3 inches thick. Prior to cooking, the grill must be heated to the desirable temperature, which may take up to 30 minutes. When cooking the meat, the meat can be placed directly on the grilling surface, in a grill pan, or in a griddle.

During the grilling process, excessive exposure of the meat to temperatures above 500°F (260°C) can cause the Maillard reaction to occur. The **Maillard reaction**, named after chemist Louis-Camille Maillard, is a heat-mediated reaction between an amino acid and a reducing sugar, and it causes nonenzymatic browning, which commonly occurs during grilling.

Maillard reaction Chemical reaction that occurs between reducing sugars and amino groups of amino acids and proteins; results in a brown color and change in flavor.

Grilling has been cause for concern in recent years because the Maillard reaction is known to produce heterocyclic amines, benzopyrenes, and polycyclic aromatic hydrocarbons. All of these chemicals have been recognized as potential cancer-causing agents (see **Special Topic 5.2**).[17] It has been demonstrated, however, that marinating meats before grilling will significantly reduce the formation of these potential carcinogens, particularly the heterocyclic amines.[18]

Special Topic 5.2

Heterocyclic Amines and Grilling Meat

Isabel Smith

Heterocyclic amines (HCAs) are mutagenic agents found in meat products that are cooked at high temperatures. HCAs are formed in meat products most often when they are grilled, baked, or pan fried. When the meat is exposed to heat that is 300°F (149°C) or higher, chemical changes in the creatine and creatinine proteins present in the muscle tissue may cause formation of HCAs. Once the HCAs are formed, the person who eats the meat may be at a greater risk for DNA mutation. The potential for DNA mutation differs from person to person and depends on the presence of certain enzymes. In a process called *bioactivation*, DNA may be mutated by the HCAs; these changes in DNA structure may lead to development of cancer.[1]

Studies have found that eating high amounts of HCAs may be specifically associated with breast, prostate, and colorectal cancers.[2] Although most studies thus far have examined the effects of HCAs in animals, current studies are looking to identify the results of eating high amounts of HCAs in humans.

HCAs are found mostly in beef and chicken, although fish that is cooked at very high temperatures may contain HCAs, too. The National Cancer Institute recommends the following techniques to avoid high amounts of HCAs in meat:[1]

1 Avoid exposing meat directly to the flame or to the hot surface, such as the grill grates.
2 Use the microwave to precook meat so that it is exposed to the open flame for less time.
3 Turn meat continuously on a hot surface so that HCA formation is reduced.
4 Remove charred portions of the meat and refrain from eating the drippings from meat that has been cooked at very high temperatures.

References

1 National Cancer Institute. Chemicals in Meat Cooked at High Temperatures and Cancer Risk. October 5, 2011. Available at: http://www.cancer.gov/cancertopics/factsheet/Risk/cooked-meats.
2 Norrish A, Ferguson L, Knize M, et al. Heterocyclic Amine Content of Cooked Meat and Risk of Prostate Cancer. *J Natl Cancer Inst.* 1999;91(23):2038–2044.

Frying

Frying, unlike grilling and broiling, requires the addition of fat or oil to the meat that is being cooked. Fats and oils can transfer heat at much higher temperatures than water. Vegetable oils also have relatively high smoke points, meaning that they will not begin to form acrolein and smoke until they have reached 400–500°F (204–260°C). Frying techniques include sautéing, stir-frying, pan frying, and shallow and deep fat frying. All are considered dry heat techniques for cooking meats.

Sautéing is a technique similar to pan-broiling in that the thinly sliced meat is added to a heavy pan over high heat on a range. The only difference is that when sautéing a small amount of fat, usually in the form of clarified butter or vegetable oil, is also added to the pan. The addition of the fat allows the meat to brown and retain the flavor of the fat. Stir-frying is also conducted over high heat on a stovetop range. For this technique, bite-sized portions of meat are placed in wok or sloped-edge pan coated in a small amount of oil. As heat is applied to the pan, the meat is constantly stirred to promote thorough and even cooking. In both sautéing and stir-frying, vegetables, seasonings, and sauces may be added to add additional flavors and textures to the dish.

Like sautéing and stir frying, pan frying (or shallow frying) takes place in a heavy pan on the range; however, more fat is typically added. Up to 1/2 inch of oil or fat is added to the pan, and as a result, the meats prepared using this technique can be larger and thicker than those used in sautéing or stir-frying. The temperature used in pan frying is lower than the temperature used for sautéing—pan frying temperatures never exceed 375°F (191°C). Meats prepared using pan frying may be unseasoned and raw, or they may be coated with flour or breading. When adding raw or cool uncooked meats to a hot pan and oil, the temperature of the oil will drastically decrease, limiting the oil's ability to cook the meat and causing the oil to infiltrate the meat. The final product will then be greasy and oil-laden. Instead, it is best to add room-temperature or slightly warmed raw meats to the oil. This will keep the oil's temperature high, cook the meat internally, and allow the steam from within the meat to push out and keep the oil from penetrating the meat's surface.

Deep fat frying usually involves submerging food in oil or fat and is done in a large pot over the stovetop or by a separate appliance called a deep fat fryer. Food is usually deep fat fried in the 345–375°F (175–191°C) range.

In this range, the water in food repels the oil and does not allow for seepage inside. Deep fat frying at too low of a temperature will cause unwanted retention of fat in the food.

Roasting

Roasting is a dry heat cooking method (using indirect heat) commonly used in the preparation of large portions of meat. Typically, a roast will be a minimum of 2 to 3 inches thick and will yield more than four servings of meat per roast. Center-cut pork loin, leg of lamb, and veal are commonly prepared using the roasting technique. Roasting is performed in an oven heated to a minimum of 300°F (149°C). Lower temperatures of 300–350°F (149–177°C) will produce uniform and tender, juicy products, whereas higher temperatures of 350–500°F (177–260°C) will produce roasts with a seared crust and a slightly smaller product due to shrinkage. In general, roasts take approximately 18 to 30 minutes per pound to cook, but a meat thermometer should be used in order to verify that the desired internal temperature has been reached.

When roasting, meats are arranged in the center of an open pan and placed in the oven. The open pan allows the drippings and liquid to evaporate during cooking and prevents simmering from occurring. Once the roast has reached the desired internal temperature, it is allowed to stand for an additional 20 to 30 minutes prior to carving to allow redistribution of juices.

Moist Heat Methods

Moist heat cooking methods are the preferred techniques for preparing meats that are lean and that contain more collagen. When using moist heat methods, the proteins in the meat become denatured, and the tough collagen will begin to break down. However, moist heat methods do not reach temperatures as high as those reached in dry heat methods and do not cause browning or excessive fluid loss. The fluid used in moist heating may reach a slight boil, but the cooking environment is slower and more controlled than with the dry heat methods. As a result of these conditions, the lean muscle tissue becomes juicy and tender, making the overall final product more palatable than if a dry heat method was employed. The most commonly utilized moist heat cooking methods include braising, stewing, simmering, pressure cooking, and steaming.

moist heat cooking methods
Meat preparation methods that include the addition of a liquid (e.g., water), such as braising, stewing, simmering, and steaming.

Braising

Braising often is used on lean cuts of meat such as shoulder of lamb and beef chuck. Braising is most well known for its use in preparing beef pot roast. Braising is done by placing a large piece of meat in a covered pan, searing the outside, and then adding a set amount of liquid, broth, or stock to the pan. The amount of liquid added should be minimal to prevent the dilution of flavors. Although braising can be carried out on a stovetop range, it is most commonly done in an oven preheated to between 300–350°F (149–177°C). The meat is allowed to simmer in liquid for several hours. As it simmers, the collagen begins to denature and melt, causing the meat to become more tender and increasing the thickness of the liquid. The moisture from the liquid is also incorporated into the muscle fibers, making the final product more juicy and palatable. Braised meat is considered done when the meat can be easily pulled apart with a fork.

Prior to braising, steps can be taken to ensure that the final product has the desired taste and texture. Because of the presence of liquid, braising does not allow for the Maillard reaction to occur; thus, if a crisp outer consistency is desired, it must be achieved prior to braising. The meat cut may be dusted with seasoned flour and browned on the stovetop range in order to sear the outside edges of the meat before it is placed in the braising pan. In addition to the prebraising browning of meat, other desirable flavors can be incorporated into the meat by the addition of seasonings and vegetables to the braising pan. Vegetables, such as potatoes, carrots, onions, and celery, often are sautéed and added to the braising pot to help add flavor and color to the final dish.

Stewing

Although similar to braising, stewing is typically done using more liquid and is carried out for a longer period of time than braising. Stewing is a popular way of preparing cuts of meats that contain a high percentage of collagen and connective tissue because the meat is exposed to the moist, heated conditions for a long period of time. During this time, the collagen will have sufficient time to melt. The proteins within the meat will also cook, but they will not become denatured and toughen very quickly. Thus, by the time the collagen has broken down, the meat has not overcooked, and the final product will be palatable. To increase the meat's exposure to heat and moisture, the chef may cut the meat into smaller pieces in order to increase the overall surface area. The internal temperature of meats that are stewed or braised rarely exceeds 210°F (99°C); to ensure food safety, the product must be kept at this temperature for approximately 25 minutes.

Simmering

Meats prepared by simmering are submerged in liquids kept just below the boiling point of water, usually around 180–200°F (82–93°C). The liquid is first brought to a boil, then its temperature is lowered before the meat is added. As in stewing and braising, the meat never reaches a high internal temperature, thus it must be kept in the simmering liquid long enough to fully cook and for the collagen to convert to gelatin. The liquid used to simmer the meat is typically made of a water base; if the chef uses a milk base, the resulting dish may be referred to as "creamed" instead of "simmered."

Steaming

This form of indirect heating is not used frequently when preparing meats. However, some meats that have already been cooked and refrozen may be reheated using this method. Steaming is considered a moist heat method because the meat is placed above a boiling liquid, and it is the steam created from this boiling liquid that heats the meat. The time needed for the steaming techniques to reheat cold or frozen meats will depend on the size and weight of the meat product.

Nutritional Properties

Nutritional Value Of Meats

Meats add a tremendous amount of nutritional value to the typical American diet. Not only are beef, lamb, and pork a significant source of high-quality protein, but they also provide an abundance of vitamins and minerals that are easy to digest and absorb. However, meats also are primary source of saturated fats and cholesterol in the American diet and should, therefore, be eaten in moderation.

Protein

A 3-ounce portion of meat provides roughly 21 grams of protein, although the actual value may be somewhat less in untrimmed cuts of meat. Because this protein originates from animal sources, meat is a source of complete protein, meaning that it contains the essential amino acids that the human body is unable to synthesize. The effect of excessive animal protein on human health remains unclear;[19] however, some research has shown that excessive protein intake from animal sources may be contributing factor to diabetes mellitus.[20]

Fats

Meats are a significant source of dietary fat. In particular, meat is one of the largest sources of saturated fat in the American diet. Saturated fatty acids are hydrocarbon chains, approximately 12 to 20 carbons in length, bound together by single bonds. Much research has examined the effects of consuming a diet high in saturated fat; to date, the general conclusion has been that such diets are associated with multiple chronic health conditions, including heart disease, hypertension, and hyperlipidemia. The current recommendation put forth by the *Dietary Guidelines for Americans* is to limit saturated fat intake to less than 10% of the overall daily caloric intake, or less than approximately 22 grams of saturated fat per day when following a 2,000 calorie diet.[21]

Several factors influence the amount of dietary fat obtained from meat consumption.[22] Lean cuts of meat that are trimmed and have little marbling will contain significantly less fat than untrimmed, well-marbled cuts. Cooking and preparation methods also affect the amount of total and saturated fat found in meats. Meats prepared by grilling and broiling often have less fat; as the meat cooks, the fat liquefies and drains away from the meat. Although this reduces the fat content, it also makes the meat less tender.

Cholesterol

Meats also are a source of dietary cholesterol. Cholesterol is a sterol-based molecule found in animal products, and the current recommendation is to limit cholesterol consumption to less than 200–300 mg per day. Because sterols are fat-based molecules, the cholesterol content of meats usually increases as the fat content increases. For example, a 3-ounce serving of 95% lean ground beef will contain approximately 5.5 grams of fat and 65 mg of cholesterol, whereas a 3-ounce serving of a lamb rib chop will contain 11.1 grams of fat and almost 80 mg of cholesterol.

Carbohydrates

Most of the carbohydrate found in the muscle tissue of animals is converted to lactic acid shortly after slaughter. As a result, meat does not provide a significant amount of carbohydrate to human dietary intake. Some prepared meats, however, may be battered and fried, and the batter (i.e., cornmeal, flour) will provide a small amount of carbohydrate.

Vitamins and Minerals

Meats contribute a number of different vitamins and minerals to the human diet. Because of the biological similarities between animals and humans, many nutrients found in animal-based products, such as meat, are readily digested and absorbed by the human body.

Iron

The iron content of meat products depends on the type of meat as well as the fat and muscle content of the cut. In general, a 3-ounce portion of beef, lamb, or pork contains 4–7 mg of iron. Iron found in meat products is known as heme iron. This type of iron is readily absorbed by cells in the intestine and does not have to be converted before it can be utilized in the human body.

Zinc

Zinc is another mineral found in high concentrations in red meats. In the human body, zinc helps to catalyze enzyme-dependent reactions and is also important in the maintenance of body proteins and cellular membranes. The average 3-ounce serving of beef will contain 6 mg of zinc; an equivalent serving of pork will contain 2.2 mg of zinc. The Recommended Dietary Allowance (RDA) for adult males is 11 mg/day; the RDA for adult females is 8 mg/day. Individuals consuming red meat usually meet these recommended amounts without needing additional supplementation.

Phosphorus and Copper

Red meats are also high in minerals such as phosphorus and copper. Phosphorus, which is found in high concentrations in the human body, helps to maintain bones and teeth. Meats are an excellent source of phosphorus, with a 3-ounce serving of beef containing 90–400 mg of phosphorus. Copper, an essential trace element, plays an active role in human metabolism and the formation of connective tissue. Although adults only need 900 μg of copper per day, 1 ounce of beef liver contains over 4,000 μg of this element.

B-complex Vitamins

The B-complex vitamins (thiamin, riboflavin, niacin, B_6, folate, and B_{12}) are the most abundant vitamins found in red meats. Vitamin B_{12}, a vitamin essential for brain function and blood formation, is found almost exclusively in animal-based products. A 3-ounce portion of top sirloin beef contains almost 100% of the recommended daily intake of vitamin B_{12}. Because this vitamin is not found in many plant-based foods, vegetarians and vegans sometimes get B_{12} injections to avoid developing a deficiency.

Nutrient Retention in Dry Heat Methods

Dry heat methods tend to preserve the nutritional value of meats better than moist heat methods because there is no addition of liquid, which can dissolve water-soluble vitamins. Nonetheless, some of the nutritional content of meats will be lost during any type of cooking simply due to heat exposure and the loss from drippings. **Table 5.3** describes the percentage of various nutrients retained from the raw product once the meat has been prepared.

In meats that are broiled, approximately 80–100% of the iron and 100% of the zinc is retained. Eighty-five to 90% percent of the phosphorus is retained, and 75–100% of the copper is retained (ground broiled lamb only retains 75% of the copper from the raw product). The B-complex vitamins are not as well retained during broiling. As little as 60% of thiamin and vitamin B_6 is retained by broiled meat, and only 75–90% of vitamin B_{12} is retained. Many broiled meats are ground prior to cooking, such as ground beef; however, this type of physical change does not contribute to a substantial loss of nutrients.

Frying meats also causes some nutrient loss, but in veal it appears that the amount lost often depends on whether the meat was coated prior to frying. For example, uncoated, fried veal retains 75% of its riboflavin and 45% of its vitamin B_6, whereas coated, fried veal retains 90% of its riboflavin and 65% of its vitamin B_6. Pork, beef, and lamb appear to have similar nutrient retention values regardless of coating. Although most coated meats do retain most of their nutritional value, they also contain more calories and carbohydrate due to the coating.

TABLE 5.3
Percentage of Select Nutrients Retained (Nutrient Retention Factor) After Specified Preparation Methods of Meats

Type of Meat	Iron (%)	Zinc (%)	Thiamine (%)	Riboflavin (%)	Niacin (%)	Vitamin B_6 (%)	Folate (%)	Vitamin B_{12} (%)
Beef								
Roasted	100	100	55	95	75	50	95	70
Broiled, cut	95	100	70	90	80	60	85	80
Broiled, ground	95	100	80	95	90	60	85	80
Fried, without coating	95	100	70	90	80	60	85	80
Fried, with coating	95	100	70	90	80	60	85	80
Veal								
Broiled	90	100	65	90	80	65	75	80
Fried, without coating	90	100	65	75	85	45	85	95
Fried, with coating	90	100	65	90	80	65	75	80
Roasted	85	100	60	90	80	50	85	85
Lamb								
Broiled	95	100	60	90	80	65	70	80
Ground, broiled	95	100	70	80	85	75	70	75
Roasted	100	100	60	90	80	75	85	75
Pork								
Fresh, broiled	80	100	70	100	80	65	85	90
Fresh, fried without coating	80	100	70	100	80	65	85	90
Fresh, fried with coating	80	10	70	100	80	65	85	90
Fresh, roasted	100	100	60	95	85	85	95	80

Source: Modified from U.S. Department of Agriculture. Table of Nutrient Retention Factors, Release 6, 2007. Available at: http://www.nal.usda.gov/fnic/foodcomp/Data/retn6/retn06.pdf. Accessed January 3, 2011.

Roasted meats retain 100% of their iron and zinc, with the exception of roasted veal, which only retains 85% of its iron. Only 55–60% of the thiamin is retained in roasted meats, whereas up to 95% of the riboflavin and 90% of the niacin is retained. Roughly half of the vitamin B_6 is retained in roasted beef and veal, whereas 75% is retained in roasted lamb and 85% is retained in roasted pork. Seventy to 85% of vitamin B_{12} is retained in roasted meats, with the highest retention being in roasted veal.

Nutrient Retention in Moist Heat Methods

Nutrient retention in moist heat methods is highly dependent on whether the drippings and liquid are retained. Many of the vitamins and minerals contained in these meats will be forced from the meat and into the drippings as a result of the moist heat cooking method. After cooking, if the liquid is consumed many of the nutrients are retained; however, if the liquid is discarded after cooking, then over 50% of some nutrients may be lost due to their water solubility.

Regardless of whether the drippings are consumed, roughly all of the iron and zinc are retained from beef, veal, lamb, and pork when prepared using any of the moist heat methods. Only 5% of the iron is lost when the drippings from veal are not consumed. For most of the B-complex vitamins, the percentage lost is about 15% greater in meat products without the drippings as compared to products with the drippings. For example, simmered roast beef that is consumed along with its drippings retains 60% of the thiamin from the original product. If the same product is consumed without its drippings, only 45% of the thiamin is retained. The largest percent difference is seen in niacin retention. Consumption of the drippings from braised roast beef can result in a retention factor of 90%, whereas avoiding the drippings results in a retention factor of only 55%.

Going Green with Meats

Impact of Meat Production on the Environment

Green Point

50,000 Hogs It is estimated that the waste generated from 100 animal feeding operations containing at least 50,000 hogs is equal to the same amount of waste generated by a city with a population of 150,000 individuals.

Because meats are produced from animals high on the food chain and therefore have a large carbon footprint, the consumption of animal products has received scrutiny from environmental groups and organizations. Agricultural operations, including the breeding and raising of cattle and other animals, have caused major problems with water and land contamination in the United States. It is estimated that 59% of rivers and 31% of lakes, ponds, and reservoirs have been impacted and polluted due to such operations.[23] Odorous air emissions from animal feeding operations contain over 330 compounds, including ammonia, hydrogen sulfate, methane, and carbon dioxide; animal manure; and organic waste. These compounds can pollute the air, and the ammonia can be deposited in surface waters, causing eutrophification. Animal manure can pollute land and water surrounding animal feed lots with contaminants such as nitrogen, nitrates, phosphorus, antibiotics, pesticides, and hormones. Nitrogen from animal manure can be found in forms such as ammonia or organic nitrogen, neither of which can be used by plants and are only readily utilized via microbial processes.

methane Greenhouse gas produced by livestock.

Animals produce gaseous pollutants such as nitrous oxide and the greenhouse gases carbon dioxide and **methane**. Methane has been estimated to have an environmental impact roughly 15 times that of carbon dioxide, and nearly one-third of all methane produced comes from animals and agriculture operations.[24] In 2008, enteric fermentation (digestion of carbohydrate, which results in the release of methane gas) and manure management were responsible for 25% and 8%, respectively, of all methane emissions from human activity.[25]

Because society is more concerned than ever with environmental health issues, government departments such as the Environmental Protection Agency (EPA) have developed recommendations and standards to minimize the impact that agriculture has on the environment.[26] As one example, the EPA recommends containing cattle and keeping them from having direct access to surface waters. It also recommends using concrete ditches to control wastewater runoff and to drain it to a safe holding area. As a regulatory measure, the EPA also requires farming operations with more than 300 cattle or veal to comply with standards set forth in the Concentrated Animal Feeding Operations Clean Water Act requirements. According to these requirements, animal feeding operations must demonstrate environmentally protective nutrient management systems before being granted the appropriate permits to start operations.

Changing the Environmental Impact of Meats

Meat production requires numerous steps, from breeding and slaughtering to transport and cooking, and each one affords an opportunity for producers and consumers to make wise environmental decisions. Ideally, producers should contain the animals in a large area so the animals' gases (e.g., methane), manure, and other emissions do not build up and become concentrated in the soil and water. Likewise, ensuring that the animals do not have direct access to surface water will also prevent contamination of local waters.

The type of feed on which an animal is raised provides another opportunity for greener options. Corn-based feed require a large input of energy due to the fertilizer and irrigation systems used to produce the corn. In addition, the transportation of the corn to the feedlot also burns fossil fuels and emits pollutants into the air. Grass-fed cattle are therefore considered to be more environmentally friendly. Cattle can also be fed with feeds rich in urea; such feeds may improve the animal's digestion and, in turn, decrease fermentation and methane emissions by 25–75%.[27]

Several other aspects of livestock maintenance also contribute to greenhouse gas emissions. The clearing of trees, grass, and other natural structures during the building of farm and livestock operation facilities contributes greatly to greenhouse gas emissions and the deterioration of the environment. As a result, many farming operations have attempted to minimize the clearing of land prior to building such operations. In addition, the combustion of fossil fuels to generate energy contributes to agricultural gas emissions. Although only small amounts of fossil fuels may be burned on the actual farmland, fossil fuels are heavily utilized in the transport of livestock to final feedlots and slaughterhouses. Thus, many operations have "gone green" by limiting the frequency and distance of transportation of their livestock.

Green Point

Eating Local Meat Eating local livestock that are minimally transported definitely reduces one's carbon footprint.

Finally, because the producing, slaughtering, and processing of animal meats is so energy intensive, many environmental organizations urge consumers to simply cut back on their overall meat intake. The National Resources Defense Council states that if every American reduced their weekly intake of beef by one-quarter of a pound, it would reduce greenhouse gas emissions by the same magnitude as taking 6 million cars off the highway.[28] Reducing the consumption of processed meats (i.e., sausage, bacon, luncheon meats) also is considered a green decision because of the large amount of energy and resources it takes to preserve, process, and package these products.

Food Safety and Foodborne Illness

Raw meats are considered to be potentially hazardous foods, thus they must be handled cautiously in any food preparation environment. Foodborne illness is caused by dangerous pathogens that can multiply quickly in environmental conditions conducive to their growth. Like many foods, meat provides the ideal environment for bacterial growth because it is not very acidic and contains a substantial amount of protein and moisture. In order to reduce the risk of foodborne illness, meats should be cooked until the innermost portion reaches a safe temperature (see **Table 5.4**).

Fresh and cured meats, meat substitutes, and other animal by-products can harbor a variety of foodborne pathogens. See **Special Topic 5.3** for information on *E. coli* 0157:H7, the bacterial cause of an extremely common foodborne illness associated with meats. *C. botulinum* is another bacterium that can be fatal when ingested; however, the addition of nitrites to preserved meats limits this bacteria's ability to survive in such foods. *T. spiralis*, commonly referred to as "pork worm," is a foodborne pathogen often found in undercooked or raw pork products. In order to reduce the

TABLE 5.4
Required Internal Cooking Temperatures and Holding Times for Meats for Food Safety Purposes

Product	Type	Minimum Internal Temperature and Rest Time
Beef	Ground Steak, chops, and roasts	160°F (71°C) 145°F (63°C) and allow to rest for at least 3 minutes
Chicken and turkey	Breasts Ground, stuffing, and casseroles Whole bird, legs, thighs, and wings	165°F (74ºC) 165°F (74ºC) 165°F (74ºC)
Eggs	Any type	160°F (71ºC)
Fish and shellfish	Any type	145°F (63°C)
Leftovers	Any type	165°F (74ºC)
Ham	Fresh or smoked (uncooked)	145°F (63°C) and allow to rest for at least 3 minutes
	Fully cooked ham (to reheat)	Reheat cooked hams packaged in USDA-inspected plants to 140°F (60°C) and all others to 165°F (74°C)

Source: Reproduced from U.S. Department of Agriculture, Food Safety and Inspection Service. Keep Food Safe! Food Safety Basics. Available at: http://www.fsis.usda.gov/factsheets/Keep_Food_Safe_Food_Safety_Basics/index.asp.

risk of foodborne illness, consumers should follow these guidelines when preparing meats:

- Use separate cutting boards for raw meats. Avoid cross-contamination by never placing raw meats on the same surface as raw poultry or ready-to-eat foods such as fruits, vegetables, or starches.
- Thoroughly wash and disinfect utensils, knives, and food preparation equipment after use. Never use cutlery for both raw meats and ready-to-eat foods.
- Do not thaw raw meat by allowing it to sit in the "danger zone"—temperatures between 41–135°F (5–57°C). If a meat appears to be spoiled or damaged, discard it immediately.
- Only purchase meats that have been inspected by the USDA.

Special Topic 5.3

E. coli 0157:H7

Courtney P. Winston, MPH, RD, LD, CDE

Escherichia coli (or *E. coli*) are a group of bacteria that commonly inhabit the intestinal tract of livestock, including cattle. Because these bacteria are found in animal guts, they can be easily passed on to humans through animal products that have been contaminated with fecal matter. One of the most fatal *E. coli* strains, 0157:H7, is estimated to kill more than 60 people each year[1] and to cause more than $1 billion annually in damages.[2] As a result, cattle producers and food inspection officers closely monitor the processing and packaging of all meat products to minimize potential *E. coli* contamination.

Meats and other food products may become contaminated with *E. coli* through several mechanisms. Ground beef, a common source of *E. coli*–related foodborne illness outbreaks, can become tainted with these deadly bacteria if portions of the cattle intestine are accidentally integrated into the ground product. In addition, cattle "shed" *E. coli* when they defecate, so their manure is often laden with these organisms. As a result, anything coming in contact with the manure (e.g., rainwater, plants, other animals, humans) can become contaminated. It is via this process that drinking and irrigation water may easily become contaminated.

Whereas animals that harbor *E. coli* show fairly mild symptoms, such as loose stools, humans have much more severe reactions, even when infected by as few as 10 individual *E. coli* bacteria. Hemorrhagic colitis, or bloody diarrhea accompanied by severe abdominal cramps and a high fever, is the common result of an *E. coli* infection. This condition should immediately be addressed by a medical doctor; without physician care, the infection can become fatal. All reports of *E. coli* and hemorrhagic colitis should be reported to the local public health department so investigators can identify the source of the infection and remove any other contaminated products from the market.[3]

To reduce the risk of foodborne illness from *E. coli* contamination, producers and consumers are advised to practice proper hand hygiene and to handle and prepare foods with extreme caution. Meat packing and processing plants are regularly and vigilantly monitored by state and federal inspectors—these inspectors ensure that meat products are not coming into contact with manure or other cattle by-products that may harbor *E. coli*. When purchasing meat products, consumers should only buy products that are tightly sealed in appropriate packaging and are stored at the correct temperatures (e.g., frozen meats should be frozen solid, not slightly thawed). Consumers are also urged to fully cook all animal products, especially ground beef. Furthermore, because fruits and vegetables can become tainted with *E. coli*–containing irrigation water, consumers should prevent infection by thoroughly washing and rinsing these items.

References

1 Mead PS, Slutsker L. Food-related illness and death in the United States. *Emerging Infectious Diseases*. 1999;5(5):607.

2 Buzby JC, Roberts T, Jordan Lin CT, MacDonald JM. Bacterial Foodborne Disease: Medical Costs and Productivity Losses. Food and Consumer Economics Division, Economic Research Service, U.S. Department of Agriculture. Agricultural Economic Report No. 741. August 1996. Available at: http://www.ers.usda.gov/publications/aer741/aer741.pdf. Accessed January 3, 2011.

3 U.S. Department of Agriculture. Food Safety Advice for Everyone. http://www.mypyramid.gov/tips_resources/foodsafety.html. Updated February 9, 2011. Accessed February 12, 2011.

Meat Regulations and Quality

Meat Inspection

The USDA mandates that meats from beef, veal, pork, and lamb go through **inspection** prior to being sold. The federal-level Food Safety and Inspection Service (FSIS) maintains responsibility for inspecting all meats brought into the United States from foreign countries and all meats that are sold interstate within the United States. Meats that are both produced and sold within one state may inspected by that state's inspection program, but such state-level programs are closely and regularly monitored by FSIS. In accordance with the 1967 Wholesome Meat Act, state-level inspection programs must regulate with the same or more stringent guidelines than the federal program. Although the FSIS and state agencies are primarily responsible for meat inspections, they also work closely with the Food and Drug Administration (FDA), the U.S. Department of Health and Human Service (DHHS), and the Environmental Protection Agency (EPA). All funds for meat inspection, both on the federal and state levels, are secured from taxpayer dollars.

inspection A federally mandated process whereby trained officials inspect meat processing plants to ensure food safety.

The primary purpose of meat inspection is to ensure that meat being sold on the market is "wholesome," free of disease and contamination, and safe for human consumption. Because raw meats can potentially be a major source of foodborne illness, inspectors do more than just visual inspections. Inspectors

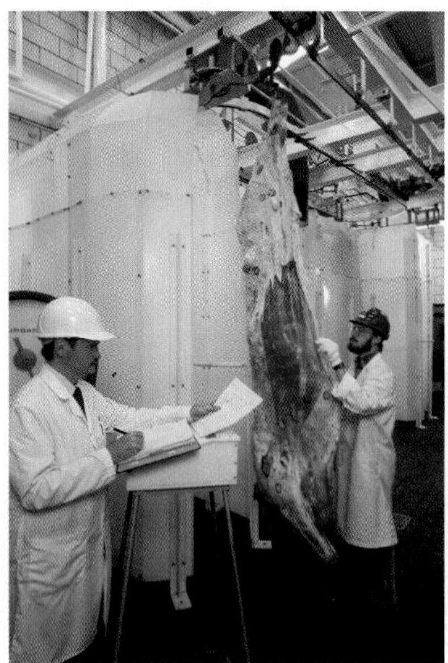

FIGURE 5.11 As part of the inspection process, a microbiologist gathers carcass samples for microbial analysis.

Courtesy of the USDA Agricultural Research Service. Photo by Keith Weller.

will test for potential biological and chemical hazards (see **Figure 5.11**), and they also critically investigate the meat packing plant's Hazard Analysis and Critical Control Point (HACCP) plan.

The HACCP plan is basically a seven-step management plan put together by the manufacturers of food products to ensure that their food products do not become contaminated with bacteria, viruses, or other foreign materials.[29] The seven HACCP steps are outlined in **Table 5.5**.

Part of the meat inspection process involves making sure that all meats are correctly labeled and packaged. One of the important labels that must be placed on all raw, uncooked, or not fully cooked meat is the "Safe Food Handling" label. This label conveys safe food handling information directly to purchasers of the product, and it reminds them to fully cook the meat prior to consuming it (see **Figure 5.12**).

TABLE 5.5
The Seven-Step Process of a Hazard Analysis and Critical Control Point (HACCP) Plan

Principle	Action
1	Conduct a hazard analysis.
2	Determine the critical control points.
3	Establish critical limits.
4	Establish monitoring procedures.
5	Establish corrective actions.
6	Establish verification procedures.
7	Establish record-keeping and documentation procedures.

Source: Reproduced from the U.S. Department of Agriculture, U.S. Food and Drug Administration. *Hazard Analysis and Critical Control Point Principles and Application Guidelines*, 1997. Available at: http://www.fda.gov/food/foodsafety/HazardAnalysisCriticalControlPointsHACCP/ucm114868.htm. Accessed January 3, 2011.

(a)

Nutrition Facts

Serving Size 4 oz (112g)
raw, as packaged.
Servings per container varied

Amount Per Serving	
Calories 150	Calories from Fat 50
	% Daily Value*
Total Fat 6g	9%
Saturated Fat 2.5g	13%
Cholesterol 70mg	23%
Sodium 75g	3%
Total Carbohydrate 0g	0%
Protein 24g	48%
Iron 15%	*

Not a significant source of dietary fiber, sugars, vitamin A, vitamin C, and calcium

* Percent Daily Values are based on a 2000-calorie diet

(b)

Nutrition Facts

Serving Size 4 oz (112g)
raw, as packaged.
Servings per container varied

Amount Per Serving	
Calories 210	Calories from Fat 110
	% Daily Value*
Total Fat 12g	19%
Saturated Fat 3.5g	18%
Cholesterol 75mg	25%
Sodium 75g	3%
Total Carbohydrate 0g	0%
Protein 23g	45%
Iron 6%	*

Not a significant source of dietary fiber, sugars, vitamin A, vitamin C, and calcium

* Percent Daily Values are based on a 2000-calorie diet

FIGURE 5.12 In addition, the Nutrition Facts label seen on most processed foods must now be on all packages of raw ground beef, turkey, and chicken. (a) Beef, ground, 95% lean/5% fat, raw. (b) Chicken, ground 89% lean/11% fat, raw.

Source: Reproduced from the U.S. Department of Agriculture, Food Safety and Inspection Service. Examples of Nutrition Facts Panels for Ground Products. Available at: http://www.fsis.usda.gov/PDF/Nutrition_Panel_Format.pdf.

Once the meat has met all of the inspection requirements, it will be stamped with a round, purple mark. There is one inspection mark for fresh meat and another inspection mark for processed meat, and both of these marks are slightly different than the inspection mark used for poultry (see **Figure 5.13** and **Figure 5.14**). The mark is placed directly on the carcass and all other major cuts of that particular meat. The purple dye used for the inspection mark is made from food-grade vegetable dye and does not taint or contaminate the meat. One of the goals of meat inspection is to prevent the spread of diseases such as Bovine Spongiform Encephalopathy (BSE), or "mad cow disease," described in **Special Topic 5.4**.

Other meats, such as elk, buffalo, rabbit, and deer, are not subject to mandatory inspection; however, the U.S. Secretary of Agriculture still reserves the right to take necessary precautions to ensure that these meats are safe for consumption. Plants that process meats other than beef, pork, and lamb and that request voluntary inspection are inspected by a trained FSIS inspector who is privy to that specific meat's inspection requirements. Funding for these voluntary inspections is secured from the plant being inspected, not from taxpayer dollars.

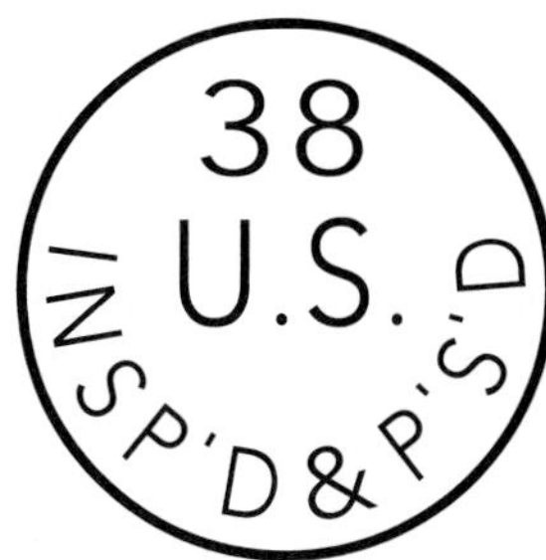
38
U.S.
INSP'D & P'S'D

FIGURE 5.13 All raw meats must be inspected by the USDA and stamped with the USDA inspection mark.

Source: Reproduced from U.S. Department of Agriculture, Food Safety and Inspection Service. Inspection and grading of meat and poultry: What are the differences? Available at: http://www.fsis.usda.gov/Factsheets/Inspection_&_Grading/index.asp. Accessed June 1, 2012.

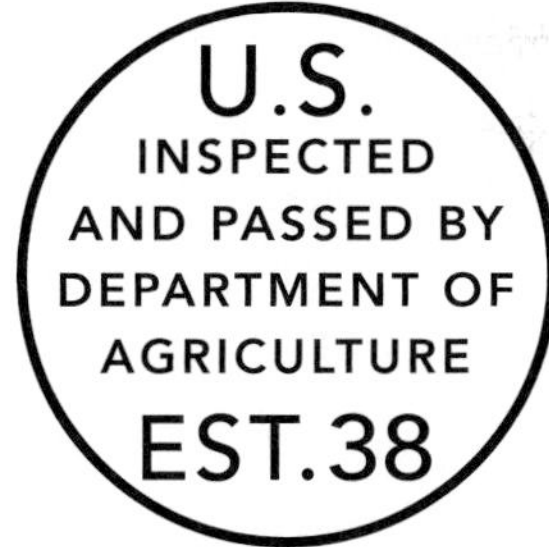
U.S.
INSPECTED
AND PASSED BY
DEPARTMENT OF
AGRICULTURE
EST.38

FIGURE 5.14 The inspection mark for processed meats, shown here, differs from the inspection mark for raw meats.

Source: Reproduced from U.S. Department of Agriculture, Food Safety and Inspection Service. Inspection and grading of meat and poultry: What are the differences? Available at: http://www.fsis.usda.gov/Factsheets/Inspection_&_Grading/index.asp. Accessed June 1, 2012.

Meat Grading

Whereas meat inspection is mandatory, meat grading is not. Grading is done solely at the discretion of meat producers and processors. Because of this, they must pay for this service using their own funds. **Grading** is a process by which the quality of meat is assessed; all meat grading is done by the USDA Agricultural Marketing Service (AMS). AMS uses federal standards of quality to assess meat products and gives a corresponding grade based on its findings. Part of the grading process involves assessing the meat's tenderness, juiciness, and flavor characteristics. Poultry is graded similarly; however, criteria for poultry are slightly different than those for meat. Grades for meat differ depending on the type of meat.

Beef

After being assessed as an entire carcass, beef receives two grades: a quality grade and a yield grade. The quality grade indicates palatability traits (i.e., marbling, age, pigmentation), whereas the yield grade indicates the amount of usable lean meat.

The top-quality grade of beef is Prime, and meats with this grade are typically from young cattle and are generally well-marbled. The next grade, Choice, also is considered high quality, but Choice meats tend to have less marbling and may be less tender. Choice meats are still appropriate for dry heat cooking methods, but some cuts may have better palatability if braised.

grading A voluntary process in which meat products are rated for their quality.

Special Topic 5.4

Bovine Spongiform Encephalopathy, or "Mad Cow Disease"

Jennifer Stallings

In 1986, a farmer in Great Britain noticed peculiar behaviors in one of the cows in his cattle herd before its eventual death. Other animals on the farm began to show similar nervous and aggressive behaviors coupled with difficulty standing, decreased body weight, and decreased milk production. A laboratory examination of the brain of a deceased cow showed hole formations, which caused a spongelike appearance. Researchers recognized these cases as Bovine Spongiform Encephalopathy (BSE), commonly known as "mad cow disease."[1] Scientists at the Central Veterinary Laboratory in Weybridge, England, identified BSE in many more of the symptomatic cattle and began to search for the cause. A common factor between all of the infected animals was their feed—a mixture made from the carcasses of dead animals that died due to BSE. Once a stop was placed on this practice the incidence of BSE decreased.[2]

In 1982, Stanley B. Prusiner, an American neurologist, had discovered the cause of BSE—protein particles without DNA or RNA, called prions. Once inside the host, prions traverse the spinal cord, entering the brain. Upon reaching the brain, prions cause a chain reaction in which normal proteins begin to stick together, forming plaques and eventually holes in the central nervous system.[3]

Prion diseases such as BSE belong to the family of transmissible spongiform encephalopathies (TSEs). According to the Centers for Disease Control and Prevention, TSEs are progressive neurodegenerative disorders affecting both humans and animals. Human consumption of contaminated products causes variant Creutzfeldt-Jakob Disease (vCJD), which is characterized by memory loss, headaches, and changes in gait. Clinical symptoms arise an average of 5 years after infection. As damage progresses, cognitive ability and motor skills deteriorate, eventually leading to death. Prions are resistant to viral inactivation techniques, making TSEs resistant to treatment. Currently, a cure for TSEs does not exist.[2]

Following the 2003 discovery in Washington of the first BSE-infected cow in the United States, the USDA has focused on the effectiveness of current policies. Because the infected dairy cow had been imported from Canada, the International Review Team (IRT) addressing the issue recommended a surveillance program for BSE in North America. Two additional discoveries were made a year later: a Texas born-and-raised beef cow in November 2004 and an Alabama cow in February 2006.[4] A statement from the USDA following a recall of beef after the first discovery stated that some of the contaminated meat may have been consumed but that the highest-risk tissues of the cow had not entered the food supply. Although the first discovery was in a cow from Canada, Japan, Mexico, South Korea and other countries banned imports of U.S. beef and cattle.[3]

Since 1989, the USDA Animal Plant Health Inspection Service (APHIS) and the U.S. Department of Health and Human Services have implemented various safeguards and restrictions to prevent the spread of BSE in the United States.[5] First, an import control was created to prevent entrance of ruminant animals and their meat products from countries where BSE had been found. Then APHIS began testing cattle that were considered higher risk in that they displayed suspicious neurological symptoms, were not ambulatory, or had died before slaughter. Use of organs that could accumulate BSE, such as the spinal cord, brain, or nerve tissues, was banned from the meat supply through meat plant regulations made by the USDA Food Safety and Inspection Service (FSIS). Along with this ban, the production of meat from nonambulatory cattle was prohibited. The Federal Drug Administration (FDA) prohibited the presence of mammalian proteins in animal feed in 1997. Seven years later poultry and plate waste as well as blood from cattle were also banned in cattle feed.[5]

Other measures put into place by the FSIS include an inspection of cattle for disease signs and symptoms. Suspect cattle undergo examination by an FSIS veterinarian for determination as to whether the animal is safe to enter the human food supply. Removal techniques have been developed that separate parts of the animal presenting increased risk, such as the brain, spinal cord, and eyes. FSIS maintains strict testing procedures and requires slaughter and processing establishments to develop similar procedures.[5]

Cattle production represents the largest sector of U.S. agriculture and one-fifth of total U.S. farm sales. As of 2006, an estimated 1 billion pounds of beef and veal is exported to other countries. Adequate food safety measures allow for continued import and export of meat products and prevent the consumption of TSE-contaminated food, by animals and humans both. These safeguards represent scientific and policy practices by the U.S. government to protect the food supply.[5]

References

1 Becker GS. 2006. *BSE ("mad cow disease"): A brief overview.* CRS Report for Congress. Order Code: RS22345.

2 Centers for Disease Control and Prevention. BSE (Bovine Spongiform Encephalopathy, or Mad Cow Disease). 2011. Available at: http://www.cdc.gov/ncidod/dvrd/bse.

3 Donnelly CA. Bovine Spongiform Encephalopathy in the United States: An epidemiologist's view. *N Eng J Med.* 2004;350(6):539–542.

4 Richt JA, Kunkle RA, Alt D, et al. Identification and characterization of two bovine spongiform encephalopathy cases diagnosed in the United States. *J Vet Diag Investigation.* 2007;19(2):142–154.

5 Abramson MB. Mad cow disease: An approach to its containment. *J Health Care Law Policy.* 2004;316:334–337.

Select grade beef is less marbled than Prime and Choice grade meats and often lacks the juiciness and flavor associated with higher grades. Standard or Commercial grades of beef follow behind Select. Finally, Utility, Cutter, and Canner grades of beef are the lowest grades given by the AMS. These low grades are often given to meats that are only used for ground beef or other processed meat-based products. **Figure 5.15** shows the stamps used to identify different quality grades of beef.

Yield grades of beef range from 1 to 5. Beef carcasses that receive a yield grade of 1 will have a high ratio of lean meat to fat, whereas carcasses with a yield grade of 5 will have only have a small amount of lean meat relative the rest of the carcass.

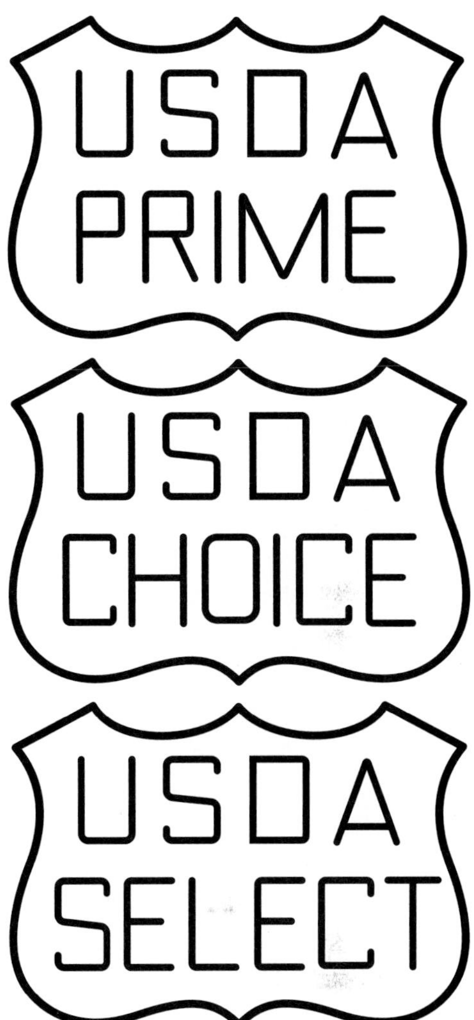

FIGURE 5.15 Producers can voluntarily agree to have the quality of their meat product graded by the USDA. These seals indicate the quality of the meat. Prime, Choice, and Select cuts are acceptable for human consumption.

Source: Reproduced from U.S. Department of Agriculture, Food Safety and Inspection Service. Inspection and grading of meat and poultry: What are the differences? Available at: http://www.fsis.usda.gov/Factsheets/Inspection_&_Grading/index.asp. Accessed June 1, 2012.

Veal

From highest to lowest quality, the grades used for veal are Prime, Choice, Good, Standard, and Utility. As with beef, the Prime and Choice grades of veal indicate a highly palatable product. These two grades of veal will be juicy and flavorful. Veal with a Prime or Choice grade will also have a fairly firm texture and will be light grayish-pink to light pink in color. Lower grades of veal are not as commonly marketed.

Lamb

Similar to veal, lamb grades include Prime, Choice, Good, Utility, and Cull. Prime and Choice are the two grades most often seen in restaurants and stores because the lower grades have poor palatability (the lower grades usually come from older sheep). Prime grade lamb is highly marbled, which increases its juiciness, tenderness, and flavor. Choice grade lamb is not quite as tender as prime grade but can still be cooked using dry heat methods if an appropriate cut (i.e., chops, roasts, leg) is used. Other choice cuts (i.e., breast, neck, shank) should be prepared by braising. The overall nutritional content of lamb cuts remains similar across all five grades.

The quality of lamb meat also can be affected by the aging process. After slaughtering, lamb meat may undergo an aging process as a means to bolster the meat's flavor and texture. Lamb ribs and loins are the only cuts of lamb that are usually aged. This process must be performed under very specific temperature and humidity requirements, and is therefore not a process that should be done in a consumer's home or kitchen. The overall aging process can take from 10 days to 6 weeks depending on the desired outcome; most aged lamb then is sold to fine dining establishments.

Pork

Unlike beef, veal, and lamb, pork is not eligible for grading by the AMS because swine are typically raised and bred to produce uniform and tender meat. Although there is little variation in pork, appearance is an appropriate indicator of the quality of meat. Palatable cuts of pork should be covered in only a small amount of fat and should be grayish pink in color. A firm texture with small amounts of marbling also is desirable because this indicates tenderness.

Chapter Review

Red meat plays a significant role in the culture, diet, and health of individuals around the world. Structurally, meat is composed of water, protein, fat, and connective tissue. Because of its chemical composition, meat makes a significant contribution to the overall nutritional status of individuals who consume it. When preparing meat, consumers may use dry or moist heat cooking methods. Dry heat cooking methods are more appropriate for well-marbled, tender cuts of meat, whereas moist heat cooking methods are more appropriate for lean and tough cuts of meat. Meat can be preserved through processes such as curing, and it can also be frozen for extended storage.

The meat industry has received criticism in recent years for its sizeable carbon footprint. A plethora of resources (e.g., fossil fuels, water) are required for the production of livestock feed, and even more resources are utilized in the maintenance of livestock ranges, farms, slaughterhouses, and processing plants.

Although meat producers have the option of having their products graded for quality, all meat processing and production facilities must be inspected by the federal government to ensure that the conditions under which these foods are produced are safe and sanitary.

Learning Portfolio

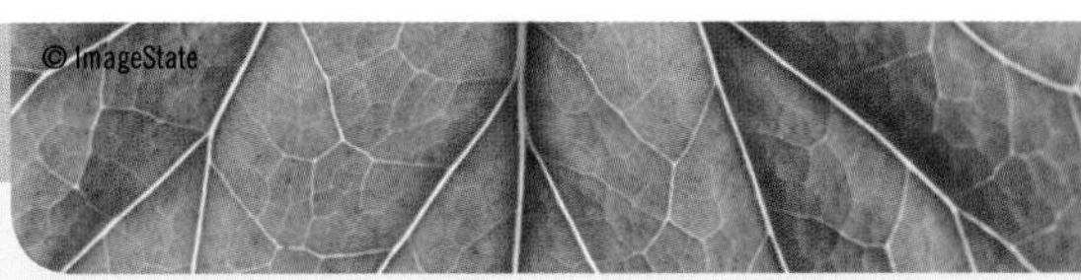

Study Points

1. The most commonly consumed meat products in the United States come from cattle (young cattle are sold as veal), sheep younger than 1 year of age (sold as lamb), and domesticated hogs (sold as pork).
2. Beef, lamb, and pork are commonly referred to as red meat because they contain myoglobin pigment, which turns to oxymyoglobin when exposed to oxygen, giving the meat a red coloration.
3. Approximately 6 to 24 hours after an animal is slaughtered, the carcass enters the state of rigor mortis. During this time, the meat maintains a low pH because of the lactic acid in the muscle tissue. If an animal is stressed or exercised immediately prior to slaughter, the meat will not maintain a low pH during rigor mortis, and, as a result, the muscle tissue will not be as palatable or desirable to the consumer.
4. Many different methods can be used to prepare meats, but the most important consideration is the meat's tenderness. If a meat is tender and well marbled, it can usually be prepared using a dry heat method, such as roasting, broiling, or baking. If a meat is not tender and has little fat, it is best prepared using a moist heat method, such as braising, stewing, or simmering.
5. Meats can be preserved through the process of curing. This process requires the addition of sodium nitrite, which prevents the growth of *Clostridium botulinum* and gives the meat product a longer shelf life.
6. Meat makes a substantial contribution to the overall human diet. Meats are an excellent source of complete protein, and they are also rich in minerals (iron, zinc, phosphorus, and copper) as well as vitamins (thiamin, riboflavin, niacin, B_6, folate, and B_{12}). While most of the proteins and minerals are retained during cooking, many of the water-soluble vitamins are lost.
7. In recent years, meat producers have taken steps to make their processing and production steps more green. Many producers raise grass-fed animals instead of grain-fed animals, reducing the amount of fossil fuel required to produce the feed. Other producers allow their animals to roam on large ranges so that the animal by-products do not build up in the nearby soil and waters. Because of the amount of resources it takes to raise, transport, slaughter, and prepare animal products, some individuals limit their meat intake and elect to consume fewer meat-based meals and more vegetarian meals (e.g., meals containing textured soy proteins and other soy-based foods).
8. Meats should be prepared and consumed under sanitary conditions. To reduce the risk of foodborne illness, food handlers must take precautions such as cooking meat to a safe internal temperature, separating raw meats from uncooked foods, and only purchasing meats that have been inspected by the FSIS.
9. *Escherichia coli* (or *E. coli*), a group of bacteria which commonly inhabit the intestinal tract of livestock animals, is a common source of foodborne illness. To prevent bacterial infection, consumers need to prepare foods appropriately and avoid cross-contamination.
10. The USDA monitors the integrity of the meat processing industry by requiring the Food Safety and Inspection Service (FSIS) to inspect all meat-processing facilities.
11. Meat manufacturers may elect to have their meat products (beef, veal, and lamb only) graded by USDA's Agricultural and Marketing Service. Grading evaluates the quality of meat, whereas inspection evaluates the safety of meat.

Key Terms

	page
actin	165
collagen	166
curing	170
dry heat cooking methods	174
elastin	166
finishing diet	161
grading	187
hormonal growth promotants (HGPs)	161
inspection	185
lactic acid	167
Maillard reaction	175
marbling	166
meat extenders	172
methane	182
metmyoglobin	167
moist heat cooking methods	177
myoglobin	167
myosin	165
nitric oxide myoglobin	167
oxymyoglobin	167
textured soy protein (TSP)	172

Issues for Discussion

1. Immediately prior to slaughter, it is important to ensure that the animal is not stressed or excited. Explain why this is, and describe the physiological and biochemical reactions that may occur if the animal is stressed prior to slaughter. How might this impact the final meat product?
2. A wide variety of cuts of beef, veal, lamb, and pork are available, and each cut may be prepared using different cooking techniques. Explain why the leaner cuts of meat should be prepared using a moist heat method and why the well-marbled cuts of meat should be prepared using a dry heat method. What are the advantages and disadvantages of each preparation method? How does the preparation method affect nutrient retention in the final product?
3. If you were in charge of a food service establishment that served beef, lamb, and pork, what steps would you take to ensure that your product had a small carbon footprint? How would you market your product so that consumers knew that your establishment was "going green?"

Research Areas for Students

1. The health and financial benefits and drawbacks of using organic animal feed versus synthetic animal feeds
2. The biochemical changes that occur during rigor mortis
3. The public health significance of recent foodborne illness outbreaks related to ground beef and other meat products
4. The carbon footprints of beef, veal, lamb, and pork production
5. The Clean Water Act's impact on animal feeding operations (AFOs)
6. Food safety practices recommended by the National Restaurant Association and other related organizations with regards to the serving of meat and meat products in restaurants

References

1. Thompson JM, Polkinghorne R, Watson R, et al. Effects of hormonal growth promotants (HGP) on growth, carcass characteristics, the palatability of different muscles in the beef carcass and their interaction with aging. *Aust J Exp Agric.* 2008;48(11):1405–1414.
2. Key N, McBride W. The changing economics of U.S. hog production. *Economic Research Service Report*, Number 52. December 2007. Available at: http://www.ers.usda.gov/media/244843/err52.pdf. Accessed July 16, 2012.
3. Beaulieu AD, Patience JF, Williams NH, Aalhus JL. Impact of piglet birth weight, birth order, and litter size on subsequent growth performance, carcass quality, muscle composition, and eating quality of pork. *J Anim Sci.* 2010;88(8):2767–2778.
4. Cannata S, Green MD, Bass PD, et al. Effect of visual marbling on sensory properties and quality traits of pork loin. *Meat Sci.* 2010;85(3):428–434.
5. Wiener P, Wood JD, Nute GR, et al. The effects of a mutation in the myostatin gene on meat and carcass quality. *Meat Sci.* 2009;83(1):127–134.
6. Smith RD, Miller RK, Griffin DB, et al. Dry versus wet aging of beef: Retail cutting yields and consumer palatability evaluations of steaks from US Choice and US Select short loins. *Meat Sci.* 2008;79(4):631–639.
7. Kilara A, Wagner FW, Shahani KM. Preparation and properties of immobilized papain and lipase. *Biotechnol Bioeng.* 1977(11):1703–1714.
8. Kemp JD, Fox JD, Montgomery RE. Chemical, palatability and cooking characteristics of normal and low quality pork loins as affected by freezer storage. *J Food Sci.* 1976(1):1–3.
9. Lind ML, Kropf DH, Harrison DL. Freezing and thawing rates of lamb chops: Effects on palatability and related characteristics. *J Food Sci.* 1971(4):629–631.
10. Smith GC, King GT, Carpenter ZL. Considerations for beef tenderness evaluations. *J Food Sci.* 1969(6):612–618.
11. Lagerstedt A, Enfält L, Johansson L, Lundström K. Effect of freezing on sensory quality, shear force and water loss in beef *M. longissimus dorsi*. *Meat Sci.* 2008;80(2):457–461.
12. Ziegler PT. *The Meat We Eat.* Danville, IL: The Interstate, Printers & Publishers; 1962.
13. Berry BW. Sodium alginate plus modified tapioca starch improves properties of low-fat beef patties. *J Food Sci.* 1997;62(6):1245.
14. Berk Z. Technology of production of edible flours and protein products from soybeans. *FAO Agricultural Services Bulletin*; 97. Rome, Italy: Food and Agriculture Organization of the United Nations; 1992.
15. Erickson DR. *Practical Handbook of Soybean Processing and Utilization.* Champaign, IL: AOCS Press; 1995.
16. Katayama M, Wilson LA. Utilization of soybeans and their components through the development of textured soy protein foods. *J Food Sci.* 2008;73(3):S158–S164.
17. Sugimura T, Wakabayashi K, Nakagama H, Nagao M. Heterocyclic amines: Mutagens/carcinogens produced during cooking of meat and fish. *Cancer Sci.* 2004;95(4):290–299.
18. Smith JS, Ameri F, Gadgil P. Effect of marinades on the formation of heterocyclic amines in grilled beef steaks. *J Food Sci.* 2008;73(6):T100–T105.
19. Preis SR, Stampfer MJ, Spiegelman D, et al. Lack of association between dietary protein intake and risk of stroke among middle-aged men. *Am J Clin Nutr.* 2010;91(1):39–45.
20. Sluijs I, Beulens JW, Spijkerman AM, et al. Dietary intake of total, animal, and vegetable protein and risk of type 2 diabetes in the European Prospective Investigation into Cancer and Nutrition (EPIC)-NL study. *Diabetes Care.* 2010;33(1):43–48.
21. U.S. Department of Agriculture. *Dietary Guidelines for Americans, 2010.* Available at: http://health.gov/dietaryguidelines/dga2010/DietaryGuidelines2010.pdf. Accessed July 16, 2012.
22. Keenan JM, Morris DH. Hypercholesterolemia: Dietary advice for patients regarding meat. *Postgrad Med.* 1995;98(4):113.
23. U.S. Environmental Protection Agency. *National Water Quality Inventory: 1998 Report to Congress.* Washington, DC: Author; 2000.
24. Cooperative State Research, Education, and, Extension Service, Midwest Plan Service. Livestock and Poultry Environmental Stewardship Curriculum/Developed by Land-grant University Faculty and Staff and USDA Research and Technical Support Staff. Ames, IA: Midwest Plan Service, Iowa State University; 2001.

25. U.S. Environmental Protection Agency. *Inventory of U.S. Greenhouse Gas Emissions and Sinks: 1990–2008*. EPA 430-R-10-006. Washington, DC: Author; April 15, 2010. Available at: http://epa.gov/climatechange/emissions/usinventoryreport.html. Accessed January 2, 2011.
26. U.S. Environmental Protection Agency, Office of Enforcement and Compliance Assurance. *Beef Cattle and Environmental Stewardship*. EPA 305-F-03-004. Washington, DC: Author; April 2003. Available at: http://www.epa.gov/agriculture/beef.pdf. Accessed January 2, 2011.
27. U.S. Environmental Protection Agency. Animal Feeding Operations: Best Management Practices, Methane. January 2011. Available at: http://www.epa.gov/agriculture/anafobmp.html#Methane. Accessed January 3, 2011.
28. National Resources Defense Council. Eat Green: Our Everyday Food Choices Affect Global Warming and the Environment. February 2010. Available at: http://www.nrdc.org/lobalWarming/files/eatgreenfs_feb2010.pdf. Accessed January 2, 2011.
29. U.S. Food and Drug Administration. Hazard Analysis and Critical Control Point Principles and Application Guidelines. Washington, DC: U.S. Food and Drug Administration; August 14, 1997. Available at: http://www.fda.gov/Food/FoodSafety/HazardAnalysisCriticalControlPointsHACCP/HACCPPrinciplesApplicationGuidelines/default.htm. Accessed January 2, 2011.

CHAPTER 6

Poultry and Fish

Bonnie Gerald, PhD, DTR

Chapter Objectives

THE STUDENT WILL BE EMPOWERED TO:

- Describe the cultural background of poultry and fish in the human diet.
- Recognize the various types of poultry, finfish, and shellfish.
- Summarize the physiological and nutritional properties of poultry and fish.
- Discuss the importance of omega-3 fatty acids on human health.
- Identify appropriate cooking techniques for poultry and fish.
- Summarize industry trends and ecological impacts of the poultry and fishing industries over the past century.
- Discuss technological innovations in processing and packaging used for poultry and fish.
- Describe the impact of environmental factors on the safety and quality of poultry and fish.

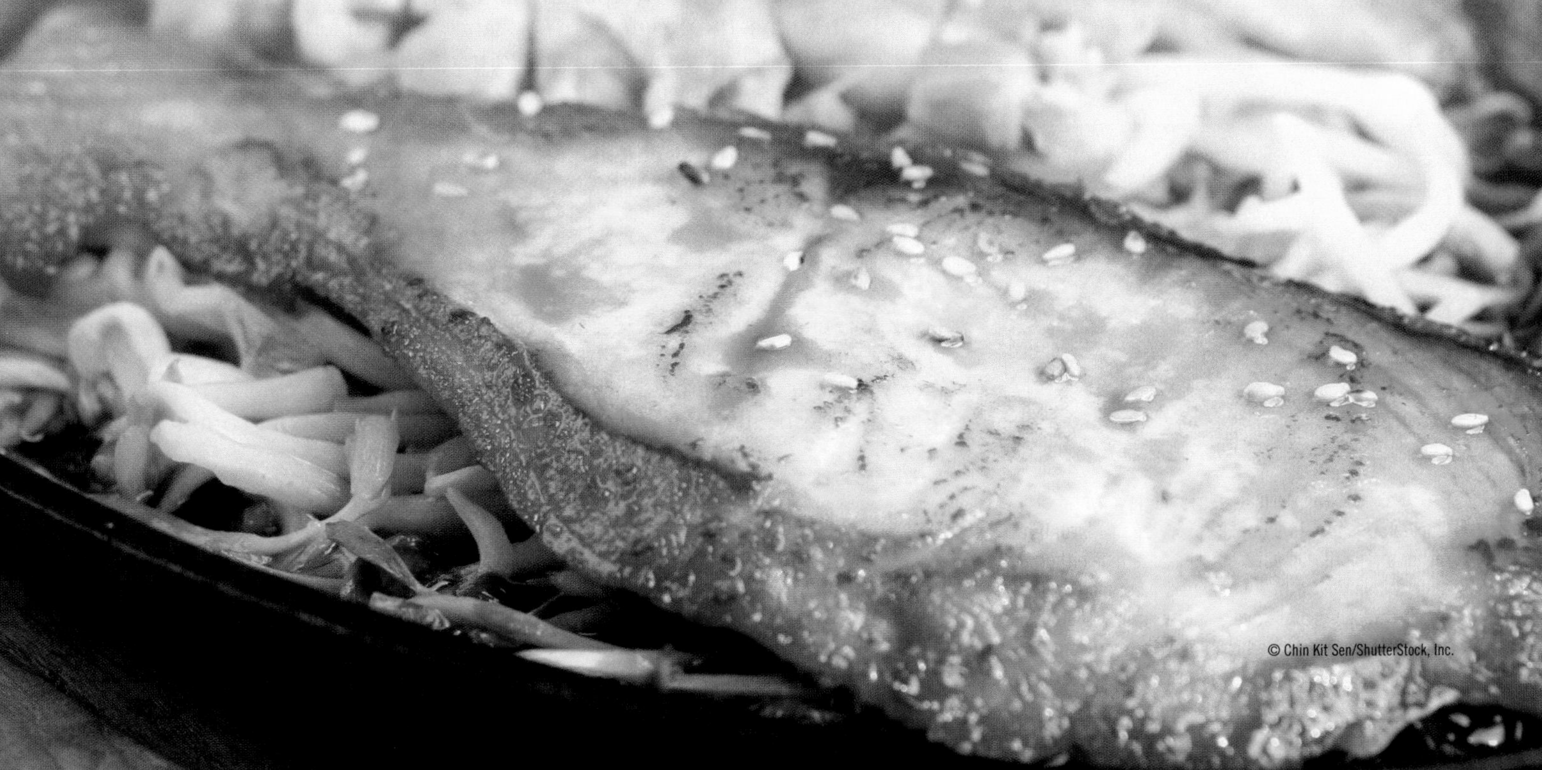

Historical and Cultural Significance

Poultry

The chicken was first domesticated in India approximately 2,000 years ago. In India, Hindus believed consumption of chicken contributed to aggressive behavior, although it also was considered to have medicinal properties.[1] The domesticated bird spread from Asia through Europe and was valued mainly for cockfighting and egg production. By the 5th century, Romans had built elaborate fight rings, or cockpits. Turkeys, native to the Americas, were introduced to Europe in the 15th century by the Spanish explorers. They replaced wild birds used in feasts hosted by European nobility because they yielded more meat than peacocks or quail.

The consumption of chicken in the Europe and North America was limited until the 18th century;[2] however, hens were valued for their egg production. Chicken was considered a luxury for Americans until the mid-20th century, when intensive animal husbandry practices made chicken a plentiful and inexpensive source of protein. Consumption of chicken rose dramatically as a result of decreased production costs and increased marketing to consumers. In 1980, chicken consumption per person was approximately 33 pounds per year. By 2000, average annual consumption of chicken per person had risen to 82 pounds.[3]

Other forms of poultry, such as turkey, duck, and goose, were considered game animals until the 19th century. Turkey did not migrate, which made it part of the American colonists' year-round diet. Despite the turkey's excellent eyesight, it was easy to hunt because when one bird was shot the remaining turkeys froze in place.

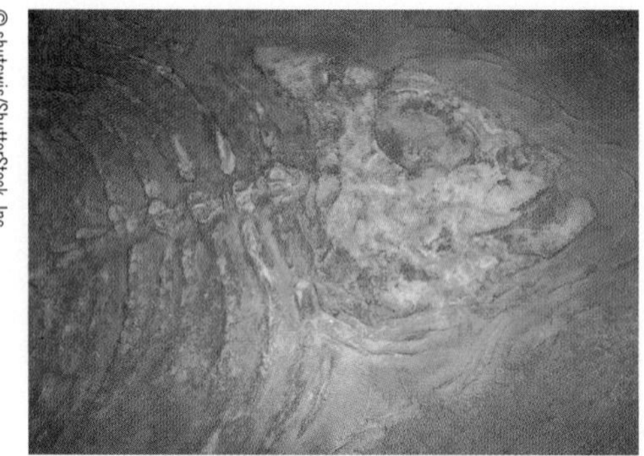

FIGURE 6.1 Fishing is an ancient practice, dating back to approximately 60,000 years ago. Archaeological evidence such as shell middens, discarded fish bones, and cave paintings suggests that fish and other seafood were important sources of food in the diet of early humans.

Fish and Shellfish

Fish and shellfish have been part of the diet of people living near the sea since humans evolved (see **Figure 6.1**). Archaeologists have found fossilized mollusk shells and fish bones in middens, or early garbage dumps, dating from 60,000 to 120,000 years ago.[4] In Mesopotamia, the first evidence of writing, dating from approximately 5000–3000 B.C., was in the form of clay cuneiform tablets. These records show that fish was prepared for feasts as well as offered to the gods.[4] Recipes for salting fish also were part of cuneiform records. In China, the precursor of soy sauce was fish fermented in salt, dating to around 1300 B.C. Recipes contained in the first known cookbook, written in Roman times, were entirely for fish. Evidence of fish consumption dating from thousands to hundreds of years ago has been found from Norway to South America to the Pacific Islands.

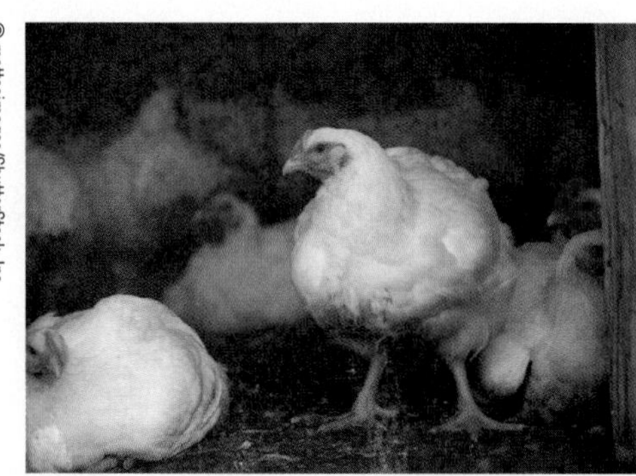

FIGURE 6.2 The Cornish game hen is a hybrid chicken. Despite its name, it is not a game bird, but rather a type of domestic chicken. It can be either male or female. Cornish game hens cost more than regular chickens and have a shorter growth period of 28 to 30 days, compared to 42 days or more for regular chicken.

Types of Poultry, Fish, and Shellfish

Poultry

Poultry is classified by species, age, and sex. In general, younger birds of any species are more tender and have less fat than older birds, but older birds have more flavor. Game birds such as pheasants and quail may be sold if raised domestically. Wild-caught game birds cannot be sold commercially.

Chicken

Chickens sold in stores may be male or female. Broiler/fryers are slaughtered at younger than 10 weeks of age and weigh from 3 to 5 pounds. Roasters weigh 6 to 7 pounds and are slaughtered when they are 9 to 11 weeks old. Neutered male chickens, called capons, are 4 months old at slaughter and weigh 12 to 14 pounds. Female chickens older than 10 months old may be referred to as hens, fowls, or baking or stewing chickens. Older male chickens are called cocks or roosters. Hens and cocks have outlived their breeding capability and are mainly used in processed foods. Their flesh is coarser (it contains enlarged muscle fibers) and has more fat deposited under the skin. Cornish game hens are a cross of a Cornish hen and another breed of chicken, such as White Plymouth Rock (see **Figure 6.2**).[5]

Turkey

Present-day turkeys are descended from turkeys domesticated by the Aztecs. The most common breed raised for food is the broad-breasted white turkey. Confined birds are raised on a diet of corn and soybean meal. No hormones are approved for their feed, but antibiotics may be added to improve feed efficiency and to impart disease resistance. Fryer-roasters are younger than 12 weeks old and weigh about 7 pounds. Young hens and toms are processed at 14.5 to 17.5 weeks of age (see **Figure 6.3**). Toms average about 26 pounds and hens about 15 pounds at slaughter.

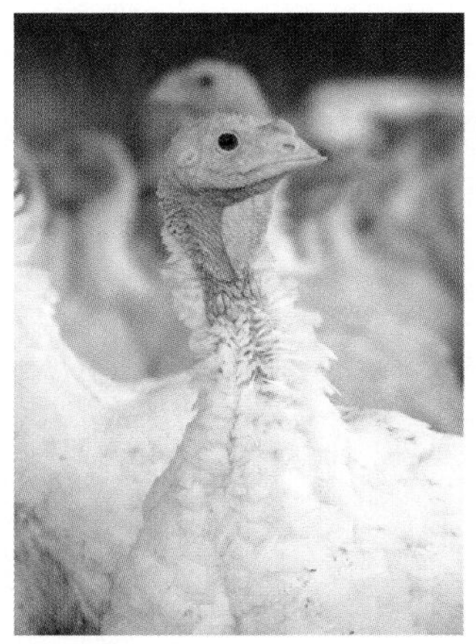

© ene/ShutterStock, Inc.

FIGURE 6.3 Male turkeys are slaughtered at 14.5 to 17.5 weeks of age. Since 1970, turkey consumption has increased 102%. In 2010, U.S. consumption of turkey was 16.4 pounds per person.

Duck

White Peking ducks were introduced to the United States from China in 1873. Ducks are raised in confinement and fed a diet of corn and soybean meal. According to Food and Drug Administration (FDA) regulations, hormones may not be added to their feed, and antibiotics are not routinely added.[6] Either sex may be sold as broiler/fryers, roasters, or mature duck. Broiler/fryer ducks are younger than 8 weeks old and weigh from 3 to 6 pounds. Roasting ducks are younger than 16 weeks old and range from 4 to 7 pounds. Both broiler/fryers and roasters have tender flesh. Mature ducks are older than 6 months and can no longer produce eggs. Their tough flesh is best suited for processed foods.

Geese

Geese were first bred in India and China. They later became popular in Europe and were then exported to the United States. Geese are raised in confinement until they are 6 weeks old. They are allowed to range outdoors, eating grass and some grains. FDA regulations for hormones and antibiotics are the same as for ducks. Young geese or goslings are 11 weeks old at slaughter and weigh 6 to 12 pounds. Mature geese have similar characteristics to mature ducks and are used in processed foods.

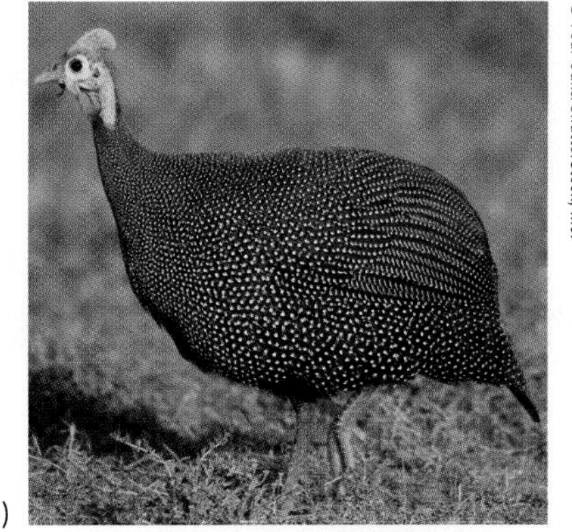

(a)

© Four Oaks/ShutterStock, Inc.

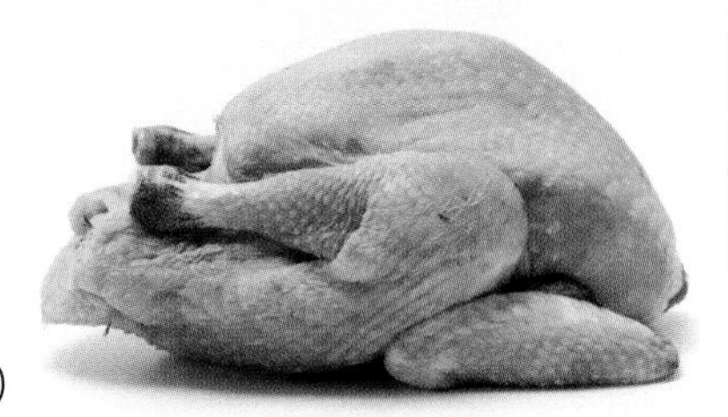

(b)

© gaffera/iStockphoto.com

FIGURE 6.4 (a) Although small birds, guinea fowl are an important food throughout much of Africa. They are found in every region of the world. These hardy birds forage for food and often are farmed in free-range or semi-wild facilities where they also perform a valuable pest-control function by eating insects. (b) The meat of a young guinea fowl is tender and tastes similar to that of wild game. It often is substituted for game birds such as grouse, partridge, quail, and pheasant. Guinea fowl meat is high in protein and low in cholesterol. It is a good source of vitamin B_6, selenium, and niacin.

Guinea Fowl

The guinea fowl is a small bird that is related to chicken and partridge (see **Figure 6.4**). Both sexes of guinea fowl are marketed, although the female is more tender than the male. Guinea fowl are 11 weeks old at time of slaughter. Their flesh is red and slightly dry when cooked. They weigh 2 to 3 pounds and are sold whole.

Pheasant

The pheasant originated in Asia and was introduced into the United States in the 1880s. Farm-raised pheasants are generally younger than 1 year old at slaughter. The age of wild-caught birds can be determined by the shape of the wing feathers or length of the spurs (the bony protrusion above the feet). Young birds have pointed wing tip feathers, which become rounded as the bird ages. Males with prominent spurs are mature birds. Drumsticks are generally not eaten from young or old birds due to the tough tendons, which are hard to remove. Females weigh 3 pounds and have more tender, juicy meat than the 5-pound males. Older birds are tough and must be cooked using moist heat.

Quail

Quail is a favorite game bird of hunters. It can also be raised commercially. The quail weighs 3 to 7 ounces and is prepared whole. The mild-flavored meat is mostly dark.

ratite Flightless bird such as ostrich and emu.

finfish Aquatic vertebrate with gills, fins, and an internal skeleton.

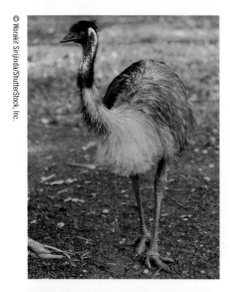

© Worakit Sirijinda/ShutterStock, Inc.

FIGURE 6.5 Emus are farmed primarily for their meat, leather, and oil. Emus produce highly nourishing red meat, with no fat marbled through the muscles.

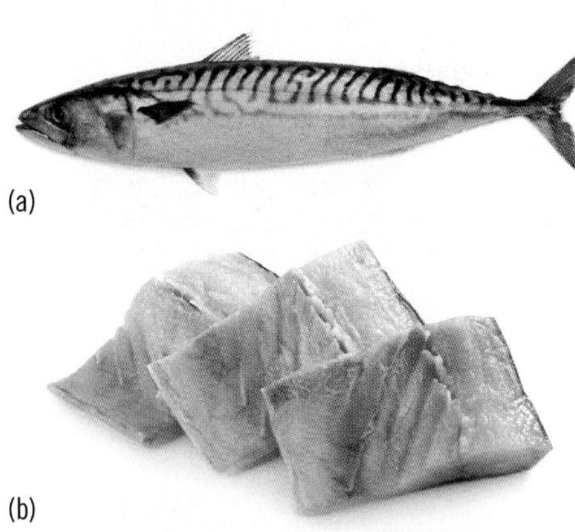

(a)

(b)

FIGURE 6.6 (a) Mackerel are found worldwide. They live along coasts or offshore in the ocean. (b) Mackerel is an oily fish and a good source of omega-3 fatty acids.

(a) © Migel/ShutterStock, Inc.; (b) © Magone/ShutterStock, Inc.

Squab and Pigeon

Squabs are immature pigeons about 4 weeks old. They weigh from 12 to 16 ounces and have tender meat. Pigeons are mature birds and have tougher meat. Both squabs and pigeons are cooked whole.

Wild Turkeys

Wild turkeys are raised and marketed similarly to domestic turkeys. Wild turkeys are smaller than their domesticated counterparts, and their flesh is leaner, less tender, and more strongly flavored than domesticated breeds. The age of wild-caught birds is determined using the same method as for pheasants.

Ratites

Ratites are a group of flightless birds that includes ostrich, emu, and rhea. Ostriches are the largest of these birds, weighing 300 to 400 pounds and standing up to 8 feet tall. Emus are 6 feet tall and weigh 125 to 140 pounds (see **Figure 6.5**). Rheas are 5 feet tall and weigh 60 to 100 pounds. Ostrich is native to Africa, emu is from Australia, and rhea originates from South America. Young birds are raised in confinement but then allowed to range. Their lean flesh is red and has a beefy flavor.

Fish

Vertebrates that breathe through gills and navigate by use of fins are called **finfish**, or often just *fish*. Approximately 160 fish species are sold in the United States. The most common are cod, salmon, tuna, haddock, halibut, flounder, catfish, whiting, red snapper, and perch. These species account for 80% of all fish sold.[7]

Fish are characterized by their habitat, appearance, and fat content. They may live in saltwater or freshwater and may either be relatively flat or round in cross-section. Flat fish, such as flounder, have eyes on the same side of the body and have an oval shape. These fish will spend most of their lives swimming near the bottom; thus the eyes are needed only on one side.

Fish can be classified by their fat content. A fatty fish has 5–10 grams of total fat per 3-ounce cooked portion. Fatty fish include mackerel (see **Figure 6.6**), lake trout (see **Figure 6.7**), and Atlantic salmon (see **Figure 6.8**). A fish is

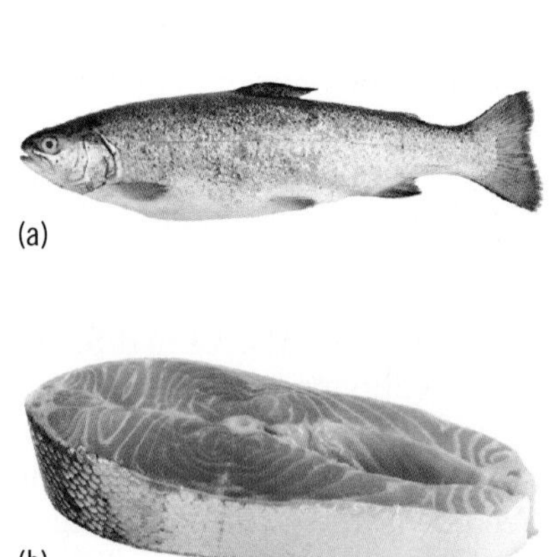

(a)

(b)

FIGURE 6.7 (a) Lake trout is a freshwater fish found primarily in northern lakes in North America. (b) Lake trout is also a good source of omega-3 fatty acids. It also is an excellent source of iron, calcium, selenium, and vitamins A, B_1, B_2, B_6, and B_{12}.

(a) © Wolna/ShutterStock, Inc.; (b) © Lu Mikhaylova/ShutterStock, Inc.

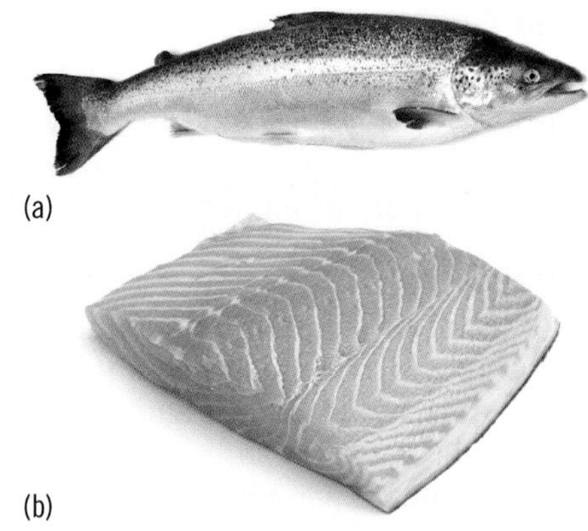

(a)

(b)

FIGURE 6.8 (a) Atlantic salmon is found in the northern Atlantic Ocean and in rivers that flow into the north Atlantic. It has freshwater and saltwater stages in its lifecycle. Due to overfishing, the large majority of Atlantic salmon is from commercial fish farms. (b) Atlantic salmon is high in omega-3 fatty acids. It is also a very good source of protein, vitamin B_{12}, and selenium.

(a) © Edward Westmacott/ShutterStock, Inc.; (b) © Alex Staroseltsev/ShutterStock, Inc.

TABLE 6.1
Characteristics of Common Fish

Type of Fish	Fat Content	Body Shape (in cross-section)	Habitat
Cod	Lean	Round	Ocean
Haddock	Lean	Round	Ocean
Halibut	Lean	Flat	Ocean
Salmon	Fat	Round	Ocean
Tuna	Fat	Round	Ocean
Flounder	Lean	Flat	Ocean
Red snapper	Lean	Round	Ocean
Perch	Fat	Round	Freshwater
Catfish	Lean	Round	Freshwater
Trout	Fat	Round	Freshwater

Source: Data from Environmental Protection Agency. Freshwater Fish Identification. Available at: http://www.epa.gov/bioiweb1/html/fish_id.html. Accessed June 1, 2012.

shellfish Freshwater or saltwater invertebrate with a hard external skeleton or shell.

crustacean Invertebrate with a jointed external skeleton.

mollusk Invertebrate with a hardened shell.

bivalve Mollusk characterized by having two shells attached by a hinge.

cephalopod Mollusk with a small internal shell.

considered lean if a 3-ounce cooked serving has less than 5 total grams of fat. Lean fish include haddock (see **Figure 6.9**), cod, tilapia, and catfish. **Table 6.1** lists some characteristics of common fish.

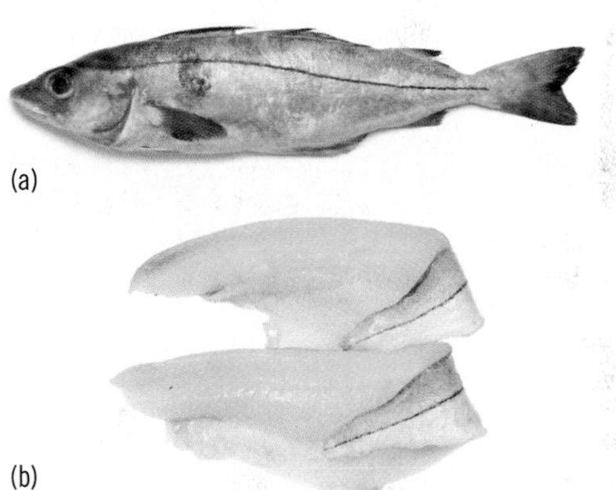

FIGURE 6.9 (a) Haddock is a marine fish that lives primarily in the north Atlantic ocean. Haddock is one of the most popular fish used in British fish and chips. (b) It is a lean fish that is very low in saturated fat. It is a very good source of protein, niacin, vitamin B_{12}, phosphorus, and selenium.

(a) © picturepartners/ShutterStock, Inc.; (b) © Richard Griffin/ShutterStock, Inc.

Shellfish

The distinguishing feature of **shellfish** is a hard external skeleton or shell. Shellfish are invertebrates that may live in freshwater or saltwater.

Crustaceans

Crustaceans have a hard, jointed external skeleton that is able to flex at the joints. Examples include shrimp, lobster (see **Figure 6.10**), crab (see **Figure 6.11**), and crawfish (see **Figure 6.12**).

Mollusks

Mollusks are invertebrates characterized by their hard external shell. The **bivalves**, including scallops, oysters (see **Figure 6.13**), clams (see **Figure 6.14**), and mussels, have two shells attached by a hinge. The univalves, which include conch and snails, have a single external shell. **Cephalopods** have a small internal shell. Examples of cephalopods are squid (see **Figure 6.15**) and octopus.

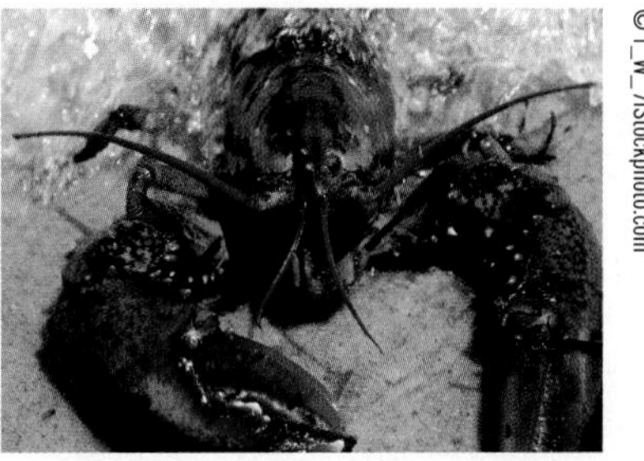

© T_W_/iStockphoto.com

FIGURE 6.10 Lobsters are found in all oceans. They live on rocky, sandy, or muddy bottoms from the shoreline to beyond the edge of the continental shelf, generally living crevices or in burrows under rocks. As a food, they are low in saturated fat and are a good source of protein, zinc, copper, and selenium.

Physical and Chemical Properties

Poultry

Poultry meat encompasses the animal's skeletal system, muscle tissues, and muscle pigments. This section elaborates on the physical properties of poultry meat.

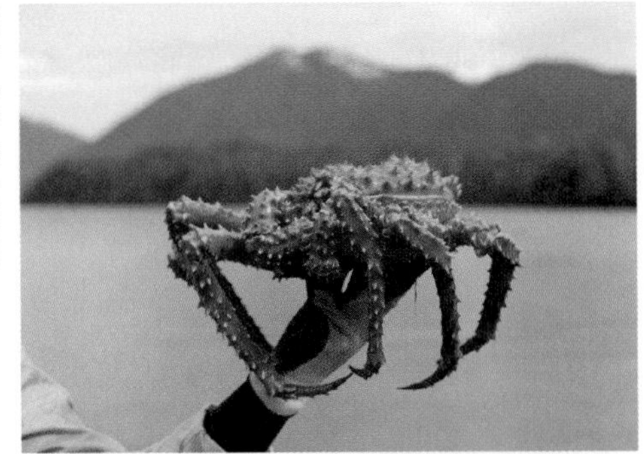

FIGURE 6.11 A number of different species of crab are used as food sources. Crabs can be found in all of the world's oceans and in various freshwater environments. Crabs make up 20% of all marine crustaceans caught, farmed, and consumed worldwide. One species, *Portunus trituberculatus*, accounts for one-fifth of that total. Crab is low in saturated fat but high in cholesterol. It is a good source of protein, vitamin B_{12}, zinc, copper, and selenium.

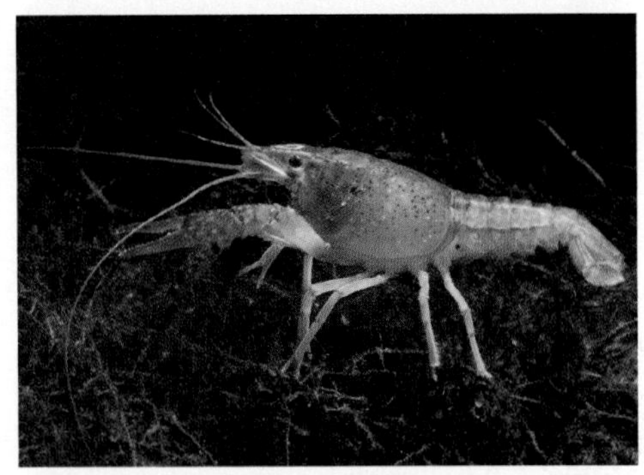

FIGURE 6.12 Crawfish are freshwater crustaceans that look like small lobsters. They are most commonly found in small freshwater brooks and streams. They are good sources of vitamin E, protein, vitamin B_{12}, phosphorus, copper, and selenium.

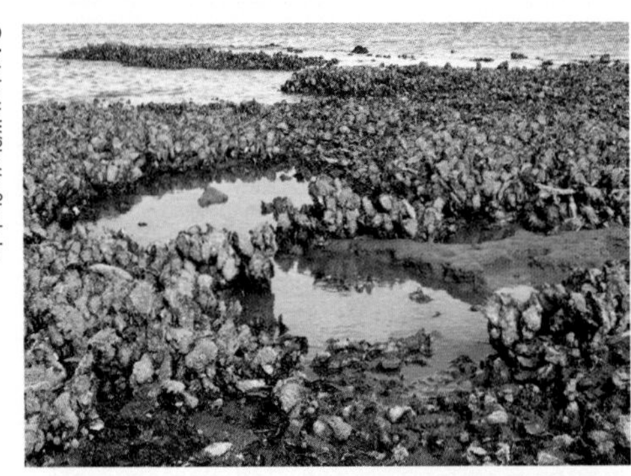

FIGURE 6.13 Oysters include a number of bivalve species that live in marine or brackish habitats. The largest oyster-producing body of water in the United States is located in Chesapeake Bay. Large beds of edible oysters also are found in Japan and Australia. Oysters are a good source of protein, vitamin D, vitamin B_{12}, iron, zinc, copper, manganese, and selenium.

Muscle

The structure of poultry muscle is similar to that of cattle and hogs. Muscles are composed of sarcolemma attached to bones by ligaments. Connective tissue is composed of collagen and elastin. Collagen is located between poultry muscles, whereas elastin is located in the ligaments and tendons. The prominent tendon located within the "tenderloin" part of the breast should be removed prior to cooking to maximize sensory characteristics of the cooked chicken "tender." Tendons are generally removed from processed chicken tenders used by the restaurant industry.

Pigments

Poultry meat is frequently categorized as either white or dark meat. Dark-colored meat is due to the large number of blood vessels found in more exercised parts of the body, such as the legs. The dark color of the muscle is not due to the blood itself but rather because of the muscle pigment myoglobin within the muscle cells. Myoglobin stores oxygen, which is needed by active muscles. Chickens and turkeys raised in confinement do not use their breast muscles for flight, therefore reducing the need for stored oxygen in the breast muscles, resulting in a decreased amount of dark meat. In contrast, wild birds such as ducks or geese will have dark-colored breast meat because they fly.

Protein and Fats

Poultry is considered a source of high-quality protein because of its large proportion of unsaturated fat, which can be decreased by removing the skin or cutting away visible fat. Unlike the marbling seen in beef or pork, poultry fat is deposited under the skin and on the outside of the muscles. It is therefore easy to remove.

Fat content increases with age; broilers/fryers that are 6 weeks old at time of slaughter have the least amount of fat. Poultry 1 year or older, such as fowl, have the most fat. Poultry undergoes rigor mortis after slaughter; however, rigor mortis is short, about 6 hours, due to poultry's small muscle size compared to the size of beef muscle.[8]

Effect of Heat

Poultry undergoes several changes when cooked. The skin changes from white or yellow to brown due to carmelization of carbohydrates on the skin's surface. Fat deposits beneath the skin melt, and the proteins in the muscles denature and coagulate. The flesh color changes from pink to white for breast meat. Dark meat also will lighten slightly as the muscle pigment myoglobin is oxidized and the iron atom at the center of the myoglobin molecule loses an electron, creating hemichrome. Hemichrome accumulates as the temperature of the meat increases, causing the color change. Myoglobin may also leak from bones, causing dark spots on flesh adjacent to bones.

Fish

Fish meat consists of muscle, connective tissue, and pigments. This section elaborates on the physical properties of fish meat.

Muscle and Connective Tissue

Fish have short muscle fibers called myotomes and little connective tissue. The myotomes are connected to thin sheets of connective tissue called myocomatta. The myocomatta is about 3% of the fish's body weight; by comparison, connective tissue comprises 15% of the body weight of cattle. An extensive skeletal and connective tissue system is unnecessary for fish because they are not affected by gravity to the same degree as animals that live on land.

Pigments

Like poultry muscle, fish muscle also contains myoglobin pigments. Fish that engage in continuous slow movement will tend to have dark-colored muscle. Dark-colored muscle is mainly composed of slow-twitch muscle fibers. Dark muscle fibers burn fats as fuel and require oxygen. In contrast, light-colored muscle has fast-twitch fibers that use carbohydrates as fuel. This type of muscle is used for short bursts of movement.[8]

Effect of Heat

During cooking, fish muscle will change in appearance from translucent to opaque as the proteins denature and coagulate. The myocomatta will gelatinize, contributing to the "flaky" texture of cooked fish. Color changes in both slow-twitch (red) or fast-twitch (white) muscle will be slight. In contrast, shellfish will have a pronounced change of color during cooking as the muscle proteins denature and coagulate. Dark black-green pigments will become less apparent as whitish-red astaxanthin pigments become more visible.

Effect of Additives

A phosphate solution may be added to fish before they are processed. The phosphate solution helps the fish retain natural moisture and retard spoilage. If fish are not treated with this solution, they can lose the majority of their water within days, resulting in dry and stringy flesh when cooked. The downside is that treated raw fish may appear slimy. Processors are not required to list phosphates as ingredients. Therefore, consumers should be aware of the characteristics of fresh fish, such as a clean nonfishy odor, so a slimy appearance is not mistaken for spoilage.

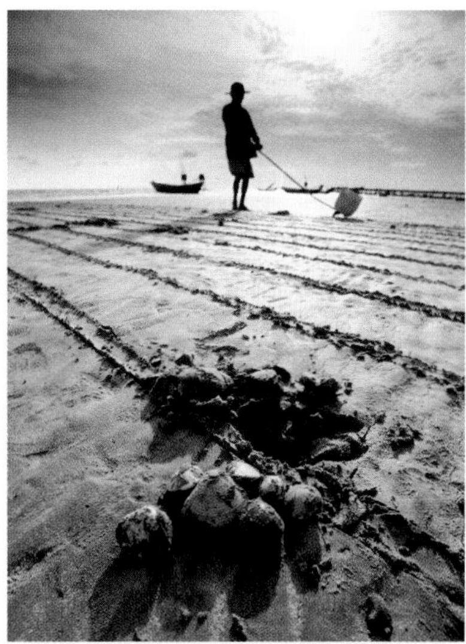

FIGURE 6.14 Clams are bivalves that burrow in sediment, as opposed to bivalves that attach themselves to a substrate (e.g., oysters, mussels). They live in marine and freshwater environments. Clams can be eaten raw, steamed, boiled, baked, or fried. Clams are very low in saturated fat and are good sources of vitamin B_{12}, phosphorus, potassium, copper, and selenium.

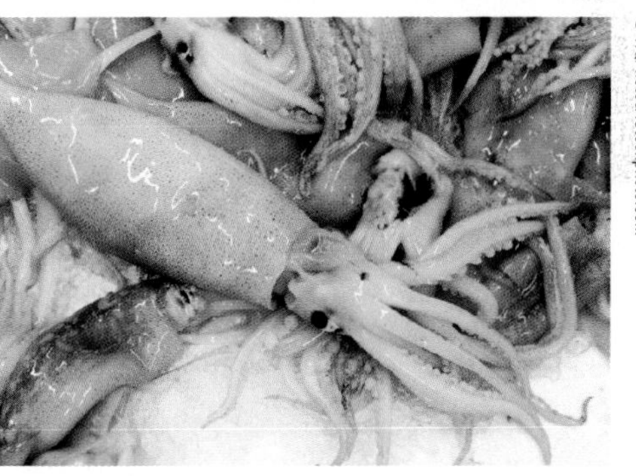

FIGURE 6.15 Squid, a cephalopod, is popular in various cuisines, including Chinese, Greek, and Japanese. In most English-speaking countries, squid is commonly consumed as calamari. Squid are abundant in certain areas and are fished commercially. It is a good source of copper, selenium, vitamin B_{12}, and riboflavin.

Nutritional Properties

Poultry

Poultry consumption has increased in part due to its perceived health benefits compared to red meat. However, poultry's nutrient profile is similar to red meat. A 3-ounce serving of skinless chicken breast has 140 calories and 3 grams of fat (see **Figure 6.16**) compared to beef sirloin steak, which has 160 calories and 6 grams of fat. A serving of pork tenderloin nearly matches the nutrient content of skinless chicken breast with 140 calories and 4 grams of fat. Poultry does have more unsaturated fat than does red meat. The fat content can be reduced by removing the skin before consumption.

Fish

Finfish and shellfish are good sources of protein, vitamins, minerals, and polyunsaturated fats. In particular, they are a good source of long-chain, polyunsaturated **omega-3 fatty acids**. Research supports many benefits of consuming fish containing omega-3 fatty acids. Omega-3 fatty acids have been shown to reduce the risk of arrhythmias and atherosclerosis and to decrease blood pressure, inflammation, and triglyceride levels. The American Heart Association (AHA) recommends eating at least two servings of fish, preferably fatty fish, twice a week.[9] Good fish sources of omega-3 fatty acids include salmon, albacore tuna (see **Figure 6.17**), lake trout, mackerel, herring, and sardines. Nutrient content varies by species and whether the fish was farmed or wild caught.

omega-3 fatty acids Long-chain polyunsaturated fatty acids found in fish that have been shown to have a positive impact on human health.

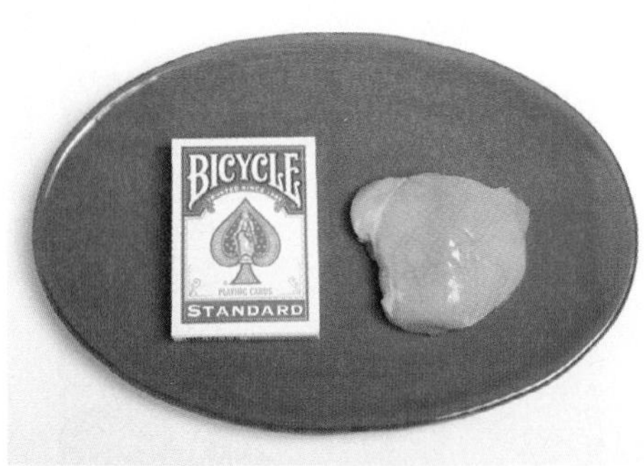

FIGURE 6.16 A 3-ounce serving of cooked chicken breast has 140 calories and 3 grams of fat.

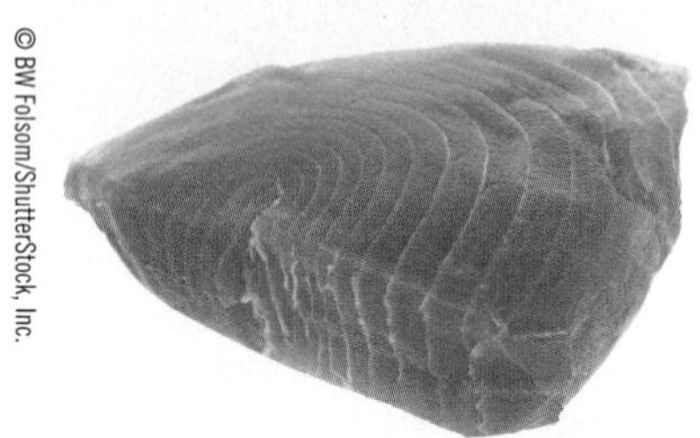

FIGURE 6.17 Fatty fish, such as tuna, salmon, and herring, contain the most omega-3 fatty acids. Fresh blue fin tuna has the highest amount of omega-3 fatty acids of any of the tuna varieties.

Cooking methods also influence the availability of omega-3 fatty acids. Eating fish that has been baked or simmered has been shown to decrease risk of cardiac disease. Fried fish consumption does not support the health benefits of omega-3 fatty acids.[10,11] **Special Topic 6.1** offers more information about the fatty acid content of various fish.

Cooking Methods

Poultry

Poultry can be purchased fresh, frozen, canned, dehydrated, or sliced. Highly processed forms of poultry are also available, including dressed, ready-to-cook, and convenience cuts, such as boneless, skinless breasts or thighs and chicken nuggets or sausage.

Age is the determining factor for the choice of cooking method. Young birds such as broiler/fryers are naturally tender and may be prepared by either moist or dry cooking methods. Older poultry has tougher flesh and should be cooked using moist heat or roasted at low temperatures to tenderize the meat. All poultry must be cooked to an internal temperature of 165°F (74°C) to destroy harmful microorganisms.

Fish

Fish have short muscle fibers that denature and coagulate faster than other types of animal muscle. Fish have less collagen than other meats, and the chemical structure of the connective tissue is different from that of red meat or poultry. Fish also has less of the amino acid hydroxyproline, which causes the proteins to denature more easily and undergo gelation when cooked.[8] Overcooking or cooking at high temperatures will create stringy, dry flesh that falls apart.

The fat content of the fish is the determining factor when choosing a cooking method. A fatty fish can be baked, broiled, poached, or steamed to maximize its firm texture and stronger flavor. A lean fish's more delicate

Special Topic 6.1

Omega-3 Fatty Acid Content of Fish

Brina Kelly

Fish are the primary sources in the human diet for omega-3 fatty acids, which have been shown to benefit the brain and nervous system as well as the cardiovascular system. The two types of omega-3 fatty acids are docosahexaenoic acid (DHA) and eicosapentaenoic acid (EPA).[1] DHA is essential for maintaining the structure of the central nervous system and brain health. EPA is important for the synthesis of prostaglandins for inflammatory control, thromboxanes to regulate platelet aggregation, and leukotrienes to help regulate allergic reactions. EPA is also known to reduce effects of depression and other mood disorders.[2] Each omega-3 fatty acid is important for various bodily functions.

Currently, experts recommend that people eat 12 ounces of fish at least twice a week.[3] For people who do not eat fish out of personal preference or for health reasons, omega-3 fatty acids are best obtained by consuming flaxseed, nuts (walnuts and almonds), and some cereals and legumes. Those fish species most rich in omega-3 fatty acids are salmon, tuna, and mackerel. DHA and EPA levels vary among fish species, so it is important to eat a variety of different types of fish.

High DPA Fish

DPA is very important in early brain development, so it is important that pregnant women, nursing mothers, and young children look for fish rich in DPA. The following are some of the fish highest in DPA:[4]

- Atlantic salmon: 950 mg/serving
- Pacific sardines: 740 mg/serving
- Sockeye salmon: 600 mg/serving
- Canned tuna: 540 mg/serving
- Rainbow trout: 440 mg/serving

High EPA Fish

EPA may benefit people with joint problems or bone loss. The following are some of the best fish sources of EPA:[4,5]

- Pacific herring: 1.06 g/serving
- Chinook salmon: 860 mg/serving
- Pacific oysters: 750 mg/serving

Other types of seafood high in EPA include eel, sturgeon, and Dungeness crab.

References

1 Academy of Nutrition and Dietetics. What Fish Are Rich in Omega-3 Fatty Acids? Available at: http://www.eatright.org/Public/content.aspx?id=6442452549&terms=fish. Accessed July 16, 2011.

2 Academy of Nutrition and Dietetics. Heart and Health Diet. Available at: http://www.eatright.org/Public/content.aspx?id=6820. Accessed July 16, 2011.

3 Academy of Nutrition and Dietetics. Feed Your Brain. Go Fish! Available at: http://www.eatright.org/Public/content.aspx?id=6442463963&terms=fish. Accessed July 16, 2011.

4 LiveStrong. Fish Containing High Levels of EPA and DHA. Available at: http://www.livestrong.com/article/309847-fish-containing-highest-levels-of-epa-dha. Accessed July 16, 2011.

5 Omega-3 Institute. Dietary Sources of Omega-3 Fatty Acids. Available at: http://www.dhaomega3.org/Overview/Dietary-Sources-of-Omega-3-Fatty-Acids. Accessed July 16, 2011.

muscle structure and mild flavor benefits from frying, broiling, poaching, or steaming (see **Figure 6.18**). Fish is done when it just flakes when touched and has reached 145°F (63°C). Sauces are a great complement to fish and poultry; see **Special Topic 6.2** for information on how to enhance the flavors of food with sauces.

Shellfish

Shellfish must always be cooked to the well-done stage because they carry more potentially hazardous microorganisms than fish. When shellfish is cooked at high temperatures, such as during deep fat frying, it can overcook, becoming tough and rubbery. It is easier to maintain a tender texture by using moist cooking methods over lower temperatures. Steaming and simmering are good moist cooking methods for shellfish.

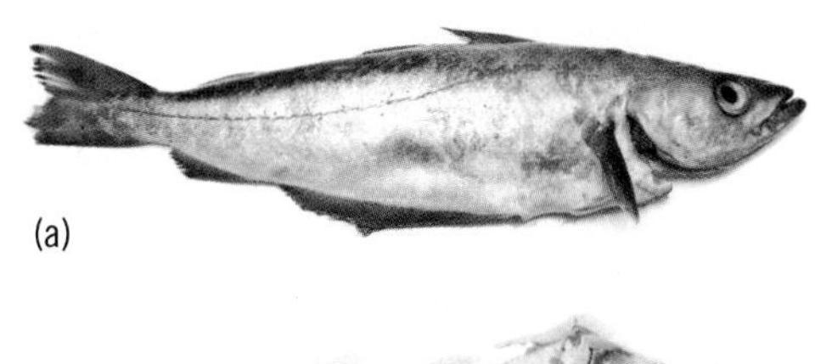

(a)

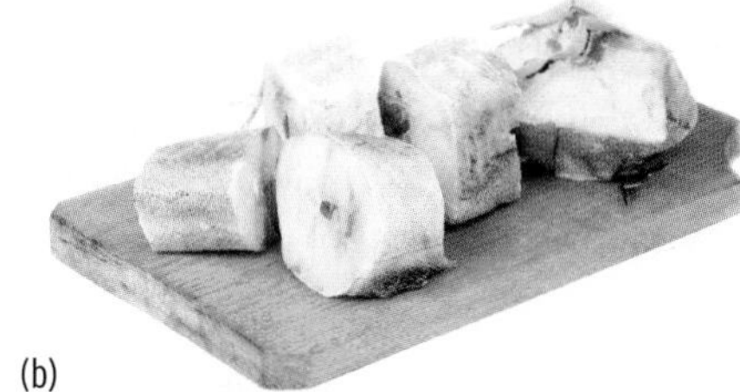

(b)

FIGURE 6.18 (a) Pollock is a popular lean fish with a very mild taste that is popular in American restaurants. (b) When cooking lean fish, cook until the fish just flakes and has an internal temperature of 145°F (63°C).

Special Topic 6.2

Sauces for Chicken and Fish

Maura Grimes

Sauces provide a flavorful component to chicken and fish dishes. Different ingredients result in the different tastes and textures of sauces. Cream, milk, and flour can be used to create thick sauces. Egg yolks help the sauce to emulsify, giving it a creamy texture. Vinegar provides an acidic taste and helps to tenderize fish or chicken. Butter provides a delicious fatty flavor that goes especially well with fish. Wine has a delicious flavor that enhances the overall dish. Overall, the different tastes in sauces are directly influenced by the ingredients included. The key to making a good sauce is having an understanding of the different ingredients and the effect they will have.

Roux-based sauces are white sauces that typically contain butter, flour, and milk. A basic roux is made by sautéing butter and slowly adding flour. Once the flour is dispersed, milk is slowly added to thicken the mixture into a sauce. The thickness of the sauce depends on the flour-to-milk ratio.[1,2] Different spices, such as nutmeg, can be combined with the sauce to create a variety of flavors to go with different types of dishes. Roux is typically served best with chicken and meat. One variety of roux is Mornay sauce, which has butter, flour, milk, egg yolks, gruyere cheese, and ground nutmeg. This sauce is good with chicken and fish. Another variety is supreme sauce, which is best served with chicken. It has butter, flour, chicken stock, and heavy cream. Another variety that goes well with chicken is caper sauce. This sauce has butter, flour, chicken stock, egg yolks, heavy cream, and capers. The capers add a sharp flavor to this sauce.

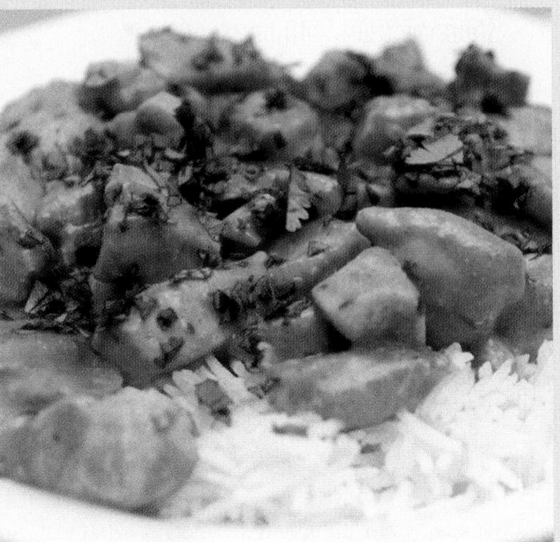

FIGURE A The term *curry* is a Western term used to describe a variety of Southeast Asian and Indian dishes that use a complex combination of spices and/or herbs and yogurt. Curry sauces can be used to complement meat, poultry, seafood, and vegetable dishes.

Yogurt-based sauces can be served with fish or chicken. Asian-Indian cultures incorporate yogurt into many of their sauces; the acidity of the yogurt helps to tenderize the meat.[1,2] The most popular yogurt-based sauce are curries, which come in many different varieties and can be served well with almost anything (see **Figure A**). Cumin, coriander, chili powder, fenugreek, cinnamon, clove, cardamom, and turmeric are all popular spices used in curries. The spices used in curries provide have many antioxidant properties.[1,2]

Butter-based sauces have a nice fatty taste and go well with just about anything. Mouselline sauce is a common type of buttery sauce that incorporates butter, egg yolks, cayenne pepper, lemon juice, and whipping cream. This delicious and easy-to-make sauce goes well with whitefish fillet. The lemon juice provides a nice acidic taste that goes well with fish, and the egg yolks help to combine the sauce.[1,2] Butter can be combined with many different herbs, spices, and vegetable purees for different varieties of flavorful sauces.

Vinegar-based sauces supply acidity, which helps tenderize meat.[1,2] Balsamic vinegar is very flavorful and goes well with fish and chicken. It is delicious when combined with tomatoes. Balsamic vinegar can be very tasty when it is served as a glaze or when it is reduced, which brings out more of the flavor. Béarnaise sauce is another variety of a vinegar-based sauce. It is typically served with chicken and contains butter, fresh tarragon, fresh chrivel, shallot, peppercorn, white wine vinegar, egg yolks, and cayenne. The butter and egg yolks in the sauce provide a delicious creamy flavor.

Barbeque sauce is a very popular vinegar-based sauce. In its use as a marinade, it is a good example of how an acidic sauce can act as a tenderizer.[1,2] Barbeque sauce contains balsamic vinegar, Worcestershire sauce, and other ingredients and is commonly served with chicken that is grilled or baked. Red wine also can be added to barbeque sauce for a delicious and unique flavor.

Wine-based sauces can flavor all kinds of meats. Wine is often added to enhance the flavors of creamy sauces and gravy. Red wine typically goes well with red meat, and white wine goes well with poultry and fish. A popular white wine sauce that goes well with both chicken and fish is a creamy mushroom sauce. This sauce includes butter, shallots, mushrooms, fresh tarragon, white wine, brown stock, and whipping cream. The mushrooms provide a nice earthy taste, and the wine combines well with the onion flavor from the shallots. Mustard sauce is another popular variety of sauce that contains white wine. This sauce has Dijon mustard, white wine, heavy cream, brown stock, butter, and shallot. The smoothness of this sauce goes well with chicken and other meats.[1,2]

References

1 Halsey K. *Sauces.* Boston, MA: Periplus Editions; 1998.
2 Sheasby A. *The Book of Sauces.* New York: HP Books; 2002.

Going Green with Poultry and Fish

Both fish and poultry consumption have increased from the mid-20th century to the first decades of the 21st century. This is part of a trend in increasing overall per capita energy intake from proteins, fats, and carbohydrates. In 1970, the average caloric intake per capita per day was 3,300 calories. By 1994, this had increased to 3,800 calories per capita per day.[12] Three demographic trends that will impact fish and poultry consumption are the aging population, increased diversity, and the overall global population increase. Consumers appear willing to pay for quality and convenience throughout all market segments. By 2020, fish consumption is projected to increase by 26% from 2000 levels.[13] Fish and poultry consumption patterns are summarized in **Table 6.2, Table 6.3**, and **Table 6.4**.

TABLE 6.2
Poultry Consumption (Pounds per Capita)

Year	All Turkey	All Chicken	Broilers	Other (Boneless) Poultry	Total Consumed
1950	3.3	14.3	21.9[a]	2.5[b]	42.0
2000	13.7	54.2	53.7	0.6	122.2
2008	13.9	58.8	58.1	0.7	131.5

[a] Includes nonbroiler chicken.
[b] Consumption for 1966. No data available prior to this date.
Source: Data from Economic Research Service, U.S. Department of Agriculture. Food Availability (Per Capita) Data System. Available at: http://www.ers.usda.gov/Data/FoodConsumption. Accessed June 8, 2012.

TABLE 6.3
Fish and Shellfish Consumption (Pounds per Capita)

Year	Fish, Fresh and Frozen	Shellfish, Fresh and Frozen	Canned	Cured	Total Consumed
1950	4.7	1.6	4.9	0.6	11.9
2000	5.6	4.6	4.7	0.3	15.2
2008	6.2	5.6	3.9	0.3	16.0

Source: Data from Economic Research Service, U.S. Department of Agriculture. Food Availability (Per Capita) Data System. Available at: http://www.ers.usda.gov/Data/FoodConsumption. Accessed June 8, 2012.

TABLE 6.4
Red Meat, Poultry, and Fish Consumption (Pounds per Capita)

Year	Beef	Veal	Pork	Lamb	Poultry	Fish
1950	44.6	5.6	43.0	2.6	42.0	11.9
2000	64.5	0.5	47.8	0.8	122.2	15.2
2008	61.2	0.3	46.0	0.7	131.5	16.0

Source: Data from Economic Research Service, U.S. Department of Agriculture. Food Availability (Per Capita) Data System. Available at: http://www.ers.usda.gov/Data/FoodConsumption. Accessed June 8, 2012.

Poultry Industry Trends

Producers raising poultry such as chicken and turkey have used several methods to maximize meat yield. Until the 1950s, poultry was housed in "coops" and had access to the outdoors. After World War II, poultry was raised in large confinement structures, which kept the birds indoors their entire lives. Feed technology improved poultry meat gain efficiency during the postwar years—from requiring 4 pounds of feed to produce 1 pound of meat to requiring just 1.5 pounds of feed to produce 1 pound of meat. The amount of time needed to raise a day-old chick to market-ready broiler or turkey also declined by more than 20%. The result of increased meat production efficiency led to lower retail prices for consumers. Processors were confronted with the need to increase the amount of poultry meat in order to compensate for lower profits. The result was industry consolidation into a few very large corporations.

Until the 1980s, most poultry was consumed as whole birds or packaged parts such as breasts and drumsticks prepared from fresh or frozen meat. Processors and retailers responded to consumer desire for more processed poultry as more women entered the workforce and fewer meals were prepared at home. Processors also added value (and increased their profits) by including poultry in products such as franks, sausage, and bologna and by chopping and reforming it into hams, loaves, and breaded patties. In 1983, McDonald's introduced the Chicken McNugget. It was an immediate success, resulting in McDonald's becoming the second largest user of chicken in the fast-food industry, after Kentucky Fried Chicken, a remarkable achievement for a hamburger restaurant.

Gastronomy Point

Low-Temperature Cooking Cooking with moist heat at low temperatures over a long period of time tenderizes older poultry.

Several ecological criticisms have been raised with regard to the poultry industry. First, the large quantities of waste generated by high-volume poultry production can migrate underground to aquifers, causing pollution of drinking water supplies. Second, some question whether keeping animals under such confined conditions is humane. Third, concerns are increasing with regard to the impact of poultry feed—which is typically enriched with subclinical levels of antibiotic additives—on overall quality and human health.

Shifts in consumer demand for less processed food have led to small-scale alternative production methods. Poultry is now available as "free range," meaning it has access to the outdoors. "Cage free" poultry may still be raised in confinement but without the use of restrictive cages. USDA certified organic chicken must be raised without the use of drugs and have a diet of organic feed. It should be noted that, despite these steps, the majority of poultry consumed in the United States is still highly processed.

Fishing Industry Trends

Fish have traditionally been prepared fresh or preserved by smoking or salting. Modern fish harvesting methods, whether from marine or freshwater, generally involve freezing the fish shortly after they have gone through rigor mortis. The process of rigor mortis for fish is completed in 1 hour to several days, depending on the species and the holding temperature. Fish become flexible again after rigor mortis because the muscles have relaxed, which also gives them better texture and flavor. Fish that are frozen immediately after harvest and not allowed to go through rigor mortis have a tough texture when cooked. Fish cooked immediately after capture also will be tough.

If fish or shellfish is to be sold as "fresh, not frozen," it must be brought to market within 24 hours and processed for sale. Fish and shellfish are highly perishable due to their unsaturated fat content and must be kept chilled and on ice as soon as they are caught if they are to be sold as fresh. High-end restaurants may purchase whole fish from a *fish monger* (seller of fish), because it gives the chef many options for preparation as well as an assurance of quality. Due to consumer demand for fresh fish, inland restaurants now have the option of air-freighting fish. Fish caught in quantity are kept in the ship's hold until brought to a processing center nearby. The fish are cleaned and processed in a variety of forms, including canned, IQF (individual quick frozen) fillets, and breaded frozen fish sticks. Fresh shellfish may be sold "as is," such as live oysters, or lightly processed, such as headless shrimp. Fresh fish sold at retail must be labeled "previously frozen."

Declining fish stocks have been noted worldwide. The cause may be due to overfishing, habitat change, or pollution. International agreements such as the International Convention for the Conservation of Atlantic Tuna (ICCAT) help to control overfishing but may not prevent it if all nations harvesting the particular fish do not sign the agreement.[14] The United Nations Food and Agriculture Organization estimates that 70% of the world's fish stocks are depleted or fully exploited. If the current trend continues, all ocean fish species used for food will be gone by 2050.[15]

One potential solution to overfishing is **aquaculture**, or fish and aquatic food farming. It is one of the fastest growing segments in the global food supply and now produces 46% of the world's total fish supply.[16] Aquaculture is used to farm mollusks, salmon, cod, grouper, and shrimp. Saltwater aquaculture farms are set up as a matrix of confinement pens connected by platforms for the workers to dispense feed and antibiotics. These structures may be located near the shoreline or in open waters. Freshwater fish such as catfish also are produced through aquaculture and may be farmed in a series of manmade ponds, frequently located in rural areas adjacent to field crops such as soybeans or corn (see **Figure 6.19**). Harvested fish are then transported by truck to a nearby processing center. Similar to land farmers' use of practices that minimize soil erosion and pesticide runoff, fish farmers use practices to reduce pollution and preserve natural habitats. However, concerns have been raised over waste management failures, diseases resulting from overcrowding, and overuse of antibiotics.

The habitats of some endangered species of birds and sea mammals have been negatively impacted by intensive marine aquaculture. Several initiatives have been implemented by nonprofit groups to promote sustainable fish farming.[17] For example, Fair Trade International (FTI) and the Aqua Stewardship Council (ASC) work with aquaculture companies to use practices that ensure the safety of the fish produced and to minimize the environmental impact of intensive aquaculture. Another hazard to the oceans' fisheries is oil spills, as described in **Special Topic 6.3**.

aquaculture The farming of fish and other aquatic species.

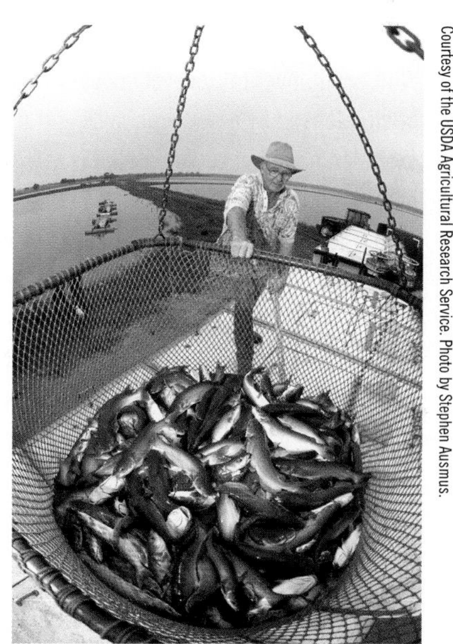

Courtesy of the USDA Agricultural Research Service. Photo by Stephen Ausmus.

FIGURE 6.19 Catfish farming started in the United States in the 1960s. Catfish are raised in inland tanks or channels and are fed a grain-based diet that includes soybean meal and pellet-shaped floating feed. Mississippi leads the nation in catfish ponds, with over 100,000 acres devoted to catfish.

Green Point

Sustainable Harvesting Companies that comply with Aqua Stewardship Council (ASC) practices may have their fish certified as being produced sustainably. Companies that comply with the group's recommendations can use the ASC label as a marketing tool.

Special Topic 6.3

Oil Spills: The Economic and Environmental Impact

Jacqueline Minichiello, MS, RD, LDN

As long as oil remains an important source of fuel around the world, fisheries and the natural environment will face the potential threat of oil spills. A single oil spill can leak millions of gallons of oil into the ocean. The amount, type, and quality of the oil spilled; the season and weather; the shoreline characteristics; and wave and tidal energy where the oil is spilled dictate the severity of an oil spill's economic and environmental impact.[1]

Due to the innate properties of oil, even if a spill occurs over a small area the area ultimately affected may be vast. According to the Oregon State Marine Board, 1 quart of oil will create an oil slick over 2 acres in size—the equivalent of nearly three football fields.[2] Large areas can be affected by any size spill.

Several massive oil spills have occurred in recent American history. The Exxon Valdez oil spill of 1989 caused 10.8 million gallons of oil to spill into the waters off the coast of Alaska.[3] This spill affected approximately 1,300 miles of shoreline, with 200 miles considered heavily oiled and 1,100 miles considered lightly oiled.[3] In 2010, a British Petroleum (BP) oil platform in the Gulf of Mexico exploded, causing oil to flow unabated into the ocean for several months. Over a year later, almost 500 miles of coastline were still contaminated.

With environmental recovery usually taking between 2 and 10 years,[4] the copious amounts of oil released by a spill can pose initial damage as well as continued harm over an extended period of time. Wildlife is affected by oil through physical contact, ingestion, inhalation, and absorption.[1] Contact with oil negatively impacts the insulating properties of feathers and fur, which can cause hyperthermia and consequently death in furred mammals. The weight of the oil can make it impossible for birds to fly, causing them to drown (see **Figure A**).[1,5] Determining the number of seabird deaths can be difficult, with the only reliable method being counting the carcasses. This method often results in an underestimate of the actual numbers of deaths, because many birds do not end up reaching the coast to be included in the count. For example, while 35,000 seabird carcasses were found after the Exxon Valdez oil spill, it was estimated that the actual number of deaths may have been closer to 250,000.[4]

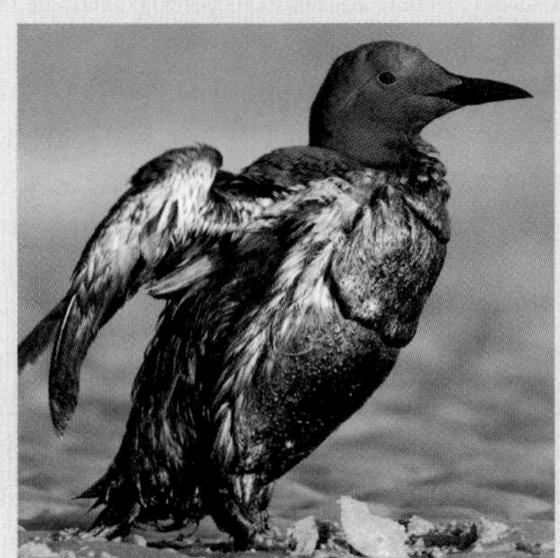

FIGURE A Oil-covered birds often are unable to fly. When the birds try to clean themselves, they ingest the oil, which irritates their digestive tract and damages their liver and kidneys, leading to dehydration and metabolic imbalances. Most birds that become covered in oil will die without human intervention.

In a spill area, oil can impact indigenous populations of fish in many ways. The fish can take in the oil either through the gills or through consumption of oil or oiled prey. This, in turn, can cause decreased growth, enlarged livers, changes in heart and respiration rates, fin erosion, and reproductive impairment.[1] Oil also decreases the survival rates of eggs and larvae. The larval stages of many fish species, including salmon, are highly sensitive to oil toxins.[1] All these effects can reduce the supply of fish. By decreasing the supply of fish, oil spills reduce an important source of omega-3 fatty acids in the human diet.

Oil spills also impact the fishing industry by affecting the safety, availability, and price of fish. In the Gulf of Mexico, for example, fishing is one of the largest industries and a major source of employment.[6] States that border the Gulf of Mexico produce around 1.3 billion pounds, or $700 million worth, of seafood annually. The Gulf of Mexico provides 73% of the country's shrimp catch and 60% of U.S. oyster landings.[7] With about one-third of the Gulf closed after the BP spill, the Gulf of Mexico saw a 39% decline in commercial fishing catches in 2010 versus 2009, representing a $62 million loss in dockside sales.[8] Similarly, after the Exxon Valdez spill, there was a huge decline in commercial fishing due to the closure of fisheries for salmon, herring, crab, shrimp, rockfish, and sablefish throughout the region.[9]

It remains unclear whether fish populations can be fully restored after an oil spill. In 2009, 20 years after the Exxon Valdez oil spill, the herring population of Prince William Sound still had not recovered. The herring harvest is not only necessary for the human communities in the region, it also provides the food-chain connection between algae and zooplankton and large predators, such as other fish, birds, and marine animals.[9]

Food safety after an oil spill is a public health concern. Oil contains polycyclic aromatic hydrocarbons (PAHs). Consumption of seafood containing large amounts of PAHs over a prolonged period of time can be toxic. Hence, the FDA has a process to determine if an area exposed to oil can reopen for harvesting. Samples of the species taken from contaminated waters need to pass a sensory examination and a chemical analysis in an approved laboratory. To pass the sensory evaluation, a minimum of 70% of the expert assessors must find no detectable petroleum or dispersant odor or flavor from each sample. If harmful levels of PAHs are found in the samples during the chemical examination, the site from which the sample was collected fails and remains closed. Even if a site does reopen, testing needs to continue to be certain that long-term contamination does not exist.[10]

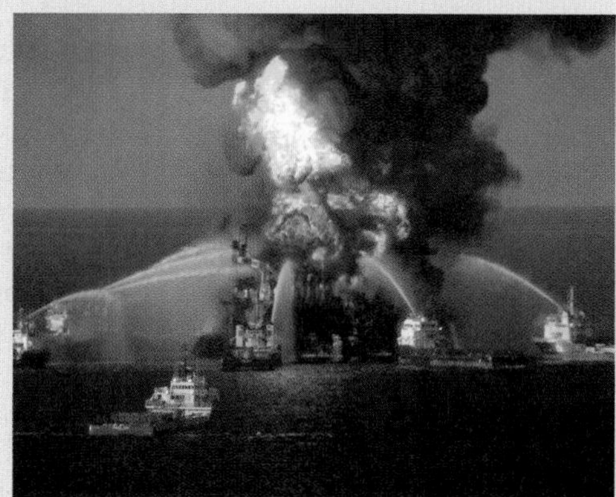
Courtesy of the U.S. Coast Guard.

FIGURE B In just the 6 months after the BP oil spill in the Gulf of Mexico, more than 8,000 birds, sea turtles, and marine animals were found dead or injured. The long-term damage caused by the oil, as well as the chemical dispersants used to contain the oil, may not be known for years.

The cost of an oil spill to the environment and the economy is widespread and long lived. Cleanup alone for the Exxon Valdez oil spill cost about $2 billion.[9] By June 2010, the cost of the response for the BP oil spill was approximately $2 billion (see **Figure B**).[11] Adding in the losses for the fishing industry and tourism, the actual economic impact of oil spills is even greater. In March 2011 a report by the Food and Drug Administration (FDA), the National Oceanic and Atmospheric Administration (NOAA), and the state of Louisiana assured that there were no safety concerns about the fish supply in the Gulf.[12] However, looking back with the 20-year perspective of the Exxon Valdez oil spill, it is clear that although some animal populations have recovered and appear healthy, others have not. This should be a cautionary tale, indicating that although initially it may appear that populations are healthy and viable, many years of continuous oil exposure can lead to persistent declines. The only way to ensure the safety of our environment is to prevent oil spills from occurring.

References

1 U.S. Fish and Wildlife Service. *Effects of Oil Spill on Wildlife and Habitat: 2004.* Washington, DC: U.S. Fish & Wildlife Service; 2004.

2 Oregon State Marine Board. *Oregon Clean Marina Guidebook: 2005.* Salem, Oregon: Oregon State Marine Board; 2005.

3 Incident News. Ten Famous Spills. Available at: http://www.incidentnews.gov/famous. Accessed March 15, 2011.

4 Kingston P. Long-term environmental effects of oil spills. *Spill Science & TechnologyBulletin.* 2002;7:53–61.

5 Peterson C, Rice S, Short J, et al. Long-term ecosystem response to the Exxon Valdez oil spill. *Science.* 2003;302:2082–2086.

6 National Oceanic and Atmospheric Administration. *Fishing Industry in the Gulf of Mexico: 2010.* Washington, DC: U.S. Department of Commerce; 2010.

7 Food and Water Watch. U.S. Seafood and the BP Gulf Disaster. Available at: http://www.foodandwaterwatch.org/factsheet/seafood-gulf-disaster. Accessed March 22, 2011.

8 The Natural Resource Defense Council. The BP Oil Disaster at One Year: A Straightforward Assessment of What We Know, What We Don't, and What Questions Need to Be Answered. Available at: http://www.nrdc.org/energy/files/bpoildisasteroneyear.pdf. Accessed April 21, 2011.

9 Exxon Valdez Oil Spill Trustee Council. 2009 Status Report. Available at: http://www.evostc.state.ak.us/Universal/Documents/Publications/AnnualStatus/2009AnnualReport.pdf. Accessed March 15, 2011.

10 U.S. Food and Drug Administration. Overview of Testing Protocol to Re-open Harvest Waters That Were Closed in Response to the Deepwater Horizon Oil Spill. Available at: http://www.fda.gov/Food/ucm217598.htm. Accessed on April 21, 2011.

11 BP. Update on Gulf of Mexico Oil Spill Response, June 21. Available at: http://www.bp.com/genericarticle.do?categoryId=2012968&contentId=7063006. Accessed April 21, 2011.

12 U.S. Food and Drug Administration. Consumers Can Be Confident in the Safety of Gulf Seafood. Available at: http://www.fda.gov/Food/ucm217598.htm. Accessed April 21, 2011.

Food Technology

A number of steps are needed for fish and poultry to make their way from the producer to the consumer's dinner table.

Poultry Processing

Poultry are first stunned to render them unconscious and then bled to complete slaughter. The carcasses are then scalded so the feathers can be removed. Next the feet and viscera are removed from the carcass. To control pathogens, poultry is chilled rapidly to 40°F (4.4°C) before it is further processed into parts, cured, or smoked.[18] Fresh and frozen poultry may be injected with a salt solution to help produce tender, moist cooked meat. The USDA allows processors who inject poultry with salt solutions to label their products as "natural."

Commercial processors use low-temperature long-time (LTLT) cooking methods to minimize moisture losses and maintain acceptable sensory properties. Mechanically deboned chicken (MDC) is widely used in food products such as soups, nuggets, luncheon meats, and tenders. MDC may be further processed into comminuted meat. **Comminution** is the reduction in muscle particle size through chopping, dicing, emulsifying with gelatin, and then grinding the tissue so that it can be formed into value-added products. The USDA permits up to 15% poultry meat to be included in comminuted red meat products such as sausages and luncheon meats.

comminution The process of finely dicing meat during industrial food processing.

In the 1960s, consumer demand for convenience products shifted poultry processing from whole-bird slaughter and packaging lines to cut-up lines. The shift enabled processors to use poultry that would not meet USDA inspected Grade A requirements to be cut into pieces for retail or for further processing. Beginning in 1977, marketers introduced new products—including chicken nuggets, patties, tenders, filets, and popcorn chicken—to the foodservice industry. Similar products also became available in the frozen-food sections of grocery stores.[19]

Innovation Point

Thermal Processing Methods Cooked poultry products undergo thermal processing in a combined system of equipment such as steam chambers, infrared devices, and microwave ovens to achieve efficiency and sensory attributes desired by consumers. Traditional frying techniques are being replaced with processes such as passing meat and seafood on a conveyor belt through a curtain of hot oil.

Fish Processing

Approximately 70% of fish are sold as fresh, frozen, or canned. The remainder are either cured or incorporated into comminuted products. Cured fish may be salted, pickled, or smoked. A brine solution is used to produce cured fish. The fish are then sold as salted dry or canned.

Most harvested fish are not intended to be marketed fresh. In these cases, rapid freezing of fish to –22°F (–30°C) within 2 hours of harvest is key to preserving the quality and safety of the fish. After being transported to the processing facility, whole fish are thawed at refrigerator temperature. Once thawed, the fish are eviscerated, their exterior surfaces cleaned, and they are sorted by muscle size. The final product determines further processing. Fish may be filleted or cut into steaks and refrozen. Canned fish are precooked by steam to facilitate deboning and then compacted into cylindrical chunks.[20] Comminuted fish are run through a specialized deboning machine that removes the spine and scales while chopping the muscle into pieces. The comminuted fish muscle is processed in a manner similar to that for poultry meat. Typical products are IQF fillets, breaded frozen fish sticks, and surimi. Surimi is a fish-based food product that has been pulverized to a thick paste and has the property of a dense and rubbery food item when cooked. Imitation crabmeat is a common surimi product.

Packaging

After cleaning and removal of internal organs and external layers, poultry and fish must be packaged. The packaging provides for protection, preservation, and storage. The quality of packaged food is related to the food itself and to the material attributes of the packaging.[21] Packaging for poultry and fish products ranges from cans to pouches. A **retort pouch** is a plastic and metal foil laminate pouch that is used as an alternative to traditional industrial canning methods.

retort pouch A flexible container that is aseptic or void of microorganisms.

Market demands for fresh products with reduced sodium present challenges for shelf life and food safety. High-pressure processing (HPP) creates a form of retort packaging that preserves the fresh qualities of foods, because no heat or preservatives are used. Foods are packaged in flexible pouches and loaded into a high-pressure chamber containing water. The fluid is pressurized up to 87,000 psi for 3 to 5 minutes. Because bacteria are inactivated at 60,000 psi, the product's microbiological shelf life is extended while the nutrient content and food texture remain unchanged. The packaged food is then refrigerated to maintain flavor quality. Shelf life of HPP foods is similar that resulting from thermal pasteurization.[22]

Innovation Point

Retort Packaging Retort packaging for poultry and fish products involves high-pressure processing (HPP), which inactivates bacteria and extends the product's shelf life.

Food Safety

As with all foods, pathogens are a potential problem with the production and processing of poultry and seafood.

Pathogens Common to Poultry

Poultry confinement creates an environment for pathogens to flourish if control measures are not taken. Limiting surface moisture of the confinement houses and providing potable water and pelletized feed are best practices to control growth of *Salmonella* and *Campylobacter* bacteria. Reducing the amount of feed prior to transport and slaughter decreases fecal material contamination of the carcass during processing.[23]

Salmonella Spp.

Poultry is considered a major source of *Salmonella*. *Salmonella* can be passed from bird to bird. It can also be passed from an infected hen's intestines to its eggs because fecal material contaminated with *Salmonella* can pass through the porous developing eggshell.[24] People who eat chicken or eggs contaminated with *Salmonella* can develop salmonellosis, a bacterial infection causing abdominal cramps, nausea, fever, and diarrhea.[25]

Clostridium Perfringens

Clostridium bacteria are present in soil. The bacterium produces spores dispersed by wind, which can then be dispersed on poultry and other meats. Consumption of improperly cooked or cooled poultry can cause foodborne illness. Symptoms of *Clostridium* infection include nausea, diarrhea, abdominal pain, and dehydration lasting 12 to 24 hours.[25]

Campylobacter Jejuni

Campylobacter jejuni spreads from bird to bird through contaminated water or infected feces. Poultry becomes contaminated at slaughter as the bacteria from the intestines come into contact the meat. *C. jejuni* also may be transmitted to the carcass during evisceration and defeathering.[18] It often is found in undercooked poultry. *Campylobacter* infections are characterized by symptoms of diarrhea, vomiting, fever, nausea, and abdominal pain lasting 2 to 10 days. Purchasing irradiated poultry and cooking poultry thoroughly can reduce the risk of infection.

Listeria Monocytogenes

Listeria monocytogenes is responsible for 20% of all foodborne illness fatalities. It causes 2,500 illnesses and 500 deaths annually. Growth media include soil, water, animal feed, and the intestinal tracts of animals. The bacteria can survive refrigeration temperatures as well as acidic, saline environments. The elderly, pregnant women, infants, and immune-compromised individuals are vulnerable to invasive-type listeriosis. The typical incubation period is 3 weeks. Symptoms range from nausea to persistent backache. Severe cases may result in meningitis, septicemia, encephalitis, and cervical infections of indefinite duration. *L. monocytogenes* has been traced to poultry deli meats and sausages and cooked and smoked seafood. The bacteria can persist in **biofilms**, aggregates of microorganisms in which cells adhere to each other, on processing equipment despite sanitation practices; therefore, the most effective measures of control are cooking to the appropriate temperature or pasteurization.[26]

biofilm A collection of microorganisms that form a surface-like lining.

Pathogens Common to Fish and Shellfish

Increased fish consumption has expanded the market for both domestic and imported fish products. Over 75% of fish consumed is imported.[27] The FDA inspects fish products at the port of entry, processing operations in countries exporting to the United States, and importer facilities. However, the use of antibiotics, vaccines, and feed additives in foreign countries may not be as strictly controlled as it is in the United States. Imported fish may have high levels of histamines from storage methods used while the ships are at sea. See **Special Topic 6.4** for more on the longer-term storage of fish for transportation purposes.

Salmonella Spp.

FDA studies show that *Salmonella* spp. is the most common contaminant of imported fish and fish products. Food safety practices such as Hazard Analysis and Critical Control Points (HACCP) techniques can be used to prevent *Salmonella* infection.[27]

Anisakis Simplex and Pseudoterranova Decipians

Anisakis simplex and *Pseudoterranova decipians* are parasitic roundworms found in raw or undercooked fish. *A. simplex* and *P. decipians* can be missed when preparing fish. Currently, no reliable method of detection is available. Symptoms of infection, including nausea, abdominal pain, and cramping, can appear 1 hour to 2 weeks after ingesting contaminated fish. The roundworms can live in the human stomach wall for several weeks or can be removed by forceps. *A. simplex* and *P. decipians* can be destroyed by freezing fish at 4°F (–16°C) or colder for at least 7 days. Cooking fish to at least 145°F (63°C) also kills the roundworms.[18]

Gastronomy Point

Boiled Shellfish Contrary to popular terminology such as "shrimp boil," shellfish such as shrimp and lobster are not "boiled" but simmered at 180°F (82°C).

Yersinia Intercolitica

Oysters may be contaminated with *Yersinia intercolitica*. *Y. intercolitica* can survive low temperatures and a pH below 4.5. Symptoms of illness from the bacteria can mimic appendicitis and persist for 2 weeks or more.

Special Topic 6.4

Fish Storage Principles and Products

Maria Belloso

Fish can be purchased fresh, frozen, canned, or cured. Fresh fish can be highly perishable and requires special attention and care in order to ensure freshness and reduce the risk of foodborne illness. The spoilage of fish flesh results from the action of enzymes, natural toxins, and contaminants. A number of techniques have been developed to decrease the deterioration rate of fish, thus preserving the quality of the fish as well as its shelf life.

Controlling Temperature

When fresh raw fish is properly frozen and then kept at a sufficiently low temperature, spoilage can be stopped almost entirely. The lower the holding temperature, the longer the fish can be stored safely. Fish must be kept at 32–40°F (0–4.4°C) when chilled and at 0°F (−17.8°C) or lower when frozen to avoid deterioration. The chill room should be equipped with a calibrated thermometer.

Depending on the type, fish can be stored in the freezer up to 9 months at an optimal temperature of −20°F (−29°C). Lean fish tend to last longer than fatty fish because the fish oils found in fat readily combine with oxygen, contributing to rancidity. Some of the enzymes normally present in fish muscle assist this reaction. Whole fresh fish can be stored by gently placing it on a bed of flaked ice. Each single layer of fish should be covered with a layer of ice.[1]

Limiting Water Activity

Water activity (a_w) is a measure of the availability of water in fish flesh. Water is required for microbial and enzymatic reactions. Preservation techniques such as drying, salting, smoking, and freeze-drying bind or remove water, thereby reducing the product's water activity.[2]

Reducing Oxygen Availability

Some bacteria responsible for spoilage require oxygen. Lipid oxidation also requires oxygen. Thus, reducing the oxygen around the fish will increase its shelf life. The amount of oxygen in the environment can be reduced through vacuum packaging or by controlling or modifying the atmosphere around the fish. Oxygen-limited storage is often combined with refrigeration for fish preservation.

Physical Methods

Methods such as ionization or microwave heating are used to inactivate microorganisms present in fish. Cooking or pasteurizing techniques often need to be combined with refrigeration to preserve fish products and to increase their shelf life. However, sterilized products are stable at room temperature and can be packaged in metal cans or retortable pouches before the heat treatment.[2]

Chemical Methods

Chemical preservation methods are designed to add antimicrobial agents to the fish or to decrease the pH of the fish muscle to levels that inhibit microbial growth and proliferation. The pH can be lowered through fermentation or through the addition of marinades or acids (e.g., acetic acid, citric acid, lactic acid) to fish products. Other preservatives include nitrites, sulfites, sorbates, and benzoates. Natural preservatives include essential oils.[3]

References

1 Brown AC. Fish and shellfish. In: *Understanding Food: Principles and Preparation.* 4th ed. Belmont, CA: Wadsworth; 2011.

2 Torry Research Station. Cold Storage of Frozen Fish. FAO Corporate Document Repository. Available at: http://www.fao.org/wairdocs/tan/x5907e/x5907e01.htm. Accessed November 30, 2011.

3 Food and Agriculture Organization of the United Nations, Fisheries and Aquaculture Department. Preservation Techniques. Available at: http://www.fao.org/fishery/topic/12322/en. Accessed November 30, 2011.

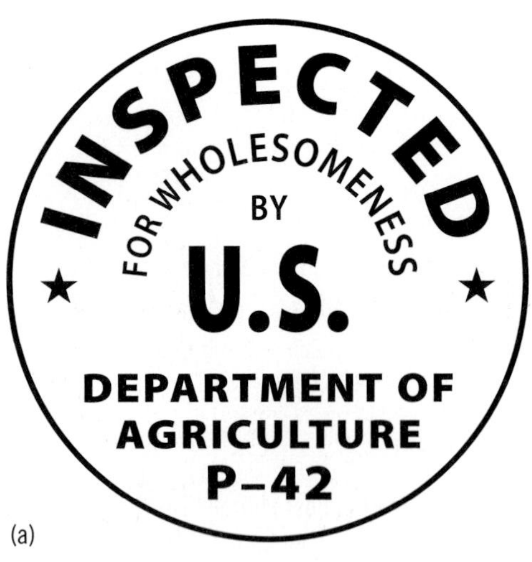

(a)

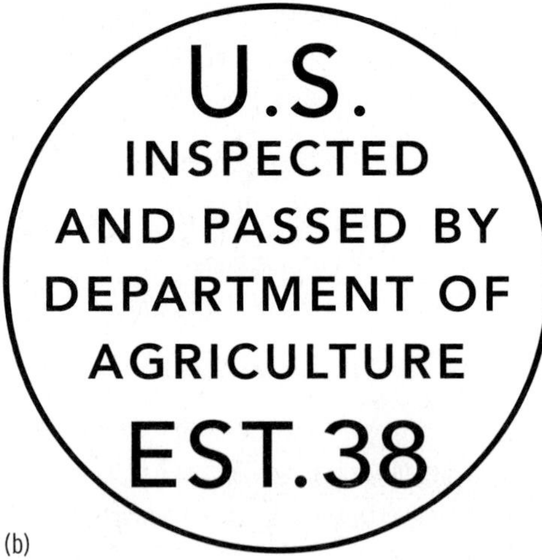

(b)

FIGURE 6.20 The FSIS, the public health agency of the USDA, inspects all raw and partially cooked poultry to ensure that it is safe, wholesome, and labeled correctly. Poultry that passes inspection is then marked with a purple stamp to indicate that it has passed the FSIS inspection. (a) Inspection stamp for raw poultry. (b) Inspection stamp for processed products.

Source: Reproduced from U.S. Department of Agriculture, Food Safety and Inspection Service. Inspection and Grading of Meat and Poultry: What Are the Differences? Available at: http://www.fsis.usda.gov/Factsheets/Inspection_&_Grading/index.asp. Accessed June 1, 2012.

Vibrio Vulnificus

Oysters and other shellfish can harbor *Vibrio vulnificus* bacteria. Shellfish from the Gulf of Mexico are frequently contaminated with *V.vulnificus*. Freezing does not destroy the bacteria. Symptoms of illness from *V. vulnificus* include fever, headache, chills, cramps, and diarrhea. Duration of the illness ranges from a day to several weeks.

Norovirus

Norovirus has been associated with oyster consumption. Freezing the contaminated shellfish or cooking it does not destroy the virus. Ingestion of contaminated shellfish results in viral gastroenteritis, an inflammation of the stomach and large and small intestines.

Hepatitis A

The hepatitis A virus is found on foods that are not heated prior to service, such as seafood, salads, and sandwiches. Good sanitation practices can control the spread of the virus.

Inspection and Grading of Poultry

The Poultry Products Inspection Act requires that raw poultry sold interstate, imported poultry, and poultry for foreign commerce be inspected by the USDA Food Safety and Inspection Service (FSIS). The 1968 Wholesome Poultry Products Act requires states to inspect poultry sold intrastate. A state's inspection program must be "at least equal to" the federal program. States may choose to end their poultry inspection program and let FSIS assume responsibility.

The USDA requires that raw or partially cooked poultry be labeled with safe-handling instructions to minimize the risk of microbial contamination. After passing inspection, the raw or partially cooked poultry is stamped with a round purple stamp made from vegetable dye (see **Figure 6.20**).

Grading of poultry is voluntary and the service is paid by the processor. The USDA's Agricultural Marketing Service (AMS) has licensed federal graders for poultry. The poultry is evaluated for conformity to normal shape and to confirm that it is fully fleshed and free of defects. The grader then gives the product a grade of A, B, or C. Grades are based on nationally uniform standards of quality. Wing tips, ground poultry, tails, necks, and giblets are not inspected for quality.

Grade A is the highest grade of poultry and the most common grade at the retail level. The product must be nearly free of defects such as feathers, bruises, and discolorations. It should have no broken bones or tears in the skin. To receive Grade A poultry must be fully fleshed and meaty (see **Figure 6.21**). Grades B and C poultry are usually in processed products such as ground, chopped, or cut up meat.[6]

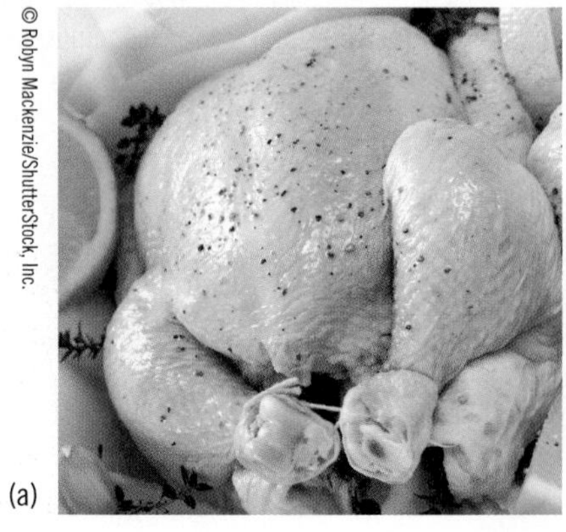

© Robyn Mackenzie/ShutterStock, Inc.

(a)

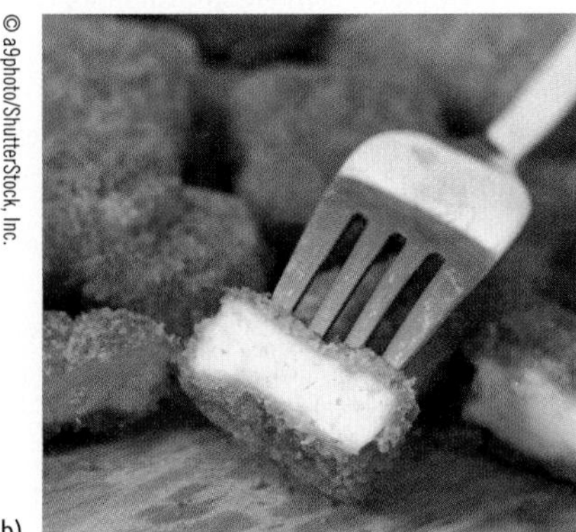

© a9photo/ShutterStock, Inc.

(b)

FIGURE 6.21 (a) The highest quality grade and the only one likely seen at retail level is Grade A. This grade offers the assurance that that the poultry products are free from bruises, discoloration, and features. It also means that no broken bones are present. For skin-on products, it assures that the skin is not torn and that there is a good covering of fat under the skin. (b) Grades B and C poultry are usually only used in highly processed products where the poultry is chopped, cut up, or ground. The grade of such products is usually not identified in the retail setting.

Inspection and Grading of Fish

Inspection and grading of fish are voluntary and are paid for by the processor. The National Marine Fisheries Service of the U.S. Department of Commerce conducts inspections of processing facilities. During an inspection, the fish are evaluated for wholesomeness and the facility is evaluated for its sanitation.

Inspected fish also may be graded. Grades are A, B, and Substandard. The quality standards are specific to each species. Fish and shellfish quality standards are based on flavor and odor and presence or absence of physical defects. Shellfish may only be harvested in waters certified by the U.S. Department of Commerce as meeting guidelines for safe levels of microorganisms or pollutants. See **Special Topic 6.5** for more about pollutants that may be found in fish.

Special Topic 6.5

Mercury and Polychlorinated Biphenyls in Fish

Bonnie Gerald, PhD, DTR

Mercury and polychlorinated biphenyls (PCBs) are chemicals that can accumulate in fish tissue. They have potentially toxic effects in people who consume the contaminated tissue. Mercury, a heavy metal, is naturally occurring in the environment; however, its levels may be amplified by industrial pollution. In saltwater, mercury changes to methylmercury, which fish ingest. The methylmercury then accumulates in their bodies. Fish higher up on the food chain—predators of smaller fish—are especially prone to accumulating high levels of methylmercury via a process called *bioaccumulation.* These fish include albacore tuna, swordfish, and king mackerel.

High levels of mercury in fish were first detected in 2004. Children and infants are particularly susceptible to mercury's harmful effects. Accumulated mercury in the bloodstream may take over 1 year to be eliminated from the body. Therefore, pregnant women, children, and women planning to become pregnant are advised not to consume fish with high mercury levels, including shark, swordfish, king mackerel, and tilefish. These populations should also eat no more than 12 ounces (two servings) of shrimp, canned light tuna, salmon, pollock, and catfish, or 6 ounces (one serving) of albacore tuna per week.[1,2] See the EPA website for the latest news on mercury levels in fish at www.epa.gov/mercury.

PCBs also may accumulate in fish at levels considered dangerous for human consumers. PCBs were manufactured from 1930 to 1977, when they were used in the production of electrical transformers, hydraulic fluid, lubricants, and carbonless paper. These chemicals are stable and nonflammable and have with high boiling points and electrical-insulating properties. PCBs have persisted in the environment because they are slow to break down, often settling in streambeds, lakes, and coastal sediments. Fish ingest the PCBs, which then accumulate in their fat tissue. Fatty predatory fish, such as bass, walleye, and white croaker, that live near industrial areas are likely to have the highest PCB concentrations. Human consumption of PCB-contaminated fish results in accumulation of PCBs in human fat tissue.

The EPA rates PCBs as "probable human carcinogens." The developing nervous systems of fetuses and young children are particularly susceptible to the harmful effects of PCBs. The risks to consumers can be reduced by removing any fat present on the fish before cooking and avoiding deep fat frying.[1] More information on fish advisories and environmental PCB issues is available at http://www.epa.gov/pcb/pubs/effects.html.

References

1 U.S. Food and Drug Administration and Environmental Protection Agency. What You Need to Know About Mercury in Fish and Shellfish. EPA-823-F04-009. 2009.

2 Environmental Protection Agency. Polychlorinated Biphenyls Update: Impact on Fish Advisories. Bigler J (ed.). U.S. EPA Fact Sheet. 2009.

Farm-to-Fork System

Farm-to-fork is an approach to safety that encompasses all aspects of food production through to distribution. Processes such as harvesting, storage, processing, packaging, sales, and consumption are the major parts of a farm-to-fork system.[28] Good agricultural practices (GAPs) such as clean water and feed help prevent the spread of microorganisms. The processed product stage is the point at which poultry and fish are most vulnerable to microbial contamination. Facilities can reduce the presence of foodborne illness–causing pathogens by using good manufacturing practices (GMPs), such as preventative maintenance and employee training. GMPs combined with a HACCP program will minimize risk of producing unsafe food.[18]

Chapter Review

Poultry and fish have been part of the human diet for thousands of years. They are excellent sources of protein and unsaturated fats. Fish is an especially good source of omega-3 fatty acids. Poultry are classified by age and sex; fish are classified by fat content, body shape, and habitat. Poultry younger than 6 months old can be cooked by moist or dry heat. Older birds are tougher and need moist heat to tenderize them. Fish have short muscle fibers and little connective tissue, thus requiring only short cooking periods.

Market demand for processed fish and poultry such as chicken nuggets, fish sticks, boneless skinless chicken, and fish fillets compared to consumption of whole birds and fish has increased since the mid-20th century. Most poultry are raised in confinement, although there has been a trend toward increased free-range pasturing. Fish may be wild caught or raised by aquaculture. Habitat destruction, overfishing, and pollution have significantly reduced populations of some fish species.

Inspection of poultry is mandatory. In contrast, inspection of fish is voluntary. Time and temperature abuse during poultry and fish preparation and cooking can result in foodborne illness. Using a farm-to-fork approach to safety can minimize the risk of producing unsafe food.

Learning Portfolio

Study Points

1. Fish is classified by its fat content and structure. Finfish are vertebrates characterized by having an internal skeleton, breathing through gills, and navigating by fins. Fish may live in saltwater or freshwater and may have flat or cylindrically shaped bodies. Flat fish have both eyes on the same side of the body and have an oval shape.
2. Fat content is one method of classification for fish. A fish is considered lean if a cooked serving has less than 5 total grams of fat. Lean fish include haddock, cod, catfish, and shrimp. A fatty fish has 5 to 10 grams of total fat per 3-ounce cooked portion. Fatty fish include mackerel, Atlantic salmon, and lake trout.
3. Poultry's nutrient profile is similar to red meat. A 3-ounce serving of skinless chicken breast has 140 calories and 3 grams fat compared to beef sirloin steak, which has 160 calories and 6 grams fat.
4. Fish have short muscle fibers called myotomes and little connective tissue. The myotomes are connected to thin sheets of connective tissue called myocomatta. The myocomatta composes about 3% of body weight compared to 15% of body weight for cattle. Fish muscle also contains myoglobin pigments.
5. Fish are good sources of protein, vitamins, and minerals. Although finfish and shellfish contain fat and cholesterol, their fat content is high in polyunsaturated fats. Long-chain, polyunsaturated omega-3–fatty acids are prevalent in fish.
6. Mechanically deboned chicken (MDC) is widely used in food products such as soup, nuggets, luncheon meats, and tenders. MDC may be further processed into comminuted meat.
7. Poultry confinement creates an environment for pathogens to flourish if control measures are not taken. Limiting surface moisture in the confinement houses and providing potable water and pelletized feed are best practices to control growth of *Salmonella* and *Campylobacter*.
8. The Poultry Products Inspection Act requires that raw poultry sold interstate, imported poultry, and poultry for foreign commerce is inspected by the Food Safety Inspection Service (FSIS). The 1968 Wholesome Poultry Products Act requires states to inspect poultry sold intrastate. If states do not chose to inspect poultry, then the federal government inspects poultry sold within the state's borders.
9. Grade A is the highest grade of poultry and the most common grade at the retail level. The product must be nearly free of defects such as feathers, bruises, and discolorations. There should be no broken bones or tears in the skin. To be designated as Grade A, poultry must be fully fleshed and meaty. Grades B and C poultry are typically used in processed products such as ground, chopped, or cut-up meat.
10. FDA studies indicate *Salmonella* is the most common contaminant of imported fish and fish products. Food safety practices such as HACCP can be effective in controlling *Salmonella*.

Issues for Class Discussion

1. Would it be possible for all large poultry operations to switch from raising chickens in confinement to raising free-range chickens?
2. Should more fish species be produced by aquaculture? Would this preserve fresh and saltwater environments from overfishing, or would more environmental damage occur?
3. Discuss the differences between preparing a whole chicken compared to using a precooked, frozen boneless skinless chicken breast. Think of as many resources needed to prepare both foods.

Key Terms

	page
aquaculture	207
biofilm	212
bivalve	199
cephalopod	199
comminution	210
crustacean	199
finfish	198
mollusk	199
omega-3 fatty acids	201
ratite	198
retort pouch	211
shellfish	199

4. Discuss the potential risks and benefits of consumption of raw fish or shellfish and consumption of partially cooked fish (i.e., "rare" or "medium.")
5. Producer associations for chicken, ostrich, and beef promote their product as "healthier" than other meats. Search online to investigate these claims to sort out the truth from hype.

Research Topics for Students

1. Sustainability and overfishing
2. Environmental impact of large poultry confinement operations
3. Poultry cooking methods that minimize cooking losses
4. Safety of imported fish
5. Nutrient comparison and safety comparison of free range, "cage free," and confined poultry
6. Active and passive packaging of fish and poultry
7. Ratite processing and marketing

References

1. Raj S. India (southern region). In: Edelstein S (ed.). *Food, Cuisine, and Cultural Competency*. Burlington, MA: Jones & Bartlett Learning; 2011.
2. McGee H. The chicken and the egg. In: *On Food and Cooking*, New York: Simon & Shuster; 2004.
3. Striffler S. Love that chicken! In: *Chicken: The Dangerous Transformation of America's Favorite Food*. New Haven, CT: Yale University Press; 2005.
4. Civitello L. The ancient agricultural revolution. In: *Cuisine and Culture: A History of Food and People*. New York: John Wiley & Sons; 2008.
5. AllCookingTips.com. Classification of Poultry. 2008. Available at: http://allcookingtips.com/2008/01/19/poultry-classification.
6. Food Safety and Inspection Service. Inspection and Grading of Meat and Poultry: What Are the Differences? 2008. Available at: http://www.fsis.usda.gov/factsheets/inspection_&_grading/index.asp.
7. Purdue University. Fin Fish. 2002. Available at: http://www.fourh.purdue.edu/foods/Fin%20fish.htm.
8. Brown A. Fish and shellfish. In: *Understanding Food: Principles and Preparation*. Belmont, CA: Thomson Wadsworth; 2008.
9. American Heart Association. Fish and Omega-3 Fatty Acids. 2011. Available at: http://www.heart.org/HEARTORG/GettingHealthy/NutritionCenter/HealthyDietGoals/Fish-and-Omega-3-Fatty-Acids_UCM_303248_Article.jsp. Accessed October 20, 2012.
10. American Heart Association. How Fish Is Cooked Affects Heart-Health Benefits of Omega-3 Fat. American Heart Association Meeting Report, Abstract 1404, Poster 2071. 2009. Available at: http://www.newsroom.heart.org/index.php?s=43&item.
11. Chung H, Nettleton JA, Lemaitre RN, et al. Frequency and type of seafood consumed influence plasma (n-3) fatty acid concentrations. *J Nutr.* 138(2008):2422–2427.
12. Putnam JJ, Allshouse JE. Nutrients. In: *Food Consumption, Prices, and Expenditures, 1970–1997*. Washington, DC: Economic Research Service; 1997.
13. Ballenger N, Blaylock J. Consumer-driven agriculture: Changing U.S. demographics influence eating habits. *Amber Waves.* 2003;1(2):28–33.
14. National Marine Fisheries Service. International Convention for the Conservation of Atlantic Tuna (Basic Instrument for the International Commission for the Conservation of Atlantic Tuna). 2010. Available at: http://www.nmfs.noaa.gov/ia/docs/international_agreements_2010.pdf.
15. Bedard M. Forecast: No Fish by 2050. Time for Aquaculture. 2011. Available at: http://www.takepart.com/article/2010/06/22/forecast-no-fish-2050-time-aquaculture. Accessed October 20, 2012.
16. Bedard M. Farmed Fish or Wild Caught: New Labels Are on the Way. 2011. Available at: http://www.takepart.com/article/2011/03/02/farmed-fish-or-wild-caught-new-labels-are-way. Accessed October 20, 2012.
17. Jacquet J, Pauly D. Seafood stewardship in crisis. *Nature.* 2010;467:28–29.
18. Dharhmarha V. A Focus on *Campylobacter Jejuni*. 2010. Available at: http://www.fsrio.nal.usda.gov/nal_web_fsrio/fsheet.php.
19. Ollinger M, MacDonald J, Madison M. Structural changes in U.S. chicken and turkey slaughter. In: *Poultry Demand Changes*, AER/787. Washington, DC: USDA Economic Research Service; 2001.
20. Murano P. Understanding food processing and preservation: Animal products. In: *Understanding Food Science and Technology*. Belmont, CA: Wadsworth/Thomson Learning; 2003.
21. Galic K, Scetar M, Kurek M. The benefits of processing and packaging. *Trends Food Sci Tech.* 2011;22:127–137.
22. Ramaswamy R, Balasubramaniam VR, Kalatunc M. High-Pressure Processing. Fact Sheet for Food Processors. The Ohio State University Extension Fact Sheet. FSE-1-04. 2004.
23. Food Safety Inspection Service (FSIS). *Compliance Guideline for Controlling Salmonella and Campylobacter in Poultry.* 3rd ed. 2010. Available at: http://www.fsis.usda.gov/compliance_guide_controlling_salmonella_poultry.pdf.
24. Dharmarha V. A Focus on Salmonella—Updated Version. 2010. Available at: http://fsrio.nal.usda.gov/nal_webfsrio/fsheet.php?id=2237printer=1.
25. Edelstein S, Gerald B, Crutchley T, Gunderson C. Foodborne illness causing pathogens. In: *Food and Nutrition at Risk in America.* Sudbury, MA: Jones and Bartlett Publishers; 2009.
26. Dharhmarha V, Smith T. A Focus on *Listeria Monocytogenes*. 2008. Available at: http://www.fsrio.nal.usda.gov/nal_web_fsriofact_sheet.
27. Allhouse J, Buzby J, Harvey D, Zorn D. Food safety and trade. Agriculture Information Bulletin 789-7. Washington, DC: USDA/Economic Research Service; 2004.
28. Domenich E, Esriche I, Yen GC. Quantification of risks to consumers' health and to companies' incomes due to failures in food safety. *Food Control.* 2007;18:1419–1427.

CHAPTER 7

Milk and Dairy Products

Toby Amidor, MS, RD, CDN

Chapter Objectives

THE STUDENT WILL BE EMPOWERED TO:

- Summarize the history of dairy products and their influence on various cultures.
- Describe the physical and chemical properties of milk, with particular reference to the milk proteins casein and whey.
- Explain the process and purpose of both pasteurization and homogenization.
- Define the various types of milk and dairy products.
- Summarize the basics of how to shop for, select, and cook with various milk and dairy products.
- Describe the benefits of milk with regard to the nutrients it provides and its impact on human health.
- Explain some of the environmental concerns surrounding the dairy industry, and summarize potential green solutions.
- Discuss various forms of food technology and dairy substitutes that are used in the dairy industry.
- List common pathogens of milk, and explain the concerns about raw milk.
- Summarize the grading systems used for butter and milk.
- Explain lactose intolerance, and describe strategies to cope with it.

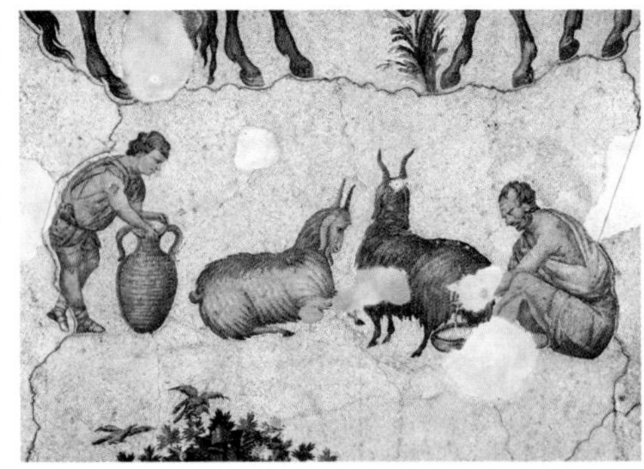

FIGURE 7.1 Because of their small size and ease of pasturing, goats were one of the earliest animals to be domesticated. Humans have been using the milk products of goats for approximately 10,000 years.

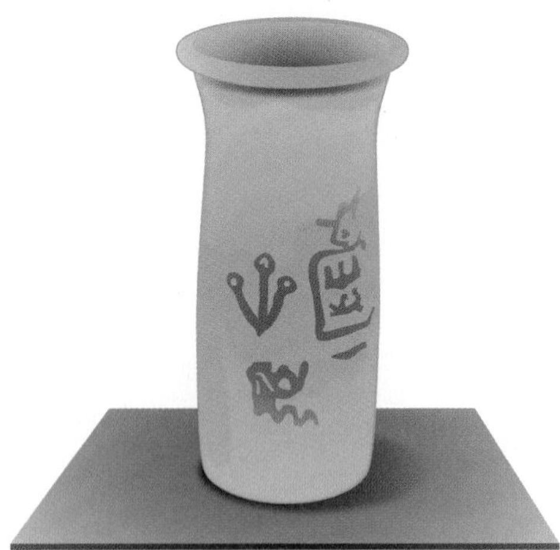

FIGURE 7.2 Archaeological evidence, such as this cylindrical jar from ancient Egypt, suggests that the ancient Egyptians bred domesticated animals for their milk, which they then processed into butter and cheese that would last longer in storage.

Historical and Cultural Significance

It is the biological nature of mammals to consume their mother's milk as their first food—humans included. One of the defining characteristics of mammals is that they nurse their young. Humans first domesticated animals for their meat and skin, and it is thought that humans began drinking the milk of animals soon after animals were domesticated. Archeological evidence suggests that sheep and goat's milk were the first to be consumed, around 11,000 and 9,500 years ago, respectively (see **Figure 7.1**).[1] Cattle, domesticated about 8,500 years ago, were less manageable and tougher to milk than the smaller animals. Archeological evidence of cylindrical jars in the First Dynasty tombs of Abydos suggest that the ancient Egyptians consumed milk obtained from domesticated animals (e.g., cattle, sheep, goats) and turned it into butter and cheese (see **Figure 7.2**). The early diet of the Phoenicians and the Carthaginians also included milk from goats, sheep, and cattle.[1]

In early Europe, milk and dairy products were an important part of the diet, but there were regional differences as to which forms were consumed. For example, cheese was very popular in Greece and Rome, whereas fresh milk and butter were not.[2] In northern Europe, fresh milk and butter were preferred over cheese. Some of these preferences were based on environmental factors. For instance, in the Mediterranean region fresh milk and butter would have spoiled quickly due to the hot climate, and thus were not a practical food source. In contrast, the cooler temperatures in northern Europe made it possible to store such items for longer periods of time.[2]

The adventurer Marco Polo traveled to and from China between 1271 and 1295 and wrote a book about his experiences.[2] He observed the nomadic Tartars creating butter from horse milk and drying the milk into a hard paste. Tartars also fermented milk to create *koumiss*, a beverage similar to what the people of the Balkans had been making for centuries, a sour beverage called *kefir*.

From the Middle Ages through the eighteenth century, changes in the handling of milk slowly evolved. Historically, milking, churning, and cheese making were all done by hand and were almost always performed by women.[2] The production of cheese, yogurt, and other fermented products was not well controlled, and microbes from the air or from previous batches commonly colonized the milk. Milk is seldom mentioned in nineteenth-century sources, and references to it rarely appear in old ledgers of working-class household budgets. Due to the fact that milk was so difficult to preserve, sales were confined to small farming villages. However, cheese became a commodity in national and international trade. Historians think that in France cheese consumption quadrupled within a century and a half—from 4.4 pounds per person per year between 1815 to 1824 to 23.3 pounds per person per year between 1960 and 1964.[3]

In North America, dairy products were unheard of until the arrival of Europeans. The European colonists established the first herd of dairy cows around 1625. The early American farmers had fresh cow's milk, but city dwellers usually consumed watered-down, disease-ridden milk that was typically hauled through the streets in open containers by the local cowmen.[3]

With the arrival of railroads and the invention of refrigeration, the Industrial Revolution changed the way milk was produced and transported, making it available to the masses. Increased demand for fresh milk and dairy products led to the creation of milking machines and automatic churners in the 1830s; specialized cheese factories in the 1850s; and margarine, which kept longer than butter, in the 1870s. By 1860, the first factory for canned milk had been built in New York by Gail Borden.[3] The milk was not very good, but it gained in popularity when the Civil War broke out in 1861. By 1900, purified bacterial cheese cultures allowed for better control of the cheese-making process, which improved the quality of cheese. By the mid-1920s, "vitamania" hit the nation. Advertisers, to help boost sales of processed foods, heralded the benefits of vitamins, which were invisible, weightless, and tasteless and could be added to a variety of foods. This was especially true for the dairy industry, which added vitamin D to canned milk. Vitamin D was soon added to butter and fresh milk as well.[2]

Between 1935 and 1938, consumption of dairy products was highest (in descending order) in Switzerland, Sweden, Ireland, Norway, Australia, the Netherlands, Denmark, Austria, the United States, and Germany. Dairy consumption was lowest (in descending order) in Greece, Italy, Turkey, Spain, and Portugal. Since the late eighteenth century, the image of milk had changed from a beverage fit for an infant to one that was good for adults, too.[3]

Physical and Chemical Properties

Cow's milk is composed of various molecules, including milk fat, proteins, salts, sugars, vitamins, and water. Cow's milk includes salts of sodium, potassium, magnesium, calcium, chloride, phosphate, sulfate, and citrate. It has a pH between 6.5 and 6.7, making it slightly acidic.[5] A number of different vitamins are found in milk, including vitamins C and A and riboflavin. Vitamin C is found in minimal quantities. The fat-soluble vitamin A and carotene (the vitamin A precursor) travel in the fat globules and give milk its buttery, yellowish color. Riboflavin has a greenish color and can sometimes be seen in nonfat (skim) milk and in the whey that separates during cheese making.[5] **Lactose**, the sugar found in milk, is not very soluble in water. Because of its relative insolubility, it crystallizes easily, aiding in the production of items such as ice cream and condensed milk.[6]

The flavor of milk is due to the mildly sweet lactose sugar, salts, fatty acids, and sulfur compounds. Sour or other undesirable flavors can result from the environment in which the cow was raised, especially if the air was foul or if the feed was contaminated. An overgrowth of bacteria that produce lactic acid can result in sour milk.[7] The presence of pathogenic microorganisms also can cause stale, bitter, or vomit-like off flavors.[7]

Milk fat has a multitude of functions, including carrying the fat-soluble vitamins and essential fatty acids. It also contributes to milk's texture, mouth feel, and taste. About half the calories of milk are found in the fat. When fresh milk stands for a while, the fat begins to rise and form a layer at the top, a process called **creaming**. The fat rises because it is lighter than water.[1]

Casein and Whey

The two main groups of proteins found in milk are curds and whey.[3] They can be differentiated by how they react with the acids and enzymes used in cheese making. The curd protein, known as **casein**, consists of various components, including calcium and phosphate ions that are found in bundles about one-tenth of a micron (approximately a few millionths of an inch) in diameter. These miniscule bundles are known as micelles. Together with the fat globules, the micelles help give milk its whitish, opaque color by deflecting light as it passes through the liquid. A protein subunit within the casein keeps the micelles separated. When milk is exposed to rennin, this protein subunit is removed from the casein micelles, and they react with the free calcium ions. This reaction enables the micelles to clump together, helping to form **curd**, which is then treated to make cheese (see **Figure 7.3**). The process of casein clumping, or coagulation, also is called **curdling**.[3]

lactose Milk sugar composed of glucose and galactose.

creaming The process by which milk fat begins to rise and form a layer at the top when fresh milk stands for a while

casein The main protein found in milk. Under certain conditions it coagulates, forming clumps; this is a key step in making cheese.

curd The semisolid portion created when milk coagulates.

curdling The process by which milk separates into its solid and liquid components, typically caused by overcooking, high heat, or the presence of acids or salt.

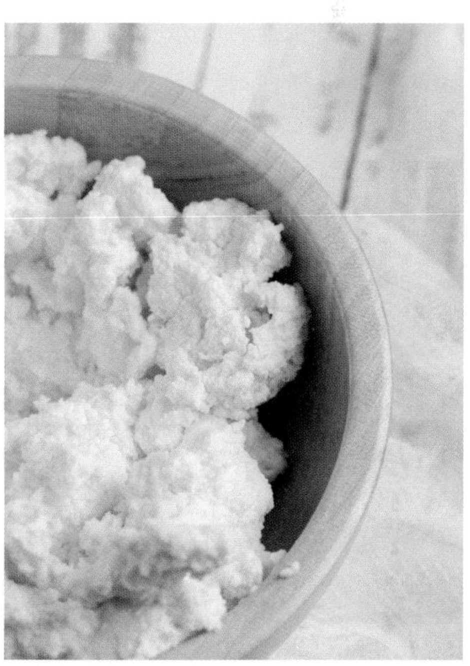

FIGURE 7.3 A variety of products are derived from curd, including cottage cheese and Indian paneer. In parts of Quebec, Canada, a dish called poutine is eaten—cheese curds on french fries topped with gravy.

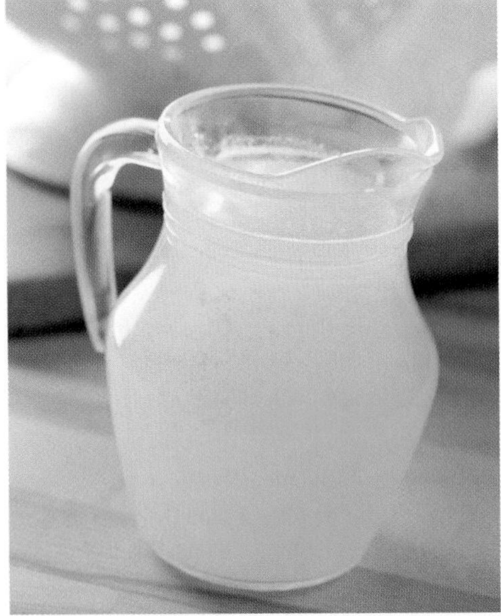

FIGURE 7.4 Whey is found in the liquid part of curdled milk. Whey is used in the production of ricotta cheese. It also is used as a food additive in baked goods and animal feed.

pasteurization The process of heating a food or beverage to a high enough temperature to destroy harmful pathogenic bacteria.

homogenization A process whereby the fat globules in milk are reduced in size and evenly distributed throughout the liquid.

whey The liquid portion of coagulated (curdled) milk.

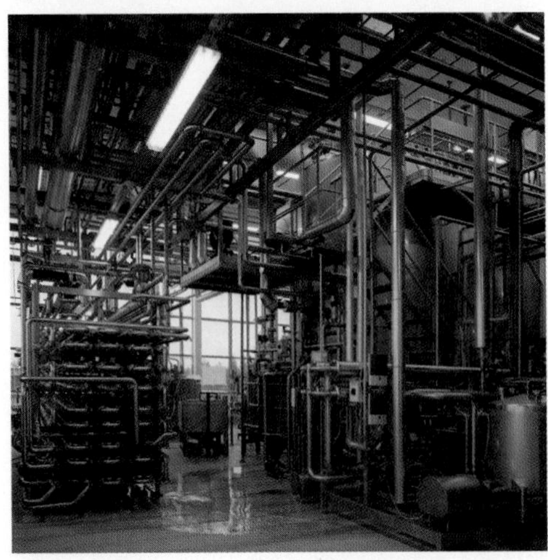

FIGURE 7.5 In the industrial pasteurization process used for dairy products, milk is forced between heated metal plates to a temperatures of 161°F (72°C) for 15 to 20 seconds. This heating destroys pathogenic bacteria without changing the nutritional quality of milk or causing the milk to curdle.

Casein also can coagulate without the removal of the protein subunit when exposed to acids, salt, or heat. For example, milk normally has a pH of around 6.5, but if the acidity is increased to a pH of 5.3 by the addition of lactic acid (produced by some bacteria), the milk will curdle.[3] The increased acidity causes the micelles to lose their negative charge and stop repelling one another, and curdling is the result. Heat alone will not usually cause milk to curdle, but if a small amount of acid or salt is present, too, then curdling may occur.

The milk proteins found in the liquid portion of curdled milk are called **whey** (see **Figure 7.4**). Unlike casein, whey is very resistant to coagulation and denaturation. A pH of 4.6 is needed for whey to coagulate, and it can sustain temperatures close to boiling (212°F/100°C) without denaturing.[3] Slight heat, however, does affect the composition of whey. Whey contains lactoglobulin, which includes sulfur atoms; when a temperature of 165°F (73.8°C) is reached, the sulfur atoms react with surrounding hydrogen atoms. The result is hydrogen sulfide (H_2S), a gas released in small quantities during cooking that contributes to the cooked aroma of many foods. At around this same temperature, the lactoglobulin unfolds into a form that interferes with the coagulation of casein micelles, which results in a slowing of clotting. The result is a final product with a softer curd.[3]

Pasteurization

Milk spoils quickly, and it can transmit diseases such as tuberculosis. The French scientist Louis Pasteur developed a heat treatment (originally for beer and wine) to prevent spoilage of foods and beverages.[8] **Pasteurization** is the process of heating a food or beverage to a high enough temperature to destroy pathogenic bacteria. Another benefit of pasteurization is the destruction of enzymes that cause spoilage, resulting in a longer shelf life. Pasteurization was first applied to milk at the turn of the nineteenth century, and by the 1940s all states required that milk undergo this process. Today, all grade A milk is required by law to be pasteurized before being sold. Milk is pasteurized by heating it to a temperature of 161°F (72°C) for 15 to 20 seconds (see **Figure 7.5**).[2,8] Note that the nutritional quality of milk is not destroyed by the pasteurization process.

Homogenization

As described earlier, when fresh milk is allowed to stand it separates naturally in a process called creaming: the fat rises to the top of the liquid and forms cream. **Homogenization** was developed around the turn of the nineteenth century to prevent creaming.[2] In this process, the fat globules are reduced in size and evenly distributed throughout the liquid, which prevents the fat globules from clumping and rising to the top (see **Figure 7.6**). Homogenized milk is whiter and has a more uniform texture than raw (unprocessed) milk; however, it is less stable to heat and is more sensitive to spoilage from light.[2]

Storage and Cooking

Milk is a highly perishable product. Even top-quality pasteurized milk contains tens of millions of bacteria per half-gallon; it must be refrigerated properly or spoilage results. Milk reacts upon exposure to sunlight, heat, and acidity. Sunlight can alter the flavor of milk, either by direct or indirect exposure. With enough exposure to direct sunlight, milk develops a cabbage-like or burnt flavor as a result of a reaction between riboflavin and the amino acid methionine. Because milk is so easily affected by sunlight, clear glass or plastic containers of milk should be kept in a dark storage area.[9] See **Table 7.1** for storage guidelines for milk and other dairy products.

During cooking, the casein proteins may curdle from the addition heat, which can cause issues during the cooking of soups and sauces. To prevent curdling, use fresh milk and carefully control the heat level of the burner.[3]

When cooking milk, a skin may form on the surface. This skin is a combination of casein and calcium. The skin results as water evaporates from the milk, leaving concentrated protein at the top. Unfortunately, skimming the skin results in the removal of the majority of nutrients found in milk. To minimize skin formation, cover the pan when cooking or whip up a little foam (like for hot chocolate) to slow down evaporation.[9]

Scorching (or burning) of milk occurs when casein micelles and whey protein drop to the bottom of the pan, stick, and burn. This easily occurs when heating up milk; the best way to prevent scorching is to use a medium-to-low flame or a double broiler.

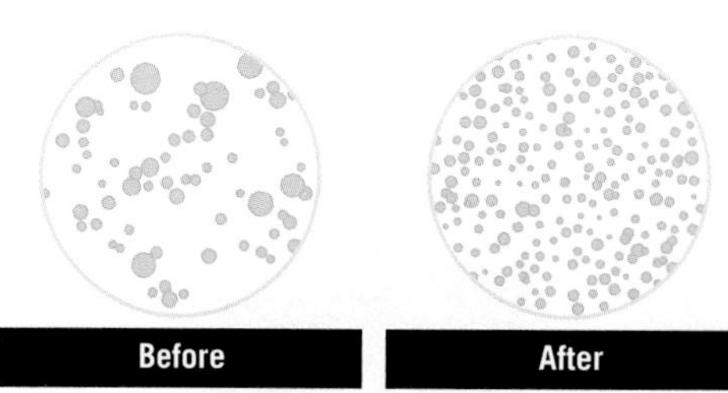

FIGURE 7.6 To produce a consistent, stable product, the milk industry uses homogenization. In this process, the milk from numerous herds or dairies is combined and then forced through small holes. This process decreases variation among milk from different sources and delays the separation of the cream from the milk

scorching Burning of milk that occurs when casein micelles and whey protein drop to the bottom of the pan, stick, and burn.

Milk and Dairy Products

A number of milk and dairy products are available on the market today. Items range from a variety of processed milks to cheeses and yogurts.

TABLE 7.1
Storage Guidelines for Milk and Dairy Products

Food	Recommended Storage Temperatures	General Storage Guidelines
Fresh milk	Keep refrigerated at or below 41°F (5°C).	Keep milk in a closed container to prevent odors and flavors from being absorbed.
Canned, aseptically packaged and dry milk powders	Store in pantry (50–70°F; 10–21°C) until opened. Then store in the refrigerator at or below 41°F (5°C).	Do not store in the original container once opened.
Ultra-pasteurized cream	Keep refrigerated at or below 41°F (5°C).	Store for up to 6 to 8 weeks. Do not freeze unwhipped cream. Keep cream away from strong odors and flavors to prevent them from being absorbed and/or affecting the cream's flavor.
Cultured dairy products (i.e., buttermilk, sour cream, crème fraîche, yogurt)	Keep refrigerated at or below 41°F (5°C).	If held at proper temperatures, sour cream can last up to 4 weeks, yogurt up to 3 weeks, and buttermilk up to 2 weeks. Do not freeze cultured dairy products; however, dishes prepared with these ingredients typically can be frozen.
Butter	Store in refrigerator at 32°–35°F (0°–2°C). Unsalted butter keeps best if frozen at 0°F (–18°C) until used.	Due to its high fat content, butter is more prone to rancidity (spoilage) than other dairy products and can develop a strong, bitter taste if not stored properly. Wrap well before storing. Unsalted butter will keep for up to 9 months in the freezer.
Cheese	Most can be stored in the refrigerator at or below 41°F (5°C).	Wrap well to prevent odors and loss of moisture. Keep firm cheeses for several weeks and fresh cheeses for 7 to 10 days. Do not freeze.
Ice cream	Store in freezer between –10°F and 0°F (–23°C to –18°C).	Store in covered container to prevent odors and large crystals from forming.

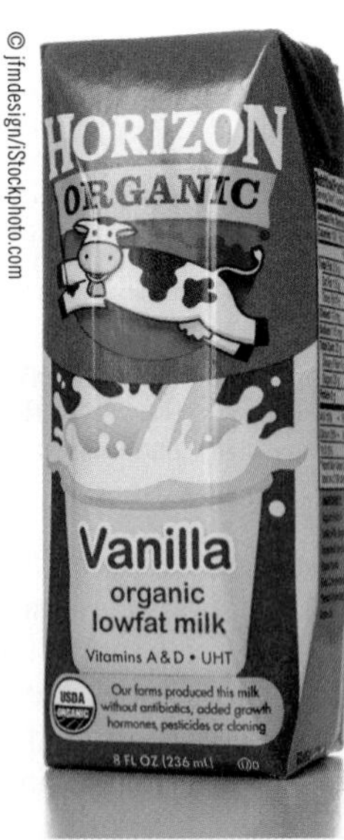

© jfmdesign/iStockphoto.com

Milk

Cow's milk is a popular beverage and is used in many recipes. Several types of milk with varying amounts of milk fat (see **Table 7.2**) can be found on the market:[5]

- *Whole milk*: Milk as it comes from the cow is called **whole milk**. It is composed of water (88%), milk fat (3.5%), and other milk solids (8.5%), including proteins, lactose, and minerals.
- *Reduced-fat milk*: Milk fat rises naturally to the top of nonhomogenized milk. Therefore, to reduce its fat content, whole milk is processed in a centrifuge to remove some or all of the milk fat. **Reduced-fat milk** contains 2% milk fat.
- *Low-fat milk*: Milk containing 1% milk fat is called **low-fat milk**.
- *Nonfat milk*: Also referred to as skim milk or fat-free milk, **nonfat milk** has as much of the milk fat is removed as possible. In order to be labeled as nonfat, it must contain less than 0.5% milk fat.

whole milk Milk as it comes from the cow; composed of water (88%), milk fat (3.5%), and other milk solids (8.5%), such as protein, lactose, and minerals.

reduced-fat milk Milk in which some of the fat has been removed; contains 2% milk fat.

low-fat milk Milk in which some of the fat has been removed; contains 1% milk fat.

nonfat milk Also referred to as skim milk and fat-free milk, this milk has as much of the milk fat removed as possible. In order to be labeled as nonfat, it must contain less than 0.5% milk fat.

cream A rich, liquid form of milk that contains at least 18% milk fat. It is more viscous than milk and is an off-white or yellowish color.

half and half A combination of cream and whole milk with more than 18%, but less than 30%, milk fat.

light cream Cream containing more than 18%, but less than 30%, milk fat; also called table cream or coffee cream.

whipping cream Cream with enough fat content to be whipped into a foam; it comes in two varieties: light whipping cream, which contains between 30% to 36% milk fat and is used in ice cream and as a thickener in soups and sauces, and heavy cream, which is better for whipping and contains at least 36% milk fat.

Cream

Cream is a rich, liquid form of milk in which the fat globules are more concentrated; it contains at least 18% fat (see Table 7.2). The proportion of fat determines the cream's consistency and versatility. Cream is richer than milk, with a smoother texture and an ivory or yellowish color. It is processed into various products:[5]

- *Half and half*: A mixture of equal parts cream and whole milk, **half and half** contains 18–30% milk fat. It is typically used in coffee or cereal. Half and half does not contain enough fat that to be whipped into foam.
- *Light cream*: Also called coffee cream or table cream, **light cream** typically contains about 20% milk fat and is used in coffee, baked goods, and soups.
- *Whipping cream*: The thickest cream is called **whipping cream** because it can be whipped into foam and used to garnish desserts or to add flavor and lightness to custards and mousses. Light whipping cream contains 30–36% milk fat. It is traditionally used as a thickener in soups and sauces and for making ice cream. It can be whipped but not as readily as heavy whipping cream, or heavy cream, the richest cream readily available. Heavy cream contains at least 36% milk fat and is used to thicken sauces and for making desserts. Due to the higher fat content, it whips up easily and holds its whipped texture longer than light whipping cream.

Cultured Dairy Products

To create cultured dairy products, specific bacterial cultures are added to fluid milk. The bacteria convert the lactose into lactic acid, which produces a tangy flavor and velvety consistency. The lactic acid produced also helps protect the product against unwanted growth of pathogens. The following are some of the more popular cultured dairy products:[5]

- *Buttermilk*: Originally, buttermilk was the liquid that remained when fresh cream was churned into butter, hence the name. Today,

TABLE 7.2
Percent Milk Fat in Various Forms of Milk and Cream

Milk or Dairy Product	Percent Milk Fat
Whole milk	3.5%
Reduced-fat milk	2.0%
Low-fat milk	1.0%
Nonfat milk	Less than 0.5%
Half and half	18–30%
Light cream, coffee cream, and table cream	18–30%
Whipping cream (light whipping cream)	30–36%
Heavy cream (heavy whipping cream)	At least 36%

buttermilk is produced by adding a harmless bacterial culture called *Streptococcus lactis* to fresh, pasteurized low-fat or nonfat milk (see **Figure 7.7**). Low-fat buttermilk is available in many markets across the United States. Buttermilk is traditionally used in baked goods (e.g., biscuits), in pancakes, or as a beverage. It also can be used as a marinade for lean meats such as chicken and fish.

- *Sour cream*: Adding a harmless culture (the same as in buttermilk) to pasteurized, homogenized light cream results in a tangy, white, gel-textured product called **sour cream** (see **Figure 7.8**). It is used in baked goods and as a condiment. Regular sour cream has a milk fat content no less than 18%. Light sour cream contains around 40% less fat than the regular version due to the fact that it is made with half and half. Nonfat sour cream also is available; it is thickened with stabilizers.
- *Crème fraîche*: This cultured dairy product made from unpasteurized cream and bacteria is popular in French cuisine.[3] **Crème fraîche** is thinner and richer than sour cream but has a similarly tart and tangy flavor (see **Figure 7.9**). The Americanized version of crème fraîche is made from pasteurized cream; buttermilk and sour cream are added to supply the necessary fermenting agents. Crème fraîche is sold in specialty markets around the United States, or you can make your own (see **Table 7.3**).
- *Yogurt*: Adding cultures of the bacteria *Lactobacillus bulgaricus* and *Streptococcus thermophiles* to milk produces **yogurt** (see **Figure 7.10**).[3] The bacteria consume the lactose as an energy source and release lactic acid as a result. The result is a creamy product with a slightly tart aftertaste. Plain yogurt is made from whole, low-fat, or nonfat milk without adding flavors (such as fruit or sugar). Flavored yogurt contains added sugar and either natural fruit and/or artificial flavorings. Some flavored yogurts have gelatin and stabilizers added in order to give them a thicker, custard-like texture. Fruit-flavored yogurts can have fruit at the bottom or have the fruit already mixed in (also known as Swiss-style). Yogurt is labeled to indicate the type of milk used.

buttermilk A cultured dairy product made by adding a harmless bacterial culture to fresh, pasteurized low-fat or nonfat milk. Once heated, lactic acid is produced, resulting in a liquid with a thick texture and tangy flavor.

sour cream A cultured dairy product made by adding a harmless bacterial culture to pasteurized, homogenized light cream. Sour cream has a milk fat content no less than 18%.

crème fraîche A thin sour cream made from unpasteurized cream and bacteria that is popular in French cuisine.

yogurt A cultured dairy product made by combining bacterial cultures to milk; it is creamy and has a slightly tart aftertaste.

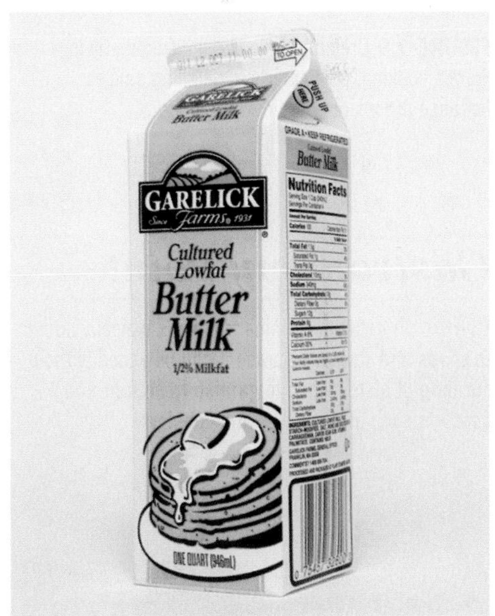

FIGURE 7.7 Why is buttermilk so tart? During the fermentation process, lactic acid is produced. This decreases the acidity of the liquid, resulting in the tart taste of buttermilk.

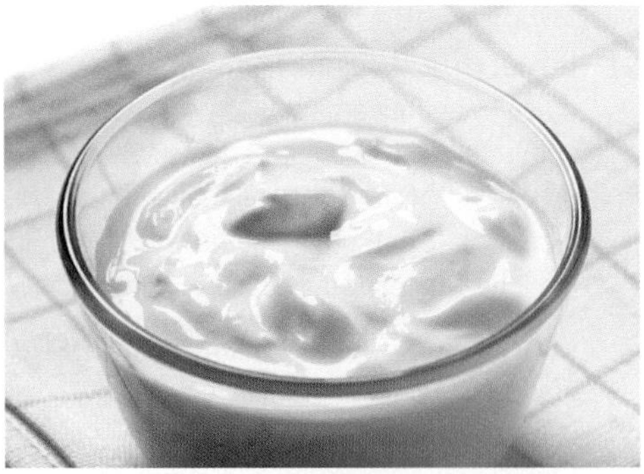

FIGURE 7.8 The term *souring* refers to the production of lactic acid by bacterial fermentation, thus the name *sour cream*. Sour cream is actually not very sour tasting.

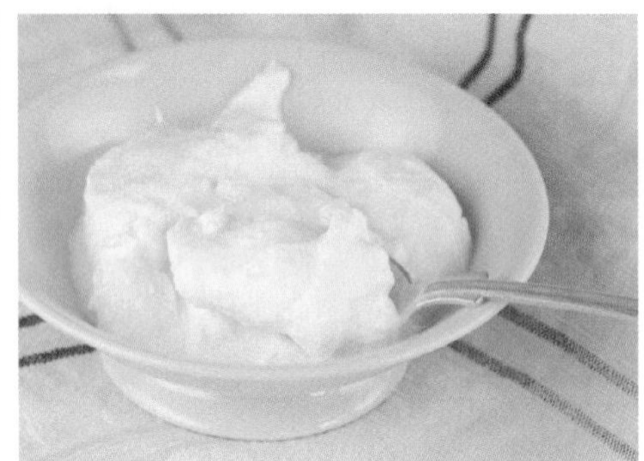

FIGURE 7.9 Crème fraîche is used frequently in French cooking, particularly in finishing sauces because it does not curdle when heated.

TABLE 7.3
Make Your Own Crème Fraîche

Ingredients	
1 cup whipping cream	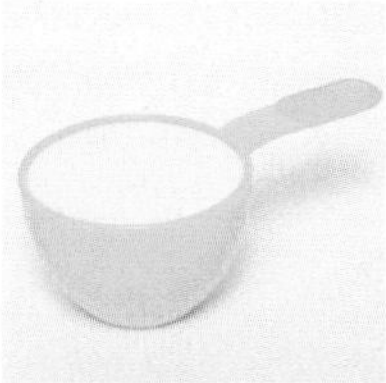
2 tablespoons buttermilk	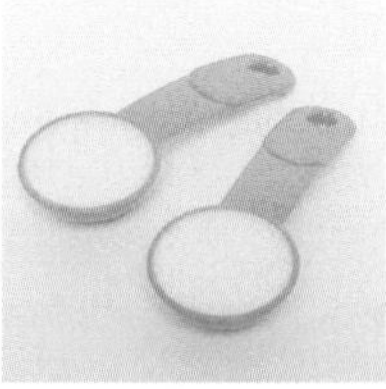
Procedure	
In a small glass container combine the whipping cream and buttermilk.	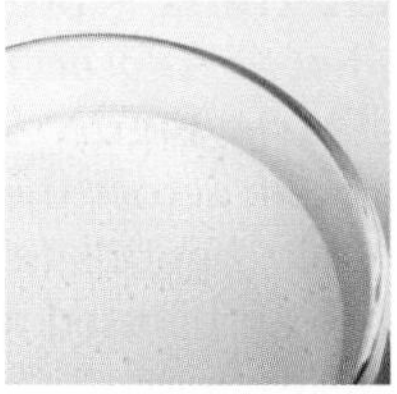
Cover the mixture and it let stand at room temperature for 8 to 24 hours or until very thick. Stir well, cover, and refrigerate for up to 10 days.	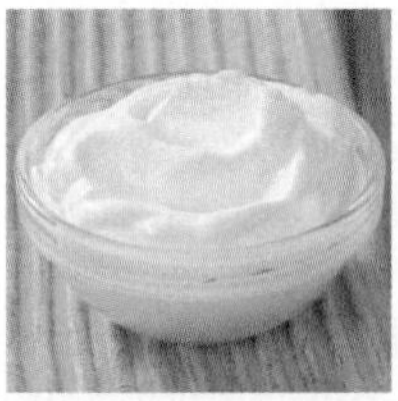

Gastronomy Point

Crème Fraîche Crème fraîche is typically added to soups and sauces because it can be added without curdling. It also is used to garnish fresh fruit and desserts such as puddings and cobblers.

butter A milk product made by churning cream until it reaches a semisolid state.

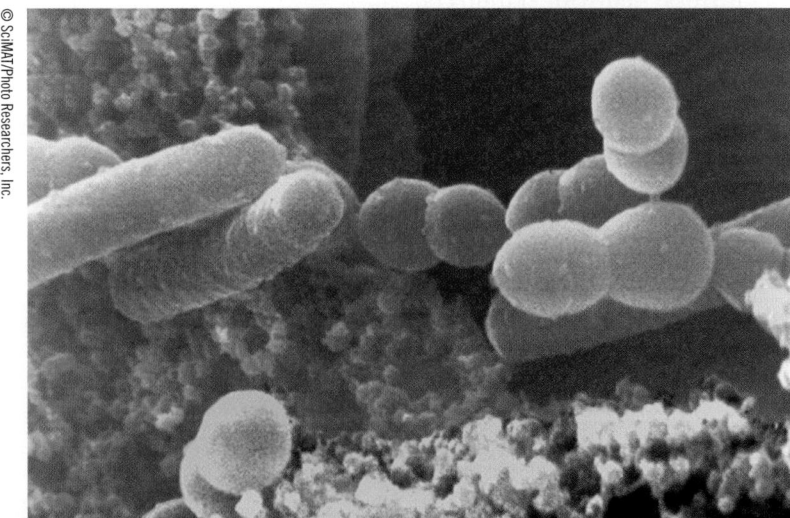

FIGURE 7.10 *Lactobacillus bulgaricus* is one of several bacteria used for the production of yogurt. It is a gram-positive rod-shaped bacteria that may appear long and filamentous. It is regarded as acidophilic because it requires a low pH (between 5.4 and 4.6) to grow effectively. *Streptococcus thermophilus* is a gram-positive bacteria used in the production of yogurt. Many of the yogurts sold in grocery stores today do not contain many live cultures of *S. thermophilus* because pasteurization destroys these beneficial organisms. However, by law *S. thermophilus* must be present in yogurt.

Butter

Butter is made by churning cream until it reaches a semisolid state (see **Figure 7.11** and **Figure 7.12**). By law, it must contain at least 80% milk fat, no more than 16% water, and 2–4% milk solids. Butter is solid when refrigerated and softens at room temperature. It melts into a liquid form at 93°F (33°C) and reaches its smoke point at 260°F (127°C). Several styles of butter are available:[5]

- *Salted butter*: This form of butter has up to 2.5% salt added. The salt adds flavor and also acts as a preservative.
- *Unsalted butter*: As the name implies, unsalted butter does not have salt added. Typically used for baking and as a condiment, unsalted butter has a shorter shelf life than its salted counterpart and can oftentimes be found in the freezer section in the local market.
- *European-style butter*: This form of butter typically contains 82–86% milk fat and has little or no added salt. Traditionally, it is churned from cultured cream, which produces a more intense, buttery flavor. It can be used in place of regular butter in baking and cooking.
- *Whipped butter*: Available salted or unsalted, whipped butter has air beaten into it to increase its volume so that it has a more spreadable consistency when cold. The addition of air also makes it turn rancid more quickly than regular butter, thus decreasing its shelf life.
- *Light or reduced-calorie butter*: Containing about half the fat of regular butter through the addition of water, skim milk, and gelatin, light or reduced-calorie butter is used as a spread. It should not be used for cooking because it does not hold up well during frying and baking.

Cheese

Although a multitude of different kinds of cheeses are available with different flavors, aromas, ages, and textures, all types of cheese are produced in a similar manner. Most cheese begins as milk, typically from a sheep, goat, or cow. The milk protein casein is then coagulated by the addition

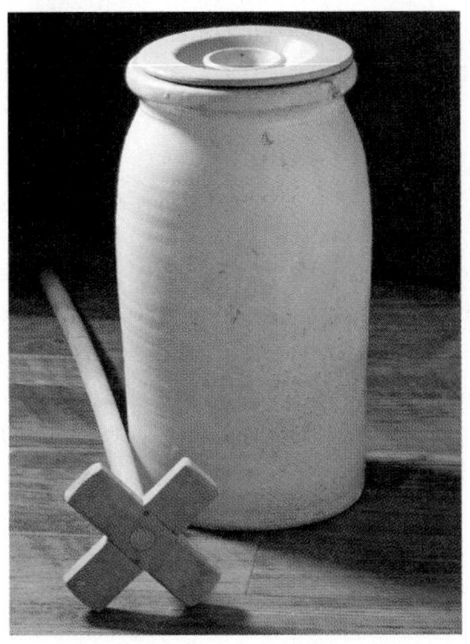

FIGURE 7.11 Until the Industrial Revolution, butter churns were basically barrels with plungers. The plunger was moved by hand to agitate the cream inside the barrel until butter formed.

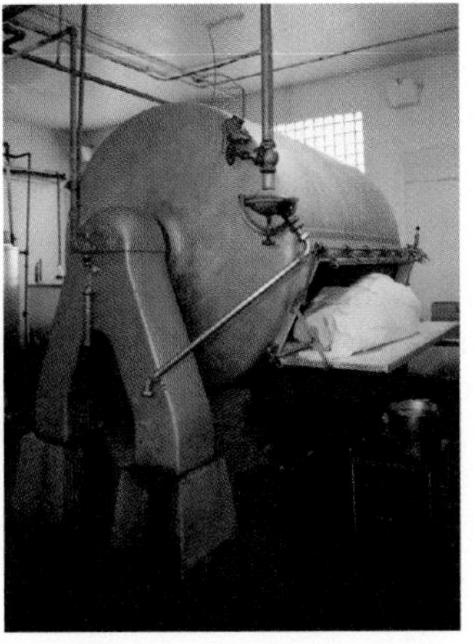

FIGURE 7.12 Today, industrial butter production uses centrifugal cream separators to separate the cream from the milk. The cream is then pasteurized and cooled. The cooled cream is placed in a large, mechanical churn that tumbles the cream until butter forms.

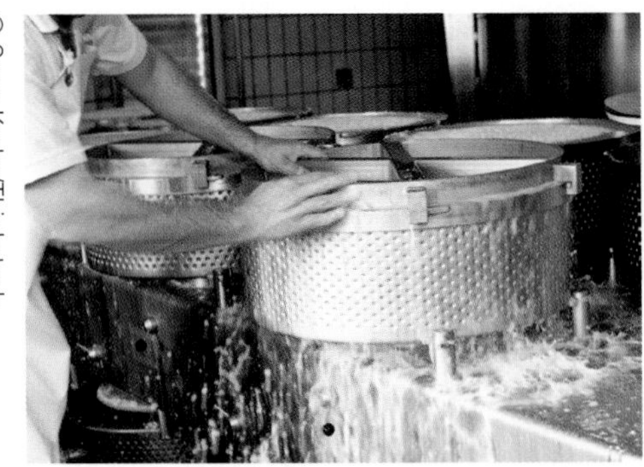

FIGURE 7.13 The final shape of a cheese is based on the type of mold or form the curds are pressed into. Pressure is applied to the forms to drive out moisture. The harder the cheese, the more pressure that was applied, and the more water that was removed.

rennin An enzyme derived from calves' stomachs that is used to coagulate the milk protein casein.

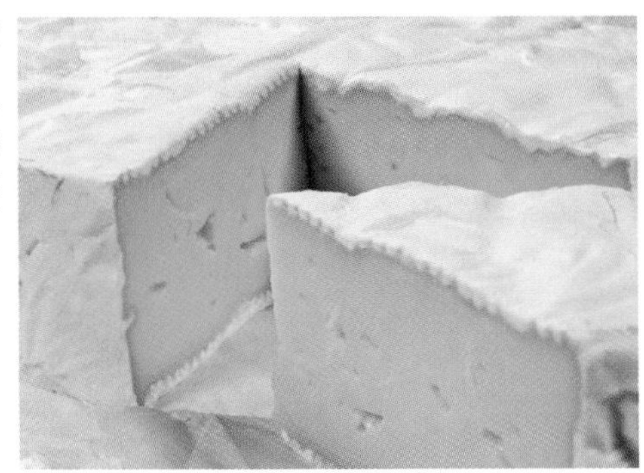

FIGURE 7.14 Before processing, soft cheeses are chalky in texture. They are then sprayed with a culture of mold. The mold reacts with the cheese from the exterior toward the interior, aging the cheese so that it forms a smooth, runny, or gooey texture. The mold forms a flexible white crust on the outside of the cheese.

of an enzyme. The added enzyme is typically **rennin**, which is derived from the stomach of a calf. As the milk coagulates, it separates into solid curds and liquid whey. After draining off the whey, the curds can be made into fresh cheese, which is unripened, or pressed into different shapes and ripened.[1,3]

To ripen (or age) cheese, the drained curds are cured by various methods, including heating, adding bacteria, and/or soaking (see **Figure 7.13**). The curds are sometimes flavored with salt, herbs, or spices. After curing, the cheese is allowed to ripen under controlled conditions until the desired texture, color, and flavor results.[1,3]

The hundreds of natural cheeses produced worldwide can be categorized by their texture and firmness as fresh cheese or as one of four categories of ripened cheese (see **Table 7.4**).

Fresh Cheeses

The most popular fresh cheeses include cottage cheese, cream cheese, pot cheese, and ricotta. For these simple cheeses, the milk is curdled and then drained. Little additional processing is applied. Without the addition of preservatives, fresh cheeses can spoil within days. Fresh cheeses are soft and spreadable and have a mild flavor.[1,3]

Soft-Ripened Cheeses

Also called *surface-ripened cheese* or *bloomy-rind cheese*, soft-ripened cheese is neither cooked nor pressed.[1,3] Soft-ripened cheeses are characterized by their creamy centers, mild flavor, and thin outer coating (or skin). They also are moist, with a typical moisture content between 50 and 75%. Soft-ripened cheeses are most often made from cow's milk and a starter culture. A mold called *Penicillium candidum* or *P. camemberti* is added, which gives this category of cheese its distinctive white bloomy rind. The mold serves to help to break down the cheese and ripen it over time from the outside in.[1,3] Compared with other cheese varieties, soft-ripened cheeses ripen quickly (within 2 to 8 weeks). The outside color is always white, sometimes with splotches of yellow or light red. The inside color ranges from ivory to yellow. The texture is soft and creamy under the rind, getting creamier towards the center as it ages. Examples of soft cheeses include Brie, Boursin, and Camembert (see **Figure 7.14**).

Semisoft Cheeses

Semisoft cheeses also are called *monastery* or *Trappist cheeses* because their origins can be traced back to monasteries. Semisoft cheeses are mild, buttery cheeses with smooth, creamy textures. They are typically aged less than 2 months. Due to the fact that they are not aged for long, they maintain an ivory color and a moisture level between 40 to 50%.[1,3] Examples include Cabrales, Fontina, Gorgonzola, Gouda, Havarti, Port-Salut, Roquefort, and Stilton (see **Figure 7.15**).

Firm Cheeses

Firm cheeses also are called semihard cheeses due to the fact that they are hard but not brittle; they contain between 30 to 40% moisture.[1,3] Their colors are varied, ranging from ivory to light brown, light gold, yellow, or orange. The interior has a smooth texture. Some varieties have tiny eyes (holes).

TABLE 7.4
Types of Cheese

Type of Cheese	Characteristics
Fresh (Unripened) Cheeses	
Cream cheese	A soft cow's milk cheese from the United States containing about 35% milk fat.
Feta	A Greek or Italian semisoft cheese made from sheep and/or goat's milk. It has a white, flaky color and is pickled and stored in brine, giving it a shelf life of 4 to 6 weeks.
Mascarpone	A soft cow's milk cheese originally from Italy. It contains 70–75% milk fat and is highly perishable. It has a smooth and creamy texture and is ivory in color with a rich, sweet flavor.
Mozzarella	An Italian firm cheese originally made with water buffalo milk but now more commonly made with cow's milk. It contains 40–45% milk fat.
Queso Oaxaca (also called quesillo or asadero)	A popular cow's milk cheese from Mexico that contains 45% milk fat. The cheese is kneaded, wound into balls, and then soaked in brine. It has a semisoft, smooth texture and is white in color. It is available in braids, balls, or rounds.
Ricotta	An Italian soft cheese similar to American cottage cheese that is made from whey. It contains 4–10% milk fat and has a mildly sweet flavor. It is white in color and has a smoother texture than cottage cheese.
Soft Cheeses	
Bel Paese	An Italian cheese made with cow's milk that contains about 50% milk fat. It has a thin, pale yellow rind that is covered with wax and a pale yellow interior. It has a mild, buttery flavor.
Brie	A French cheese made with cow's milk that contains about 60% milk fat. It has a white rind and an ivory, buttery-soft center.
Boursin	A French cheese made with cow's milk that contains about 75% milk fat. It is usually flavored with herbs, peppers, or garlic. It is rindless and has a smooth, creamy texture.
Camembert	A French rind-ripened cheese made with cow's milk that contains about 45% milk fat. It has a bloomy rind and is shaped like a small round or oval disc. The inside is smooth and creamy. It has a milder flavor than Brie.
Taleggio	An Italian cheese made with cow's milk that is about 48% milk fat. It ranges in flavor from mild-sweet to nutty-rich, depending on how long it has been aged. The rind also varies in color from yellow to pink to orange to spots of gray. The inside has a creamy texture and a pale yellow color.
Semisoft Cheeses	
Cabrales	A blue cheese from Spain traditionally made from a combination of cow, goat, and ewe's milk. It contains 45–48% milk fat, resulting in a soft, creamy texture. It has a zesty flavor, a crumbly interior with purplish-blue veins, and a rough rind. It is typically aged for 3 to 6 months.
Fontina	An Italian cheese made with cow's milk containing 45% milk fat. It has a thin rind that ranges in color from goldish-yellow to reddish-brown. The interior ranges from pale to dark yellow with little holes (called eyes). The flavor is rich, buttery, and slightly nutty.
Gorgonzola	Originally from Italy, this cow's milk cheese contains about 48% milk fat. It has an ivory interior that is lightly or thickly streaked with blue-green veins. The texture is rich and creamy. It has a slightly pungent flavor. When aged longer than 6 months, the flavor becomes very strong and has been described as stinky.
Gouda	Originally from Holland, this cow's milk cheese contains about 48% milk fat. It comes in large wheels with a rind that may or may not be covered with red or yellow wax. The interior has a yellow color, and the flavor ranges from mild in younger cheeses to full, rich, and nutty in aged versions.

(*continues*)

TABLE 7.4
Types of Cheese (*continued*)

Type of Cheese	Characteristics
Havarti	This Danish cheese is made from cow's milk and contains 45–60% milk fat. It has a mild flavor and creamy texture. It is a pale yellow color and contains small holes.
Port-Salut	This French cheese is made from cow's milk and contains about 50% milk fat. It has a mild, savory flavor and smooth texture. The interior is a pale yellow, and it has a bright orange rind.
Roquefort	This French blue-veined cheese is made from sheep's milk and contains about 45% milk fat. It has a creamy, rich texture; a pungent aroma; and a piquant, salty flavor.
Stilton	Originally from Great Britain, this cow's milk cheese contains 45% milk fat. The interior is white or pale yellow with blue veins. The texture is rich and creamy but slightly crumbly. The flavor is rich and tangy.
Firm Cheeses	
Cheddar	This cow' milk cheese is produced in the United States and Great Britain and contains 45–50% milk fat. It has a smooth, dense texture and varies in flavor from mild to sharp. The color varies from white to bright orange.
Emmenthaler	This Swiss cheese is made from cow's milk and contains about 45% milk fat. The rind varies from light tan to dark brown in color; the interior is light yellow. It has a nutty, rich flavor and a smooth texture.
Gruyere	This Swiss cheese is made from cow's milk and contains 45–50% milk fat. The rind is brown; the interior ranges from ivory to a light yellow color. It has a sweet, nutty, earthy flavor.
Jarlsberg	The cow's milk cheese from Norway contains about 45% milk fat. The rind is pale yellow to brownish-yellow with an ivory to light yellow interior. It has a smooth texture and a slightly nutty, buttery flavor.
Manchego	This Spanish sheep's milk cheese contains 45–57% milk fat. The edible rind ranges in color from black to beige, and the interior is pale yellow with a crumbly texture. It has a buttery flavor that is a bit piquant.
Monterey Jack	A California cow's milk cheese that contains 50% milk fat. It has a pale ivory color, smooth interior, and mild flavor. As the cheese ages, the rind becomes wrinkly brown and the interior becomes more yellow and firm. The flavor becomes nutty and sharp.
Provolone	An Italian cheese made from cow's milk that contains about 45% milk fat. The rind is pale to golden yellow and the mild form (aged 2 to 3 months) has a pale yellow color and mild flavor. Aged provolone has a darker yellow color, a flaky or stringy texture, and a stronger flavor.
Hard Cheeses	
Asiago	An Italian cheese made with cow's milk that is about 30% milk fat. It has a rich flavor that can be sharp in aged versions. The interior color ranges from ivory to pale yellow to deep gold. The rind color ranges from elastic and tan-colored to hard and brownish-gray.
Parmesan	A cow's milk cheese made in Argentina, Australia, and the United States that contains 32–35% milk fat. The Italian Parmigiano-Reggiano variety, which is typically aged for at least 2 years, is the most famous variety. The cheese has a hard, pale-golden rind and tan-colored interior with a rich, sharp flavor.
Pecorino Romano	An Italian cheese made from sheep's milk containing about 35% fat. It is more brittle and sharper than other cheeses. The interior is grainy and whiter in color than Parmesan or Asiago. It has a yellow rind.

Examples include Cheddar, Emmenthaler, Gruyere, Jarlsberg, Monterey Jack, and Provolone (see **Figure 7.16**).

Hard Cheeses

Hard cheeses are aged for long periods of time and have a moisture content of about 30%. They are commonly referred to as *grana* cheeses due to their grainy texture.[1,3] They have an intense flavor and often are quite salty—typically a small amount goes a long way. The color ranges from yellow to bright gold or light tan, and the cut surface looks like rough granite. Examples include Asiago, Parmesan, and Pecorino Romano (see **Figure 7.17**).

© Alexandralaw1977/iStockphoto.com

FIGURE 7.15 Semisoft cheeses have a texture that is only slightly firmer than the soft category. They have a relatively high moisture content, but they have a longer shelf life than their softer counterparts. Many cheese styles fall within this popular group.

Ice Cream and Ice Milk

Ice cream is made from a combination of various products. It typically includes cream mixed with fresh, condensed, or dry milk; a sweetening agent (e.g., honey, corn syrup, sugar); and sometimes solid ingredients such as chocolate pieces, fruit, or nuts. According to Food and Drug Administration (FDA) guidelines, plain ice cream (without solids) must contain at least 10% milk fat; ice cream with solid additions must contain a minimum of 8% milk fat.[10] Many commercial brands contain stabilizers to help create a creamier texture and a fuller mouth feel and to help slow down melting. Ice milk is made using the same basic method to make ice cream except that the result contains less milk fat and milk solids. The product is thus lower in fat and calories and has a lighter, less creamy texture (see **Figure 7.18**).[10] More information about ice cream and frozen dairy products can be found in **Special Topic 7.1**.

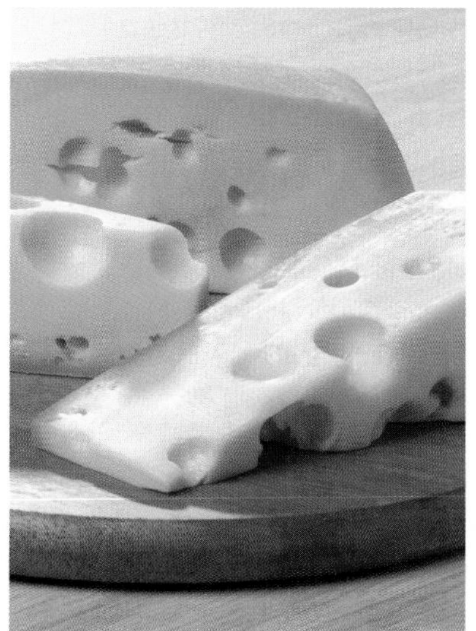

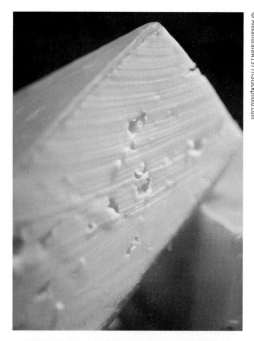

© Gustavo Toledo/ShutterStock, Inc.

FIGURE 7.16 Firm cheeses are ideal for melting and are often used on deli sandwiches, as quick snacks, or as simple meals.

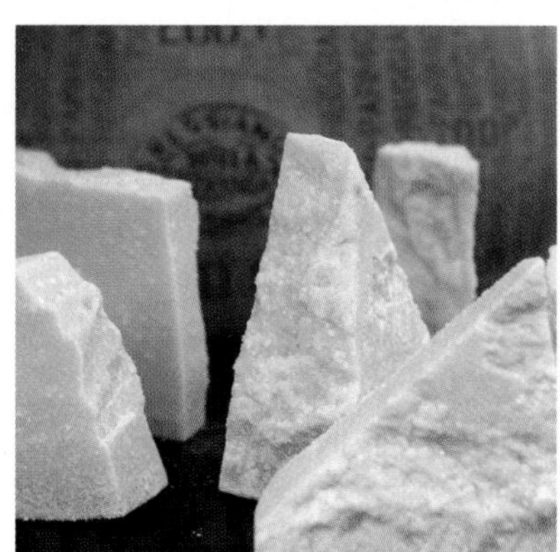

© Michael Blann/Thinkstock

FIGURE 7.17 Parmigiano-Reggiano, more commonly called Parmesan cheese in English, is named after the area where it is produced—the Italian provinces of Parma, Reggio Emilia, Modena, Bologna, and Mantova. Italian law mandates that only cheese produced in these provinces can be labeled "Parmigiano-Reggiano." The European Union classifies the name as a protected designation of origin.

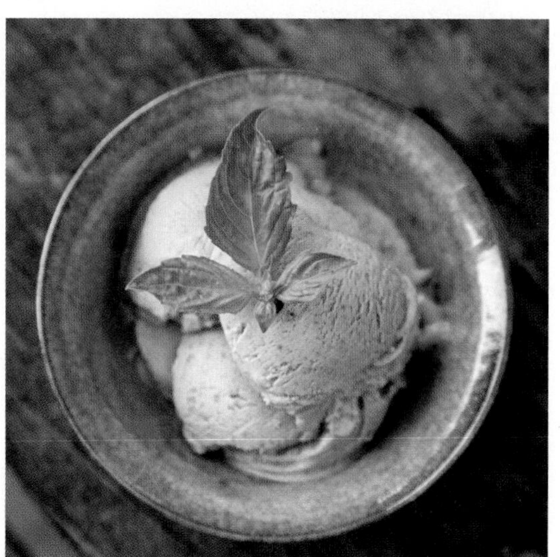

© wyndy25/iStockphoto.com

FIGURE 7.18 Ice milk has 10% fat and the same sweetener content as ice cream. In 1994, the USDA changed its labeling guidelines so that ice milk could be labeled as low-fat ice cream.

Special Topic 7.1

Ice Cream and Frozen Dairy Desserts

Mary McAvoy

More ice cream is consumed in the United States than in any other country.[1] But ice cream is not the only frozen dairy dessert option on the average American's grocery list; other frozen dairy options include gelato, bombe, frozen yogurt, frozen custard, sherbet, parfaits, and ice milk. Ice cream and other frozen dairy desserts are popular because their cool, sweet, creaminess creates a pleasing taste for most consumers. Each type of frozen dairy dessert is prepared in a similar fashion.

Ice cream is made of a mixture of dairy products such as milk, cream, butter, MSNF (milk solid, nonfat) and nondairy products that run the gamut from sugar, eggs, and fruit to added flavorings and colors.[2] The MSNF contributes to ice cream's viscosity, richness, firmness, resistance to melting, and nutritive value, as it can add protein, calcium, and vitamins. The federal government regulates the general names of ice creams that are available to consumers in the United States.[1] By law, ice cream is defined as having at least 10% milk fat by weight. Super-premium ice cream is prized for its creaminess due to its composition of up to 20% milk fat. Light ice cream contains 50% less fat and 33% fewer calories than regular ice cream but has more added sugar.[2] Low-fat ice cream contains 3 grams of fat per serving, and nonfat ice cream contains less than 0.5% fat per serving.[3]

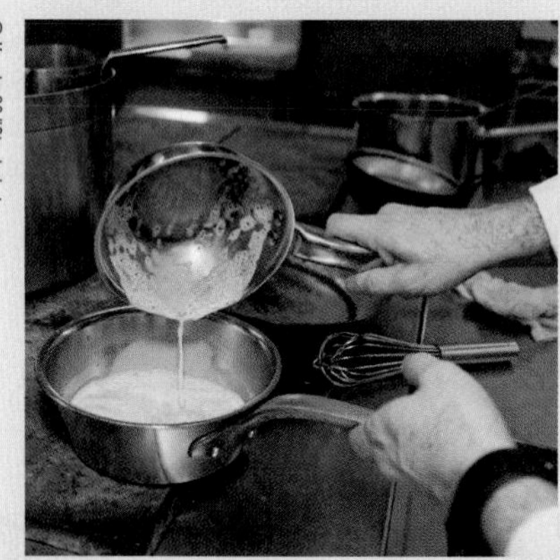

FIGURE A The first step in making ice cream.

Gelato, which hails from Italy, has become a popular frozen dairy dessert. Gelato is denser than ice cream because it contains more milk and less cream. It also is churned more slowly and at higher temperatures, creating a very smooth and creamy texture.[1] Sherbets contain less than 2% milk fat. Sherbets are made with frozen sweetened fruit juices or purees. Gelatin and/or eggs are added to make it creamier. Sherbet often has a higher sugar content than ice cream to make up for the lower fat content. Sherbet also tastes colder. Why is this? Sugar depresses the freezing point and causes lower-fat frozen dairy desserts to have a more solid form, which conveys a colder sensation to the tongue.[3]

Cooking or Heating

The first step in ice cream preparation involves cooking or heating the ingredients (see **Figure A**). The cooking method of making ice cream creates a custard-like base. The eggs and sugar are beaten until smooth and subsequently added to the heated cream.[1] The mixture is then removed from the heat and flavors are added. It is then aged in a refrigerator for several hours until it is ready to be churned and frozen.[3]

With the heating method, the liquid ingredients are heated to 104°F (40°C) to dissolve the sugar. Stabilizers and emulsifiers such as lecithin, guar gum, and glycerol monosterate may be added before the mixture is aged. (Homemade ice cream is generally grainier because it does not contain these commercial additives that add viscosity to the unfrozen part of the water, making it firmer to the chew.[2]) During the aging process, the body and texture of the ice cream is improved as the fat begins to solidify.[3]

Freezing and Churning

Next, the freezing and churning process takes place. The creamy texture of most frozen dairy desserts comes from the incorporation of air into the mixture during the churning process. Ice crystals are often formed from the water content and create a smooth and creamy texture.[1] To create the optimal texture, the ice cream is churned so that small ice crystals form throughout the mixture rather than in large clumps, which would result in a coarser texture.[1] The more air molecule nuclei in the mixture, the creamier the texture.[3]

During churning, fat cells are broken down and reformed into larger masses, which also improves the ice cream's texture and body (see **Figure B**). The initial churning of the mixture takes place slowly and then is sped up toward the end of the churning process in order to increase the number of air molecule nuclei.[1] The canister that holds the ice cream mixture is two-thirds full and surrounded by a mixture of crushed ice and rock salt.[1] The ice and rock salt absorb heat from the ice cream mixture, which allows it to freeze faster. The churning process takes about 20 minutes. The ice cream is frozen at 0°F (32°C) overnight so that the mixture hardens and does not have a grainy texture.

Other forms of frozen dairy desserts are prepared in a similar fashion, but the ingredients are altered slightly.[1] Some frozen dairy desserts are "still frozen" and require no churning; they maintain their creaminess through ingredients such as egg white foams or whipped cream.[1]

Storage

Ice cream and other dairy desserts will shrink over time and the texture will deteriorate. Heat shock deteriorates the texture by resulting in the formation of large ice crystals. Therefore, frozen dairy products should be stored at a consistently cold temperature.

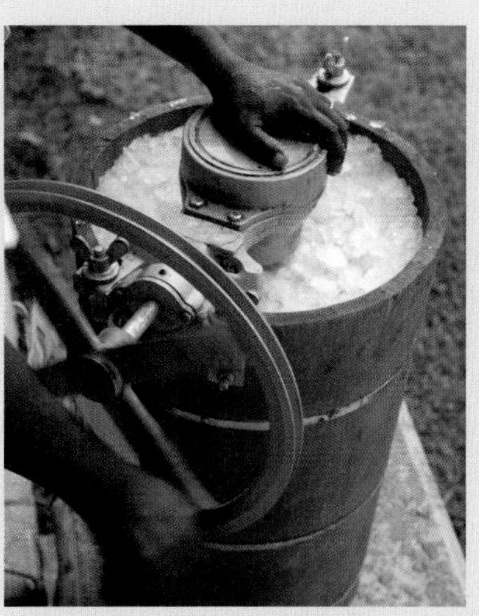

© Susanne Kischnick/Alamy

FIGURE B The second step in making ice cream.

References

1 Brown A. *Understanding Food: Principles and Preparation.* 4th ed. New York: Wadsworth; 2011.

2 University of Guelph. Dairy Science and Technology. Available at: http://www.foodsci.uoguelph.ca/dairyedu/overrun.html. Accessed November 24, 2011.

3 Goff D. Finding Science in Ice Cream. University of Guelph. Available at: http://www.physics.uoguelph.ca/STAO/icecream.html. Accessed November 24, 2011.

Food Selection, Menu Planning, and Basic Food Preparation Techniques

Purchasing Milk and Dairy Products

Purchase dairy products such as cream, dried milk, cottage cheese, butter, cream cheese, and ice cream that have a Grade A label and are made with pasteurized milk.[7] Fresh milk should have a sweet flavor and should not be consumed if it tastes sour, bitter, or moldy or if it has any off odors. Make sure to check the sell-by date; do not purchase milk after that date. Butter should have a sweet flavor; a firm texture; and a uniform, yellowish color. Reject if it has signs of mold, specks, or other foreign materials or if the container is dirty or damaged. Cheese should resemble the variety purchased in terms of odor, texture, and color. If it has a rind, make sure it is unbroken and clean. It should not contain signs of unnatural mold (mold that was not intentionally added). Check for clean and undamaged packaging.

Menu Planning

According to the 2010 Dietary Guidelines for Americans, 3 cups of low-fat milk is recommended per day for individuals 9 years and older.[4] For children between the ages of 2 to 8, the recommendation is 2 cups. One cup equals 8 fluid ounces. Alternatively, other dairy products can be consumed in place of milk. Serving equivalents are listed in **Table 7.5**.

Basic Food Preparation Techniques

Milk and dairy products are used in a variety of recipes, from soups and sauces to desserts and baked goods. They help provide these dishes with a creamy texture and rich flavor. Keep the following guidelines in mind when preparing dishes that contain milk:[1,3]

TABLE 7.5
Equivalent Serving Sizes for Dairy Products

Food	One Serving
Nonfat (skim) or low-fat (1%) milk	1 cup
Yogurt	1 cup (or 8-fluid ounce container)
Natural cheese (e.g., cheddar, Swiss, Parmesan)	1½ ounces
Processed cheese (e.g., American)	2 ounces
Ricotta cheese	½ cup
Cottage cheese	2 cups
Pudding made with milk	1 cup
Frozen yogurt	1 cup
Ice cream	1½ cups (though ½ cup servings are the recommended portion to keep fat and calories under control)

Source: Data from U.S. Department of Agriculture. ChooseMyPlate. Available at: http://www.choosemyplate.gov.

- *Prevent curdling.* Slowly add acidic ingredients such as citrus juice, vinegar, or tomato sauce while stirring.
- *Prevent scorching.* Make sure to use low heat and stir frequently. Heat just until the milk begins to steam.
- *Prevent skin from forming.* Place plastic wrap over the surface of cooked milk as it cools.
- *Prevent foaming.* Make sure to stir milk slowly as it is cooking.

Several guidelines apply when cooking with cheese:

- Ripened and processed cheeses melt well, but processed cheeses melt quickly and can burn.
- Cheese should be heated at low temperatures for a short period of time. High temperatures can cause cheese to become rubbery.
- Cheese should be added to hot white sauce towards the end of the cooking process.
- Cheese melts better when between layers of other food, as in lasagna.
- Add cheese toppings (as in ziti) at the end of baking or broiling, and monitor closely so the cheese does not burn.

Nutritional Value

Cow's milk is 87% water and contains all three energy-yielding nutrients: carbohydrates, fats, and proteins. The carbohydrates found in milk are in the form of lactose, a disaccharide (double sugar) that is categorized as a simple sugar. Lactose is digested with the help of the enzyme lactase, which separates the double sugar into its single sugar counterparts, glucose and galactose.[11] Once digested, these single sugars are easily absorbed into the body. Most of the fat found in cow's milk is saturated and has been linked to increased low-density lipoproteins (LDL; "bad") cholesterol levels. The nutritional value of whole milk and skim (nonfat) milk is compared in **Table 7.6**. The amount of saturated and total fat is significantly lower in skim milk. However, note that otherwise the nutritional content is not much different between whole and skim milk. Cow's milk also is a good source of protein, with 1 cup of whole or skim containing 12% of the daily recommended amount.[11]

TABLE 7.6
Comparison of 1 Cup of Whole Versus 1 Cup of Skim Milk

Nutritional Content	Amount in Whole Milk	Percent of Recommended Daily Value for Whole Milk	Amount in Skim Milk	Percent of Recommended Daily Value for Skim Milk
Calories	146		91	
Calories from fat	71		5	
Total fat	8 g	12%	1 g	1%
Saturated fat	5 g	23%	0 g	2%
Sodium	98 mg	4%	130 mg	5%
Protein	8 g	16%	8.7 g	17%
Calcium	276 mg	28%	316 mg	32%
Vitamin D	97.6 IU	24%	98 IU	24%
Vitamin A	249 IU	5%	497 IU	10%
Potassium	349 mg	10%	419 mg	12%
Riboflavin	0.4 mg	26%	0.4 mg	26%
Vitamin B_{12}	1.1 mg	18%	1.0 mg	16%
Phosphorus	222 mg	22%	255 mg	25%

Source: Data from U.S. Department of Agriculture. USDA National Nutrient Database for Standard Reference, Release 24. Available at: http://www.ars.usda.gov/ba/bhnrc/ndl. Accessed April 19, 2011.

Milk provides at least 10% of the FDA recommended daily allowance (RDA) of numerous essential nutrients; obtaining these nutrients at the same level from nonmilk sources would take some effort. Additionally, milk contains various bioactive ingredients that have been shown to benefit numerous health conditions, including low bone mass, metabolic disorders, stroke, and some forms of cancer.[12–23]

Milk, cheese, and yogurt contain nine essential nutrients: calcium, potassium, phosphorus, protein, vitamin A, vitamin D, vitamin B_{12}, riboflavin, and niacin.[5] Only milk and dairy products contain all nine of these nutrients on their own. Cheese is an excellent source of calcium, providing at least 20% or more of the RDA for calcium per serving. Cheese also is a good source of phosphorus, providing 10–12% of the RDA.[5] Yogurts are an excellent source of several nutrients, including calcium, phosphorus, and riboflavin, and they are a good source of protein and potassium.[5]

Calcium

Dairy products are one of the best dietary sources of calcium. Calcium is an important mineral; the body needs it to maintain healthy bones and teeth.[11] The nervous and circulatory systems also need calcium to function.[24,25] Calcium aids in the release of hormones and enzymes and helps the muscles to function. Inadequate calcium intake can lead to osteoporosis, causing weak and brittle bones.[13,21] **Table 7.7** lists the recommended calcium intake for various age groups.

Among adults ages 19 and older, 88% of women and 63% of men do not the daily calcium recommendations.[26] Among teenage girls and boys, 91% and 69%, respectively, do not meet the daily calcium recommendations.[26] Based on these statistics and other studies showing the need for more calcium in the American diet, the National Dairy Council began the 3-Every-Day® initiative to educate people on how to incorporate more dairy into their diet.[27] **Table 7.8** lists various dietary sources of calcium.

TABLE 7.7
Recommended Calcium Intake Based on Age

Age	Recommended Calcium Intake (mg/day)
0 to 6 months	200
7 to 12 months	260
1 to 3 years	700
4 to 8 years	1,000
9 to 13 years	1,300
14 to 18 years	1,300
19 to 50 years	1,000
Adult men 51 to 70 years	1,000
Adult women 51 to 70 years	1,200
Adults 71 years and older	1,200
Pregnant and breastfeeding teens	1,300
Pregnant and breastfeeding adults	1,000

Source: Reproduced from Office of Dietary Supplements, National Institutes of Health. Dietary Supplement Fact Sheet: Calcium. Available at: http://ods.od.nih.gov/factsheets/Calcium-QuickFacts. Accessed March 1, 2011.

TABLE 7.8
Dietary Sources of Calcium

Food	Portion	Amount of Calcium (in mg)
Whole milk	1 cup	276
Reduced-fat milk (2%)	1 cup	293
Low-fat milk (1%)	1 cup	305
Skim milk (nonfat)	1 cup	316
American cheese	1 ounce	162
Cheddar cheese	1 ounce	204
Cottage cheese	1 cup	174
Cream cheese	1 tablespoon	14
Feta cheese	1 ounce	140
Swiss cheese	1 ounce	224
Yogurt, fruit, low fat	8-ounce container	345
Frozen yogurt, soft serve, chocolate	½ cup	106

Source: Data from U.S. Department of Agriculture. USDA National Nutrient Database for Standard Reference, Release 22. Available at: http://www.ars.usda.gov/SP2UserFiles/Place/12354500/Data/SR22/nutrlist/sr22a301.pdf. Accessed March 2, 2011.

Vitamin D

Commercial cow's milk is fortified with the fat-soluble vitamins A and D. In the late 1920s, the dairy industry began fortifying canned milk with vitamin D. This practice was soon expanded to butter and fresh milk. Because the main food sources of vitamin D are limited to egg yolks and fish liver oils, it was only logical to add vitamin D (which works with calcium to help build healthy bones) to milk and dairy products.

Based on a study that showed that fluid milk and milk beverages provided between 50% and 66% of total vitamin D intake for those 2 years of age and older; it appears that milk and dairy products are the primary sources of vitamin D in the American diet.[28] Sun exposure is another way to help activate vitamin D, but the average American does not get enough daily exposure. (About 30 to 45 minutes of sun exposure are needed, depending on a person's skin color and the amount of skin exposed.)

Impact of Milk and Dairy Products on Health

Milk and dairy products have been found to have a number of benefits to human health, including the ability to maintain a healthy weight, improved bone health, and many others.

Weight

Numerous studies have linked milk and dairy consumption with a healthier weight. A 2-year weight loss study published in 2010 in the *American Journal of Clinical Nutrition* examined more than 300 overweight and at-risk men and women who followed a low-fat, a Mediterranean, or a low-carb diet for 2 years. Regardless of the type of diet followed, those who consumed the greatest amount of dairy (nearly two glasses of milk a day on average) lost approximately 12 pounds by the end of the 2-year period, compared to 7 pounds for those consuming a low dairy diet (about half a glass of milk on average).[29] In a 2006 study published in *Obesity*, researchers found that young, normal weight women who consumed diets high in dairy (1,000–1,400 mg dairy calcium per day) gained less body fat over 18 months than those who consumed low-dairy diets (less than 800 mg dairy calcium per day).[30] The authors concluded that increasing dietary calcium through dairy products may prevent the accumulation of fat in young, healthy women.

Muscle Mass and Recovery After Exercise

According to a 2007 study in the *American Journal of Clinical Nutrition*, healthy young men ages 18 to 30 who drank milk over a 12-week period gained 40% more muscle than those who drank soy protein beverages and 60% more muscle compared to those who drank carbohydrate beverages.[11] In addition, the milk drinkers also lost an average of 2 pounds of fat; the soy beverage drinkers lost no fat.

Milk has been shown to be an effective way to refuel, rehydrate, and recover after exercise. A 2008 study found both white and chocolate milk to be effective following both resistance and endurance exercise.[25] The composition of milk is ideal in providing nutrients the body needs, including carbohydrates to refuel muscles, protein to reduce muscle breakdown and promote growth, and fluid and electrolytes to help rehydrate and replace fluids lost through sweat.

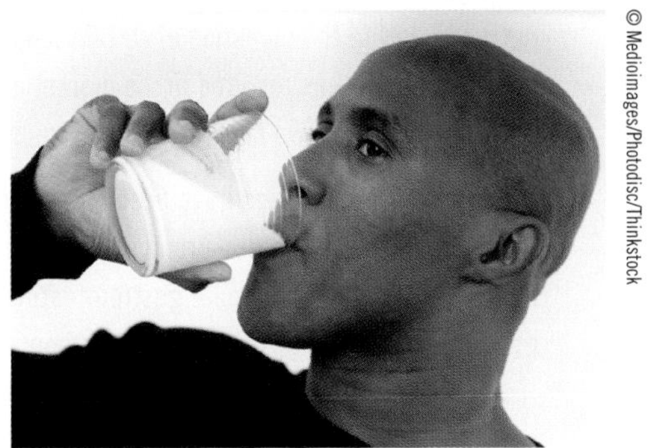

Bone Health

The connection between calcium and bone health (including dental health) has been well established. The U.S. Surgeon General's Report on Bone Health and Osteoporosis identifies eating calcium-rich foods such as milk, yogurt, and cheese as a way to maintain bone health.[31] In order to prevent overconsumption of fat, however, low and nonfat dairy products are suggested.

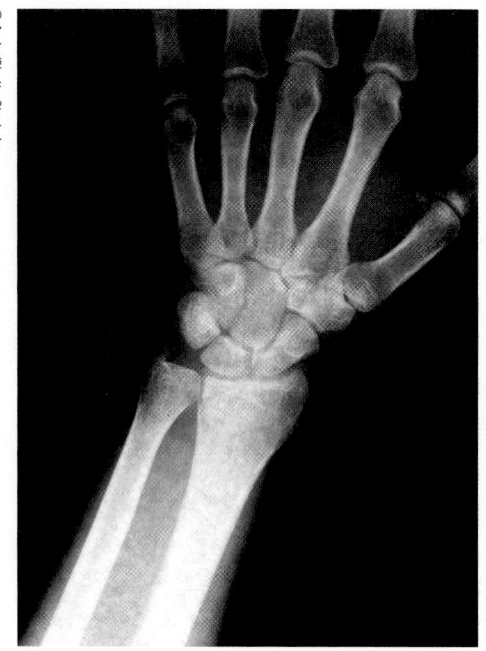

FIGURE 7.19 In osteoporosis, bone density decreases, the bone architecture deteriorates, and bone proteins are altered. These changes make the bone more susceptible to fracture.

Osteoporosis is a degenerative bone disease that is characterized by weak and brittle bones (see **Figure 7.19**). Typically, fractures occur in the hip, spine, and wrist. Compression of weakening bones in the spine can cause some people to lose height or to develop a hunched posture. Eighty percent of those affected by the disease are women. According to the National Osteoporosis Foundation, more than 44 million American are at risk for developing osteoporosis and more than 1 in 10 women are either at risk or have been diagnosed with bone disease. The associated costs related to fractured bone are $12 to $18 billion each year and rising. Statistics also reveal that 20% of older adults who fracture a bone die within the first year, either from problems associated with the broken bone or during the surgery needed to repair it. Many studies link low calcium intake with low bone density, bone loss, and a higher number of broken bones. Increasing one's intake of calcium and vitamin D has been shown to help reduce bone loss.[13]

Dairy also plays a role in dental health. A 2008 study published in *The Journal of Periodontology* revealed that consumption of foods containing lactic acid, including yogurt, was associated with improved gum health.[32]

Digestive Health

Probiotics have been gaining in popularity, especially those found in yogurt. Probiotics are live microorganisms that when consumed in adequate amounts can provide health benefits. Research suggests a link between consumption of probiotics and the prevention of gastrointestinal infections; however, further research is needed. Probiotics also have been shown to help breakdown the milk sugar lactose, which can cause flatulence, diarrhea, bloating, and other gastrointestinal discomforts to those who are lactose intolerant.[8] See more about probiotics in **Special Topic 7.2**.

Special Topic 7.2

Prebiotics and Probiotics

Colleen Lynch

The human body contains between 10^{12} and 10^{14} bacteria, outnumbering human cells by 10 to 1. The gut, predominately the colon, is rapidly colonized from birth with 400 to 500 species of bacteria (see **Figure A**).[1] These bacteria are critical to the development of a healthy immune system and are referred to as the body's normal flora. They protect against invasions of pathogenic strains of bacteria, promote normal bowel contractions, and are crucial to the release of vitamins and nutrients during the digestion of certain foods.[1] The importance of these bacteria to digestive health has resulted in the marketing of products that promote their growth and maintenance. Two such products of importance are prebiotics and probiotics.

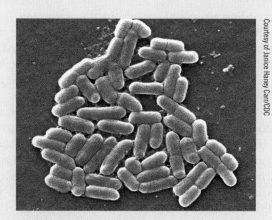

FIGURE A Magnified gut flora.

Prebiotics and probiotics have been identified as functional foods—foods or food additives that have health-promoting or disease-preventing properties beyond the function of solely supplying nutrients. Consumption of both is thought to promote gastrointestinal health. Probiotics are live bacteria believed to be beneficial to the host organism, whereas prebiotics are nondigestible food ingredients that serve as nutrients to these bacteria and stimulate their growth and/or activity.[1]

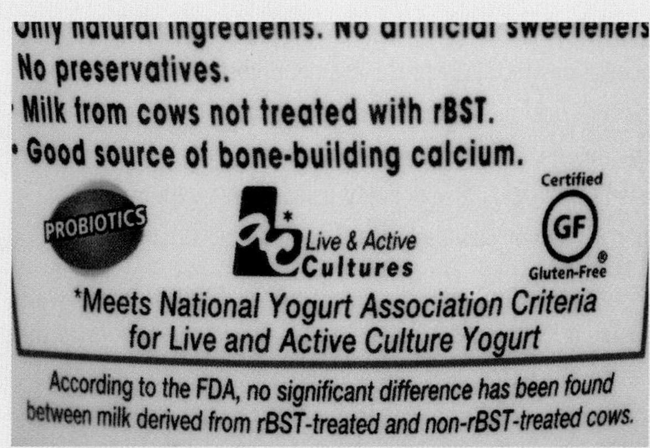
No preservatives.
Milk from cows not treated with rBST.
Good source of bone-building calcium.
PROBIOTICS
Live & Active Cultures
Certified
GF
Gluten-Free
*Meets National Yogurt Association Criteria for Live and Active Culture Yogurt
According to the FDA, no significant difference has been found between milk derived from rBST-treated and non-rBST-treated cows.

FIGURE B The LAC seal.

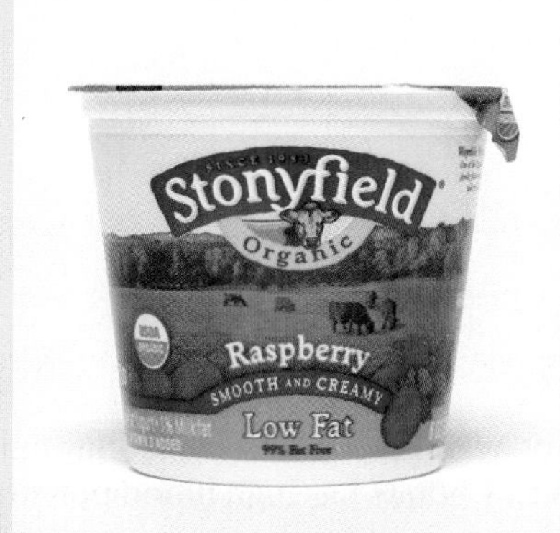

FIGURE C A certified LAC yogurt.

When taken together, prebiotics and probiotics are called *synbiotics* or *eubiotics* because both work together to enhance probiotic benefits. Synbiotics may improve the survival of the bacteria crossing the upper part of the gastrointestinal tract, thereby enhancing their effects in the large intestine.[2] When consumed as synbiotics, the benefits may be greater than when prebiotics and probiotics are consumed separately.

Probiotics

In 2001, the Food and Agriculture Organization (FAO) of the United Nations, in conjunction with the World Health Organization (WHO), defined *probiotics* as "live microorganisms, which, when administered in adequate amounts, confer a beneficial health effect on the host."[2] After passage through the stomach and the small intestine, some probiotics survive and become established in the large intestine.[2] Probiotics aid the gut by increasing the number of helpful bacteria (normal flora) and inhibiting harmful bacteria, therefore strengthening the body's immune response.

Several types of probiotics have been identified. The amount needed for positive health effects varies by genus, species, and strain. The three most common probiotic bacterial groups seen in the marketplace are *Lactobacillus* spp., *Bifidobacterium* spp., and *Streptococcus thermophilus*. These bacteria are found in various supplements and in naturally and commercially fermented foods as well as in yogurts, cereals, breads, and juices. Studies suggest that probiotics may have a therapeutic effect on people with certain gastrointestinal conditions, such as lactose intolerance, rotavirus-induced diarrhea, and irritable bowel syndrome (IBS). *Lactobacillus* spp., for example, was found to reduce the duration of diarrhea and the frequency of stools compared to placebo in a meta-analysis of its use in children.[1] The symptoms of bloating in IBS have shown to be reduced by *Bifidobacterium* spp. as well. Other claims of probiotic benefits include decreased cholesterol and blood pressure, prevention of colon cancer, and faster healing of infections.

Although evidence suggests the benefits of probiotics, much is still unknown. Currently, no evidence suggests that healthy individuals benefit from consuming probiotics on a regular basis. The gut is good at maintaining homeostasis with regard to its natural flora.[1] However, there is no evidence that regular consumption of probiotics is harmful either. Probiotic preparations increase the number of anti-inflammatory bacteria in the gut. Some experts think that this may act as an additional barrier to pathogenic invasion, thereby preventing gastroenteritis.

Yogurt is one of the products being intensely marketed as a probiotic powerhouse. However, only certain types of yogurt have probiotic benefits. Yogurts bearing the Live and Active Cultures (LAC) seal are certified by the National Yogurt Association, which holds manufacturers to very strict criteria (see **Figure B** and **Figure C**). All probiotics are LAC, but not all LAC are probiotics. Therefore, when a yogurt has this seal, you should read the label to make sure that it contains probiotics. Consumers also should be aware that probiotics are time sensitive. Bacterial activity declines the longer a product sits unused.

Prebiotics

Unlike probiotics, prebiotics are not live sources of bacteria. Prebiotics are complex carbohydrates (such as oligosaccharides) that the human body is unable to metabolize. They act as a food source for beneficial probiotic bacteria and enhance their activity. In addition, prebiotics have been found to offer other health benefits. They encourage the absorption of some minerals, such as calcium, magnesium, and zinc, due to the way they are digested by the body. They also increase the concentration of short-chain fatty acids in the large intestine. In some studies, oligosaccharides with mannose side chains have been shown to block receptors on the intestinal wall available for interaction with pathogenic bacteria such as *Escherichia coli*.[3]

The only prebiotic forms for which sufficient data have been produced are inulin-type fructans, which include native inulin and enzymatically hydrolyzed inulin and oligofructose, and synthetic fructooligosaccharides (FOS). Because it is not digested within the gastrointestinal tract, inulin-type fructans have been associated with constipation relief due to fecal bulking and with the suppression of diarrhea. Other health claims of prebiotics require further research. For example, one claim is that inulin-type fructans can reduce the risk of osteoporosis because it improves the bioavailability of calcium.[2] The use of probiotics also is being investigated with regard to decreasing risks for type 2 diabetes, obesity, and atherosclerotic cardiovascular disease associated with dyslipidemia.

Prebiotics are available in supplement and food forms; they can be naturally occurring or artificial. The most common types of prebiotics added to foods are FOS, inulin, and galactooligosaccharides (GOS). Natural food sources include whole grains, almonds, honey, and certain fruits and vegetables, including bananas, asparagus, garlic, tomatoes, onions, chicory, garlic, leeks, and artichokes. Prebiotic ingredients can be found in baked goods, chocolate, and flavored waters. Prebiotics are less sensitive than probiotics and can be stored at room temperature for months. General dosage recommendations also exist for prebiotics. The scientific consensus is that 4 to 8 grams per day promote beneficial bacteria in the colon.

References

1 Parkes GC. An overview of probiotics and prebiotics. *Nursing Standard.* 2007;21:43–47.
2 Roberfroid M. Prebiotics and probiotics: Are they functional foods? *AJCN.* 2000;71:16825–16875.
3 Tomasik P, Tomasik PJ. Review: Probiotics and prebiotics. *Cereal Chem.* 2003;20:113–117.

Hypertension and Heart Disease

High blood pressure can lead to coronary heart disease, stroke, kidney failure, and other diseases. Approximately 1 in 3 U.S. adults has high blood pressure.[33] One of the key recommendations to help control blood pressure is diet. The Dietary Approaches to Stop Hypertension (DASH) study has shown that a diet that is low in fat, high in fruits and vegetables (8 to 10 per day), and that contains two to three servings per day of low or nonfat dairy foods can help reduce blood pressure in prehypertensive and hypertensive adults.[9] According to a 2006 study published in *Hypertension*, participants who consumed more low-fat dairy foods had lower blood pressure, which may help lower the risk of heart attacks or stroke.[14] A 2008 study published in the *American Journal of Clinical Nutrition* found that adults who consumed at least one serving of low-fat milk or milk products a day were 37% less likely to have poor kidney function linked to heart disease compared to those who drank little or no low-fat milk.[34] The National Heart, Lung, and Blood Institute recommends following a healthy eating plan in order to help prevent high blood pressure.[33] This includes consumption of low-fat or nonfat dairy products, as outlined by the DASH diet.

Cancer

Thus far, the research has been inconclusive regarding the effects of milk and calcium consumption on cancer, a disease that affects an estimated 10.5 million Americans. According to the American Cancer Society, numerous studies have shown an association between milk consumption and a decreased risk of colorectal cancer.[15] A 2003 study published in *Cancer Causes and Controls* followed over 120,000 men and women and found that those with the highest calcium intakes through both supplements and diet had a slightly reduced risk of colorectal cancer as compared to those with the lowest calcium intakes.[16] However, several studies have indicated that calcium intake may actually increase the risk of prostate cancer.[6]

Diabetes

A 2006 study published in the *Archives of Internal Medicine* studied the relationship between dairy intake and incidence of type 2 diabetes in 41,254 male participants with no history of diabetes, cancer, or heart disease over a 12-year period. The study found that greater dairy consumption was linked to a 9% lower risk for type 2 diabetes. Lower-fat dairy products may be linked to a decreased incidence of type 2 diabetes in men.[17]

Other Health Conditions

Researchers have examined the relationship between milk and premenstrual syndrome (PMS). According to a 2006 study published in the *Archives of Internal Medicine*, which used data from the Nurses' Health Study, women who consumed the highest amounts of calcium and vitamin D from food (1,280 milligrams calcium and 380 IUs of vitamin D on average) reported fewer PMS symptoms compared to women who consumed little to no calcium or vitamin D.[35] In addition, the study found that women who drank at least two servings of nonfat or low-fat milk per day had a significantly lower risk of developing PMS symptoms compared with those who consumed one or fewer servings of non- or low-fat milk per day.

The link between acne and consumption of dairy products is not as clear. Acne is the most common skin disorder, affecting 70–87% of U.S. teenagers. Although diet has been implicated in the past, the American Academy of Dermatology has found that the research does not support a link between dairy products and acne at this time.[36]

Food Technology

Various types of food technology can be applied to the processing and packaging of milk and dairy products to increase their shelf life. In addition, the food industry has developed a number of dairy substitutes that offer many of the same nutritional benefits as dairy products to lactose-intolerant individuals and to those with dairy allergies or who otherwise prefer not to consume dairy products.

Concentrated Milk Products

In concentrated milks, most or part of the water from whole milk is removed, resulting in products with a high concentration of milk fat and milk solids. Concentrated products include the following:[5]

- *Dry milk powder*: This concentrated milk product is created by removing almost all of the moisture from pasteurized milk. Its low moisture content helps prevent the growth of microorganisms and allows for long-term storage at room temperature. To reconstitute, it is combined with water and used like fresh milk. Dry milk powder can be found as whole milk, nonfat milk, and buttermilk.
- *Sweetened condensed milk*: To make this product, 60% of the water is removed from the milk and extra sweetener is added. The result contains 40–45% sugar. Once canned, the milk darkens in color and takes on a caramel flavor. Sweetened condensed milk has a distinctive flavor. It is typically used in desserts and cannot be substituted with fresh milk.
- *Evaporated milk*: During the processing of evaporated milk, 60% of the water from homogenized whole milk is removed. The remainder of the liquid is canned and sterilized by heat. The result

is a darker-colored milk with a cooked flavor. Evaporated milk also can be produced from skim milk; this product is defined as having a milk fat content of 0.5%. Evaporated milk should be stored in a cool, dry place and, once opened, stored in the refrigerator. Evaporated milk should be mixed with equal parts of water to reconstitute it for use as whole milk.

pasteurized processed cheese Products created by combining shredded or ground pasteurized cheeses with emulsifiers and flavors; they are less expensive than natural cheeses and have a longer shelf life because they do not ripen with age.

processed cheese food A product containing less real cheese than processed cheese; it typically has added water, milk solids, and/or vegetable oil to make it softer and more spreadable. It must have a minimum fat content of 23% and a maximum of 44%.

imitation cheese A product similar to processed cheese, but the butterfat is replaced by vegetable oil, nonfat milk, or whey solids mixed with water.

Processed Cheese

Processed cheeses are less expensive than natural cheeses and have a longer shelf life because they do not ripen or age. They have a consistent texture and flavor, and they melt without separating. By law, most processed cheeses must contain no more than 43% moisture and at least 47% fat.[5] A **pasteurized processed cheese** is created by combining shredded or ground pasteurized cheese with emulsifiers and flavorings such as salt. The mixture is cooked and then molded to solidify. **Processed cheese food** contains less real cheese than processed cheese; it typically has added water, milk solids, and/or vegetable oil to make it softer and more spreadable. Processed cheese food must have a minimum fat content of 23% and maximum of 44%. **Imitation cheese** is similar to processed cheese, but the butterfat is replaced by vegetable oil, nonfat milk, or whey solids mixed with water. Compared to natural cheese, imitation cheese has little flavor and a dense, rubbery texture. However, it is much less expensive and has a longer shelf life than real cheese and does not require refrigeration.

Dairy Substitutes

In recent years, dairy substitutes have gone mainstream. Soy, almond, rice, and hemp milk have found their way into the marketplace. These alternatives are all made from plant sources and therefore contain no saturated fat or cholesterol. The following are some of the more popular dairy substitutes:[5]

- *Soy milk*: Made from ground, soaked soybeans, soy milk has a taste and texture similar to cow's milk. The color is off-white or yellowish. It is typically fortified with vitamin D and calcium. It also contains protein, vitamin A, thiamin, and riboflavin. Soy flour and soy oil are used in many processed foods, and small quantities can add up quickly.
- *Almond milk*: Made from ground, soaked almonds, almond milk has a texture similar to low-fat (1%) cow's milk and a sweet aroma. Almond milk tastes good in whole grain cereal and even on its own.
- *Rice milk*: Made from unsweetened brown rice, rice milk has a mild flavor and a watery texture that is most similar to fat-free milk. Rice milk is very low in fat and is fortified with vitamins A and D, some B vitamins, iron, and calcium in order to enhance its nutritional benefits.
- *Hemp milk*: Made from ground, soaked hemp seeds, hemp milk has a creamy, nutty flavor.

Phytonutrient Point

Almond Milk and Hemp Milk Almond milk is naturally packed with vitamins and minerals, including magnesium, potassium, iron, zinc, and calcium. Hemp milk contains proteins and heart-healthy omega-3 fatty acids.

Going Green with Milk Products

According to the International Dairy Federation, the main environmental issues associated with the dairy industry are greenhouse gas (GHG) emissions, nonrenewable energy use, and water use.[37] Others are concerned about the effect of some of the industry's practices on human health. Hormones, such as estrogen, are naturally secreted by lactating cows in small amounts into the milk, which has no effect on those who consume it. However, in order to increase a cow's milk production by 10–20% some farmers inject the cow every 2 weeks with growth hormone.[38] The most common synthetically produced hormone used is recombinant bovine somatotropin (rBST). Although the 1993 FDA approval of rBST was controversial, dairy farmers injected the hormone into 22% of the U.S. dairy herd.[2]

An issue that arises with hormone injections is the need for antibiotics. Multiple injections of rBST to the cow increases the incidence of skin infection. Additionally, the increased milk production causes udder infections (called *mastitis*). The more infections a cow has, the more antibiotics that are used, and these antibiotics go into the milk that humans ingest.[39] See **Special Topic 7.3** for more on rBST and **Special Topic 7.4** for more on antibiotic-resistant bacteria.

Special Topic 7.3

Bovine Somatotropin in Cow's Milk

Bridget Mahoney

Cow's milk has been an excellent source of nutrition for centuries, but over the last two decades it has become a topic of tremendous controversy. Many consumers are beginning to ask questions about how dairy farming is being impacted by advancements in biotechnology and genetically engineered foods. Specifically, how are synthetic hormone injections affecting the safety of milk? Unfortunately, there is no clear-cut answer; more research needs to be done.

Somatotropin is a protein hormone that is produced by the pituitary gland of all mammals (including humans). It regulates body growth, cell replication, lactation, and nutrient metabolism. During lactation, somatotropin is responsible for mobilizing body fat for fuel as well as directing energy toward producing milk instead of tissue. Bovine somatotropin (BST) occurs naturally in cattle in small quantities, but it also can be engineered and injected in larger amounts. Recombinant DNA technology and gene splicing are used to produce a synthetic BST—recombinant BST (rBST). Injecting cows with rBST can increase milk production by 10–20%.[1]

All milk has BST in some form or other. The naturally occurring form of BST varies only slightly in chemical structure from rBST and cannot be distinguished from rBST in milk. During pasteurization, 90% of BST (and rBST) is destroyed, and the rest is digested just like a regular protein; it is not consumed as the active form of the hormone. BST and rBST are not able to bind to human somatotropin receptors, and therefore have no effect on humans when consumed. These qualities led to FDA approval of rBST in 1993.[1]

Although rBST-treated animal products are FDA approved, consumers are not completely convinced of the safety of rBST. One major concern is that large quantities of rBST could potentially increase the presence of insulin-like growth factor I (IGF-I). This hormone has been linked to possible tumor growth. Unlike rBST, IGF-I is not denatured by pasteurization, and if it is consumed it can potentially be absorbed in its active form. In addition to IGF-I, milk treated with rBST has been shown to have higher amounts of antibiotics, bacteria, and infection.[2] Recombinant DNA technology is relatively new, and thus there are no long-term studies on the effects of rBST in humans. However, some studies show that injecting cattle with rBST can be harmful to the animals' health and well-being. The consequences of boosting their milk production with rBST include udder infections (mastitis), reproductive problems, digestive disorders, sores, and foot and leg ailments. Cows suffering from these illnesses are given antibiotics, which leads to an additional consumer concern about human consumption of these antibiotics.[3]

Products treated with rBST are banned in all industrialized nations except the United States, where products containing rBST do not need to be labeled. In addition to the potential harm to humans, many countries banned rBST because of the detrimental effects it has on animal health. Since the FDA approved rBST, about one-third of American dairy farmers have gone out of business, leaving milk production to larger companies, all of which use rBST injection treatments. About 15% of the 10 million American dairy cows are treated with rBST.[2,3]

Over the past few years, the demand for organic milk products has increased exponentially due to consumer apprehension and awareness of rBST; however, some studies suggest that the worry isn't warranted. As it stands today, the use of rBST in cattle has certainly been proven to be harmful to the animals; however it is unclear that it is hazardous to human health. More research needs to be done to confirm or deny concerns about the effects of rBST on human health. The FDA and numerous other scientific and medical organizations, including the American Medical Association (AMA), the Academy of Nutrition and Dietetics, and the National Institutes of Health (NIH), among others, state that rBST is safe for the cow and that the milk produced is safe for human consumption.

References

1 Holstead J. Recombinant bovine growth hormone. *Office of Legislative Research Report.* 2007. Available at: http://www.cga.ct.gov/2007/rpt/2007-R-0159.htm.

2 Khanal AR. Adoption of technology, management practices, and production systems in U.S. milk production. *J Dairy Sci.* 2010;93(12):6012–6022.

3 Tucker HA. Safety of Bovine Somatotropin. UMass Extension. 2010. Available at: http://www.extension.org/pages/Safety_of_Bovine_Somatotropin_(bST).

Special Topic 7.4

Antibiotic Resistance

Michelle Boutet

Following their successful use in human medicine, antibiotics are increasingly being used to treat and prevent diseases in animals. Besides disease prevention, subtherapeutic doses of antibiotics have been shown to have growth-enhancing effects (although the link remains unclear) and have been used in animal-rearing practices for decades.[1]

However, research has identified a link between administering antibiotics to animals and the development of antibiotic-resistant bacteria in humans. Some of these antibiotic-resistant strains of bacteria cause humans to become sicker for longer periods of time than their antibiotic-susceptible counterparts. They are responsible for the physical and emotional burden of prolonged illnesses and sometimes death while also creating a major financial strain on the healthcare system. Doctors, scientists, and journalists have watched and protested as drug-resistant strains of bacteria have become increasingly prominent in hospitals and areas surrounding livestock operations. Congress has repeatedly tried to pass legislation to restrict the use of subtherapeutic antibiotic dosing in livestock, but no real changes have been made. Meanwhile, the FDA has done little to prevent antibiotic-resistance in human bacteria from becoming a critical public health issue.[2]

Prevalence of Antibiotic Use in the Food Industry

The Union of Concerned Scientists states that 70% of all antibiotic types important to human medicine are given in subtherapeutic doses to livestock. Livestock producers administer 13.5 million pounds of these antibiotics each year. Antibiotics that are commonly used in human medicine, such as tetracycline and penicillin, are used extensively in livestock. This practice has caused a rise in strains of drug-resistant bacteria, the most notable being *Campylobacter* spp., *Salmonella* spp., and *Escherichia coli*.[2]

The move from small, family-owned farms to large, industrial factory farms—also known as animal feeding operations (AFOs)—has resulted in farmers keeping their animals in close confinement in order to increase their production and, therefore, profit. These cramped quarters, along with other stresses of their unnatural lives on factory farms, puts animals in greater danger of becoming diseased and behaving in aggressive ways that lead to further injury and illness. Antibiotics were introduced into animal feed to fight disease and infection in order to maximize health and growth. Animals living in confinement are particularly susceptible to diseases such as pneumonia and diarrhea, the major causes of calf mortality. Antibiotic compounds can currently be detected in liquid waste at animal feedlots and fish-breeding locations and in lakes and groundwater supplies.[2]

Aimed at prevention of disease, subtherapeutic doses are low levels of antibiotics that are not strong enough to actually suppress a bacterial infection but are able to prevent a bacterial infection from occurring. Subtherapeutic antibiotics for disease prevention are usually used during high-risk periods for the animal, such as when it is being weaned from its mother. The main problem is that the ability to mass medicate through animal feed allows farmers to continue giving animals the antibiotics for growth enhancement over the course of the animals' lives. Subtherapeutic doses of antibiotics administered over long periods of time to a large group of animals encourages natural selection for drug-resistant bacterial strains. This natural selection happens when an antibiotic used to treat an infection kills off the bacteria most susceptible to that antibiotic, leaving behind the most resistant bacteria to multiply and spread.[2]

The CDC and the AMA have known about the connection between antibiotic use in livestock since at least 1984 and antibiotic resistance in humans since at least 2001. According to a 2002 study by the Alliance for the Prudent Use of Antibiotics (APUA) and other medical scholars who have written on the subject, direct, temporal, and circumstantial evidence proves that antibiotic use in livestock causes drug-resistant infections in humans.[2]

In addition, scientists have uncovered evidence that directly ties human infections back to specific livestock operations. An obvious fact is that the animal antibiotics that threaten the health of humans the most are the ones that are important in human medicine. One of the most notable examples of an antibiotic used in animals that has caused antibiotic resistance in humans is fluoroquinolone, a critical antibiotic used in treating *Campylobacter* spp. and *Salmonella* spp. infections. Because it has been used extensively in poultry farming, it is no longer as effective in humans. Two years after the FDA approved fluoroquinolone for animal use, the percentage of fluoroquinolone-resistant bacteria in chickens rose to 14%. During the same period, the amount of fluoroquinolone-resistant bacteria in humans rose from 1.3% to 10.2%. The resistant strain caused more hospitalizations, longer illnesses, and more costly treatment for infected patients than a nonresistant strain of the same bacteria.[3]

The Spread of Antibiotic Resistance to Humans

The three main ways that antibiotic-resistant bacteria are transferred from animals to humans are contact with livestock, food consumption, and the environment.

Contact with Livestock

Livestock workers can become infected with resistant bacteria by touching the animals, animal feed, or animal manure. Once the drug-resistant bacteria strain infects a farm worker, it can be easily transferred to the rest of the community.[1]

Food Consumption

Another method of animal-to-human transference is through the food products themselves. Throughout an animal's life on a factory farm, drug-resistant bacteria build-up in its intestines. During slaughter and processing, these bacteria are spread to the processed and packaged meat. Consumers then ingest the drug-resistant bacterial strains, which then colonize their intestines. The resistance gene thrives in the intestines, where it can eventually spread to other species, creating new resistant strains across different bacterial species. A 2002 Consumer Reports study about this danger found that 42% of supermarket broiler chickens were contaminated with *Campylobacter* spp. Of the 42% that were infected, 20% carried an antibiotic-resistant strain of the bacterium.[1]

The Environment

Humans contract drug-resistant bacteria through the environment primarily by consuming contaminated water. Antibiotics pass through treated animals' intestines, such that as much as 75% of the antibiotics consumed end up in manure. Approximately 2.7 trillion pounds of manure is generated annually by AFOs in the United States alone. This manure is kept in open manure lagoons and then leaks into nearby groundwater. In addition, animal waste in the lagoons mixes with rainwater, becoming runoff that ends up in lakes and streams, many of which are major water sources for human consumption.[1]

Global Concern

Antibiotic resistance is a growing international problem that affects both current and future generations. No country is safe from the spread of antibiotic-resistant bacteria. Resistance that develops in one area of a country may easily spread nationwide, and eventually to other countries. Globalization, with its increased migration of human populations, trade, and travel, has made more areas susceptible to infectious diseases, especially in the developing world. Although cutting-edge therapies for treating drug-resistant infections are researched in depth in industrialized countries, they are often not readily available or affordable in many developing countries.[3]

References

1 Dushoff J, Morris JG Jr, Smith DL. Agricultural antibodies and human health: Does antibiotic use in agriculture have a greater impact than hospital use? *Int J Risk Safety Med.* 2005;17(3/4):147–155.

2 Lessing A. Killing us softly: How sub-therapeutic dosing of livestock causes drug-resistant bacteria in humans. *Boston Coll Env Affairs Law Rev.* 2010;37(2):463–491.

3 Richwine A, Shryock TR. The interface between veterinary and human antibiotic use. *Ann NY Acad Sci.* 2010 Dec;1213(1):92–105.

Green Point

GHG Emissions Based on studies conducted by the International Dairy Federation, organic farming does not seem to lower GHG emissions, possibly due to the nature of the forage and the lower productivity of organic systems compared with conventional ones.

Greening the Industry

One way to reduce the environmental impact of milk production is to decrease GHG emissions. This can be done by altering the cow's diet to reduce its production of methane gas. Additionally, fodder production can utilize organic practices. As for dairy processing, modifying the order in which the equipment is used can help reduce its environmental impact. Some products require equipment to be cleaned completely before moving on to the next, whereas others require a quick rinse or even no cleaning. Having the most efficient order of production can help reduce the environmental impact of milk collection and processing.[37]

Milk that is labeled as organic means that the milk is from dairy cows that have been pastured for at least half the year so that they can graze on grass. The FDA's organic guidelines also mandate that the cows do not receive synthetic hormones, such as rBST, and that they are not administered antibiotics unless needed to treat a disease or infection. Note that many local farmers may practice organic farming techniques but cannot afford to become certified organic due to the high costs involved. Local organic options can be found at farmers' markets and some supermarkets.

Food Safety and Potential Foodborne Illness

Each year in the United States, almost 76 million cases of foodborne illness are reported, resulting in about 325,000 hospitalizations and 5,000 deaths.[8] Milk is considered a potentially hazardous food due to its neutral pH, nutrient-rich composition, and high water activity—conditions that allow for the growth of pathogenic microorganisms.

Common Pathogens

Common pathogenic microorganisms that can be introduced into milk upon production include *Salmonella enterica*, *Listeria monocytogenes*, *E. coli*, and *Campylobacter jejuni*. Foodborne pathogens are especially dangerous to very young children, pregnant or lactating women, and older adults. *L. monocytogenes* especially has been known to affect pregnant women in their third trimester, sometimes resulting in spontaneous abortions or stillbirth.

The Pasteurized Milk Ordinance

Dairy farmers work closely with the FDA and state officials in order to minimize the risk of milk and dairy pathogens reaching consumers. The federal Pasteurized Milk Ordinance (PMO) provides guidelines for milk production, milk hauling, pasteurization, product safety, equipment sanitation, and labeling. Milk is routinely tested by state regulatory agencies to ensure its quality and safety. Both the FDA and the Environmental Protection Agency (EPA) monitor milk producers' compliance with milk safety guidelines.[7] The PMO guidelines have been effective, as less than 1% of foodborne illness outbreaks are due to pasteurized dairy products.[40]

Concerns About Raw Milk

The risk of illness is much higher when drinking **raw milk**. The sale of raw milk sale is allowed in some states. However, the FDA does not recommend the consumption of raw milk. From 1998 to 2008, the CDC reported 85 outbreaks from the consumption of raw milk, with 1,614 reported cases of illness and 2 deaths.[40] It is very likely that this number is higher because many foodborne illnesses go unreported. Symptoms of foodborne illness from raw milk include vomiting, diarrhea, abdominal pain, fever, and headache. Although some people will have a short recovery time, others may develop more severe, even life-threatening, symptoms. Pasteurization destroys the pathogenic microorganisms while still maintaining healthy bacteria and nutrients. In the United States, pasteurization of milk is required if milk is moved from one state to another.

Food Regulation and Food Quality

Food quality monitoring is a voluntary service that is paid for by dairy manufacturers and producers. It is done in a variety of ways, due to the various methods used to prepare and produce dairy products.

Butter is one dairy product that is graded. The U.S. Department of Agriculture (USDA) grades the quality of butter based on its flavor, texture, body, color, and salt. Butter packages contain a shield with a letter grade (and sometimes the numerical equivalent) to indicate its quality. Grading standards for butter can be AA (93), A (92), B (90), or C (89). The most commonly sold grades in the market are AA and A. USDA grade AA butter indicates superior quality, a fresh flavor and aroma, a smooth and creamy texture, and good spreadability. USDA grade A butter is very good quality with a pleasant flavor and a smooth texture. USDA grade B butter is most often used for food manufacturing. The butter is of standard quality and is made from sour cream. The flavor, texture, and body does not match that of grades AA and A butter.

Milk is graded—as A, B, or C—based on standards set forth by the U.S. Public Health Service. Grades vary based on the milk's bacterial load, with grade A having the highest quality and the lowest bacterial count. Grades B and C are typically not sold for retail or commercial use.[5]

Lactose Intolerance

Lactose intolerance is a fairly common condition. Hippocrates first described lactose intolerance around 400 B.C. However, our knowledge of the condition has been limited, and only over the past 25 years have we begun to understand its causes. The National Institutes of Health (NIH) has concluded that the true prevalence of lactose intolerance in the United States is unknown (most people self-diagnose). However, it is known that its prevalence varies across racial and ethnic groups. In the United States, it is most common among Native Americans, Asian Americans, Hispanic Americans, and African Americans; it is less

Innovation Point

Ultra-pasteurization **Ultra-pasteurization** is a process whereby milk is heated to even higher temperatures (275°F or 135°C) for a shorter time period (2 to 4 seconds). With one form of ultra-pasteurization, known as **ultra-high-temperature (UHT) processing**, milk is heated to 280°–300°F (138°–150°C) for 2 to 6 seconds. After heat treatment, UHT products are packed into sterile containers that are sealed aseptically. Once sealed, the container can be stored unrefrigerated for up to 3 months.

raw milk Milk in its natural form that has not undergone processing such as pasteurization and homogenization.

ultra-high-temperature (UHT) processing A high-heat pasteurization method where milk is heated to 280–300°F (138–150°C) for 2 to 6 seconds.

ultra-pasteurization A high-heat pasteurization method where milk is heated to 275°F (135°C) for 2 to 4 seconds.

common in European Americans.[6] According to a study based on self-reported lactose intolerance, 8% of European Americans, 10% of Hispanic Americans, and 19.5% of African American consider themselves to be lactose intolerant. Many people who have self-diagnosed themselves lactose intolerance are not actually lactose malabsorbers; their discomfort may be due to other physiological conditions, a learned aversion, or social and cultural perceptions.[6]

Lactose malabsorption is due to insufficient levels of the enzyme lactase, which breaks down lactose into glucose and galactose. Lactose malabsorption can be diagnosed by the hydrogen breath test, an intestinal biopsy, or genetic testing.[6] Not everyone with malabsorption exhibits symptoms of lactose intolerance. Gastrointestinal symptoms of lactose intolerance include bloating, abdominal cramps, and diarrhea after consuming milk or milk products containing the lactose. These symptoms result when the consumption of lactose is greater than the body's ability to digest and absorb it.

Most individuals with lactose intolerance can tolerate a small amount of lactose at a time. Complete avoidance is unnecessary, although commonly practiced. Because milk is the major contributor of calcium, vitamin D, potassium, protein, vitamin A, phosphorus, magnesium, zinc, vitamin B_{12}, and riboflavin, completely eliminating dairy can result in a higher risk of osteoporosis due to insufficient calcium and vitamin D in the diet.[6]

The NIH recommends that those with lactose intolerance should be able to ingest 12 grams of lactose in a single dose. This is equivalent to 1 cup of milk or yogurt. It also has been found that lactose is more easily digested on a full stomach. Other strategies for those with lactose intolerance to include dairy's nutritional benefits in their diet is to consume small amounts of dairy throughout the day, to choose lactose-free dairy products, to take lactase pills before the consumption of dairy products, or to find alternative sources of calcium and vitamin D (e.g., sardines with bones, calcium-fortified breads and juices, and green leafy vegetables). People with lactose intolerance are usually able to tolerate yogurt better than other dairy products due to the production of lactase by the yogurt starter cultures. Natural cheeses such as Swiss and cheddar also contain minimal lactose due to the fact that much of the lactose is removed during processing.

Chapter Review

Mammals, including humans, consume their mother's milk as their first food. Archeological evidence suggests that sheep and goat's milk were first consumed around 11,000 and 9,500 years ago, respectively. Today, milk, cheese, and yogurt are enjoyed throughout the world.

According to the 2005 Dietary Guidelines for Americans, 3 cups of low fat milk is recommended for the general population. Milk provides at least 10% of the RDA of numerous essential nutrients, including calcium, vitamin D, magnesium, phosphorus, riboflavin, protein, and carbohydrates.

Milk and dairy products include milk, cream, cultured dairy products, butter, and cheese. Several types of milk can be found in the market, including whole, reduced-fat, low-fat, and nonfat milk. Cultured dairy products include buttermilk, sour cream, crème fraîche, and yogurt. They are created by adding bacterial cultures to milk or cream. Butter is made by churning cream until it reaches a semisolid state. By law, it must contain at least 80% milk fat, no more than 16% water, and 2–4% milk solids.

Cheese can be categorized as unripened (or fresh) or ripened. The four categories of ripened cheese are soft, semisoft, firm, and hard. Most cheese begins as milk (typically sheep, goat, or cow). The milk protein called casein is coagulated by the addition of an enzyme (typically rennet). As the milk coagulates, it separates into solid curds and liquid whey. After draining off the whey, the curds can be made into fresh cheese or pressed into different shapes and aged, depending on the variety.

Milk is composed of an various molecules, including milk fat, proteins, salts, sugars, vitamins, and water. Milk has a pH between 6.5 and 6.7, making it a slightly acidic. The flavor of milk is due to the mildly sweet sugar lactose, salts, fatty acids, and sulfur compounds. Sour or other undesirable flavors can result if the cow was raised in poor unfavorable environmental conditions. An overgrowth of bacteria that produce lactic acid can result in sour milk.

Milk fat carries fat-soluble vitamins (e.g., vitamin A) and essential fatty acids. It contributes about half the calories to the milk and gives milk its characteristic texture, mouth feel, and taste. When fresh milk stands for a while, the fat begins to rise and form a layer at the top, which is called creaming.

The two main groups of proteins found in milk are curds and whey. The curd protein, casein, forms small bundles called micelles. A protein subunit keeps the micelles separated. When this protein subunit is removed through the addition of the rennin, the casein reacts with free calcium ions, which causes the micelles to clot. This helps form curd, which is then treated to make cheese.

Pasteurization is the process of heating a food or beverage to a high enough temperature to destroy harmful pathogenic bacteria. All grade A milk is required by law to be pasteurized before being sold. Milk is pasteurized by heating it to a temperature of 161°F (72°C) for 15 seconds.

Milk, cheese, and yogurt contain nine essential nutrients: calcium, potassium, phosphorus, protein, vitamin A, vitamin D, vitamin B_{12}, riboflavin, and niacin. Only milk contains all nine of these nutrients on its own. Many cheeses are an excellent source of calcium, providing at least 20% or more of the RDA, and a good source of phosphorus, providing 10–12% of the RDA. Most yogurts are excellent sources of several nutrients, including calcium, phosphorus, and riboflavin, and good sources of protein and potassium.

Milk and dairy products are a great source of calcium. Calcium is needed to maintain healthy bones and teeth. Inadequate calcium intake can lead to osteoporosis. The 2010 Dietary Guidelines for Americans recommend 3 cups of nonfat or low-fat dairy products each day for individuals 9 years and older and 2 cups for children between the ages of 2 to 8.

The main environmental issues associated with the dairy industry are greenhouse gas (GHG) emissions, nonrenewable primary energy use, and water use. One recommendation to help reduce the environmental impact of milk production is decreasing GHG emissions. This can be done by altering the cow's diet in order to reduce its production of methane gas. Fodder production can utilize organic practices that require fewer fertilizers and pesticides.

© ImageState

Learning Portfolio

Key Terms

	page
butter	227
buttermilk	225
casein	221
cream	224
creaming	221
crème fraîche	225
curd	221
curdling	221
half and half	224
homogenization	222
imitation cheese	242
lactose	221
light cream	224
low-fat milk	224
nonfat milk	224
pasteurization	222
pasteurized processed cheese	242
processed cheese food	242
raw milk	247
reduced-fat milk	224
rennin	228
scorching	223
sour cream	225
ultra-high-temperature (UHT) processing	247
ultra-pasteurization	247
whey	222
whipping cream	224
whole milk	224
yogurt	225

Study Points

1. The two main groups of proteins found in milk are casein and whey.
2. Cultured dairy products include buttermilk, sour cream, crème fraîche, and yogurt. They are created by adding specific cultures to milk or cream. Buttermilk is produced by adding a harmless bacterial culture called *Streptococcus lactis* to fresh, pasteurized low-fat or nonfat milk.
3. Yogurt is cultured by adding *Lactobacillus bulgaricus* and *Streptococcus thermophiles* to milk (either whole, low fat or nonfat).
4. Hundreds of natural cheeses are produced worldwide. They can be categorized as unripened (fresh) or ripened. Ripened cheeses can be further categorized as soft, semisoft, firm, and hard.
5. Casein is coagulated by the addition of an enzyme (typically rennin, which is derived from the stomach of a calf) to make cheese.
6. Pasteurization is the process of heating a food or beverage to a high enough temperature to destroy harmful pathogenic bacteria. All grade A milk is required by law to be pasteurized before being sold. Milk is heated to a temperature of 161°F (72°C) for 15 to 20 seconds.
7. Milk contains nine essential nutrients: calcium, potassium, phosphorus, protein, vitamin A, vitamin D, vitamin B_{12}, riboflavin, and niacin.
8. Scorching (or burning) of milk occurs when casein micelles and whey protein drop to the bottom of the pan, stick, and burn.
9. Common pathogenic microorganisms that can be introduced into milk during production include *Salmonella enterica*, *Listeria monocytogenes*, *Escherichia coli*, and *Campylobacter jejuni*.
10. Research on bovine somatotropin and antibiotics given to cows has given rise to much discussion about their risks versus benefits.

Issues for Discussion

1. How does the public view organic milk? Is this view accurate?
2. Do you think that today's milking methods are humane?
3. What are the health risks and benefits of consuming milk products?
4. Are milk substitutes worse than or superior to milk?
5. How can a lactose-intolerant person get enough calcium and vitamin D without the use of vitamin supplements?

Research Ideas for Students

1. Risks and benefits of raw milk consumption
2. Alternate feeds that will reduce methane gas emission from cows
3. Potential of irradiation as an alternative to pasteurization
4. Risks and benefits of using bovine somatotropin
5. Risks and benefits of using antibiotics in animals

References

1. McGee H. *On Food and Cooking: The Science and Lore of the Kitchen*. New York: Collier Books; 1984.
2. U.S. Department of Agriculture. Early Developments in the American Dairy Industry. Available at: http://www.nal.usda.gov/speccoll/images1/dairy.htm. Accessed June 1, 2012.
3. Sonnenfeld A. *Food: A Culinary History*. New York: Penguin Books; 1999.
4. U.S. Department of Agriculture. *Dietary Guidelines for Americans, 2010*. 7th ed. Washington, DC: U.S. Government Printing Office; 2010.
5. U.S. Department of Agriculture. National Nutrient Database. Reference Standard. Available at: http://www.nal.usda.gov/fnic/foodcomp/search. Accessed April 19, 2011.

6. National Dairy Council. Lactose intolerance: New understandings. *Dairy Council Digest*. 2010 Aug;81(4):19–24. Available at: http://www.nationaldairycouncil.org/SiteCollectionDocuments/research/dairy_council_digests/2010/DCD1043r.pdf. Accessed October 20, 2012.
7. National Dairy Council. Dairy Food Safety. Available at: http://www.nationaldairycouncil.org/SiteCollectionDocuments/footer/FAQ/food_safety/FoodSafetyFactSheetPDF.pdf. Accessed March 24, 2011.
8. Mead, PS Slutsker L, Dietz V, et al. Food-related illness and death in the United States. *Emerging Infectious Diseases*. 1999;5(5):607–625.
9. National Dairy Council. *Dairy Council Digest*. 2009 Jan–Feb;80(1):1–6.
10. U.S. Department of Agriculture. United States Department of Agriculture Standards for Ice Cream. Available at: http://www.ams.usda.gov/AMSv1.0/getfile?dDocName=STELDEV3004477. Accessed June 1, 2012.
11. Office of Dietary Supplements, National Institutes of Health. Dietary Supplement Fact Sheet: Calcium. Available at: http://ods.od.nih.gov/factsheets/Calcium-QuickFacts. Accessed March 1, 2011.
12. Elwood PC, Pickering JE, Givens DI, Gallacher JE. The consumption of milk and dairy foods and the incidence of vascular disease and diabetes: An overview of the evidence. *Lipids*. 2010 Oct;45(10):925–939.
13. National Osteoporosis Foundation. Available at: http://www.nof.org. Accessed March 1, 2011.
14. Djousse L, Pankow JS, Hunt SC, et al. Influence of saturated fat and linolenic acid on the association between intake of dairy products and blood pressure. *Hypertension*. 2006;48:335–341.
15. National Cancer Institute. Calcium and Cancer Prevention: Strengths and Limits of the Evidence. Available at: http://www.cancer.gov/cancertopics/factsheet/prevention/calcium. Accessed March 21, 2011.
16. McCullough ML, Robertson AS, Rodriguez C, et al. Calcium, vitamin D, dairy products, and risk of colorectal cancer in the Cancer Prevention Study II Nutrition Cohort (United States). *Cancer Causes Control*. 2003;14(1):1–12.
17. Choi HK, Willett W, Stampfer MJ, et al. Dairy consumption and risk of type 2 diabetes mellitus in men: A prospective study. *Arch Int Med*. 2005;165:997–1003.
18. McCarron DA, Heaney RP. Estimated healthcare savings associated with adequate dairy food intake. *Am J Hyperten*. 2004;17:88–97.
19. Alonso A, Beunza JJ, Delgado-Rodriquez M, et al. Low-fat dairy consumption and reduced risk of hypertension: The Sequimiento Universidad de Navarra (SUN) cohort. *AJCN*. 2005;82:972–979.
20. Greer FR, Krebs NF, the American Academy of Pediatrics Committee on Nutrition. American Academy of Pediatrics: Optimizing bone health and calcium intakes of infants, children, and adolescents. *Pediatrics*. 2006;117(2):578–585.
21. Heaney RP. Calcium, dairy products, and osteoporosis. *JACN*. 2000;19(suppl):83s–99s.
22. Huncharek M, Muscat J, Kupelnick B. Colorectal cancer risk and dietary intake of calcium, vitamin D, and dairy products: A meta-analysis of 26,335 cases from 60 observational studies. *Nutri Cancer*. 2009;61:47–69.
23. Larsson SC, Bergkvist L, Rutegard J, et al. Calcium and dairy food intakes are inversely associated with colorectal cancer risk in the cohort of Swedish men. *AJCN*. 2006;83:667–673.
24. Hartman JW, Tang JE, Wilkinson SB, et al. Consumption of fat-free fluid milk following resistance exercise promotes greater lean mass accretion than soy or carbohydrate consumption in young novice male weightlifters. *AJCN*. 2007;86:373–381.
25. Roy BD. Milk: The new sports drink? A review. J Int Soc Sports Nutri. 2008;2:5–15.
26. U.S. Department of Agriculture. What We Eat in America, NHANES 2001–2002: Usual Nutrient Intakes from Food Compared to Dietary Reference Intakes. Available at: http://www.ars.usda.gov/foodsurvey. Accessed March 1, 2011.
27. National Dairy Council. 3 Every Day of Dairy. Available at: http://www.nationaldairycouncil.org/EducationMaterials/HealthProfessionalsEducationKits/Pages/3EveryDayofDairy.aspx. Accessed March 1, 2011.
28. Keast DR, Fulgoni VL, Quann EE, Auestad N. Contributions of milk, dairy products, and other foods to vitamin D intakes in the U.S.: NHANES, 2003–2006. *FASEB*. 2010 Apr;24:274–279.
29. Shahar DR, Schwarzfuchs D, Fraser D, et al. Dairy calcium intake, serum vitamin D, and successful weight loss. *AJCN*. 2010 Nov;92(5):1017–1022.
30. Eagan MS, Lyle MN, Gunther CW, et al. Effect of 1-year dairy product intervention on fat mass in young women: 6-month follow-up. *Obesity*. 2006;14:2242–2248.
31. U.S. Department of Health and Human Services. Bone Health and Osteoporosis: A Report of the Surgeon General. Available at: http://www.surgeongeneral.gov/library/reports/bonehealth. Accessed March 1, 2011.
32. Shimazaki Y, Shirota T, Uchida K, et al. Intake of dairy products and periodontal disease: The Hisayama Study. *J Periodontology*. 2008;131–137.
33. National Heart, Lung and Blood Institute. Available at: http://www.nhlbi.nih.gov. Accessed March 21, 2011.
34. Nettleton JA, Steffen LM, Palmas W, et al. Associations between microalbuminuria and animal foods, plants foods, and dietary patterns in the Multiethnic Study of Atherosclerosis. *AJCN*. 2008;87:1825–1836.
35. Bertone-Johnsom ER, Hankinson SE, Bendich A, et al. Calcium and vitamin D intake and risk of incident of premenstrual syndrome. *Arch Int Med*. 2005;165:1246–1252.
36. American Academy of Dermatology. Food Does Not Cause Acne. Available at: http://www.skincarephysicians.com/acnenet/acne_and_diet.html. Accessed April 12, 2011.
37. World Dairy Summit 2010. Environmental/ecological impact of the dairy sector. *Bull Int Dairy Fed*. 2009;436. Available at: http://www.wds2010.com/PDF/Enviro-bulletin.pdf. Accessed March 21, 2011.
38. Innovation Center for U.S. Dairy. Available at: http://www.usdairy.com/sustainability. Accessed March 22, 2011.
39. Nestle M. *What to Eat*. New York: North Point Press; 2006.
40. National Environmental Health Association Position Regarding Sale or Distribution of Raw Milk. January 28, 2008. Available at: http://www.neha.org/position_papers/position_raw_milk.htm. Accessed October 20, 2012.

CHAPTER 8

Eggs and Egg Replacements

Debra King, MS, RD, LD

Chapter Objectives

THE STUDENT WILL BE EMPOWERED TO:

- Summarize the history of eggs as an important food source, both around the world and in the United States.
- Identify the components of an egg and the physical properties that affect freshness.
- Discuss the nutritional properties of eggs and their impacts on human health.
- Summarize basic safety precautions that should be taken when cooking with eggs.
- Identify uses of whole eggs, egg whites, and egg yolks in food preparation.
- Identify the characteristics of eggs as a protein source for all meals, including their uses as leavening agents, binders, coagulants, and emulsifiers.
- Identify different means of substituting for eggs in recipes.
- Summarize the development of various egg products, including dried egg mixes.
- Define the various types of housing for laying hens.
- Discuss the measures that protect consumers from the dangers of *Salmonella* and other pathogens.
- Describe methods of egg grading, sizing, dating, and labeling.

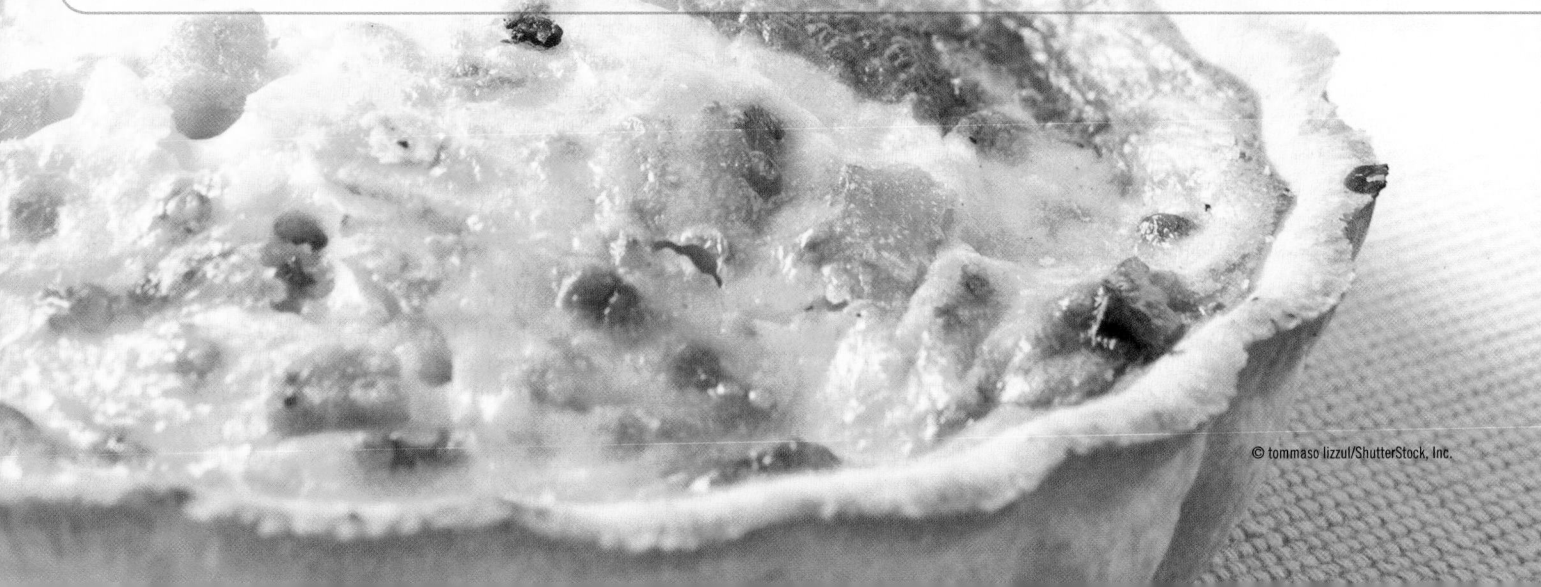

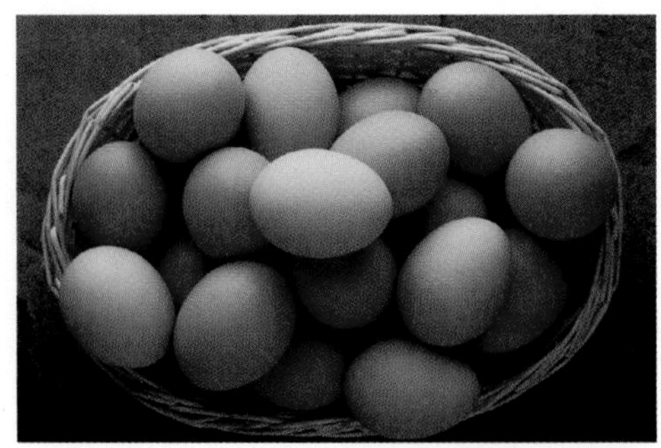

FIGURE 8.1 Eggs have been an important food since the dawn of civilization. The egg often is used as a symbol of creation, fertility, and new life, as evidenced by its use in Easter and other spring rituals. Today, eggs are an essential ingredient in many foods.

Historical and Cultural Significance

Eggs, which are often called the perfect food, provide a sustainable source of protein and many other nutrients. Historical records provide information showing that eggs from fowl became part of human diets at least as early as 3200 B.C. (see **Figure 8.1**). Hens were domesticated in Europe for centuries before they were brought to the Americas in 1493 on the second trip made by Christopher Columbus. Chickens on this cross-Atlantic adventure were a lightweight, economical food source for the crew and an important foundation food in the New World.[1]

Eggs Around the World

The domestic chicken, *Gallus domesticus*, had the same genetic code 4,000 to 5,000 years ago as it does today.[1] The properties of eggs allow for low-cost, simple production, and their varied uses in meals make them a highly desirable food in many cultures. For example, many Asian cultures improve the protein content of vegetable and pasta dishes by adding eggs, and the French have long worked at perfecting the art of using eggs in pastries and sauces.

Eggs in the American Diet

Over the last few centuries, eggs have become an integral part of the American diet. They are now used as an important protein source for breakfast, as a binder and leavening agent in baking, and as an emulsifier in many food items, including sauces and dressings. Through artificial selection, farmers produced better **laying hens**, also called **pullets**, increasing egg production and their income. In the 1940s, farmers developed large egg production farms by housing hens to control their access to food and water and to protect them from predators. Such housing also offered weaker hens protection from more aggressive ones, further increasing egg production.

As the demand for eggs grew, farmers continued to find ways to increase production and decrease costs. Over time, the concept of mass production took hold. Laying hens are now routinely placed in wire cages raised above the ground. The eggs that they lay roll onto conveyor belts that transport them through cleaning, grading, and packaging.

In the 1950s, egg consumption in the United States reached an all-time high, with the average American eating almost eight eggs per week. A downward slide in egg consumption followed due to concerns that egg consumption contributed to heart disease. Egg consumption began to increase again in 1990s, as shown in **Table 8.1**, as more accurate information about the health effects of egg consumption was ascertained. Since then, egg consumption has continued to increase. The current average is about five eggs per person per week, which includes not only whole-shell eggs but also **egg products** used in baked items, sauces, and dressings.

laying hens Domesticated chickens raised solely for the purpose of egg production.

pullets An alternate term for laying hens.

egg product The result of removing eggs from their shells and processing them into liquid, frozen, and dried forms.

air cell The pocket of air usually found at the large end of an egg between the outer and inner shell membranes.

yolk The yellow, usually spherical, portion of an egg surrounded by the albumen that serves as nutrition for the developing chick in a fertilized egg; the yolk is a major source of vitamins and minerals. It contains almost half the egg's protein and all of the fat and cholesterol.

albumen The clear substance consisting of water-soluble protein that surrounds the yolk of an egg.

egg white Common name used for the albumen that surrounds the yolk of an egg.

shell Outer covering of the egg, composed mainly of calcium carbonate; may be white or brown depending on the breed of chicken.

Physical and Chemical Properties

The minute a hen lays the egg it begins to decrease in quality; the **air cell** grows, and the firmness of the **yolk** and **albumen** (or **egg white**) diminish. Over time, whether refrigerated or not, the yolk absorbs water from the white. Moisture evaporates from the white through the **shell**'s pores, and air moves into the shell, enlarging the air cell. The size of the air cell in an egg determines the age of the egg: the smaller the air cell, the fresher the egg; the larger the air cell, the older the egg. You can test the age of an egg by submerging it into a bowl of water. A small air cell will cause the egg to sink to the bottom

TABLE 8.1
Average Per Capita Consumption of Eggs, United States

Year	Eggs per Person
2009	248
2005	257
1990	236
1950	389

Source: Data from Economic Research Service, U.S. Department of Agriculture. Food Availability (Per Capita) Data System. Available at: http://www.ers.usda.gov/Data/FoodConsumption. Accessed June 8, 2012.

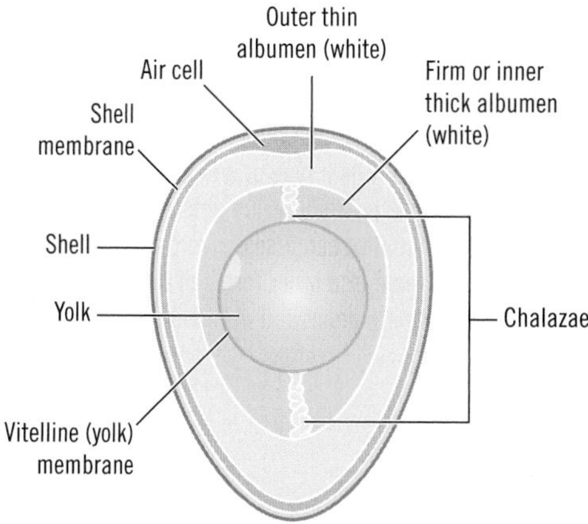

FIGURE 8.2 The structure of the egg serves to protect and nourish the developing embryo (chick) until it is ready to hatch.

Source: Adapted from How to Buy Eggs, *Home and Garden Bulletin* No. 264. U.S. Department of Agriculture, Agricultural Marketing Service, December 1981.

of the bowl, meaning that the egg is fresh. A large air cells will keep the egg floating, meaning that the egg is old.

Other indicators of freshness become apparent when the egg is cracked open. When a fresh egg is cracked, the egg white is thick and the yolk is firm and round. The volume of liquid released from a broken egg will be greater the older the egg. With age, the albumen becomes thinner, losing some of its thickening and leavening powers. The yolk also grows flatter, larger, and is more easily broken. In addition, the **chalazae** (kah-LAY-zuh), the twisted cordlike strands of egg white that anchor the yolk in the center of the white, become less prominent and weaker, allowing the yolk to move off center. Storing eggs at 40–45°F (4–7°C) helps to maintain freshness and decreases the risk of foodborne illness. The parts of an egg are labeled in **Figure 8.2**.

Nutritional Properties

Eggs are a great source of protein and a host of essential nutrients. A large egg provides about 72 calories, 50% of which comes from fats in the yolk. It has more than 6 grams of protein: 3.6 grams come from the egg white, and about 2.7 grams come from the yolk. Eggs are also loaded with vitamins. They are excellent sources of vitamin B_{12}, riboflavin, folate, and the fat-soluble vitamins A, D, and K. Eggs are also a good source of the minerals calcium, iodine, iron, phosphorus, selenium, and sodium. Eggs also contain **lutein** and **zeaxanthin**. These two carotenoids act as antioxidants and are thought to be important to eye health, reducing the risk of cataracts and age-related macular degeneration.

Finally, eggs contain more **choline**, a micronutrient essential for breaking down fats to produce energy and maintain cell membranes, than any other single food.[2] Choline also plays a role in nerve signaling and may assist the body in maintaining lower blood levels of **homocysteine**, an amino acid naturally produced by our bodies and a potential contributor to heart disease.[3]

Cooking eggs alone or in prepared dishes removes a only minimal amount of nutrients. Minerals, fat-soluble vitamins, and antioxidants in eggs remain stable whether the eggs are baked, fried, hard-boiled, poached, or reheated. The only slight loss of nutrients comes from water-soluble vitamins, which are sensitive to heat. Cooking causes losses of between 5% and 20% of the raw egg values for water-soluble vitamins.[4]

Impact on Health

Consumption of eggs in the United States dropped significantly in the 1970s and 1980s when leading health authorities touted reports about the negative health effects of cholesterol. When news first spread that cholesterol caused heart disease, scientists believed that eggs contained 274 milligrams of cholesterol; today, we know that the average large egg contains only

chalazae The twisted cordlike strands of egg white that anchor the yolk in the center of the white.

lutein A carotenoid found in eggs and green leafy vegetables that may act as an antioxidant, protecting the eyes from cataracts and age-related macular degeneration.

zeaxanthin A carotenoid found in eggs and green leafy vegetables that may act as an antioxidant, protecting eyes from cataracts and age-related macular degeneration.

choline A micronutrient essential for breaking down fats to produce energy and maintain cell membranes.

homocysteine An amino acid produced in the body and a potential contributor to heart disease and certain age-related diseases when blood levels are elevated.

ovalbumen The main protein found in the albumen or egg white; it makes up 60–65% of the total protein in an egg.

vitelline membrane A colorless membrane that surrounds the yolk.

Phytonutrient Point

Omega-3 Fatty Acids Eggs can be fortified with omega-3 fatty acids by including flaxseed in chicken feed. Flaxseed contains a type of omega-3 fatty acid called alpha-linolenic acid, which gets deposited in the egg yolk. Hens fed flaxseed also convert some of the alpha-linolenic acid into other forms of omega-3 fatty acids; these also are deposited in the egg yolk.

Gastronomy Point

Eggs As early as 550 B.C., followers of the Jain religion in India did not consume eggs because it was against their philosophy of "do no harm." It was not as easy then as now to distinguish between fertilized and unfertilized eggs. The early influence of Jainism is still reflected in traditional Indian recipes today, which use eggs sparingly, even in baking and bread making.

187 milligrams of cholesterol. Another fact that influenced the negative image of eggs was that often the research did not control for the effects of other high-fat food items commonly eaten with eggs, such as bacon, sausage, and butter. It is now known that the saturated fat in these accompanying foods also contributes to human cholesterol levels. Today, experts believe that eggs, when consumed in moderation, can play an important role in the American diet. **Table 8.2** compares the cholesterol content of different foods.

Effects of Cholesterol from Eggs

Research has shown that consuming an average of one egg per day from all sources, including baked foods and prepared dishes, does not contribute to heart disease or stroke in healthy adults. However, this finding does not mean that eggs should be eaten without limit. Research also reveals that eating more than seven eggs per week increases the possibility of high blood cholesterol, which increases the risk of related diseases. Caution on consuming eggs is still advised for individuals with type 2 diabetes, where any increase in dietary cholesterol from eggs and other sources increases the risk of cardiovascular disease.[5]

Egg Allergies

The Food, Drug, and Cosmetic Act classifies eggs as a major food allergen.[6] It is the most common food allergen in infants and children. Food allergy results from an abnormal reaction of the body to a food it determines to be harmful. The food causes the release of antibodies, leading to increased levels of serum immunoglobulin levels and one or more of the following symptoms:

- Hives
- Tingling in the mouth
- Swelling in the tongue and throat
- Difficulty breathing
- Abdominal cramps
- Vomiting or diarrhea
- Eczema or rash
- Coughing or wheezing
- Loss of consciousness
- Dizziness

Some of these symptoms can have serious consequences, including death, so an egg allergy cannot be taken lightly.[7] The diagnosis of an egg allergy comes from tracking immediate reactions after eggs are consumed. In homes

Table 8.2
Comparison of Cholesterol in Foods

Food	Serving Size	Cholesterol
Egg, hard boiled	1 whole	187 mg
Cheddar cheese	1 ounce	30 mg
Chicken, baked	½ breast	73 mg
80% lean beef patty, broiled	3 ounces	77 mg
Pork bacon, broiled	3 medium slices	21 mg
Salmon, dry heat	3 ounces	54 mg

Source: Data from U.S. Department of Agriculture, Agricultural Research Service. 2011. USDA National Nutrient Database for Standard Reference, Release 24. Nutrient Data Laboratory Home Page, http://www.ars.usda.gov/ba/bhnrc/ndl.

with children or adults allergic to eggs, anyone preparing food must be vigilant about hand washing and keeping all egg products separate from any food served to the allergic individual. Similarly, restaurants, school lunch programs, and day care centers also must track how foods are prepared and provide information to parents of children with egg and other food allergies.[8]

Since 2006 food manufacturers have been required to use plain language on labels to define definite or possible contents of the top eight food allergens, which include eggs. A strict policy of reading food labels is essential for ongoing prevention of allergic reactions. At the end of 2010, the FDA Food Safety Modernization Act allowed for the creation of voluntary guidelines by the Secretary of Education, which will help early childhood and school programs develop programs to manage egg and other food allergies presented by the children in their care.[9]

Innovation Point

The Flu Vaccine Most flu vaccines are grown in chicken eggs, which can be a problem for people who are allergic to eggs. People with egg allergies may not be able to receive the flu vaccine.

Special Topic 8.1

Avian Influenza

Debra King, MS, RD, LD

Described in 1878 as the "fowl plague" by the Italian physician Edoardo Perroncito, avian influenza, or avian flu as it is more commonly called, is a disease of poultry. Symptoms range from completely mild or unnoticeable to catastrophic, with a mortality rate that can reach up to 100% in some avian species.

The natural hosts of the virus are ducks, shorebirds, and other species of wild aquatic birds. In the natural hosts, influenza infections cause almost no symptoms, and the infection is established mostly in the intestinal tract. The virus is excreted with the feces into the water, promoting a cycle of fecal–oral transmission. Outbreaks in poultry occasionally occur when the the virus "jumps" from wild birds to domestic birds. These outbreaks sometimes stay under the radar for a while before becoming more obvious as they increase in virulence.

Strains of avian influenza have caused problems in U.S. turkey flocks and live poultry markets since the 1960s. In 1983, a virus originally characterized as relatively nonpathogenic began to produce avian flulike symptoms with high poultry death losses in Pennsylvania.[1] The next pathogenic avian influenza outbreak among poultry was in 2004 in south-central Texas. In neither outbreak was there any report of transmission of the virus to humans.[2]

Most avian influenza viruses do not infect humans. Avian influenza viruses from wild birds are so well adapted to these species that the chances of humans becoming infected are very small. Avian influenza viruses that become adapted to domestic flocks also are not likely to "jump" to humans.[3] However, infections of non-life-threatening avian influenza viruses do occur in humans, mostly in association with conjunctivitis (pink eye).

The H5N1 Outbreak

However, avian flu does affect humans every now and then in a much more serious way. The highly publicized outbreak of H5N1 avian influenza in chickens and people in Hong Kong illustrates the potential public health concerns that such an outbreak can cause.

In the rare cases where domesticated poultry develop a strain of avian flu that can be transmitted to humans, the people most likely to get sick are those in direct contact with the birds. The H5N1 virus experience in Asia taught poultry handlers that letting influenza viruses circulate in domestic bird species for extended periods can lead to strains of avian flu becoming more and more efficient at making the transition to humans and other animals. Being vigilant, identifying potential disease signs, and learning more about the disease and its interactions with the host are keys to preventing future outbreaks. Putting strict biosecurity measures in place can also help. For example, in 2004 the U.S. government issued a ban on importation of poultry from countries affected by avian influenza viruses. Through the combined effort of poultry farmers, poultry veterinarians, government agencies, diagnosticians, and scientists, the likelihood of future outbreaks is reduced.[3]

Eggs and Avian Influenza

People cannot become infected with avian flu by eating safely handled and properly cooked poultry or eggs. Most cases of avian flu in humans have resulted from direct or close contact with infected poultry or surfaces contaminated with secretions and excretions from infected birds. Studies show that the cooking methods recommended by the U.S. Department of Agriculture and the Food and Drug Administration for poultry and eggs to prevent other infections will destroy avian flu viruses as well.[4]

To learn more about avian influenza, visit http://www.pandemicflu.gov.

References

1 U.S. Department of Agriculture. Agriculture Research Service. Avian Influenza. Updated April 23, 2009. Available at: http://www.ars.usda.gov/Research/docs.htm?docid=8638. Accessed December 22, 2010.

2 Centers for Disease Control and Prevention. Avian Influenza: A Virus Infections of Humans. Updated May 23, 2008. Available at: http://www.cdc.gov/flu/avian/gen-info/avian-flu-humans.htm. Accessed December 21, 2010.

3 U.S. Department of Agriculture. Information Resources on Avian Influenza. Introduction by Daniel R. Perez, PhD. Updated October 2005. Available at: http://www.nal.usda.gov/awic/aflu/Avian%20Influenza.htm Accessed December 20, 2010.

4 Centers for Disease Control and Prevention. Questions and Answers About Avian Influenza (Bird Flu) and Avian Influenza A (H5N1) Virus. Updated May 28, 2008. Available at: http://www.cdc.gov/flu/avian/gen-info/qa.htm. Accessed December 21, 2010.

Food Preparation Principles

Eggs provide a versatile source of protein for any meal, not just breakfast. Try eggs in a sandwich for lunch, or top off a salad with a hard-boiled egg to increase your satiety. Need a snack for hungry children? Keep hardboiled eggs in the refrigerator and use them to make funny faces on whole grain bread. Eggs also can easily star in one-dish meals for family dinners. For example, a frittata filled with veggies, an Asian egg-drop soup, or a fancy mushroom soufflé are all great ways to serve eggs as a main course.

Roles of Eggs in Recipes

Eggs have a number of roles in recipe preparation. Because the protein in eggs coagulates upon heating, eggs help to thicken mixtures and create structure. For example, a meatloaf recipe may use eggs to bind the rest of the ingredients together so that it stands firm when baked. Eggs act as a leavening agent in baked goods, making them lighter and fuller, and provide moisture. Eggs also create **emulsions**, which are used in salad dressings.

emulsion A mixture of two liquids that cannot easily blend together unless an emulsifier is present.

Cooking Safely with Eggs

The key to cooking with eggs is to cook them so they are safe to eat.

Take Basic Precautions

When cooking with eggs, practice these basic safety tips:

- Wash hands, utensils, equipment, and work areas with hot, soapy water.
- Remove only the number of eggs needed from the carton for the meal or recipe being prepared, and immediately return the carton to the refrigerator.
- Cook eggs until the white is completely firm and the yolk begins to thicken but is not hard. Scrambled eggs should be cooked until no visible liquid remains, and fried eggs should be cooked on both sides or in a covered pan.

- Recipes that call for a stirred egg custard base must first be cooked to 160°F (71°C).
- If a recipe calls for adding raw eggs to a previously cooked dish, the dish must be cooked further until it reaches 160°F (71°C).
- The USDA does not recommend eating shell eggs that are raw or undercooked due to the possibility that *Salmonella* bacteria may be present.
- When preparing any recipe that contains eggs, resist the temptation to taste-test the mixture during preparation.
- Egg-containing foods should be thoroughly cooked before eating.
- Never allow egg-containing foods to be out the refrigerator more than 2 hours total, not including cooking time.
- If hot egg-rich foods are not going to be served immediately after cooking, put them into shallow containers and refrigerate at once so they will cool quickly, then reheat them as needed.
- Once eggs are cooked, use them within 3 days.
- If your recipe calls for uncooked eggs (such as for Caesar salad, Hollandaise sauce, eggnog, homemade mayonnaise, ice cream, and key lime pie), use of pasteurized eggs is recommended.
- If you do use raw eggs in a recipe, heat the eggs in one of the recipe's other liquid ingredients over low heat, stirring constantly, until the mixture reaches 160°F (71°C).
- Raw eggs and other ingredients, combined according to recipe directions, should be cooked immediately or refrigerated and cooked within 24 hours.
- When preparing foods for high-risk persons, such as infants and young children, pregnant women, older adults, and people with weakened immune systems (such as those with HIV/AIDS, cancer, diabetes, kidney disease, and transplant patients) cook egg products to 160°F (71°C) (just as you would raw eggs). Even though the egg products are required to be pasteurized, showing extra caution provides the highest food safety standard.
- Use a thermometer to determine the temperature inside egg dishes to ensure the safety of all cooked egg products.[10]

Take Note of Color Cues

Variations in the color of eggs can be caused by many factors. The following guidelines describe how color variations in raw and cooked eggs may (or may not) indicate a problem:

- *Blood spots* occur due to a rupture of one or more small blood vessels in the yolk at the time of ovulation. They do not affect the safety of the egg.
- A *cloudy white* (albumen) indicates freshness. A clear white indicates that the egg has aged.
- A *pink* or *iridescent white* (albumen) indicates spoilage due to *Pseudomonas* bacteria. Some of these microorganisms, which produce a greenish, fluorescent, water-soluble pigment, are harmful to humans.
- The *color of yolk* varies in shades of yellow based on the hen's diet. For example, a hen eating plenty of yellow-orange plant pigments from marigold petals and yellow corn will produce a darker yellow yolk than a hen eating a white cornmeal. Artificial color additives are not permitted in egg production.
- A *green ring* around the yolk of hard-cooked egg means that the egg was overcooked, but that it is still safe to consume (see **Figure 8.3**).

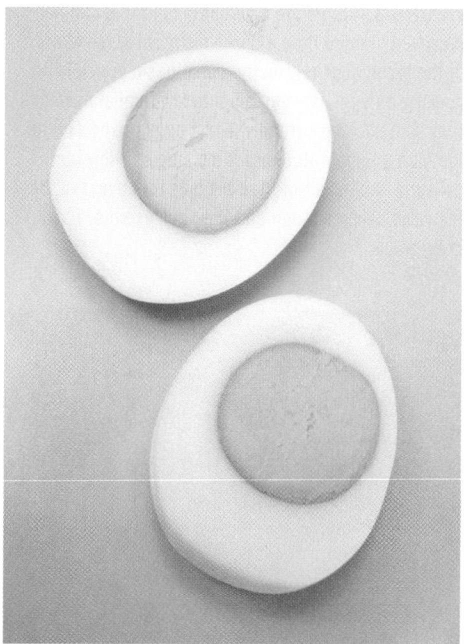

FIGURE 8.3 Hard-boiled eggs with a green ring around the yolk are safe to eat. The green ring is just an indication that the egg was cooked too long, causing the sulfur and iron compounds in the egg to react on the surface of the yolk.

The green color results from sulfur and iron compounds in the egg reacting on the surface of the yolk. The green color may also result from boiling the eggs in water with a high concentration of iron. Scrambled eggs cooked at too high a temperature or held on a steam table too long may also develop a greenish cast. These eggs are safe to consume, provided they are held at 160°F (70°C).[1]

Safety of Cracked Eggs

Bacteria enter eggs through cracks in the shell; it is never acceptable to purchase cracked eggs. However, if eggs crack on the way home from the store they can be broken into a clean container, covered tightly, kept refrigerated, and used within 2 days. If cracks occur while boiling for hard-cooked eggs, the eggs are safe to eat.[1]

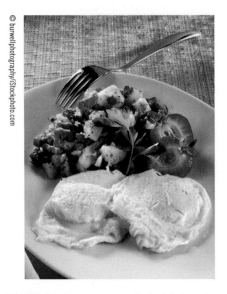

FIGURE 8.4 Eggs are a versatile food that can be prepared in more than a dozen different ways. Many of the techniques rely on the same basic principle of cooking an egg: use a medium to low temperature and time your cooking carefully. When eggs are cooked at too high a temperature or for too long at a low temperature, whites shrink and become tough and rubbery; the yolks become tough and their surface may turn gray-green.

Storing Hard-Cooked Eggs

When fresh eggs are boiled to produce hard-boiled eggs for making egg salad, tossing in a salad, or eating as a snack, the protective coating in the shell washes away. This leaves no protection over the pores in the shell, which means that bacteria can enter and contaminate the egg. Refrigerate hard-cooked eggs with 2 hours of cooking and use them within a week of cooking.[1]

Whole Egg Preparation Techniques

Eggs lend themselves to many preparation techniques, each resulting in a slightly different presentation. All result in appetizing high-protein additions to any plate. The following are some of the more common preparation techniques:

- *Coddled:* The egg is cracked and emptied into an egg coddler, a container typically made of porcelain, which is then placed into a boiling pot of water and cooked until done. Coddled eggs are a delicacy in Great Britain.
- *Fried:* The egg is cracked and placed on a skillet with butter or oil and cooked slowly. For safety reasons, a sunny-side up egg (with the yolk on top) should be cooked until the yolk is firm, which can be achieved by using a covered pan. An over-easy egg is flipped just as the white of the egg coagulates, and the egg yolk is cooked until firm (see **Figure 8.4**). (The critical prerequisite to flipping an egg without breaking the yolk—besides a steady hand—is a fresh egg.)
- *Hard boiled:* Shelled eggs are cooked in boiling water until the egg white coagulates and the yolk it is cooked through.
- *Frittata:* Cracked eggs are beaten, which adds air; this creates a fluffy texture when baked. Cooked meat, cheese, vegetables, and/or herbs are stirred into the eggs, and the mixture is baked.
- *Omelets:* The eggs are cracked and whipped until the yolk and white are blended together. Then the egg is spread over a hot skillet, filled with any combination of cheese, cooked meat, and vegetables, and then folded in half (see **Figure 8.5**).
- *Pickled:* Pickled eggs are considered by many to be a delicacy. To prepare pickled eggs, hard-boiled eggs are marinated in vinegar and pickling spices, spicy cider, or juice from pickles or pickled beets.[1]
- *Poached:* Eggs are cracked and emptied into lightly boiling water, then cooked at low heat until the egg white and yolk are firm.
- *Quiche:* Beaten eggs and a variety of eggs, cheeses, herbs, or cooked meats are mixed together and then baked in an unbaked crust.

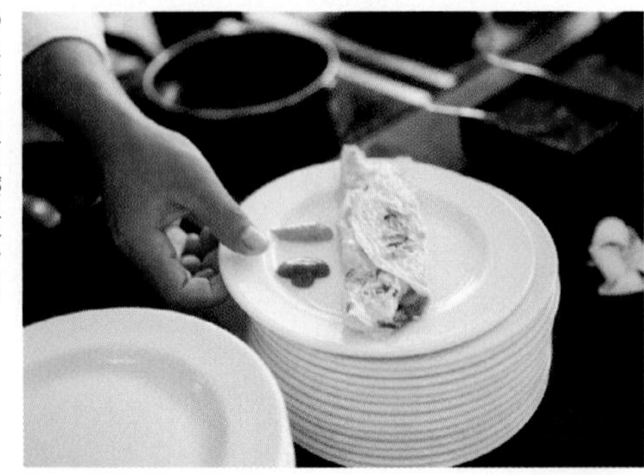

FIGURE 8.5 Omelets are a quick and easy way to prepare eggs. They also are a great way to incorporate meat and vegetables into a breakfast dish. Omelets should be cooked in a nonstick omelet pan for best results.

- *Scrambled:* Eggs are cracked and whipped until the yolk and white are blended together. Water, milk, and other ingredients are then mixed in. The mixture is slowly cooked until no visible liquid remains.
- *Shirred:* Eggs are cracked and placed in a ramekin with cream or butter and then baked. This procedure may be adapted to create baked eggs, or custard.
- *Soft boiled:* With a soft-boiled egg, the egg is boiled whole until the white of the egg is firm and the yolk is lightly runny.
- *Soufflé:* A French word meaning "puffed," a soufflé is a savory or sweet dish with a light, airy texture provided by stiffly beaten egg whites (see **Figure 8.6**). Eggs are cracked and the yolks and whites separated; the yolks are mixed with cream, cheese, vegetables, and/or other ingredients to provide the base and flavor of a soufflé. The whites are whipped into a stiff foam to create the lightness. The stiff whites are then folded into the yolk mixture. The mixture then is baked. The soufflé rises high, becoming a light and airy dish.

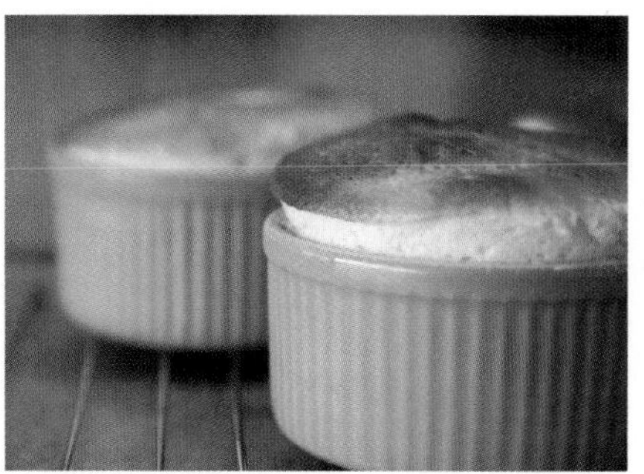

FIGURE 8.6 All soufflés have two basic components: a flavored cream sauce or puree and egg whites beaten into a meringue. One of the most popular types of soufflé is chocolate soufflé.

Uses of Egg Whites

Egg whites provide texture and volume to a variety of food items, from candy to meringues. Caution must be taken when preparing items such as meringue shells, divinity candy, and 7-minute frosting to ensure the safe consumption of egg whites. Meringue-topped pies should be safe if baked at 350°F (177°C) for 15 minutes (see **Figure 8.7**). Avoid chiffon pies and fruit whips made with raw, beaten egg whites. If you want to make these items, substitute with a pasteurized dried egg whites product or use a whipped cream topping. Do not use recipes for icings that require uncooked eggs. To ensure food safety, instead use recipes that start with a hot sugar syrup followed by adding beaten egg whites.

Egg Foams

Egg whites create **egg foam** through friction and incorporation of air. Any time friction—such as that caused by beating egg whites—intersects with air and protein, a change in the texture of the liquid results, which increases its volume. Egg foams enhance egg dishes, including such items as divinity candy, soufflés, frittatas, angel food cake, and other cake batters. Using clean, dry bowls and mixers provides the key to the best egg foam. Contamination from a drop of oil or a poorly removed yolk changes the texture of the albumen and can significantly reduce foam volume (see **Figure 8.8**).

egg foam Created when the albumen (egg white) is whipped; when heated, the air expands and the protein in the egg foam solidifies, creating a light texture for soufflés, cakes, and meringues.

Candy

Certain types of candy are made by combining food crystals with eggs. The results are candies and frozen desserts with the perfect texture and taste. The most common crystal in foods is sugar. Another common crystal is ice. Because of eggs' ability to form foam and to act as an emulsifier, they can be used to prepare a number of different sweets.

In making candy, the properties of eggs contribute to air incorporation, water binding, and product structure. For example, eggs control the growth of sugar crystals: The fat and protein from eggs reduces the size and number of sugar crystals that form in the candy by interfering with the orientation of the sucrose molecules, resulting in a smooth, creamy texture. Crystalline candies that may use eggs include fudge, fondant, and divinity.[11]

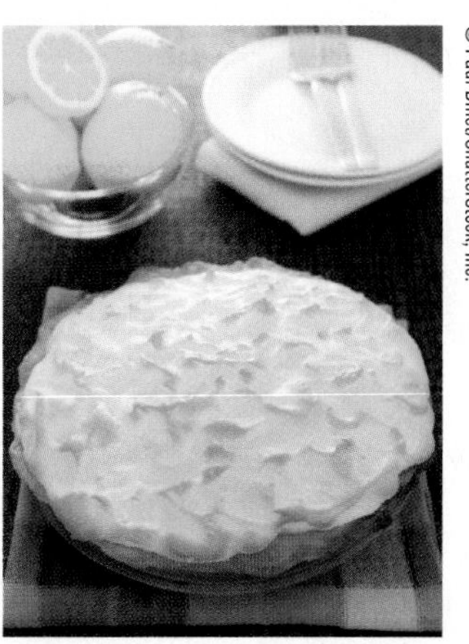

FIGURE 8.7 A meringue is made from whipped egg whites and sugar. Oftentimes a bit of acid is added, such as vinegar or cream of tartar. These light, sweet, airy confections are often flavored with vanilla and a small amount of almond or coconut extract.

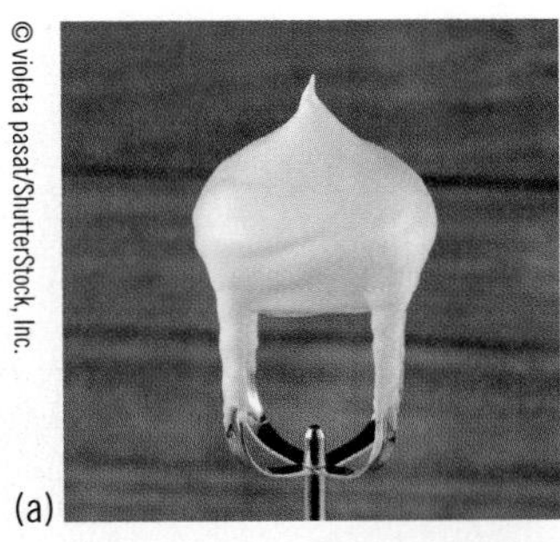

(a)

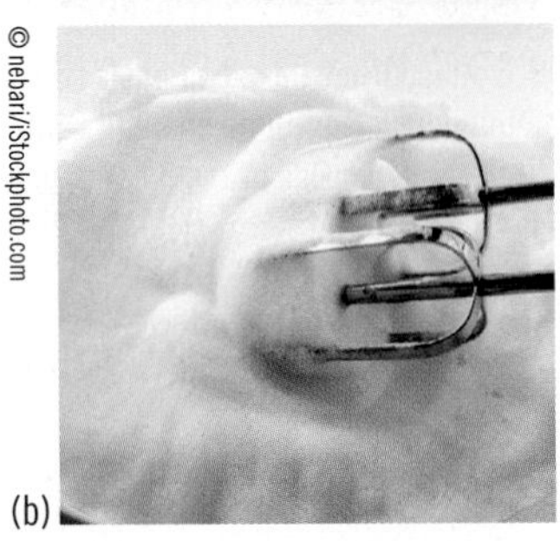

(b)

FIGURE 8.8 (a) When an egg white is beaten, air bubbles become trapped in the albumen. This causes the white to increase in volume, forming a foam. Heating the foam causes the air cells to expand. Egg proteins then coagulate around the air cells, which give the foam permanence. (b) Use of egg whites that are underbeaten will result in a flat product. Overbeaten egg whites will form clumps that are difficult to blend in with other ingredients and will not have the elasticity needed to expand properly when heated. Products made with underbeaten or overbeaten eggs may be dry and flat or collapse.

lecithin A phospholipid found in the cell membrane of egg yolks; used as an emulsifier in cooking.

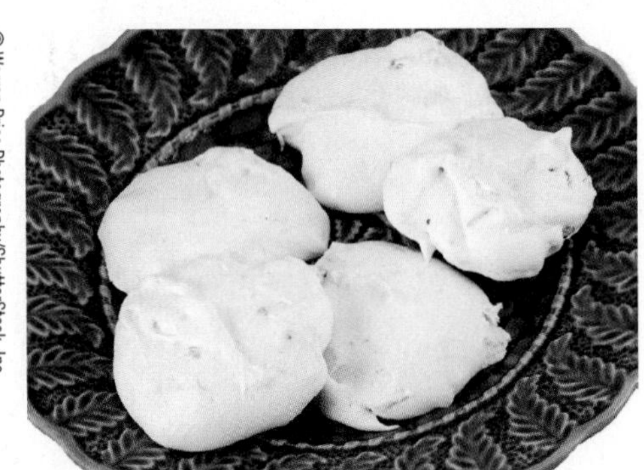

FIGURE 8.9 Divinity is one of the easiest candies to make. All you need is sugar, water, light corn syrup, and vanilla. You will also need two egg whites beaten stiff to hold the ingredients together.

Divinity candy's distinctive texture is provided by its unique use of egg foam to disperse sugar crystals (see **Figure 8.9**). The small crystal size of the sugar and the foamy texture makes this candy melt in the mouth. Using too little albumen can lead to dense, coarse candy due to the presence of larger sugar crystals and denser foam. The addition of too much albumen can create a "chalky" texture due to excessive foam formation for the amount of sucrose syrup present.

Egg Yolks in Desserts

Egg yolks serve many functions in frozen desserts. For example, egg yolks impart flavor, especially to frozen custards, where they help to add "richness." The **lecithin** present in egg yolks acts as an emulsifier, improving the whipping ability and the formation of fat structure in ice cream and other frozen desserts. By using egg yolks as the emulsifier (instead of other chemicals), a frozen dessert can be labeled as "all natural." The egg yolks also increase the viscosity of ice cream, giving it a creamy mouthfeel. A film forms around the fat in the ice cream mixture, enabling the fat molecules to more readily adhere to other solids in the mixture (see **Figure 8.10**). The interaction of solids in the mixture reduces the formation of ice crystals, and fat clumping makes it easier to whip the product, making it smooth.

Generally, eggs are added to frozen dessert mixes before they are pasteurized to ensure food safety. Keeping frozen desserts out of the freezer for short periods of time and storing at 0°F (–18°C) will prevent them from developing off-flavors and melting. Slight melting can give the frozen dessert a foamy look, which consumers often view as a negative quality. Furthermore, refreezing after melting will lead to ice crystal formation, which can destroy a dessert's creamy texture.

When preparing eggnog, ice cream, or custard, always heat the egg mixture to 160°F (71°C) to kill potential bacteria and protect the integrity of the food. The following steps will assist in reducing the risk of foodborne illness from egg-containing frozen desserts:

- Heat milk and/or cream slowly in a sauce pan on the stovetop, but do not let the milk boil.
- When the milk/cream becomes heated, beat together eggs and sugar in a bowl, then slowly add the milk/cream to the egg mixture, stirring constantly.
- After combining the eggs and milk/cream, pour the mixture back into the saucepan. Use low heat, and stir constantly with a whisk until the mixture thickens and just coats a spoon. At that point, use a food thermometer. It should read 160°F (71°C); if it does not, continue heating the mixture until it reaches the desired temperature.
- Remove the pan from the stovetop and stir in the remaining ingredients. If the recipe does not require further cooking, cool the egg/milk mixture quickly by setting the saucepan in a bowl of ice or cold water and stirring for about 10 minutes.
- Keep egg foods safe by storing them in the refrigerator. Never leave them at room temperature for more than 2 hours.[12]

Cooking Eggs at High Altitudes

Cooking eggs at high altitudes takes more time than when cooking at sea level. This is especially true when cooking poached or hard-boiled eggs.

At high altitudes water boils at a lower temperature, so eggs cooked in boiling water may take longer to reach doneness.

For best results, when cooking eggs at high temperatures simply increase the cooking time but not the temperature. At high altitude make sure eggs cook thoroughly by ensuring that the yolks are firm; in egg dishes, always use a food thermometer to determine that the temperature has reached 160°F (71°C).[10]

When a recipe calls for an egg, it means one large egg (at sea level). If baking a cake at high altitude, you may need to increase the amount of eggs (or use extra-large eggs) to augment the air cell structure of the cake. Using smaller eggs in baked dishes at sea level, but especially at high altitude, may result in a batter that is less stable and more likely to fall during the cooking process.[10]

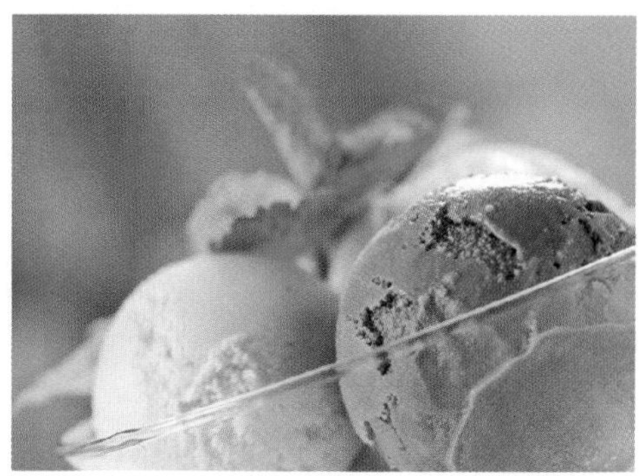

FIGURE 8.10 Because of its emulsification abilities, egg yolks play an important role in the production of ice cream. The viscosity of the ice cream mix is increased when egg yolks are added. Generally, only yolks are used in ice cream making.

Cooking with Egg Substitutes

For vegans and others who prefer to cook without eggs or without their high-cholesterol yolks, a number of other ingredients can take on the role of eggs in most dishes. Making substitutions for eggs can be accomplished in a variety of ways.

Yolk-Free "Eggs"

One type of substitute egg product uses only the albumin, which is then modified with color and flavorings to look like beaten eggs (see **Figure 8.11**). This reduced-fat and cholesterol-free egg substitute can be cooked as scrambled eggs or used in place of eggs in most recipes, as directed on the package.

Commercial Powdered Egg Replacers

Powdered egg replacers require the addition of water or other liquids to supply the full requirements of an egg substitute (see **Figure 8.11**). They use a combination of ingredients to provide the binding and leavening properties required for baking cookies, pancakes, muffins, cakes, brownies, and waffles. Commercial egg replacers are usually a combination of potato starch, tapioca flour, and a leavening agent or whole soy flour, wheat gluten, corn syrup solids, and algin (from brown algae/seaweed).

Plant-Based Egg Substitutes

For people allergic to eggs or those who choose not to eat any part of the egg, the plant world offers a variety of other substitutes to aid in eliminating eggs all together:

- *Flax seed:* Grind three level tablespoons of flax seed in a blender for several minutes to produce a fine powder. Then add ½ cup of cold water, and blend until the mixture is frothy and viscous, with a texture similar to that of well-beaten whole eggs. This mixture provides the equivalent of about two large eggs and can be added to batter whenever the recipe calls for the addition of eggs. It can be stored in the refrigerator for up to 5 days.
- *Soy flour:* Soy flour contains unique properties not found in other legume or grain flours that help serve some egglike functions in baked goods. For each egg called for in a recipe, substitute one heaping tablespoon of soy flour and one tablespoon of water.
- *Mashed fruits:* The addition of mashed banana, applesauce, or pureed prunes can replace the moisture of an egg; however, note that it will make the product somewhat heavier and change its flavor. Use ¼ cup of mashed banana, applesauce, or pureed prunes (plus ½ teaspoon of baking powder to enhance lightness) to replace each egg omitted from the baked good recipe.

If you are feeling adventurous, it is easy to make your own egg substitute (see **Table 8.3**).

Gastronomy Point

The Power of the Yolk A single raw egg yolk is capable of emulsifying many cups of oil. Cooks take advantage of the natural emulsifying ability of egg yolk phospholipids in products such as mayonnaise (oil and vinegar emulsion) and hollandaise sauce (butter and lemon juice emulsion). Food producers use phospholipid emulsifiers in processed foods, which today provide much of our intake.

Source: Reproduced from Insel P, Ross, D, McMahon K, Bernstein M. *Nutrition.* 4th ed. Burlington, MA: Jones & Bartlett Learning; 2011:231.

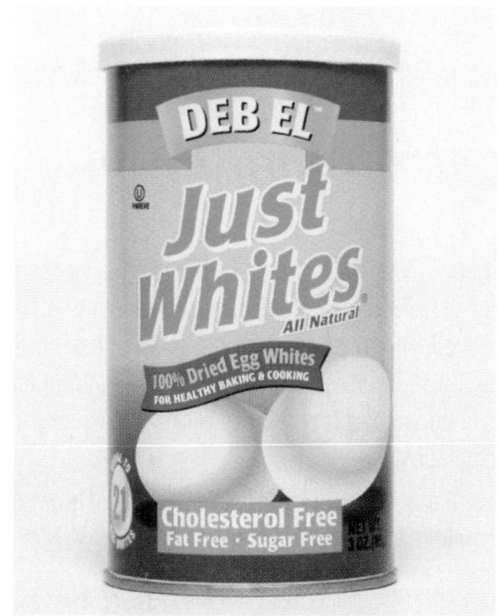

FIGURE 8.11 Note the difference between an egg *replacement* and an egg *substitute.* Egg substitutes are in the dairy portion of the grocery store. They contain egg whites and are unsafe for those with egg allergies. In contrast, commercial egg replacement products do not contain eggs and can be used by vegetarians and those with egg allergies.

TABLE 8.3
Make Your Own Egg Substitute

To prepare the equivalent of one egg, whisk together:	
2 tablespoons white flour	
½ tablespoon vegetable oil	
2 tablespoons water	
½ teaspoon baking powder	

Omitting the Egg

Another alternative for those who seek to avoid eggs is to simply omit eggs from recipes that call for them. In recipes that call for one egg but that do not require a great deal of leavening, it is usually acceptable to leave the egg out and add two to three additional tablespoons of liquid to the batter.

Gastronomy Point

How to Beat the Stiffest Egg Whites Whenever you want the greatest possible lightness or fluffiness, beat egg whites alone. A single drop of yolk or fat may reduce the foam's maximum volume by as much as two-thirds. Also, avoid plastic bowls because plastics tend to retain fatty material on their surfaces.

Source: Reproduced from Insel P, Ross, D, McMahon K, Bernstein M. *Nutrition.* 4th ed. Burlington, MA: Jones & Bartlett Learning; 2011:231.

Substitute Binders

When preparing eggless loaves or burgers, binding agents can be found from a variety of alternate sources:

- *Tomato paste:* Thin the tomato paste with a few drops of water and combine it with the other ingredients. (Use caution when adding water because too much will result in the tomato paste losing its ability to bind.)
- *Tahini (sesame seed paste):* Mix tahini with tomato paste and combine with other ingredients.
- *Blended tofu:* Blend silken tofu in the blender and add ¼ to ½ cup to replace each egg. Adding a tablespoon of white flour to each blended tofu egg equivalent will improve the binding capacity of the blended tofu.

- *White cream sauce:* A thick white cream sauce prepared with flour, margarine, and a milk alternative will supply the binding needed. Use ¼ cup of thick white cream sauce to replace each egg.
- *Mashed potatoes:* Add ¼ cup of mashed potato to replace each egg. This is a great way to use leftover mashed potatoes.
- *Flour, matzo meal, or quick oats:* Add one tablespoon at a time to achieve the binding necessary. If you use too much, the burgers and loaves will become heavy and dense.
- *Moistened bread crumbs:* Add one tablespoon at a time to achieve the desired binding.[13]

Food Technology

Basic egg processing traditionally just resulted in the whole egg as the product, as you would buy in the carton. Today, various technologies are used to process eggs into a number of different types of products. Egg products are derived from just the whites or yolks, or from various blends, with or without nonegg ingredients.

History of Egg Product Development

Commercial egg drying began in St. Louis, Missouri, in the 1880s. The first commercially produced frozen whole eggs were sold in 1903, and separated eggs were sold as early as 1912. Invention and use of commercial egg-breaking machines started in 1951. Following the development of health concerns about high-cholesterol diets in the 1960s, no-cholesterol refrigerated or frozen egg substitutes became available to consumers in 1973. The initial product consisted of egg whites, artificial color, and other nonegg additives.

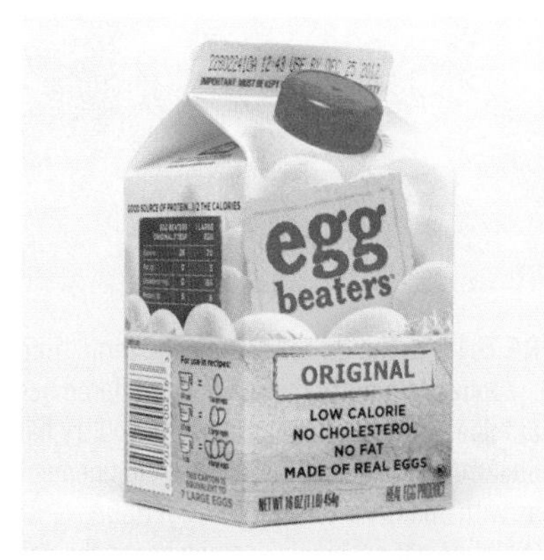

FIGURE 8.12 Low-cholesterol egg products are predominantly made of egg whites. Coloring, salt, spices, and thickeners are then added. Some of these products also contain vegetable oil.

Processing of Egg Products

Processing eggs into egg products includes breaking, filtering, mixing, stabilizing, blending, pasteurizing, cooling, freezing or drying, and packaging the eggs. Processing is performed only at USDA-inspected plants. Processed products go through pasteurization before being packaged and sold in liquid, frozen, and dried forms (see **Figure 8.12**).

Dried Egg Mixes

A number of dried egg mixes have been developed. USDA Dried Egg Mix, initially developed for the military in the 1930s, contains a blend of dried whole eggs, nonfat dry milk, soybean oil, and a small amount of salt. It is has very little moisture. It can be reconstituted by blending 2 tablespoons of Dried Egg Mix with ¼ cup water to make the equivalent of one large whole egg. The Dried Egg Mix is packaged in 6-ounce pouches, equivalent to about 6 eggs each. It is distributed by USDA to food banks, Indian reservations, and others in need. It also is used to feed victims of natural disasters, such as hurricanes and floods.

A similar product called All Purpose Egg Mix, contains a greater proportion of eggs, and was designed for the USDA. It is reconstituted by mixing one part egg mix with two parts of water (by weight). All Purpose Egg Mix is available to schools as part of the national School Lunch Program and is packaged in 10-pound bags.[14]

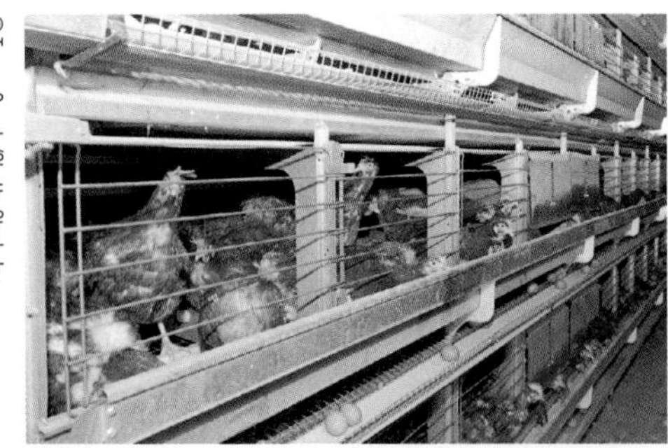

FIGURE 8.13 The majority of eggs in the United States come from hens raised in battery cages. Critics complain that the cages are inhumane because the cages are so small that the birds cannot spread their wings and are unable to perch, nest, or bathe in dust.

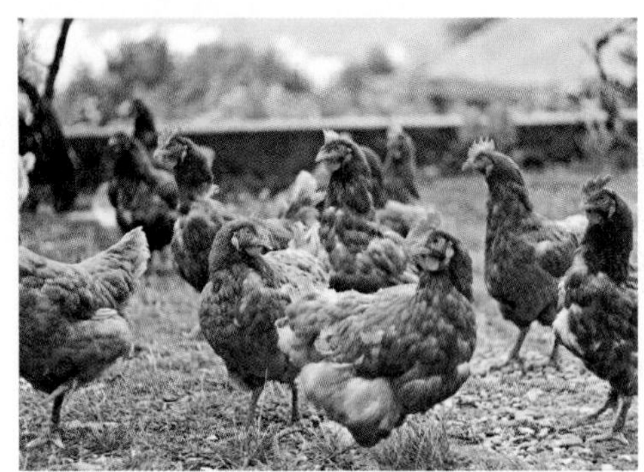

FIGURE 8.14 In the United States, the term "free range" applies to poultry that has been offered access to go outside. It does not mean that the poultry has been allowed to roam freely outside of confinement, such as with "pasture-raised" poultry. USDA regulations do not specify how much space the poultry are offered outside or the amount of time the chicken must have access to the outside for either term.

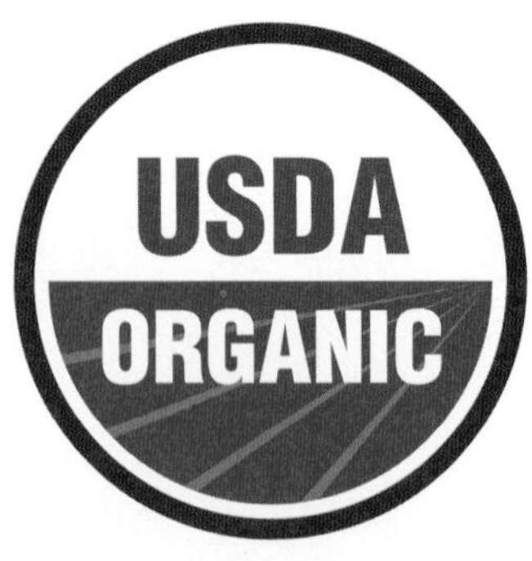

FIGURE 8.15 In the United States, for eggs to be labeled organic the poultry may only be fed organic feed. The laying hens must have access to the outdoors and cannot be raised in cages. Organic egg producers cannot use antibiotics. If needed for the welfare of the birds, the birds must be diverted to non-organic production.

Source: Courtesy of the USDA.

Going Green with Eggs

For centuries eggs have provided a sustainable, ecological, and low-cost source of protein in the American diet. But as demand for eggs increased, the process of raising hens became more and more mechanized. Today, the housing and treatment of hens pose important ecological and ethical concerns.

The Lives of Laying Hens

Laying hens (pullets) are raised for the sole purpose of egg production. Each hatched female is a future egg producer and is put to work at 5 months of age. The kind of life the hen will lead depends in large part on her housing.

Battery Cages

Battery cages are the most commonly used housing system for hens in conventional commercial egg production (see **Figure 8.13**). Battery cages consist of layered wire cages with sloping floors. The cages are in large buildings with controlled environments. The layout of the cages ensures that any eggs produced immediately drop to a conveyor belt, which transports them away for cleaning, sorting, and packaging.

Cage-Free and Free-Range

Most cage-free and free-range hens also live in large buildings with a controlled environment, but instead of living in cages they live on the floor and have the ability to move more freely and climb to raised nesting roosts. They typically have at least some access to the outside or, at a minimum, vents with fresh air. Because the USDA does not provide regulations for cage-free or free-range housing systems, wide variations in living conditions exist.

Pasture-Raised or Pasture-Based

Hens said to be pasture-raised or pasture-based may live on smaller farms similar to those common a hundred years ago, where limited confinement provides the hens seasonal temperatures, natural light, a choice of nesting roosts, and the ability to take dust baths and scratch for bugs and worms (see **Figure 8.14**). Again, the USDA does not provide regulations for the "pasture-raised" label, so the consumer cannot be certain what conditions the hens actually experience.

Organic

When it comes to labels found on eggs that describe the hens' living conditions, the term *organic* is the only one that is backed up by regulations. Organic eggs must come from laying hens that are only fed certified organic feed, and are not permitted to be fed any poultry or mammal slaughter by-products. The hens must live in cage-free environments with access to the outdoors, including direct sunlight and living conditions that accommodate the health and natural behavior of the hens. Furthermore, the eggs must be processed in plants certified to handle organic eggs. A certifier evaluates each farm's system to decide whether the density of hens is appropriate (as specific rules for the number of hens per square foot do not exist).[15] **Figure 8.15** shows the USDA Organic Seal used for eggs.

The Debate

About 90% of the eggs produced in the United States come from hens living in large buildings with multilevel cages where control of heat, light, and temperature follows strict standards to maximize egg production. Routine procedures include trimming the hens' beaks and claws to reduce injuries. Humanitarians and many small egg farmers believe these practices do not place adequate value on the hens. They argue that a more ecological and humane environment produces better eggs, and that the higher cost is supported by consumer demand for environmental protection and the humane treatment of animals.[16] Concerns such as these led California voters to approve a statewide ban of eggs from caged laying hens beginning January 2015. The European Union enacted a similar initiative that will begin in 2012.

Egg producers counter that hens in safe, clean environments produce more eggs, and that proper care of laying hens demands reducing the risk of injury between the hens held in close proximity. They are not convinced that ecological concerns trump economics. In fact, one study showed that only 15% of consumers choose the higher cost eggs for reasons of food safety, the ethical treatment of hens, the work environment, or the quality of the eggs.[16]

Quality

As far as egg quality is concerned, advocates for more humane hen housing have not decisively proven an advantage. When the USDA Agricultural Research Service (ARS) studied the quality of eggs from various hen housing systems, they found that, on average, "there was no substantial quality difference between many types of eggs available in supermarkets in the United Sates. So, no matter which specialty egg is chosen, it will be nearly the same quality as any other egg."[17] Growth in sales of organic eggs therefore stems less from concern over egg quality and more from concern over the health and welfare of animals.

Alternative Purchasing

In an attempt to get the best price for eggs from hens raised in more human environments, some consumers have begun to consider alternatives from mainstream purchasing, such as purchasing eggs directly from local farmers or from farmers' markets. These eggs are not always certified organic, but the consumer can be sure of where the eggs are coming from and can learn how the hens are kept. Some people even establish hen houses in their own backyards or on apartment roof tops (where local ordinances allow).

Food Safety

Keeping Eggs Fresh and Bacteria-Free

The temperature of a just laid egg is about 105°F (41°C), and it normally does not contain an air cell. Immediately after it is laid, the egg starts to cool and an air cell forms. The air cell usually forms in the large end of the egg, developing between the two **shell membranes** as a result of the different rates of contraction between the shell and its contents.[1]

Eggs usually grow in a sterile place but may become contaminated as they exit the hen's body or come into contacted with contaminated surfaces. Fortunately, cleansing procedures are used to protect consumers from bacteria. Eggs are washed with water that is between 90°F (32°C) and 120°F (49°C) and then rinsed with hot water and chlorine. After they have been washed, the eggs are placed in cold storage for shipping.

The USDA requires that all shell eggs reach their storage temperature of 45°F (7°C) as soon as possible after laying. This reduces the growth of bacteria and protects the quality of the eggs. ***Salmonella***, the organism most often associated with foodborne disease from eggs, does not grow well at refrigerated temperatures.[18]

Green Point

Egg Consumption Egg consumption in the United States generally remains constant regardless of price fluctuations. With the implementation of statewide ecological hen housing systems in California, economists predict a 40% increase in the price of eggs and estimate a reduction in consumption of less than 10%.

shell membranes Two membranes, outer and inner, that surround the albumen (white) of an egg; they provide a protective barrier against bacterial penetration.

Salmonella Rod-shaped bacteria responsible for many foodborne illnesses.

Regulating Agencies

Federal and state governments, the egg industry, and the scientific community collaborate together on issues of egg safety. Monitoring of egg production and distribution is handled by various agencies within the USDA:

- *Agricultural Marketing Service (AMS):* The AMS administers a voluntary egg-quality grading program for shell eggs. The service is paid for by processing plants. This is the agency that places the USDA grade symbol on egg cartons, assuring consumers that eggs in the marketplace are as good as or better than U.S. Consumer Grade B quality standards (see section on grading of eggs).
- *Animal and Plant Health Inspection Service (APHIS):* The APHIS conducts activities to reduce the risk of disease in flocks of laying hens, including the APHIS voluntary National Poultry Improvement Plan (NPIP), which certifies that poultry breeding stock and hatcheries are free from certain diseases.
- *Food Safety and Inspection Service (FSIS):* The FSIS's responsibility includes the import of eggs destined for further processing and for assuring that imported shell eggs destined for the retail market are transported at temperatures no greater than 45°F (7°C). The FSIS also ensures that eggs packed for consumers use labels that instruct consumers to "Keep Refrigerated." This agency also provides English and Spanish education materials on food safety.
- *Agricultural Research Service (ARS):* The ARS provides food safety research through a program administered by USDA's National Institute of Food and Agriculture (NIFA).
- *National Agricultural Statistics Service (NASS):* The NASS provides the processing and distribution information for the economic analysis of the egg products industry for the USDA.
- *FSIS/FDA Cooperation:* The FSIS and the FDA share authority for egg safety and work together to solve the problem of *Salmonella* in eggs and to strengthen the *Food Code* and encourage its adoption by states and local jurisdictions.
- State departments of agriculture and state and local departments of health also play a valuable role in ensuring the safety of eggs.[1]

Gastronomy Point

Egg Whites Although cooking food in a copper pot is inadvisable, copper mixing bowls can be a plus. Meringues made in ceramic or steel bowls tend to be snowy white and drier than those made in copper bowls. Making meringue in a copper bowl leads to a creamier, yellowish foam that is harder to overbeat into a lumpy liquid. The copper bowl also contributes copper ions to conalbumin, a metal-binding egg protein, thus stabilizing the whipped egg whites.

Source: Reproduced from Insel P, Ross, D, McMahon K, Bernstein M. *Nutrition.* 4th ed. Burlington, MA: Jones & Bartlett Learning; 2011:534.

Salmonella on the Rise

The summer of 2010 added the word *Salmonella* to the vocabulary of most Americans due to the massive egg recall caused by a *Salmonella enteritidis* (SE) outbreak linked to two egg farms in the state of Iowa. In May through November of 2010, almost 2,000 illnesses linked to this outbreak were reported. Consumers became reluctant to purchase eggs unless they were familiar with the origin of the eggs, which led to increased sales at farmers' markets and small farms. Interest in raising chickens for eggs also increased.[19,20]

Salmonella serotype *enteritidis* (SE) is one of the most common serotypes of *Salmonella* bacteria reported worldwide. Beginning in the 1980s, SE emerged as an important cause of human illness in the United States. The number of outbreaks rose dramatically, beginning in the northeastern states and then spreading west during the 1990s. SE illness now occurs in most regions of the country.[21]

Eggs are the most common food source linked to SE infections. Consuming raw or lightly cooked eggs (runny egg whites or yolks) contaminated with SE always presents the potential for illness. This ever-present risk requires vigilance from both the commercial chef and home cook to follow egg safety guidelines.

Symptoms of Infection

A person infected with SE usually experiences fever, abdominal cramps, and diarrhea beginning 12 to 72 hours after consuming a contaminated food or beverage. The illness typically lasts 4 to 7 days, and most people recover without antibiotic treatment. However, the diarrhea can be severe, and hospitalization may be required for the elderly, infants, and those with impaired immune systems. These groups often exhibit symptoms of a more serious illness, with the infection spreading from the intestines to the bloodstream and then to other body sites. This more serious illness can potentially cause death unless the person is treated promptly with antibiotics.

Repercussions of the 2010 Outbreak

Epidemiologic investigations conducted by public health officials in 11 states identified 29 restaurants or event clusters where more than one ill person with the outbreak strain purchased and consumed a meal. Data from these investigations suggest that shell eggs probably provided the source of infections in many of these restaurants or event clusters. Wright County Egg, in Galt, Iowa, supplied eggs in 15 of the 29 restaurants or event clusters.

A formal investigation into the SE outbreak commenced. It included state partners in California, Colorado, and Minnesota, where the illness also was found. These agencies collaborated with Food and Drug Administration (FDA) and the Centers for Disease Control and Prevention (CDC) to find a common source of the infected shell eggs. The FDA completed on-site investigations of two farms that showed a substantial risk for *Salmonella* to have persisted in the environment and contaminated the eggs.[19,20]

On July 9, 2010, FDA issued a rule requiring shell egg producers to implement measures to prevent SE from contaminating eggs. Eggs from commercial flocks known to be infected would no longer will be sold as grade A. The ruling also identified requirements for refrigeration during storage and transportation.[20]

Following this outbreak, the United Egg Producers (UEP)—which represents 95% of egg producers in the United States—developed a "U.S. Egg Industry Sustainability Vision," which aims to provide egg producers adoptable concepts for their operations to advance social responsibilities. According to the UEP, producers are committed to working toward a "sustainable future" for egg producers, their communities, customers, consumers, and the planet.[22]

Egg Product Inspection

Congress passed the Egg Products Inspection Act (EPIA) in 1970, which mandated continuous inspection of the processing of liquid, frozen, and dried egg products. For 25 years, the Poultry Division of the USDA's AMS inspected egg products to ensure they were wholesome, not otherwise adulterated, properly labeled, and packaged to protect the health and welfare of consumers.

In 1995, the USDA's FSIS became responsible for the inspection of egg products. The FSIS inspects all egg products, with the exception of those products exempted under the act that are used by certain food manufacturers, food services, institutions, and retail markets. The EPIA specifies that egg products may not be imported into the United States except from countries that have an egg products inspection system equivalent to that used in the United States. Currently, Canada is the only active exporter of egg products to the United States.

The Inspection Process

Egg products are processed in sanitary facilities under continuous inspection by the USDA. Eggs move through automated equipment that first washes and sanitizes the shells and then breaks the eggs. The whites are separated from the yolks or a mixture is made from the whites and yolks, depending on the desired end product. The liquid egg product is filtered, mixed, and then chilled prior to additional processing.

Pasteurization

According to the EPIA, all egg products distributed for consumption must be pasteurized, which involves rapidly heating the eggs and holding them at a minimum required temperature for a specified time. Pasteurization of dried egg whites similarly involves heating egg in the dried form for a specified time and at a minimum required temperature. Pasteurization destroys *Salmonella* but does not cook the eggs or affect their color, flavor, nutritional value, or use. The EPIA guidelines do not consider freeze-dried egg products, imitation egg products, and egg substitutes to be egg products, thus making them exempt from pasteurization. However, because they are foods, they are still under the jurisdiction of the FDA.

Egg product manufacturers use pasteurized eggs when producing their products. Companies may decide to repasteurize these products following formulation and before packaging. With many new and different types of egg products currently under development, government and industry are continually evaluating the effectiveness of the pasteurization processes used. Ongoing research will determine if supplemental or different safety measures need to be implemented to continue to provide safe egg products for food service, industry, and consumers.

Green Point

Egg Shells Ground egg shells can be used as bone meal for plants.

Recommendations for Safe Storage

The USDA recommends these safe storage and handling guidelines for all egg products to prevent bacterial contamination:

- For best quality, frozen egg products should only be stored for up to 1 year. They should remain frozen at 0°F (18°C) or lower. After thawing, do not refreeze.
- Thaw frozen egg products in the refrigerator or under cold running water. Do not thaw them on the counter at room temperature.
- If the container for liquid products bears a "use-by" date, observe it. Follow the storage and handling instructions provided by the manufacturer.
- For liquid products without an expiration date, store unopened containers at 40°F (4°C) or below for up to 7 days (not to exceed 3 days after opening). Do not freeze opened cartons of liquid egg products.
- Unopened dried egg products and egg white solids can be stored at room temperature as long as they are kept cool and dry. After opening, store in the refrigerator.
- Reconstituted egg products should be used immediately or refrigerated and used that day.
- USDA Commodity Dried Egg Mix should be stored at less than 50°F (10°C), preferably in the refrigerator. After opening, use within 7 to 10 days. Reconstitute only the amount needed at one time. Use reconstituted egg mix immediately or refrigerate and use within 1 hour.[14]

Table 8.4 offers additional guidelines for appropriate refrigerator and freezer storage for various forms of eggs, egg substitutes, and egg dishes.

TABLE 8.4
Egg Storage Chart

Product	Refrigerator*	Freezer†
Raw eggs in shell	3 to 5 weeks	Do not freeze.
Raw egg whites	2 to 4 days	Discard after 1 year.
Raw egg yolks	2 to 4 days	Yolks do not freeze well alone, but, when combined with sugar, salt, and/or corn syrup, they do freeze well.
Raw egg accidentally frozen in shell	Use immediately after thawing.	Keep frozen; then refrigerate to thaw.
Hard-cooked eggs	1 week	Do not freeze.
Egg substitutes, liquid, unopened	10 days	Do not freeze.
Egg substitutes, liquid, opened	3 days	Do not freeze.
Egg substitutes, frozen, unopened	After thawing, 7 days, or refer to "use-by" date on carton	Discard after 1 year.
Egg substitutes, frozen, opened	After thawing, 3 days, or refer to "use-by" date on carton	Do not freeze.
Casseroles made with eggs	3 to 4 days	After baking, use within 2 to 3 months.
Eggnog, commercial	3 to 5 days	Discard after 6 months.
Eggnog, homemade	2 to 4 days	Do not freeze.
Pies, pumpkin or pecan	3 to 4 days	After baking, 1 to 2 months.
Pies, custard and chiffon	3 to 4 days	Do not freeze.
Quiche with any kind of filling	3 to 4 days	After baking, 2 months.

*Optimum refrigerator temperature is 40°F (4°C).
†Optimum freezer temperature is 0°F (–17°C).
Source: Reproduced from U.S. Food and Drug Administration. FoodSafety.gov: Egg Storage Chart. Available at: http://www.foodsafety.gov/keep/charts/eggstorage.html. Accessed May 29, 2012.

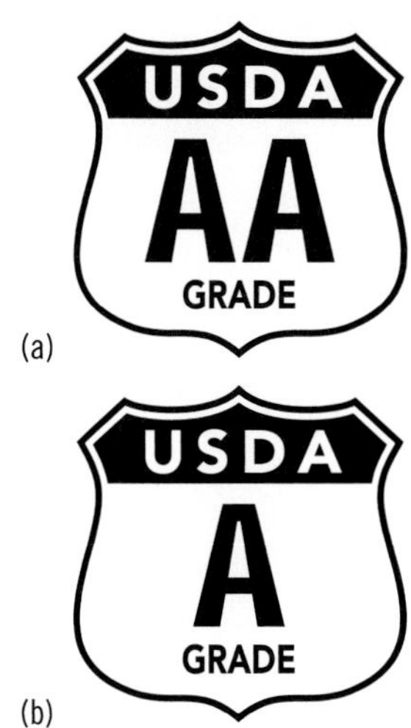

FIGURE 8.16 The two main grades of eggs that consumers will encounter in the retail environment are grades AA and A. (a) Grade AA eggs are the highest quality eggs. (b) Grade A eggs are similar to grade AA eggs except that the egg whites are "reasonably" firm.

Source: Reproduced from How to Buy Eggs, *Home and Garden Bulletin* No. 264. U.S. Department of Agriculture, Agricultural Marketing Service, December 1981.

Food Regulations

Egg Grading

The USDA's public health agency, the Agricultural Marketing Service (AMS), is responsible for inspecting eggs for wholesomeness. Egg producers voluntarily choose to have their eggs graded and pay for this service. The USDA grade shield on the carton means that the eggs have been graded for quality and checked for weight (size) under the supervision of a trained USDA grader. Compliance with quality standards, grades, and weights is monitored by the USDA AMS. State agencies that monitor compliance for egg packers do not use the USDA grading service. Eggs sold to consumers monitored by state agencies will bear a term such as "Grade A" on their cartons, without the USDA shield.[23]

The interior quality of the egg, the appearance, and the condition of the egg shell determine the grade. Eggs of any quality grade may differ in weight or size. **Figure 8.16** shows examples of the grading shields found on egg cartons. Eggs are graded as AA, A, or B:

- U.S. Grade AA eggs have thick and firm whites; yolks that are high, round, and practically free from defects; and clean, unbroken shells.

Innovation Point

Graded Eggs As an alternative to candling, eggs may be graded by way of advanced technologies that use computerized integrated cameras and sound waves.

Choose Grade AA and Grade A eggs for frying and poaching where appearance is important.

- U.S. Grade A eggs have the same characteristics of Grade AA eggs except that the whites are "reasonably" firm. Grade A is the quality most often sold in stores.
- U.S. Grade B eggs have thinner whites and yolks that appear wider and flatter than the egg yolks of higher grades. For eggs to earn this grade, the shells must be unbroken, but they may show slight stains. This quality is seldom found in retail stores because these eggs are typically reserved for making liquid, frozen, and dried egg products.[1]

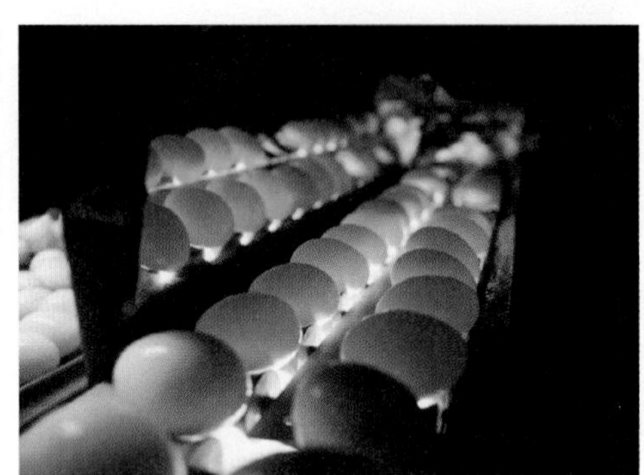

FIGURE 8.17 Eggs are candled to determine the condition of the air cell, yolk, and white. By passing the egg in front of a bright light, the egg grader can see bloody whites or blood spots in an unfertilized egg. In a fertilized egg, candling can be used to determine the stage of embryonic development.

Candling

Egg grades are determined by a method called **candling**, whereby a light is shined through the shell to help visualize the quality of an egg (see **Figure 8.17**). Today, most egg packers use automated mass-scanning equipment to detect eggs with cracked shells and interior defects. During the candling process, eggs travel along a conveyor belt and pass over a light source where any defects become visible. Defective eggs are removed. Hand candling—holding a shell egg directly in front of a light source—is done to spot check and determine accuracy in grading.

candling A process that uses light to help determine the quality of an egg.

Assigning Haugh Units

Another method of assessing the quality of eggs is the use of Haugh units. Raymond Haugh developed the Haugh unit in 1937, and it has become the most widely used measurement of the albumen, which is used as an indicator of egg quality. To determine the Haugh unit, the egg is weighed and then broken onto a flat surface. A micrometer is then used to measure the height of the albumin that surrounds the yolk. The Haugh unit is a correlation between the weight of the egg and the height of the thick albumen. The higher the number, the better the quality of the egg (fresher, higher quality eggs have thicker whites). From the Haugh unit, it is possible to determine the protein content and freshness of the egg.

Egg Sizing

Sizing eggs ensures that the minimum ounces required for a dozen eggs is met. Although some eggs in the carton may look slightly larger or smaller than the rest, the weight class does not refer to the dimensions of an individual egg but rather to the total weight of the dozen eggs in the carton. A carton of eggs is classed based on the total weight of the 12 eggs in the carton (see **Table 8.5**).[1]

TABLE 8.5
Egg Sizes

Size or Weight Class	Minimum Net Weight per Dozen
Jumbo	30 ounces
Extra Large	27 ounces
Large	24 ounces
Medium	21 ounces
Small	18 ounces
Peewee	15 ounces

Source: Reproduced from Food Safety and Inspection Service, U.S. Department of Agriculture. Fact Sheets: Egg Products Preparation, Shell Eggs from Farm to Table, 2011. Available at: http://www.fsis.usda.gov/Fact_Sheets/Focus_On_Shell_Eggs/index.asp#2.

Egg Dating

The dating code used by egg processors for controlling inventory and rotating stock provides information about how long eggs have been sitting in a carton. Terminology for coding egg cartons include: *EXP*, *Sell By*, *Not to be Sold After*, and *Best Used Before*. Egg cartons are dated based on rules outlined by the USDA, but egg processors can opt-out and not use any dates at all. Following the USDA rules, an expiration date must be printed in month/day format and preceded by the appropriate prefix (see **Figure 8.18**). A maximum 30-day expiration date must be calculated from the day the eggs were packed into the carton.[24]

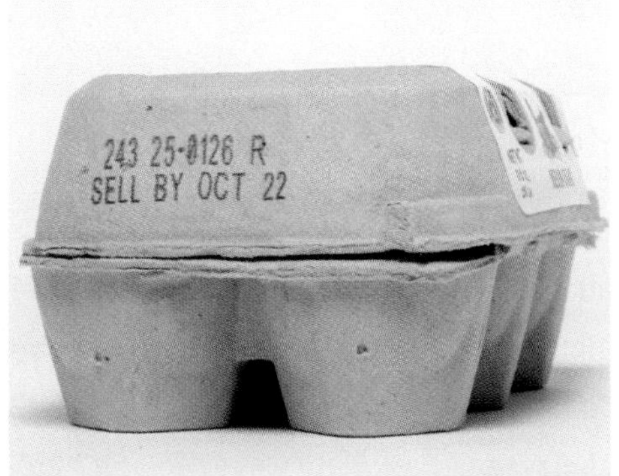

FIGURE 8.18 Most egg cartons have a "Sell-By" or "EXP" date on the carton. Always purchase eggs that have not passed their expiration date. After taking the eggs home from the store, refrigerate the eggs in their original carton and place them in the coldest part of the refrigerator. For best quality, use the eggs within 3 to 5 weeks of purchase.

Labeling Egg Products

In addition to nutrition information on consumer packages, other labeling information is required for egg products. All egg products must be labeled with the following:

- The common or usual name of the product and (if the product is composed of two or more ingredients) the ingredients listed in the order of descending proportions
- Name and address of the packer or distributor
- Date of packing, which may be shown as a lot number or production code number
- The net contents
- Official USDA inspection mark and establishment number[1]

Chapter Review

Eggs provide a sustainable, economical, and nutritious food source in the United States. Eggs were once obtained from small producers, but now the majority of eggs come from large producers that keep hens in battery cages to speed production and decrease costs. Today, many are concerned with the humane treatment of laying hens. In addition, large-scale production practices were cited in the 2010 massive egg recall from *Salmonella*–infected foods served to a large group of people from several states.

The USDA is responsible for keeping the egg supply safe. Several different USDA agencies enforce regulations for safe handling, determining the size and quality of eggs, and the monitoring the treatment and health of hens. The USDA's goal is to work with industry for results that benefit consumers. At the same time, the food service industry requires affordable, pasteurized egg products and seeks to speed the production of eggs in ways that are not always humane or environmentally friendly.

Eggs, which were once the main course at breakfast, were targeted as a food to avoid due to scientists finding a link between egg consumption and cardiovascular disease. However, current research has redeemed the egg, showing that most people can average one egg a day. Today, consumers are eating eggs and are becoming more interested in where their eggs come from. Eggs from large-scale farms as well as from backyard farms offer a great food source to the home or restaurant chef and are a delicious addition to any meal.

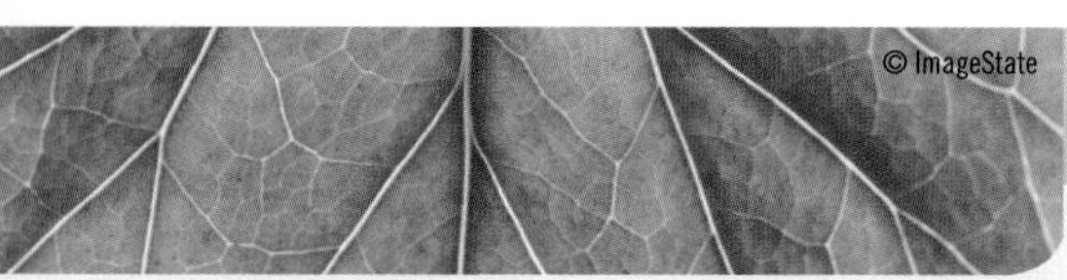

Learning Portfolio

Key Terms

	page
air cell	254
albumen	254
candling	272
chalazae	255
choline	255
emulsion	258
egg foam	261
egg product	254
egg white	254
homocysteine	255
laying hens	254
lecithin	262
lutein	255
ovalbumen	255
pullets	254
Salmonella	267
shell	254
shell membranes	267
vitelline membrane	255
yolk	254
zeaxanthin	255

Study Points

1. Eggs are an integral part of the American diet. They are an important source of dietary protein, act as a binder and leavening agent in baking, and are used as an emulsifier in many food items, including sauces and dressings.
2. Increased demand for eggs led to the rise of industrial egg farming, which has led to debate about the humane treatment of hens.
3. Vigilance in food preparation for the elderly, infants, and those with impaired immune systems must be maintained to prevent bacterial infections from food.
4. Albumen or egg whites provide texture and volume to a variety of food items, from candy to meringues, through the use of friction, which adds air to the protein, changing the albumin's texture and increasing its volume.
5. Ecological egg farming means treating laying hens humanely and providing a bacteria-free egg with minimal impact on the environment.
6. The Egg Products Inspection Act (EPIA) of 1970 requires pasteurization of all egg products distributed for consumption. Eggs are pasteurized and then held at a minimum required temperature for a specified time to destroy bacteria such as *Salmonella*.
7. The USDA, through the Agricultural Marketing Service (AMS), mandates the inspection of eggs for cleanliness, yet egg farmers can voluntarily choose not to use the service to grade the quality of eggs.
8. Through the process of candling, the USDA provides three grade levels of eggs, AA, A, and B.
9. The net weight of a dozen eggs determines the size designation of a carton of eggs.

Issues for Discussion

1. Would you vote to change the housing for laying hens knowing that nontraditional housing would increase the cost of eggs by 40%?
2. How might you recommend increasing the use of eggs in the American diet?
3. Suppose you were the food service manager in a restaurant that served eggs resulting in multiple patrons visiting emergency rooms and receiving a diagnosis of *Salmonella* infection. What kitchen procedures would you review, and what cleaning techniques would you implement to stop the spread of these bacteria?
4. Discuss the options for using raw or partially cooked eggs and/or egg whites in food preparation and the food safety procedures required for a bacteria-free result.
5. Discuss how a family's cultural background can affect how eggs are incorporated into family meals.

Research Ideas for Students

1. The ethical treatment of laying hens
2. Recent laws that allow community allows residents to raise chickens for eggs
3. Increased use of eggs and the reduction of our carbon footprint

References

1. U.S. Department of Agriculture. Shell Eggs from Farm to Table. Updated September 7, 2010. Available at: http://www.fsis.usda.gov/Fact_Sheets/Focus_On_Shell_Eggs/index.asp.
2. U.S. Department of Agriculture. USDA Database for the Choline Content of Common Foods. Updated August 2008. Available at: http://www.ars.usda.gov/SP2UserFiles/Place/12354500/Data/Choline/Choln02.pdf.
3. U.S. Department of Agriculture, Agricultural Research Service. Homocysteine—The New "Bad Guy." Updated October 23, 2006. Available at: http://www.ars.usda.gov/News/docs.htm?docid=10678.

4. U.S. Department of Agriculture. USDA Table of Nutrient Retention Factors, Release 6. Updated December 2007. Available at: http://www.ars.usda.gov/SP2UserFiles/Place/12354500/Data/retn/retn06.pdf.
5. U.S. Department of Agriculture, Nutrition Evidence Library. What Is the Effect of Dietary Cholesterol Intake on Risk of Cardiovascular Disease? Available at: http://www.nutritionevidencelibrary.com/conclusion.cfm?conclusion_statement_id=250193.
6. U.S. Department of Agriculture. Food Allergen Labeling and Consumer Protection Act of 2004 (Public Law 18-282, Title II). Updated August 21, 2009. Available at: http://www.fda.gov/Food/LabelingNutrition/FoodAllergensLabeling/GuidanceComplianceRegulatoryInformation/ucm106187.htm.
7. U.S. Department of Health and Human Resources. Food Allergy: An Overview. Updated November 2010. Available: http://www.niaid.nih.gov/topics/foodallergy/documents/foodallergy.pdf.
8. National Center for Chronic Disease Prevention and Health Promotion, Division of Adolescent and School Health. Healthy Youth, Food Allergies. Updated November 19, 2010. Available at: http://www.cdc.gov/HealthyYouth/foodallergies.
9. GovTrack.us. Senate Bill 510 FDA Food Safety Modernization Act. Voted November 30, 2010. Available at: http://www.govtrack.us/congress/billtext.xpd?bill=s111-510.
10. U.S. Department of Agriculture. Safe Food Handling, High Altitude Cooking and Food Safety. Updated September 9, 2010. Available at: http://www.fsis.usda.gov/Fact_Sheets/High_Altitude_Cooking_and_Food_Safety/index.asp#9.
11. U.S. Department of Agriculture, Agricultural Research Service. Food Crystals: The Role of Eggs. Updated December 26, 2010. Available at: http://www.ars.usda.gov/research/publications/publications.htm?seq_no_115=231468.
12. U.S. Department of Agriculture. Food Safety for Those Glorious Holiday Goodies! Available at: http://www.fsis.usda.gov/OA/pubs/holiday_goodies1.pdf.
13. Mangels R, Messina V, Messina M. Using egg substitutes. In: Mangels R, Messina V, Messina M (eds.). *The Dietitian's Guide to Vegetarian Diets.* 3rd ed. Burlington, MA: Jones & Bartlett Learning; 2011.
14. U.S. Department of Agriculture. Egg Products Preparation. Updated August 21, 2006. Available at: http://www.fsis.usda.gov/Fact_Sheets/Egg_Products_and_Food_Safety/index.asp.
15. Oberholtzer L, Greene C, Lopez E. Organic Poultry and Eggs Capture High Price Premiums and Growing Share of Specialty Markets, Outlook Report from the Economic Research Service. 2006. Available at: http://usda.mannlib.cornell.edu/usda/ers/LDP-M/2000s/2006/LDP-M-12-27-2006_Special_Report.pdf.
16. Mesías FJ, Martínez-Carrasco F, Martínez JM, Gaspar P. Functional and organic eggs as an alternative to conventional production: A conjoint analysis of consumers' preferences. *J Sci Food Agric.* 2011 Feb;91(3):532–817.
17. U.S. Department of Agriculture, Agricultural Research Service. Study Eyes Egg Quality and Composition. Updated August 26, 2010. Available at: http://www.ars.usda.gov/is/pr/2010/100707.htm.
18. U.S. Department of Agriculture, Food Safety and Inspection Service. *Salmonella* Questions and Answers. Modified October 22, 2010. Available at: http://www.fsis.usda.gov/PDF/Salmonella_Questions_and_Answers.pdf.
19. Centers for Disease Control and Prevention. Investigation Update: Multistate Outbreak of Human *Salmonella enteritidis* Infections Associated with Shell Eggs. Updated December 2, 2010. Available at: http://www.cdc.gov/salmonella/enteritidis.
20. Centers for Disease Control and Prevention. Recall of Shell Eggs. Updated October 18, 2010. Available at: http://www.fda.gov/Safety/Recalls/MajorProductRecalls/ucm223522.htm.
21. U.S. Department of Agriculture, Food Safety and Inspection Service. *Salmonella* Questions and Answers. Modified October 22, 2010. Available at: http://www.fsis.usda.gov/PDF/Salmonella_Questions_and_Answers.pdf.
22. United Egg Producers. Plenty to Think About. The Thinking Person's Guide to Feeding a Hungry Planet. 2010. Available at: http://www.unitedegg.org/information/homeNews/EggsProteinandConsumerChoice.pdf.
23. U.S. Department of Agriculture. United States Standards, Grades, and Weight Classes for Shell Eggs. Updated July 20, 2000. Available at: http://www.ams.usda.gov/AMSv1.0/getfile?dDocName=STELDEV3004376.
24. U.S. Department of Agriculture. An Egg Story: Does the Date Mean "Too Late"? Updated May 27, 2004. Available at: http://www.ars.usda.gov/is/AR/archive/jun04/egg0604.htm.

CHAPTER 9

Vegetarianism

Tim Radak, DrPH, RD

Chapter Objectives

THE STUDENT WILL BE EMPOWERED TO:

- Define the various types of vegetarian diets and explain how they differ.
- Discuss the history of vegetarianism and identify current trends.
- State reasons why people choose to eat a vegetarian diet.
- Summarize the results of research on the health effects of vegetarian versus meat-based diets, including strengths and weaknesses of each dietary plan.
- Cite specific examples of how vegetarian diets may be recommended in the treatment or prevention of disease.
- Explain how to ensure that a vegetarian diet is nutritionally adequate.
- Compare and contrast the potential impacts that food production for vegetarian versus meat-based diets have on the environment.

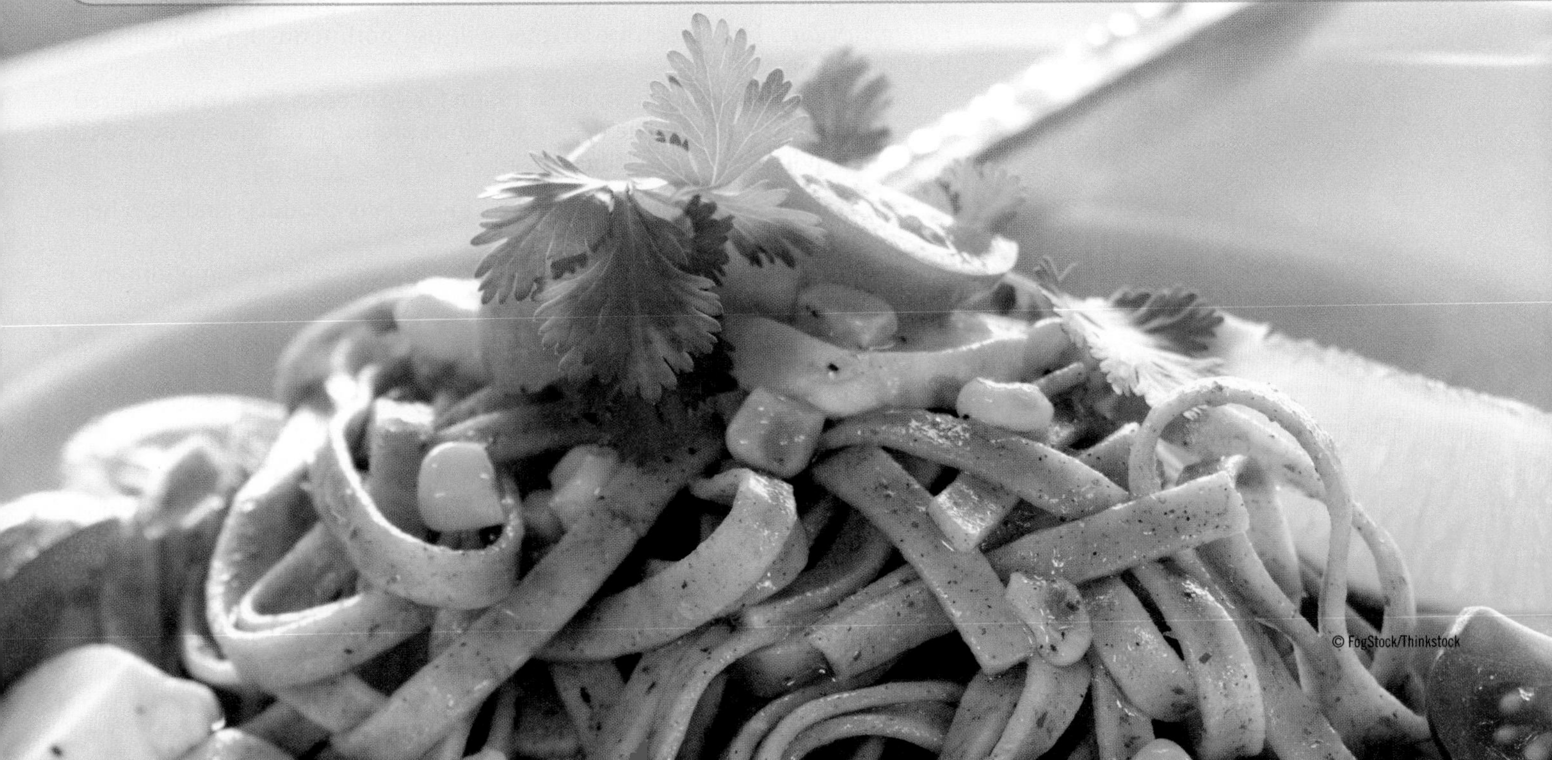

Introduction

Vegetarianism has been practiced for thousands of years in many parts of the world, and its roots can be traced back to a number of religions and philosophies. **Vegetarian diets** are characterized by the absence of meat, poultry, and fish. Those following a vegetarian diet, including its many variations, comprise a very small segment of the U.S. population; however, vegetarianism has increased in popularity and prominence in the United States in recent years. Although it was once a challenge to find vegetarian options outside of the home, vegetarian foods and menu options are becoming increasingly more available. Individuals may choose a vegetarian diet for a number of reasons, including ethical, moral, health, religious, and environmental concerns.

Every type of diet has nutritional implications and issues that should be considered, and the vegetarian diet is no exception. This chapter will explore the history of vegetarianism, some of the reasons for adopting it, and its relationship to health. Our food choices affect our health. Currently, in the developed world the number of people suffering from diet-related diseases, such as atherosclerosis, cancer, diabetes, and obesity, is reaching epidemic proportions.

In some areas of the world, crises are occurring over food prices, water, and energy.[1] Measuring the exact influence of our diets on the environment is complex and controversial. However, continued research into the health and environmental effects of how we grow, process, and transport food can help inform our future food choices. This chapter will also explore whether a meat-based or vegetarian diet may be considered a "green diet."

vegetarian diet Diet characterized by the consumption of plant-based foods with some (eggs and/or dairy) or no animal products.

omnivore diet Diet characterized by the consumption of both plant-based foods and animal products.

plant-based diet A diet that is primarily made up of plant food sources but may include some animal products.

lacto-ovo vegetarian diet Diet characterized by the consumption of plant-based foods and the addition of dairy products and eggs.

lacto vegetarian diet Diet characterized by the consumption of plant-based foods and the addition of dairy products.

ovo vegetarian diet Diets characterized by the consumption of plant-based foods and the addition of eggs.

vegan Diet characterized by the consumption of exclusively plant-based foods and lifestyle habits that strive to exclude any animal derived products.

Classification

Vegetarian diets are characterized by the fact that they include few or no animal products. Today, the word *diet* implies an eating style designed for weight loss purposes. Thus, the vegetarian diet could more aptly be described as a *vegetarian dietary plan* because weight loss is not the main reason for adopting this eating style. Nonetheless, the use of the term *vegetarian diet* is widely accepted. This is less the case when describing the **omnivore diet**, the dietary pattern where individuals eat both animal and plant foods. The term *omnivore diet* is less commonly encountered in common parlance than *vegetarian diet*. However, this chapter will use both terms for convenience in comparison.

It is becoming more and more common for vegetarian diets to be referred to as **plant-based diets**. The degree to which animal products are excluded varies depending on the specific diet adopted:

- A **lacto-ovo vegetarian diet** includes dairy products and eggs in addition to plant-based foods.
- A **lacto vegetarian diet** includes only dairy products in addition to plant-based foods.
- An **ovo vegetarian diet** includes only eggs in addition to plant-based foods.
- A **vegan diet** includes plant-based foods exclusively; individuals following this diet strive to exclude any animal-derived products from their diet and lifestyle.

Table 9.1 compares the composition of an omnivore diet and the various vegetarian dietary plans. **Figure 9.1** depicts the plant-based food pyramid.

Occasionally the terms *semi* and *partial vegetarian* are used, but these are technically misnomers because these individuals occasionally consume meat or seafood. The following are the more appropriate designations for

TABLE 9.1
Composition of Omnivore and Plant-Based Diets

	Type of Dietary Plan				
Type of Food	Omnivore	Lacto-ovo Vegetarian	Lacto Vegetarian	Ovo Vegetarian	Vegan
Meats*	✓				
Eggs	✓	✓		✓	
Dairy products	✓	✓	✓		
Grains	✓	✓	✓	✓	✓
Legumes	✓	✓	✓	✓	✓
Fruits	✓	✓	✓	✓	✓
Vegetables	✓	✓	✓	✓	✓
Nuts/seeds	✓	✓	✓	✓	✓

*Includes beef, pork, chicken, turkey, lamb, wild game, and fish/seafood.

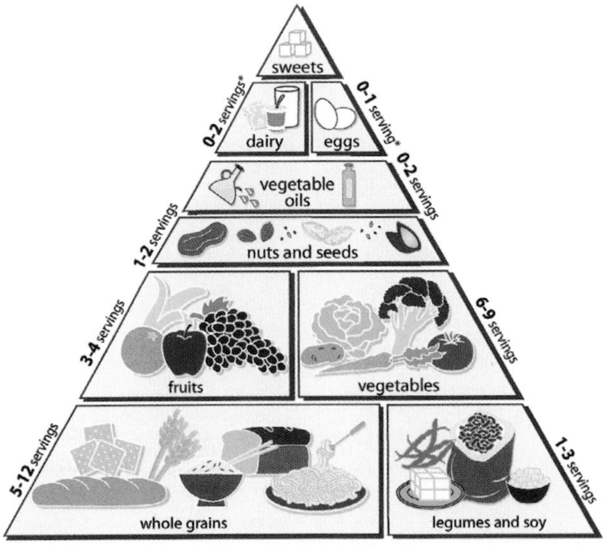

FIGURE 9.1 Vegetarian Food Guide Pyramid. The vegetarian food guide pyramid includes the five major plant-based food groups: whole grains, legumes, vegetables, fruit, and nuts and seeds. These groups form the largest part of the pyramid. Optional food groups that may be avoided by some types of vegetarians, such as vegetable oils, dairy, eggs, and sweets, form the smaller triangle-shaped top portion of the pyramid.

people who follow a mostly vegetarian diet but occasionally include certain types of meats:

- A **pescatarian**, or **pesco-vegetarian, diet** excludes all meat except fish; it may include eggs or dairy products.
- A **flexitarian diet** is primarily vegetarian, but its adopters occasionally eat meat.
- A person following a **macrobiotic diet**, an eating regimen first popularized in Japan, eats a predominantly vegetarian diet that is based on grains and supplemented with local vegetables. People following this diet avoid highly processed or refined foods and most animal products.
- A **raw food diet** may or may not consist entirely of vegetarian foods and comprises mostly uncooked or unprocessed foods.
- A **fruitarian diet** consists mainly fruits, nuts, seeds, and in some cases legumes. **Legumes**, sometimes referred to as pulses, are a class of vegetables that contains edible seed pods. Beans, peas, lentils, and peanuts are all legumes.

In some cases, the diets just described, as well as some of the other plant-based diets listed in Table 9.1, may represent transitional diets for individuals who wish to change from omnivorous diets but are but not quite ready to become fully vegetarian.

pescatarian (pesco vegetarian diet) Diet characterized by the exclusion of all meat except from fish and may include eggs or dairy products.

flexitarian diet A primarily vegetarian eating plan, but its adopters occasionally eat meat.

macrobiotic diet An eating regimen first popularized in Japan; a predominantly vegetarian diet that is based on grains and supplemented with local vegetables. People following this diet avoid highly processed or refined foods and most animal products.

raw food diet Diet that may or may not consist entirely of vegetarian foods; comprises mostly uncooked or unprocessed foods.

fruitarian diet Diet characterized by consumption of fruits, nuts, seeds, and, in some cases, legumes.

legumes A class of vegetables that have edible seed pods, including beans, peas, lentils, and peanuts. Sometimes referred to as *pulses*.

History of Vegetarianism

The term *vegetarian* is likely derived from the word *vegetable* and the suffix *-arian*, which is a person who has a connection to or belief in something. It is a relatively recent term, dating back only to the mid-1800s, when the first "vegetarian societies" were formed in Britain and the United States.[2,3] However, the concept of vegetarianism—the avoidance of meat—dates back thousands of years (as early as 600 B.C.) as parts of various philosophies and religions.[2] In the Western world, Pythagoras, the famous Greek mathematician, could perhaps be considered the father of philosophical vegetarianism and was among its earliest advocates.[4]

Food is an important part of worship and social life across many religions, with some religions placing a greater importance on dietary protocol

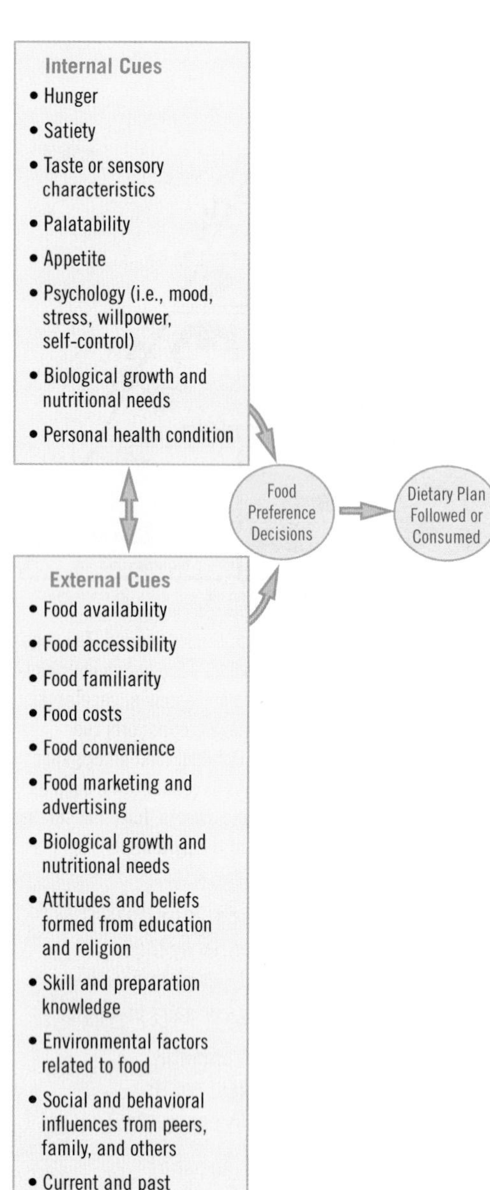

FIGURE 9.2 Determinants of food intake. A number of internal and external cues determine a person's food consumption patterns.

Gastronomy Point

Restaurants Creative and groundbreaking vegetarian restaurants have played a key role in generating interest in vegetarianism. One of the early innovators, the Moosewood Restaurant in Ithaca, New York, was named one of the 13 most influential restaurants of the 20th century by *Bon Appétit* magazine.

than others.[5] A number of Eastern and Indian religions advocate or prescribe vegetarian or plant-based diets, including Hinduism, Jainism, and Buddhism.[6] India even had a Buddhist vegetarian emperor named Emperor Ashoka the Great (265 B.C.) who encouraged his followers to follow a vegetarian diet by decree of abstention from killing animals or living beings.[7] Some Christian denominations advocate vegetarianism, the most notable being the Seventh-day Adventists, a Protestant denomination originating in the United States in the 19th century. Seventh-day Adventists have suggested abstinence from meat to promote health for the past 140 years.[8] Some followers of the Christian Protestant Quaker religion, which originated in the 17th century, also are adherents to a vegetarian diet, based on their belief of nonviolence toward all living beings.

In addition to the religious and philosophical influences of the past millennia, other factors have contributed to an expanded interest in vegetarianism worldwide over the last century and a half. These include ethical, moral, health, nutrition, and, more recently, environmental influences.

Reasons for Choosing a Vegetarian Diet

What we eat is guided by much more than just simply hunger. Numerous factors are at play in what determines our food choices and dietary preferences, as shown in **Figure 9.2**. The last few decades have seen tremendous growth in the public's interest in food systems and politics, including the production, transport and handling, labeling, safety, and nutritional quality of food products. Coverage of these topics via radio and television, news articles, popular and trade magazines, academic and industry research, books, the Internet, and movie documentaries has helped fuel this interest. Public awareness extends to dietary choices, including vegetarianism.[2]

The increase in the number of vegetarian cookbooks published over the past few decades has been exponential. As early as 1998, a vegetarian cookbook was selected as the top cookbook of the year, attesting to the popularity of vegetarian cuisine; more recently, a vegan cookbook was a number one best seller.[9,10] One recent cookbook, *How to Cook Everything Vegetarian: Simple Meatless Recipes for Great Food*, demonstrates the interest in cooking vegetarian; furthermore, it is intended to appeal to both vegetarians and omnivores who wish to reduce their meat intake.[11]

Wide-ranging interest in healthy eating has helped spur the public's interest in vegetarianism. This should come as no surprise given the recent spotlight on some of the negative health implications of consuming a typical Westernized diet. Consider the following facts:

- Diet and activity are implicated in at least 3 of the 10 leading causes of death in the United States.[12]
- At least one-third of adult men and women in the United States are classified as being obese, a risk factor for many chronic diseases.[13]
- One research study spanning 52 countries suggested that the globalization of the Western diet, which is high in animal products, fried foods, and salty snacks, is responsible for one-third of the risk for heart attacks worldwide.[14]
- Recent reports of foodborne illnesses and numerous food scares—mad cow disease, *E. coli*–contaminated ground beef, chicken and pork recalls, H1N1 (avian) flu, and Q fever in goats—have contributed to a perception that animal products threaten health.[2]

These health considerations have affected the popularity of vegetarian diets, making vegetarianism less of a trend and more of a mainstay.[15] In fact, a recent survey of vegetarians across all age groups suggested that health is the top reason for each age group adopting vegetarianism.[16]

Other reasons for choosing a vegetarian diet include concerns about animal welfare, ethics, and the environment. For example, a 2010 survey listed reducing intake of meat as one of the "most compelling trends" of the year and reported that 19% did so for environmental reasons.[17] In addition, a recent U.S. study found that a rising interest in animal welfare has been correlated with reduced demand for meat intake.[18]

Influences from friends or family members also play a role, particularly if one is born into a vegetarian family.[19,20] Simple economics may play a role, too, as vegetarian diets are perceived as costing less. Finally, some people may choose vegetarian diets as a form of restrictive diet, with a goal of weight reduction. However, it is important to note that some individuals may mask an underlying eating disorder behind their vegetarianism. Others may be singularly focused on reducing animal product consumption.

Green Point

Vegetarian Day The city of Ghent in Belgium recently made history in becoming the first city in the world to declare every Thursday "Vegetarian Day," suggesting that its citizens try eating vegetarian one day per week as a way to address environmental issues relating to global warming. In the United States, "Meatless Mondays," an initiative of the Johns Hopkins School of Public Health, is gaining momentum as a strategy to provide environmentally friendly meatless meals; "Meatless Mondays" have been adopted by a number of major food service providers and restaurants.

Prevalence of Vegetarianism

Quantifying how many vegetarians there are in a given population is challenging for a number of reasons, including how individuals define their diet as well as uncertainty around the various classifications of vegetarian diets. The number of vegetarians in Western countries varies by country and may comprise anywhere from less than 1% to as much as 10% of the population, depending on how the term vegetarian is defined.[15,21–24]

Innovation Point

Fake Meat The interest in reducing meat intake has spurred interest in the development of fake meat that can be grown in a test tube in a lab.

In some parts of the world, such as India, vegetarian diets are commonplace. In fact, India has more vegetarians than everywhere else in the world combined. In India, meat consumption is discouraged mainly for religious reasons, but there are large populations there that do consume meat and seafood. Approximately 80% of India's population of 1.2 billion is believed to eat mostly a plant-based or vegetarian diet, with the traditional Indian dietary plan being lacto-vegetarian.[2,7] It is estimated that lacto-ovo, ovo, and strict vegetarians comprise 30–42% of the Indian population.[25–27]

A survey by the Israeli government reported that 8.5% of its population, or 595,000 people, are vegetarians or vegans, making Israel the country with the second largest percentage of vegetarians.[28] Studies carried out in the United Kingdom suggest rates of vegetarianism that are highest among Western countries, with roughly 3–7% defining themselves as vegetarian.[29–31] Surveys conducted in both Canada and Australia suggest that approximately 4% of adults consider themselves vegetarian; similar numbers are found in Finland, with 1–4% being vegetarian.[32–34]

In the United States, two recent surveys from nationwide samples estimated that 3.0–3.2% of the adult population (6 to 8 million people) never eat meat, poultry, fish, or seafood. One percent (or 1 million adults) identify themselves as vegan.[21,23] Ten percent, or 22 million adults, claim to follow a vegetarian-inclined diet, and approximately 20–25% of U.S. adults report usually or sometimes maintaining a vegetarian diet or eating meatless meals at least four times weekly.[35]

Earlier surveys from the 1990s through 2006 estimated that the number of adult vegetarians in the United States ranged between 1% and almost 7%. This broad range suggests some uncertainty around the various classifications for those who described themselves as vegetarians.[15,22] More recent surveys provide evidence of an increase in those who consider themselves vegetarian.[24]

Some surveys have focused on specific population groups. For example, a study investigating the prevalence of vegetarianism among U.S. female physicians found that approximately 8% considered themselves vegetarian.[36]

Other studies have focused on Seventh-day Adventists. This religious group is estimated to be approximately 30–35% lacto-ovo vegetarian, with another 20% eating meat less than once per week.[8,37,38] In the large studies that have looked at the health characteristics of Seventh-day Adventists, roughly 3% were described as vegans.[37]

One of the groups with the fastest growing rate of vegetarianism is young adults and youth.[39] Recent estimates from a Centers for Disease Control and Prevention survey found that 1 in 200 children, or 367,000 youths, aged 17 and younger are vegetarian.[24] College students have shown an increase in describing themselves as vegetarian; a recent survey across college campuses in the United States found 12% to be vegetarian and almost 2% to be vegan, up significantly from the same survey 3 years earlier.[40] One study of college students in Australia found that 13% of female students considered themselves vegetarian and 17% semi-vegetarian.[33] One recent U.S. survey indicated that a significant number of young adults are vegetarian, with 12% of females aged 18–34 saying they "never eat meat."[23]

Impact on Health

Food provides energy and nutrition for the body; an adequate intake of a variety of foods is necessary to sustain health. We have all heard the adage "you are what you eat"; in terms of proper nutrition, health promotion, and disease prevention, this is certainly true. In his Report on Nutrition and Health, the former Surgeon General Dr. C. Everett Koop stated that "For the two out of three adult Americans who do not smoke or drink excessively, one personal choice seems to influence long-term health prospects more than any other: what we eat."[41]

Vegetarianism Through the Life Stages

Each stage of the human life cycle has distinct nutritional requirements. A healthy diet should contain all of the required nutrients in recommended amounts and sufficient calories to balance energy intake with expenditure. The inclusion of animal products can be an important source of energy-dense nutrition, but it is not necessary to obtain adequate nutrition. Although animal-derived protein content is of high biological value and contains essential nutrients, animal products contain saturated fats and cholesterol and are devoid of dietary fiber. According to the position paper by the Academy of Nutrition and Dietetics, appropriately planned vegetarian and vegan diets are healthful and nutritionally adequate for all stages of the life cycle, including during pregnancy and lactation, infancy, and childhood.[42] See **Special Topic 9.1** for more on the use of vegetarian diets in childhood. A number of respected organizations support or encourage the use of plant-based diets (see **Figure 9.3**), including the American Heart Association,[43] the Academy of Nutrition and Dietetics,[42,44] the American Institute for Cancer Research,[45] the World Health Organization and Food and Agriculture Organization of the United Nations,[46] the World Watch Institute,[47] and the Center for Science for the Public Interest.[48]

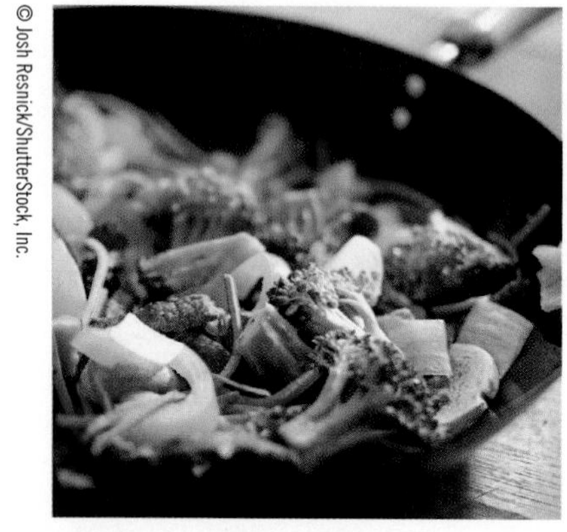

FIGURE 9.3 A growing number of nonprofit and governmental agencies are advocating the vegetarian diet because of its well-documented health benefits. In addition to the health benefits, vegetarian diets also can play an important role in promoting environmental health and improving animal welfare.

Comparing Health Effects of Vegetarian Versus Omnivore Diets

A well-planned vegetarian diet can provide health benefits and help prevent many of the chronic diseases affecting Western cultures today. Over the past few decades the research focus on vegetarian dietary plans has shifted from examining deficiencies and adequacy of vegetarian diets to determining their

Special Topic 9.1

Nutrition and Growth for Vegetarian Children

Tim Radak, DrPH, RD

Vegetarian and vegan dietary plans can contain fewer calories and in some cases fewer vitamins and minerals than omnivore diets. Although there are demonstrated health benefits from following a vegetarian or vegan diet in adults, what are the implications of the vegetarian or vegan diet for infants, children, and adolescents? Will children who follow a vegetarian or vegan diet from birth grow at that same rate as those who include meat and/or dairy and eggs in their diets? Can they reduce their risk of childhood obesity?

Important physical changes take place during childhood. Some of the most rapid growth takes place during this time, and caloric and nutrient demands are significant. Monitoring growth, weight, and height are standard during this part of the lifecycle to ensure adequate nutrition and to identify health issues or diseases. Children need the same variety of foods as adults do, but have different nutritional goals. Childhood also is a time when picky eaters may refuse many kinds of foods, which could put them at risk for nutritional deficiencies, regardless of whether they are vegetarian.

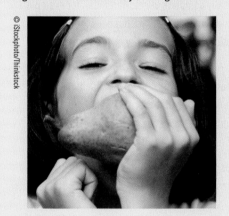

A healthy diet helps children grow and learn. In addition, a healthy diet can prevent obesity and weight-related diseases, such as diabetes. Vegetarian diets can be a healthful option for children and promote positive, lifelong eating habits.

During childhood, habits are being formed that can last a lifetime. Eliminating animal products from children's diets may pose special concerns for meeting dietary adequacy if proper planning and equivalent substitutes are not provided. Both the Academy of Nutrition and Dietetics and the American Academy of Pediatrics support vegetarian or vegan diets for normal infant and child growth.[1] Unfortunately, deficiencies can occur in any kind of diet, whether vegetarian, vegan, or omnivore. Poor dietary planning, poverty, and other lifestyle influences can jeopardize a child's health and growth.

Nutritional Intake

Vegetarian or vegan infants consume milk as a primary source of nutrition in the form of either breast milk or formula. Studies reviewing the composition of breast milk have shown that the breast milk of most vegan and vegetarian women contains adequate nutrients. However, some studies have indicated somewhat lower concentrations of vitamin B_{12}, eicosapentaenoic acid, and docosahexaenoic acid in the breast milk of vegan and vegetarian mothers.[2–4]

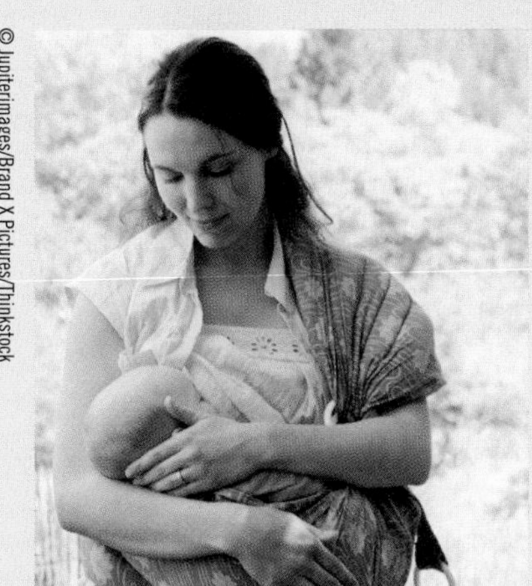

Vegetarian or vegan mothers who breastfeed must ensure that their diet contains adequate amounts of vitamin B_{12}, calcium, and zinc. Breastfed infants of vegetarian mothers grow and develop normally while obtaining all of the benefits of breast milk.

Studies of vegetarian or vegan children or adolescents indicate nutrient intakes similar to those of omnivores, although in some instances total energy intake, protein, or calcium were lower and intake of iron was higher.[5] Several studies have suggested that vegetarian adolescents have better overall diets than their omnivore counterparts, and a recent large study suggested that they were more likely to meet the Healthy People 2010 objectives than adolescents who followed an omnivore diet.[6,7]

Growth Rates

Vegetarian or vegan infants have been shown to have growth rates within normal limits. Any differences between vegetarian or omnivore infants have been attributed to length of time being breastfed.[4] Multiple studies of vegetarian or vegan children or adolescents indicate that they grow normally on properly designed vegetarian or vegan diets.[1,8–15]

One large study in the United Kingdom looked at differences between lifelong vegetarians and those who adopted a vegetarian diet after age 20. Results suggested that there were no differences in height or adult weight between the groups for both men and women.[16]

Although growth does not appear to differ among vegetarian, vegan, and omnivore children, some studies evaluating nutrition intake have found differences in nutrient status. Some indicators, such as consumption of lower amounts of total fat, saturated fat, and cholesterol and higher fiber and fruit and vegetable intake in vegetarian and vegan children, are beneficial to health. However, lower intakes of calcium and essential fatty acids may suggest that better planning is needed by those making the food choice decisions for children and adolescents.[1]

Additional Considerations

Families that are predominantly composed of omnivores but that have a vegetarian or vegan child are becoming more common.[3] Some families may find this an extra challenge when providing meals within the home.

Some are concerned that food options outside of the home may be inadequate for vegetarian and vegan children. Many children get at least one meal, and sometimes more, while at school. The available vegetarian options must be nutritionally equivalent to the standard meat- and dairy-based offerings. A salad, french fries, and a piece of fruit are not a nutritionally complete vegetarian meal, for example. Many schools cafeterias may not offer vegetarian or vegan options because the student population with these preferences may be too small to make it feasible to provide alternatives. However, for those children given the option, the acceptability of the vegetarian alternatives at schools has been high.[17–19]

Peer pressure or other societal influences may encourage unhealthy eating habits in vegetarians and vegans, just as with omnivores. Note that adolescents adopting vegetarian diets could be masking an underlying eating disorder. However, because most children and adolescents benefit from good health while they are vegetarian, care should be taken not to interpret the cause of an eating disorder as coming from an individual's choice of dietary plan.

In conclusion, as long as adequate nutrients are provided, which can be achieved with proper planning, there appears to be no significant difference in overall growth of children who adopt vegetarian or vegan diets. Furthermore, these diets may offer substantial health benefits that could last into adulthood.

References

1 Dunham L, Kollar LM. Vegetarian eating for children and adolescents. *J Pediatr Health Care.* 2006;20(1):27–34.

2 Mangels AR, Messina V. Considerations in planning vegan diets: Infants. *J Am Diet Assoc.* 2001;101(6):670–677.

3 Moilanen BC. Vegan diets in infants, children, and adolescents. *Pediatr Rev.* 2004;25(5):174–176.

4 Messina M, Mangels R, Messina V. Vegetarian diets in infancy. In: *The Dietitian's Guide to Vegetarian Diets: Issues and Applications.* Sudbury, MA: Jones and Bartlett Publishers; 2004.

5 Messina V, Mangels AR. Considerations in planning vegan diets: Children. *J Am Diet Assoc.* 2001 June;101(6):661–669.

6 Perry CL, McGuire MT, Neumark-Sztainer D, Story M. Adolescent vegetarians: How well do their dietary patterns meet the Healthy People 2010 objectives? *Arch Pediatr Adolesc Med.* 2002;156(5):431–437.

7 Messina M, Mangels R, Messina V. Vegetarian diets for adolescents. In: *The Dietitian's Guide to Vegetarian Diets: Issues and Applications.* Sudbury, MA: Jones and Bartlett Publishers; 2004.

8 Sabaté J, Lindsted K, Harris R, Sanchez A. Attained height of lacto-ovo vegetarian children and adolescents. *Eur J Clin Nutr.* 1991;45:51–58.

9 Sabaté J, Lindsted KD, Harris RD, Johnston PK. Anthropometric parameters of schoolchildren with different lifestyles. *Am J Dis Child.* 1990;144(10):1159–1163.

10 Sanders, TAB, Manning J. The growth and development of vegan children. *J Hum Nutr Diet.* 1992;5:11–21.

11 Sanders TAB, Reddy S. Vegetarian diets and children. *Am J Clin Nutr.* 1994;59(5 Suppl):1176S–1181S.

12 Renda M, Fischer P. Vegetarian diets in children and adolescents. *Pediatr Rev.* 2009;30(1):e1–e8.

13 Nathan I, Hackett, AF, Kirby S. A longitudinal study of the growth of matched pairs of vegetarian and omnivorous children, aged 7–11 years, in the north-west of England. *Eur J Clin Nutr.* 1997;51:20–25.

14 Hebbelinck M, Clarys P, De Malsche A. Growth, development, and physical fitness of Flemish vegetarian children, adolescents, and young adults. *Am J Clin Nutr.* 1999;70(3 Suppl):579S–585S.

15 O'Connell JM, Dibley MJ, Sierra J, et al. Growth of vegetarian children: The Farm Study. *Pediatrics.* 1989;84(3):475–481.

16 Rosell M, Appleby P, Key T. Height, age at menarche, body weight and body mass index in lifelong vegetarians. *Public Health Nutr.* 2005;8(7):870–875.

17 Lazor K, Chapman N, Levine E. Soy goes to school: Acceptance of healthful, vegetarian options in Maryland middle school lunches. *J Sch Health.* 2010;80(4):200–206.

18 Endres J, Barter S, Theodora P, Welch P. Soy-enhanced lunch acceptance by preschoolers. *J Am Diet Assoc.* 2003;103(3):346–351.

19 Reilly JK, Lanou AJ, Barnard ND, et al. Acceptability of soymilk as a calcium-rich beverage in elementary school children. *J Am Diet Assoc.* 2006;106:590–593.

health benefits, both preventive and therapeutic.[49] Studies evaluating vegetarian and vegan dietary patterns generally suggest decreased risk for many diseases; furthermore, much of the controversy surrounding adequacy of vegetarian diets has been resolved.

Many of the chronic diseases seen in Westernized countries today have been examined in relation to various dietary patterns, including vegetarian and vegan diets. Some of the most significant studies have come from the Seventh-day Adventists, who have a large number of followers who practice a vegetarian diet. A number of large observational studies that have compared Seventh-day Adventists in the United States to individuals who consume meat have found a reduced risk in all-cause mortality, ischemic heart disease, and colon and prostate cancers.[50] Some large studies in Europe support this conclusion; however, others have shown that the differences were small or the same when compared to omnivores who followed a healthy lifestyle.[51,52]

A large prospective study of over half a million people found that high intakes of red meat or processed meat increased the risk for overall mortality and mortality from cancer. Red meat and processed meat also increased cardiovascular disease risk and the risk for cerebral infarction (a type of stroke) in women.[53] However, white meat intake in another study was found to decrease the risk for overall mortality and cancer.[54] Taken together, these studies suggest that either choosing a vegetarian eating pattern or reducing red and processed meat intake (or doing both) has important health benefits.

Cardiovascular Disease

Compared to omnivores, vegetarians tend to weigh less and have lower saturated fat intake, lower total cholesterol and LDL levels, and higher fiber intake and are less likely to suffer from hypertension.[42,55,56] Compared to vegetarians, vegans tend to have lower total and LDL cholesterol and blood pressure.[56,57] Studies looking at various diets suggest overall energy intake to be significantly greater from meat-based diets compared to vegetarian or vegan diets.[58] As expected, vegetarians and vegans have a lower overall body mass index.[57]

Cancer

Food and nutrition modify the risks for many kinds of cancers.[45] Some studies show a decrease in certain cancers in vegetarians,[50,59] whereas others do not.[60] Generally, rates of many cancers are only moderately lower in vegetarians; however, there is stronger evidence of risk reduction from consuming particular food groups that comprise a vegetarian or vegan diet, such as fruits and vegetables, particularly for cancers of the lung, stomach, esophagus, and mouth.[45,61]

The American Institute for Cancer Research (AICR) and the World Cancer Research Fund advise following a plant-based diet and limiting intake of red meat and processed meat as a public health goal in reducing cancer risk in general.[45] Convincing evidence supports a link between red meat consumption and colorectal cancer risk.[45] Furthermore, a recent large worldwide review of dietary patterns and colorectal cancer risk found meat-based diets to elevate the risk of cancer more than any other dietary pattern.[62] High consumption of meat and processed meat by both pre- and postmenopausal women has been shown to be associated with increased breast cancer risk; however, the risk for premenopausal women who had low intakes of meat was actually less than for vegetarians.[63]

Insulin-like growth factor-I (IGF-I) is a hormone involved in cellular growth and stimulation of growth hormone. It may play a role in reproductive cancers[58] and appears to be affected by dietary intake.[64] A study evaluating the status of IGF-I found similar levels between omnivores and vegetarians, but found levels in vegans to be 9–13% lower than those in the other two groups.[64] Furthermore, both vegetarians and vegans have been found to have lower levels of secondary bile acids compared to omnivores.[65] Secondary bile acids are potentially carcinogenic; higher levels have been found to increase the risk for colorectal cancer.[65,66]

Diabetes

The number of Americans with diabetes is expected to increase from roughly 23 million to 44 million over the next 25 years.[67] Vegetarians have a lower risk of developing type 2 diabetes than omnivores,[61,68,69] and vegans have been found to have less risk than both vegetarians and omnivores.[70] Studies investigating insulin resistance among omnivores and vegans found no difference in insulin sensitivity but did find a significant increase in beta cell function and intramyocellular lipid levels in vegans.[71,72] Both of these factors have been suggested to be protective for type 2 diabetes.[72]

Osteoporosis

Osteoporosis is a disease of low bone mass that predominantly affects women. Approximately 40% of women at 50 years of age will experience an osteoporotic fracture during their lifetimes.[73] Fracture rates as well as bone mass measurements and bone markers are used to evaluate bone health and have been studied in relation to diet. A large European study found similar fracture rates between vegetarians and omnivores but an increase in fracture rates for vegans.[74] However, the study did find that vegans whose calcium intake was above a certain level (525 mg/day) did not show any increase in fracture risk compared to omnivores.

A review of available vegetarian studies concluded that vegetarians have similar bone indices compared to omnivores and have normal bone mass.[75] This is despite the fact that some known characteristics that negatively affect bone occur in vegetarians, such as lower body weights and lower circulating levels of estrogen. The majority of studies that have looked at bone mineral density of vegans compared to that of omnivores have shown lower bone mass measurements in vegans.[76–78] Other studies have shown no difference between these groups.[79–81] Because vegans tend to be slimmer than individuals following other dietary plans,[57] this would be expected. Perhaps the only health benefit to those who are obese is the advantage of having extra mass to support load-bearing pressures on bones, which is beneficial to bone integrity.

Other Health Considerations

Other health benefits observed in vegetarians compared to omnivores include decreased risk for diverticulitis (an inflammation of the bowel that is one of the most common disorders of the colon among the elderly) and gallstones.[42] Vegetarians also have been shown to benefit from longer life expectancies than nonvegetarians.[82,83]

Research Caveats

Determining the actual significance of vegetarian and vegan diets on health and interpreting true benefits or risks is complex because a number of dietary and nondietary differences and patterns exist between omnivores and vegetarians. Because vegetarians tend to be healthier, they may smoke less, consume alcohol less frequently, and exercise more, making for a more health-conscious lifestyle.[30] Indeed, surveys of vegetarians suggest that they are more health conscious than nonvegetarians.[84]

Among vegetarians and vegans, dietary choices of particular foods, food groups, and individual nutrients, in addition to other lifestyle choices, can vary considerably. These complicating variables can make the terms *vegetarian* and *vegan* somewhat subjective. For example, some vegetarians consume low quantities of fruits and vegetables compared to others, who may far exceed dietary recommendations. Even the types of fruits and vegetables consumed can differ among vegetarians. Consider that a diet of mostly processed vegetarian fast food with little whole fruit or vegetable intake technically constitutes a "vegetarian diet," but one would hardly call it a healthy or adequate diet. Despite the presence of complicating variables, research studies continue to find associations between following a vegetarian or vegan diet and good health (see **Figure 9.4**).

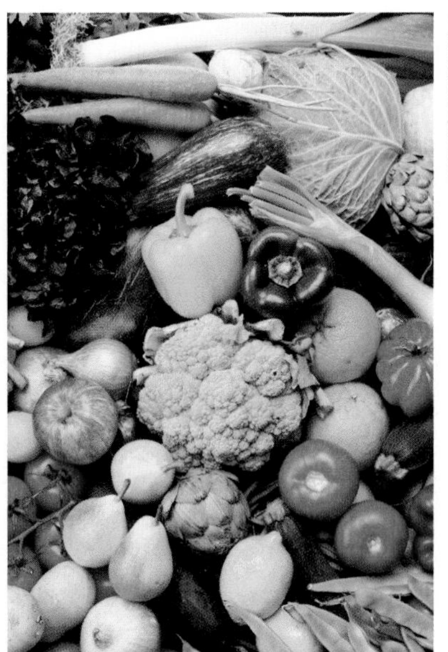

FIGURE 9.4 Numerous studies have demonstrated the health benefits of vegetarian eating patterns. In general, vegetarians have lower rates of heart disease and diabetes. In addition, studies have found that diets that are high in fruits and vegetables may be protective against the development of certain types of cancers.

Vegetarian Diets in the Treatment of Disease

Vegetarian, vegan, and plant-based dietary plans have been used in the treatment and management of specific diseases and for reducing specific disease risk factors. However, the success of such diets depends on the patient's perception: The diet needs to be both acceptable and relatively easy to follow.[85,86]

Treatment of Cardiovascular Disease

Plant-based diets reduce known risk factors for cardiovascular disease, such as total cholesterol and LDL cholesterol,[87–89] and can be used to help control and even reverse heart disease,[88,90,91] the leading cause of death in the United States. Treatment of hypertension has been shown to be favorably influenced by following vegetarian or vegan diets.[92]

Diabetes Control

In the treatment of type 2 diabetes, vegan diets may be equal to and in some instances even preferable to the diet recommended by the American Diabetes Association. Vegan diets have been demonstrated to be an effective strategy of diabetes control.[93] Vegan diets have also been shown to be of benefit in influencing the regression of painful diabetic neuropathy.[94]

Weight Loss

Opting for a plant-based diet can certainly be an important component of an effective weight loss plan (see **Special Topic 9.2**). Vegetarian diets used in weight loss programs have shown similar success rates when compared to other weight loss diets.[39,95]

Arthritis and Asthma Control

Studies examining rheumatoid arthritis suggest a possible benefit from following a vegetarian or vegan diet.[96] Another study investigating patients with long-term asthma found significant improvement from following a vegan diet, including a reduction in medication use and asthmatic attacks.[97]

Treatment of Prostate Cancer

In studies investigating cases of prostate cancer, some therapeutic benefit has been shown from following a plant-based or vegan diet.[98–100]

Special Topic 9.2

Vegetarian Diets for Obesity Prevention

Tim Radak, DrPH, RD

The current state of obesity or overweight in children has reached a level to where it is now a serious public health concern. Risk factors for diseases such as type 2 diabetes and heart disease, which were previously thought to be diseases of adulthood, are now seen frequently in young people. These diseases are strongly associated with obesity, poor diet, and physical inactivity.[1]

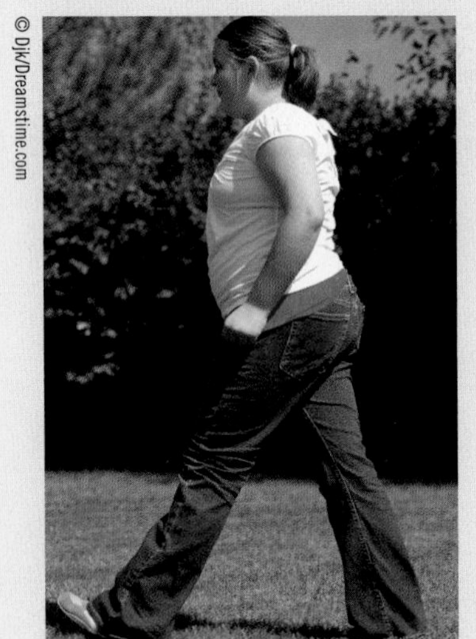

Childhood obesity has more than tripled in the past 30 years. Healthy lifestyle habits, including healthy eating and physical activity, can lower the risk of becoming obese and developing related diseases, such as cardiovascular disease, type 2 diabetes, and hypertension.

It is well documented that children who are obese or overweight strongly tend to keep that characteristic into adulthood. Most weight loss treatments have not shown success over the long term. Clearly, new approaches are needed. Some researchers have proposed that adopting and following a vegetarian diet can be a tool in addressing childhood obesity.[2] Adult vegetarians tend to weigh less than omnivores, and a number of studies in vegetarian youth suggest that they are at decreased risk for overweight and obesity.[2,3]

Well-planned vegetarian diets are plentiful in grains, legumes, fruits, and vegetables, which are high in fiber and low in fat. Eating foods that are high in fiber and low in fat can make a person feel full sooner, therefore ingesting fewer calories overall. High-fiber, low-fat diets have been shown to reduce the risk for many chronic diseases, including type 2 diabetes and heart disease. Vegetarians also tend to adopt other healthy lifestyle behaviors, which could have a positive effect on reducing risk for obesity over the long term. Taken together, these reasons present a strong case for having children adopt a vegetarian diet as a practical step in reducing their risk for becoming obese or overweight or in reducing weight for those already obese or overweight.

Other researchers have critically reviewed the idea of using plant-based diets to address childhood obesity. They have expressed concerns over whether this recommendation is ethical given the perceived cost constraints of a plant-based diet.[4] Fruits, vegetables, and dairy products can be costly. However, plant-based proteins such as beans, legumes, and grains generally cost less than animal protein sources. A recent study reviewing the cost of adopting a plant-based diet found it to be minimal.[5]

A large review assessing the impact on health from *not* consuming adequate fruits and vegetables suggested that, independent of anything else, consumption of more fruits and vegetables could play a role in reducing incidence of and death from most chronic diseases affecting us today.[6] The author suggests that these diseases add extraordinary healthcare costs and should prompt national strategies to promote population-based programs to increase fruit and vegetable intake.[6] For example, populations that are at or near the poverty line may find recommendations to eat adequate amounts of fruits and vegetables an extra economic burden or otherwise impractical; therefore, population-based programs targeting them might encourage increased intake through school food programs or by providing better access to fruits and vegetables in those areas where such options are minimal.

References

1 Stroup DF, Johnson V, Hahn RS, Proctor DC. Reversing the trend of childhood obesity. *Prev Chronic Dis.* 2009;6(3):A83.

2 Sabaté J, Wien M. Vegetarian diets and childhood obesity prevention. *Am J Clin Nutr.* 2010;91(5):1525S–1529S.

3 Robinson-O'Brien R, Perry CL, Wall MM, et al. Adolescent and young adult vegetarianism: Better dietary intake and weight outcomes but increased risk of disordered eating behaviors. *J Am Diet Assoc.* 2009;109:648–655.

4 Newby PK. Plant foods and plant-based diets: protective against childhood obesity? *Am J Clin Nutr.* 2009;89(5):1572S–1587S.

5 Hyder JA, Thomson CA, Natarajan L, et al. Adopting a plant-based diet minimally increased food costs in WHEL Study. *Am J Health Behav.* 2009;33(5):530–539.

6 Bazzano LA. The high cost of not consuming fruits and vegetables. *J Am Diet Assoc.* 2006;106(9):1364–1368.

Nutritional Considerations

Vegetarian diets need to include ample amounts of fruits, vegetables, whole grains, legumes, seeds, and nuts from a wide variety of sources to meet all of the body's nutritional needs. The key to successful vegetarian diets is to not only replace the nutrition that would have been included from animal products but to also meet the other established recommendations for general nutrition. This may be a particular challenge if the contribution of animal products to the diet is large, as in the case of the standard American diet.

Nutritional Deficiencies of the Typical American Diet

Data from national dietary and nutrition intake surveys show that many Americans are not meeting recommendations for many nutrients (see **Table 9.2**).[101] Survey data suggest that up to 66% of adult Americans have eating patterns that "need improvement" and another 16% are considered "poor."[102] Approximately 50–60% of adults consume the recommended number of servings for grains, 40–50% for vegetables, and 30% for fruits.[103] In addition, some groups are not meeting protein intake recommendations.[101,104]

Nutritional Benefits of Switching to a Plant-Based Diet

Studies looking at vegetarians in comparison to omnivores in relation to established nutritional recommendations indicate that vegetarians have increased intakes of fruits, vegetables, grains, legumes, nuts and seeds, fiber, vitamins C and E, folic acid, potassium, magnesium, copper, antioxidants, and phytonutrients and that they have decreased intakes or levels of cholesterol and saturated fat. Taken together, these factors are likely to be responsible for the positive health benefits seen in both small and large-scale research studies.[30,57,105–108] Numerous studies have identified various health benefits from consuming fruits, vegetables, grains, legumes, nuts, and seeds.

TABLE 9.2
Percentage of Americans Meeting Required Nutrient Intakes

Vitamin or Mineral	Percent Meeting Required Intake
Vitamin A	46%
Vitamin B_{12}	79%
Vitamin C	51%
Vitamin E	13%
Folate	59%
Magnesium	43%
Zinc	70%
Calcium	30%

Source: Data from U.S. Department of Agriculture. Community Nutrition Mapping Project: CNMap, Version 2. Available at: http://ars.usda.gov/Services/docs.htm?docid=15656. Accessed January 2, 2011.

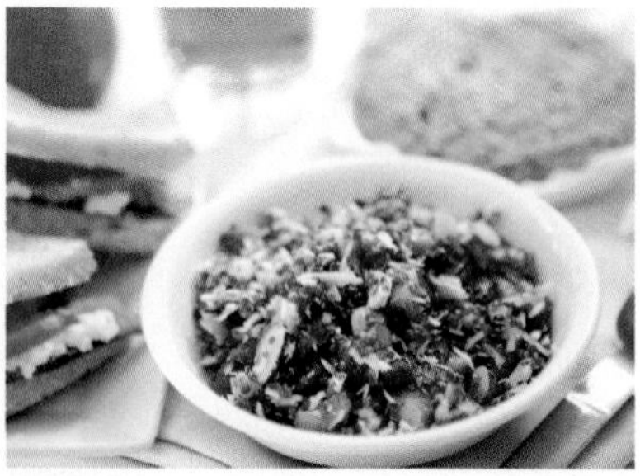

FIGURE 9.5 Plants and plant-based foods are an important source of dietary fiber. Dietary fiber has important health benefits, such as lowering blood cholesterol levels, controlling blood glucose levels, andaiding in weight loss.

Consider just one of these factors that is vastly different in the typical American omnivore diet versus a vegetarian diet—fiber. Adults and children in the United States do not meet even half the recommended intake for fiber (see **Figure 9.5**), which is not supplied by any animal products.[109] A recent study looking at thousands of American adults found that high fiber intake from grains was associated with a reduced risk for death from all causes, including heart, infectious, and respiratory diseases.[110]

Planning a Successful Vegetarian Diet

Although the overwhelming majority of research suggests the healthfulness of vegetarian diets, a number of nutritional and cultural factors must be considered when defining and interpreting what constitutes a balanced vegetarian diet. Vegetarian diets that are poorly planned may not contain adequate amounts of certain critical nutrients or they may contain excessive amounts of nutrients that could pose a health risk. Also, individual needs must be considered because nutrient requirements can vary from person to person. Some population groups—such as older adults, children and adolescents, pregnant or lactating women, and those who suffer from poverty—face extra challenges in meeting their nutritional needs. Being aware of these potential challenges will ensure the best chance of achieving nutritional adequacy and optimal health from a vegetarian diet.

Protein

The total available protein from vegetarian diets tends to be less than that from omnivore diets. However, although animal proteins are more digestible, proteins from plant sources are adequate and generally meet dietary recommendations. The USDA's Recommended Daily Allowance (RDA) is the same regardless of the whether plant or animal protein is consumed.[111] Although protein malnutrition is rare, what may be more important is low energy intake, such that low protein intake could lead to inadequate energy levels. Beans, chickpeas, lentils, tempeh, soy (for example, tofu), nuts, and certain grains (for example, quinoa) are all good sources of plant protein. Quinoa is especially recommended because it is a complete plant protein, meaning that it contains all of the essential amino acids. In addition, low-fat dairy products and eggs are good sources of animal protein for those vegetarians that incorporate these foods into their diets.

Calcium

Most vegetarians have adequate calcium intake. In fact, vegetarians may have higher calcium intake than omnivores, as well as better absorption.[42,112] However, vegans risk having a lower calcium intake unless they are careful in their choices of calcium-containing alternatives to dairy products. Calcium needs from nondairy sources can be met by a variety of calcium-containing plant sources complemented with calcium-fortified or enriched foods and beverages. Good sources of dietary calcium include tofu; certain green vegetables, such as collards, turnips, bok choy, and kale; sesame seeds; dried figs; fortified apple or orange juices; and most dairy-free milks made from soy, rice, or almonds. Recent research suggests that taking calcium supplements in addition to getting calcium from the diet may not be recommended; fortunately, adequate intake for those who exclude dairy products can be supplied via calcium-containing foods and beverages.

Vitamin D

Synthesis of vitamin D can be achieved from adequate exposure to sunlight in combination with consumption of fortified foods or supplements. Food is a poor source of vitamin D, which is why fortified dairy products are the main source for most of the population. Those who do not live in climates with abundant sun exposure should make extra effort to meet their requirements through fortified foods and beverages or supplementation. Vegans and ovo-vegetarians can get vitamin D the same way most omnivores do: from fortified products and sunshine. Good sources of vitamin D include fortified dairy-free milks made from soy, rice, or almonds, some breakfast cereals, and some juices and margarines.

Vitamin B_{12}

Although it is required in smaller amounts than other vitamins, vitamin B_{12} is a very important vitamin—deficiencies may cause irreversible health problems. There are no reliable plant sources, but vegans can meet their B_{12} requirement by consuming fortified foods and beverages. Vegetarians who consume dairy products and eggs, which contain vitamin B_{12}, are more easily able to meet their vitamin B_{12} needs. Although reported deficiencies are rare, some vegetarians and vegans may not be meeting dietary recommendations for vitamin B_{12}. It is important to meet the recommended intake to avoid potential elevations in homocysteine levels, a risk factor for cardiovascular disease. Homocysteine levels have been shown to be elevated in some vegetarians and vegans in countries other than the United States.[113–115] Good sources of vitamin B_{12} include some breakfast cereals, some dairy-free milks, Red Star brand nutritional yeast, and some types of veggie burgers and other meat substitutes.

Iron

Two types of iron are available in foods: heme and nonheme. Nonheme iron is found in plant foods. Nonheme iron is typically less well absorbed than heme iron, especially due to other substances found in plant foods, such as fiber and phytate. Although some vegetarians may need more iron than omnivores, most studies report adequate intake by vegetarians despite their having lower iron stores.[106] In fact, a number of studies have reported higher iron intake by vegetarians than by omnivores, and the intake by vegans higher still.[116] Studies also suggest that there is no difference in risk for anemia (caused by blood iron deficiency) among omnivores, vegetarians, and vegans.[57]

Good sources of iron include soybeans and other beans, lentils, enriched breakfast cereals, blackstrap molasses, pumpkin seeds, and Swiss chard. Combining iron intake with vitamin C–containing foods or beverages can enhance absorption.

Zinc

Plant sources of zinc are less well absorbed than those from animal sources, and studies assessing intakes by vegetarians and vegans have shown less, equal, or in some cases greater levels than in omnivores.[106,116] Whether a decreased absorption rate is responsible is still unresolved because functional indicators of zinc status in humans are variable and may lack sensitivity. One study showed that although zinc absorption was lower in vegetarians, the actual bioavailability was the same as in omnivores.[117] Good sources of zinc include some breakfast cereals, pumpkin seeds, tahini (made with ground sesame seeds and olive oil), beans such as adzuki or chickpeas, wheat germ, and some soy products.

Omega-3 and Omega-6 Fatty Acids

Omega-3 fatty acids are essential fats that cannot be derived from other fats in the diet; they are associated with cardioprotective and anti-inflammatory health effects. The long-chain fatty acids, including eicosapentaenoic acid (EPA) and docosahexaenoic acid (DHA), are particularly healthful. (See **Special Topic 9.3** for information on plant compounds that have been shown to have positive health effects.) Studies examining omega-3 fatty acid have tended to report lower levels of EPA and DHA in vegetarians and vegans;[70,118] however, a recent study reported that EPA and DHA blood levels in vegetarians and vegans were similar to omnivores.[119]

Vegetarians and vegans predominantly derive EPA and DHA from the conversion of alpha-linolenic acid (ALA), another omega-3 fatty acid found in plants, in the body. Good food sources of ALA include flaxseed, flaxseed oil, canola oil, tofu, soybeans, and walnuts. Omnivores obtain EPA and DHA from the conversion of ALA, too, but they also derive it directly from animal sources, particularly fish. (Fish obtain EPA and DHA from the algae they consume.) Sources of plant-based EPA and DHA are available in some fortified soy milks. It also is available directly from algae in the form of supplements.

The other essential fats are known as omega-6 fatty acids, which are found in similar plant sources as omega-3 fatty acids, but also in other foods, particularly vegetable oils and processed foods.[120] When consumed in moderate amounts along with omega-3 fatty acids, omega-6 fatty acids help regulate metabolism, stimulate growth of skin and hair, and maintain bone health. However, excessive intakes of omega-6 fatty acids have been implicated in the promotion of pathogenesis of cardiovascular disease, cancer, and inflammatory and autoimmune diseases. The important thing is the ratio of omega-6 to omega-3: a low omega-6/omega-3 ratio suppresses pathogenesis.[10] Avoiding excessive consumption of processed foods and vegetable oils, in which omega-6 is abundant but omega-3 is not, is a good way to keep this ratio low.

Some, but not all, studies have shown levels of omega-6 fatty acids to be higher in vegetarians and vegans than in omnivores.[120] Although few studies have attempted to determine whether there are health consequences of this (or of lower intakes of EPA and DHA), it is recommended that vegetarians and vegans achieve an appropriate ratio of omega-3 to omega-6 fatty acids. Moderating intake of omega-6 fatty acids may be more important than ensuring intake of omega-3 fatty acids.[119,120]

Special Topic 9.3

Phytonutrients

Tim Radak, DrPH, RD

Phytonutrients are chemicals found in many plant foods that are believed to confer certain protective effects on health. The term *phytochemical* is sometimes used interchangeably with *phytonutrient*. Phytonutrients differ from vitamins and minerals in that they are not necessarily essential nutrients. Literally thousands of phytonutrients have been identified, whereas there are only a few dozen vitamins and minerals. Phytonutrients are found in almost all plant foods, including fruits, vegetables, grains, legumes, nuts, seeds, spices, and herbs. Phytonutrients have also been identified in beverages such as teas and coffee and in chocolate (from cocoa). Many phytonutrients act as antioxidants, protecting the body from free oxygen radical damage to cell membranes, DNA molecules, and other important structures and processes of the body.

Numerous vegetables and fruits, and berries in particular, are believed to have cancer-prevention properties,[1] in part because of their high antioxidant concentrations. Vitamins and minerals such as beta-carotene, vitamins C and E, copper, zinc, and selenium also act as antioxidants, and many of these antioxidants are found in both plant and animal foods.

Certain phytonutrients, such as those in soy and soy products, may have positive effects on hormonal processes. Phytonutrients in vegetables such as cabbage and broccoli may positively affect enzymes and help with the body's detoxification systems. Intake of foods rich in certain phytonutrients has been associated with a reduced risk of heart disease and certain cancers.[2–6]

Well-planned vegetarian diets would be expected to contain high levels of phytonutrients because literally all whole foods and food groups that comprise a vegetarian diet, including fruits, vegetables, grains, legumes, nuts, and seeds, contain them. In fact, studies comparing omnivores and vegetarians have reported that vegetarians have higher intakes of antioxidants and phytonutrients[2,7] and higher plasma antioxidant levels.[8] These results may help to explain the lower incidence of some chronic diseases in vegetarians and vegans. Phytonutrient intake has also been hypothesized as a potential mechanism of longevity in vegetarians.[7] It is rare to find a research study identifying health risks for particular fruits, vegetables, or grains, and it is no coincidence that their health benefits have resulted in their promotion and emphasis in various dietary guidelines. Many studies in the last few decades have tried to identify and determine the type of benefit that can be provided from the intake of particular kinds of phytonutrients.

Animal products do not contain phytonutrients, but that does not mean that they do not contain important nutrients beyond vitamins and minerals. The term *zoochemicals* has been coined to describe the non-nutritive chemicals found in some animal foods. Some antioxidants are found in both. Some examples are lutein and zeaxanthin, which occur in green leafy vegetables as well as in egg yolks.[9]

Some phytonutrients have been added to animal products to increase the products' health benefits. For example, phytonutrients have been added to meats,[10] including hamburger, to influence cholesterol levels in hypercholesterolemic individuals.[11]

Phytonutrients can be placed into various categories. There are literally too many phytonutrients and phytochemicals to list them all here, but some common examples of classes and representative sources are shown in **Table A**. More and more researchers are investigating phytonutrient compounds and their mechanisms of action and relationship to health. To further the research process, the U.S. Department of Agriculture (USDA) maintains a number of phytonutrient databases and tables that list foods high in carotenoids, proanthocyanidins, flavonoids, and isoflavones.

TABLE A
Classes of Phytonutrients and Representative Sources

Classes	Sources
Carotenoids	Dark green leafy vegetables; red, yellow, and orange vegetables; cantaloupe, watermelon, and citrus fruits
Flavonoids	Berries, grapes, citrus fruits, onions, broccoli, cranberries, cocoa, peanuts, cinnamon, green and black tea
Phytoestrogens	Soy and soy products, such as tofu and tempeh; flaxseeds; sesame seeds; rye
Sulfides and thiols	Onions, garlic, scallions
Phytosterols	Wheat and wheat germ, corn, soy, peanuts, black and green teas, vegetable oils, green and yellow vegetables
Isothiocyanates	Broccoli, cauliflower, kale, Brussels sprouts

Source: Data from U.S. Department of Agriculture, Agricultural Research Service. USDA National Nutrient Database for Standard Reference, Release 18. Available at: http://www.nal.usda.gov/fnic/foodcomp/Data.

Fruits and vegetables are thought to be phytonutrient powerhouses. Some, like spinach, which are already plentiful in nutrients, are being marketed as "superfoods" because of their high phytonutrient content. Perhaps in the fight against disease, fruits and vegetables should be considered as our front-line defense because of their association with health promotion and disease reduction.

References

1 Mangat I. Do vegetarians have to eat fish for optimal cardiovascular protection? *Am J Clin Nutr.* 2009;89(5):1597S–1601S.

2 Rajaram S. The effect of vegetarian diet, plant foods, and phytochemicals on hemostasis and thrombosis. *Am J Clin Nutr.* 2003;78(3 Suppl): 552S–558S.

3 Lin J, Rexrode KM, Hu F, et al. Dietary intakes of flavonols and flavones and coronary heart disease in US women. *Am J Epidemiol.* 2007;165(11):1305–1313.

4 Omoni AO, Aluko RE. Soybean foods and their benefits: Potential mechanisms of action. *Nutr Rev.* 2005;63(8):272–283.

5 Adebamowo CA, Cho E, Sampson L, et al. Dietary flavonols and flavonol-rich foods intake and the risk of breast cancer. *Int J Cancer.* 2005;114(4):628–633.

6 Messina M, Messina V. The role of soy in vegetarian diets. *Nutrients.* 2010;2:855–888.

7 Burri BJ. Antioxidant status in vegetarians versus omnivores: A mechanism for longer life? *Nutrition.* 2000;16(2):149–150.

8 Haldar S, Rowland IR, Barnett YA, et al. Influence of habitual diet on antioxidant status: A study in a population of vegetarians and omnivores. *Eur J Clin Nutr.* 2007;61(8):1011–1022.

9 Thurnham DI. Macular zeaxanthins and lutein: A review of dietary sources and bioavailability and some relationships with macular pigment optical density, and age-related macular disease. *Nutr Res Rev.* 2007;20(2):163–179.

10 Andrés Nieto AI, O'Grady MN, Gutierrez JI, Kerry JP. Screening of phytochemicals in fresh lamb meat patties stored in modified atmosphere packs: Influence on selected meat quality characteristics. *Int J Food Sci Tech.* 2010;45:289–294.

11 Matvienko OA, Lewis DS, Swanson M, et al. A single daily dose of soybean phytosterols in ground beef decreases serum total cholesterol and LDL cholesterol in young, mildly hypercholesterolemic men. *Am J Clin Nutr.* 2002;76(1):57–64.

Dietary Planning Resources

A number of resources are available that have been designed to help vegetarians and vegans select foods and determine the amounts to consume in order to have a nutritionally complete diet, including ones that follow MyPlate and the *Dietary Guidelines for Americans*.[121] Food guides are even available for specific ethnic groups, such as the Japanese Vegetarian Food Guide Pyramid.[122] The focus of MyPlate is on plant-based foods. The *Dietary Guidelines for Americans, 2010* includes a number of sections detailing vegetarian and vegan diets and their health-promoting aspects; it also suggests eating patterns that adapt the guidelines to 12 different calorie-intake levels.[123]

Going Green with Vegetarianism

Over half a century ago the famous scientist Albert Einstein was quoted as saying, "Nothing will benefit human health or increase chances for survival of life on Earth as much as the evolution to a vegetarian diet."[124] One of the first people to encourage widespread thought about the relationship between food and the environment, and particularly animal products, was France's Moore Lappé, who in the early 1970s published the book *Diet for a Small Planet*.[125] Another influence was an increasing public awareness of shifts in agricultural practices, especially from small farms to large-scale agribusiness. In recent decades, the trend has been toward increased awareness of the link between one's food choices and the local and global environment. This awareness happened concomitantly with the environmental movement, which emphasized resource conservation.

Nutritional Ecology

A recent University of Chicago study made headlines and generated controversy by estimating the impact of diet on greenhouse gas emissions. The study found that the average American could do more to reduce global warming emissions by going vegan than by switching to a hybrid car.[126] Determining the environmental effects of choosing to eat a particular food, food group, or diet involves the analysis of a complex and dynamic set of factors. Research estimates vary widely in terms of influence of food choices on climate change and air, soil, and water quality. Where food is grown can be as important as what is grown, making it even more challenging for scientists to draw conclusions. A relatively new field—*nutritional ecology*—has developed that explores the complex interactions among nutritional and food production issues and their impact on the environment.[127]

Food production and consumption can influence the environment in a number of different ways:

- The methods and scale of agriculture for either plant or animal production (including the type of land used, the particular farming method and technique, fertilizers, feed composition, other chemicals used, and water and electricity usage)
- Harvesting, processing, preservation, packaging, transportation, and storage methods
- Wastes or energy use between retail purchases and home (and wholesale purchases and restaurant or other facility) and waste and disposal during and after preparation and consumption

All forms of agriculture, whether for plant or animal production, impact the environment. Growing crops and raising animals each carries specific types of pollution and environmental impacts. Numerous methods have been developed for estimating and modeling the effects of the food production and different diets, including vegetarian, vegan, and omnivore eating patterns. Several studies have attempted to quantify the differences in environmental impact among these diets, as well as among specific foods or food groups:

- *A U.S. study used a model to generate comparisons in the production and processing of various protein sources and the impact on the environment.*[128] Researchers calculated the impacts in order of smallest to greatest: soybeans, cheese, fish, and meat. They suggested the environmental impact from meat-based diets may be 1½ to 2 times greater than for vegetarian diets.
- *Another U.S. study assessed the impact of 11 foods in vegetarian and nonvegetarian diets on water, energy, pesticide, and fertilizer use.*[129] Results suggested that foods found in vegetarian diets have significantly less impact on the environment than foods of animal origin. They found some of the greatest differences in water usage.
- *A study by researchers in Italy evaluated the environmental impact of omnivore, vegetarian, and vegan diets and for conventional farming versus organic methods of production.*[130] The vegan diet was found to have the smallest overall impact and the omnivorous diet the greatest. Organic farming was found to be more environmentally friendly than conventional farming. The researchers also analyzed the impacts for specific foods and found beef to be the single food with the greatest negative impact on the environment. The study concluded that "vegetarian and vegan diets could play an important role in preserving environmental resources and in reducing hunger and malnutrition in poorer nations."

- *A study in Finland estimated greenhouse gas emissions from agricultural production of various plant and animal product foods.*[34] The conclusion was that a vegan diet would reduce greenhouse gas emissions by nearly half compared to the standard diet.
- *A study in Sweden estimated greenhouse gas production in 22 food items common to the Swedish diet.*[131] The study accounted for all aspects of emissions from "farm to table" and found that most plant foods had fewer total emissions than animal foods, with a few exceptions: Fresh oranges shipped from overseas had greater total emissions than those from milk, and fresh tropical fruit flown from overseas tied for the second highest of all foods in total greenhouse gas emissions. These exceptions illustrate the impact of food transportation on greenhouse gas emissions.

Air Quality

In addition to the contribution of food production to greenhouse gases, other effects on the air have been investigated. Factory farms can house tens of thousands of animals in one location, posing special environmental challenges. For example, levels of ammonia, a byproduct of manure, have been found to be significantly higher around areas where factory farms exist. Unhealthy concentrations of ammonia can lead to respiratory and other health conditions and contribute to smog and acid rain.[48] In some, but not all, studies, individuals living downwind or near areas where large numbers of animals are confined have experienced compromised health.[132–134]

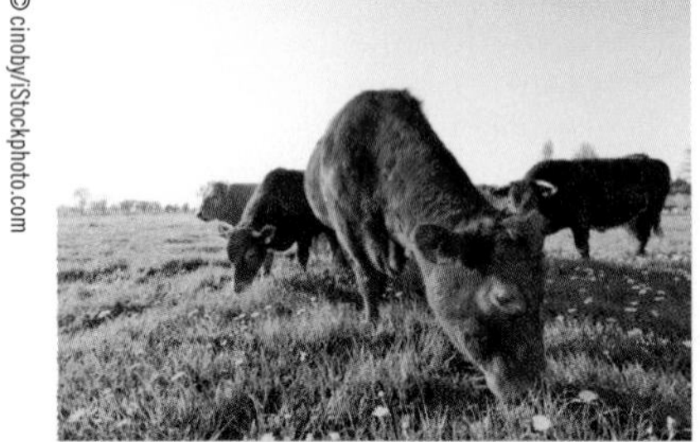

FIGURE 9.6 Overgrazing can lead to soil compaction and decreased plant cover, which can cause the topsoil to blow away.

Soil Quality

The enormous demand for grain and feed for animal agriculture can result in soil erosion and topsoil depletion in cropland, affecting soil fertility. Pastureland can suffer from overgrazing when densities of animals are high (see **Figure 9.6**). Overgrazing can cause degradation or erosion of the land due to soil compaction and decreased plant cover. In turn, poor soil quality can reduce air quality as dust is carried by winds.[135]

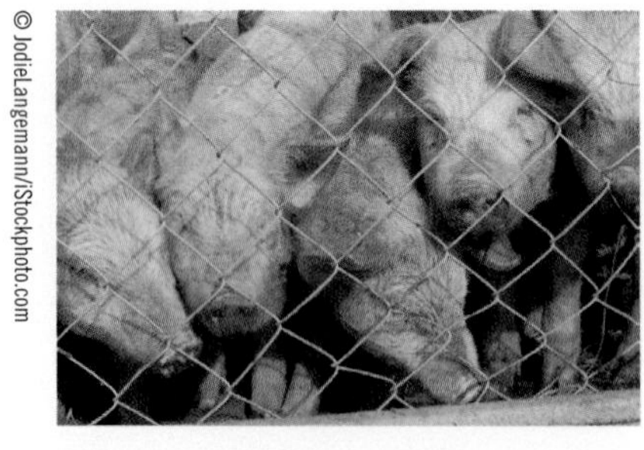

FIGURE 9.7 Animal waste from factory farms can degrade the quality of the surrounding air and water. In addition, the production of the huge amounts of grain and feed needed to raise these animals can result in soil degradation.

Challenges in the Study of Environmental Impacts

Agricultural methods for animal production and plants vary in growing or rearing techniques, geography, and available natural resources. These variables make it difficult to interpret results and draw comprehensive conclusions across multiple studies. A scientific consensus has not yet emerged as to the extent of the impact of food production and consumption on the environment. For example, in some areas of the world clearing land for growing plants may be less environmentally friendly than using it for animal production.[34,136] However, other studies suggest that an affluent meat-based diet requires more than three times as much land as a vegetarian diet.[137] Almost one-third of the entire land surface of the planet is used by livestock,[138] and in the United States 35% of cropland is used for feed grain production (see **Figure 9.7**).[139] Some suggest that more land could become available if a shift in consumption from animal foods to plant food occurred.[139] However, animal production, whether on pastures or factory farms, has generated controversy in terms of actual effect on the environment.[140,141]

Climate Change

Globally, it is estimated that the total contribution of all livestock represents 18% of the total greenhouse gas emissions.[142] A recent report comparing developing and developed countries suggested that developing countries are using more intensive livestock production methods, resulting in epidemic animal diseases and loss of important food sources.[143] Some reports have expressed concern about deforestation for agriculture of any kind due to its influence on greenhouse gases. Increases in greenhouse gases may lead to global climate change, which may impact the geographic suitability of various crops and animals, the lengths of growing seasons, and other variables important to food production. Climate change may create great challenges for land use if coastal areas are flooded or if droughts become more persistent or widespread.

Government Guidelines for Greener Diets

The Institute of Food Production and Sustainability is a section of the USDA whose mission includes the promotion of sustainable natural resources use. The USDA is concerned about the impact global warming will have on agriculture and land use in the United States and has studied adaption to climate change.[144] The USDA also developed standards for organic food in 2002 and is expected to facilitate more growth and research in organic food production that does not use non-natural fertilizers or pesticides and promotes ecological balance.[145,146]

The United Kingdom also offers progressive suggestions and tips regarding the relationship between food choices and the environment. For example, the main U.K. central government website (http://www.nidirect.gov.uk/index/information-and-services/environment-and-greener-living/greener-lifestyles/greener-shopping-and-products.htm) offers advice on "Greener Food and Drink" and suggests climate-friendly foods choices that have a lower carbon footprint. It also features advice on specific food groups.

Chapter Review

The word *vegetarian* is a relatively new one, but the practice of vegetarianism—the avoidance of meat in the diet—has existed for well over a thousand years. Vegetarianism is practiced by a relatively small percentage of the population today, but there are some groups where vegetarianism is well represented. People choose to follow vegetarian dietary patterns for a number of reasons, including an interest in healthy eating; a desire to reduce the specific risks for chronic diseases; as a treatment of some diseases; for its decreased impact on the environment; as well as for religious, moral, or ethical reasons.

Although they are a source of good nutrition, certain animal products have been identified to have some health risks. Vegetarian and vegan diets have been shown to promote health and reduce risk for many diseases; however, such diets are not automatically healthy. Care in planning a diverse, well-rounded diet with appropriate total calories can help vegetarians meet and maintain the demonstrated health effects. Many resources and food guides exist for vegetarians. Carefully planned vegetarian and vegan diets are adequate and nutritionally complete for all life stages.

Food production, because of its sheer scale, may have many environmental impacts, including effects on global warming, energy consumption, and the quality of air, water, and land resources. Determining the true impact of different types of food production is complicated due to the many complex relationships involved. Can choosing a vegetarian or vegan diet reduce the environmental impact of food production? Although some of the data are inconclusive, a number of studies suggest better outcomes for the environment, especially for land and water usage, and to an extent, pollution when compared to large-scale animal production and inefficiencies related to conversion of grain to meat in animal production. Yet, other environmental outcomes are not improved by eliminating meat from the diet.

While the environmental issues continue to be debated, focusing on the positive aspects of what constitutes a vegetarian diet—increased intakes of fruits and vegetables, whole grains, legumes and purchasing them while they are in season and from local sources—would seem to have a beneficial effect on some aspects of the environment and certainly on many aspects of one's health. Remember that there is a lot of room in between the strict categories of "vegetarian" and "omnivore," and one may find a comfortable and healthy dietary plan somewhere in the middle.

Learning Portfolio

Study Points

1. Reasons for choosing vegetarian diets include health benefits; religious or spiritual convictions; cost or economics; concerns about animal welfare, ethics, or the environment; or cultural influences from family, peers, or well-known figures in society.
2. Determinants of food intake involve a number of internal and external cues that drive our decision making.
3. The inclusion of animal products in the diet can provide an important source of energy-dense nutrition, but animal products are not necessary to obtain adequate nutrition. Some animal products carry health risks because they contain saturated fats and cholesterol and are devoid of dietary fiber.
4. Appropriately planned vegetarian and vegan diets are healthful and nutritionally adequate for all stages of the life cycle. Vegetarian or vegan diets can support normal infant and child growth; however, poor dietary planning may jeopardize a child's health and growth.
5. Food and nutrition modify the risks for many kinds of diseases. Studies and research evaluating vegetarian and vegan dietary patterns generally suggest decreased risk for many diseases.
6. Dietary standards and values for some nutrients and food groups are not being met by many Americans; improvement is needed. For example, adults and children in the U.S. do not meet even half the recommended intake for fiber.
7. Phytonutrients are chemicals found in many plant foods including fruits, vegetables, grains, legumes, nuts, and seeds, as well as in spices and herbs. They are believed to confer certain protective effects on health.
8. Our dietary choices make an environmental impact, but measuring the exact influence is complex and controversial. There are many considerations—including whether a food was bought fresh, frozen or processed, in or out of season, and how far it traveled to reach the supermarket or farmers' market—that influence the actual environmental impact.

Issues for Class Discussion

1. What factors could make a vegetarian or vegan diet unhealthy?
2. What issues should a person consider when deciding whether to renounce animal products and become a vegan or vegetarian?
3. Should vegetarian diets become part of a solution for the obesity epidemic in adults? In children?
4. How do proteins from animals and plants differ?
5. Should dietary recommendations account for environmental health in addition to human health?

Research Areas for Students

1. Foods that have health risks
2. The impact of dietary food choices on the environment
3. The possibility of environmentally friendly meat-based diets
4. The carbon footprint or water footprint of meat- versus plant-based diets
5. Efficiency of meat production compared to plant production
6. Use of vegetarianism to fight the obesity epidemic
7. Healthfulness of processed vegetarian foods

Key Terms

	page
flexitarian diet	279
fruitarian diet	279
lacto vegetarian diet	278
lacto-ovo vegetarian diet	278
legumes	279
macrobiotic diet	279
omnivore diet	278
ovo vegetarian diet	278
pescatarian (pesco vegetarian diet)	279
plant-based diet	278
raw food diet	279
vegan	278
vegetarian diet	278

References

1. Popkin BM. Reducing meat consumption has multiple benefits for the world's health. *Arch Intern Med.* 2009;169(6):543–545.
2. Spencer C. *Vegetarianism: A History.* New York: Fourth Walls Eight Windows; 2002.
3. *Cambridge Advanced Learner's Dictionary.* 3rd ed. Cambridge, UK: Cambridge University Press; 2008.
4. Dombrowski DA. *The Pythagoreans: The Philosophy of Vegetarianism.* Amherst, MA: University of Massachusetts Press; 1984.
5. Nath J. 'God is a vegetarian': The food, health and bio-spirituality of Hare Krishna, Buddhist, and Seventh-day Adventist devotees. *Health Sociol Rev.* 2010;19(3):356–368.
6. Johnson P. Nutritional implications of vegetarian diets. In: Shils ME, Olson JA, Shike M, Ross AC (eds.). *Modern Nutrition in Health and Disease.* 9th ed. Baltimore, MD: Lippincott Williams and Wilkins; 1998: 1755–1767.
7. Jayanthi V. Vegetarianism in India. *Perit Dial Int.* 2001;21(Suppl 3):S322–S325.
8. Fraser GE. *Diet, Life Expectancy, and Chronic Disease: Studies of Seventh-day Adventists and Other Vegetarians.* New York: Oxford University Press; 2003.
9. McDaniel L. Operators Unearth the Possibilities of Vegetarian Cuisines. Restaurants USA, January 1999. Available at: http://www.restaurant.org/profitability/openrestaurant/businesstopics/fandb/articles/article/?ArticleID=324. Accessed December 20, 2010.
10. Hill M (Associated Press). Vegan diets becoming more popular, more mainstream. *Washington Post,* January, 5, 2011. Available at: http://www.washingtonpost.com/wp-dyn/content/article/2011/01/05/AR2011010503153.html. Accessed January 10, 2011.
11. Bittman M. *How to Cook Everything Vegetarian: Simple Meatless Recipes for Great Food.* Hoboken, NJ: Wiley; 2007.
12. Minino A, Smith L. Deaths: Preliminary data for 2000. *National Vital Statistics Report.* 2001;49(12). Washington, DC: National Center for Health Statistics, Centers for Disease Control and Prevention, U.S. Department of Health and Human Services.
13. Flegal KM, Carroll MD, Ogden CL, Curtin LR. Prevalence and trends in obesity among US adults, 1999–2008. *JAMA.* 2010;303(3):235–241.
14. Ahmed F. Edible advice. *Nature.* 2010;468:S10–S12.
15. Krizmanic J. Here's who we are: A new survey reveals some surprises about America: 12 million plus (and counting) vegetarians. *Vegetarian Times.* 1992 Oct;182:73–80.
16. Pribis M, Pencak RC, Grajales T. Beliefs and attitudes toward vegetarian lifestyle across generations. *Nutrients.* 2010;2(5):523–531.
17. Avni R. AllRecipes.com. What American Families Are Eating and Cooking: 2011 Insights and Trends. The Measuring Cup. Available at: http://www.slideshare.net/AllrecipesPR/ar-2011-trendsnewsletter. 2010. Accessed January 20, 2011.
18. Tonsor GT, Olynk NJ. U.S. Meat Demand: The Influence of Animal Welfare Media Coverage. Kansas State University, September 2010. Available at: http://www.agmanager.info/livestock/marketing/AnimalWelfare/MF2951.pdf. Accessed February 1, 2011.
19. Winders B, Nibert D. Consuming the surplus: Expanding "meat" consumption and animal oppression. *Int J Sociol Social Policy.* 2004;24(9):76.
20. Iacobbo K, Iacobbo M. *Vegetarians and Vegans in America Today(American Subcultures).* Westport, CT: Praeger; 2006.
21. Vegetarianism in America. 2008. *Vegetarian Times.* Available at: http://www.vegetariantimes.com/features/archive_of_editorial/667. Accessed December 5, 2010.
22. Stahler C. How many adults are vegetarian? *Veg J.* 2006;4(25):14–5.
23. Stahler C. How many vegetarians are there? *Veg J.* 2009;4(28):12–13.
24. Barnes PM, Bloom B, Nahin RL. Complementary and alternative medicine use among adults and children: United States, 2007. *Natl Health Stat Report.* 2008 Dec;12:1–23.
25. Kala A. The flesh-eater of India: A recent trend. *The Times of India,* October 25, 2005. Available at: http://timesofindia.indiatimes.com/articleshow/msid-1273309,curpg-1.cms. Accessed January 2, 2011.
26. Yadav Y, Kumar S. The food habits of a nation. *The Hindu,* August 14, 2006. Available at: http://www.hindu.com/2006/08/14/stories/2006081403771200.htm. Accessed January 15, 2011.
27. Delgado C, Narrod C, Tiongco M. Growth and concentration in India. In: *Project on Livestock Industrialization, Trade and Social-Health-Environment Impacts in Developing Countries.* Food and Agriculture Organization. 2003. Available at: http://www.fao.org/WAIRDOCS/LEAD/X6170E/X6170E00.HTM. Accessed January 2, 2011.
28. Israel Center for Disease Control and the Food and Nutrition Services. MABAT, First Israeli Health and Nutrition Survey, 1999–2001. Publication No. 225. Tel Hashomer, Israel. Israeli Ministry of Health; October 2003.
29. Social Surveys (Gallup Poll). The 1988 Survey into Meat Eating and Vegetarianism. Realeat Company Ltd; 1988.
30. Phillips F. Vegetarian nutrition. *Nutr Bull.* 2005;30:132–67.
31. UK Food Standards Agency. Public Attitudes to Food Survey 2009. Available at: http://www.food.gov.co.uk. Accessed February 1, 2011.
32. American Dietetic Association; Dietitians of Canada. Position of the American Dietetic Association and Dietitians of Canada: Vegetarian diets. *J Am Diet Assoc.* 2003;103:748–765.
33. National Health and Medical Research Council. Dietary Guidelines for Australian Adults. Canberra, Australia: NHMRC; 2003. Available at: http://www.nhmrc.gov.au/_files_nhmrc/publications/attachments/n29.pdf. Accessed October 28, 2012.
34. Risku-Norja H. Dietary choices and greenhouse gas emissions: Assessment of impact of vegetarian and organic options at national scale. *Progress in Industrial Ecology—An International Journal.* 2009;6(4):340–354.
35. Ginsberg C, Ostrowski A. The market for vegetarian foods. *Veg J.* 2002;4:25–29.
36. White RF, Seymour J, Frank EJ. Vegetarianism among US women physicians. *J Am DietAssoc.* 1999;99(5):595–598.
37. General Conference of Seventh-day Adventists. *Three Strategic Issues: A World Survey.* Institute of Church Ministry, Seventh-day Adventist Theological Seminary, Andrews University; 2002.
38. Montgomery S, Herring P, Yancey A, et al. Comparing self-reported disease outcomes, diet, and lifestyles in a national cohort of black and white Seventh-day Adventists. *Prev Chronic Dis.* 2007;4(3):A62.

39. Barr SI, Broughton TM. Relative weight, weight loss efforts and nutrient intakes among health-conscious vegetarian, past vegetarian and nonvegetarian women ages 18 to 50. *J Am Coll Nutr.* 2000;19(6):781–788.
40. Nguyen A. Meatless eating is hot on Philadelphia college campuses. *Philadelphia Daily News,* October 14, 2010. Available at: http://articles.philly.com/2010-10-14/entertainment/24982387_1_vegan-college-students-graduate-student. Accessed January 2, 2011.
41. U.S. Department of Health and Human Services. *The Surgeon General's Report on Nutrition and Health: Summary and Recommendations.* Public Health Service: Publication No. 88-50211. Washington, DC: U.S. Government Printing Office; 1988.
42. Craig WJ, Mangels AR, American Dietetic Association. Position of the American Dietetic Association and Dietitians of Canada: Vegetarian diets. *J Am Diet Assoc.* 2009;109(7):1266–1282.
43. American Heart Association. Vegetarian Diets. Available at: http://www.heart.org/HEARTORG/GettingHealthy/NutritionCenter/Vegetarian-Diets_UCM_306032_Article.jsp. Accessed May 20, 2010.
44. Eldridge B, Hamilton K. Adopting a plant-based diet. In: *Management of Nutrition Impact Symptoms in Cancer and Educational Handouts.* Chicago, IL: American Dietetic Association; 2004.
45. World Cancer Research Fund/American Institute for Cancer Research. *Food, Nutrition, Physical Activity, and the Prevention of Cancer: A Global Perspective.* Washington DC: AICR; 2007.
46. Food and Agriculture Organization, World Health Organization. Human Vitamin and Mineral Requirements. A report of a joint FAO/WHO expert consultation, Bangkok, Thailand. Rome, Italy: World Health Organization and Food and Agriculture Organization of the United Nations; 2002: 7–25.
47. Goodland R, Anhang J. Livestock and climate change. *World Watch.* 2009;22(6):10–19.
48. Jacobson M, Center for Science in the Public Interest. *Six Arguments for a Greener Diet: How a More Plant-Based Diet Could Save Your Health and the Environment.* Washington, DC: Center for Science in the Public Interest; 2006.
49. Sabate J. The contribution of vegetarian diets to health and disease: A paradigm shift? *Am J Clin Nutr.* 2003;78(suppl):502S–507S.
50. Fraser GE. Associations between diet and cancer, ischemic heart disease, and all-cause mortality in non-Hispanic white California Seventh-day Adventists. *Am J Clin Nutr.* 1999;70(3 Suppl): 532S–538S.
51. Appleby P, Key TJ, Thorogood M, et al. Mortality in British vegetarians. *Public Health Nutr.* 2002;5:29–36.
52. Key T, Fraser G, Thorogood M, et al. Mortality in vegetarians and nonvegetarians: A collaborative analysis of 8300 deaths among 76,000 men and women in five prospective studies. *Public Health Nutr.* 1998;1(1):33–41.
53. Larsson SC, Virtamo J, Wolk A. Red meat consumption and risk of stroke in Swedish women. *Stroke.* 2011;42(2):324–329.
54. Sinha R, Cross AJ, Graubard BI, et al. Meat intake and mortality: A prospective study of over half a million people. *Arch Intern Med.* 2009;169(6):562–571.
55. Appleby PN, Davey GK, Key TJ. Hypertension and blood pressure among meat eaters, fish eaters, vegetarians and vegans in EPIC Oxford. *Public Health Nutr.* 2002;5:645–654.
56. Key TJ, Appleby PN, Rosell MS. Health effects of vegetarian and vegan diets. *Proc Nutr Soc.* 2006;65(1):35–41.
57. Craig WJ. Health effects of vegan diets. *Am J Clin Nutr.* 2009;89(5):1627S–1633S.
58. Williamson CS, Foster RK, Stanner SA, Buttriss JL. Red meat in the diet. *Nutr Bull.* 2005;30:323–355.
59. Kiani F, Knutsen S, Singh P, et al. Dietary risk factors for ovarian cancer: The Adventist Health Study (United States). *Cancer Causes Control.* 2006;17(2):137–146.
60. Key T, Fraser G, Thorogood M, et al. Mortality in vegetarians and nonvegetarians: Detailed findings from a collaborative analysis of 5 prospective studies. *Am J Clin Nutr.* 1999;70(3 Suppl):516S–524S.
61. Craig WJ. Nutrition concerns and health effects of vegetarian diets. *Nutr Clin Pract.* 2010;25(6):613–620.
62. Randi G, Edefonti V, Ferraroni M, et al. Dietary patterns and the risk of colorectal cancer and adenomas. *Nutr Rev.* 2010;68(7):389–408.
63. Allen NE, Appleby PN, Davey GK, et al. The associations of diet with serum insulin-like growth factor I and its main binding proteins in 292 women meat-eaters, vegetarians, and vegans. *Cancer Epidemiol Biomarkers Prev.* 2002;11(11):1441–1448.
64. Brodsky I. Hormone, cytokine, and nutrient interactions. In: Shils ME, Olson JA, Shike M, Ross AC (eds). *Modern Nutrition in Health and Disease.* 9th ed. Baltimore, MD: Lippincott Williams and Wilkins; 1998: 699–724.
65. van Faassen A, Hazen MJ, van den Brandt PA, et al. Bile acids and pH values in total feces and in fecal water from habitually omnivorous and vegetarian subjects. *Am J Clin Nutr.* 1993;58(6):917–922.
66. Pearson JR, Gill CI, Rowland IR. Diet, fecal water, and colon cancer: Development of a biomarker. *Nutr Rev.* 2009;67(9):509–526.
67. Huang ES, Basu A, O'Grady M, Capretta JC. Projecting the future diabetes population size and related costs for the U.S. *Diabetes Care.* 2009;32(12):2225–2229.
68. Snowdon DA, Phillips RL. Does a vegetarian diet reduce the occurrence of diabetes? *Am J Public Health.* 1985;75(5):507–12.
69. Trapp C, Barnard N, Katcher H. A plant-based diet for type 2 diabetes: Scientific support and practical strategies. *Diabetes Educ.* 2010;36(1):33–48.
70. Marsh K, Miller-Brand J. Vegetarian diets and diabetes. *Am J Lifestyle Med.* November 19, 2010. Available at: http://ajl.sagepub.com/content/early/2010/11/10/1559827610387393.abstract. Accessed February 2, 2011.
71. Barnard ND, Scialli AR, Turner-McGrievy G, et al. The effects of a low-fat, plant-based dietary intervention on body weight, metabolism, and insulin sensitivity. *Am J Med.* 2005;118(9):991–997.
72. Goff LM, Bell JD, So PW, et al. Veganism and its relationship with insulin resistance and intramyocellular lipid. *Eur J Clin Nutr.* 2005;59(2):291–298.
73. Melton LJ 3rd. How many women have osteoporosis now? *J Bone Miner Res.* 1995;10:175–177.
74. Appleby P, Roddam A, Allen N, Key T. Comparative fracture risk in vegetarians and nonvegetarians in EPIC-Oxford. *Eur J Clin Nutr.* 2007;61:1400–1406.
75. New SA. Do vegetarians have a normal bone mass? *Osteoporos Int.* 2004;15:679–688.
76. Parsons TJ, van Dusseldorp M, van der Vliet M, et al. Reduced bone mass in Dutch adolescents fed a macrobiotic diet in early life. *J Bone Miner Res.* 1997;12(9):1486–1494.

77. Outila TA, Kärkkäinen MU, Seppänen RH, Lamberg-Allardt CJ. Dietary intake of vitamin D in premenopausal, healthy vegans was insufficient to maintain concentrations of serum 25-hydroxyvitamin D and intact parathyroid hormone within normal ranges during the winter in Finland. *J Am Diet Assoc.* 2000;100(4):434–441.
78. Chiu JF, Lan SJ, Yang CY, et al. Long-term vegetarian diet and bone mineral density in postmenopausal Taiwanese women. *Calcif Tissue Int.* 1997;60:245–249.
79. Lau EMC, Kwok T, Woo J, Ho SC. Bone mineral density in Chinese elderly female vegetarians, vegans, lacto-ovo vegetarians and omnivores. *Eur J Clin Nutr.* 1998;52:60–64.
80. Ho-Pham LT, Nguyen PL, Le TT, et al. Veganism, bone mineral density, and body composition: A study in Buddhist nuns. *Osteoporos Int.* 2009;20(12):2087–2093.
81. Wang YF, Chiu JS, Chuang MH, et al. Bone mineral density of vegetarian and non-vegetarian adults in Taiwan. *Asia Pac J Clin Nutr.* 2008;17:101–106.
82. Singh PN, Sabaté J, Fraser GE. Does low meat consumption increase life expectancy in humans? *Am J Clin Nutr.* 2003;78 (3 Suppl):526S–532S.
83. Fraser GE, Shavlik DJ. Ten years of life: Is it a matter of choice? *Arch Intern Med.* 2001;161:1645–1652.
84. Bedford JL, Barr SI. Diets and selected lifestyle practices of self-defined adult vegetarians from a population-based sample suggest they are more 'health conscious'. *Int J Behav Nutr Phys Act.* 2005;2(1):4.
85. Berkow SE, Barnard N, Eckart J, Katcher H. Four therapeutic diets: Adherence and acceptability. *Can J Diet Pract Res.* 2010;71(4):199–204.
86. Barnard ND, Scialli AR, Turner-McGrievy G, Lanou AJ. Acceptability of a low-fat vegan diet compares favorably to a step II diet in a randomized, controlled trial. *J Cardiopulm Rehabil.* 2004;24(4):229–235.
87. Ferdowsian HR, Barnard ND. Effects of plant-based diets on plasma lipids. *Am J Cardiol.* 2009;104(7):947–956.
88. Ornish D, Brown SE, Scherwitz JHB, at el. Intensive lifestyle changes for reversal of coronary heart disease. *JAMA.* 1998;280(23):2001–2007.
89. Barnard ND, Scialli AR, Bertron P, et al. Effectiveness of a low-fat vegetarian diet in altering serum lipids in healthy premenopausal women. *Am J Cardiol.* 2000;85:969–972.
90. Ornish D, Brown SE, Scherwitz LW, et al. Can lifestyle changes reverse coronary heart disease? The Lifestyle Heart Trial. *Lancet.* 1990;336:129–133.
91. Esselstyn CB Jr. Updating a 12-year experience with arrest and reversal therapy for coronary heart disease: An overdue requiem for palliative cardiology. *Am J Cardiol.* 1999;84(3):339–341, A8.
92. Berkow SE, Barnard ND. Blood pressure regulation and vegetarian diets. *Nutr Rev.* 2005;63(1):1–8.
93. Trapp CB, Barnard ND. Usefulness of vegetarian and vegan diets for treating type 2 diabetes. *Curr Diab Rep.* 2010;10(2):152–158.
94. Crane MG. Regression of diabetic neuropathy with total vegetarian (vegan) diet. *J Nutr Med.* 1994;4:431–439.
95. Burke LE, Hudson AG, Warziski MT, et al. Effects of a vegetarian diet and treatment preference on biochemical and dietary variables in overweight and obese adults: A randomized clinical trial. *Am J Clin Nutr.* 2007;86(3):588–596.
96. Messina M, Mangels R, Messina V. Health consequences of vegetarian diets. In: *The Dietitian's Guide to Vegetarian Diets: Issues and Applications.* Sudbury, MA: Jones and Bartlett Publishers; 2004.
97. Lindahl O, Lindwall L, Spångberg A, et al. Vegan regimen with reduced medication in the treatment of bronchial asthma. *J Asthma.* 1985;22(1):45–55.
98. Nguyen JY, Major JM, Knott CJ, et al. Adoption of a plant-based diet by patients with recurrent prostate cancer. *Integr Cancer Ther.* 2006;5(3):214–223.
99. Daubenmier JJ, Weidner G, Marlin R, et al. Lifestyle and health-related quality of life of men with prostate cancer managed with active surveillance. *Urology.* 2006;67(1):125–130.
100. Flynn MM, Mega A. Treating recurrent prostate cancer with a plant-based, olive oil diet. *J Am Diet Assoc.* 2010;110 (9 Supp):A12.
101. Community Nutrition Mapping Project, CNMap, Version 2. United States Department of Agriculture. http://ars.usda.gov/Services/docs.htm?docid=15656. Accessed January 2, 2011.
102. Basiotis PP, Carlson A, Gerrior SA, et al. *The Healthy Eating Index: 1999–2000.* CNPP-12 2002 Washington, DC: U.S. Department of Agriculture, Center for Nutrition Policy and Promotion; 2002.
103. Cook A, Friday J. CNRG Table Set 3.0: Pyramid Servings Intakes in the United States, 1999–2002, 1 Day. USDA, Agricultural Research Service, Community Nutrition Research Group; March 21, 2005. Available at: http://www.ars.usda.gov/Services/docs.htm?docid=8503. Accessed January 2, 2011.
104. Kerstetter JE, O'Brien KO, Insogna KL. Dietary protein, calcium metabolism, and skeletal homeostasis revisited. *Am J Clin Nutr.* 2003;78(3 Suppl):584S–592S.
105. Haddad EH, Tanzman JS. What do vegetarians in the United States eat? *Am J Clin Nutr.* 2003;78:626S–632S.
106. Gibson RS. Content and bioavailability of trace elements in vegetarian diets. *Am J Clin Nutr.* 1994;59(5 Suppl):1223S–1232S.
107. Rauma AL, Mykkänen H. Antioxidant status in vegetarians versus omnivores. *Nutrition.* 2000;16(2):111–119.
108. Szeto YT, Kwok TC, Benzie IF. Effects of a long-term vegetarian diet on biomarkers of antioxidant status and cardiovascular disease risk. *Nutrition.* 2004;20(10):863–866.
109. Anderson JW, Baird P, Davis RH Jr, et al. Health benefits of dietary fiber. *Nutr Rev.* 2009;67(4):188–205.
110. Park Y, Subar AF, Hollenbeck A, Schatzkin A. Dietary fiber intake and mortality in the NIH-AARP Diet and Health Study. *Arch Intern Med.* 2011;(0):181–188. Published online February 14, 2011.
111. Institute of Medicine, Food and Nutrition Board. *Dietary Reference Intakes for Energy, Carbohydrate, Fiber, Fat, Fatty Acids, Cholesterol, Protein, and Amino Acids.* Washington, DC: National Academies Press; 2002.
112. Nnakwe N, Kies C, Fox HM. Calcium and Phosphorus Utilization by Omnivores and Vegetarians. Proceedings of Nebraska Academy of Sciences and Affiliated Societies. 1982;92:29.
113. Leitzmann C. Vegetarian diets: What are the advantages? *Forum Nutr.* 2005;(57):147–156.

114. Elmadfa I, Singer I. Vitamin B_{12} and homocysteine status among vegetarians: A global perspective. *Am J Clin Nutr.* 2009;89(5):1693S–1698S.
115. Yen CE, Yen CH, Cheng CH, Huang YC. Vitamin B_{12} status is not associated with plasma homocysteine in parents and their preschool children: Lacto-ovo, lacto, and ovo vegetarians and omnivores. *J Am Coll Nutr*. 2010;29(1):7–13.
116. Messina M, Mangels R, Messina V. Minerals. In: *The Dietitian's Guide to Vegetarian Diets: Issues and Applications.* Sudbury, MA: Jones and Bartlett Publishers; 2004.
117. Kristensen MB, Hels O, Morberg CM, et al. Total zinc absorption in young women but not fractional zinc absorption, differs between vegetarian and meat-based diets with equal phytic acid content. *Br J Nutr.* 2006;95(5):963–967.
118. Rosell MS, Lloyd-Wright Z, Appleby PN, et al. Long-chain n-3 polyunsaturated fatty acids in plasma in British meat-eating, vegetarian, and vegan men. *Am J Clin Nutr.* 2005;82(2):327–334.
119. Welch AA, Shakya-Shrestha S, Lentjes MA, et al. Dietary intake and status of n-3 polyunsaturated fatty acids in a population of fish-eating and non-fish-eating meat-eaters, vegetarians, and vegans and the precursor-product ratio of α-linolenic acid to long-chain n-3 polyunsaturated fatty acids: Results from the EPIC-Norfolk cohort. *Am J Clin Nutr.* 2010;92(5):1040–1051.
120. Davis BC, Kris-Etherton PM. Achieving optimal essential fatty acid status in vegetarians: Current knowledge and practical implications. *Am J Clin Nutr.* 2003;78(3 Suppl):640S–646S.
121. U.S. Department of Health and Human Services, U.S. Department of Agriculture. *Dietary Guidelines for Americans, 2005.* Washington, DC: U.S. Government Printing Office; 2005.
122. Nakamoto K, Arashi M, Noparatanawong S, et al. A new Japanese vegetarian food guide. *Asia Pac J Public Health.* 2009;21(2):160–169.
123. U.S. Department of Agriculture, U.S. Department of Health and Human Services. *Dietary Guidelines for Americans, 2010.* 7th ed. Washington, DC: U.S. Government Printing Office; December 2010.
124. Albert Einstein quotes. Available at: http://thinkexist.com/quotation/nothing_will_benefit_human_health_and_increase/15538.html. Accessed October 28, 2012.
125. Lappé FM. *Diet for a Small Planet.* New York: Ballantine Books; 1971.
126. Eshel G, Martin PA. Diet, energy, and global warming. *Earth Interact.* 2006;10:1–17.
127. Metz M, Hoffmann I. Effects of vegetarian nutrition: A nutrition ecological perspective. *Nutrients.* 2010;2(5):496–504.
128. Reijnders L, Soret S. Quantification of the environmental impact of different dietary protein choices. *Am J Clin Nutr.* 2003;78(3 Suppl):664S–668S.
129. Marlow HJ, Hayes WK, Soret S, et al. Diet and the environment: Does what you eat matter? *Am J Clin Nutr.* 2009;89(5): 1699S–1703S.
130. Baroni L, Cenci L, Tettamanti M, Berati M. Evaluating the environmental impact of various dietary patterns combined with different food production systems. *Eur J Clin Nutr.* 2007;61(2):279–186.
131. Carlsson-Kanyama A, González AD. Potential contributions of food consumption patterns to climate change. *Am J Clin Nutr.* 2009;89(5):1704S–1709S.
132. Schiffman SS, Miller EA, Suggs MS, Graham BG. The effect of environmental odors emanating from commercial swine operations on the mood of nearby residents. *Brain Res Bull.* 1995;37(4):369–375.
133. Wing S, Wolf S. Intensive livestock operations, health, and quality of life among eastern North Carolina residents. *Environ Health Perspect.* 2000;108(3):233–238.
134. Villeneuve PJ, Ali A, Challacombe L, Hebert S. Intensive hog farming operations and self-reported health among nearby rural residents in Ottawa, Canada. *BMC Public Health.* 2009 Sept;9:330.
135. University of Wyoming. Grazing Livestock on Small Acreages. Campbell County Conservation District. Available at: http://www.cccdwy.net/Livestock%20Brochure.pdf. Accessed February 1, 2011.
136. Del Grosso SJ. Climate change: Grazing and nitrous oxide. *Nature.* 2010;464(7290):843–844.
137. Gerbens-Leenes PW, Nonhebel S, Ivens WPMF. A method to determine land requirements relating to food consumption patterns. *Agriculture, Ecosystems, & Environment.* 2002;90:47–58.
138. Food and Agriculture Organization Newsroom. Livestock a Major Threat to Environment. November 29, 2006. Available at: http://www.fao.org/newsroom/en/news/2006/1000448/index.html. Accessed February 1, 2011.
139. Duxbury JM, Welch RM. Agriculture and dietary guidelines. *Food Policy.* 1999; 24:197–209.
140. Hopp SL, Fussow JD. [Comment on] Food miles and the relative climate impacts of food choices in the United States. *Environ Sci Technol.* 2009;43(10):3982–3983.
141. Weber CL, Matthews HS. [Response to Comment on] Food miles and the relative climate impacts of food choices in the United States. *Environ Sci Technol.* 2009;43(10):3984.
142. Food and Agriculture Organization. *Livestock's Long Shadow: Environmental Issues and Options.* Rome, Italy: Food and Agriculture Organization of the United Nations; 2006.
143. Karaimu P. Livestock Boom Risks Aggravating Animal 'Plagues,' Poses Growing Threat to Food Security and Health of World's Poor. International Livestock Research Institute. February 10, 2011. Available at: http://www.ilri.org/ilrinews/?p=4535&utm_source=feedburner&utm_medium=feed&utm_campaign=Feed%3A+ilrinews+%28ILRI+News%29. Accessed February 14, 2011.
144. Malcolm S, Marshall E, Aillery M, et al. Agricultural Adaptation to a Changing Climate: Economic and Environmental Implications Vary by U.S. Region. Economic Research Report No. (ERR-136). July 2012. Available at: http://www.ers.usda.gov/publications/err-economic-research-report/err136.aspx. Accessed August 7, 2012.
145. Economic Research Service, U.S. Department of Agriculture. Recent Growth Patterns in the U.S. Organic Foods Market: Summary. Available at: http://www.ers.usda.gov/media/255728/aib777a_1_.pdf. Accessed August 7, 2012.
146. U.S. Department of Agriculture. National Organic Program. Available at: http://www.ams.usda.gov/AMSv1.0/nop. Accessed August 7, 2012.

CHAPTER 10

Fruits and Vegetables

Catherine Frederico, MS, RD, LDN

Chapter Objectives

THE STUDENT WILL BE EMPOWERED TO:

- Summarize the historical, cultural, and ecological significance of fruits and vegetables.
- Define fruits and vegetables and describe their classification.
- Describe the physical and chemical properties of fruits and vegetables.
- Summarize the key nutritional and health benefits of fruits and vegetables and the healthful effects of various phytonutrients.
- Review menu planning, food-selection criteria, and basic food preparation of fruits and vegetables.
- List innovations in food technologies relating to fruits and vegetables.
- Discuss green initiatives in growing, choosing, and cooking fruits and vegetables.
- Identify important food safety considerations relating to the production and preparation of fruits and vegetables.

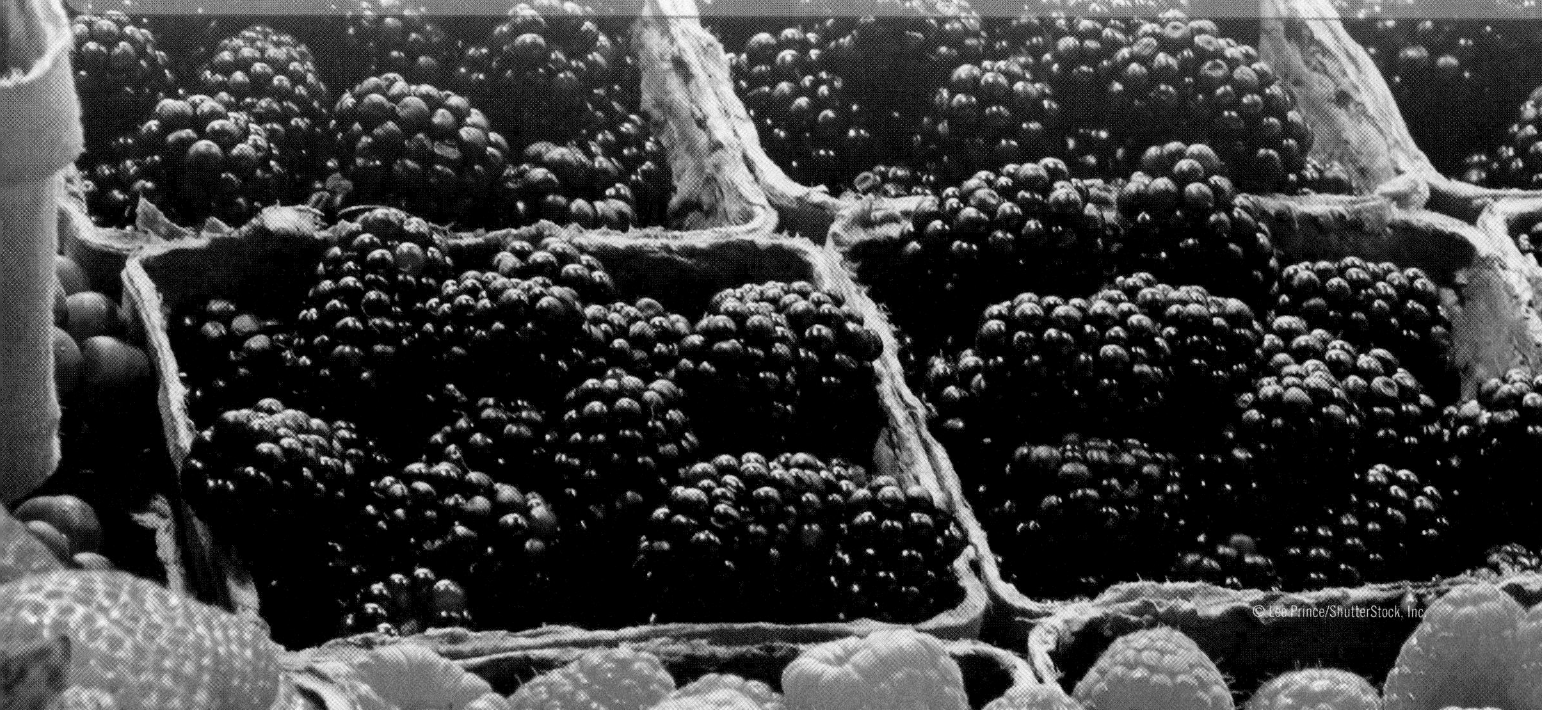

Historical, Cultural, and Ecological Significance

The earliest humans were hunter-gatherers who ate wild plants and animals. Agriculture was developed about 11,000 years ago, and it has taken thousands of years to develop the plant species and farming practices that we know today. Archeological evidence suggests that farming was first developed in the Near East around 8500 B.C., in China around 7500 B.C., and in Central and South America around 3500 B.C. Nomadic people and farmers influenced each other as the farming practices that we know today developed. Agriculture had the obvious benefit of providing a stable, reliable food source with efficient yields, as long as the weather cooperated and a sufficient number of people had settled in one place to tend crops. However, based on dental and skeletal remains, it appears that the people living in these early agricultural settlements were more susceptible to diseases and were more malnourished, as evidenced by their shorter stature, than their hunter-gather counterparts. The diets of early agriculturists were not as varied as those of hunter-gatherers because they relied on only the few crops they cultivated. Today, the few remaining hunter-gatherer cultures left in the world enjoy the benefit of working fewer hours to acquire food to fuel their active lifestyles compared to farming cultures. However, they need to move often to seek ready food supplies over large areas of land.[1]

Grains such as wheat and barley supported early Near East and Asian civilizations, whereas maize and potatoes supported those in the Americas. Maize, the ancestor of today's corn, was developed from a wild Mexican grass called teosinte. Teosinte has only two rows of kernels on half-inch cobs. As humans intervened to farm it, larger ears were most likely replanted each year, leading to the rise of the 8-inch-long, multirowed cob we know today (see **Figure 10.1**). Columbus' crew first enjoyed maize on the island of Hispaniola in 1492, when they mistakenly thought they were in Asia. Maize was then introduced to Europe, and its cultivation quickly spread as far as China by the mid-1500s.[1]

(a) (b)

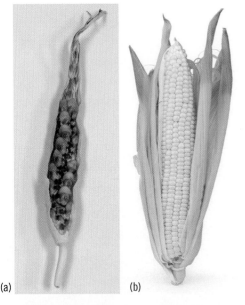

FIGURE 10.1 (a) Although teosinte does not look much like today's modern corn, at the DNA level the two are surprisingly alike. They have the same number of chromosomes and a remarkably similar arrangement of genes. (b) Over time, farmers selected for a variety of different traits that we now see in modern maize. Farmers selected for larger, starchier kernels and longer cobs, among other traits. Today, maize is one of the most important food sources in our modern world.

(a) Courtesy of the U.S. Department of Agriculture.; (b) © iStockphoto/Thinkstock

In the Andes of South America, the Spanish conquistadores found Incan societies cultivating hundreds of varieties of white, purple, and yellow potatoes of various shapes and sizes. In the 1500s, the Spanish conquistadores carried this new crop back to their European homes; however, initially, potatoes did not share the same quick popularity as corn. Potatoes did not grow as well in European seasonal climates, and their irregular shapes and colors were foreign to Europeans. Rumors quickly spread that they caused leprosy. It was not until famines in the 1600s and 1700s in England, France, and Germany that potatoes were cultivated, proving their worth in curbing starvation and becoming a daily staple by 1800. In Ireland, especially, the potato become a major dietary staple, with ruinous consequences when approximately a million people in Ireland died of starvation when a devastating fungal blight ruined the 1845 and 1846 potato crops.[1]

As trade routes became well established, other vegetables and fruits traveled from one continent to another. Fruits and vegetables that reached England from South America were then introduced to North America. Christopher Columbus' travels between the Old and New Worlds brought bananas west from Africa and tomatoes and potatoes east from South America. Botanical study became popular, and movement of new crops was swift. The Japanese were glad to find that sweet potatoes were not affected by typhoons, and Africans pleasantly found that locusts did not like cassava. Peanuts were added to menus in Africa and India.[1] An English King received a rare and valuable pineapple from the West Indies in the 1600s in an effort to persuade him to rule favorably on sugar trade prices.[1] In the mid-1800s, British sailors were nicknamed Limeys because the Royal Navy found that if limes were included in their diet they would be spared the symptoms of scurvy.[2] Rhubarb was carried on the Silk Road during the 1800s.

Ancient and colonial travel and commerce stirred the "global food pot" as indigenous foods crossed land and waterways as plants and seeds. Food historians and anthropologists have worked hard to trace the history of different foods. It is estimated that 50% of the food crops eaten in the world today originated in the Americas.[3] **Table 10.1** lists the origins of several commonly cultivated fruits and vegetables.[1,4–6]

Botanical Definitions of Fruits and Vegetables

Thousands of varieties of fruits and vegetables are known to food cultures all over the world. Often what is thought to be a vegetable is really a fruit, and vice versa. This is due to the botanical definitions of these two food groups and how they are prepared and served. Consider the definitions of fruits and vegetables found in the *American Heritage Science Dictionary*:[7]

- *Fruit*: "The ripened ovary of a flowering plant that contains the seeds."
- *Vegetable*: "Part of a plant that is grown primarily for food. Thus, the leaf of spinach, the root of a carrot, the flower of broccoli, and the stalk of celery are all vegetables."

Strictly speaking then, rhubarb is really a vegetable, but it is most often thought of and served as a fruit. Conversely, cucumbers, tomatoes, squashes, avocados, and olives are really fruits by nature of their seeds and having developed from flowers but are typically served as vegetables because of their less sweet taste. (Fruits are generally regarded as being sweeter than vegetables.) Overall, what matters most is not their proper botanical category but that people include them in their diets because of their nutrient composition and contributions to good health.

TABLE 10.1
Origins of Popular Fruits and Vegetables

Food	Region of Origin
Fruits	
Apple	Caucasus
Avocado	Central America
Banana	India
Grapefruit	Indonesia
Lemon	India
Lime	India
Tomato	South America
Vegetables	
Carrot	Central Asia (Afghanistan)
Corn	Central America
Potato	South America
Sweet potato	South America
Yam	Africa
Zucchini	Europe

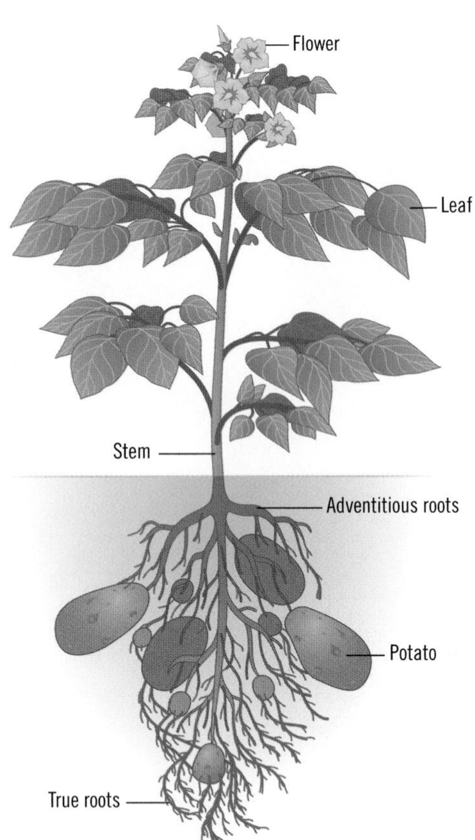

FIGURE 10.2 Plants have roots, stems, leaves, flowers, and fruits. The part of the plant that is eaten varies based on the species. For example, we eat the stems and flowers of broccoli, the fruits of tomatoes, the leaves of lettuce, and the roots of potatoes.

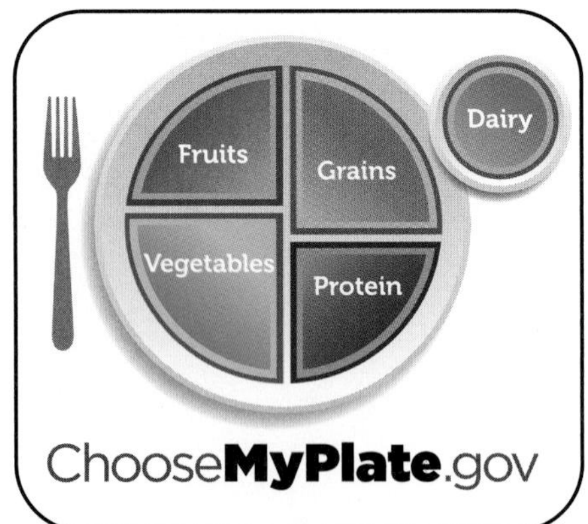

FIGURE 10.3 The U.S. Department of Agriculture developed MyPlate to help Americans make better food choices. As indicated by the MyPlate graphic, half of a person's daily intake should be fruits and vegetables. For more information on MyPlate, visit http://www.choosemyplate.gov.

Source: Courtesy of the U.S. Department of Agriculture.

Most food plants have roots, stems, leaves, flowers, and fruit, as shown in **Figure 10.2**. The parts of the plant that are eaten varies based on the species. **Table 10.2** offers examples of the various edible plant parts.[8]

Cultural Assimilation

As transportation improved, fruits and vegetables crossed oceans and continents at an expedited pace. Memories of food origins faded as the foreign foods became assimilated into various cultures. Many foods that originated in one geographic region were often studied, developed, and cultivated to thrive in another. Hardier and more flavorful varieties were bred that would yield more food per acre. Plants were bred for different soils and climates. Culinary food traits were changed and improved.

Today, many fruits and vegetables are firmly ensconced in cultural menus and have become signature culinary icons in countries where the produce did not originate. Few people today know that carrots originated in Afghanistan and were originally white and purple. The orange variety of carrots that we are familiar with today was created by the Dutch to honor William I, Prince of Orange.[1] Potatoes originated in South America, but today they are associated with Irish and French dishes. Likewise, tomatoes originated in the South American Andes but are most associated with southern Italian fare. Bananas are associated with Central America but are thought to originate from India. **Table 10.3** lists fruits and vegetables commonly associated with different food traditions.

Fruits and vegetables comprise two of the five major food groups in the U.S. Department of Agriculture's MyPlate guidelines (see **Figure 10.3**).[9] In fact, fruits and vegetables are the primary components of dietary food guidance systems all over the world, including those of Canada, Great Britain, Germany, China, Mexico, South Korea, Australia, Portugal, Sweden, Puerto Rico, and the Philippines.[10] The Food and Agriculture Organization of the United Nations maintains a substantial database of food guidance systems for six major geographic areas of the world (see http://www.fao.org/ag/humannutrition/nutritioneducation/fbdg/en). All include fruits and vegetables.[11]

A variety of resources are available to learn more about how different fruits and vegetables are used in various cuisines:

- Many foods used in different cultures and cuisines are available in U.S. supermarkets. When grocery shopping, choose an unfamiliar

TABLE 10.2
Edible Plant Parts

Part of the Plant	Examples
Roots	Beet, carrot, parsnip, radish, sweet potato, manioc
Stems, stalks, tubers, or rhizomes	Asparagus, broccoli, celery, turnip, celery root, potato, yam, ginger
Leaves	Arugula, basil, cabbage, collard greens, lettuce, spinach
Flowers	Artichoke, broccoli, cauliflower
Seeds	Beans, corn, soy
Bulbs	Garlic, onion
Fruits	Tomato, pepper, cucumber
Bark	Cinnamon

TABLE 10.3
Fruits and Vegetables Prominent in Different Cuisines

Culture	Associated Fruits and Vegetables
African	Onion, kiwano-horned melon
American	Apples, carrot, celery, corn, cranberry, onion, peach, potato fries, pumpkin, strawberry
Arabic	Kousa, eggplant, onion, cucumber, carrot, chili, spinach, tomato, banana
Asian	Baby corn, bamboo shoots, bok choy, daikon radish, lotus root, snow pea pod, soy, tofu
Caribbean	Bananas, cherimoya, coconut, mango, papaya
French	Green beans, potato
German	Cabbage, potato, sauerkraut
Greek	Apricots, figs, olives
Indian	Cauliflower, eggplant, lentil, lychee, mango
Italian	Eggplant, nuts, salad, tomato
Mediterranean	Olive, fig, apricots, tabouli, hummus
Pacific Islander	Pineapple, taro poi
Spanish	Avocado guacamole, bean, corn tortilla, plantain, tomatillo, tomato salsa

food from the "International" or "Around the World" aisle each week to experience a new flavor adventure.

- The *American Dietetic Association Complete Food and Nutrition Guide* includes a section that surveys some of the more uncommon fruit and vegetable and offers suggestions for how to prepare them. It also suggests asking a friend for a recipe, checking out a cultural cookbook from the library, dining at local ethnic restaurants, or attending a local cultural festival or cooking class.[3]
- The book *Cultural Food Practices* surveys 15 different American cultural diets, including American Indian, Alaska Native, African American, Hmong American, Asian Indian, and Korean American.[12]
- In *What I Eat: Around the World in 80 Diets*, photojournalists chronicle the calories people eat in one day from countries throughout the world. Entries are presented by the number of calories, ranging from 800 to 12,300.[13]
- *Culinarias*, or food and cooking travel tours, are available to many countries, including Italy, France, Spain, and Mexico. Oldways, a nonprofit organization that promotes healthy eating based on regional cuisines, has sponsored culinarias to Morocco, Turkey, Normandy, Italy, and China.[14]
- In the United States, local tours of ethnic neighborhoods and markets are popular in many large cities.[15]

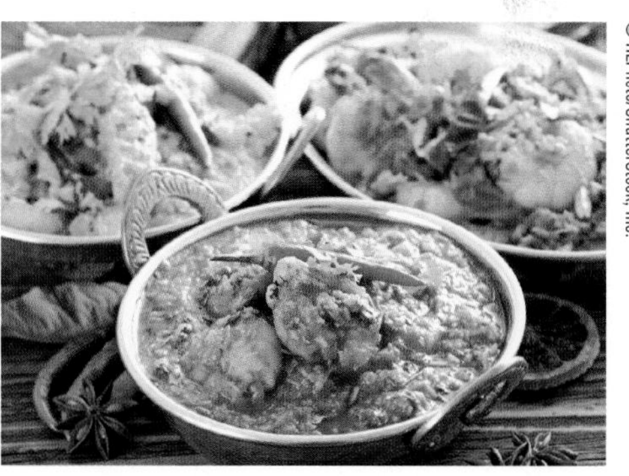
© HLPhoto/ShutterStock, Inc.

Physical and Chemical Properties

Carbohydrates comprise the bulk of the tissues of fruits and vegetables. Plants produce these carbohydrates through the reaction of water, carbon dioxide, and the sun's energy via **photosynthesis** (see **Figure 10.4**). Photosynthesis

photosynthesis Process whereby plants use sunlight, water, and carbon dioxide to create oxygen and glucose.

cytoplasm Fluid inside a plant or animal cell that contains the organelles.

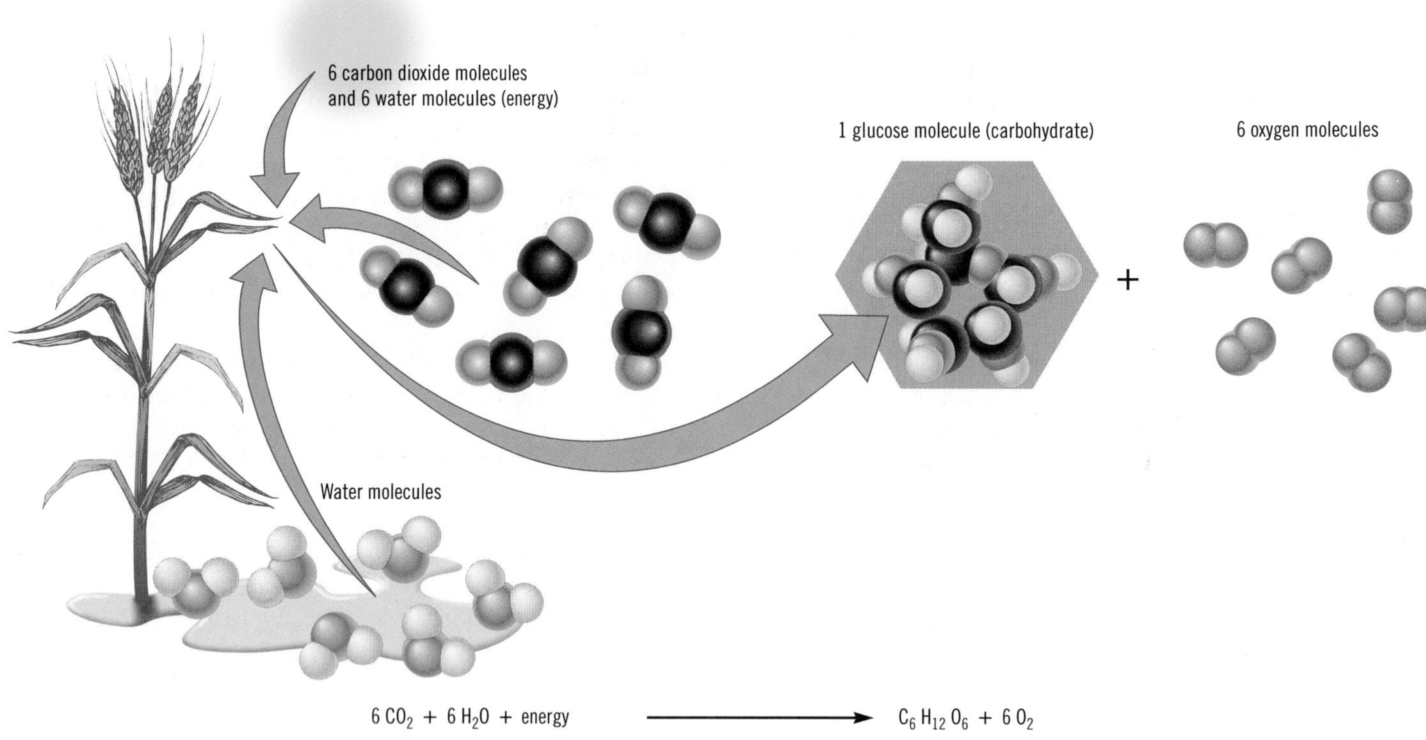

FIGURE 10.4 Photosynthesis is a process used by plants to capture the sun's energy to split off water's hydrogen from oxygen. The hydrogen then is combined with carbon dioxide (absorbed from air or water) to form glucose. Oxygen is released as a by-product.

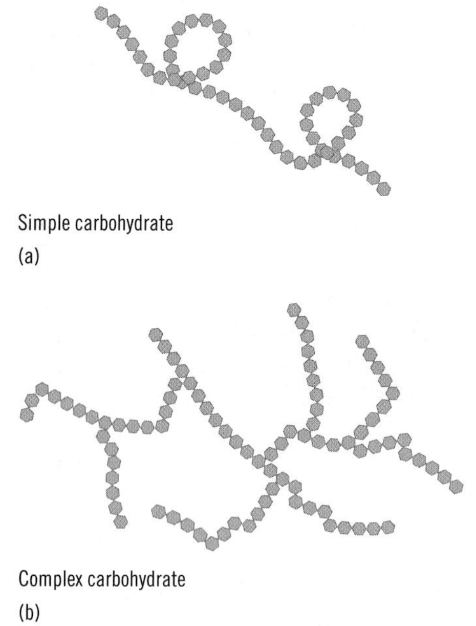

FIGURE 10.5 (a) Simple monosaccharides have a linear and unbranched carbon skeleton with one carbonyl (C=O) functional group and one hydroxyl (OH) group on each of the remaining carbon atoms. (b) Polysaccharides are long chains of monosaccharide units that are bound together by glycosidic bonds. Starch is one of the most important polysaccharides in plants. Plants store most of their energy in the form of starch.

harnesses the sun's energy to split six molecules each of water and carbon dioxide and then recombines the atoms to form glucose and oxygen:

$$\text{water} + \text{carbon dioxide} \Rightarrow \text{glucose} + \text{oxygen}$$

$$6\ H_2O + 6\ CO_2 \Rightarrow C_6H_{12}O_6 + 6\ O_2$$

Carbohydrates are composed of carbon, hydrogen, and oxygen atoms. Glucose is a simple carbohydrate and is classified as a monosaccharide. Fructose and galactose are other important monosaccharides. Various combinations of two molecules of glucose, fructose, and galactose form disaccharides. Complex carbohydrates (polysaccharides) contain many sugar molecules in long, branched chains. The structure of simple and complex carbohydrates is compared in **Figure 10.5**.

Because simple carbohydrates have short, single-branched chains, they are easier to digest than complex carbohydrates. Plants use complex carbohydrates for storage and structure. For example, the fiber found in many plant tissues and organs is a complex carbohydrate that adds rigidity. Plant fiber is either soluble or insoluble in water. Insoluble fiber is not digested well, but it adds bulk to stool. In recent years, insoluble fiber has been marketed as a prebiotic to aid bowel regularity and promote growth of "good" digestive bacteria.[16]

Plant Cell Structure

Unlike animal cells, plant cells have strong cell walls made of cellulose. The cells are lined by a lipid–protein membrane that is permeable to water. **Figure 10.6** shows the organelles and other components that float in the fluid—the **cytoplasm**—inside the cell.

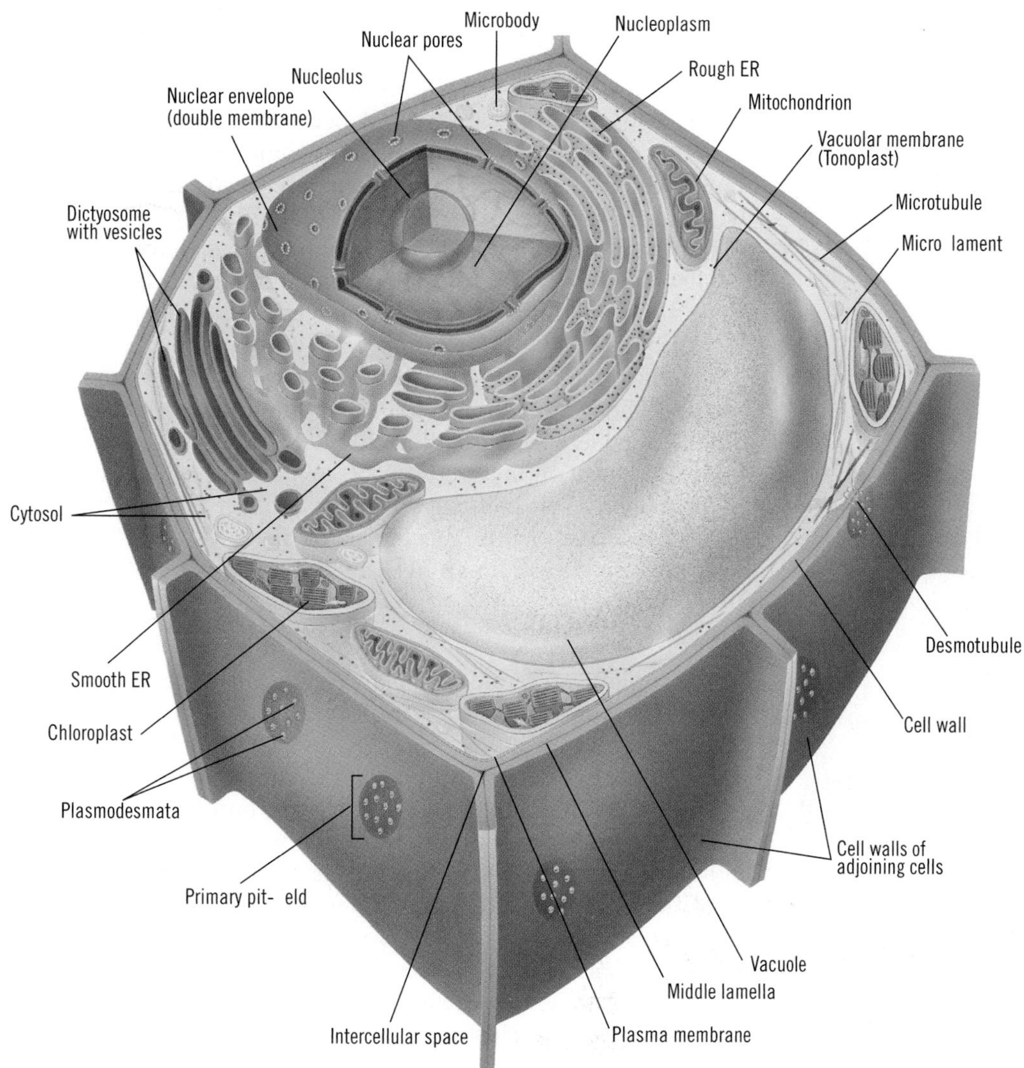

FIGURE 10.6 Unlike animal cells, plants have cell walls composed of cellulose and protein. Inside the plant cell are various organelles, including the chloroplast, which is where photosynthesis takes place.

The **vacuole** is the largest structure in most plant cells; it can contain a mixture of sugars, enzymes, pigments, and other compounds that contribute to a food's flavor. The vacuoles may also contain **phenolic compounds**, which are thought to play a role in defending the plant against predators. An important group of phenolic compounds is flavonoids, which are thought to confer positive health benefits. When filled with fluid, the vacuole can get so big that the plant cell nucleus is squished to one side.

Elongated **chloroplasts**, which are the site of photosynthesis in the plant, contain chlorophyll, the light-harvesting pigment in photosynthesis. The cells in the plant's leaves are arranged so there is space between the cells so they can easily obtain the carbon dioxide gas required for photosynthesis.[8] Leaves, which are usually long, flat, thin structures, have evolved to maximize a plant's light-gathering, photosynthetic capacity.

In animals, the storage form of glucose is glycogen; in plants, it is starch. In animals, glycogen is stored in liver and muscle tissue. In plants, the starch produced during photosynthesis is stored in the chloroplasts and in structures called **amyloplasts**.[17] Plants also have proteins in their cell walls; the enzymes used to facilitate the various chemical reactions in plants are also proteins.[18]

vacuole The largest structure in the plant cell; it holds a mixture of sugars, enzymes, pigments, and other compounds that contribute to a food's flavor.

phenolic compounds Substances that affect the taste, aroma, mouthfeel and nutrient content of the fruits and vegetables that contain them.

chloroplasts Organelles in plant cells where photosynthesis takes place; contains the green pigment chlorophyll.

amyloplast An organelle in some plant cells that stores starch; commonly found in starchy plants such as tubers and fruits.

chromoplasts Plant cell organelles that contain colored compounds other than chlorophyll.

carotenoids Plant compounds known for their yellow-orange color and antioxidant properties.

In addition to the chlorophyll required for photosynthesis, plants produce many other pigments. The plant pigments in **chromoplasts** are responsible for the colors of fruits and flowers. Important classes of plant pigments are **carotenoids**, anthocyanins, and betalains. **Table 10.4** lists some of the colors of various phytochemicals and some examples of where they can be found. Many of these plant pigments are *phytochemicals* or *phytonutrients*, which are chemicals that may have biological significance with regards to human health. More than 4,000 phytonutrients have been identified, many of which have proven health benefits relating to antioxidant functions, cancer prevention, inflammation inhibition, cardiovascular health, and eye health. For example, the dark greens and oranges found in vegetables such as spinach and sweet potatoes are due to phytonutrients that confer important health benefits. The Produce for Better Health Foundation, in partnership with the U.S. Department of Agriculture (USDA), maintains an extensive interactive online database of phytonutrients (see http://pbhfoundation.org/about/res/pic/phytolist).[19] In contrast to natural sources of color additives, artificial coloring added to fruits, vegetables, or other food products may actually be disadvantageous to human health (see **Special Topic 10.1**).

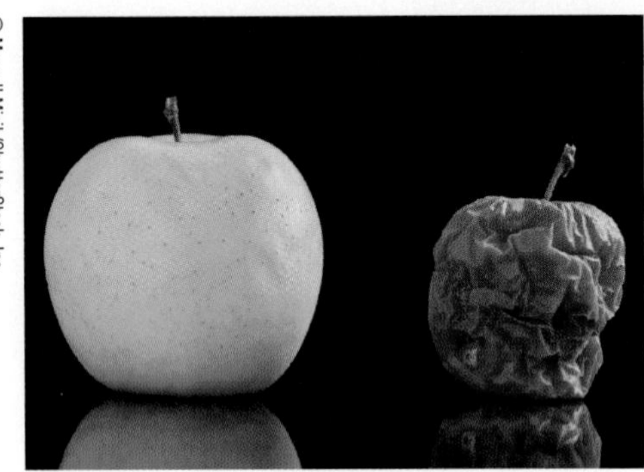

FIGURE 10.7 (left) In a ripe fruit, the cell walls are rigid because they are full of moisture. (right) As the fruit passes its peak, water evaporates from the cell walls, resulting in the breakdown of the cell wall structure.

Ripening and Aging

Microscopic examination of plant cell walls of fruits shows rigid, fibrous strands of compact glucose molecules, called cellulose, intertwined with other less rigid forms of fiber, such as pectin or hemicellulose as well as a water bath of minerals and proteins. As long as the cell wall is vibrant and strong, the hydrous material stays in place and the fruit is plump. As the cell wall loses moisture to evaporation, the wall structure begins to collapse, as shown in **Figure 10.7**. The grainy texture of an aging apple is due to the evaporation of moisture from between the cell walls. The mushy, soft texture of aging cantaloupe or watermelon is caused by cell walls that have begun to disintegrate, allowing the intercellular fluid to easily escape.

The cells of some vegetables, such as potatoes, have a dryer vacuole and a more compact starch structure. When potato cell walls age and break down, the potato becomes granular with escaped starch molecules. Starch absorbs water, so if old potatoes are cooked they become glue-like because the cell walls are no longer able to hold moisture inside the cell.

Structural changes to the cell wall are also responsible for other texture changes that occur during ripening:

- Pectin is lost as enzymes alter the cell walls, which causes the cell walls to break down. This contributes to the mushy texture of overripe fruit.

TABLE 10.4
Phytochemicals in Produce

Phytochemical	Color	Plants Containing
Carotenoids	Orange, yellow, red	Apricot, butternut squash, cantaloupe, carrot, collard, kale, pumpkin, spinach, sweet potato
Anthocyanins	Red, blue, purple	Radish, potato, tomato, apple, raspberries, blackberries, blueberries, red cabbage
Anthoxanthins	Pale yellow to nearly colorless	Cauliflower, onion, potato
Betains	Red, yellow	Beet, chard, cactus pear

Sources: Data from McGee H. *On Food and Cooking: The Science and Lore of the Kitchen.* New York: Scribner; 2004:266–269; and U.S. Department of Agriculture. USDA National Nutrient Database for Standard Reference, Release 20. Available at: http://www.ars.usda.gov/Main/docs.htm?docid=15869. Accessed July 27, 2011.

Special Topic 10.1

Natural and Artificial Food Coloring

Lauren Mudgett

For thousands of years, many different cultures all over the world have used and still use food coloring to enhance the color of certain foods. The ancient Romans and Egyptians used natural food colorings from vegetable and mineral sources, such as paprika, turmeric, saffron, and copper sulfate. William Henry Perkin discovered the first synthetic organic dye, called mauve, in 1856. Following this discovery, many more dyes and colorings were discovered, and they rapidly came to be used in foods, drugs, and cosmetics to make these products more appetizing or appealing. Artificial food coloring started to become popular in the 1900s when it was first used in butter and cheese.

Throughout the years, the federal government has passed a variety of laws and guidelines regarding artificial food coloring, including the prohibition of the "use of poisonous or deleterious colors in confectionery and the coloring or staining of food to conceal damage or inferiority."[1] The FDA maintains a list of safe and harmless food dyes that can legally be used and sold.

Natural food colorings are derived from fruits, vegetables, other plant organs, and spices, but they are not as common as artificial food colorings. However, there are many natural ways to get similar colors as one would with artificial dye. For example, caramelized sugar can produce a brown color; many cola products contain caramelized sugar. Another common and vibrant natural food color is betanin, which is extracted from beets. Boiled red cabbage leaves can produce a beautiful blue color. Natural food coloring runs a very low risk of being toxic or hazardous.[2]

Artificial food coloring comes in many different hues and is used in a huge number products and foods. Currently, seven artificial dyes are approved for use by the FDA: Blue E133, Indigotine E132, Fast Green E143, Allura Red E129, Erythrosine E127, Tartazin E102, and Sunset Yellow E110. Artificial food dyes are most commonly found in candy, cereals, and baked goods. Artificial food colorings have recently been scrutinized for being possibly linked to cancer, hyperactivity, and allergies.[3,4]

Consumers need to be aware of the possible health risks and concerns regarding artificial food coloring. Children, especially, have a greater risk of adverse effects from artificial food colorings because their bodies are still growing and developing; artificial food dyes can have a greater effect on them, even when consumed in small amounts. The European Food Safety Authority has added warning labels to foods containing artificial food dyes; however, as of 2011 the FDA does not require any warning labels.

Natural and artificial food colorings have been used for years to make foods more appealing and enticing. They guarantee a more colorful food product that catches consumers' eyes. Both natural and artificial food dyes are being closely studied, regulated, and monitored regarding their potential safety and health hazards. Consumers should be aware of what they are eating and consume artificially colored products in moderation.

References

1 U.S. Food and Drug Administration. Food Ingredients and Colors. 2009. Available at: http://www.fda.gov/food/foodingredientspackaging/ucm094211.htm. Accessed December 8, 2011.

2 Beil L. The color of controversy. Science News. 2011;180(5):22–25.

3 U.S. Food and Drug Administration. Summary of Color Additives for Use in the United States in Foods, Drugs, Cosmetics, and Medical Devices. 2007. Available at: http://www.fda.gov/forindustry/coloradditives/coloradditiveinventories/ucm115641.htm. Accessed December 8, 2011.

4 U.S. Food and Drug Administration. Color Additives: FDA's Regulatory Process and Historical Perspectives. 2007. Available at: http://www.fda.gov/ForIndustry/ColorAdditives/RegulatoryProcessHistoricalPerspectives/default.htm. Accessed December 8, 2011.

- Glucose molecules that were stored as starch are converted back to sugar, making the fruit more and more sweet. Bananas, grapes, and pears ripen this way.
- Other fruits and vegetables stop ripening when picked, and their sugars combine to make more complex starches. If broccoli or asparagus is permitted to grow for too long, the stalk will actually become woodier as more complex cellulose strands (lignin) form.[8]

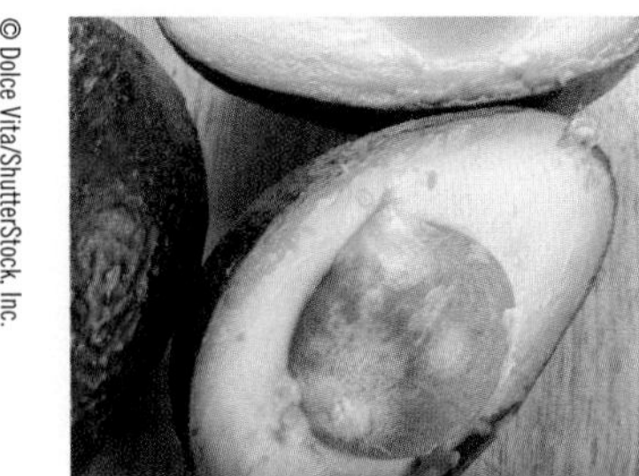
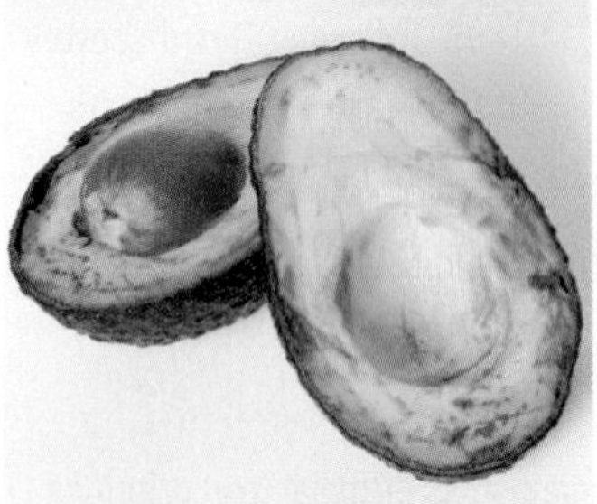

FIGURE 10.8 Why does guacamole turn brown? Avocados are sensitive to enzymatic browning. When the avocado is sliced, enzymes from the cell cytoplasm and phenols from the vacuole react with oxygen. This oxidation reaction results in browning of the fruit. Enzymatic browning can be slowed by adding lemon juice to a fruit. Lemon juice is an antioxidant that reduces the speed of oxidation. It also is acidic, which decreases the pH of the surface of the fruit, making it more difficult for the oxidation reaction to occur.

Enzymatic Browning

After being cut open, some produce turns brown as the cells inside the plant are exposed to oxygen in the air. This is true of apples, quinces, bananas, pears, potatoes, and avocados (see **Figure 10.8**). Enzymatic browning is caused by reactions involving the plant enzymes in the cytoplasm, phenolic compounds in the vacuole, and oxygen in the air. Phenols are defensive chemicals that plants have evolved that are effective in fending off predators. In nature, if the plant were attacked by microbes or insects, the phenols released from the vacuole would damage the invader's enzymes and cell membranes.[8]

A quick way to stop enzymatic browning is to plunge freshly cut raw produce into water, limiting its contact with oxygen. Another way to prevent oxidation is to coat the cut surfaces with an antioxidant. Vitamin C is an antioxidant, thus mixing a food with lemon, lime, or orange juice will also prevent the food from turning brown. Chilling the food to below 40°F (4.4°C) will also slow the browning process.[8]

Boiling or Steaming

During cooking, especially boiling, insoluble cellulose strands remain intact, but the other cell wall materials soften or dissolve into the water. This weakens the cell walls and tenderizes the vegetable or fruit. Air also escapes when the cell wall structure is weakened during cooking (especially from leaf cells, which are about 70% air). This results in wilted leaves, such as with cooked spinach or greens.[8] (Fortunately, most fruits do not need to be cooked before being eaten, which is best for color, texture, and nutrient preservation.)

When a green vegetable such as green beans or broccoli are first plunged into boiling water or steamed, their color intensifies into a rich hue (see **Figure 10.9**). This is caused by gases escaping from between the cell walls and water then seeping into those spaces. The water acts as a refracting mirror, reflecting the vegetable's green color, just as a diamond's facets sparkle in reflected light.[20]

Because the composition of the hundreds of fruits and vegetables available varies, there is no one perfect cooking method or cooking time. Besides weakening plant cell walls, long cooking times leach plant enzymes from the cell. Hydrogen ions replace magnesium ions in the chlorophyll, which allows chlorophyll to absorb a broader range of light wavelengths. This results in the vegetable taking on a drab olive-brown color because green light is now absorbed by the vegetable rather than being reflected.[20] Carrots do not lose their color when boiled because the carotenoids that give carrots their orange color are not water soluble. Lycopene, the red color in tomatoes and red peppers, is a carotenoid; it also does not readily change color.[19,20]

(a)
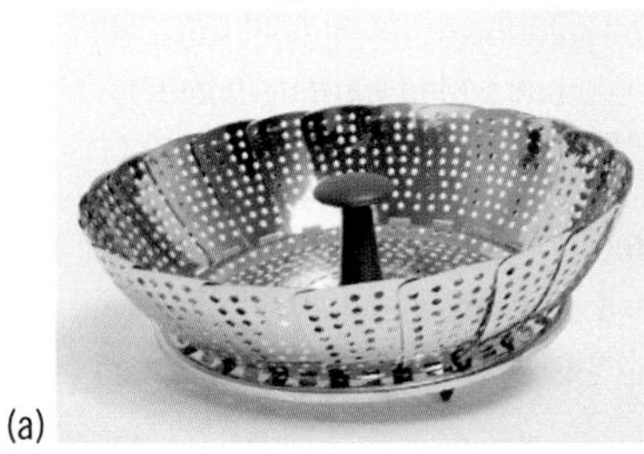

(b)
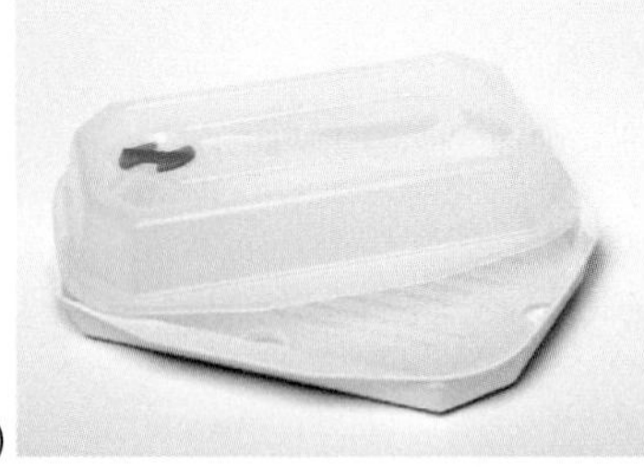

FIGURE 10.9 (a) Steaming is a great way to prepare vegetables. When steaming on the stovetop, use a steaming basket inside a pot. Fill the pot with enough water so is just barely reaches the bottom of basket. Bring the water to a boil, and then add the vegetables to the basket, placing a loose fitting lid on top so steam can escape. (b) To steam vegetables in the microwave, use a microwave steaming tray with a small amount of water in the bottom. You can also put the vegetables in a microwave-safe bowl, add a small amount of water, and cover the bowl with microwave safe plastic wrap, leaving one corner open to vent.

Acid–Base Chemistry

Changes in acidity during food preparation also can affect the color of food. Acids, such as citrus juice, vinegar, or wine, turn chlorophyll olive-brown (see **Figure 10.10**) but have no effect on flavonoids, such as anthocyanins. When acids are added, vegetables will require longer cooking times.[21] Conversely, bases, such as baking soda, cause flavonoids to lose their color but do but not affect chlorophyll. Unfortunately, bases can make vegetables mushy.

Freezing

Freezing is a wonderful way to preserve fruits and vegetables for use at a later time. Freezing stops the ripening or rotting process, but the spoilage microbes will begin their work anew when the food is thawed. When frozen, the cellular fluids turn to ice crystals, which then puncture the cell walls when thawed. Thawing produce often results in a puddle of liquid—this is the cell fluid that has escaped through the broken cell walls.

Some cell enzymes that affect a plant's color and vitamin content do not stop reacting when frozen. This causes a buildup of enzymes that may negatively affect the taste and texture of the produce. To guard against this, a vegetable can be boiled for 1 to 2 minutes and then plunged into cold water. This process, called **blanching**, stops the cooking process and destroys the active enzymes.

Fruits do not tolerate blanching well. Instead, they but can be packed in a sugar syrup solution of 1.5 pounds of sugar per quart of water. This will improve the texture of the cell wall structure during freezing. Berries freeze quite nicely without a sugar bath but should be cooked directly from their frozen state to prevent color from seeping into the batter or dish.[21]

Both fruits and vegetables should be packed in air- and water-tight containers. If produce is left uncovered in cold air, the cells will lose moisture, causing **freezer burn** that will impair its taste and texture.[8] Commercially, berries and fruit slices are individually quick frozen (IQF) with blasts of cold air. This reduces the size of the ice crystals that form in the plant cells, which results in less cell damage when the fruit is thawed.[21]

Canning

Canning is another method of preservation. During canning, fruits or vegetables are cooked in a liquid to kill microbes and destroy enzymes, packed into an airtight can or jar, and then placed in a pressure cooker bath to further ensure food safety. Most microbes are killed by the combination of high temperature and an anoxic environment. However, *Clostridium botulinum* is not killed by high temperatures, and it thrives in low-oxygen, low-acid environments. Boiling may destroy the bacteria, but the spores are hardy.[1] *C. botulinum* produces a deadly toxin that can cause botulism in humans. If present, *C. botulinum* bacteria expel gases that cause the cans to bulge. Therefore, cans with bulging or seeping tops should be discarded immediately to avoid the risk of botulism.

Drying

Drying is an ancient form of food preservation. Grapes, apples, apricots, pineapple, bananas, mangos, plums, dates, figs, and tomatoes are still dried today. Dried produce retains 16–26% of its moisture. Some types of produce may brown in the drying process; these typically have sulfur dioxide added to prevent browning.[21] Fruit leathers are popular with children but discouraged by dentists because they stick to teeth and cause dental caries. Dried produce should be stored in an airtight container.

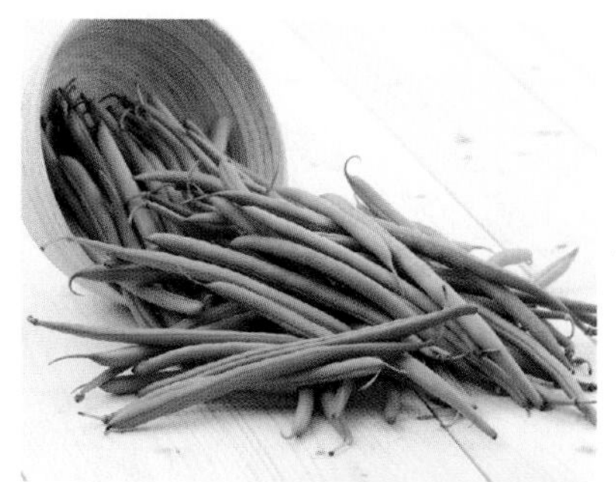

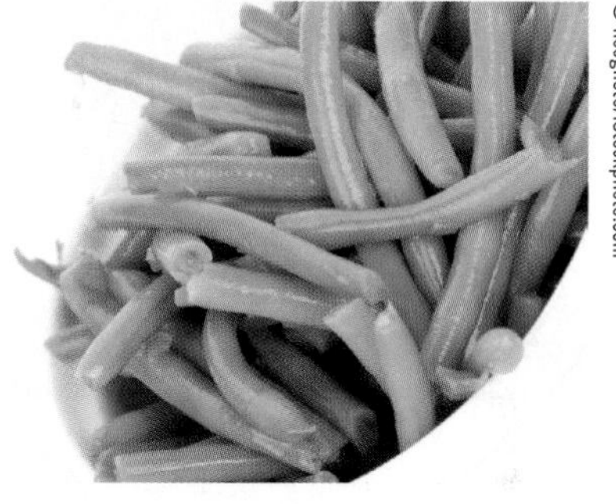

FIGURE 10.10 Some vegetables, including green beans, turn brown (bottom) when citrus juice is added because the acidity of the citrus juice causes chlorophyll to turn olive-brown.

Gastronomy Point

Steaming Vegetables To retain nutrients and color when cooking vegetables, place a steam basket into a cooking pot and add water to a level that does not reach the vegetables. Steam until slightly crisp. With a slotted spoon or tongs, immediately transfer the vegetables to a bowl of cold water to stop the cooking and to retain their bright color. With steaming, the plants enzymes do not exchange ions with the water. The food's bright color is thus preserved as well as its nutrient content.

Gastronomy Point

Frozen Blueberries Add prewashed, frozen blueberries directly to pancakes or muffin batter to prevent crystals in the fruit cells from puncturing and leaking purple fluid into the batter.

blanching Cooking produce for 1 to 2 minutes and then plunging into cold water to destroy plant enzymes that can affect color and flavor.

freezer burn Shriveled cells on food that have lost too much moisture due to sublimation.

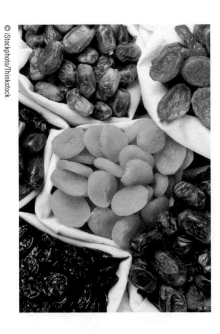
© iStockphoto/Thinkstock

Nutritional Properties

The nutritional quality of fruits and vegetables depends on the nutrient content of the soil in which they are grown. Except for nuts and legumes, fruits and vegetables tend to be low in protein and fat but high in carbohydrates. Fruits and vegetables contain fiber, starch, sugars, proteins, vitamins, minerals, water, and any combination of thousands of phytochemicals.

Carbohydrates and Fiber

Carbohydrates supply 4 calories of energy per gram. A typical piece or one-half cup of fruit provides about 50 calories from carbohydrates. Vegetables provide about 25 calories per one-half cup; starchy vegetables such as corn and potatoes provide approximately 75 calories per cup.[22]

Unlike whole grains, most fruit and vegetable fiber is of the soluble form, which binds with cholesterol that is then eliminated in the stool.[23] Pectin is a type of soluble fiber found in fruit that is used in making jams and jellies. Cellulose and lignin fibers are insoluble fibers, found in the edible skins of certain produce and in celery stalks.

Proteins and Fats

The protein content of fruit is very low. Similarly, a half-cup of most vegetables contributes only about 2 grams of protein.[22] Fruits and vegetables are low in fat when served without added sauces or oils, making them excellent choices for low-calorie snacks and meals.

Vitamins, Minerals, and Water

Table 10.5 lists some of the major vitamin and mineral nutrients that plant foods provide. Fruits and vegetables are generally high in vitamin A, vitamin C, folate, and potassium.[24] Some vegetables, such as collard greens, kale, okra, spinach, and beet greens, are also good sources of calcium, which is important for people who are lactose intolerant and unable to digest dairy products.[25]

Fruits and vegetables average about 80–90% water.[21] Melons, citrus fruits, greens, and tomatoes have a very high water content. Because it contains so much water, produce is generally very low in calories and fat. Its high water content also influences how it should be stored, served, and cooked.

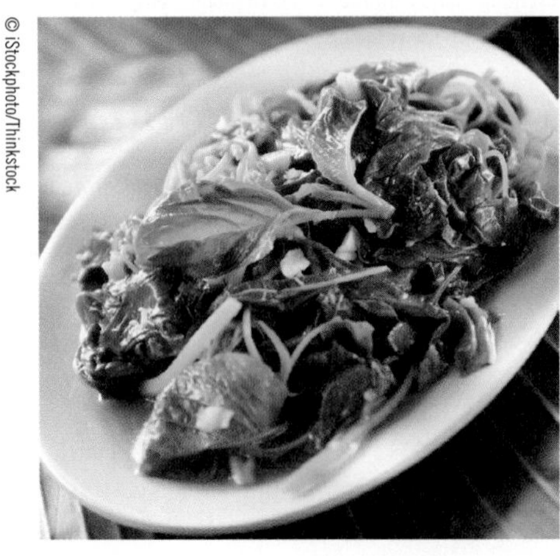
© iStockphoto/Thinkstock

Impact on Human Health

Humans have been consuming fruits and vegetables for tens of thousands of years, even though the secrets of their benefits to human health have not always been known. Many of the health benefits of fruits and vegetables were unknown until the twentieth century. For example, vitamins were not even discovered until the 1930s. Today, we know that vitamin C prevents scurvy, vitamin A prevents nightblindness, folate can prevent neural tube defects in infants, and that potassium is necessary for heart and muscle contractions and can help lower blood pressure. All of these vitamins and minerals are found in plants.

Current Areas of Research

Much current research is focused on how to get people to eat more fruits and vegetables as a disease-prevention measure. With few exceptions, such as olives and avocados, fruits and vegetables are low-calorie foods that can quell hunger and provide significant nutrients without contributing excess calories. Getting the public to eat more fruits and vegetables is seen as part

TABLE 10.5
Fruit and Vegetable Sources of Different Vitamins and Minerals

Vitamin or Mineral	Good Food Sources
Vitamin A (carotenoids)	• Bright orange vegetables, such as carrots, sweet potatoes, and pumpkins • Tomatoes and tomato products • Red sweet peppers • Leafy greens, including spinach, collard greens, turnip greens, kale, beet greens, mustard greens, green leaf lettuce, and romaine lettuce • Orange fruits, including mangos, cantaloupes, apricots, and red or pink grapefruits
Vitamin C	• Citrus fruits and juices, kiwifruit, strawberries, guava, papaya, and cantaloupe • Broccoli, peppers, tomatoes, cabbage (especially Chinese cabbage), Brussels sprouts, and potatoes • Leafy greens, such as romaine, turnip greens, and spinach
Folate	• Cooked dry beans and peas • Oranges and orange juice • Deep green leafy greens, such as spinach and mustard greens
Potassium	• Baked white or sweet potatoes, cooked greens (such as spinach), winter (orange) squash • Bananas, plantains, many dried fruits, oranges and orange juice, cantaloupe, and honeydew melons • Cooked dry beans • Soybeans (green and mature) • Tomato products (sauce, paste, puree) • Beet greens

Source: Reproduced from *Dietary Guidelines for Americans, 2005*. 6th ed. U.S. Government Printing Office; January 2005. Courtesy of U.S. Department of Agriculture and U.S. Department of Health and Human Services.

of the answer to solving the American obesity problem and also preventing heart disease and some cancers.[24]

Getting children to eat sufficient fruits and vegetables is a frequent concern of parents. A recent study concluded that "parents and caregivers should be encouraged to expose young children to a wide variety of fruits and vegetables," among other measures, to provide a nutrient-dense, calorie-controlled diet. An analysis of Feeding Infants and Toddlers Study (FITS) data for 2008 showed that of the more than 1,400 participants, approximately 70% ate at least one vegetable a day and 87% ate at least one serving of fruit a day. The most popular vegetables were potatoes, followed by green beans, corn, and broccoli. Favored fruits included apples, bananas, grapes, strawberries, and applesauce.[26]

Since 1999 public health studies managed by the CDC have examined diet and nutrition habits, among other health parameters, of 5,000 participants in all age groups, across the country each year. These studies are called the National Health and Nutrition Examination Studies, or NHANES.[27] The data are then made available to scientists to help them better understand dietary patterns and set guidelines for fruit and vegetable consumption. For example, a regression study of 2008 NHANES data on snacking trends in adolescents revealed that snacking promoted fruit consumption, which had a positive impact on vitamin C intake.[28]

Gastronomy Point

Past Their Prime Some fruits and vegetables that are slightly past their prime can still be used in cooking soups, sauces, or sautéed dishes or baked into breads. For example, banana bread is best when overripe bananas are used.

Phytonutrients

Much research is focused on discovering and documenting the phytonutrient content of different fruits and vegetables. The different brightly colored pigments of phytonutrients in fruits and vegetables is a primary reason that dietitians recommend "eating the rainbow." Thousands of phytonutrients have been identified.[29] Phytonutrients have special properties that give the produce containing them their particular smell and taste in addition to providing human health benefits through their antioxidant and anti-inflammatory properties.[30,31] As inflammation inhibitors, phytonutrients may protect against some cancers, nerve damage, and heart disease.[32] For example, the following foods may reduce the risk of cancer: broccoli, tomatoes, garlic, onions, soybeans, grapes, strawberries, raspberries, oranges, and lemons.[33]

Carotenoids, flavonoids, and a few other phytochemicals are found predominantly in fruits and vegetables. Carotenoids give foods their yellow, red, and purple color. Cooking foods with carotenoids enhances their phytonutrient content. One type of carotenoid, **lycopene**, is found in tomatoes, watermelon, pink grapefruit, and red peppers. Much has been written in recent years about lycopene's antioxidant properties and its positive effect in reducing the risk of prostate cancer.[19]

lycopene Bright red compound found in tomatoes and some other red fruits and vegetables.

resveratrol A strong antioxidant and anti-inflammatory compound found in red wine, grape juice, and peanuts.

Another phytonutrient, **resveratrol**, is found in red wine, grape juice, and peanuts. It is a strong antioxidant with anti-inflammatory properties that may help prevent heart disease and cancer.[19] Read more about resveratrol in **Special Topic 10.2**.

Special Topic 10.2

Resveratrol

Christina Molinski, MS, RD

Resveratrol is a compound synthesized by some species of plants during times of stress, particularly when exposed to ultraviolet (UV) radiation.[1,2] Resveratrol has been found in over 70 plant species, including grapes, peanuts, berries, and eucalyptus.[1,2] Its concentration has been found to be highest in *Vitis vinifera*, *V. labrusca*, and *V. muscadine* grapes and red wine.[3] In grape skin, it is produced in quantities of up to 50–100 μg per gram, which is approximately 5–10% of the grape's biomass.[2,4] After grapes are fermented into wine, the amount of resveratrol available is about 0.5 mg/L in white wine and 7 mg/L in red.[5] Resveratrol was first isolated in 1940 from *Veratrum grandiflorum O. Loes*, commonly known as white hellebore. In 1963, it was extracted from *Polygonum cuspidatum*, a plant used in traditional Japanese and Chinese medicine.[6]

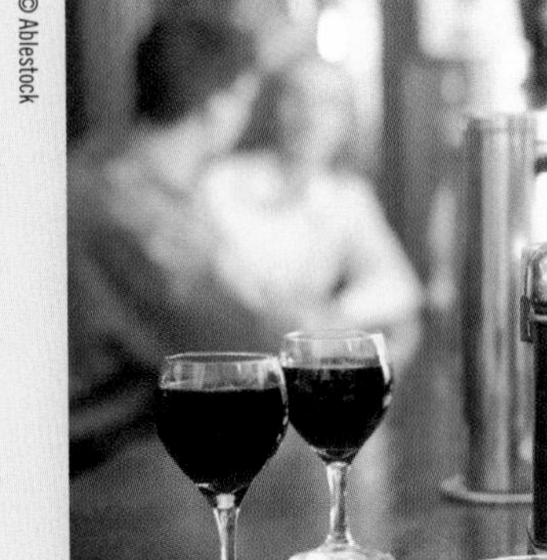

Resveratrol is found in red wine, which is why some say red wine is good for the heart.

Resveratrol was not of much interest again until 1992, when researchers began to examine its wide ranging potential health benefits.[2] It has been described as having antioxidant, antibiotic, anti-inflammatory, antitumor, cardioprotective, and anti-aging properties.[1–12] It has even been linked to the "French paradox"—the fact that the French consume a diet high in saturated fat yet have a low risk for heart disease. This has been attributed to their moderate consumption of red wine and the resveratrol found in it.[11,12] Resveratrol also has become a popular supplement, mostly due to claims of its anti-aging benefits.

One particularly well-studied application of resveratrol is its potential as a cancer deterrent. It has been found to work at three stages of tumor development: the initiation phase, the promotion phase, and the progression phase, leading to decreased cell growth and increased apoptosis (i.e., programmed cell death) in certain cancer cell lines, such as those associated with colon cancer, uterine cancer, and lymphoblastic leukemia.[1,9] Because resveratrol is synthesized by plants exposed to UV radiation, it is now being studied with regards to skin cancer.

One caveat about resveratrol is that its potential for toxicity requires further study. Although chronic consumption of low doses seems to have no harmful effects, larger doses may be lethal.[8] It is thought that it may be toxic at when amounts greater than 1 g/kg of body weight are consumed.[6]

References

1 Delmas D, Lançon A, Colin D, et al. Resveratrol as a chemopreventive agent: A promising molecule for fighting cancer. *Curr Drug Targets.* 2006 April;7(4):423–442.

2 Labinsky N, Csiszar A, Veress G, et al. Vascular dysfunction in aging: Potential effects of resveratrol, an anti-inflammatory phytoestrogen. *Curr Med Chem.* 2006;13(9):989–996.

3 Das S, Das D. Anti-inflammatory responses of resveratrol. *Inflamm Allergy Drug Targets.* 2007 Sept;6(3):168–173.

4 Rocha-González H, Ambriz-Tututi M, Granados-Soto V. Resveratrol: A natural compound with pharmacological potential in neurodegenerative diseases. *CNS Neurosci Therapeutics.* 2008 Fall;14(3):234–247.

5 Raval A, Lin H, Dave K, et al. Resveratrol and ischemic preconditioning in the brain. *Curr Med Chem.* 2008;15(15):1545–1551.

6 Baur J, Sinclair D. Therapeutic potential of resveratrol: The in vivo evidence. *Nat Rev Drug Discov.* 2006 June;5(6):493–506.

7 Baxter R. Anti-aging properties of resveratrol: Review and report of a potent new antioxidant skin care formulation. *J Cosmetic Dermatol.* 2008 Mar;7(1):2–7.

8 Knutson M, Leeuwenburgh C. Resveratrol and novel potent activators of SIRT1: Effects on aging and age-related diseases. *Nutri Rev.* 2008 Oct;66(10):591–596.

9 Pirola L, Fröjdö S. Resveratrol: One molecule, many targets. *IUBMB Life.* 2008 May;60(5):323–332.

10 Reagan-Shaw S, Mukhtar H, Ahmad N. Resveratrol imparts photoprotection of normal cells and enhances the efficacy of radiation therapy in cancer cells. *Photochem Photobiol.* 2008 Mar;84(2):415–421.

11 Shen M, Hsiao G, Liu C, et al. Inhibitory mechanisms of resveratrol in platelet activation: Pivotal roles of p38 MAPK and NO/cyclic GMP. *Br J Haematol.* 2007 Nov;139(3):475–485.

12 Udenigwe C, Ramprasath V, Aluko R, Jones P. Potential of resveratrol in anticancer and anti-inflammatory therapy. *Nutri Rev.* 2008 Aug;66(8):445–454.

The first issue of *Food and Function*, a journal of the British Royal Society of Chemistry, was published in 2010 in response to the new frontier of phytonutrient research; this journal focuses on food chemistry and physics and their effect on nutrition and health.[34] One of the first studies published examined the antioxidant content of 36 European fruit juices, identifying vitamin C as the major antioxidant in some of the juices and ellagitannins as the primary antioxidants in pomegranate juice.[32] Other researchers corroborated these finding in a study of the antioxidant properties of multiple juices using four different tests. Pomegranate juice was found to have the highest antioxidant potency.[35] More recent research has focused on fiber and its relationship to colon cancer prevention. Phytochemicals will be a focus of study for many years to come, as research continues on the learning about the benefits of known antioxidants and their effect on neutralizing free radicals and preventing age-related macular degeneration.

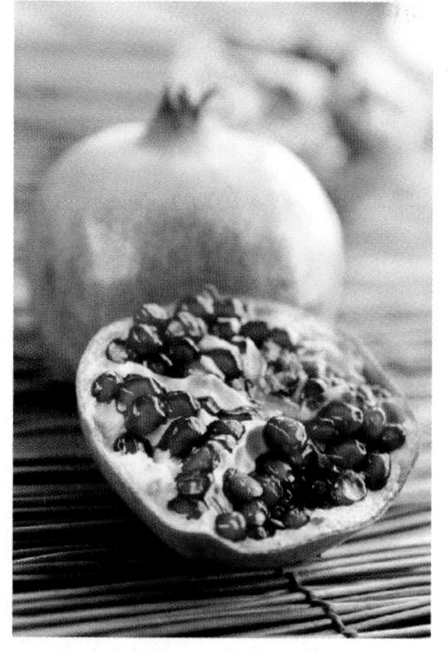

Menu Planning and Food Selection

The *Dietary Guidelines for Americans* and MyPlate

The USDA's MyPlate graphic is based on the *Dietary Guidelines for Americans*.[9,36] The *Dietary Guidelines for Americans* are reviewed and updated every 5 years. From 1995 to 2005, the USDA promoted a "Five a Day" campaign to simplify the fruit and vegetables message for adults and children. Although easy enough to remember, it was not an individualized message. In 2007, the public recommendations began using cup-size servings for fruits and vegetables.

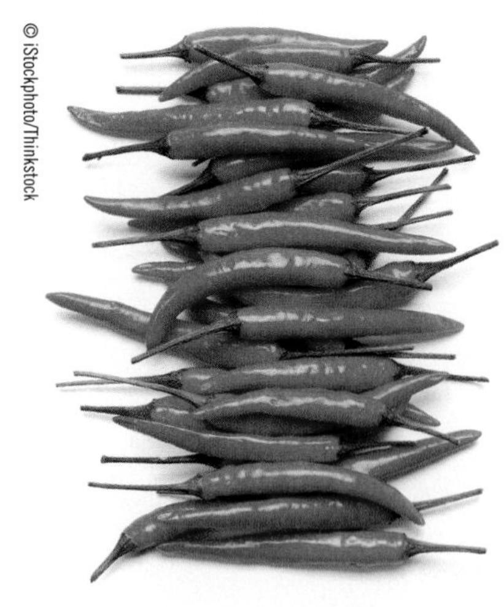

Phytonutrient Point

Capsaicin Content of Chili Peppers Capsaicin, a chemical found in chili peppers, has been found to affect both pain relief and obesity. Capsaicin has been shown to have a 50-calorie per day thermogenic (heat) effect on the resting metabolic rate. When incorporated into a cream, it has been proven to be an effective topical pain blocker on soft tissue.

Putting together a healthy menu is a daunting task to some, but the *Dietary Guidelines for Americans* and MyPlate aim to make the process as simple as possible. The most recent version of the *Dietary Guidelines for Americans*, released in 2010, offers the following suggestions:[36]

- Fruits and vegetables should be part of everyone's daily meal plan.
- As a general guide, plates should be half fruits and vegetables. A person requiring a 2,000-calorie diet should eat 2 cups of fruit and 2.5 cups of vegetables per day (see **Figure 10.11**).
- Dark green or orange-colored produce, legumes, and starchy vegetables should be consumed several times a week. They should be rich in fiber and potassium and prepared with minimal sugar and sodium.

Registered dietitians also can recommend or help design family meal plans. To find a registered dietitian, visit http://www.eatright.org and click "Find a Registered Dietitian."

Purchasing Produce

Most people buy fruits and vegetables at local groceries, farmers' markets, and supermarkets. Some people are lucky enough to grow their own! In communities where grocery stores are a rarity, traveling farmers' markets may provide an option to obtain fresh fruits and vegetables—**Special Topic 10.3** discusses such "farm-to-plate" programs in more detail.

Shopping from a list based on a week's worth of menu ideas can help in budgeting for produce and reducing waste. Leftover produce can be added to salads, sandwiches, soups, and sauces.

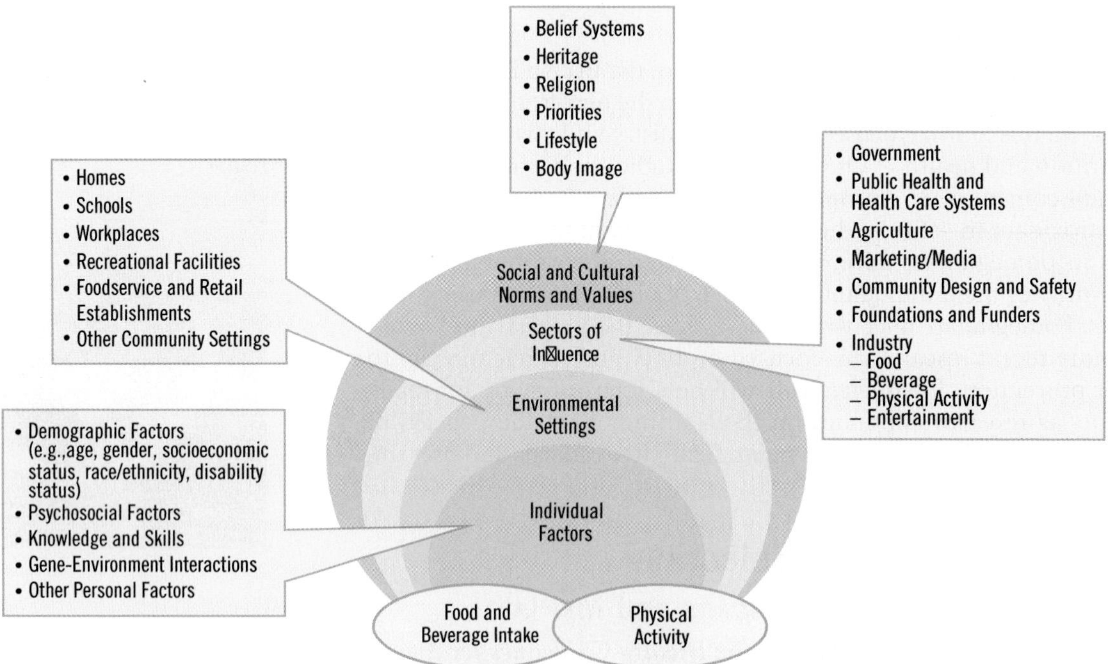

FIGURE 10.11 MyPlate, which is based on the *Dietary Guidelines for Americans, 2010*, identifies five food groups: fruits, vegetables, dairy, grains, and lean proteins. MyPlate emphasizes the consumption of fruits, vegetables, whole grains, and fat-free or low-fat milk and milk products. It recommends lean meats, poultry, fish, beans, eggs, and nuts in moderation. Saturated fats, trans fats, cholesterol, salt (sodium), and added sugars should be consumed sparingly.

Source: Reproduced from *Dietary Guidelines for Americans, 2010.* 7th ed. U.S. Government Printing Office; 2010. Courtesy of U.S. Department of Agriculture and U.S. Department of Health and Human Services.

Special Topic 10.3

Farm to Plate

Catherine Frederico, MS, RD, LDN

In the movie *Food Fight*, credit is given to chef Alice Waters of Chez Panisse fame for starting the local sustainable food movement.[1] In the 1970s, her popular restaurant in Berkeley, California, was one of the first to include location sources for the dishes on the menu. She took pride in serving fresh, local ingredients and supporting local farmers. She used primarily organic foods, just as the organic movement was sweeping the country.

Years later, in 2007, Michael Pollan wrote the *Omnivore's Dilemma*.[2] He followed this book up with *In Defense of Food* in 2009, which chronicled his personal search to discover the who, what, where, and how behind the production of his food.[3] Columbia Professor Dr. Marion Nestle has written several books and articles on the politics of food, including *What to Eat*, *Food Politics*, and *Safe Food: The Politics of Food Safety*.[4–6]

American citizens are being bombarded with messages about global climate change and the obesity epidemic in the United States. The current generation of children is on track to have shorter life spans than their parents, in large part due to obesity. The obesity epidemic also is an issue of national defense because the number of people rejected for military service because of obesity continues to rise. The medical costs resulting from health problems caused by obesity is $150 billion a year and climbing. In 2010, First Lady Michelle Obama planted a vegetable garden on the White House lawn and has made getting our children healthy the major focus of her tenure. She created the Let's Move Campaign to get children and their families moving and in better health.[7]

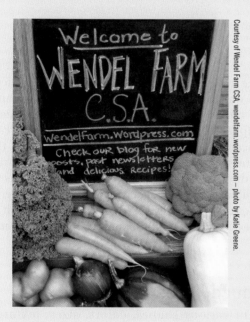

Courtesy of Wendel Farm CSA, wendelfarm.wordpress.com – photo by Katie Greene.

This confluence of issues has piqued the interest of Americans with regard to how to make the best food choices for themselves and the environment. National "farm-to-plate" programs encourage people to get to know their local farmers, support their local economy, and eat foods that are in season. Buying local assures a crisper and healthier bounty because some produce lose nutrients when shipped long distances.

Farmers' markets are increasing in popularity and are even being held indoors in the winter in northern climates. Community supported agriculture (CSA) farms sell annual and seasonal memberships ahead of the planting season to ensure customer support of their businesses. To give consumers more options, the USDA manages a website titled "Know Your Farmer, Know Your Food." Its mission is to connect consumers with producers and to foster an understanding about where food comes from on its journey to our plates.[8]

Buying local also helps the environment by decreasing the need for refrigeration and transcontinental trucking, thereby reducing the burden on our nation's energy resources. Plant-based diets have a smaller carbon footprint than animal-based diets. *Bon Appétit* hosts a calculator on its website that calculates the carbon footprint of different foods. Numerous websites provide information about farm-to-plate opportunities and other resources to help Americans eat as well and as smart as possible. **Table A** (see the next page) offers websites, books, and movies that explore these issues.

References

1 Taylor C. *Food Fight.* 2008. Available at: http://www.foodfightthedoc.com. Accessed January 5, 2011.

2 Pollan M. *Omnivore's Dilemma.* New York: Penguin; 2007.

3 Pollan M. *In Defense of Food.* New York: Penguin; 2009.

4 Nestle M. *What to Eat.* New York: North Point Press; 2007.

5 Nestle M. *Food Politics.* Berkeley, CA: University of California Press; 2007

6 Nestle M. *Safe Food: The Politics of Food Safety.* Berkeley, CA: University of California Press; 2010.

7 White House, Department of Health and Human Services, United States Department of Agriculture, Department of Education. Let's Move. Available at: http://www.letsmove.gov. Accessed February 16, 2011.

8 U.S. Department of Agriculture. Know Your Farmer, Know Your Food. Available at: http://www.usda.gov/wps/portal/usda/knowyourfarmer?navid=KNOWYOURFARMER. Accessed January 5, 2011.

TABLE A
Farm-to-Plate Resources

Websites	http://www.cnpp.usda.gov/knowyourfarmer.htm http://www.farmbasededucation.org http://www.localharvest.org http://www.eatlowcarbon.org http://www.farmtoschool.org http://www.sustainabletable.org http://www.growingpower.org http://www.sierraclub.org/truecostoffood http://www.slowfoodusa.org http://www.fieldtoplate.com http://www.sierraclub.org/truecostoffood
Movies	*Food, Inc.* (http://www.FoodIncMovie.com) *Food Fight* (http://www.FoodFightthedoc.com)
Books	Geagan K. *Go Green Get Lean.* New York: Rodale; 2009. Newgent J. *Big Green Cookbook.* Hoboken, NJ: Wiley; 2009. Bitman M. *Food Matters.* New York: Simon & Schuster; 2009.
iPhone Apps	Fresh Fruit iLocavore Food Focus: Fruits

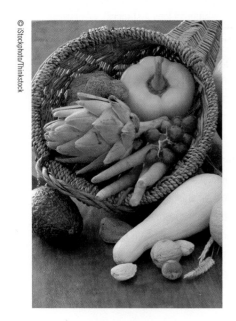

Vegetarianism

Many studies have examined the potential health benefits of vegetarian diets. One of the largest such studies was the China Study. In a book by the same name, Dr. T. Colin Campbell relates the findings of his diet and disease research of rural Chinese. Campbell concludes that the prevalence of breast and prostate cancers is significantly lower in vegetarians.[37] Similarly, the Vegetarian Resource Group states that "vegetarians are generally at lower risk than nonvegetarians for heart disease, high blood pressure, some forms of cancer, and obesity."[38,39] A position paper on vegetarianism by the Academy of Nutrition and Dietetics echoes these findings.[40] Not everyone may wish to adhere to a vegetarian diet, but everyone can still benefit from the nutrients found in fruits and vegetables.

A Cornucopia of Produce Types

Fruits and vegetables come in various shapes, colors, sizes, textures, and aromas. Some grow on trees, others on bushes, stalks, stems, or vines. Some grow above ground, and some grow beneath it. Fruits and vegetables are often encased in a protective skin. Some skins are edible, others are not. Melon, pineapple, banana, and lychee peels are not edible, whereas apple, grape, pear, peach, plum, and potato skins are edible (and contribute to dietary fiber). Except for thin-skinned kumquats, citrus skins are typically not eaten, but they can be cooked or candied, and be grated or zested into dishes to add extra flavor. When we eat produce, are eating a variety of different plant parts—fruits, leaves, stems, bulbs, and so on.

Gastronomy Point

Citrus Peels Citrus peels or slices can be floated in beverages to infuse their essence.

Fruits

By definition, fruits have seeds, some of which can be eaten. Strawberry seeds are small and are on the outside of the fruit. Most others are larger and encased within the fruit. Cucumbers, zucchini, tomatoes, and cactus fruit have edible seeds, whereas avocado, peach, plum, cherry, and olive fruits do not. There is a wide variety of fruit types available:

- *Pome fruits:* A **pome** is a fleshy fruit (such as an apple or pear) that has an outer fleshy layer surrounding a central core that encloses the seeds.
- *Citrus:* Citrus fruits have a thick rind and juicy pulp and are grown in warm regions. Orange, grapefruit, tangerine, lemon, and lime are examples of citrus fruits.
- *Stone fruits:* These are fruits that have a pit, such as a peach, plum, apricot, cherry, and mango. The hard, inedible pit or seed in this group is called a **stone**. The huge, fibrous mango stone is about 3.5 inches long by 2 inches wide. The seeds of stone and pome fruits contain cyanide and, in large quantities, may be poisonous.
- *Soft fruits:* Soft fruits include those that have flesh and a firm structure but can be easily deformed. Grape, strawberry, pineapple, banana, berry fruit, kiwi, papaya, and lychee are some examples.
- *Amorphous fruits:* These are fruits with little firm flesh structure under the skin, such as passion fruit and guava.

pome A fleshy fruit with a middle core and seeds; examples include apples and pears.

stone The pit of a fruit; found in fruits such as cherries, plums, and peaches.

Innovation Point

Squashes Squashes are botanically fruits because they have seeds and develop from flowers. However, they are often considered vegetables for cooking and menu-planning purposes. Squash is loosely grouped into summer squash or winter squash, depending on whether it is harvested as immature fruit (summer squash) or mature fruit (winter squash) (see **Figure 10.12**). Summer squashes include zucchini, yellow crooknecks, and pattypan. Winter squashes include pumpkin, butternut, acorn, and spaghetti squash as well as many others. The zucchini blossoms themselves are an edible summer delicacy.

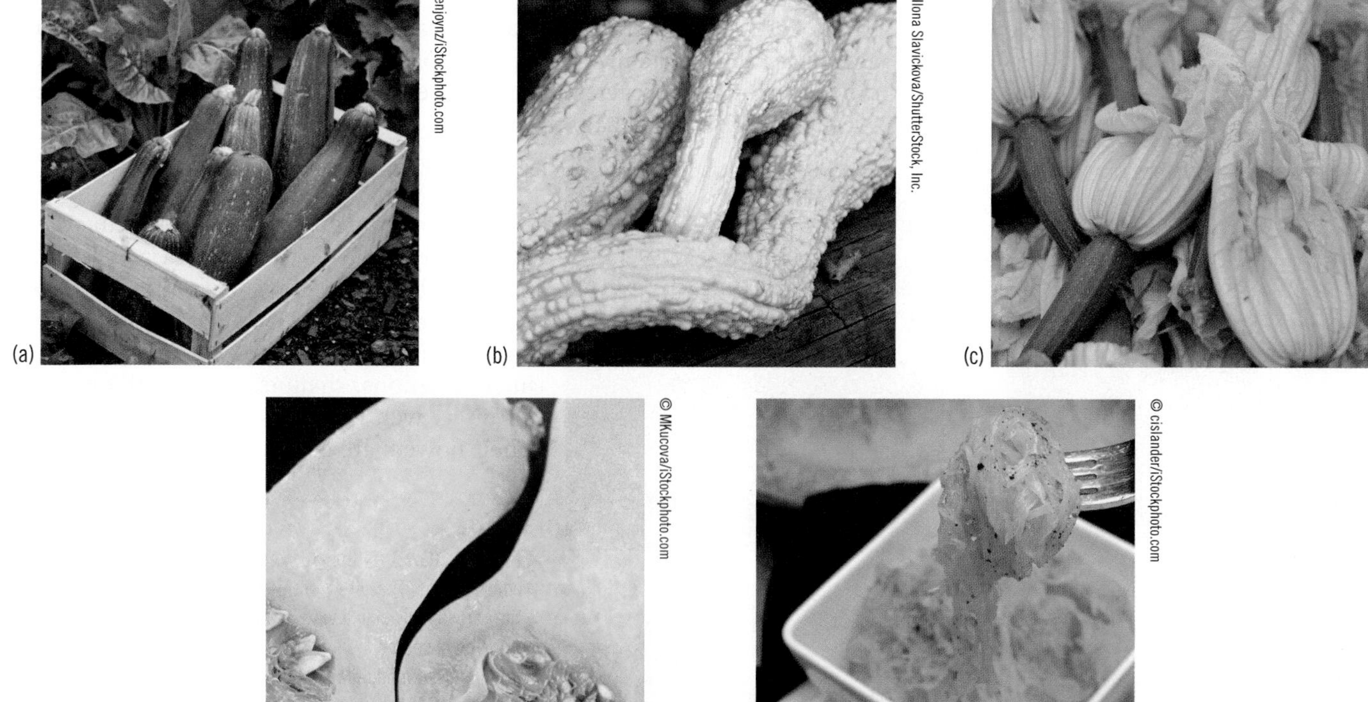

FIGURE 10.12 (a) Zucchini is a type of summer squash. It is very versatile and can be prepared in a number of different ways—steamed, boiled, grilled, or baked. It can even be incorporated into soufflés and baked goods, such as banana bread. (b) Yellow crookneck squash is a type of summer squash with a bumpy yellow skin. It has a buttery flavor and a smooth texture. It is best when boiled or sautéed. (c) Squash blossoms are edible. They can be eaten raw or be battered and fried. They can also be incorporated into casseroles and quiches. (d) Butternut squash is a type of winter squash that has a sweet, nutty flavor. It can be roasted and eaten or puréed and incorporated into soups, casseroles, or baked goods. (e) Spaghetti squash is a winter squash. The flesh of the squash flakes into strands that look like spaghetti. When cooked, these strands can be eaten as an alternative to pasta and topped with pasta sauce.

Green Point

Avoid Waste Buy only what you will use within a week to avoid waste. Root vegetables and winter squashes will keep longer.

- *Tree nuts:* Nuts grown from trees are really fruits.
- *Tropical and subtropical:* Named for the climatic conditions under which they are grown, none of these fruits can tolerate frost or grow in temperatures below 50°F (10°C). Tropical and subtropical fruits include figs, dates, kiwis, mangos, bananas, papayas, pomegranates, guava, star fruit, and passion fruit.

Leaves

Leafy vegetable greens include lettuce, spinach, collard greens, sorrel, chard, mustard greens, and turnip greens (see **Figure 10.13**). Spring green mix is a popular combination of several salad greens and can include dandelion greens, frisee, arugula, radicchio, endive, mache, and red and green lettuces. When you eat cabbages and Brussels sprouts you are also eating the leaves of plants that are spaced closely on a shortened stem.

Leafy greens are a great source of vitamins and minerals. Spring mix contains large amounts of vitamins A and C as well as several of the B vitamins. One cup provides 70% of the Daily Recommended Intake (DRI) for vitamin A and 20% for vitamin C. Leafy greens are also a rich source of iron and calcium and numerous trace minerals, including magnesium, phosphorus, and potassium. Dark leafy greens, such as spinach and kale, also are good sources of vitamins K and E.

Stems

When you eat celery, rhubarb, fennel, bamboo shoots, or asparagus you are actually eating the stem, or stalk, of the plant (see **Figure 10.14**). Oftentimes, the leaves of these vegetables are also edible. Most of these vegetables are excellent sources of dietary fiber.

Bulbs

Alliums, or onion-type vegetables, are members of the Lily family. They are characterized as having a bulb that grows beneath the ground and edible tall green slender stems. They often have stunning white or purple flowers. Alliums include onions, shallots, leeks, scallions, and garlic as well as chives (see **Figure 10.15**). Their flowers are edible.

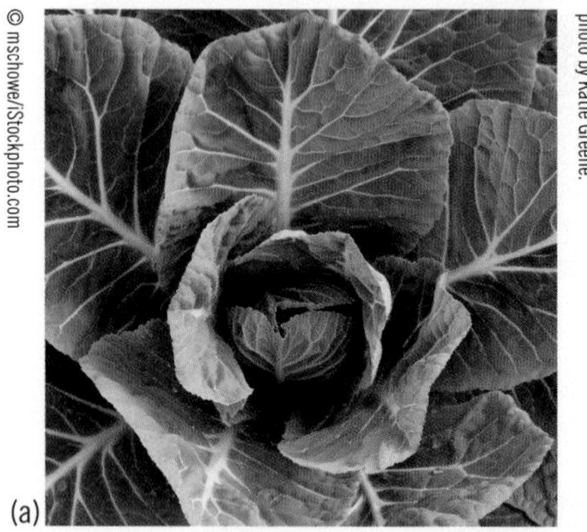

(a)

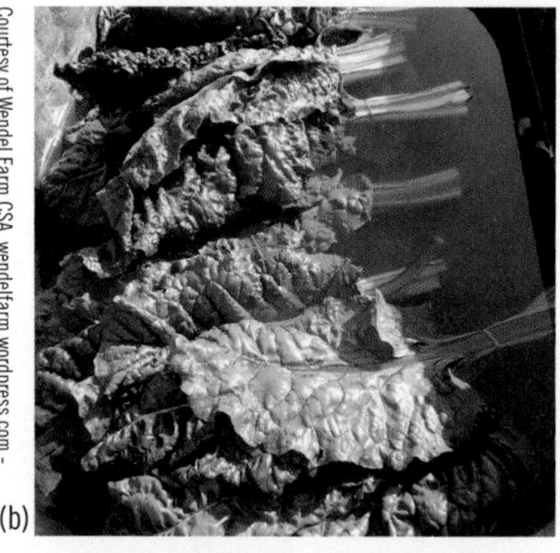

(b)

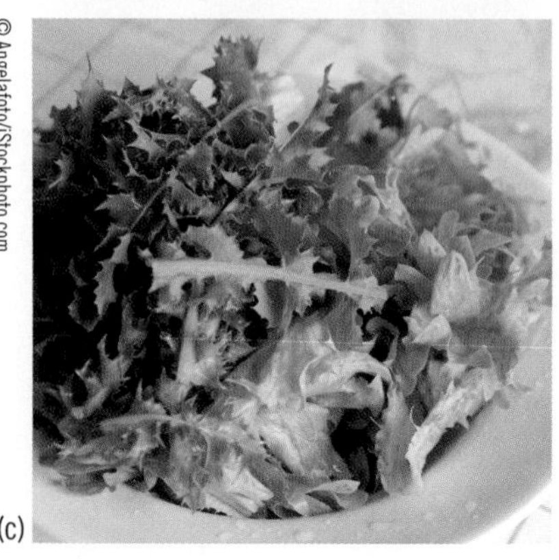

(c)

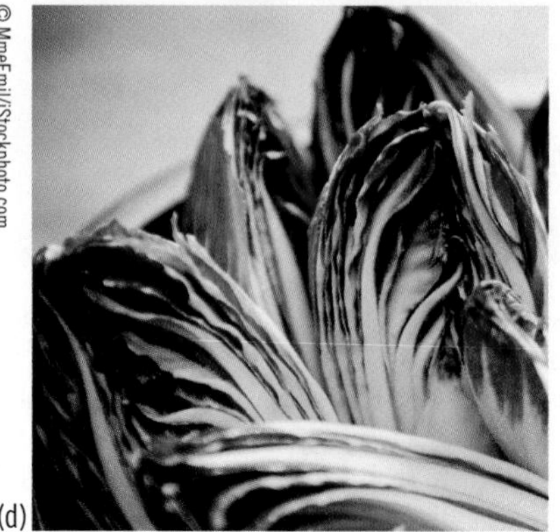

(d)

FIGURE 10.13 (a) Collard greens have large, dark-colored edible leaves. They are a staple in Southern cuisine, in which they are usually boiled with a ham hock and lots of salt. They are a good source of vitamin C and dietary fiber. (b) Chard often is used in Middle Eastern cuisines. Swiss chard is high in vitamins A, K and C. It also is rich in minerals, dietary fiber and protein. (c) The dandelions that dot so many fields and lawns are edible! In particular, the leaves are great in salads. Dandelion greens pack quite a nutritional punch, being good sources of fiber; vitamins A, C, E, K, and B_6; thiamin; riboflavin; calcium; iron; potassium; and manganese. (d) Radicchio has a bitter and spicy taste. In Italian cuisine it is often sautéed and served with risotto. In the United States, it is used as a salad green. It is a good source of vitamins C, E, and K; folate; potassium; copper; and manganese.

Roots and Tubers

Root vegetables (see **Figure 10.16**) include carrots, potatoes, sweet potatoes, yams, beets, turnips, parsnips, rutabagas, and radishes. Tubers (see **Figure 10.17**) include taro, jicama, yucca, celery root, sunchokes, and daikon.

Legumes

Beans and peas are some of the most well-known plant pods, which are known as legumes (see **Figure 10.18**). The more tender, sweet varieties of beans include green, wax, haricot verts, long, and fava. Green peas are husked from a tough shell, called a pod. Some beans, such as farmer's bean, require longer cooking times than others. Edible pea pods include snow peas and sugar snap peas. Commonly used canned or dried beans include pinto, kidney, garbanzo, cannellini, navy, soldier, lima, and black beans. Lentils, another legume, are high in protein and come in yellow, orange, and green varieties.

Other "Vegetables"

Corn is most often served as a vegetable, either on the cob or just its kernels, but corn is categorized as a grain because it is from the fruit of a grass species. (Wheat and barley also are grains.) Once corn is picked, it is best cooked and eaten as soon as possible because its sugar begins to break down to form starch and thereby taste less sweet. Three-fourths of the starch in corn is the branched glucose chain amylopectin, which forms corn's insoluble, semicrystalline granules. Unbranched amylose makes up the other quarter of corn's starch and accounts for its viscosity and gelation properties.[41]

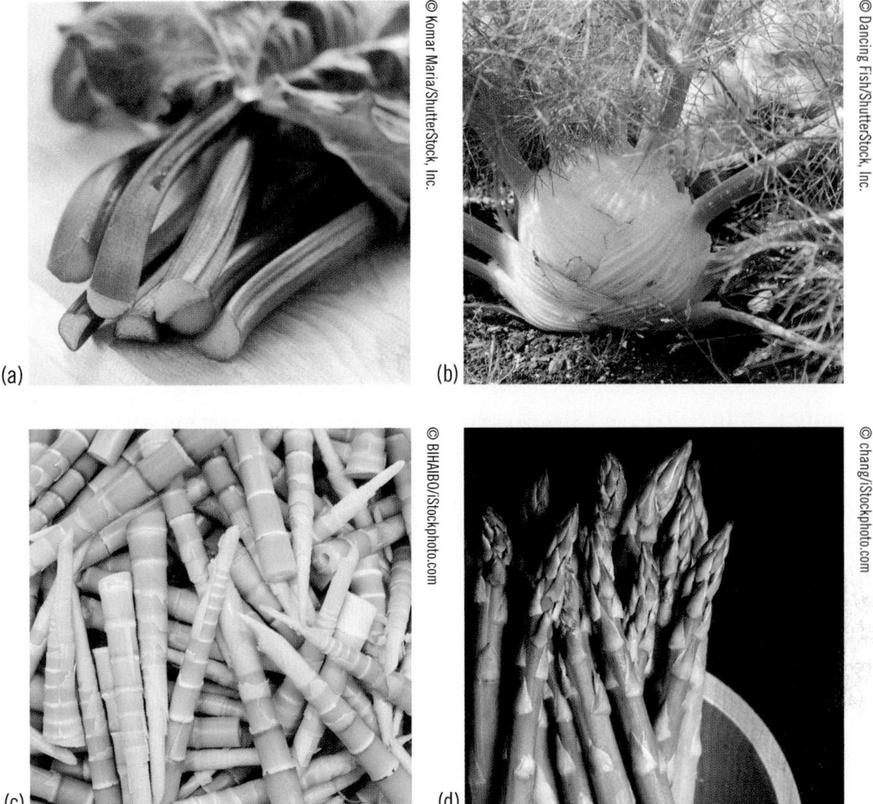

(a) © Komar Maria/ShutterStock, Inc. (b) © Dancing Fish/ShutterStock, Inc. (c) © BIHAIBO/iStockphoto.com (d) © chang/iStockphoto.com

FIGURE 10.14 (a) Rhubarb is a popular stalk vegetable. The stalks can be boiled until soft and then mixed with sugar to make a pie filling. It is a good source of fiber, vitamin C, vitamin K, calcium, magnesium, and manganese. (b) The fleshy stalk of the fennel plant is called a bulb. The bulb is eaten as a vegetable and often is used in Italian cooking. The leaves and seeds of fennel also are used a seasoning. It is a good source of vitamin C, fiber, and potassium. (c) Bamboo shoots are popular in Asian cuisines. Bamboo shoots cannot be eaten raw; they must be cooked first. They are a very good source of potassium, copper, and manganese. (d) Asparagus is a popular vegetable that must be cooked, usually by steaming, before it is eaten. It is a great source of fiber, iron, magnesium, and zinc.

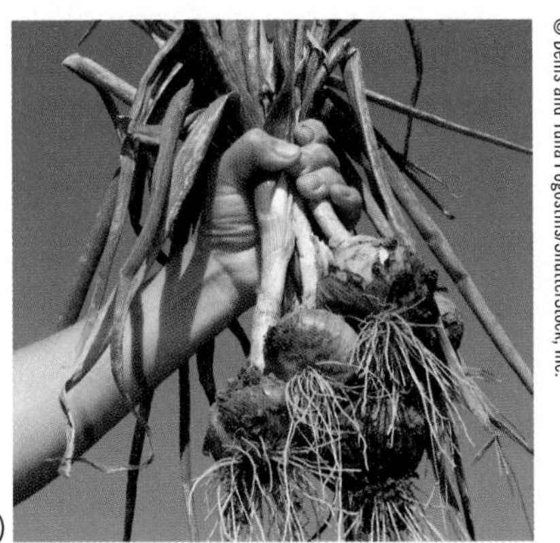

(a) © Denis and Yulia Pogostins/ShutterStock, Inc.

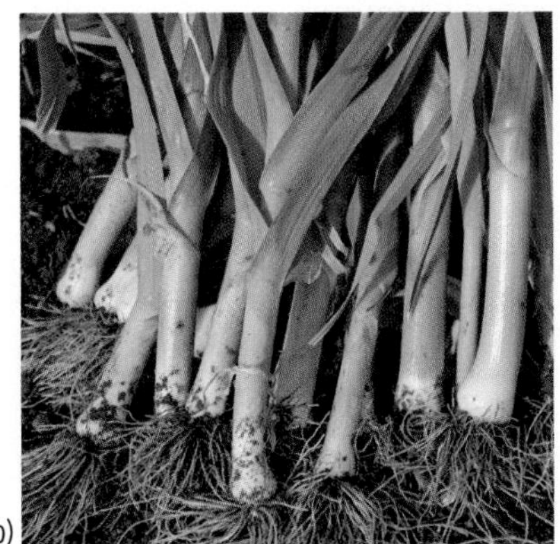

(b) © Stefan Fierros/ShutterStock, Inc.

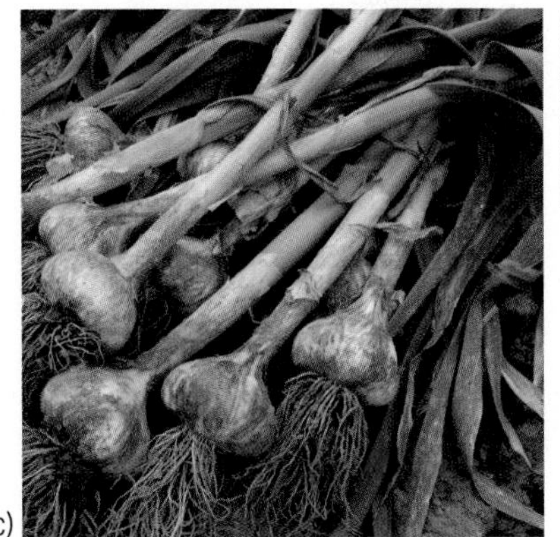

(c) © iStockphoto/Thinkstock

FIGURE 10.15 (a) Many different varieties of onion are available, including red, yellow, white, and green. They are used to flavor dips, salads, soups, spreads, stir-fry, and other dishes. They are a good source of vitamin C. (b) Leeks have a mild onion taste. They are a good source of vitamins A, C, and K; folate; and manganese. (c) Garlic is used as a seasoning in many cuisines around the world. It is a good source of antioxidants and some claim that it has medicinal properties. It is a good source of vitamin C, vitamin B_6, and manganese.

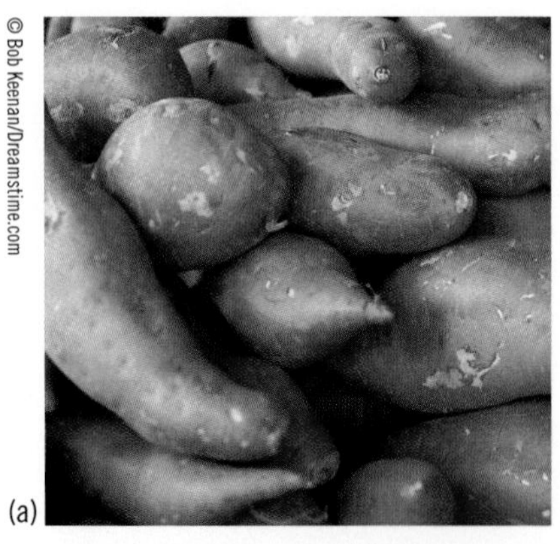

© Bob Keenan/Dreamstime.com

(a)

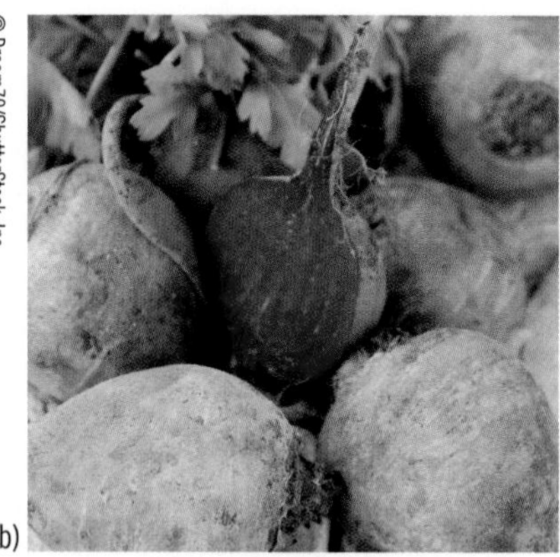

© Dream79/ShutterStock, Inc.

(b)

FIGURE 10.16 (a) Yams are a starchy root vegetable. They are an important agricultural product in West Africa, which produces 95% of the world's yam harvest. Yams are not the same as sweet potatoes, which are a different species. Yams are a good source of fiber, vitamin C, potassium, and manganese. (b) Beets are a unique source of phytonutrients called betalains, which gives beets their distinctive purple color. They are a good source of fiber, folate, potassium, and manganese.

Mushrooms are also served as vegetables, but they are fungi. Wild mushrooms should never be eaten unless they have been identified as safe by an expert. They are very tricky to identify; some poisonous mushrooms look very similar to safe mushrooms. The mushrooms sold in stores are grown in controlled conditions and are the most safe to eat. Both the caps and stems are edible.

Although nuts, which grow on trees, are technically vegetables, their chemistry—low in carbohydrates but rich in protein—is very different from most vegetables. (Of surprise to many people is the fact that peanuts are not nuts but actually legumes because they grow underground.)

Selecting the Best Produce

In general, fruits and vegetables should be dry and free of blemishes and mold. Vegetables should be crisp and not wilted. Storing produce in bags with holes for moisture to escape can help keep produce fresh.

Green Point

Climacteric Fruits When shopping for the week, buy a few ripe climacteric fruits and a few green ones to ensure having perfectly ripe fruit available all week long without needing to make another drive to the store.

climacteric fruits Fruits that continue to ripen once picked.

nonclimacteric fruits Fruits that only ripen when left on the plant.

Understanding Ripeness

Once picked, **climacteric fruits** continue to ripen. Bananas, pears, avocados, and tomatoes are climacteric, which means they can be picked green and they will continue to ripen. To speed ripening, climacteric produce can be placed in paper or plastic bags to increase their exposure to ethylene gas (produced by ripening fruit), which enhances ripening by turning starch to sugar. **Nonclimacteric fruits** stop ripening and begin to deteriorate immediately after picking. Pineapples, citrus, berries, and melons are nonclimacteric.

Table 10.6 provides information on selecting and storing fruits. **Table 10.7** offers information on selecting and storing vegetables. Additional information can be found on the CDC's Fruits and Veggies Matter website (http://www.fruitsandveggiesmatter.gov).

Food Preparation

The challenge of cooking vegetables and fruits is to create an appealing dish without compromising their color, flavor, texture, and nutrition. Accomplishing this can sometimes seem like a balancing act because each meal needs to completed, plated, and served at about the same time for multiple people.

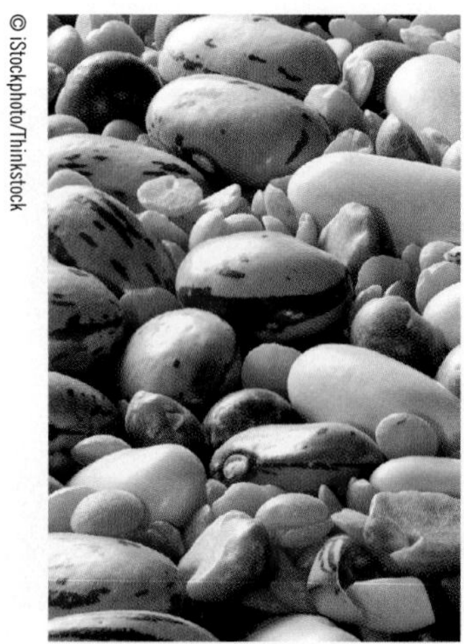

© iStockphoto/Thinkstock

FIGURE 10.18 Beans and peas are important components of cuisines around the world. They are excellent sources fiber, proteins, folate, and iron.

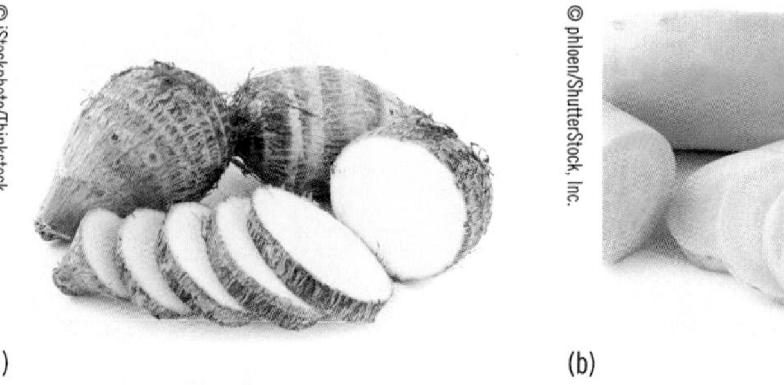

© iStockphoto/Thinkstock

(a)

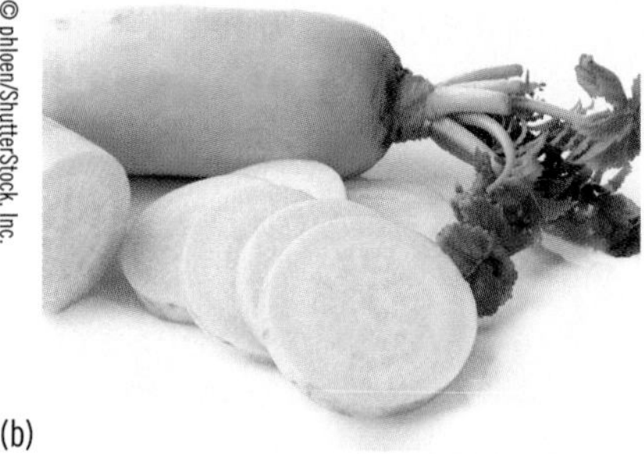

© phloen/ShutterStock, Inc.

(b)

FIGURE 10.17 (a) Taro is a starchy root vegetable that is widely used in African and Asian cuisines. It is a good source of fiber, vitamin E, vitamin B_5, potassium, and manganese. (b) Daikon is another root vegetable that is popular in Asian cuisines. It is very low in calories and is a good source of vitamin C.

Pleasing varied palettes may not be easy, especially in large institutional settings. For example, people vary in their texture preferences for fruits and vegetables. A person who likes raw tomatoes may not care for stewed tomatoes. Someone who likes raw apples may not like cooked apples.

It is also important for the home cook to consider individual needs; it is often polite to ask invited dinner guests about special food needs. Some may have food sensitivities or allergies, difficulty chewing, or need to avoid potential additives or preservatives. Despite these challenges, cooking can be a very relaxing, rewarding, educational, creative art form.

Washing and Cooking

Many fruits need only the bare minimum of preparation of washing and maybe cutting. They travel well and do not necessarily require refrigeration in their whole form when traveling short distances. Combination salads are a fabulous way to include fruit in meals.

Although fruit preparation is relatively easy, requiring just washing and drying, most vegetables (other than in raw salads) will need to be cooked. Wash, cut, and cook vegetables as close to serving time as possible to avoid discoloration and nutrient and moisture loss. To prevent cross-contamination by bacteria, use a cutting board and knife different from those used for raw meats, poultry, and fish. Except for bananas, tomatoes, potatoes, winter squash, and onions, most produce is best kept refrigerated.

Fresh vegetables are best cooked to a crisp, tender stage. Remember that water-soluble vitamins and cell structure can be destroyed by heat, and fiber can be lost if recipes call for using only using the juice of a fruit. Steaming, grilling, broiling, baking, stir-frying, and microwaving in a minimal amount of water for a short time are the best cooking methods to preserve nutrients, texture, and flavor. Cooking vegetables until they are "al dente," or slightly crisp, helps preserve vitamins. In warmer months, grilling is an option even for fruits such as pineapples or peaches.

When cooking by boiling, microwaving, or steaming, immediately "shock" vegetables by transferring them to a bowl of cold water to stop the cooking process and preserve color. Overcooking in too much water will make vegetables limp, off-color, and devoid of vitamins, minerals, and flavor.

Adding Flavoring

It is not necessary or encouraged to add salt, sodium bicarbonate, or seasoning blends to fruits and vegetables due to the detrimental health effects of added sodium. Sodium bicarbonate added to the cooking water can preserve the vegetable's color, but it adds sodium and contributes to a mushy texture. However, a multitude of herbs and spices are available that can be used to enhance flavor. Do not add too much oil when sautéing or when preparing dressings or sauces because oils add approximately 40 calories per teaspoon to a dish. Frying—as with vegetable tempuras and french fries—is discouraged to limit adding fat calories.

Finding Inspiration

Today, recipes and cooking tips can be found in books and on various multimedia platforms, including websites and smartphone apps. Hundreds of international cooking websites, blogs, videos, slideshows, and phone applications are available. Epicurious (http://www.epicurious.com) and AllRecipes (http://www.allrecipes.com) are two of the more popular recipe websites. iPhoto Cookbook and iCookbook for iPad use photos and videos to demonstrate recipe steps. iCookbook features voice control to turn pages and manage timers.

Gastronomy Point

Mushrooms Portobello, shitake, oyster, and white button mushrooms are popular varieties of mushrooms. They can add flavor and texture to vegetable, rice, and egg dishes and soups. Make sure to wipe mushrooms with a clean cloth or quickly rinse them to remove any dirt because they become soggy if soaked in water.

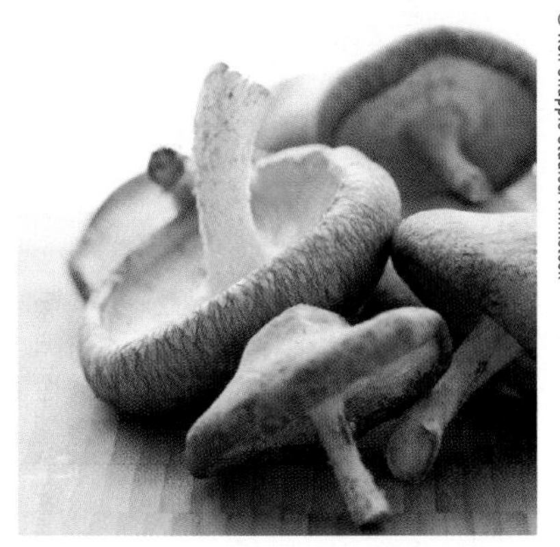

Gastronomy Point

Storing Tomatoes Store tomatoes on the counter. Refrigerated tomatoes will lose flavor. Serve tomato salads that combine multiple varieties and colors of tomatoes. Lightly dress with balsamic vinegar, extra virgin olive oil, and fresh basil.

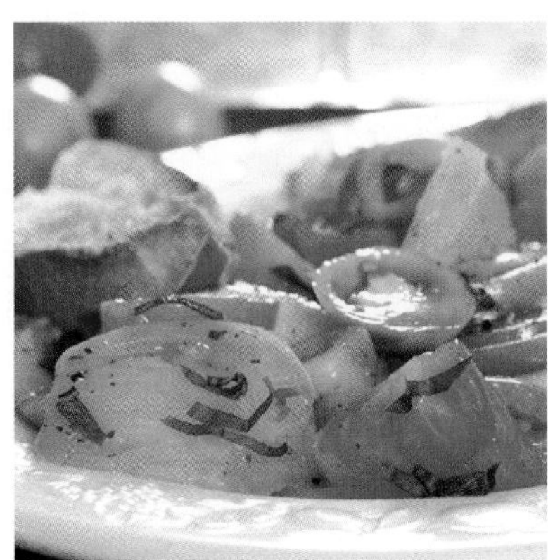

TABLE 10.6
Fruit Selection Criteria and Storage Tips

Fruit	Selection Criteria	Storage Tips
Apple	Choose apples that are firm with no soft spots. Avoid apples that are discolored for their variety. There are more than 2,500 varieties of apple!	Store apples in a plastic bag in the refrigerator after purchasing to prevent further ripening. Apples can keep for up to 6 weeks. However, check apples often and remove any that begin to decay, or the others will do the same.
Apricot	Look for plump apricots with as much golden-orange color as possible. Stay clear of fruit that is pale yellow, greenish-yellow, very firm, shriveled, or bruised. Apricots that are soft-ripe have the best flavor, but they must be eaten immediately.	Apricots will ripen at room temperature. To speed ripening, place them in a paper bag with an apple. When they yield to gentle pressure, they are ready to eat. Refrigerate ripe apricots, unwashed, in a paper or plastic bag for up to 2 days. Wash before eating. They are the perfect fast food! To cut the fruit, slice around its seam, twist it in half, and lift out the pit.
Avocado	Look for firm avocados if you are planning on using them later in the week, otherwise select fruit that yields to gentle pressure for immediate use. Color alone will not tell you if the avocado is ripe. Ripe fruit will be slightly firm but will yield to gentle pressure.	To speed the ripening process, place the avocado in a paper bag and store it at room temperature until ready to eat (usually 2 to 5 days). Placing an apple together with the avocado speeds up the process even more.
Banana	Avoid bananas with brown spots that seem very soft. Select bananas with a nice color, specific for the variety. Choose fruit that is firm and free of bruises. Best eating quality has been reached when the solid yellow skin color is speckled with brown. Bananas with green tips or with practically no yellow color have not developed their full flavor. Bananas are overripe when they have a strong odor.	To further ripen bananas, leave them at room temperature for a couple of days. Once ripe, they can be stored in the refrigerator for 3 to 5 days. The peel may turn brown in the refrigerator, but the fruit will not change.
Blackberries	Blackberries should be dry, firm, well shaped, and eaten within a week after purchase. Select blackberries that are unblemished, dry, and in an unstained container. Blackberries should be shiny and black—avoid those that are dull or reddish. Moisture will increase spoilage.	After purchasing blackberries, check the fruit and toss out any moldy or deformed berries. Immediately eat the overripe berries within 24 hours. Return the other berries back to the original container or arrange them unwashed in a shallow pan lined with paper towels and wash them just prior to use. The berries may be topped with a paper towel to absorb any additional moisture. Place plastic wrap around the entire container. This will ensure the fruit retains its freshness. Generally, berries should be eaten within 1 week. Eat at room temperature for fullest flavor.
Blueberries	Berries should be dry, firm, well shaped, and eaten within a week after purchase. Select blueberries that are firm, dry, plump, and smooth-skinned. Berries should be deep-purple blue to blue-black; reddish berries are not ripe but can be used in cooking.	After purchasing berries, check for and toss out any moldy or deformed berries. Immediately eat the overripe berries within 24 hours. Return the other berries back to the original container or arrange them unwashed in a shallow pan lined with paper towels and wash just prior to use. The berries may be topped with a paper towel to absorb any additional moisture. Plastic wrap the entire container. This will ensure the fruit retains its freshness, but generally berries should be eaten within 1 week.
Cherry	Buy cherries that have been kept cool and moist because both flavor and texture suffer at warm temperatures. Good cherries should be large (1 inch or more in diameter), glossy, plump, hard, and dark colored for their variety. Buy cherries with the stems on; they should be fresh and green. Reject undersized cherries or those that are soft or flabby. Avoid fruit that is bruised or has cuts on the dark surface.	Loosely pack unwashed cherries in plastic bags or pour them into a shallow pan in a single layer and cover with plastic wrap to minimize bruising. Store cherries in the refrigerator. Cherries in good condition should last up to a week.
Cranberry	Good, ripe cranberries will bounce, which is why they are nicknamed "bounceberries." They should be shiny and plump and range in color from bright light red to dark red. Shriveled berries or those with brown spots should be avoided. Cranberries do not ripen after harvest.	Store fresh cranberries in a tightly sealed plastic bag in the refrigerator. As with all berries, if one starts getting soft and decaying, the others will quickly soften and decay as well. Be sure to sort out the soft ones if you plan to store them for more than a few days. Fresh cranberries may last up to 2 months in the refrigerator. Cooked cranberries can last up to a month in a covered container in the refrigerator. Washed cranberries may be frozen for up to 1 year in airtight bags.

Figs	Look for figs that are soft and smell sweet. Handle carefully because their fragile skins bruise easily.	Store fully ripened figs in the refrigerator up to 2 days; bring to room temperature before serving.
Grapes	Look for firm, plump, well-colored clusters of grapes that are securely attached to the stems. Fully ripe grapes are soft and tender. Grapes showing signs of decay, shriveling, stickiness, or brown spots or dry brittle stems should be avoided.	
Grapefruit	Choose grapefruit that is glossy, round, smooth and heavy for its size. Avoid any grapefruit with brown and/or soft spots.	Store grapefruit at room temperature up to a week or up to 8 weeks in the refrigerator. Leave at room temperature for a couple of hours before eating.
Kiwifruit	Select kiwifruit with no bruises or soft spots. Avoid fruits with wrinkles or signs of exterior damage. Buy firm kiwifruit and let them ripen at home for a juicier flavor. A kiwifruit is ripe when plump and slightly soft to the touch with a fragrant smell.	Ripen kiwifruit at room temperature for 3 to 5 days. If necessary, ripe kiwifruit can be stored in the refrigerator for up to 7 days. If they need to be stored longer, put kiwis in a plastic bag in the refrigerator for up to 2 weeks.
Lemon	Lemons should be firm and have a bright yellow color. Avoid soft, shriveled lemons with spots. The best lemons will be fine textured and heavy for their size. Thin-skinned fruit tends to have more juice, whereas fruit that has a greenish cast is likely to be more acidic. One medium lemon has about 3 tablespoons of juice and 3 tablespoons of grated peel.	You may store lemons at room temperature for about 2 weeks. They will keep for up to 6 weeks in a plastic bag in the refrigerator. Use lemons as quickly as possible after cutting.
Lime	Select limes that are glossy and light to deep green in color. Limes should have a thin, smooth skin and be heavy for their size. Small brown areas on the skin should not affect flavor, but large blemishes or soft spots indicate a damaged lime. Ripe limes are firm but not hard. Avoid limes that have a yellowish skin or are too small. A hard shriveled skin is a sign of dryness, as is a coarse thick skin.	Limes may be stored at room temperature or in the refrigerator for up to 3 weeks. Limes store better in a plastic bag if placed in the refrigerator. Those stored at room temperature will yield more juice. Take care to keep limes out of direct sunlight because they will shrivel and become discolored.
Mango	Choose firm plump mangos that give slightly when pressure is applied. Avoid those with bruised or dry and shriveled skin. The ripeness of mangos can be determined by either smelling or squeezing. A ripe mango will have a full, fruity aroma emitting from the stem end. Mangos are considered ready to eat when slightly soft to the touch and yield to gentle pressure. The best-flavored fruit have a yellow tinge when ripe; however, their color may be red, yellow, orange, green, or any combination.	Store mangos at room temperature and out of the sun until ripened. The ideal storage temperature for mangos is 55°F (12.7°C). When stored properly, a mango should have a shelf life of 1 to 2 weeks. Although the mango will not ripen in the refrigerator, it can be kept chilled there once ripe. Store cut mangos in a plastic bag for no more than 3 days.
Melon	In general, melons should be shaped according to their variety. For example, cantaloupes should be round. In addition, melons should not have cracks, soft spots, or dark bruises. You should look for a clean and smooth break at the stem and for a fruity fragrance (if not chilled).	Keep uncut melons at room temperature for 2 to 4 days or until fully ripe, then refrigerate for up to 5 days. Refrigerate cut up melon in a covered container for up to 3 days. Remember that cut melons are aromatic and their smell will penetrate other foods.
Nectarine	Ripe fruit are fragrant and give, slightly, to the touch. If they are underripe, leave them at room temperature for 2 to 3 days to ripen. Look for fruit with smooth unblemished skin. Avoid extremely hard or dull colored fruits and fruit with soft, wrinkled, punctured skin.	Nectarines keep for 5 days if stored in a plastic bag in the coldest part of the refrigerator.

(*continues*)

TABLE 10.6
Fruit Selection Criteria and Storage Tips (*continued*)

Fruit	Selection Criteria	Storage Tips
Orange	All varieties should be firm, heavy for size, and have fine-textured skin. Look for fruit that is firm and heavy for its size, with bright, colorful skins. Skin color is not a good guide to quality. Fruits may be ripe even though they may have green spots. Avoid fruit with bruised, wrinkled, or discolored skins; this indicates the fruit is old or has been stored incorrectly.	Oranges can be stored at room temperature, in the refrigerator without plastic bags, or in the crisper drawer for up to 2 weeks. They do not ripen further after picking. Fresh-squeezed juice and grated peel or zest may be refrigerated or frozen, but whole citrus fruits should not be frozen.
Papaya	Look for papayas that are partly or completely yellow in color, depending on variety, and that give slightly to pressure but are not soft at the stem end. Avoid papayas that are bruised, shriveled, or have soft areas. Papayas that are hard and green are immature and will not ripen properly. Uncut papayas have no smell. Papayas that are cut should smell sweet, not bad or fermented.	Slightly green papayas will ripen quickly at room temperature, especially if placed in a paper bag. As the papaya ripens, it will turn from green to yellow. Place ripe papayas in a plastic bag and store in the refrigerator. Papayas will keep for up to a week, but it is best to use them within a day or two.
Passion fruit	Choose large, heavy, firm fruit. When ripe, it has wrinkled, dimpled, deep purple skin. Skin is old-looking, but that does not mean the fruit is rotten. Mold does not affect quality and can be wiped off. Fruit color is green when immature, changing to shades of purple, red, or yellow as it ripens.	Leave at room temperature to ripen. The skin will wrinkle, but the fruit will not soften much. Once ripe, store in the refrigerator up to 1 week.
Peach	When selecting fresh peaches, look for ones that are soft to the touch, blemish free, and have a fragrant smell. Peaches that are mildly fragrant ripen into sweet and delicious flavors. Choose fruit that has a background color of yellow or cream and has a fresh looking appearance. Peaches may have some red "blush" depending on the variety, but this isn't a sign of how the fruit will taste after it's ripened. Peaches are highly perishable, so don't buy more than you plan to use. When selecting canned peaches, choose those labeled "packed in its own juice" and "no added sugar"; these are the healthier choices.	The best way to ripen stone fruit is to place the fruit in a paper bag, fold the top of the bag over loosely, and place the bag on the counter for 1 to 3 days. Never store hard fruit in the refrigerator, in plastic bags, or in direct sunlight. Check the fruit daily. When it is ripe, it will be aromatic and will give slightly to gentle pressure. Once ripened, it can be stored in the refrigerator for about a week.
Pear	Sweet, succulent pears are perhaps the most glorious of fall fruits. Avoid pears with bruises or cuts and dark brown color; purchase pears that are slightly green; they ripen better and faster off the tree. Look for pears with a smooth unblemished skin. Ripe ones will yield slightly to gentle pressure at the stem end. If you plan to bake pears, select those that are fairly firm.	If pears are unripe, place them in a paper bag at room temperature for 2 to 3 days or store them in a ventilated fruit bowl in a cool, dark place and refrigerate as soon as they ripen. Ripe pears should be stored in the refrigerator in a plastic bag up to 3 days. They continue to ripen after harvest.
Pineapple	Select pineapples with a nice fragrant smell. If possible, choose pineapples that have been jet shipped from Hawaii or Central America because they will be the freshest. Avoid those with sour or fermented odors. It is really ripe if you can easily pull one of the leaves out of the top.	Store at room temperature for 1 or 2 days before serving to allow the pineapple to become softer and sweeter. Store in the refrigerator for 3 to 5 days or cut pineapple into chunks and store for up to 7 days. Cut up pineapple also freezes well.
Plantain	You can buy plantains at any stage (green, yellow, or black), depending on how you are going to use them and when you want to enjoy them.	Plantains need to be stored at room temperature. After the desired stage of ripeness is reached, refrigerate them 2 to 3 days before cooking to slow ripening. As with other bananas, plantains freeze well.
Plum	Plums should be plump and well colored for their variety. Plums are usually about 3–6 cm. If a fruit yields to gentle pressure, it is ready to eat; however, you can buy plums that are fairly firm, but not rock hard, and let them soften at home. They will not increase in sweetness. Ripe plums will be slightly soft at the stem and tip, but watch out for shriveled skin, mushy spots, or breaks in the skin.	To soften hard plums, place several in a loosely closed paper bag and leave them at room temperature for a day or two; when softened, transfer them to the refrigerator. Ripe plums can be refrigerated for up to 3 days.

Pomegranate	Select fruit that is heavy for its size with a bright, fresh color and blemish-free skin.	Refrigerate whole pomegranates for up to 2 months or store them in a cool, dark place for up to 1 month. Pomegranate seeds packed in an airtight container and stored in the freezer will keep for up to 3 months.
Raspberries	Berries should be dry, firm, well shaped, and eaten within a week after purchase. Select raspberries and blackberries that are unblemished, dry, and in an unstained container. Raspberries should be medium to bright red, depending on the variety.	After purchasing berries, check the fruit and toss out any moldy or deformed ones. Immediately eat the overripe berries within 24 hours. Return the other berries back to the original container or arrange them unwashed in a shallow pan lined with paper towels and wash them just prior to use. The berries may be topped with a paper towel to absorb any additional moisture. Plastic wrap the entire container. This will ensure the fruit retains its freshness, but generally berries should be eaten within 1 week. Eat at room temperature for fullest flavor.
Starfruit	Select firm, shiny, even-colored fruit. Star fruits will ripen at room temperature and have lightly brown edges on the ribs when ripe. Avoid purchasing star fruit with brown, shriveled ribs.	Nonripe star fruit should be turned often until yellow in color and ripe with light brown ribs. Store ripe star fruits at room temperature for 2 to 3 days or unwashed and refrigerated in a plastic bag for up to 1 week.
Strawberries	Berries should be dry, firm, well shaped, and eaten within a week after purchase. Strawberries should be a bright shade of red; the caps on the berries should be green and fresh looking. Berries that are green or yellow are unripe and will taste sour.	After purchasing berries, check the fruit and toss out any moldy or deformed ones. Immediately eat the overripe berries within 24 hours. Return the other berries back to the original container or arrange them unwashed in a shallow pan lined with paper towels and wash just prior to use. The berries may be topped with a paper towel to absorb any additional moisture. Plastic wrap the entire container. This will ensure the fruit retains its freshness, but generally berries should be eaten within 1 week.
Watermelon	Choose firm, symmetrical, fruit free of cracks, bruises, soft spots, or mold. Ripe watermelon will have a healthy sheen, a dry stem, and a buttery yellow underside where it touched the ground. It should have a melon-like smell. If you thump it, the sound should be dull and hollow. It should be heavy for its size.	Once picked, watermelon will not ripen easily. If unripe, try putting the whole melon in a paper bag at room temperature. This sometimes works to ripen it. Uncut watermelons can be kept for up to 2 weeks at room temperature. Wash watermelon with soap and water before cutting. Once cut, package what is not eaten in a closed plastic containers or bag and store in the refrigerator.

Source: Modified from FruitsandVeggiesMatter.gov, Centers for Disease Control and Prevention. Fruits and Vegetables of the Month. Available at: http://www.fruitsandveggiesmatter.gov/month/index.html.

TABLE 10.7
Vegetable Selection Criteria and Storage Tips

Vegetable	Selection Criteria	Storage Tips
Artichoke	High-quality artichokes are usually compact and heavy for their size. When squeezed, a fresh artichoke will make a squeak. The thickness of each stalk should correspond to the size of the artichoke. Thin stalks signal dehydration, so look for stalks that are firm.	Artichokes remain fairly constant in appearance for weeks, but flavor is adversely affected from the moment they are cut from the stalk. For maximum taste and tenderness, cook as soon as possible. Do not stock up on artichokes. Refrigerate them unwashed in a plastic bag for up to 1 week.
Asparagus	Choose firm yet tender stalks. For the green variety, choose stalks with deep green or purplish tips that are closed and compact. Avoid excessively sandy spears. Stalks with a narrow diameter are more tender than thick ones.	Store stalks with bottoms wrapped in a damp paper towel in the crisper section of the refrigerator. If you don't have a crisper, put them in plastic bags and place them in the coldest part of the refrigerator. It is best to eat asparagus the day it is purchased because the flavor lessens with each passing day.
Beans (fresh)	It is best to handpick green beans from a market that sells them loose. To ensure uniform cooking time, select beans of similar size and shape. Choose slender beans (no thicker than a pencil) that are crisp and free of blemishes. The beans should be a bright green color. Do not purchase beans that are stiff or have the seeds visible through the pod because those beans will be tough.	Keep green beans dry in a perforated plastic bag in the refrigerator. They should stay fresh for 4 to 5 days.
Beets	Young, small beets are fine textured, tender, and excellent in salads. Medium and large size beets are good for cooking. Very large roots are too woody for eating, regardless of cooking method. Whichever size you choose, look for smooth, hard, uniformly round beets that are free of cuts and bruises.	It is best to store beets that have their tops chopped off in individual plastic bags in the coolest part of the refrigerator. These should last up to 1 week. The greens should be eaten as soon as possible.
Bell pepper	Bell peppers are available and are in good supply all year, but they are more plentiful and less expensive during the summer months. Fresh bell peppers come in variety of colors, shapes, and sizes. The guidelines for selection are the same for all varieties. The skin should be firm without any wrinkles; the stem should be fresh and green. The pepper should feel heavy for its size. Avoid peppers with sunken areas, slashes, or black spots.	Store unwashed bell peppers in a plastic bag in the refrigerator. They will stay fresh for about a week. Green bell peppers will stay fresh a little longer than the yellow and red ones.
Broccoli	Choose bunches that are dark green. Good color indicates high nutrient value. Florets that are dark green, purplish, or bluish green contain more beta-carotene, an important phytonutrient, and vitamin C than paler or yellowing ones. Choose bunches with stalks that are very firm. Stalks that bend or seem rubbery are of poor quality. Avoid broccoli with open, flowering, discolored, or water-soaked bud clusters and tough, woody stems.	Store broccoli unwashed in an open plastic bag and place in the crisper drawer of refrigerator. It is best when used within a day or two after purchasing.
Broccoli rabe	Broccoli rabe can be found in a refrigerator case sprinkled with ice because it wilts very easily. Choose firm, green, small stems with compact heads and flower buds that are tightly closed and dark green, not open or yellow.	Broccoli rabe should be stored in a refrigerator crisper unwashed, either wrapped in a wet towel or in a plastic bag, for a maximum of 3 days. To keep it longer, blanch and freeze it.
Cabbage	Look for solid, heavy heads of cabbage. Avoid cabbage that has discolored veins or worm damage. Do not buy precut cabbage; the leaves may have already lost their vitamin C. Look for stems that are healthy looking, closely trimmed, and are not dry or split.	Keep cabbage cold. This helps it retain its vitamin C content. Place the whole head of cabbage in a plastic bag and store in the refrigerator. Once the head has been cut, place the remainder in plastic bags and place in the refrigerator. Try to use the remaining cabbage in the next day or two.

Carrots	Look for well-shaped carrots. Pick carrots that are deep orange in color. More beta-carotene is present in carrots that have a darker orange color. Avoid carrots that are crackled, shriveled, soft, or wilted.	Carrots are best stored between 32–50°F (0–10°C) degrees in the crisper section of the refrigerator. If you buy carrots with the green tops still on, break off the tops and rinse, place in a plastic bag, and store as described above. Storing them in the refrigerator will preserve their flavor, texture, and the beta-carotene. Do not store them with fruits. Fruits produce ethylene gas as they ripen. This gas will decrease the storage life of the carrots as well as other vegetables. This is why it is best to store fruits and vegetables separately.
Cauliflower	Look for heads that are white or creamy white, firm, compact, and heavy for their size. There should not be any speckling of discoloration on the head or leaves. Avoid cauliflower with brown patches. A medium-size head will serve four to six people.	Cauliflower will keep for up to 5 days if stored in the crisper section of the refrigerator. If the head is not purchased wrapped, store it in an open or perforated plastic bag. Keep the head stem-side up to prevent moisture from collecting on it. For the best flavor, cauliflower should be eaten as soon as possible. Precut florets do not keep well, and they are best when eaten within a day of purchase.
Celery	Select celery that is compact in shape with firm, crisp ribs and green leaves. Avoid celery that is bruised or discolored.	Celery should be refrigerated in a plastic bag and placed in the crisper for up to 2 weeks. If the ribs are wilted, separate the ribs and place them in a bowl of ice water for several minutes before use.
Chili peppers	Look for firm, glossy chili peppers with taut, unwrinkled skin and fresh green stems. Dried hot peppers should be glossy, yet unbroken.	Chilies should be stored unwashed and wrapped in paper towels in the refrigerator for up to 3 weeks. Dried chilies should be stored in airtight containers at room temperature for a maximum of 4 months. To keep dried chilies for more than 4 months, store them in the refrigerator.
Collard greens	The best collards are found in crisp bunches with the leaves still intact. Collards can also be found canned.	Fresh collards should be stored in the crisper drawer of the refrigerator or in a plastic bag with holes in it.
Corn	Make sure the husks are green, tight, and fresh looking. Pull the husk open to make sure that the ear contains tightly packed rows of plump kernels. The kernels should be smaller at the tip of each ear. Large kernels at the tip is a sign of overmaturity. If you pinch a kernel, milky juice should spurt out.	If the corn is not cooked shortly after it is purchased, then it should be stored in refrigerator. Refrigeration helps the corn retain its sugar and vitamin C content. If you buy unhusked corn, keep it in its husk until you are ready to cook it. This will help the corn retain moisture. To fully enjoy the great taste of sweet corn, cook it as soon as possible. The sooner the better is a good rule of thumb.
Cucumber	Look for firm cucumbers with a rich green color and no soft spots. Do not choose cucumbers that bulge in the middle; this most likely means it is filled with large watery seeds and tasteless flesh.	Whole cucumbers should be refrigerated in a crisper for up to a week. Unwaxed cucumbers will easily lose moisture, so keep them wrapped tightly in plastic.
Eggplant	Look for a symmetrical eggplant with smooth, uniformly colored skin. Tan patches, scars, or bruises indicate decay. Avoid eggplants with wrinkled or flabby-looking skin. Oversized purple eggplants, those greater than 6 inches in diameter, may be tough and bitter. When you press gently on an eggplant, the finger mark will disappear quickly if the eggplant is fresh. Eggplant should feel heavy; one that feels light for its size may not have a good flavor. The stem and cap should be bright green.	Both cold and warm temperatures can damage eggplant. It is best to store eggplant uncut and unwashed in a plastic bag in the cooler section of the refrigerator. Do not force the eggplant into the crisper if it is too big, as this will bruise the vegetable. Eggplant may be blanched or steamed and then frozen for up to 6 months.

(*continues*)

TABLE 10.7
Vegetable Selection Criteria and Storage Tips (*continued*)

Vegetable	Selection Criteria	Storage Tips
Fennel	Select fennel that is firm, has straight stalks, and green leaves. The bulb should be compact in shape with the stalks fairly close and not too spread out. Avoid fennel that is discolored or shows signs of splitting.	Fennel is more delicate than celery and will dry out quickly. Before storing, cut the stalks off, wrap the stalks separately from the bulb in plastic bags, and store in the crisper section of the refrigerator. Fennel should keep for 3 to 4 days, but it is best to use it as soon as possible.
Green onions/scallions	Purchase only green crisp tops and white bottoms. In general, the more slender bottoms will have a sweeter taste.	Store in a refrigerator to avoid mold, and wash thoroughly before using, as the vegetable needs to have dirt and/or sand removed before eating.
Jicama	When purchasing jicama, select tubers that are firm and have dry roots. Make sure that the jicama has unblemished skin.	Store in a refrigerator to avoid mold, and wash thoroughly before using, as the vegetable needs to have dirt and/or sand removed before eating.
Kale	It is best to select small, deep-colored kale bunches with clean leaves. Avoid kale with dry leaves as well as that with dry, browned, yellowed, or coarse stems.	Best when kept at 32°F (0°C), kale should be stored wrapped in plastic in the refrigerator crisper. Kale can only be kept for a few days.
Leeks	Select leeks with clean white bottoms. Make sure the ends are straight and not wider than 1½ inches in diameter; otherwise they will have a tough texture. The tops should be green, crisp, and fresh-looking. Leeks less than 1½ inches in diameter are the most tender.	Store in a refrigerator to avoid mold, and wash thoroughly before using, as the vegetable needs to have dirt and/or sand removed before eating.
Lettuce	Make sure that the leaves are fresh and crisp, with no signs of wilting, slime, or dark spots or edges. Remember that the darker outer leaves are the most nutritious.	Lettuce tends to keep well in plastic bags in the crisper section of the refrigerator. Iceberg lettuce keeps the best, lasting around 2 weeks. Romaine can last 10 days and butterheads types and endives approximately 4 days. The very delicate greens do not last very long, so it's best to buy only as much as you need at one time and use immediately.
Mushrooms	Buy mushrooms from a reputable grower or grocer. Do not eat mushrooms you collect from the wild because there are many poisonous mushrooms. Eating poisonous mushrooms can lead to symptoms of sweating, cramps, diarrhea, confusion, convulsions, and potentially result in liver damage or even death.	Look for firm, moisture-free (not dry), unblemished caps. Make sure they are free of mold. Place loose mushrooms in a paper bag in the refrigerator. Airtight plastic bags tend to retain moisture and will accelerate spoilage. Properly stored mushrooms will last for approximate 5 days.
Onion	Most onions are sold loose by the pound, although some types are sold in bags or small boxes. Look for onions that feel dry and solid all over, with no soft spots or sprouts. The neck should be tightly closed and the outer skin should have a crackly feel and a shiny appearance. Onions should smell mild, even if their flavor is not. Avoid onions with green areas or dark patches.	Onions should be kept in a cool, dry open space away from bright light. Onions do best in an area that allows for air circulation. Because onions absorb moisture, do not store onions under the sink. Also, do not place onions near potatoes because potatoes give off moisture and produce a gas that causes onions to spoil more quickly. Spring/summer onions usually store for about 2 weeks and storage onions for about 3 to 4 weeks.
Parsnips	Select medium-sized roots with uniform creamy beige skin. Avoid limp, pitted, or shriveled roots.	Wrap the unwashed parsnips in a paper towel, wrap them in plastic, and store them in the vegetable crisper for about 2 weeks.
Peas	Look for pods that are firm, glossy, have a slightly velvety feel, and look they are about to burst. Peas should not rattle loosely in the pod. Pods should not be dull, yellowed, or heavily speckled.	It is best to serve all types of fresh peas the day they are purchased. If they must be stored, place them in a perforated plastic bag in the refrigerator. Half of the sugar content of peas will turn to starch within 6 hours if they are kept at room temperature. Low temperatures also preserve their texture and nutrient content. Do not wash them before they are stored. Shell green peas right before you cook them.
Potato	When choosing potatoes, be sure they are firm, smooth, and the color they are supposed to be. Softness, a green tinge, or wrinkly skin may indicate a potato that is past its prime.	Store potatoes in a cool, dry place. Sunlight can cause the skin to turn green; if this occurs, the skin must be peeled off before consuming.

Radish	Radishes with their leaves intact are usually tied in bunches, while topped radishes are sold in plastic bags. If the leaves are attached, they should be crisp and green. Whether red or white, roots should be hard and solid, with a smooth, unblemished surface. Avoid soft or spongy radishes. Be sure to check bagged radishes for mold before purchasing. Black radishes should be solid, heavy, and free of cracks. This variety is often found in Russian or Polish neighborhood stores. Daikons, found in most Asian markets, should be evenly shaped and firm, with a glossy, almost translucent sheen.	If radishes were purchased with the leaves attached, remove the tops unless they will be served the same day. Place radishes in plastic bags, if they are not already packaged, and store in the refrigerator. Most varieties will keep up to 2 weeks in the refrigerator. Black radishes can be stored for months if they remain dry; store them in perforated plastic bags and keep in the refrigerator.
Rhubarb	Spring stalks are the juiciest and most-tender.	Wrap rhubarb in plastic wrap and store it in the coldest part of the refrigerator for up to 1 week. Cooked and raw rhubarb both freeze well.
Spinach	Fresh spinach is usually found loose or bagged. For the best quality, select leaves that are green and crisp, with a nice fresh fragrance. Avoid leaves that are limp, damaged, or spotted. If you are in a rush, grab a bag of fresh, prewashed spinach.	Fresh spinach should be dried and packed loosely in a cellophane or plastic bag and stored in the refrigerator crisper. If stored properly, it should last 3 or 4 days.
Summer squash	Choose squash that are firm and fairly heavy for their size, otherwise they may be dry and cottony inside. Look for squash that have bright, glossy exteriors. Avoid squash with nicks or bruises on the skin or that have soft spots.	Place summer squash in plastic bags and store in the refrigerator. Fresh summer squash should keep for up to a week. Thicker-shinned varieties, such as chayote, will stay fresh for 2 weeks or longer.
Sweet potato	Choose firm, dark, smooth sweet potatoes without wrinkles, bruises, sprouts, or decay. Even if cut away, a decayed spot may have already caused the whole sweet potato to take on an unpleasant flavor.	Sweet potatoes spoil rapidly. Store them in a dry, cool (55–60°F; 13–16°C) place such as a cellar, pantry, or garage. Do not store them in the refrigerator, where they will develop a hard core and an off taste. If stored properly, sweet potatoes will keep for a month or longer. At normal room temperature, they should be used within a week of purchase. Do not wash them before storing them because it will make the sweet potato spoil faster.
Swiss chard	Choose Swiss chard that has crisp stalks and firm, bright leaves.	Like other greens, chard should be wrapped in plastic and kept in the refrigerator for approximately 2 days. If blanched, Swiss chard greens can be frozen. Boil greens for 2 minutes, drain, chill in ice water, drain again, and then pack in an airtight container.
Turnips	Select smooth roots that are firm and heavy with some root hairs at the bottom. In general, the smaller the turnip, the sweeter the taste.	Turnips keep well; cut the greens and bag them separately from the root, placing them in the crisper section of the refrigerator for up to a week.
Winter squash	Winter squash comes in many sizes. Pick a size based on your cooking needs. For a quality squash, choose one with a smooth, dry rind that is free of cracks or soft spots. Skin that is easily nicked or scraped with a fingernail means that the squash did not reach maturity. Look for rind that has a dull appearance. A shiny rind indicates that is has been picked too early or has a wax coating, which masks the skin and makes it inedible when cooked. Choose squash that has a deep color and is heavy for its size. Make sure the stem is present; if the stem is missing, bacteria can enter the squash.	Winter squash has a long shelf life and can be stored for up to 3 months or longer in a cool, dry place (55–60°F; 13–16°C). A higher temperature will shorten the storage time, but it will not alter the flavor. Storage temperatures below 50°F (10°C) will cause squash to spoil more rapidly. If the squash needs to be refrigerated, it can be stored for 1 to 2 weeks. Cut pieces of squash should be tightly wrapped and refrigerated. Cooked, pureed squash can be frozen for use later as a side dish or to thicken, color, or flavor soups, sauces, or stews.
Yucca root	Look for firm blemish-free tubers.	

Source: Modified from FruitsandVeggiesMatter.gov, Centers for Disease Control and Prevention. Fruits and Vegetables of the Month. Available at: http://www.fruitsandveggiesmatter.gov/month/index.html.

Gastronomy Point

Spinach Salad Spinach pairs well with mixed berries. Fresh and dried fruits are fantastic additions to any salad.

heirloom Plants from seed of older times.

Innovation Point

Hardy Produce Plant scientists research ways to create hardy produce that will grow well in various climates. This had been done naturally and by astute farmers for thousands of years. In the 1960s, Dr. Norman Borlaug launched the Green Revolution, breeding crops for developing countries that had much higher yields per acre than traditional varieties. Food production soared, and today he is responsible for having saved millions of lives by increasing global food supplies. Today, modern equipment and methods use genetic engineering to introduce beneficial characteristics to various agricultural varieties.

Green Point

Local Produce Eating fresh, locally grown produce can reduce your carbon footprint by way of minimizing the energy required for processing, packaging, and transportation.

Some are concerned that young people—accustomed to fast food dining, convenience grocery items, and easy take-out venues—no longer know how to cook. Since the global economic downturn that began in 2007, interest has surged in teaching basic cooking skills to children and young adults. Healthy cooking classes have sprung up in cities large and small. Dietitians and chefs have been collaborating to develop menus featuring nutritious, easy-to-cook meals for home, work, and school. See Eating Well at http://www.eatingwell.com for a good example of such a collaboration. Group cooking classes can also be found in many communities.

Food Technology

At present, much of the food Americans eat comes from large corporate farms, both in and out of the United States. Most people are not even aware of which foods at the market are **heirloom**, meaning that they existed before industrial times, and which are genetically modified organisms (GMOs). Botanists and food scientists expend much effort in developing hybrids that combine the best of all produce traits. Such hybrids may be produced by intensive breeding or through genetic engineering.

Controlled manufacturing standards in product development, packaging, storage, and shipping mean that more and more new food products are available on grocery shelves each year. For example, in 2010, Wegman's Supermarkets introduced over 30,000 new foods into its chain of stores.[42] Computerized food sales reports keep detailed records that determine whether a store should continue to carry a particular item or if it should be removed to create space for new offerings. Over the last decade, more and more grocery stores have hired registered dietitians to help focus their brand's health message and to help educate employees and shoppers about eating well and making the best food choices for good health.

Most fruits and vegetables are still available in familiar forms such as bags, cans, boxes, crates, bushels, and bulk. Recent innovations include:

- Vegetables in sealed plastic bags that can be steamed in the microwave
- Freeze-dried vegetables
- Exotic produce options made possible because of modern, rapid, refrigerated transportation
- Edible wax on fruits such as apples, cucumbers, oranges and tomatoes (the wax keeps in moisture and keeps out microbes and dirt)

Going Green

In the United States, scientists and the public are becoming more interested in using environmentally friendly methods to grow, distribute, and cook produce. With regards to growing produce, "green" means using fewer or no pesticides or chemical fertilizers. The green philosophy encourages water, land, and energy conservation at every step of the production cycle.

Organic Produce

In recent years, organic food production has moved from small, isolated operations to large-scale commercial farms. Several grocery chains sell primarily organic foods. Many people confuse organic food with gluten-free or vegetarian foods, but *organic* simply means that the food was grown and produced without added chemicals, such as pesticides, herbicides, fertilizers, antibiotics, hormones, or food additives.

In 1990, the U.S. Congress passed the Organic Foods Production Act (OFPA). Farms that are certified organic are allowed to place the USDA organic symbol on their food products (see **Figure 10.19**).[43] However, certification requires strict adherence to federal guidelines, filing of paperwork, and payment of fees, so some farms choose to not become certified. Read more about organic certification at http://www.ams.usda.gov/AMSv1.0/nop.[43] A guide on making good choices when buying organic food products is available at http://fnic.nal.usda.gov/food-labeling/organic-foods.[44]

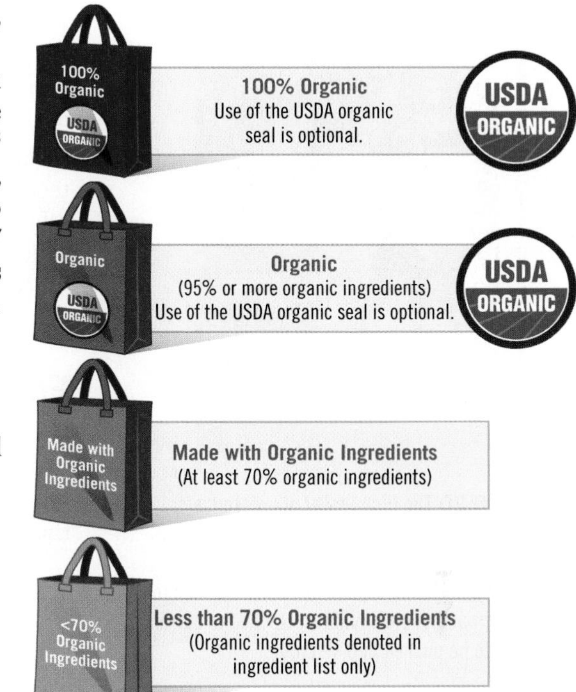

FIGURE 10.19 The USDA organic seal is backed by a set of rigorous federal production and processing standards. Products bearing the USDA seal must be overseen by a USDA National Organic Program-authorized certifying agent, following all USDA organic regulations. They must also be produced without excluded methods (e.g., genetic engineering), ionizing radiation, or sewage sludge and per the National List of Allowed and Prohibited Substances (National List).

Source: Courtesy of the USDA.

Minimizing Cost

Going green does not have to be more expensive than conventional production methods:

- If costs are contained by using fewer resources to grow, transport, and store produce, then cheaper pricing may make produce more affordable.
- Purchasing local produce in bulk or from large bins and crates decreases the cost and waste of packaging materials.
- Locally grown or even organic produce can be cheaper than conventional produce if you comparison shop carefully and buy in season.

Most grocery stores are working to employ as many green initiatives as possible, offering reusable bags and recycling bins for cans and plastics. Thanks to nature, most fruits and vegetables come in their own neat and secure packages of peels, shells, or pods. Leafy greens and smaller fruits such as grapes and berries still require some packaging, principally recyclable plastics.

Saving Energy During Cooking and Storage

Most fruits and some tender vegetables do not need to be cooked. Starchier and bitter-tasting vegetables require cooking but lend themselves well to green cooking methods. Green cooking tips include:

- Turning off the stove once a pot has boiled when boiling or steaming
- Cooking potatoes and other root or tuber vegetables in an oven along with other foods to use immediately or save for later
- Baking multiple meals at the same time
- Cooking food quickly by stir-frying or using microwaving ovens
- Using a solar oven

Canned fruits and vegetables are cooked but are shelf-stable and require no further energy to store. (In contrast, although produce is easy to freeze, it requires electricity to maintain its form.) Green storage tips include:

- Buying only as much as you will use in a week or can store without electricity
- Buying in bulk and sharing with a neighbor
- Buying shelf-stable canned fruits and vegetables instead of frozen ones
- Saving leftovers for use in soups, salads, smoothies, or sauces

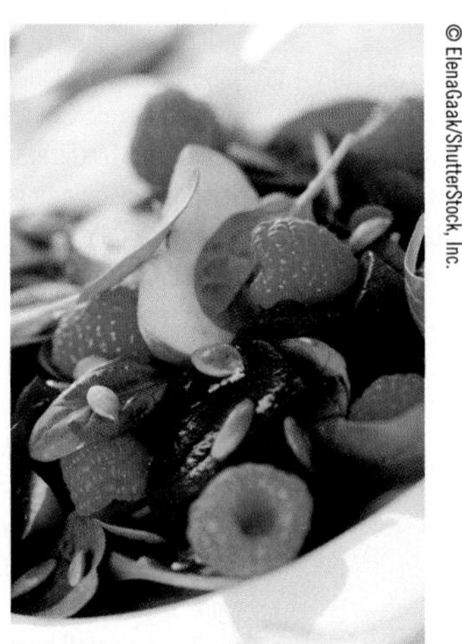

Green Point

Community Supported Agriculture Consider joining a Community Supported Agriculture (CSA) group to support local agriculture. Buying local, fresh produce conserves nutrients and minimizes travel time, resulting in a smaller carbon footprint.

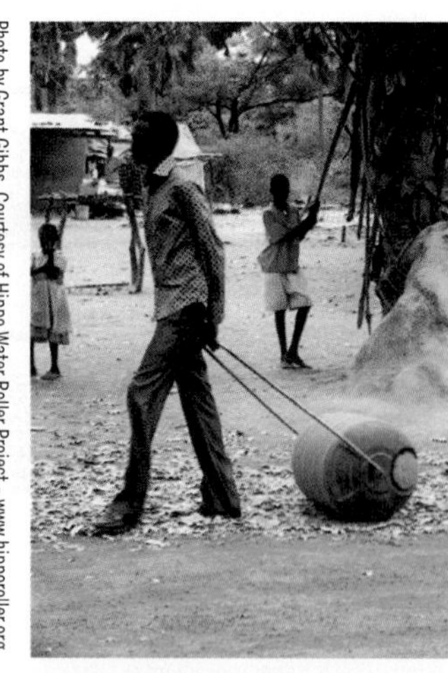
Photo by Grant Gibbs. Courtesy of Hippo Water Roller Project - www.hipporoller.org

FIGURE 10.20 The Hippo roller allows farmers, particularly in developing countries, to carry water more easily than traditional methods. The roller consists of a barrel that holds the water and can roll along the ground. A steel handle attached to barrel enables it to be pushed and steered.

Reducing the Environment Impact of Production

Major concerns with the commercial production of fruits and vegetables include global warming/climate change, acid rain, water conservation, and land preservation, especially of tropical rainforests. The United States has been a leader in helping developing countries manage agriculture with new technologies and genetically engineered crops. Some developing countries adapt to their environment with simple pieces of equipment, such as hippo rollers to carry water long distances from wells to home (see **Figure 10.20**),[45] black garden boxes that conserve irrigation water (see **Figure 10.21**),[46] clay water filters (see **Figure 10.22**),[47] and solar ovens (see **Figure 10.23**).[48]

Food Safety and Regulations

For consumers, food safety begins at the store. Keep raw meats away from fresh produce in your cart. Using a small hand basket inside a larger cart can help keep these foods separate while shopping. Insist that the person bagging the groceries pack them separately as well.

Keep the following food safety guidelines in mind when preparing produce:

- Always wash hands before and after handling foods.
- Avoid cross-contamination with raw meats. Use a special-colored cutting board just for produce, which will help prevent cross-contamination.
- Clean all prep surfaces and wash the produce.
- Chill produce that is susceptible to spoiling.
- Cook foods to appropriate temperatures.

Adhering to these guidelines is especially important whenever produce comes into contact with meats, fish, eggs, or poultry.[49]

Some other tips for produce safety include the following:

- Remove spoiled pieces of fruit or vegetables from others in a bag or package.
- Throw away any bulging or dented canned items to avoid ingesting dangerous bacteria.
- Organize canned goods in the pantry by the use-by date on the can.
- Cut away any green parts under potato skins to avoid solanine poisoning.
- Do not eat uncooked rhubarb leaves, which contain high levels of toxic oxalic acid.

Food technology has made our food system one of the safest in the world, but it takes constant vigilance by all parties along the food delivery chain to ensure that it stays safe. See **Special Topic 10.4** for more information on food safety.

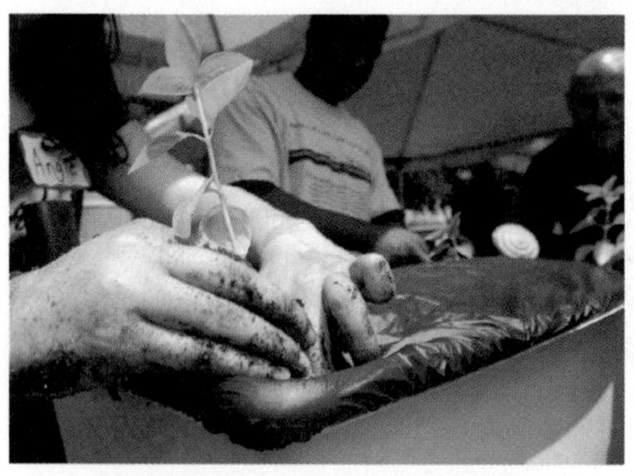
© Richard Levine/Alamy

FIGURE 10.21 Black garden boxes are an innovative way to grow produce in raised boxes. Crops grown in these boxes require less water and fertilizers than those grown in the ground. It allows people to grow food plants in places that normally would not support gardens, such as balconies in urban areas.

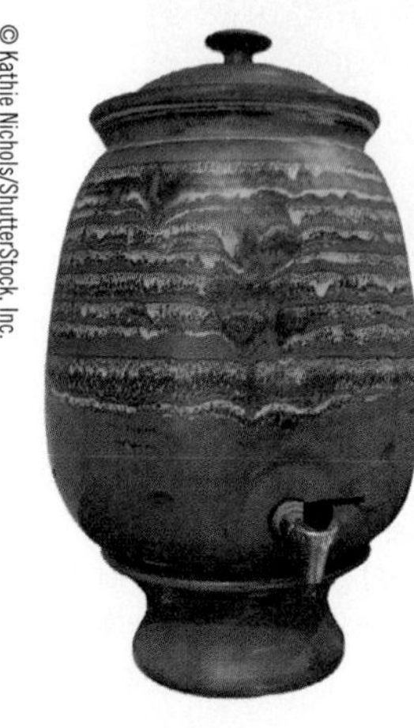
© Kathie Nichols/ShutterStock, Inc.

FIGURE 10.22 Clay water filters are a new technology where water filters are formed from clay, organic matter, and a small amount of water. They are then cooked using manure, rather than a kiln. Studies have shown that these inexpensive and easily made filters are effective in removing more than 90% of *E. coli* from water.

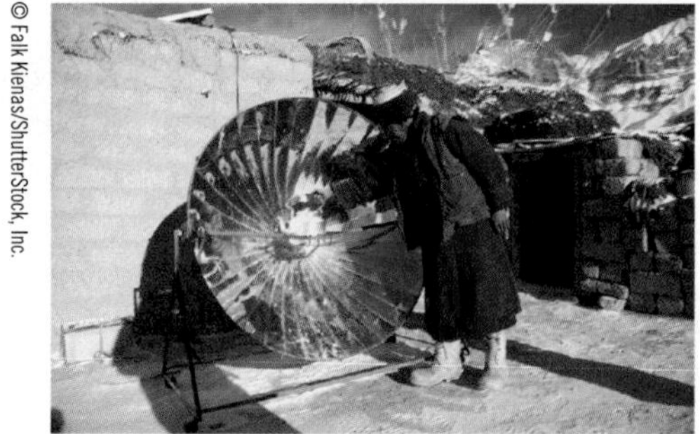
© Falk Kienas/ShutterStock, Inc.

FIGURE 10.23 Solar ovens use energy from sunlight to heat food or beverages. A variety of different types are available, ranging in price from very inexpensive box cookers to more expensive cookers that use solar cells. Solar ovens, because they do not require fuel, cost nothing to operate. Because of this, they may be a good way for people developing countries to decrease their fuel costs while at the same time reducing air pollution and deforestation that result when wood is used as a cooking fuel.

Special Topic 10.4

Food Safety

Emily Kaley

Foodborne illnesses can be prevented by following some easy safety steps when handling, cooking, and storing food. Note that the dangerous bacteria that cause such illnesses in most cases cannot be seen, tasted, or smelled.

Purchasing

The first time you come in contact with your food will be at the grocery store. As you do your shopping, you should be aware of a few things. Never buy food past the sell-by or use-by expiration dates. Check canned foods for dents or bulges. Check the packaging of meats or poultry to make sure the packaging is not torn or leaking. When choosing fresh produce, fish, poultry, or meats, be sure that there are no offensive odors, discolorations, or infestations.

Storing

The next stage of food safety begins when you return home with your groceries. Always refrigerate perishable foods within 2 hours. Especially during the warmer months, you should return home directly after grocery shopping to store food properly. How can you store your food to optimize its shelf life? As soon as you return home, the perishables should be your first priority. Some examples of perishables are high-protein foods, eggs, meats, fish, poultry, dairy, and soft cheeses. Frozen foods should not be allowed to thaw unless you plan on using them within the next few days. After you have put away the perishables, then store your fruits, vegetables, and dry foods. Save the canned goods for last.

Make sure to check the temperature of your refrigerator and freezer so your refrigerator reads 41°F (5°C) or below and your freezer 32°F (0°C) or below. The following order is recommended for storing different raw food on different shelves in the refrigerator. The order, from top to bottom, is ready-to-eat food (e.g., fruits, vegetables), whole fish, whole meat, ground meat, and poultry last. Ground meat and raw poultry are the most likely to leak fluids containing bacteria onto other foods. By storing them on the lower shelves, you can prevent cross-contamination, and therefore foodborne illness.

Most whole, raw fruits and vegetables can be stored at 41°F (5°C) or lower. To prevent fruits and vegetables from drying out, the refrigerator's humidity should be between 85% and 95%. Most produce should not be washed before storage because this can promote the growth of mold. Remember that some fruits and vegetables ripen best at room temperature, including avocados, bananas, pears, and tomatoes.

Dry food and canned goods can be stored between 50°F (10°C) and 70°F (21°C). Make sure to discard damaged cans and keep dry goods off the floor to prevent moisture from damaging the bag or container.

Preparing

Food preparation can be a smooth process by following a few simple steps. The first step in preparing your food is washing your hands. Apply soap and make sure to keep your hands under warm running water for 20 seconds. If you are switching from between meat or fish and fresh produce, you need to wash your hands in between. Cutting boards, utensils, and countertops can be sanitized by using a solution of 1 tablespoon of unscented, liquid chlorine bleach in 1 gallon of water. Make sure to assign cutting boards to different foods (e.g., a red cutting board for meats and a green cutting board for vegetables).

Thaw food in a safe way to prevent the growth of bacteria. The three ways to thaw food are in the refrigerator, submerged under running water, and in the microwave. The refrigerator allows for slow, safe thawing. Make sure that juice from thawing meat or poultry does not drip onto other food. For faster thawing, place food in a leak-proof plastic bag. Submerge the bag in cold tap water and either keep the water running or change the water every 30 minutes. Be sure to cook immediately after thawing. Microwave thawing can start cooking the product, so cook the food immediately after the thawing.

Some cooked foods must reach certain internal temperatures for a specific amount of time to ensure their safety. Use a cooking thermometer to check the internal temperatures of the following foods:

- Poultry, pasta, and food cooked in a microwave: 165°F (73°C) for 15 seconds
- Ground meat, injected meat, and mechanically tenderized meat: 155°F (68°C) for 15 seconds
- Pork, beef, veal, lamb, seafood, and shell eggs: 145°F (63°C) for 15 seconds
- Ready-to-eat-foods: 135°F (57°C)

If these foods do not reach the correct temperature, prolong the cooking process or discard the food.

Serving

Safe food handling continues during the serving process. Food must be protected from time and temperature. Hot foods need to be kept at 135°F (57°C) or hotter and cold food at 41°F (5°C) or colder. The internal temperature of the food should be checked every 4 hours. If it is not the correct temperature, it needs to be discarded. To protect food from contaminants, use covers and lids if the food is not eaten right away.

Gastronomy Point

Cinnamon A sprinkle of cinnamon or fresh mint will add extra flavor to fruits. Fresh, julienned basil strips are a fabulous addition to vegetable dishes. Use kitchen shears to snip washed herbs into dishes.

The FDA has regulatory jurisdiction over fruits and vegetables sold for human consumption. In January 2011, President Obama signed the Food Safety Modernization Act into law. The new law gives the FDA the authority to order a recall for contaminated food instead of waiting for manufacturers to do so voluntarily. Facility and import inspections will occur more frequently, and improved prevention plans will be implemented. Production and harvesting standards will be science-based and provide flexibility for small farms. A collaborative food safety approach will include federal, state, and local partners.[50,51]

Chapter Review

Fruits and vegetables are a vital part of the human diet and an important component of every culture. Over the millennia, fruits and vegetables have traveled by land, water, and air to and from every continent. Research is ongoing on the best ways to grow, store, transport, sell, and cook fruits and vegetables. Despite a few cooking challenges, only basic cooking knowledge is necessary to prepare and serve produce in a safe and healthy fashion.

At meals, half the plate should be fruits and vegetables. The USDA's MyPlate guidelines recommend 2 cups of fruit and 2½ cups of vegetables per day for a 2,000-calorie diet. Fruits and vegetables are rich sources of carbohydrates, water, vitamins, minerals, phytonutrients, and fiber.

It is easy to consider green initiatives when choosing and preparing produce. Support local farmers, eat seasonal foods with minimal packaging, and use organic produce. Also make sure to prepare, cook, and use produce efficiently.

Learning Portfolio

Study Points

1. Approximately 50% of the foods eaten in the world today had their origins in the Americas. There are roughly 300,000 edible plants in the world, but only about 2,000 are cultivated.
2. Climate, soil conditions, traditions, and religion all help determine menus for different cultures. Modern transportation, agricultural developments, adventure, and curiosity are drivers of fusion cuisine.
3. Fruits are the developed ovaries of a plant and contain the seeds. Vegetables are any other part of the plant: root, stem, or leaf.
4. The primary parts of a plant cell are the cell wall, cell membrane, cytoplasm, nucleus, chloroplasts, amyloplasts, and vacuole.
5. Plants store their energy as starch, a carbohydrate derived from the glucose made during photosynthesis in chloroplasts.
6. Fruits and vegetables are good sources of energy, fiber, vitamins, minerals, and phytonutrients, while being naturally low in calories.
7. Thousands of phytonutrients have been identified in plants. They include flavonoids, carotenoids, and other pigments, which determine a plant's color, flavor, and aroma. Some phytonutrients provide health benefits, including roles in preventing some cancers, heart disease, and inflammation and in promoting eye health.
8. Most produce should be cooked until tender, but crisp, using minimal water and time. Suggested cooking methods include: steaming, stir-frying, sautéing, microwaving, grilling, baking, broiling, and pressure cooking.
9. Fruits and vegetables are an important part of eating well for good health and should comprise about 50% of a meal. Include fruits and vegetables of a variety of colors to get the most nutrients. A 2,000-calorie diet should include 2 cups of fruit and 2½ cups of vegetables.
10. The use of green initiatives in growing, shipping, shopping, storing, cooking, and serving fruits and vegetables will help the environment and provide the most health benefits for the least cost.

Issues for Discussion

1. Discuss the pros and cons of genetically modified produce, both in developed and in developing countries.
2. Debate the positive and negative aspects of organic farming and consumption.
3. Explore the causes of hunger causes, its effects, and potential remedies in the United States and abroad. (Information can be found at http://www.who.org, http://www.fao.org, http://www.strength.org, and http://maps.ers.usda.gov/FoodAtlas).
4. Offer reasons for and against disguising fruits and vegetables in toddler meals.
5. Debate the pros and cons of using added salt and sugar on foods.
6. Watch and review a food documentary such as *Food Inc.*, *Food Fight*, or *Forks over Knives.*

Research Ideas for Students

1. Health benefits of functional foods and appropriate food-labeling laws
2. Benefits of various fiber types and sources
3. Roles of various phytonutrients
4. Symptoms and diseases caused by lack of produce intake
5. Ways to encourage the public to register to receive food safety recall alerts from http://www.foodsafety.gov
6. Seasonal grocery produce availability, promotions, and prices by region
7. The history of vitamin identification

Key Terms

	page
amyloplast	311
blanching	315
carotenoids	312
climacteric fruits	326
chloroplasts	311
chromoplasts	312
cytoplasm	309
freezer burn	315
heirloom	336
lycopene	318
nonclimacteric fruits	326
phenolic compounds	311
photosynthesis	309
pome	323
resveratrol	318
stone	323
vacuole	311

8. Ethnic differences in fruit and vegetable consumption
9. Sustainability of the produce supply
10. Pros and cons of organic produce
11. Nutrient preservation in food storage and preparation

References

1. Standage T. *An Edible History of Humanity*. New York: Walker & Company; 2009.
2. Brown S. *Scurvy*. New York: Thomas Dunne Books; 2003.
3. Duyff RL. *American Dietetic Association Complete Food and Nutrition Guide*. Hoboken, NJ: John Wiley & Sons; 2002.
4. U.S. Apple Association. Apples in History. Available at: http://www.usapple.org/consumers/all-about-apples/history-and-folklore/apple-in-history. Accessed October 30, 2012.
5. Kiple K, Ornelas KC. *Cambridge World History of Food*. Cambridge: Cambridge University Press; 2000.
6. Davidson A. *Oxford Companion to Food*. Oxford: Oxford University Press; 1999.
7. *American Heritage Science Dictionary*. Boston: Houghton Mifflin; 2005: 247.
8. McGee H. *On Food and Cooking: The Science and Lore of the Kitchen*. New York: Scribner; 2004.
9. U.S. Department of Agriculture. Choose MyPlate. Available at: http://www.choosemyplate.gov. Accessed July 27, 2011.
10. Painter J, Rah J, Lee Y. Comparison of international food guide pictorial representations. *J Am Diet Assoc.* 2002; 102(4):483–489.
11. Food and Agriculture Organization of the United Nations. Available at: http://www.fao.org/ag/humannutrition/nutrition-education/fbdg/en. Accessed January 2, 2011.
12. Goody CM, Drago L. *Cultural Food Practices*. Chicago: American Dietetic Association; 2010.
13. Menzel P, D'Aluisio F. *What I Eat: Around the World in 80 Diets*. Napa, CA: Material World Book; 2010.
14. Oldways. Oldways Culinarias: Delicious Cultural Immersion. Available at: http://www.oldwayspt.org/eventsandtours/culin-arytours. Accessed January 4, 2011.
15. Topor M. Boston North End Market Tours. Available at: http://www.bostonfoodtours.com. Accessed October 30, 2012.
16. American Institute for Cancer Research. Get the Facts on Fiber. Available at: http://www.aicr.org/site/PageServer?pagename=elements_fiber. Accessed January 10, 2011.
17. The Structure of a Plant Cell. Available at: http://www.biologie.uni-hamburg.de/b-online/e04/04a.htm. Accessed January 2, 2011.
18. Yahoo Answers. Where in a Plant Would You Find Glucose, DNA, Proteins, Lipids, Starch and Cellulose? Available at: http://answers.yahoo.com/question/index?qid=20090306172646AAdrnDe. Accessed January 2, 2011.
19. Produce for Better Health. Phytochemical Information Center. Available at: http://pbhfoundation.org/about/res/pic/phytolist/. Accessed October 29, 2012.
20. This H. *Kitchen Mysteries*. New York: Columbia University Press; 2007.
21. Labensky SR, Hause AM, Martel PA. *On Cooking: A Textbook of Culinary Fundamentals*. Boston: Pearson. 2011;592–593.
22. U.S. Department of Agriculture. My Food-A-Pedia. Available at: http://www.MyFoodapedia.gov. Accessed February 16, 2011.
23. Anderson J, Perryman S, Young L, Prior S. Dietary Fiber. Colorado State University Extension. Available at: http://www.ext.colostate.edu/pubs/foodnut/09333.html. Accessed January 2, 2011.
24. U.S. Department of Health and Human Services, US Department of Agriculture. *Dietary Guidelines for Americans, 2005*. 6th ed. Washington, DC: US Government Printing Office; January 2005.
25. U.S. Department of Agriculture. USDA National Nutrient Database for Standard Reference, Release 20, Nutrient Lists. Available at: http://www.ars.usda.gov/Main/docs.htm?docid=15869. Accessed July 27, 2011.
26. Fox MK, Condon E, Briefel R, et al. Food consumption patterns of young preschoolers: Are they starting off on the right path? *J Am Diet Assoc.* 2010 Dec;(suppl 3):S52–S59.
27. Centers for Disease Control and Prevention. About the National Health and Nutrition Examination Survey. Available at: http://www.cdc.gov/nchs/nhanes/about_nhanes.htm. Accessed January 2, 2011.
28. Sebastian RS, Cleveland LE, Goldman JD. Effect of snacking frequency on adolescents' dietary intakes and meeting national recommendations. *J Adol Health.* 2008 May;42(5):503–511.
29. Heber D. Phytochemicals beyond antioxidation. *J Nutr.* 2004;134(11):3175S–3176S.
30. Zied E. *Nutrition at Your Fingertips*. New York: Penguin; 2009.
31. Wegener D, Jansen G. Antioxidant capacity in cultivated and wild *Solanum* species: The effect of wound stress. *Food and Funct.* 2010;1:209–218.
32. Pan M, Lai C, Ho C. Anti-inflammatory activity of natural dietary flavonoids. *Food Funct.* 2010;1:15–31.
33. International Food Information Council. Functional foods: Can they reduce your risk of cancer? *Food Insight.* Available at: http://www.foodinsight.org/Newsletter/Detail.aspx?topic=Functional_Foods_Can_They_Reduce_Your_Risk_of_Cancer. Accessed January 6, 2011.
34. RSC Publishing. Food and Function. Available at: http://www.rsc.org/foodfunction. Accessed January 4, 2011.
35. Pom Wonderful. Available at: http://www.pomwonderful.com/health/poms-unique-antioxidants. Accessed October 30, 2012.
36. U.S. Department of Health and Human Services, U.S. Department of Agriculture. *Dietary Guidelines for Americans, 2010*. 7th ed. Washington, DC: U.S. Government Printing Office; 2010.
37. Campbell TC, Campbell TM II, Lyman H, Robbins J. *The China Study: The Most Comprehensive Study of Nutrition Ever Conducted and the Startling Implications for Diet, Weight Loss and Long-term Health*. Dallas, TX: Benbella Books; 2006.
38. Mangels R. Vegetarian Nutrition for Teenagers. Vegetarian Resource Group. Available at: http://www.vrg.org/nutrition/teennutrition.htm. Accessed January 2, 2011.
39. Lindbloom E. Long-term benefits of a vegetarian diet. *Am Fam Physician.* 2009 Apr;79(7):541–542.
40. Craig WJ, Mangels AR. Position of the American Dietetic Association: Vegetarian diets. *J Am Diet Assoc.* 2009 Jul;109(7):1266–1282.
41. Whitt SR, Wilson LM, Tenaillon MI, et al. Genetic diversity and selection in the maize starch pathway. *PNAS*. October 1,

2002;99(20):12959-12962. Available at: http://www.pnas.org/content/99/20/12959.full. Accessed January 2, 2011.

42. Andrews J. Wegmans: TEDxRochester. Available at: http://www.youtube.com/watch?v=P81ABzf5N4g&feature=email. Accessed February 16, 2011.
43. U.S. Department of Agriculture. Welcome to the National Organic Program. Available at: http://www.ams.usda.gov/AMSv1.0/nop. Accessed July 28, 2011.
44. U.S. Department of Agriculture. Organic Foods. Available at: http://fnic.nal.usda.gov/food-labeling/organic-foods. Accessed October 30, 2012.
45. Hippo Water Roller Project. Available at: http://www.hipporoller.org. Accessed February 16, 2011.
46. The Growing Connection of the Food and Agriculture Organization of the United Nations. Earth Box.com. Available at: http://www.thegrowingconnection.org. Accessed February 16, 2011.
47. Potters for Peace. Available at: http://www.pottersforpeace.org. Accessed February 16, 2011.
48. Solar Cookers International. Available at: http://www.solarcooking.org. Accessed February 16, 2011.
49. U.S. Department of Agriculture, Food and Drug Administration, Centers for Disease Control and Prevention. The Basics: Clean, Separate, Cook and Chill. Available at: http://www.foodsafety.gov/keep/basics. Accessed January 5, 2011.
50. Hamburg M, U.S. Department of Agriculture, Food and Drug Administration, Centers for Disease Control and Prevention. What Does the New Food Safety Law Mean for You? Available at: http://www.foodsafety.gov/blog/fsma.html. Accessed January 11, 2011.
51. Food and Drug Administration. Food Safety Legislation Key Facts. Available at: http://www.fda.gov/Food/FoodSafety/FSMA/ucm237934.htm. Accessed October 30, 2012.

CHAPTER 11

Grains, Cereals, Pasta, Flour, and Starch Cookery

Diane K. Tidwell, PhD, RD

Chapter Objectives

THE STUDENT WILL BE EMPOWERED TO:

- Describe the history of the use and cultivation of grains.
- List and describe common cereal grains, less common grains, and plants used as grains but that technically are not grains.
- Identify the structure and composition of the cereal kernel.
- Describe the process of refining cereal flours by milling, and explain how this affects the qualities of cereal foods.
- Explain the formation and importance of gluten, and give examples of gluten and gluten-free flours.
- List the three methods of cooking cereal grains.
- Describe the major classes of wheat, and list typical wheat products.
- Describe the production and cooking of pasta.
- Summarize the types of rice, corn, and other plants used as grains, and provide examples of the food products made from them.
- Discuss the invention of breakfast cereals and define the different types.
- Summarize the nutritional properties of grains.
- Discuss strategies to make the production of cereal grains and their packaging more environmentally friendly.
- Recall food safety issues and regulations specific to grains.

cereals Edible kernels from plants of the grass family.

grain General term for all cereals and cereal plants.

Historical, Cultural, and Ecological Significance

The edible seeds from members of the grass family (Gramineae) are called cereal grains, or **cereals**. Both the fruit (the seed or kernel) and the plant are referred to as a **grain**. The word *cereal* is derived from *Ceres*, the Roman goddess of agriculture and fertility. Her name is from the Latin word *creare*, or *creation*, and reflects Ceres' ability to produce food. The goddess Ceres was also a symbol of abundance, nurturance, and cultivation as well as of the harvesting and threshing of grains and the production of flour and bread. A statue of Ceres sits on top of the dome of the Chicago Board of Trade building, a major center for the trading of agricultural commodities. The ancient Romans are generally credited with being the first to turn the grinding of grain into an industry and using sifting to create refined white bread.

Cereal grains are grown in greater quantities compared to other crops and are referred to as *staple crops*. Grains are essential for sustaining animal and human life and are the most important component of the world's food supply. The main staple cereal crops worldwide are wheat, rice, corn (maize), barley, sorghum, oats, rye, and millets. Less common cereals and plants that are used as cereals but that are not technically cereals include amaranth, buckwheat, quinoa, spelt, teff, and triticale. Grains are grown worldwide. The specific grains grown in a region varies based on the physical environment. See **Figure 11.1** for world production of the major cereal crops based on land area.[1]

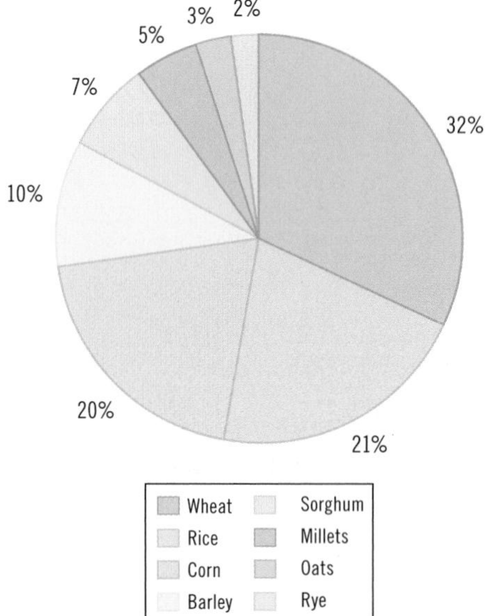

FIGURE 11.1 This map of world cereal production based on land area shows the importance of wheat, which comprises 32% of all land used for cereal production.

Source: Data from Dendy DAV, Dobraszczyk BJ (eds.). *Cereals and Cereal Products: Chemistry and Technology.* Gaithersburg, MD: Aspen Publishers; 2001.

Although there are over 50,000 edible plants, three—wheat, rice, and corn—provide over 60% of the world's food energy intake. Using grains as staple foods is an economical and ecological necessity for many nations. With 10 acres of cultivated land, approximately 24 people could be fed for 1 year with a rice crop, about 15 people with a crop of wheat, and only 1 person if the same amount of land was used for animal production.[2]

Many domesticated varieties of grains are believed to have originated in southwestern Asia many centuries ago. Cultivation spread throughout the Fertile Crescent of the Middle East around 8500 B.C. and into the Nile Valley around 4000 B.C. Some of the earliest remains of wheat crops have been found in Syria, Jordan, Turkey, and eastern Iraq.

Wheat

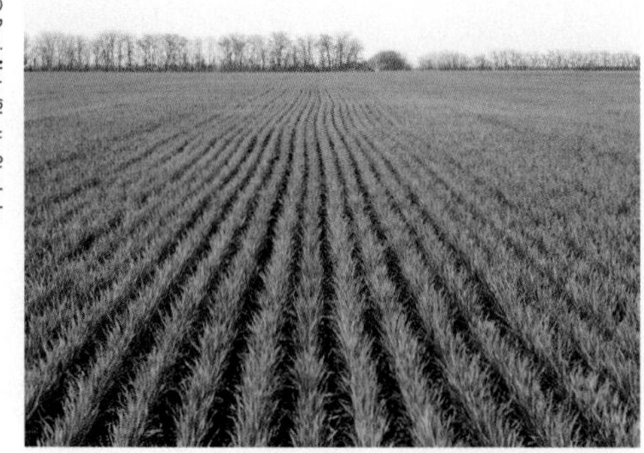

FIGURE 11.2 Modern wheat is adapted to fairly dry and mild climates. Winter wheat, which is planted from September to November, is planted in narrow channels called furrows. The snow fills the furrows and protects the plants from the cold. Spring wheat is planted from early March to mid-April. It has a shorter growing period than winter wheat.

Wheat has been cultivated for thousands of years and is grown on more land area than any other crop (see **Figure 11.2**). Wheat can be grown in harsh environments that are too dry and cold for rice and corn production.

Specialty wheat crops (*Triticum* spp.) include spelt (*T. spelta*), einkorn (*T. baeoticum*), and emmer (*T. dicoccum*). These ancient varieties of wheat are regaining in popularity, especially in Central Europe. Modern wheat (*T. aestivum*) is believed to have evolved from these three varieties. Experts believe that the ancient varieties of wheat originated in the Near East thousands of years ago and then spread to Europe and other parts of the world. Researchers have found that Asian spelt is genetically related to modern wheat.[3]

Spelt (*T. spelta*) is similar to modern wheat in that it can be used to produce bread, pasta, and other baked products. Spelt has the familiar taste and texture of modern wheat, but it differs in several ways. Modern wheat has been developed to have loose husks that can be easily removed from the kernels; in contrast, spelt kernels have tough husks that are not easily removed. Spelt is a hardier grain than wheat and can grow in a wider range of environmental conditions, although it has lower yields than wheat. The more difficult hulling and milling and lower crop yields have resulted in less interest in growing spelt in the United States.

Spelt is a popular grain in Italy, especially in the areas of Tuscany, Lazio, Umbria, and Abruzzo; in Italian it is called *farro*.[4] Spelt also is popular in regions of Germany and Switzerland, where it is called *dinkle*. Swiss immigrants in Ohio are credited for bringing spelt to the United States. Spelt was the primary grain used for flour production until approximately 1920, when modern wheat became the more popular grain to use for flour production.

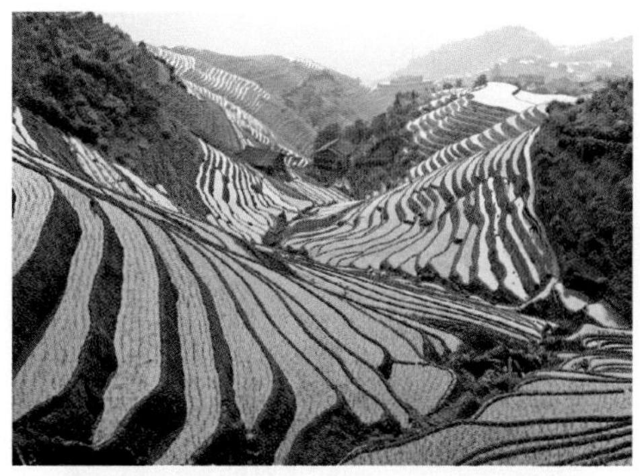

© Hung Chung Chih/ShutterStock, Inc.

FIGURE 11.3 Rice cultivation is labor intensive and requires a great deal of water. Rice is cultivated in wet fields called paddies. Varieties of rice can be grown at high altitudes, and, in some regions, paddies are terraced up the sides of hills and mountains.

Rice

Rice (*Oryza* spp.) is a staple food for billions of people (see **Figure 11.3**). The vast majority of the world's rice crop is grown in Asia, where it is a symbol of fertility. In some Asian languages and dialects, the words that refer to eating literally mean "to eat rice." Rice provides more than 50% of the daily calories for more than half of the world's population.

Corn

Corn (*Zea mays*) originated in Central America. European explorers found corn fields throughout Central America, where it had been used as a dried grain for thousands of years (see **Figure 11.4**). The European explorers brought corn back with them to Europe, and its cultivation quickly spread. Today, the majority of the world's corn crop is grown in the United States. Outside of the United States, corn is called *maize*.

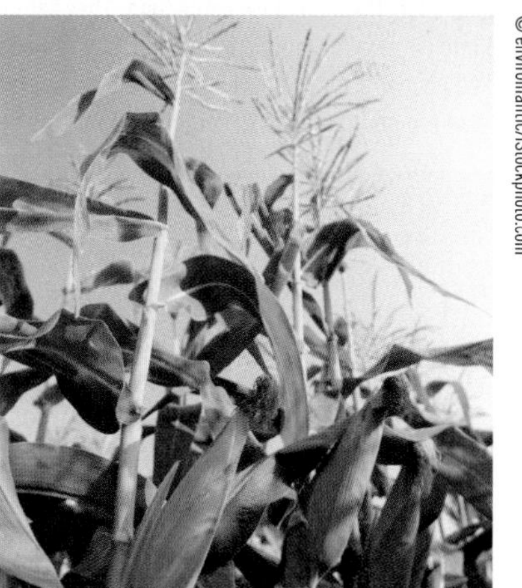

© enviromantic/iStockphoto.com

FIGURE 11.4 The corn plant has a leafy stalk that produces ears with seeds that are called kernels. Although technically a grain, corn often is consumed as a vegetable. It can grow in a variety of different climates, which has aided its spread throughout the world.

Barley

Barley (*Hordeum vulgare*) is one of the oldest cultivated cereal grains (see **Figure 11.5**). Evidence suggests that it was grown thousands of years ago in the Fertile Crescent along with wheat. In ancient times, barley was the more abundant of the two cereals. Barley was brought to North America by Columbus on his second voyage in 1494. In the United States, 65% of the barley crop is used for animal feed; 30% is used for malt and alcohol production. Barley is used as a human food product primarily in Ethiopia, India, China, and Morocco.[5]

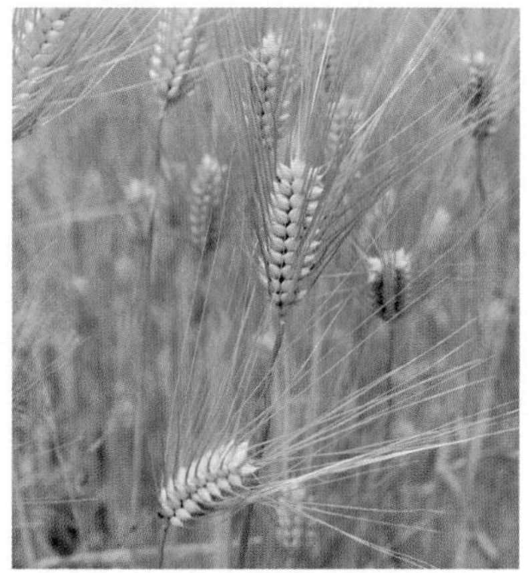

© iStockphoto/Thinkstock

FIGURE 11.5 Barley was one of the first domesticated grains in the Fertile Crescent. Humans have long used barley in the production of bread, beer, and distilled spirits.

Oats

Oats (*Avena sativa*) were not cultivated as early in history as most other cereals (see **Figure 11.6**). The oldest oat grains, which were discovered in Egypt, indicate that oats were cultivated around 2000 B.C. Oats were brought to North America in the early seventeenth century and planted in Massachusetts. Today, the middle and upper Mississippi Valley are major areas of production in the United States. Oats have been used for livestock feed and human food for centuries.

Rye and Triticale

Rye (*Secale cereale*) is related to wheat and barley (see **Figure 11.7**). Rye can grow in poorer soils and much colder climates than most other grains,

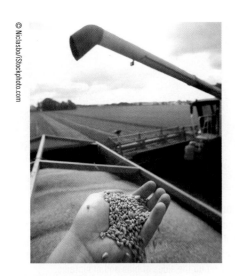

© Niclasbo/iStockphoto.com

FIGURE 11.6 Oats are a versatile food. They can be rolled into oatmeal or ground into flour. They can be used in baked goods, such as oatmeal cookies and oat breads. Oats also are an ingredient in cereals such as granola.

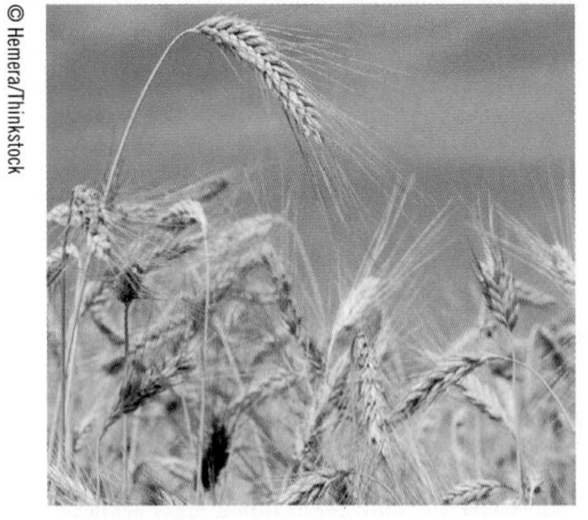

© Hemera/Thinkstock

FIGURE 11.7 Rye is most commonly grown for grain and for forage. The grain is used as a flour to produce rye bread. The grain also is used in the production of alcoholic beverages such as beer, whiskey, and vodka.

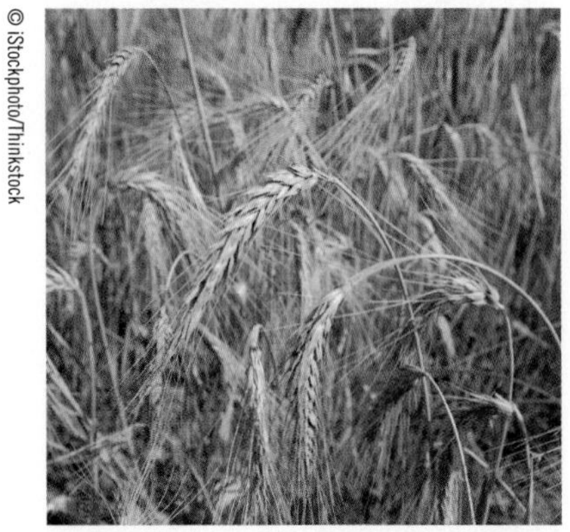

© iStockphoto/Thinkstock

FIGURE 11.8 The goal in developing and refining triticale is to improve food production and nutrition in developing countries. Triticale has a higher protein content and more lysine than wheat. Today, it is used primarily as animal fodder, but there is potential that it can be used in baked goods and cereals.

and it is a valuable crop in areas where farming conditions are too poor for grain production. Triticale (X *Triticosecale*), the first manmade cereal, is a hybrid of wheat (*Triticum* spp.) and rye (*Secale cereale*) and exhibits properties of both cereals (see **Figure 11.8**). It was first developed in 1875, but the seeds were sterile. In 1888, the first fertile triticale seeds were developed, but it was not until 1935 that the word *triticale* appeared.[4] Triticale has higher amounts of the essential amino acid lysine than wheat or other common grains, although the overall amount of protein is lower in triticale than in wheat. Triticale flour performs like soft wheat in baked products and is usually mixed with wheat flour. Triticale is used more in Europe than in the United States.

Sorghum

Sorghum (*Sorghum* spp.) is a major food crop in parts of Africa, Central America, China, India, and Pakistan (see **Figure 11.9**). It grows in hot, dry regions of the world where corn and other grains cannot be grown successfully. It is estimated that sorghum requires about one-third less water than corn.[4] Sorghum also is known as chicken corn, guinea corn, and kafficorn. As sorghum grows, it resembles the corn plant, but mature sorghum does not look like corn other than the stalk. A head containing hundreds of sorghum berries grows out of the center of the stalk. The berries range in color from light to very dark and from yellow to red or bronze, depending on the variety. The lighter berries are used for food; the dark varieties are typically used for animal feed.[4]

Sorghum is the fifth leading grain crop in the world, after wheat, rice, corn, and barley. In most parts of the world, more than 50% of the sorghum grown is used for human consumption. However, about 98% of sorghum grown in the United States is used for animal feed, with only 2% used for food and alcohol production. Cultivated types of sorghum include broomcorn, grain, grass, and sweet sorghums. Broomcorn has stiff branches that are used to make brooms. Grain sorghum (*S. vulgare*) is used in porridge, unleavened bread, and beer. Grass sorghum is grown for animal feed. Sweet sorghum is processed into molasses, syrups, and sugar; the stalks can be chewed like sugarcane. Sorghum kernels are milled into flakes, flour, or puffed and used in cereals, snacks, granola cereals and bars, and other baked goods. Many types of sorghums produce mild-flavored flours that blend well with other flours.[4]

Millets

Millets are cereal grains with small kernels that are indigenous to many areas of the world (see **Figure 11.10**). The many types of millet are well adapted to poor soil conditions, low moisture, and hot environments, conditions frequently found in the subtropics. Millets have very hard husks and lower crop yields than other cereals. However, because millets can be grown in harsh environments, they provide nourishment to many people in African and Asian countries. In the United States, millets are used mainly for animal fodder and birdseed.

Teff (*Eragrostis tef*) is a type of millet native to the northern Ethiopian highlands of northeast Africa (see **Figure 11.11**). This ancient grain is having a resurgence in popularity. Like other millets, teff grows well in poor environmental conditions. The word *teff* comes from the Amharic word *teffa*, which means "lost;" if you drop a teff seed, it is lost due to its very tiny size. The seeds vary in color from light to dark, with the lighter varieties having a milder taste.

Other Plants Used as Grains

Wild rice, buckwheat, amaranth, and quinoa (pronounced KEEN-wa) are not technically grains, but they are important plants used as grains.

Wild Rice

Wild rice (*Zizania aquatica*) is a reedlike plant that grows wild in wetlands. It is harvested in the Great Lakes region of the United States and parts of Canada. It was a traditional food of Native Americans who lived in these areas. Today, it also is being cultivated commercially.

Buckwheat

Despite its name, buckwheat (*Fagopyrum esculentum*) is not a form of wheat. Buckwheat is related to sorrels and knotweeds. The name *buckwheat* comes from the Dutch word *bockweit*, indicating the seeds' resemblance to the seeds of the beech tree and the similarity of its flour to wheat flour (see **Figure 11.12**).

Amaranth

Amaranth (*Amaranthus* spp.) is an annual herb native to Central and South America that produces large seed heads containing thousands of tiny seeds (see **Figure 11.13**). Amaranth is an ancient food of the Aztec, Incan, and Mayan peoples. It was a staple food in pre-Columbian times; however, in an attempt to conquer and demolish native cultures, Spanish conquistadors in

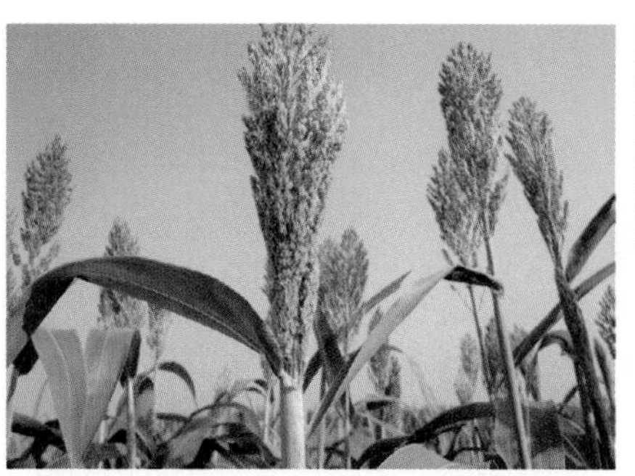

FIGURE 11.9 Sorghum is relatively drought tolerant. It is one of the most important food crops in semiarid areas in Africa and Asia and is a good source of energy, protein, vitamins, and minerals. In other parts of the world, it is primarily used as animal feed.

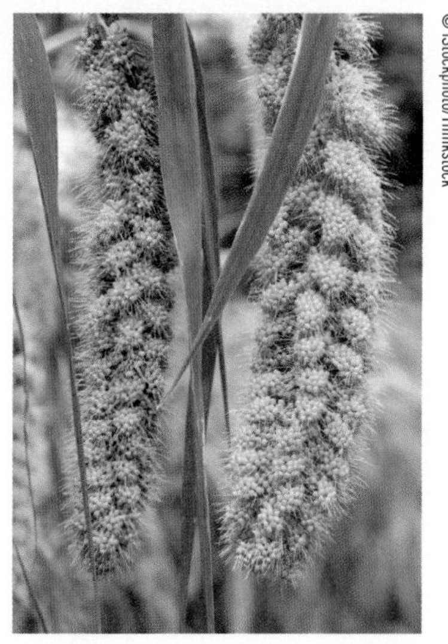

FIGURE 11.10 The most popular forms of millet are pearl millet and finger millet. The raw seeds are not suitable for human consumption; millet must be cooked before it is eaten.

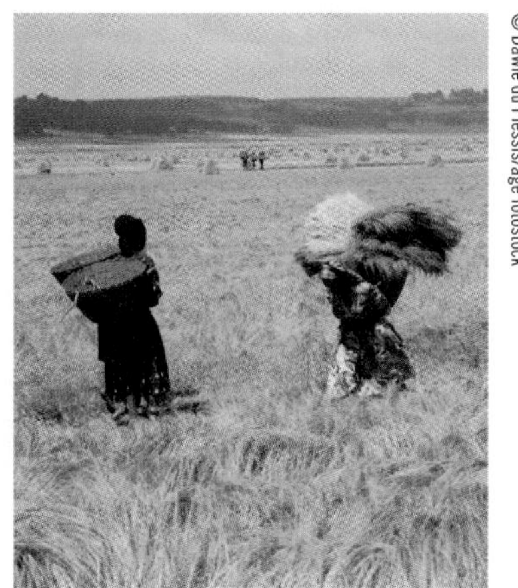

FIGURE 11.11 Teff is an important millet in Africa. In Ethiopia and Eritrea, it is used to make injera, a type of fermented flatbread with a spongy texture and a slightly sour taste.

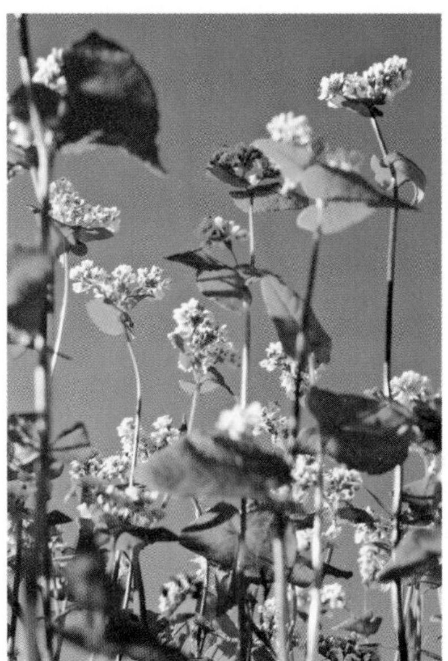

FIGURE 11.12 Buckwheat fruits can be milled to produce buckwheat flour. This flour can be used to make buckwheat noodles, also called soba noodles, which are important in Japanese and Korean cuisines.

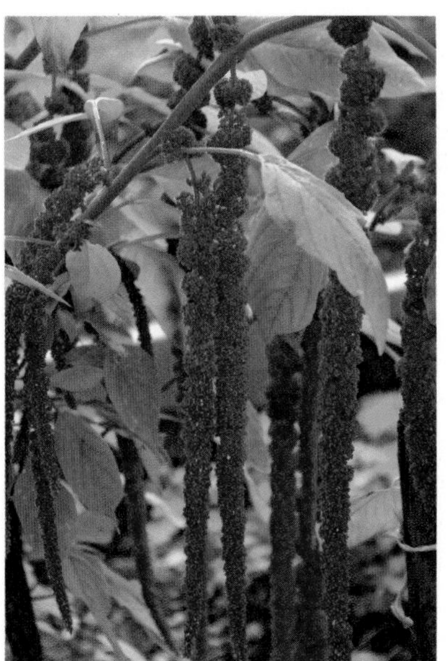

FIGURE 11.13 Amaranth is a drought tolerant plant that can be cultivated in arid environments. Amaranth seeds are a good source of protein and lysine, an essential amino acid.

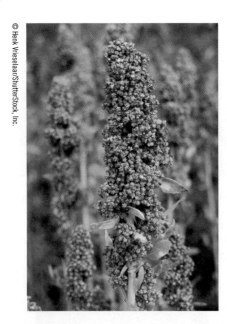

FIGURE 11.14 Quinoa was second only to the potato in nutritional importance in pre-Columbian Andean civilizations. Quinoa is an excellent source of protein and also a good source of dietary fiber, phosphorus, magnesium, and iron.

the early part of the sixteenth century burned every field of amaranth they could find and forbade the growing of amaranth. Luckily, it survived in remote areas of the Andes and Mexico and gained popularity centuries later for its high nutritional value and health benefits.[4] Amaranth, a tall plant with colorful leaves, also is a popular ornamental plant. It is easy to grow, resistant to heat, and has no major disease problems.

Quinoa

Quinoa (*Chenopodium quinoa*) is a popular food crop in many regions of South America (see **Figure 11.14**). Quinoa is native to the Andean region of South America and is botanically related to beets, spinach, and chard. The small seeds of quinoa were a staple food of the Incans, who referred to quinoa as the "mother grain," the "mother seeds," and "gold of the Incans."[4] A variety of different types of quinoa is grown, with seeds ranging from tiny and dark brown to large and almost white. As with amaranth, the Spanish conquistadors destroyed all quinoa production and killed anyone found growing it. With quinoa's rediscovery in recent years, its consumption is becoming more popular. It is very nutritious and contains all the essential amino acids.

Physical and Chemical Properties

Physical Structure of the Cereal Grain

Plants that produce cereal seeds have a similar structure. The fruit, or cereal kernel, of the plant is covered by a husk—also called the hull or chaff—which protects the kernel from environmental damage. The husk is removed after harvesting the grain. The shape and size of the kernel varies based on the particular type of cereal, but all have similar features. All cereal kernels contain three major parts: the *bran*, the *endosperm*, and the *germ*, or embryo, as shown in **Figure 11.15**. Whole grain products contain all parts of the kernel, excluding the husk.

endosperm The large inner portion of cereal kernels that contains large amounts of starch in a protein matrix.

bran The high-fiber outer layers of cereal kernels that protect the endosperm and germ.

aleurone The layer between the bran and endosperm in cereal kernels.

Endosperm

The **endosperm**—the inner portion of the kernel—is the largest part of the kernel and is where cereal plants store energy as starch in a protein matrix. The amount of starch and protein in the endosperm varies by cereal. The two components of starch are amylose and amylopectin, which have different properties. The endosperm is approximately 83% of the wheat kernel and is a rich source of starch, protein, and B vitamins.

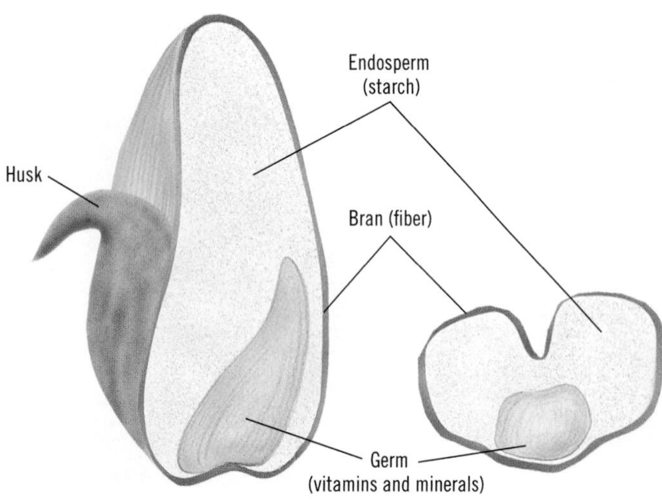

FIGURE 11.15 The bran is the outer layer of the seed. The endosperm is the nutrient-rich tissue inside the seed that surrounds the embryo, providing it with energy. The germ is the plant embryo, which upon germination will grow into a new plant.

Bran

The **bran**, also called the *pericarp*, consists of outer layers of the kernel that cover the endosperm and germ. Bran is composed of the epidermis, epicarp, and endocarp layers. It is a good source of fiber because it contains mainly cellulose. Bran also contains B vitamins, minerals, and some protein. The bran portion of the kernel is included in whole grain products and also is used in animal feed. Approximately 14.5% of the wheat kernel contains layers of bran and aleurone. The **aleurone** component of the cereal kernel, which is the layer between the bran and the endosperm, contains many nutrients but has less fiber than the bran. The aleurone layer is removed with the bran during the milling of grains into a **refined flour**.

Germ

The **germ**, or embryo, is the smallest part of the kernel and comprises approximately 2.5% of the kernel. This is the part of the kernel from which the new plant will emerge. The germ contains fat, which over time can cause rancidity, limiting the storage life of products made with germ, such as whole grain products. The germ also contains protein, B vitamins, and vitamin E.

refined flour Wheat flour that has the germ and bran removed and usually has been whitened as well.

germ The smallest part of the cereal kernel; it produces a sprout for a new plant.

milling The process of grinding grain in a mill.

Processing Cereal Grains by Milling

Prior to milling, cereal kernels are cleaned of field debris and other contaminants that may be introduced during harvesting and transporting. The objective of **milling** is to separate the endosperm from the bran and germ, with further processing of the endosperm into grits, meal, or flour, depending on the extent of the milling. Reasons for removing the bran and germ are to improve the functional properties of the endosperm in manufactured products and to increase their shelf life.

Milling of Wheat

The most commonly milled grain is wheat, which is usually dry milled. Dry milling of cereals consists of tempering and conditioning the kernels and then roller milling them. Tempering involves the addition of water to toughen the bran and soften the endosperm, making for easier separation. The tempered wheat is then put through rollers to remove the bran and germ and reduce the starchy endosperm into smaller particles.

During roller milling, kernels are put through a series of rollers that progressively move closer together. The first rollers open the kernel, breaking the bran and freeing the germ. The next rollers crush the endosperm and flatten the germ. The bran and germ are removed by air currents and sieves under the rollers. The endosperm is further pulverized by rollers set close enough to grind it into fine flour particles, with continued sifting to remove small pieces of bran and germ. With further milling, even smaller particles are produced, and the flour becomes lighter in color and lower in vitamin and mineral content.

Milling can be used to produce several different types of flours. Refined white flours from any of the wheat varieties are graded based on the streams of millings included in the final flour product. The highest grade of flour is *short-patent*, which contains refined flour from approximately 50% of the streams of endosperm, especially the middle portion of the endosperm, and is high in starch and low in protein. *Medium-patent* flour includes about 90% of the streams and is higher in protein and lower in starch than short-patent flour. *Long-patent* flour contains nearly all the flour streams and is the highest in protein and lowest in starch.

The U.S. Food and Drug Administration (FDA) defines white wheat flour as a food produced by grinding and sifting cleaned wheat. Freshly milled white flours have a creamy or yellow color due to carotenoid pigments and have better baking qualities when aged or matured for weeks or months. Ageing or maturing can be done simply by storing the flour. During storage, oxidation occurs and the flour becomes lighter in color due to oxidation of the carotenoids, resulting in flour with a lighter color. Oxidation also allows for more bonds when gluten is formed, which makes for better baking flour. This process is usually accelerated with oxidizing agents such as benzoyl peroxide and chlorine. These floors must be labeled "bleached." Both unbleached and bleached flours are available in the retail market.

Rice Milling

Rice milling also involves dry milling. It begins by placing whole grains of rice into machines that rub the outer hulls off the kernels (see **Figure 11.16**).

Innovation Point

Milling The earliest method of milling was to grind cereal kernels between two stones. In fact, flour milling was the first automated industrial system. Roller milling began around 1880 and continues today with modern equipment.

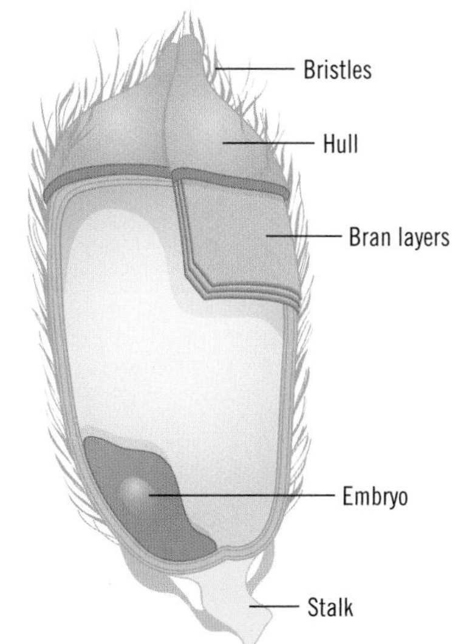

FIGURE 11.16 Rice grains are enclosed in a tough husk that must be removed. Under the husk are the bran and germ, which are high in vitamins, minerals, oil and various phytonutrients. With rice milling, the husk and bran are removed to produce an edible white rice kernel called polished white rice.

Green Point

Wheat and Rice Wheat and rice provide approximately equal amounts of calories for feeding the world's population; however, about half as much land is used to grow the world's rice crop. Farmers in the rice-producing regions of Japan, Korea, and China were early adopters of Green Revolution technologies used to increase crop yields.

gluten The protein complex formed from the fractions gliadin and glutenin when flour is mixed with water.

The most common rice huller used in milling operations is a rubber-roll sheller, which uses bursts of air to remove the outer hull, producing brown rice.[6] Brown rice can be further milled to remove the bran and germ. This additional milling produces what is called *polished white rice*—the kernels have smooth surfaces due to the action of the revolving bands of rubber-lined rollers that rub the kernels.

Corn Milling

Wet milling is used to mill corn into cornstarch and other corn products. The corn kernels are softened by steeping them in water and acid. The kernels are then broken with a milling action, forming a pasty mass. The germ floats above the endosperm and hulls, and the germ is removed. The remaining hulls are separated from the endosperm's starch–protein complex, and the starch is dried to form powdered cornstarch. In addition to cornstarch, wet milling of corn produces corn oil, corn protein, corn germ meal, corn fiber, and condensed fermented corn extracts.[6] Wet milling is a more complicated process than dry milling, but common to all milling and processing of cereals is the loss of fiber, vitamins, and minerals.

Gluten Chemistry

Wheat flour is the preferred flour for baking due to the formation of gluten (note that some other flours produce it, too). Gliadin and glutenin are the two insoluble proteins that develop **gluten** when flour is mixed with water and stirred or beaten, such as when making a batter or kneading a dough. Gluten development requires both the addition of water to the flour and the physical manipulation of the hydrated flour mixture. The protein in flour is able to absorb up to 200 times its weight in water; in contrast, starch is only able to absorb about 15% of its weight in water.[7] Because the hydration capacity of flour is influenced by its protein content, hard wheat provides more structure and higher loaf volume in breads.

Flour contains much more starch than protein, but it is the protein that gives baked products a strong structure. Gluten is responsible for the viscous and elastic characteristics and high volume of baked products. The gliadin fraction of gluten contributes to the viscosity, and the glutenin fraction is responsible for the elasticity and strength.

Celiac Disease

Individuals with celiac disease, also called celiac sprue, have an immune-mediated reaction to the gliadin fraction in gluten; they should avoid all products containing gluten. In the United States, about 1% of the population has celiac disease; another 5–10% are estimated to have gluten intolerance, a condition more recently described by the medical community. The relative frequency of celiac disease and gluten intolerance has influenced the number gluten-free products in the marketplace.[8] Gluten-free products were once thought of as a small niche market, but large food corporations have introduced gluten-free cake mixes and breakfast cereals into the retail market, making gluten-free products mainstream.[9] **Special Topic 11.1** discusses celiac disease and gluten intolerance in more detail.

Gluten-Free Flours

Flours can be produced from any plant containing starch, although nonwheat flours are less popular than wheat flours. In addition to cereals, legumes and nuts also can be used for flour production. It is important to note that not all nonwheat flours are gluten-free. Flours made from barley, rye, and triticale contain gluten. Including oats in gluten-free diets is controversial because

Special Topic 11.1

Gluten Intolerance: Celiac Disease and Nonceliac Gluten Sensitivity

Lisa S. Brown, PhD, RD

Celiac disease, also known as celiac sprue and gluten-sensitive enteropathy, is the most common genetic disease in the world, affecting approximately 1% of the gluten-consuming population.[1] The disease is characterized by inflammation in the small intestine that occurs when the body attacks gluten (more specifically gliadin), a protein found in wheat, rye, and barley. The inflammation damages the villi within the small intestine. If gluten is ingested consistently over time, chronic inflammation of the small intestine can lead to atrophy of the villi, resulting in malabsorption and malnutrition. Celiac disease is technically an intolerance to the proteins found in wheat, rye, and barley. It is not an allergy because the process is mediated by immune factors IgG and IgA, whereas an allergy is mediated by the immune factor IgE. The only treatment for celiac disease is a gluten-free diet.

Celiac disease has been described by doctors for many centuries, but the connection between gastrointestinal symptoms, failure to thrive, and ingestion of wheat, rye, and barley was only discovered as a result of the food embargo in the Netherlands during World War II. After World War II, a Dutch pediatrician noticed that children with certain gastrointestinal symptoms seemed to get better during the food shortages but relapsed after cereal supplies were restored.[2]

The original symptoms identified in the 1940s as part of the disorder included diarrhea, stomach pain, gas, and failure to thrive and are still thought of as the classic presentation of celiac disease. In the 1960s, small bowel biopsy was introduced, making possible a more accurate diagnosis of celiac disease than was achievable from symptoms alone. Subsequently, a much fuller understanding of the disease formed.[3] Symptoms not previously associated with celiac disease were proven to be caused by the disease, and populations previously thought to be unaffected were shown to be impacted.

Over the last 25 years celiac disease has been associated with a broad range of symptoms, including anemia; neurologic symptoms, such as migraine headaches and ataxia; and skin-related symptoms, which may be formally diagnosed as a variant of celiac disease called dermatitis herpetiformis.[4] Celiac disease also may be present with no outward symptoms at all, although the hallmark damage still occurs within the small intestine.[5]

Generally considered a European disease, celiac disease also has been shown to be prevalent in a number of different ethnic groups, including Brazilians, Asians, Arabs, and people from Northern India.

Recently, another condition, *gluten intolerance*, has been described. It is not diagnosable as celiac disease, although symptoms often are similar in nature and severity.[6] In sensitive individuals, symptoms appear to be related to ingestion of gluten based on patient history, but no hallmark antibodies and no damage to the villi are found. Gluten intolerance, also called *nonceliac gluten sensitivity*, has been increasingly recognized by the medical community and is diagnosed in an individual who tests negative for celiac disease but whose symptoms improve on a gluten-free diet. Work is ongoing to understand this disorder; it is currently estimated to affect 5–10% of the American population. Like celiac disease, treatment involves the complete elimination of gluten from the diet. The discovery of this new disorder suggests that the market for gluten-free products will continue to expand.

References

1 Fasano A, Berti I, Gerarduzzi T, et al. Prevalence of celiac disease in at-risk and not-at-risk groups in the United States: A large multicenter study. *Arch Intern Med.* 2003 Feb;163(3):286–292.

2 Farrell RJ, Kelly CP. Current concepts: Celiac sprue. *New Eng J Med.* 2002;346(3):180–188.

3 Green P, Stavropoulos S, Panagi S, et al. Characteristics of adult celiac disease in the USA: Results of a national survey. *Am J Gastroenterol.* 2001 Jan;96(1):126–131.

4 Cicarelli G, Della Rocca G, Amboni M, et al. Clinical and neurological abnormalities in adult celiac disease. *Neurol Sci.* 2003 Dec;24(5):311–317.

5 Agardh D, Nilsson A, Tuomi T, et al. Prediction of silent celiac disease at diagnosis of childhood type 1 diabetes by tissue transglutaminase autoantibodies and HLA. *Pediatr Diabetes.* 2001 Jun;2(2):58–65.

6 Bizzaro N, Tozzoli R, Villalta D, et al. Cutting-edge issues in celiac disease and in gluten intolerance. *Clin Rev Allergy Immunol.* 2012 Jun;42(3):279–287.

most oat products in the United States are contaminated with gluten from other grains.[10] In fact, gluten contamination can occur during harvesting, transporting, processing, or manufacturing of many food products.

Gluten-free flours include those from corn, potato, rice, soy, and others. Breads produced from gluten-free flours usually contain a mixture of flours from different sources.[11] Baking without gluten is challenging because all aspects of the finished product are affected.[12] Flours used in making gluten-free baked products must be chosen carefully for an acceptable gluten-free product, but it can be done. For example, substitution of wheat flour with rice flour did not affect consumer acceptability of baked or fried chicken nuggets.[13] The protein content of gluten-containing and gluten-free flours is compared in **Table 11.1**.

TABLE 11.1
Protein Content of Gluten-Containing and Gluten-Free Flours

Type of Flour	Protein (%)
Flours Containing Gluten	
Cake flour (white enriched)	8
Pastry flour	9
All-purpose flour (white enriched wheat)	10
Rye flour (light)	10
Rye flour (medium)	11
Bread flour (white enriched wheat)	12
Whole wheat flour	13
Durum or semolina flour (enriched)	13
Triticale flour (whole grain)	13
Oat flour (partially debranned)	15
Rye flour (dark)	16
High-gluten or gluten flour	41
Gluten-Free Flours*	
Rice flour (white)	6
Rice flour (brown)	7
Potato flour	7
Corn flour (whole grain white or yellow)	7
Corn flour (masa enriched white or yellow)	9
Corn flour (whole grain blue)	9
Teff flour	12
Sorghum flour	12
Buckwheat flour (whole groat)	13
Quinoa flour (dehulled)	16
Chickpea flour (besan)	22
Soy flour (defatted)	47

*Some legume flours are included in the gluten-free flours because they are used by people unable to tolerate gluten.

Source: Data from the U.S. Department of Agriculture. USDA National Nutrient Database for Standard Reference, Release 24. Available at: http://www.ars.usda.gov/ba/bhnrc/ndl. Accessed June 5, 2012.

Starch

Starch is the storage form of carbohydrate (energy) in plants. It is a complex carbohydrate composed of the two fractions—amylose and amylopectin—that are polymers of glucose. Plants generate glucose through photosynthesis. This glucose is used immediately by the plant for energy or converted to starch so the energy can be stored for future use.

Starch has important properties that affect its usefulness as a food:

- It is not sweet.
- It is not soluble in cold water.
- It forms pastes and gels with the aid of hot water.
- It is good source of energy.
- It is found in seeds, tubers, and other plant parts as starch granules.

Starch can be derived from many different types of plants that have good reserves of stored energy, especially cereal kernels such as corn, wheat, rice, and sorghum. Tuberous plants such as potato, cassava (tapioca), arrowroot, taro, and kudzu (kuzu) also are sources of starch, as are legumes. Cornstarch is the most common refined starch and is used in numerous industrial applications. Starches from different plants have different properties due to variation in the ratio of amylose to amylopectin and other factors such as the structure and size of the starch granules. Most starches have very little taste or flavor; however, residual protein or fat not extracted during the milling and refining process can influence the flavor.[14]

The two fractions of starch, amylose and amylopectin, do not occur free in nature but are stored in starch granules. Regardless of the botanical source, all natural starches contain glucose units linked together by α-1,4 and α-1,6 glycosidic bonds.

Amylose

Amylose is the linear fraction of starch that has α-1,4 glycosidic linkages between the glucose molecules. A small number of α-1,6 glycosidic bonds may be present for a small amount of branching on the linear glucose chain.[14] Natural starches contain less amylose than amylopectin. The main characteristic of amylose is that it can form a firm gel after starch is cooked and cooled.

Amylopectin

Amylopectin is the branched fraction of starch. It has both α-1,4 and α-1,6 glycosidic linkages among the glucose units. Amylopectin is like amylose in that it has a linear chain of glucose units connected by α-1,4 glycosidic bonds, but unlike amylose it has numerous side branches of glucose units connected to the chain by α-1,6 glycosidic bonds. The structure of amylopectin is more complex than that of amylose, and it is a much larger molecule. Amylopectin is the predominant fraction in natural starches, and it is a thickening agent, which is its main characteristic. Amylopectin does not form a gel but typically imparts a nongelling, cohesive, gummy texture to a food product.[14]

Effect of Dry and Moist Heat on Starch

When starch or flour is heated without moisture, it turns a brown color due to the formation of dextrin molecules. *Dextrinization* is the hydrolytic chemical breakdown of starch by intense dry heat. Some of the glucose linkages break via chemical reactions with the small amount of water present in the dry starch. This imparts the flavors important in some gravies and sauces. Moist heat causes starch mixtures to gelatinize, paste, and retrograde, as explained in the following sections.

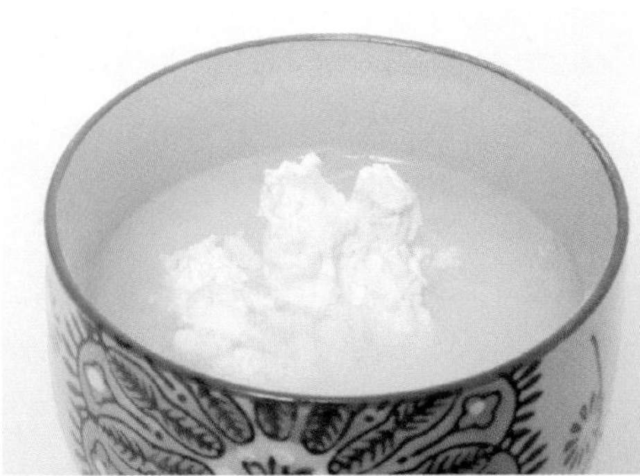

FIGURE 11.17 Cornstarch is not soluble in water or other liquids unless heat is applied. This is why heat must be applied when forming a roux, a thickening agent used in many sauces in French cuisine.

Gelatinization

Starch is insoluble in cold water. When starch granules are mixed with water, it forms a suspension, with the starch granules becoming suspended in the liquid. If left undisturbed, the starch does not stay suspended and settles at the bottom of the container (see **Figure 11.17**). When heat (at a temperature range characteristic of the particular starch) is applied to the starch and water suspension, the granules swell with water. Cornstarch granules swell at 144–162°F (62–72°C); wheat starch granules swell at 136–147°F (58–64°C); and potato starch granules swell at 138–154°F (59–68°C). As heating continues, the suspension becomes thicker, the viscosity of the mixture increases, and it becomes more translucent. This process of heating starch in water or any water-based liquid and the swelling of starch granules, which causes thickening and increased viscosity of the mixture, is called *gelatinization*.

Heating must continue beyond the gelatinization temperature to obtain a good gel and avoid a raw starch taste. During usual cooking procedures, most of the starch stays inside the swollen granules; only a small amount of amylose leaks out of the granules. Excessive stirring of the starch mixture or heating at high temperatures can cause the swollen granules to break, which can produce a lower-quality food product.

Pasting

Pasting occurs with continued heating of the starch mixture beyond gelatinization. The viscosity of the mixture increases as more of the starch granules become swollen. A starch mixture will reach peak viscosity when the number of swollen, intact starch granules is maximized. At this point, the starch mixture is fully pasted. Pasting causes the starch granules to become very swollen and soft, forming a paste. Continued, prolonged heating of natural starch mixtures results in decreased viscosity as the granules break and dissolve and the glucose polymers (starch molecules) become soluble. Pasting is not separate from gelatinization; it is a continuation of gelatinization.[14]

Most starch mixtures begin to thicken and increase in translucency at 165–190°F (74–88°C). A thickened starch mixture is called a *starch paste*. If the starch paste is fluid, it is called a sol. An example of a sol is a gravy or sauce (see **Figure 11.18**). A sol can be described as a solid (starch) dispersed in a liquid (water). If the starch paste is solid, it is a gel. An example of a gel is a firm pudding. A gel can be described as a liquid (water) dispersed in a solid (starch or a gelling agent).

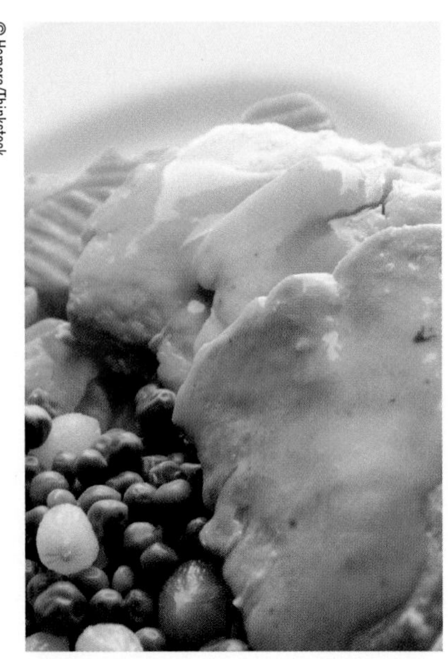

FIGURE 11.18 Gravy is an example of a sol. In gravy, the starch is dispersed in a liquid, most often the juices from cooked meats or vegetables.

Gelation

Gelatinized starch mixtures exist as sols or gels. All hot starch paste mixtures exhibit the flow properties of sols, but many convert to gels as they cool. *Gelation* is the formation of a gel. Amylose molecules that leaked out of the starch granules during gelatinization move about in the paste. As the paste cools, amylose molecules move more slowly; when they come into contact with each other, they form hydrogen bonds (junction zones). This hydrogen bonding forms a network among the amylose molecules, which results in gelation. Swollen starch granules and water become trapped in the strong amylose network and a gel forms. The concentration of amylose affects the strength of the gel; the higher the amylose concentration, the firmer the gel.

Retrogradation

Gels change with time as some of the hydrogen bonds holding the amylose network together break and form hydrogen bonds with other amylose molecules in the gel. The strong tendency for amylose molecules to reassociate back to an orderly structure causes the gel to become dense. Gelatinization disrupts the starch molecules, and following gelation the amylose molecules reassociate in an orderly structure, forming crystalline aggregates and a gelled texture. The effect of this *retrogradation* can be felt on the tongue as a gritty texture.

Amylopectin molecules also retrograde upon cooling of starch gels but not to the extent of amylose molecules. Amylopectin forms new bonds between branches at a slower rate than amylose and are weak in comparison to the strong bonds between amylose molecules. Amylopectin molecules cannot form gels.

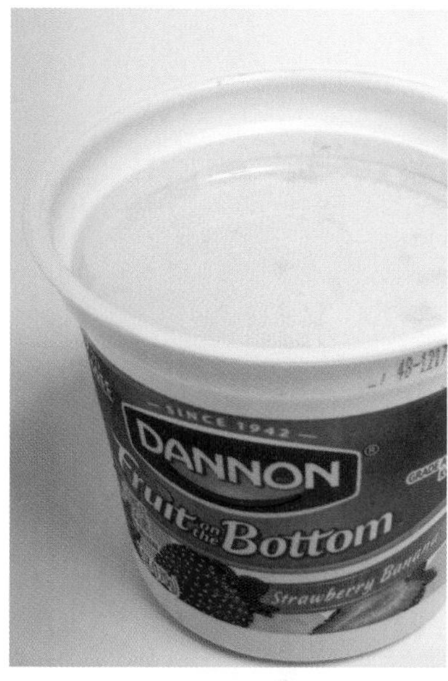

FIGURE 11.19 A good example of syneresis is the collection of whey on the surface of yogurt.

Syneresis

As retrogradation occurs over time, water molecules are released from the reordered amylose network, a process called syneresis. *Syneresis* also is defined as the separation of a liquid from a gel.[14] Retrogradation causes the gel to become opaque. When the gel is cut, water leaks out. The gel also becomes rubbery, with the release of water droplets (weeping). Syneresis often occurs in gelled foods using unmodified starches containing amylose. It is common in refrigerated and frozen products (see **Figure 11.19**). Starches from different plants retrograde at different rates and to various degrees.

The Chemistry of Cereal Starches During Cooking

Corn and wheat are common cereal starches used in cooking. Cornstarch is widely used because it is inexpensive, cooks to a smooth paste in liquid, combines well with other ingredients, and does not impart a strong flavor. It also is gluten-free, unlike wheat. Wheat flour has less thickening power and produces a more opaque gel than cornstarch.

Slurry Formation

A starch mixed in a cool or cold liquid forms a **slurry**. The cool liquid helps separate the starch granules in cornstarch or other cereal starches, allowing them to begin absorbing water without forming lumps. The slurry can be added to a hot or cold liquid. If added to a hot liquid, the mixture must be continuously stirred to avoid clumping. Cornstarch begins to thicken quickly if the mixture is hot. After gently cooking for about 5 minutes, the raw starch flavor disappears.

slurry A starch mixed in a cool or cold liquid.

Moist-Heat Cooking Methods

Cereals must be cooked so they can be digested by the human body. The most common cooking method is moist-heat cooking, which includes simmering, pilaf, and risotto.[15] (Pilaf and risotto also are the names of rice dishes, but technically they are the cooking methods used to make the dishes.)

The simmering method involves adding the grains into boiling liquid and stirring if necessary to disperse the grains, covering the pan, lowering the heat, and simmering until cooked, which is when the liquid is absorbed and the grains are tender. The cereal should not be stirred excessively because this causes rupturing of starch granules, resulting in a gummy texture.

In the pilaf and risotto methods, the cereal pieces or kernels are coated with hot fat and sautéed before adding liquid. In the pilaf method, all the liquid is added at once into the pan with the sautéed cereal, and the pan is covered and the cereal simmered until done. In the risotto method, hot liquid is gradually added over the cooking period and the cereal is stirred constantly to produce a more creamy texture.

Cereals are usually done when the liquid is absorbed, which is indicated by the appearance of small tunnel-like holes between the grains. Cooking times vary, with processed cereals requiring less time than whole grains. The required amount of water varies with the type of cereal. **Table 11.2** lists the usual amount of cooking water required per cup for different cereals.

TABLE 11.2
Approximate Amounts of Cereal and Water for Cooking

Type of Cereal (1 cup)	Water Needed (cups)
Berries, groats, and cracked cereals	3–4
Rolled and flaked cereals	2–2½
Regular and quick-cooking cereals, including regular rice	2
Instant cereals, including instant rice	1

Source: Data from Oldways Preservation Trust and the Whole Grains Council (http://www.wholegraincouncil.org).

Modified Starches

Modified starches are commonly used in processed foods because the pastes and gels produced by natural starches are often gummy, sticky, or rubbery. The functional properties of starches are greatly improved by modification. Different types of modification produce starches that can withstand heat, shear, and acids.

Starches can be modified by chemical and physical methods. The most common type of chemical starch modification is treating starches with small amounts of chemicals as approved by the FDA and published in Title 21 of the Code of Federal Regulations (Section 172.892). Starches become more stable with the chemical process of cross-linking, which changes their structure. See **Special Topic 11.2** to learn how modified starches are used as food thickeners for people who have problems swallowing.

Special Topic 11.2

Food Thickeners and Dysphagia

Leslie Rathon, MS, RD

Have you ever considered what life would be like if you could not swallow? Though it is often taken for granted, the act of swallowing liquids, purees, or semi-chewed solids generates serious problems for many. *Dysphagia* is the umbrella clinical term for the inability to swallow, which can arise from a multitude of etiologies. In fact, the mechanics of swallowing itself involve 50 muscles and many nerves,[1] and dysphagia can arise due to a malfunction in any of these muscular or neural pathways caused by stroke, head or neck injury, cancer, gastroesophageal disorders (e.g., GERD), or nervous system disorders (e.g., Parkinson's disease). Common in elderly persons, symptoms of dysphagia can span from dry mouth to the complete inability to swallow. Additionally, infants born with physical abnormalities, such as a cleft palate, have difficulty nursing due to the inability to suck properly.

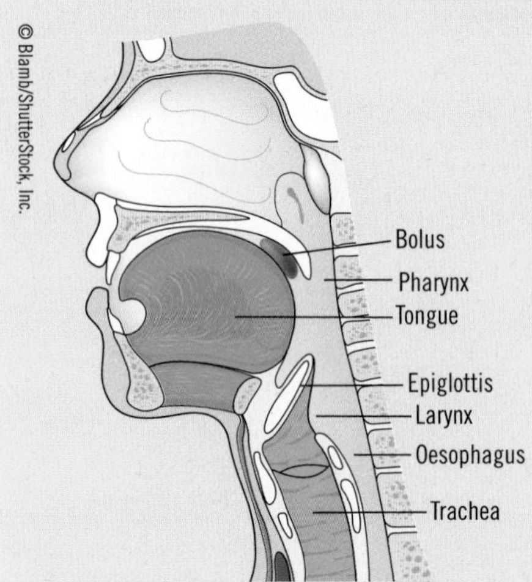

With proper swallowing, the oral cavity, the pharynx, and the esophagus ensure that food goes in one direction—to the stomach—without entering into the lungs.

For the approximately 15 million dysphagia patients in the United States,[2] the seriousness of the disorder centers on the inability to ingest adequate nutrition or hydration to sustain the body and maintain an ideal body weight. Other complications can arise from ingesting food pieces that are too large and that can block the airway or even enter the lungs (i.e., by aspiration), causing bacterial infections, such as aspiration pneumonia.

What can be done to help dysphagia patients? No clear standards of care for dysphagia are available; however, based on clinical evaluations by medical doctors and speech pathologists, it can be managed in a number of different ways. In cases of extreme dysphagia, tube feedings are the only option to supply nutrition. However, in less extreme cases food and drinks can be prepared in ways so they can be tolerated by people experiencing swallowing difficulties. Modifying the texture of foods and beverages often allows dysphagia patients safe oral intake[2,3] to maintain sufficient nutrition. Food thickeners are one way to alter the texture of foods and beverages. Thickening liquids increases their viscosity and promotes safe swallowing by creating a more cohesive bolus in the mouth.[2] Thickeners for therapeutic usage vary with regard to ingredients (e.g., starch, gum) and consistency (e.g., nectar, honey).[2] The effectiveness of dysphagia therapies depends on tailoring the level of viscosity that is appropriate for each patient.[3] Although thickeners enable safer swallowing, they can suppress or alter the flavor of the base beverage or food.[2] It is important to consider which thickener to use based on the patient's sensory preferences.[2]

Many scientific fields are involved in dysphagia research, making it an area of specialized research. Although there is no single agreed upon protocol for swallowing severity, rating scales for clinical use are available.[4] In 2002, the Academy of Nutrition and Dietetics published the National Dysphagia Diet (NDD), with the goal of standardizing terms and practices of texture modification to ensure optimal care. The evidence-based NDD is divided into four levels of semi-solid and solid foods:[4]

- *NDD Level 1:* Dysphagia-Pureed (homogenous, very cohesive, pudding-like, requiring very little chewing ability)
- *NDD Level 2:* Dysphagia-Mechanical Altered (cohesive, moist, semisolid foods, requiring some chewing)
- *NDD Level 3:* Dysphagia-Advanced (soft foods that require more chewing ability)
- *Regular:* All foods allowed

Although the NDD demonstrates a major advance in standardizing dysphagia management, more research should be conducted to guide clinicians on individualizing the diet to each patient.

References

1 National Institutes of Health, National Institute of Deafness and Other Communication Disorders. Dysphagia. Available at: http://www.nidcd.nih.gov/health/voice/dysph.aspx. Accessed January 31, 2011.

2 Chambers E, Garcia J, Helverson J, Matta Z. Sensory characteristics of beverages prepared with commercial thickeners used for dysphagia diets. *J Am Diet Assoc.* 2006 July;106:1049–1054.

3 Bulow M, Ekberg O, Ekman S, et al. Objective and quantitative definitions of modified food textures based on sensory and rheological methodology. *Food Nutri Res.* 2010 Jun;28:54.

4 National Dysphagia Diet Task Force, American Dietetic Association. National Dysphagia Diet: Standardization for Optimal Care. Chicago: American Dietetic Association; 2002.

Cereal Products

Wheat

The major use of wheat (*Triticum* spp.) is for human food; more foods are made with wheat than any other cereal. The use of wheat flour for bread production is of worldwide importance. The gluten in wheat enables leavened dough to rise and produces bread with a light texture. Wheat contains more gluten that any other grain.

As the principle cereal used in the United States, wheat is the main ingredient in most bread products, crackers, cookies, cakes, muffins, doughnuts, biscuits, pancakes, waffles, pastries, noodles, pastas, pizza and piecrusts, and many breakfast cereals. Wheat flour also is used for baking and as a thickener in gravies, sauces, soups, and stews.

Classes of Wheat

Wheat can be broken down into six classes and thousands of wheat varieties. Wheat is classified according to the time of year it is planted, the hardness of the kernels, and the color of the kernels. The classes of wheat are: (1) hard red winter, (2) hard red spring, (3) soft red winter, (4) hard white winter, (5) soft white wheat, and (6) durum. Winter wheat is planted in the fall and harvested in the spring and summer; spring wheat is planted in the spring and harvested in late summer or early fall. Hard red winter wheat is the dominant wheat grown and used in the United States.

The hard wheats, including durum wheat, are higher in protein and lower in starch than the soft wheats. Therefore, the harder types of wheat—especially hard red winter and hard red spring—are used for making bread to provide good structure. **Durum**—the hardest type of wheat—is used to make **semolina**, the flour used to make pasta products such as spaghetti, macaroni, and egg noodles. The soft, low-protein types of wheat are used for cakes, biscuits, some noodle products, pastries, and other baked products that require a soft and tender crumb.

durum A type of hard wheat that is higher in protein than other wheat types; it is used for pasta.

semolina Durum flour used for production of pasta and couscous.

wheat berry A raw, unprocessed wheat kernel.

cracked wheat Wheat berries that are crushed or cut into small pieces.

bulgur Cracked wheat produced from steamed and dried or roasted wheat berries.

couscous A semolina grain rolled into small, round pellets.

farina Coarsely ground wheat endosperm.

Forms of Wheat

Wheat is processed to different degrees to make various food products:

- A **wheat berry** is raw, unprocessed wheat kernel containing the bran, germ, and endosperm. These kernels double in volume when cooked in water and have a nutty taste, with a chewy but tender texture.
- **Cracked wheat** is created when raw, unprocessed wheat berries are crushed or cut into smaller pieces. Cracked wheat is used in the production of cereals and can be used in casseroles, salads, stuffing, and as a meat extender.
- **Bulgur** is cracked wheat produced from steamed and dried or roasted wheat berries; it has a nutty flavor. Bulgur is used in pilaf dishes and in tabouleh, which is a popular salad dish in the Middle East.
- **Farina** is coarsely ground wheat endosperm. It is used as a breakfast cereal and as a baby food cereal. Cream of Wheat is a popular commercial farina product.
- **Couscous** is a product produced by rolling and shaping moistened semolina into small granules, which are then dried. Couscous was traditionally made from the hard part of the kernel that resisted grinding when primitive grinding stones were used. Couscous is a staple food in many parts of northern Africa, especially north of the Sahara. Today, other grains also are made into a couscous product, such as coarsely ground barley and rice.

Gastronomy Point

Couscous Serve couscous as an alternative to rice or potatoes. Cooking couscous in vegetable or chicken stock and adding savory seasonings complements any meal with fish, chicken, or legumes. Fluff cooked couscous with a fork to produce a light and fluffy product. Cooked couscous should not be gritty or gummy.

Wheat Starch, Germ, and Bran

Wheat starch is produced from the carbohydrates in wheat endosperm. It is a useful thickener, but it does not have the thickening power of cornstarch. The germ component of wheat appears as tiny, crumblike grains. Wheat germ has a nutty taste and is used in hot cereals and breads. It can also be sprinkled over yogurt and salads. Wheat bran can be used in baking, as an ingredient in meatloaf, and stirred into hot cereals. Bran from all cereals can be used as a fiber supplement.

Types of Wheat Flour

Many types of wheat flour are available. **Table 11.1** compared the protein content of various wheat flours and their nonwheat counterparts:

- Whole wheat flour, also known as graham flour or entire wheat flour, contains the bran, germ, and endosperm of wheat berries and may be ground to varying degrees of fineness. Compared to white flour, whole wheat flour has a shorter shelf-life because the fat in the germ will oxidize and cause rancidity. It also is higher in fiber due to the bran component. It produces baked products that have a denser texture and a lower volume due to the bran and germ's interference with gluten development.

- Enriched flour is white flour produced from just the endosperm, with the B vitamins thiamin, riboflavin, niacin, and folic acid and the mineral iron added based on federal standards.
- All-purpose flour is white flour produced from a blend of wheat varieties. It is used to make quick breads. It contains enough protein to make homemade yeast breads and some cakes, but it has too much protein for delicate cakes. It is the most common type of flour sold in the retail market. The amount of protein in all-purpose flours varies depending on the mill, the brand, and the region where it is marketed.
- Self-rising flour is all-purpose flour to which a leavening agent and salt have been added. The leavening agent is baking powder in the form of monocalcium phosphate (an acid salt) combined with sodium biocarbonate (baking soda). One cup of self-rising flour usually contains 1½ teaspoons of baking powder and ½ teaspoon salt.
- Bread flour is long-patent flour produced from a blend of hard wheat varieties. It contains more protein than all-purpose flour. The higher protein content results in a higher loaf volume. Bread flour produces excellent yeast breads and is used by commercial bakers.
- Gluten flour, or high-gluten flour, is a specialty wheat flour produced by adding vital wheat gluten, which is dried gluten, to increase the amount of protein to approximately 41%. This flour produces a chewy and tough bread product that also is very palatable.[16] Bagels often contain high-gluten flour to give them a chewy texture. By raising the protein content, gluten flour provides good structure to baked products and improves their nutritional value.
- Cake flour is short-patent flour that is finely milled from soft wheat varieties. It is a high-starch, low-protein flour. This flour will produce delicate, fine-textured cakes. Cake flour is usually bleached with chlorine to inhibit gluten development and to allow starch to easily absorb water—desirable characteristics when making cakes. The chlorine treatment also produces flour with a very white color.
- Pastry flour is a soft wheat flour, but it includes medium-patent in addition to short-patent flour; it contains approximately 9% protein. Pastry flour is used by commercial bakers to produce tender pastry products.
- Instantized flour also is known as instant-blending or quick-mixing flour. It is produced by passing all-purpose flour through moist air to form agglomerates that are dried to produce small sandlike granules. This type of flour flows easily without a lot of dust. It blends easily with water and does not require sifting. Instantized flour is useful for thickening gravies and sauces.

Pasta

Although **pasta** may not have originated in Italy, pasta makers in Italy were well established and organized into strictly regulated trade associations by the sixteenth century, a practice that continues today. In fact, in Rome, Italy, there is even a museum devoted to pasta—the National Museum of Pasta Foods.[17] Pasta is synonymous with Italian cooking. Italians are the largest consumers of pasta and refer to pasta products as *pasta alimentare* (alimentary paste), Germans refer to them as *teigwaren* (pasta goods), and the French call them *pates alimentaires*.[18] Basic ingredients for Italian pasta

pasta General term for any macaroni or noodle product.

are simple—semolina and water. When they are combined, they form an alimentary paste, or pasta dough. In the United States, pasta is fortified with thiamin, riboflavin, folic acid, and ferrous sulfate (iron).[17]

Pasta Production

The most important factor for producing high-quality pasta is the use of durum wheat,[17] which has a higher protein content than the other varieties of wheat. Durum wheat is milled into coarse particles known as semolina, or semolina flour. It is possible to make pasta with other types of milled wheat, but they are considered lower in quality. Durum wheat contains carotenoid pigments, which gives pasta its characteristic yellow or amber color. In commercial pasta production, the alimentary paste is formed by mixing approximately 100 parts semolina to 30 parts water. The paste that forms is extruded (forced through perforated steel plates) by commercial equipment into hundreds of different shapes and sizes or extruded onto thin sheets and cut into flat pasta products. The product is dried in ovens to about 12% moisture for dried pasta.[17]

Most pasta that is produced and marketed is dried, but fresh pasta is available in the marketplace. Dried pasta offers consumers convenience, quality, and low cost. Fresh pasta is more expensive and must be kept refrigerated; its higher moisture content gives it a softer texture, shorter cooking time, and shorter shelf life than dried pasta. The general term for all types of dried pasta is **macaroni**, whereas *pasta* refers to all types of dried and fresh pasta. (Only in the United States does *macaroni* refer *only* to the elbow-shaped, hollow-tube pasta.)

macaroni General term for all dried pasta products made with wheat flour and water.

al dente Italian phrase meaning "to the tooth" used to describe cooked pasta that is tender yet firm enough to be resistant when bitten.

Cooking Pasta

The most important aspects of cooking pasta are placing the pasta in boiling liquid and not overcooking it. It is important to add the pasta to boiling water; if placed in cold water it will not cook well and become sticky. During cooking, the pasta should be stirred to separate the pieces. It should be cooked to **al dente**, which means "to the tooth" in Italian. This means cooking the pasta until it is tender but firm and resistant when biting into it. Cooking dried and fresh pasta too long will cause excessive stickiness, resulting in a sticky mass of overcooked pasta. Undercooked pasta will be unpalatable because it is too firm.

Gastronomy Point

Fresh Pasta Fresh pasta cooks very fast—in less than 1 minute it is at the al dente stage.

Types of Pasta

Hundreds of types of pastas are available in a vast array of shapes and sizes (see **Figure 11.20**). Common pastas include spaghetti, which are long, solid, round, and rod-shaped noodles. Spaghetti varies in diameter, from very small-diameter angel hair, or capellini, to medium-diameter vermicelli and spaghettini, to larger-diameter fettuccini. Linguini is like spaghetti, but flat instead of round; lasagna is a large, flat pasta with ribbon edges; rigatoni are large, ridged hollow tubes; rotini are spiral shaped, elbow macaroni; and shell pastas come in many sizes, from tiny for soups and stews to large ones for stuffing. There also are numerous pastas with unusual shapes and sizes, such as bowties (farfalle), spirals, wagon wheels, letters, and animals.

Specialty Pastas

Natural colorants, such as spinach, carrot, or tomato powder or puree, and eggs or other ingredients can be added to some alimentary pastes. Herbs and seasonings can be added. Protein sources such as soy, wheat germ, whey, or other dairy proteins can be added to produce high-protein pastas. Whole grain pasta produced from whole wheat flour—or from other whole grain flours,

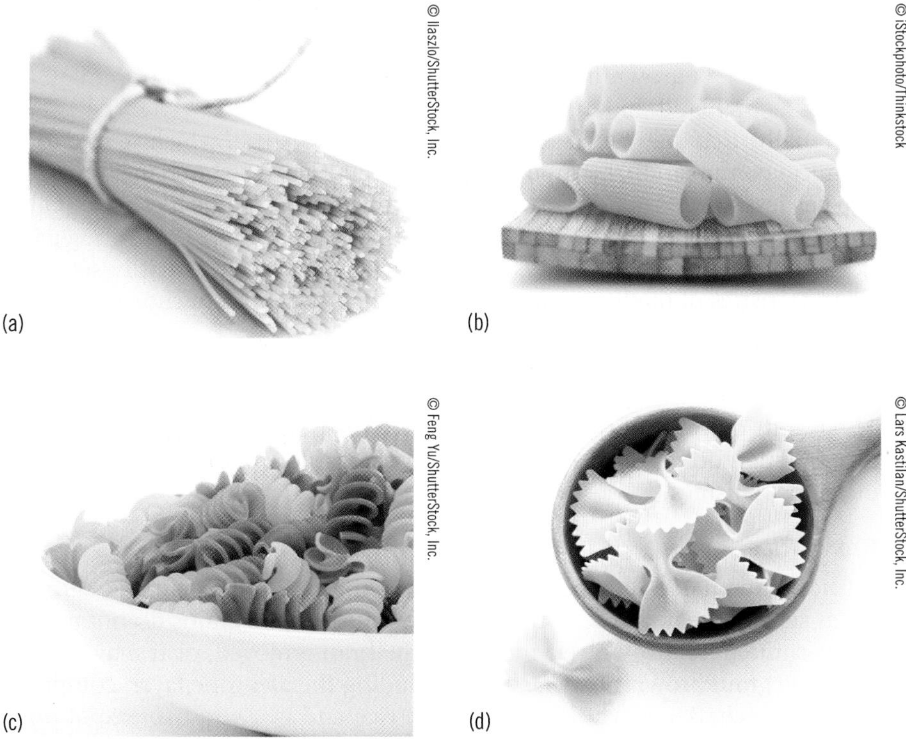

FIGURE 11.20 (a) Angel hair pasta has a diameter between 0.78 and 0.88 mm. Because it is a very light pasta, it pairs well with seafoods and light sauces. (b) Rigatoni, a tube pasta that is popular in southern Italian cuisine, comes in a variety of different sizes. It is usually ridged and has a squared-off end. (c) Rotini has a corkscrew shape that helps it hold sauces well. It often is used in pasta salads or in dishes calling for tomato sauces. (d) Farfalle is more commonly known as "bow-tie" pasta. It often is used in soups, such as chicken soup, and in dishes with cream or tomato sauces.

such as brown rice and buckwheat—are available but have a different texture and easily fall apart into small fragments if overcooked.

Gluten-free pasta products made with brown rice, corn, quinoa, and combinations of grains are available. However, it is difficult to produce a high-quality pasta product from a low-protein grain, such as rice, that will be of comparable texture to pasta made with semolina. The tendency for low-protein pastas to disintegrate into the cooking liquid is due to their weaker protein and starch matrix. When pasta is placed in boiling water, the starch molecules rapidly swell and are somewhat soluble, whereas the protein molecules are completely insoluble and coagulate, forming a network structure that traps the starch molecules. If a weak protein matrix is formed, the soluble starch molecules leak out of the matrix into the water, producing a pasta product with a sticky, gummy texture. In contrast to rice, quinoa flour is high in protein. Pasta made with quinoa and corn flours is gluten-free and similar in texture to semolina pasta.

Rice

Rice is most commonly classified based on the size of the kernel. The three rice categories are (1) short grain, (2) medium grain, and (3) long grain (see **Figure 11.21**). The relative length of the rice kernel in relationship to its width determines its classification. The length of most long-grain rice kernels is about three to four times the width. Short-grain kernels have similar lengths and widths and are oval shaped. Medium-grain kernels are longer and thinner than short-grain rice, but not as long and thin as long-grain kernels.

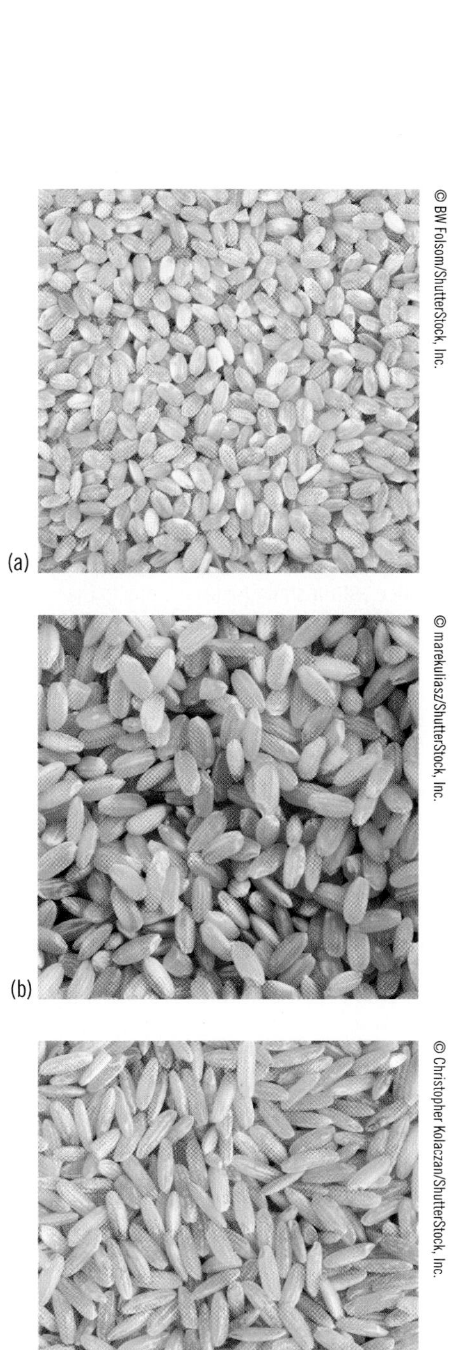

FIGURE 11.21 (a) Short grain rice is low in starch and very sticky. It is commonly used in Asian dishes, including sushi. (b) Medium-grain rice is a plump rice. It often is used in paella and risotto. (c) Long-grain rice is long and slender. Because the grains stay separate and fluffy after cooking, it is a good choice for rice served as a side dish.

Rice can also be classified according to its cultivation. Most rice is grown with the roots submerged in water and is known as lowland, wet, or irrigated rice. Rice plants grown in hilly areas receiving large amounts of rainfall are known as highland, hill, or dry rice.

Finally, rice may be classified by its cooked texture, which is due to its chemical composition. Compared to long-grain rice, the starch in short-grain rice has less amylose and more amylopectin, which explains its sticky quality and the relative ease with which it can be eaten with chopsticks. Long-grain rice cooks to a drier, fluffier texture, allowing the kernels to easily separate. Characteristics of medium-grain rice are in between those of short- and long-grain rice.

Forms of Rice

Thousands of forms of rice are available worldwide, depending on the type of rice and method of processing. Rice is very versatile and can be incorporated into most cuisines.

brown rice Hulled, unprocessed whole grain rice.

polished white rice Milled brown rice with a smooth surface due to the rubbing away of the bran and germ from the rice kernels during milling.

converted rice Long-grain rice that is parboiled before milling.

parboiling The partial cooking of food as the first step in the cooking process.

instant or quick-cooking cereal Precooked cereal that only requires rehydration.

Brown Rice

All rice when harvested and hulled is referred to as **brown rice**. Frequently, green kernels are found with brown rice because all the grains do not mature at the same time. Brown rice may have the bran removed, or it may be kept as whole grain brown rice. The bran, including the aleurone layer, comprises approximately 3% of whole grain brown rice and is a good source of fiber. The endosperm and germ comprise approximately 93% and 4% of the brown rice kernel, respectively (see Figure 11.15). Brown rice absorbs more water and requires a longer cooking time than white rice. Rice bran causes a texture that is chewier and tougher compared to white rice.

Polished White Rice

Polished white rice has a smooth surface produced by milling and is the most common type of rice produced and purchased. Along with the bran and the germ, milling removes the fiber and most of the vitamins and minerals, although some nutrients are replaced if the rice is enriched. Polished rice is sprayed with the enrichment nutrients and then coated with a waterproof edible film that hardens. The film prevents the nutrients from being easily removed if the rice is washed; however, enriched rice should not be rinsed prior to cooking.

Converted Rice

Converted rice is long-grain rice (either brown or white) that is parboiled before milling. (**Parboiling** means to partially cook a food; it is similar to blanching, but the cooking time is longer.) To parboil rice, the kernels are soaked, steamed, and dried before milling. This process removes the starch from the surface of the kernels and forces nutrients from the bran into the endosperm. Parboiled rice therefore retains more nutrients compared to white rice but has the advantage of tasting the same. Converted rice is not precooked or instant rice, and it cooks more slowly than regularly milled white rice. Food service establishments commonly use converted rice because the kernels stay firm and do not clump together.

Quick Cooking Rice

Instant or quick-cooking rice is rice that is fully cooked and then dehydrated. This form of rice is widely available and only takes a few minutes to prepare by rehydrating and heating; it is widely used for its convenience. However, it usually has a lower quality texture than other forms of rice.

In addition, problems of the kernels splitting during cooking and a dry texture are associated with instant rice.

Glutinous Rice

Glutinous rice is a short-grain rice also known as sticky rice, waxy rice, or sweet rice due to its stickiness and slightly sweet taste when cooked. This type of rice is characterized by its low amylose content. Glutinous rice is more transparent than other types of cooked rice and clumps together when cooked. This sticky quality is valued for making the rice easy to shape or mold; glutinous rice is therefore preferred for sushi and rice cakes. It also can be ground into flour and used for making dumplings and pastries. Japanese sake, Chinese shaoxing, and rice vinegars are usually produced from fermented sticky rice.

glutinous rice Short-grain rice that produces sticky clumps desired for sushi and rice cakes, also called sticky or waxy rice.

Specialty Rice

Specialty types of rice are usually not enriched and are more expensive than white and brown rices:

- Arborio rice is an oval, short-grain rice with a white color and mild flavor. Arborio rice can absorb a high quantity of liquid while cooking without becoming soggy.
- Basmati rice is considered one of the finest long-grain types of rice in the world. It is grown in the foothills of the Himalayas and is preferred in Indian cuisine. It is usually aged and highly aromatic; it should be washed prior to cooking. Basmati rice also is grown in other areas of the world, such as California, but this rice is grown from India's Basmati rice seed.[15]
- Jasmine rice is a long-grain, aromatic rice. It is grown in Thailand and used throughout Southeast Asia.
- Wild pecan rice is grown only in the bayou area of southern Louisiana. It is a long-grain rice with a rich, nutty flavor.
- Golden rice, or vitamin A rice, is a type of genetically engineered rice. It does not provide vitamin A directly; however, golden rice produces and deposits carotene (provitamin A) in the endosperm of the kernels as it grows, which is then converted to vitamin A in the human body. This is important because the risk of vitamin A deficiency is high in more than 100 developing countries where the average diet is based on rice. Golden rice has the potential to alleviate widespread vitamin A deficiency, which causes susceptibility to infections, blindness, and death. This golden-colored rice can benefit millions of children in developing countries who experience the devastating effects of vitamin A deficiency.[19]

Asian Noodles

Asian noodles are produced using rice, mung bean, taro, soy, or other flours. (They do not usually contain semolina or egg.) Most of these noodles, especially rice noodles, are transparent or opaque in color. Quick-cooking or instant noodles are produced by steaming the noodle paste and then frying it to remove the moisture. The precooked noodles only require rehydration in a hot liquid for preparation.

Rice Flour, Starch, and Bran

Flour and starch milled from rice is gluten-free and available in the marketplace. Rice bran is usually a mixture of the bran and germ; it is high in soluble fiber. Full-fat rice bran has been shown to be as effective as oat bran in

Gastronomy Point

Arborio Rice Arborio rice has a creamy and chewy texture. It makes wonderful rice puddings and paella and risotto dishes.

lowering high blood cholesterol levels.[20] Another study determined that rice bran oil was responsible for the decreased cholesterol levels, not the fiber.[21] Rice bran has a different taste and shorter shelf life compared to oat bran.

Corn

Corn (*Zea mays*) kernels grow in rows on a cob, which is partially covered by "corn silk" and enclosed in a husk. Corn is the only grain that can also be eaten as a fresh vegetable. Corn oil extracted from the germ is high in polyunsaturated fatty acids.

Types of Corn

Corn is classified according to the color and type of kernel. Yellow and white colors predominate. Other colors are red, blue, pink, black, and striped. Common types of corn include sweet, flint, flour, popcorn, and dent; all of these are varieties of *Zea mays*. The majority of corn eaten as a vegetable is yellow or white sweet corn, which is commonly eaten fresh or canned or is frozen for future consumption.

Flint Corn

Flint corn, also known as Indian corn, has extremely hard kernels and produces good quality cornmeal.

Flour Corn

Flour corn produces a softer kernel that can be easily ground into flour. It is usually white or blue. Commonly used by Native Americans in the southwest United States and Mexico, this corn flour has been used for over a thousand years to make staples such as tortillas and tamales. Blue corn chips are sold in the retail market with the more familiar yellow corn chips.

> ***Gastronomy Point***
>
> **Popcorn** Popcorn has been eaten for centuries and is considered the oldest snack food. For a salt-free, low-fat treat, season plain popcorn with savory, sweet, or hot and spicy seasonings.

Popcorn

Popcorn is grown for the snack food of the same name. The kernels have a soft starchy center surrounded by a hard, thick-walled exterior. Popping corn involves heating popcorn kernels to a temperature that causes the moisture inside the kernels to change to steam, which increases the pressure inside the kernels. This causes the kernels to burst, which pops the kernels open and exposes the puffed starch. Not all cereals will pop; popcorn pops well due to its pericarp (bran) withstanding high temperatures before bursting. The United States is the largest producer and consumer of popcorn.[22]

Dent Corn

Dent corn, also known as field corn, has a small, discernable dent on each kernel and accounts for the vast majority of all corn grown in the United States. About 50% of dent corn is used for livestock feed; the remainder is used by manufacturers for production of corn syrup, starch, alcohol, and canned or other processed corn; exported; or stored as reserves for future use to safeguard against the possibility of next year's corn crop failing or producing inadequate yields to meet current needs.

Corn Products

Corn is prepared in various ways and transformed into a multitude of products. Fresh sweet corn is eaten in its original form as corn on the cob. Ears of corn are shucked, cleaned, cooked, and eaten directly off the corn cob. Kernels that are removed from the cobs are cooked and eaten as kernel corn (a starchy vegetable) or combined with other foods and used in various dishes.

Hominy

Hominy is the endosperm of white or yellow sweet corn kernels. Dried corn is soaked in hydrated lime or lye, which causes the kernels to swell and loosens the hulls. The hulls and germs are removed, and the remaining endosperms are washed and dried. Hominy is available in canned and frozen forms and can be used as a side dish or in stews and soups. *Masa harina*, a finely ground flour produced from dried hominy, is used in breads, tamales, tortillas, and other Mexican and southwestern dishes.[15]

Hominy Grits

Hominy grits are dried hominy that has been coarsely ground. Grits are boiled with water and commonly eaten as a hot breakfast dish in the southern United States with butter, salt, or cheese added for flavor. Grits can also be used in baked dishes. Quick-cooking and instant grits are commercially available. Polenta is a popular northern Italian dish prepared from hominy grits.

Cornmeal

Cornmeal is produced by drying and grinding dent corn. **Meal** is more coarsely ground than grits, but not as fine as flour, which is produced by sifting or further grinding the cornmeal. Products made with meal have a grittier texture than products made with flour, which is usually ground to a fine powder. Cornmeal has a higher fat content than wheat flour. Therefore, cornbread has a shorter shelf life due to the speed of fat oxidation and resulting rancidity compared to wheat bread. **Degermed cornmeal** is cornmeal produced with the bran and germ removed prior to milling the endosperm. This produces a drier meal with less fat and more starch than cornmeal produced from whole corn kernels.

Cornstarch

Cornstarch is obtained from processed corn endosperm and is the most common culinary starch in the United States. Cornstarch is used to thicken gravies, puddings, and sauces.

Corn Syrup

Corn syrup is produced by treating cornstarch with hydrolytic enzymes. Corn syrups are viscous liquids of varying consistency and color and contain mainly fructose, glucose, maltose, and dextrins. Dark corn syrup has a stronger flavor than light corn syrup.

Barley

Barley (*H. vulgare*) is a versatile grain. Worldwide production of barley is right behind that for wheat, rice, and corn. The nutritive content is similar to corn, but unlike corn, barley contains the B vitamin niacin. Barley contains gluten and has a rich, nutty flavor. Barley is found in various food products:

- Barley **groats** are whole barley kernels, which also are called barley berries. Barley berries are rolled flat for whole grain flaked barley.
- Pearled barley is milled and polished to remove the bran and germ and usually some of the endosperm. It is used in soups, stews, and baby foods. Pearled barley also is milled to make barley grits and flour or rolled into flakes for use in hot breakfast cereals.

An important use of barley is for the production of **malt**, which is sprouted, dried barley. Whole barley kernels are steeped in water to allow the germ to sprout. The sprouted, or germinated, barley produces

hominy Corn endosperm.

hominy grits Coarsely milled hominy.

meal Coarsely ground cereal milled finer than grits but not as fine as flour.

degermed cornmeal Cornmeal produced with the bran and germ removed prior to milling the corn endosperm.

groats Whole cereal kernels, such as oat groats.

malt Sprouted, dried barley.

starch-digesting amylase activity. The sprouted barley is gently heated to promote browning and the creation of a malt flavor. Malt, with its enzymatic activity, provides a source of carbohydrates for yeast to produce alcohol in the production of alcoholic beverages, as described in **Special Topic 11.3**. Malt also is incorporated into many bakery products for flavor and dough

Special Topic 11.3

History of Beer Making

Caitlin Portrie

Beer is the most consumed alcoholic beverage in the world; it also happens to be one of the oldest. Whether by accident or on purpose, beer making dates back to 9500 to 8000 B.C., coincident with the domestication of cereals. Debate continues over where beer making first originated, but the earliest documentations is from Ancient Egypt and Sumeria, circa 4000 B.C. Beer was first recognized in writing in a 4,000-year-old Sumerian poem dedicated to Ninkasi, the Sumerian goddess of brewing. The recipe in the poem describes beer as being produced from barley via bread and being a thicker beverage than that consumed today. People drank it from a straw to avoid consuming the precipitate. In the brewing process, fermentation stoppers were placed on the mouth of a jar. When cloth was packed inside the clay stopper's hole, it allowed gasses to escape during the fermentation process but prevented microorganisms from entering that would spoil the brew.[1]

Beer was introduced to Europe by the Egyptians, who brought it to Greece. In 450 B.C., Sophocles wrote about beer and the need for drinking it in moderation. Citizens of Ancient Rome and Ancient Greece drank it, but wine was much more favored in this time period. Beer made a resurgence in popularity in the Middle Ages. In the seventh century, the Christian faith adopted beer, making it in their monasteries. It was only sold domestically because the shelf life of beer was still only a few days.

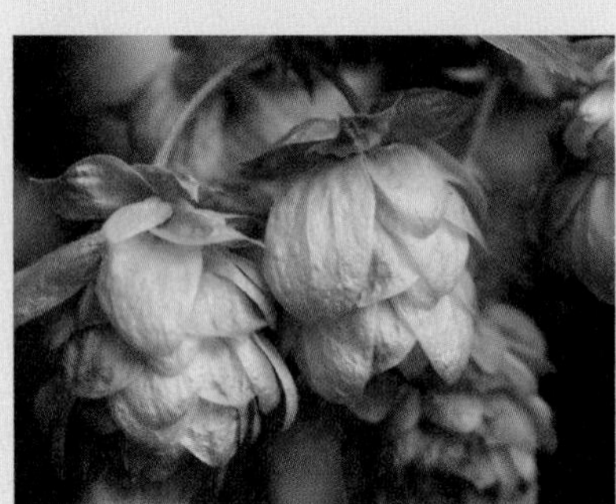

FIGURE A Hops (*Humulus lupulus*) is used a flavoring agent in beer, giving it a bitter, tangy flavor. It also has an antibacterial agent, lengthening the shelf life of beer.

The discovery of hops in 822 was a breakthrough. Hops was used as a preservative and to add flavor (see **Figure A**).[2] After the introduction of hops, the flavor of beer differed greatly and its shelf life improved. One of the oldest food-quality regulations still in use today, the "German Purity Law," was adopted in 1516 by William IV, Duke of Bavaria. It stated that the ingredients that made beer were water, hops, and barley malt. Brewer's yeast was added to the list in 1857—after Louis Pasteur's discovery—to preserve the fermentation of the beer. If the beverage did not include all of these ingredients, it would have to be called something else.[3]

Great strides were made in beer making with the Industrial Revolution because beer could finally be produced on a larger scale. Beer making moved from being brewed by artisans in small breweries to mass production on an industrial scale. The steam engine, hydrometers, and thermometers increased precision and allowed for more control over the brewing process. Pasteurization of beer meant it could be shipped safely and in large quantities. In fact, the beer industry adopted pasteurization long before it was applied to milk. For example, Anheuser-Busch began pasteurizing beer in 1872.[2]

Today, beer making is an art form. Each country and each brewery has its own style of making beer. Dark beers, light beers, wheat beers, and lagers now can be found all over the world. The brewing industry has become an enormous global business and a great source of commerce in international trade.

References

1 Homan M. Beer and its drinkers: An ancient near eastern love story. *Near Eastern Archaeology*. 2004;67(2):84–95.

2 Nelson M. *The Barbarian's Beverage: A History of Beer in Ancient Europe*. London: Routledge; 2005.

3 Wolf A, Bray GA, Popkin BM. A short history of beverages and how our body treats them. *Obes Rev*. 2008 Mar;9(2):151–164.

improvement, and it is used for flavor in malted milk additives and breakfast cereals.

Oats

Oats (*A. sativa*) are a popular hot breakfast cereal in the United States, in addition to being used in breads, muffins, cookies, baby foods, granola bars, and other baked and snack food items. The components of oat kernels are strongly attached; when the husks are removed, the bran and germ tend to remain with the oat kernels. This property of oats may help account for its health benefits. For example, the water-soluble fiber in oat bran has been shown to help prevent heart disease. Because most of the germ is usually present, oats are higher in polyunsaturated fat than most other grains products. Dry quick-cooking oats contain approximately 7% fat, dry instant corn grits have about 2%, and dry wheat farina has about 1%.[23]

A variety of different oat products are available:

- Oat groats are whole oat kernels. They also are known as whole grain oats or oat berries.
- Steel-cut oats, also known as Irish oats, are toasted groats cut into small pieces with steel blades, which creates a denser, chewier texture. Steel-cut oats are more popular in Ireland and Scotland than in the United States.
- Rolled oats are groats that have been heated and then flattened with steel rollers.

Commercial oat products include regular old fashioned, quick-cooking, and instant oatmeal. Regular old fashioned oatmeal is just rolled groats. Quick-cooking oatmeal is produced by cutting the groats into tiny pieces before rolling them to reduce cooking time. Instant oatmeal contains oats that have been steamed to pregelatinize the starch; this allows immediate hydration in hot water for fast and easy preparation. Rolled and quick-cooking oats can be used interchangeably in recipes, but instant oats should not be substituted for rolled or quick-cooking oats.[15]

Rye

Rye (*S. cereale*) has a number of uses. It can be ground into a flour for making bread. It also can be used in the production of alcoholic beverages, such as beer and whiskey. Rye also is grown for animal feed.

Rye is found in various forms:

- Whole rye kernels are available as rye berries. Rolled, flat rye berries are processed into flakes and used for hot breakfast cereals, flat Swedish rye bread, and rye crisp wafers.
- Rye meal is coarsely milled rye berries. It is used for making crisp bread and pumpernickel bread. Pumpernickel is a dense rye bread that contains a high proportion of dark rye flour.
- Rye flour is available in three varieties: white, medium, and dark. The flour can be used to make bread and other baked goods. White rye flour has a milder flavor than medium rye flour; dark rye flour has the strongest flavor. Rye flour is lower in gluten protein than wheat flour and contains a higher proportion of soluble fiber. Due to its low gluten content, bread made with rye flour is dense and compact. Rye flour is used in breads because of its unique flavor; however, most rye breads contain a combination of wheat and rye flours for better acceptability.

Phytonutrient Point

Beta-Glucan Beta-glucan is a cell wall component of cereal grains that can help lower cholesterol. Barley is higher in beta-glucans than oats.

Innovation Point

Fermentation The fermentation by yeast of the carbohydrates in grain produces many alcoholic beverages.

Millets

Millets used as cereals have a nutty flavor; they are cooked and eaten as porridge and used to make unleavened bread and beer. Because millets do not contain gluten, millet flour is mixed with wheat flour or other flours when used for baking leavened products. There are thousands of types of millets. Pearl millet (*Pennisetumg laucum*) is the most widely grown millet.[24] Other common types are foxtail millet (*Setaria italica*); proso millet, also called hog, common, or broomcorn millet (*Panicum miliaceum*); finger millet (*Eleusine coracana*); and teff (*Eragrostis tef*).

Teff has very tiny seeds, less than 1 millimeter across, or about the size of a poppy seed. The seeds are cooked as a hot cereal product or milled into flour for making pancakes, flat breads, and other products. Teff seeds are too small to allow separation of the bran, endosperm, and germ components, so it is always consumed as a whole grain. It is very nutritious and contains high levels of iron and calcium compared to other grains. Teff is ground into flour and fermented to make the sourdough bread in Ethiopia known as "injera." Injera is used as an edible plate—food is piled on the bread, and pieces of bread are torn off for wrapping food to be eaten. In addition, the leaves of the teff plant can be eaten as a vegetable.

Breakfast Cereals

The breakfast cereal industry as we know it today began in the late nineteenth century in Battle Creek, Michigan, at the Battle Creek Sanitarium of the Seventh-day Adventist Church. There, the Kellogg brothers invented flaked cereals as a healthful food. Dr. John Harvey Kellogg filed a patent application in 1894 for the processing of flaked cereals from grains, including wheat, corn, oats, and barley. Also in 1894, C.W. Post—a former patient of the Battle Creek Sanitarium—invented a coffee substitute using roasted wheat, bran, and molasses. He called it Postum and formed The Postum Cereal Company. Post made another coffee substitute, but it was poorly accepted—he sold it in granular form as a breakfast food and called it Grape Nuts. More than a hundred years later, Grape Nuts cereal is still being produced and eaten. Another important person in the history of the breakfast cereal industry is C.C. Washburn, who began a flour mill in Minneapolis, Minnesota, and formed the General Mills Company. He introduced a wheat flake that became Wheaties in the 1920s and is still popular today.

Gastronomy Point

Grits Corn grits are a common ready-to-cook or instant cereal in the southern United States.

Most breakfast cereals are produced from the endosperm of wheat, corn, rice, or oats. In all the cereal categories, different cereals may be combined together. Additives, such as sugar, malt, and flavorings, may be used to improve taste; however, many breakfast cereals have few additives other than vitamins and minerals. The five categories of cereals recognized by the U.S. cereal industry are (1) traditional cereals that require cooking, or hot, ready-to-cook cereals; (2) instant traditional hot cereals; (3) ready-to-eat cereals; (4) ready-to-eat cereal mixes; and (5) miscellaneous cereal products.[25]

Ready-to-Cook Cereals

Wheat or oat cereals consumed hot can take various forms, such as whole, cracked, ground, or rolled cereals. (Rice is not commonly used in this category.) Grinding or rolling cereal kernels allows for a quicker cooking time than for whole kernels.

Instant Traditional Hot Cereals

Instant traditional hot cereals—such as wheat, oats, and corn—are ground, cut, or rolled into smaller particles compared to cereals labeled as regular or quick-cooking. Instant cereals are fully cooked and dehydrated and only need the addition of hot liquid to prepare the cereal.

Ready-to-Eat Cereals

Ready-to-eat cereals are produced from endosperm particles that are broken and ground into a mash, cooked, and converted into flakes by squeezing the broken grits or mash between rollers. The mash can also be extruded, or formed, into numerous shapes and sizes. Puffed cereals are produced by heating intact endosperm under high pressure; when the pressure is suddenly released, the steam inside the endosperm forces the cell walls to break and puffs the cereal to about eight times its original size. Whether flaked, extruded, puffed, or shredded, all cereals are roasted in ovens to develop toasted flavors and reduce moisture, which is approximately 3–5% in most cereals. Many ready-to-eat breakfast cereals are fortified with vitamins and minerals to improve their nutritional content. The largest market for breakfast cereals is convenient, ready-to-eat cereals.

Ready-to-Eat Cereal Mixes

Ready-to-eat cereal mixes are cereals combined with other grains, legumes, seeds, or dried fruits. Granola cereal mixes are an example of ready-to-eat cereal mixes.

Miscellaneous Cereal Products

Cereal products that cannot be included in the other breakfast categories due to specialized processes or end uses—such as baby foods and cereal nuggets—may be put in this miscellaneous category.

Other Plants Used as Grains

Earlier in the chapter, several seeds of nongrass plants were introduced as grains, although technically they are not grains.

Wild Rice

Wild rice (*Z. aquatica*) has long, slender kernels that are dark brown to black in color. It has a nutty flavor and a chewy, fibrous texture. Compared to white rice, wild rice is much higher in fiber, protein, and B vitamins. Wild rice is generally served with game, used as a poultry stuffing, or combined with white or brown rice and served as a side dish.[15]

Buckwheat

Buckwheat flour is used to make griddle cakes, or pancakes. Buckwheat groats are roasted to form **kasha**, which has a nutty flavor and is used in many types of dishes and as a breakfast cereal, especially in Slavic countries and Eastern Europe. The endosperm of buckwheat contains a protein similar to the gluten found in some of the true grains.

kasha Roasted buckwheat groats.

Amaranth

Seeds from the amaranth plant can be ground into flour or puffed for a cereal product. The whole grain flour contains fairly high levels of polyunsaturated fat and should be stored at cold temperatures to prevent spoiling. Amaranth does not contain gluten and is usually mixed with wheat when used for baking. Amaranth is high in fiber and contains many vitamins and minerals at higher levels than wheat and other grains; additionally, it is high in protein and contains the essential amino acids lysine and methionine, which are lacking or insufficient in other grains. A complete source of protein is provided when amaranth seeds are combined with wheat, rice, or barley.

Like other whole seeds, amaranth should be rinsed with water before cooking. Amaranth can be cooked and served as a side dish, but toasting the seeds first for a few minutes in a hot dry pan promotes the nutty flavor. It can be used as a thickener in soups and stews; it congeals as it cools. The amaranth plant's broad leaves with red markings can be cooked and eaten as a vegetable and taste somewhat like spinach.[15]

Quinoa

Quinoa is used as a grain product, in that the whole seeds are milled into flour for use in baked products. It does not contain gluten and is usually mixed with other flours for baking purposes. The outer portion of quinoa seeds contains a bitter-tasting natural compound that protects the seeds from insects and birds. To remove this taste, the seeds should be rinsed well in cool water using a fine-mesh colander prior to cooking. Quinoa can be cooked similar to rice. For a nuttier flavor, toast quinoa seeds in a hot dry pan for a few minutes before adding liquid. Quinoa can be used as a hot breakfast cereal and as an ingredient in soups, stews, salads, casseroles, breads, and desserts. Quinoa flour is used for dried pasta production by mixing it with corn flour for a gluten-free pasta product. The nutritional composition of quinoa is excellent; it contains carbohydrate, fat, vitamins, minerals, and all the essential amino acids. It is an excellent source of protein for vegans. The leaves of the quinoa plant can be eaten as a vegetable.[15]

Nutritional Properties and Impact on Health

Grains have an impact on human health perhaps greater than any other food group because of the large quantity found in the typical diet. These are some of the nutritional aspects of grains that impact human health:[26]

- Grains are important sources of many nutrients, including dietary fiber, several B vitamins (thiamin, riboflavin, niacin, and folate), and several minerals (iron, magnesium, and selenium).
- Dietary fiber from whole grains may help reduce blood cholesterol levels and may lower risk of heart disease, obesity, and type 2 diabetes. Fiber is important for proper bowel function, and it helps reduce constipation and diverticulosis. Fiber-containing foods such as whole grains help provide a feeling of fullness with fewer calories.
- The B vitamins thiamin, riboflavin, and niacin play a key role in metabolism. These nutrients help the body release energy from protein, fat, and carbohydrates. B vitamins also are essential for a healthy nervous system. Many refined grains are enriched with these B vitamins.
- Folate (folic acid), another B vitamin, helps the body form red blood cells. Women of childbearing age who may become pregnant should consume adequate folate from foods, and in addition 400 mcg of synthetic folic acid from fortified foods or supplements. This reduces the risk of neural tube defects, spina bifida, and anencephaly during fetal development.
- Iron is used to carry oxygen in the blood. Many teenage girls and women in their childbearing years have iron-deficiency anemia. They should eat foods high in heme-iron (meats) or eat other iron containing foods along with foods rich in vitamin C, which can improve absorption of non-heme iron. Whole and enriched

refined grain products are major sources of non-heme iron in American diets.
- Whole grains are sources of magnesium and selenium. Magnesium is a mineral used in building bones and releasing energy from muscles. Selenium protects cells from oxidation. It also is important for a healthy immune system.

Most refined grains are *enriched*. This means certain B vitamins (thiamin, riboflavin, niacin, and folic acid) and iron are added back after processing. Fiber is not added back to enriched grains. Check the ingredient list on refined grain products to make sure that the word "enriched" or "fortified" is included in the grain name. Some food products are made from mixtures of whole grains and refined grains.

Whole Grains

Whole grains—such as brown rice, oats, barley, wheat berries, amaranth, quinoa, teff, and bulgur—are nutritious sources of complex carbohydrates that provide many nutrients and fiber. Increasing intakes of whole grains is associated with lower visceral adipose tissue in adults.[27] Whole grains include all parts of the cereal kernel—bran, germ, and endosperm—whereas refined grains include only the starchy endosperm.

Fortified Grains

Fortified grains have nutrients added to improve their nutritional content. Fortification is the process of adding nutrients that were not available in the food before processing. (This differs from enrichment, where original nutrients are added back to foods that processing may have filtered out.) Many breakfast cereals are fortified with nutrients and are important sources of micronutrients, such as vitamin B_{12}; this is especially important for vegans because they do not have a food source for this vitamin. Cereal bars and power energy bars may be fortified with protein and many other nutrients. The United Nations World Food Program has several cereal-based fortified food products that are used as emergency supplemental foods in times of famine and disasters to provide individuals with nutrient-dense calories (protein, fat, and carbohydrate), and essential vitamins and minerals.

Going Green with Grains

The United Nations World Commission on Environment and Development has defined sustainable development as "meeting the needs of the present generation without compromising the ability of future generations to meet their own needs."[28] This can be accomplished, in part, through the greening of cereal grains cultivation.

Farming Practices

Farming practices that promote green agriculture for cereal grains include:

- Restoring and enhancing soil fertility through increased use of natural and sustainable nutrient inputs
- Diversifying crop rotations
- Reducing soil erosion and improving water use efficiency by incorporating cover crop cultivation techniques
- Producing crops using minimum tillage[28]

Packaging

Packaging is another area that the cereal industry must address in terms of reducing waste. The three Rs of green packaging are reduce, reuse, and recycle. In many cases, the amount of materials used for packaging could be reduced. Industry-wide reduction in the amount of material used to package cereal products could save millions of pounds of waste from landfills. Reusing means using a food package for other uses after its use as a food package has been fulfilled. Most plastic packaging from food items is disposed in landfills, which causes environmental problems. Recycling is a potential solution; however, the industrial processes required to recycle paperboard and plastics into other products create greenhouse gas emissions and other environmental pollutants. Using recycled plastics or other recycled materials to create more food packaging presents food safety (contamination) concerns.[29]

An ideal food package does not exist. Food safety and other issues, such as cost, mechanical strength, and marketing appeal, must be considered. Ideally, a package should decay without polluting the environment once its function has been accomplished. The packaging industry is challenged with developing reusable, recyclable, environmentally friendly disposable packaging that appeals to consumers and also keeps food safe during shipping and storage.[29]

Green Point

Rice Packaging Some rice producers have reduced packaging material by about 15% by removing the reusable zippers in their 2-pound rice bags, saving 35,000 pounds of plastic from entering landfills yearly.

Food Safety and Regulations

Storage

Dry cereals are low in water content and more shelf stable than other foods, such as dairy and meat products and fresh vegetables and fruits. Whole grain cereals should be stored at cool temperatures because they contain more fat than processed cereal products and deteriorate more rapidly. Leftover cereal dishes should be handled like any type of cooked food containing protein is handled. Leftovers should be cooled quickly and stored at refrigerated temperatures of 41°F (5°C) or lower and reheated thoroughly to 165°F (74°C) or higher. Cooked rice is very perishable due to its neutral pH and protein content and is considered a potentially hazardous food. To avoid the risk of foodborne illness, keep hot rice, or any hot food, at 140°F (60°C) or higher and store leftovers quickly in the refrigerator.

Enrichment and Fortification

The word *enriched* is often listed on the label or packaging of grain products. Enriched grains are those that have nutrients added back—based on federal guidelines—after they have been processed or refined. Enrichment is important because nutrients are lost during the processing of cereal grains into refined products such as white flour and white rice. After processing and refinement of grains became prevalent in the early part of the twentieth century, nutrient deficiencies became more common. In response to this problem, the U.S. Congress passed the Enrichment Act of 1942, which required the addition of thiamin, riboflavin, niacin, and iron to refined white flour. In 1996, the enrichment standards were amended to include folic acid.

Chapter Review

Edible seeds from the grass (Gramineae) family are called cereal grains. Common cereals are wheat, rice, corn (maize), oats, barley, sorghum, rye, and millets. Less common cereals are spelt, triticale, and teff (which is a millet). Wild rice, amaranth, buckwheat, and quinoa are used as cereals in many parts of the world (although they are not technically cereals because they are not in the grass family). The top three cereal crops are wheat, rice, and corn—they provide the majority of the world's energy intake.

Cereals are available as whole grains and in many refined and processed forms. Whole grain products contain all parts of the cereal kernel—the bran, endosperm, and germ. Refined grains have been milled to remove the bran and germ. This improves the shelf life but removes nutrients and fiber. Many grains are enriched by adding thiamin, riboflavin, niacin, folic acid, and iron after processing based on federal guidelines. Fortification is the process of adding nutrients to foods to improve the nutritional content.

A general term for all types of dried pasta is macaroni. *Pasta* is a general term for all types of dried and fresh pasta commonly known as spaghetti, macaroni, and noodles. Pasta is produced from semolina flour milled from durum wheat, which is higher in protein than other types of wheat. There are hundreds of pasta shapes and sizes. Pasta should be added to boiling water for proper cooking.

The three cooking methods used to prepare grains or cereals are simmering, pilaf, and risotto. Simmering is adding the cereal to boiling water and simmering until cooked and tender. The cereals are sautéed in fat before adding liquid in the pilaf and risotto methods. All the liquid is added at one time in the pilaf method. Hot liquid is gradually added over the cooking time and the cereal is constantly stirred in the risotto method to produce a more creamy texture.

Many cereal and flour products contain gluten, which is the protein formed when the proteins gliadin and glutenin are mixed with water to form a dough or batter. Gluten is responsible for the viscous and elastic characteristics and high volume of baked products. Individuals with celiac disease have gluten intolerance and must avoid consuming gluten. There are many gluten-free cereals and flours available in the marketplace.

Starch is the storage form of energy in plants and is a complex carbohydrate. Natural starches contain amylose and amylopectin, which have different properties. Amylose will form a firm gel when cooked but amylopectin will not. Amylopectin contributes to thickening of products. The most common starch is cornstarch.

The cereal industry can provide green products to the public by focusing on green agriculture practices and green packaging. An ecological focus on packaging is occurring with consumers becoming more aware of environmental issues. The three Rs of green packaging are reduce, reuse, and recycle; that is, reduce the amount of material used for packaging, reuse packages, and recycle packaging instead of disposing it in landfills.

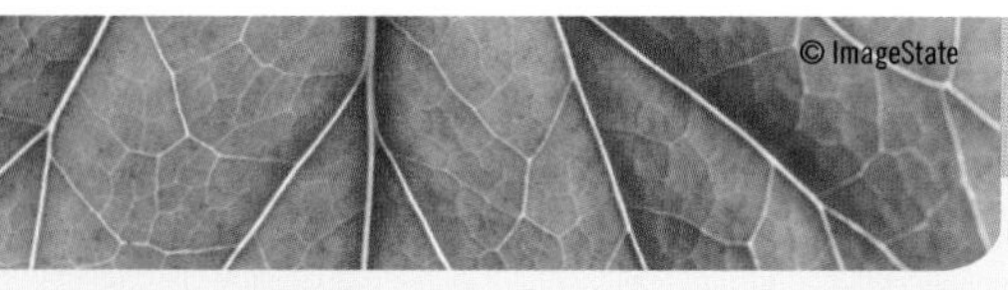

© ImageState

Learning Portfolio

Key Terms

	page
al dente	362
aleurone	350
bran	350
brown rice	364
bulgur	360
cereals	346
converted rice	364
couscous	360
cracked wheat	360
degermed cornmeal	367
durum	360
endosperm	350
farina	360
germ	351
gluten	352
glutinous rice	365
grain	346
groats	367
hominy	367
hominy grits	367
instant or quick-cooking cereal	364
kasha	371
macaroni	362
malt	367
meal	367
milling	351
parboiling	364
pasta	361
polished white rice	364
refined flour	351
semolina	360
slurry	357
wheat berry	360

Study Points

1. Edible seeds from the grass (Gramineae) family are cereal grains. Both the fruit (the seed or kernel) and the plant are referred to as a grain. The terms *cereal* and *grain* are often used interchangeably.
2. Cereal grains are grown in greater quantities compared to other crops and are referred to as *staple crops*. Grains are essential for sustaining animal and human life and are the most important source of the world's food supply. The main staple cereal crops are wheat, rice, corn (maize), barley, sorghum, oats, rye, and millets. Less common cereals or plants used as cereals include amaranth, buckwheat, quinoa, teff, and triticale.
3. The main structural parts of all cereal kernels are (1) the outer bran portion, which is high in dietary fiber; (2) the middle endosperm, which is the largest part of the kernel and contains stored starch that can be processed into flour; (3) the germ or embryo, which is the smallest part of the kernel and produces a sprout for a new plant to grow; and (4) the aleurone component, which is the layer between the bran and the endosperm and contains many nutrients but less fiber than the bran. Most grains are processed, or milled, to separate the kernel parts to improve storage quality. Processing also improves the functional properties of the endosperm in manufactured products.
4. Many types of flours are available, including whole wheat, all-purpose, bread, and cake flour. All flours are high in starch. Gluten protein is formed when wheat flour or other gluten-containing flour is mixed with water. Gluten imparts good structure and texture to baked products. Gluten-free flours such as rice and corn flours are available. Enriched flour contains thiamin, riboflavin, niacin, and folic acid, and the mineral iron, all added based on federal standards.
5. Three basic methods of cooking grains are simmering, pilaf, and risotto. Pilaf and risotto methods include coating the cereal kernels with fat and sautéing prior to adding liquid.
6. The six classes of wheat are (1) hard red winter, (2) hard red spring, (3) soft red winter, (4) hard white winter, (5) soft white wheat, and (6) durum. Hard wheat varieties are higher in protein and lower in starch compared to soft wheat varieties. Hard wheat varieties are used for making bread because the protein provides good structure in baked products. Durum wheat is the hardest wheat and is used for pasta production.
7. There are many types and forms of cereals/grains, such as whole berries or groats, and processed forms, such as cracked, rolled, or flaked cereals; grits; and flour. Corn is the only grain eaten as a fresh vegetable (corn on the cob). Hominy is the endosperm of corn kernels. Dried hominy is ground to make grits.
8. Durum wheat is milled into coarse semolina flour used for pasta production. Pasta can be formed into hundreds of different shapes and sizes. All pastas are made of the simple ingredients of semolina and water.
9. The most common classification of rice is based on kernel size: short grain, medium grain, and long grain. Long-grain rice cooks to a fluffier, drier texture than short- or medium-grain rice. Cooked short-grain rice sticks together and is good for making sushi and rice cakes and for eating with chopsticks. Instant rice is precooked and only requires rehydration with hot water for preparation.
10. Most breakfast cereals are produced from the endosperm of wheat, corn, rice, or oats. The five categories of breakfast cereals are (1) traditional cereals that require cooking, or hot, ready-to-cook cereals; (2) instant traditional hot cereals; (3) ready-to-eat cereals; (4) ready-to-eat cereal mixes; and (5) miscellaneous cereal products.

Issues for Discussion

1. Discuss how the cereal industry can make its packages more environmentally friendly.
2. Discuss the origins of your favorite grains and explain why they are your favorite. Describe how you prefer to consume your favorite grains/cereal products.
3. Discuss gluten and why it has become a marketplace trend to offer gluten-free products. Evaluate some of the culinary concerns about using gluten-free flours for baked products.

Research Ideas for Students

1. The nutrient content of various grains
2. How grains are commonly prepared in different cultures
3. The marketing and pricing of whole grains versus refined grains

References

1. Cai Y, Corke H. Cereals: Biology, pre- and post-harvest management. In: Hui Y-H (ed.). *Handbook of Food Science, Technology, and Engineering*. Vol 1. Boca Raton, FL: CRC Press; 2006.
2. United Nations Food and Agriculture Organization. Staple Foods: What Do People Eat? Available at: http://www.fao.org/docrep/u8480e/u8480e07.htm.
3. Blatter RHE, Jacomet S, Schlumbaum A. About the origin of European spelt (*Triticum spelta* L.): Allelic differentiation of the HMW glutenin B1-1 and A1-2 subunit genes. *Theor Appl Genet*. 2004;108:360–367.
4. Murray M, Pizzorno J, Pizzorno L. *The Encyclopedia of Healing Foods*. New York: Atria Books/Simon and Schuster; 2005.
5. Newman CW, Newman RK. A brief history of barley foods. *Cereal Foods World*. 2006;51(1):4–7.
6. Mahapatra AK, Yubin L. Postharvest handling of grains and pulses. In: Rahman MS (ed.). *Handbook of Food Preservation*. 2nd ed. Boca Raton, FL: CRC Press; 2007.
7. Vail GE, Griswold RM, Justin MM, Rust LO. *Foods*. 5th ed. Boston: Houghton Mifflin; 1967.
8. Ludvigsson JF, Montgomery SM, Ekbom A, et al. Small-intestinal histopathology and mortality risk in celiac disease. *JAMA*. 2009;302(11):1171–1178.
9. Aranowski AL. Looking ahead: Most-mentioned food and ingredient trends for 2009. *Cereal Foods World*. 2009;54(1): 15–17.
10. Thompson T. Gluten contamination of commercial oat products in the United States. *N Eng J Med*. 2004;351:2021–2022.
11. Sanchez HD, Osella CA, De La Torre MA. Optimization of gluten-free bread prepared from cornstarch, rice flour, and cassava starch. *J Food Sci*. 2002;67:416–419.
12. Gallagher E, Gormley TR, Arendt EK. Recent advances in the formulation of gluten-free cereal-based products. *Trends Food Sci Tech*. 2004;15:143–152.
13. Jackson V, Schilling MW, Falkenberg SM, et al. Quality characteristics and storage stability of baked and fried chicken nuggets formulated with wheat and rice flour. *J Food Qual*. 2009;32:760–774.
14. Thomas DJ, Atwell WA. *Starches*. St. Paul, MS: Eagan Press; 1999.
15. Labensky SR, Hause AM, Martel PA. Potatoes, grains, and pasta. In: *On Cooking: A Textbook of Culinary Fundamentals*. 5th ed. New York: Pearson; 2011.
16. McWilliams M. *Foods: Experimental Perspectives*. 7th ed. Upper Saddle River, NJ: Prentice Hall; 2008.
17. Kill RC, Turnbull K. *Pasta and Semolina Technology*. Oxford, England: Blackwell Science; 2001.
18. Donnelly BJ. Pasta: Raw materials and processing. In: Lorenz KJ, Kulp K (eds.). *Handbook of Cereal Science and Technology*. New York: Marcel Dekker; 1991.
19. Tang G, Qin J, Dolnikowski GG, et al. Golden rice is an effective source of vitamin A. *Am J Clin Nutri*. 2009;89:1776–1783.
20. Gerhardt AL, Gallo NB. Full-fat rice bran and oat bran similarly reduce hypercholesterolemia in humans. *J Nutri*. 1998;128: 865–869.
21. Most MM, Tulley R, Morales S, Lefevre M. Rice brain oil, not fiber, lowers cholesterol in humans. *Am J Clin Nutri*. 2005; 81: 64–68.
22. Johnson LA. Corn: Production, processing, and utilization. In: Lorenz KJ, Kulp K (eds.). *Handbook of Cereal Science and Technology*. New York: Marcel Dekker; 1991.
23. U.S. Department of Agriculture. National Nutrient Database for Standard Reference, Release 23. Food Group: 08 Breakfast Cereals. 2010. Available at: http://www.ars.usda.gov/SP2UserFiles/Place/12354500/Data/SR23/reports/sr23_doc.pdf. Accessed August 22, 2011.
24. Serna-Saldivar SO, McDonough CM, Rooney LW. The millets. In: Lorenz KJ, Kulp K (eds.). *Handbook of Cereal Science and Technology*. New York: Marcel Dekker; 1991.
25. Tribelhorn RE. Breakfast cereals. In: Lorenz KJ, Kulp K (eds.). *Handbook of Cereal Science and Technology*. New York: Marcel Dekker; 1991.
26. U.S. Department of Agriculture. Choose My Plate. Why Is It Important to Eat Grains, Especially Whole Grains? Available at: http://www.choosemyplate.gov/food-groups/grains-why.html. Accessed June 14, 2012.
27. McKeown NM, Troy LM, Jacques PF, et al. Whole- and refined-grain intakes are differentially associated with abdominal visceral and subcutaneous adiposity in healthy adults: the Framingham Heart Study. *Am J Clin Nutri*. 2010;92(5):1165–1171.
28. United Nations Environment Programme. 2011. Agriculture Investing in Natural Capital. Available at: http://www.unep.org/greeneconomy/Portals/88/documents/ger/GER_2_Agriculture.pdf.
29. Rahman MS. Packaging as a preservation technique. In: Rahman MS (ed.). *Handbook of Food Preservation*. 2nd ed. Boca Raton, FL: CRC Press; 2007.

CHAPTER 12

Yeast Breads, Quick Breads, and Cakes

Jeannie Houchins, MA, RD

Chapter Objectives

THE STUDENT WILL BE EMPOWERED TO:

- Summarize the historical, cultural, and ecological significance of bread.
- Explain the role of each key ingredient used in the preparation of yeast breads.
- Summarize the process of making yeast breads and contrast the three mixing methods.
- Contrast the production process for quick breads and cakes with that of yeast breads.
- List the different types of quick bread batters.
- Contrast the three methods of mixing used in quick bread preparation.
- List examples of the various types of quick breads and cakes.
- Discuss the changes that occur when bread stales, including ways to slow the staling process.
- Discuss different types of spoilage and identify the responsible microorganisms.
- Discuss the effects of processing on the nutritive value of breads.
- Explain the goals of food technologists with regard to bread packaging.
- Identify two initiatives for greening the bread industry.

Historical, Cultural, and Ecological Significance

The use of bread as food staple has deep roots and permeates nearly every culture. Some historians speculate that the first unleavened bread appeared in the Neolithic era.[1,2] Along with the discovery of yeast, fermented bread originated in Egypt more than 5,000 years ago. Throughout the ages, every culture created its own type of bread based on the types of ingredients that were available.[1,3–5]

Wheat, the grain most often used in breads, has evolved as a species under the strong influence of humankind. The evolution of wheat took different paths in different parts of the world, based on local climates, soils, and human factors—from economic to political to industrial.[5,6] Wheat types and classes have, in turn, affected the types of bread produced by different cultures. Wheat is grown everywhere in the world but in the tropics. It is one of the most important food crops in the world.[2,7–9]

Wheat, in the form of bread, is nutrient dense, supplying carbohydrates, proteins, and B vitamins as well as vitamin E. Bread is typically categorized as leavened, flat, or steamed, based on the quality of the grain, how it is processed, and the desired end product (see **Figure 12.1**).[3,10,11] Bread in its simplest form of flour and water may have arisen from free-floating natural **yeasts**. In early civilizations, bread leavening and beer making were connected, stemming from the use of **barm**, the yeast foam produced in beer making.[2,5,12] The barm was skimmed, dried, and then dehydrated for use in bread. Louis Pasteur was the first to describe how the fermentation of carbohydrates by yeast creates the carbon dioxide that causes dough to rise (leaven).[1,2,5] **Fermentation** is the general transformation of organic substances, such as simple sugars, into smaller molecules by the action of microorganisms.

yeasts Microscopic one-celled fungi used as leavening agents. *Saccharomyces cerevisiae* is the species most commonly used in baking.

barm Foam at of the top of fermenting beer that was used as yeast for bread.

fermentation The general transformation of organic substances, such as simple sugars, into smaller molecules by the action of microorganisms.

The types of bread used in the Western world vary based on how the yeast is used and the type of wheat. The process of globalization is spreading traditional European-style breads to distant countries and is bringing a variety of other culture's breads to the United States. **Table 12.1** lists some of the more popular breads enjoyed around the world.

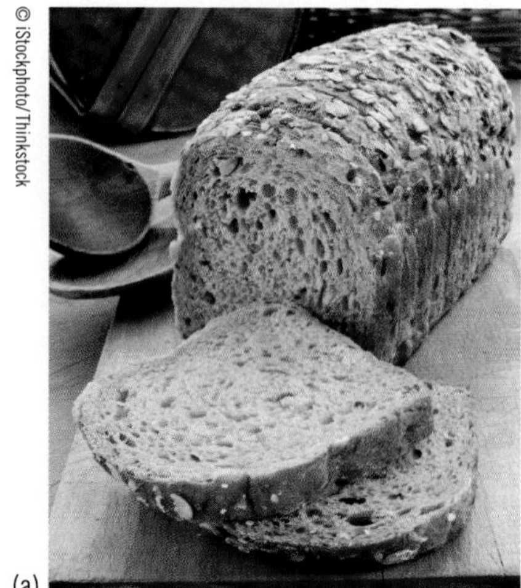

(a)

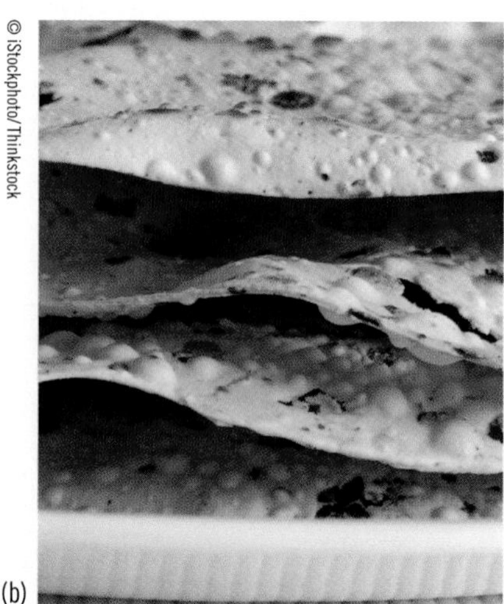

(b)

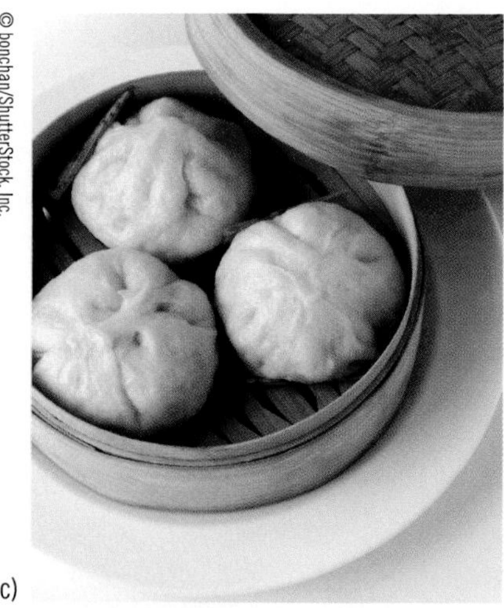

(c)

FIGURE 12.1 (a) Leavened bread is bread that contains a leavening agent, usually yeast. The leavening agent produces gas bubbles that are incorporated into the dough, which causes the dough to rise. Upon baking, it results in bread that has tiny air pockets. Most of the breads at the store, such as French bread, loaf bread, and rolls, are leavened breads. (b) Unleavened breads do not use a leavening agent. Most are a simple recipe of flour, water, and salt. Such breads are flat and are very crisp and crunchy, examples include crackers and matzos. (c) With steamed bread, the steam produced when baking the bread leavens the bread. Chinese buns are a good example of steamed bread.

TABLE 12.1
Breads from Around the World

Country	Popular Indigenous Breads
Afghanistan	Naan, chapati 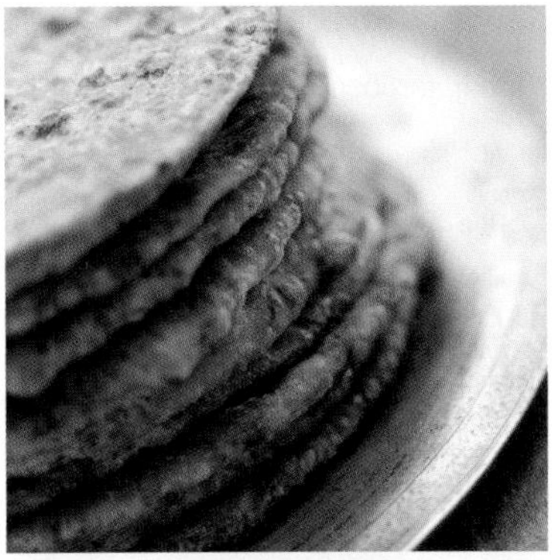 © Hemera/Thinkstock
Algeria	Matlowa, Khobz El-daar 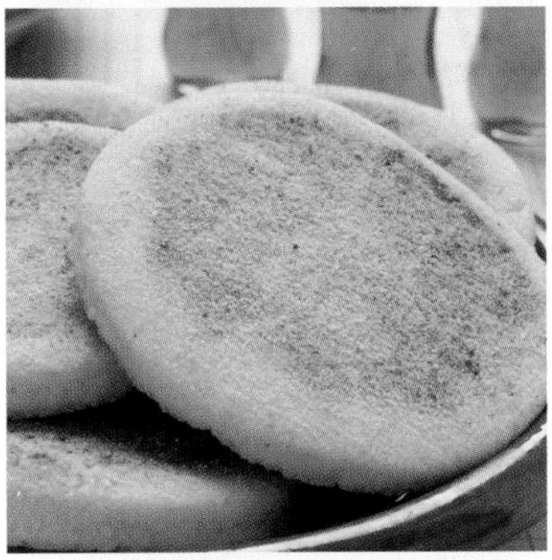 © picturepartners/ShutterStock, Inc.
Iran	Barbari, tanoor, lavash, teeri, suage, sangak 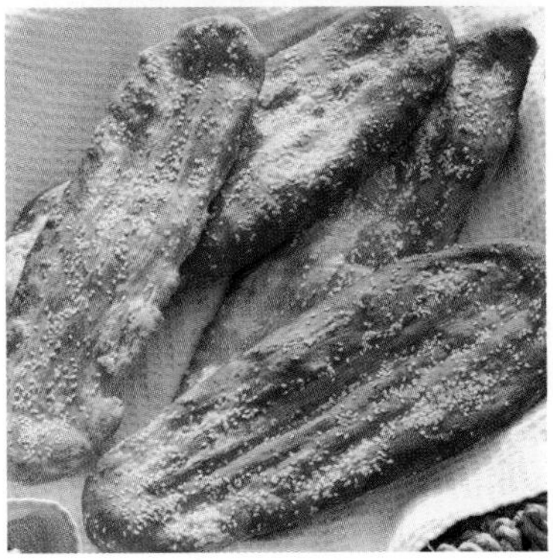 © iStockphoto/Thinkstock
Egypt	Baladi, shami, samoon, fatier, shamsi, bataw
Bahrain	Tanoor, Arabic, chapati, samoon
Ethiopia	Injera
Lebanon	Lebanese, suaj 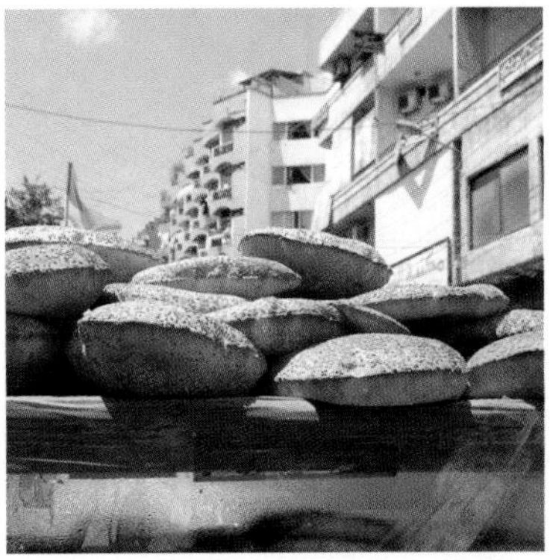 © Eliane Haykal/ShutterStock, Inc.

(*continues*)

TABLE 12.1
Breads from Around the World (*continued*)

Country	Popular Indigenous Breads
Jordan	Armani, nafrood, sauj
Israel	Sadj, tarboon, kimaj
Morocco	Moroccan Khobz El-daar
Somalia	Injera 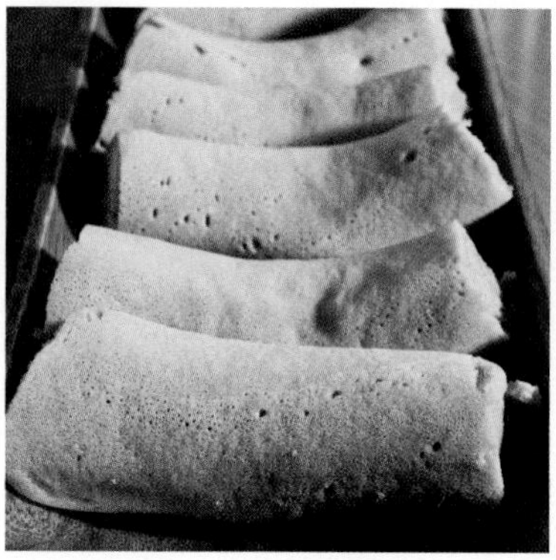 © Otokimus/ShutterStock, Inc.
Syria	Mafrood, armani, samoon, suaj
Tunisia	Trabilsi
Turkey	Balzuma, gomme, yafka 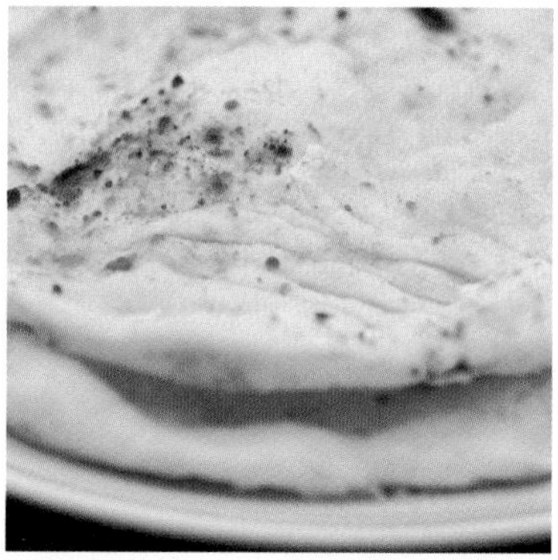 © Taratorki/ShutterStock, Inc.
Yemen	Roti, malouge
Mexico	Pan, corn tortillas, bolillo roll, pan dulce 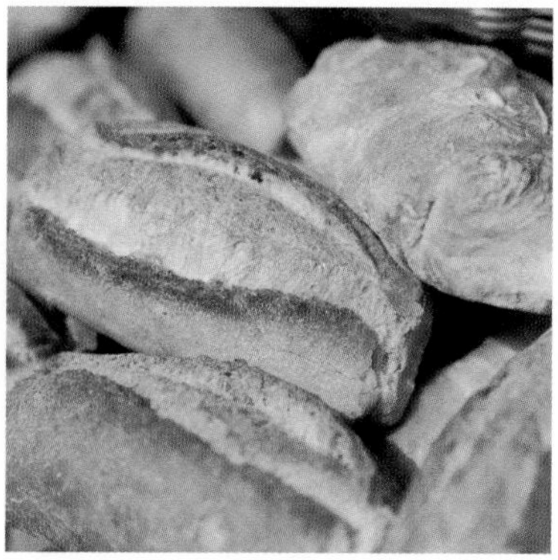 © Jesus Cervantes/ShutterStock, Inc.

Country	Popular Indigenous Breads
India	Naan, roti, chapati, puri © Hemera/Thinkstock
Philippines	Pandesal © Glenn Young/ShutterStock, Inc.
Peru	Pan de piso, pan serrano
China	Mantou, char siu bao
Vietnam	Bahn mi © iStockphoto/Thinkstock
Yemen	Roti, malouge

Source: Data from Edelstein S (ed.). *Food, Cuisine, and Cultural Competency for the Culinary, Hospitality, and Nutrition Professions.* Sudbury, MA: Jones and Bartlett Publishers; 2010.

Physical and Chemical Properties

Yeast Breads

Yeast breads are leavened by the action of yeast, which converts the fermentable sugars present in the dough into carbon dioxide gas. This causes the dough to expand, or rise, as the gas forms pockets or bubbles. When the dough is baked, the yeast dies, and the air pockets "set," giving the baked product a soft, spongy texture. The essential ingredients for yeast-leavened dough are flour, liquid, yeast, and salt. Some yeast doughs also contain additional fat, sugar, and substances called dough conditioners.

yeast breads Breads that are leavened by the action of yeast, which converts the fermentable sugars present in dough into the gas carbon dioxide. This causes the dough to expand or rise as the gas forms pockets or bubbles. When the dough is baked, the yeast dies and the air pockets "set," giving the baked product a soft and spongy texture.

leavening agent An ingredient in leavened bread that incorporates gas bubbles into the dough, causing it to rise.

gluten The protein in wheat flour that gives dough its stretchiness. If dough is leavened with yeast, fermentation produces carbon dioxide bubbles, which, trapped by the gluten network, cause the dough to rise.

Yeast

The microscopic one-celled organism *Saccharomyces cerevisiae*, commonly called bread yeast, is used as the biological **leavening agent** in yeast breads. The yeast is available in a number of different forms for use in bread making:[13–15]

- *Active dry yeast:* Loose yeast granules sold in envelopes and jars. The yeast must be reactivated with warm water (100–115°F or 43–46°C) before it is added to the flour (see **Figure 12.2**).
- *Instant quick-rising active dry yeast:* Dried yeast that can be mixed directly into other ingredients without being reactivated first.
- *Bread machine yeast:* Instant yeast that can be added directly to dry ingredients.
- *Compressed or fresh cake yeast:* Sold as moist foil-wrapped cakes, fresh cake yeast is highly perishable and must be refrigerated and revived with warm water.
- *Starters:* Yeast preparations that have been growing prior to incorporation into the dough; versions include sourdough, sponge, polish (wet sponge), and biga (dry sponge), with each type producing a different bread texture, flavor, and aroma.

Flour

Flour is one of the main ingredients necessary to produce yeast bread. Flour provides protein for bread in the form of glutenin and gliadin, which combine with water to produce **gluten**. Gluten's sheetlike structure traps air and gases made by the yeast, causing the bread to rise.[13,16,17] The amount of flour needed to make bread dough varies based on the type of flour, the type of liquid, and level of humidity present in the surrounding environment. The type of flour used and its protein content dictate how much water the flour will absorb.[13,18–20] The following types of flour are best for yeast breads:[18–20]

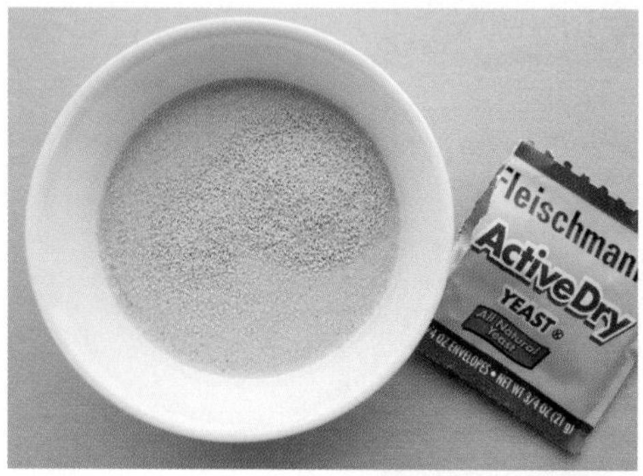

FIGURE 12.2 Dry yeast must be reactivated in warm water before it can be used. Yeast must be activated in order for it to act as a leavening agent. If the yeast is not active, the bread will not rise.

- *Bread flour:* Made from hard wheat, it has more protein than other flours.
- *All-purpose flour:* Protein content varies and adjustments to bread recipes may be necessary.
- *Whole wheat flour:* Provides more vitamins, minerals, and antioxidants than other types of flour.
- *Rye, barley, or rice flour:* Can be mixed with wheat flour to add flavor.

Liquid

Another essential component in bread making is the liquid. The liquid-to-flour ratio varies by recipe. The liquid used in the bread recipe serves several purposes, including hydrating the flour proteins, contributing to gluten development, and dissolving ingredients such as sugar and salt.[13,19,20] The following liquids may be used in bread:

- *Water:* The mineral content of the water will affect dough. Alkaline water creates a more elastic dough, whereas acidic water creates weaker gluten.
- *Milk:* Adds flavor and nutrients and aids in browning by contributing lactose.
- *Egg:* Weakens the gluten structure, resulting in a tenderer end product.

Salt

Salt adds flavor and balances the taste of the bread. It retards yeast fermentation, making the dough less sticky and the gluten more elastic, resulting in a lighter product.[13,19,20]

Fat

Fat is not called for in all bread recipes, but it is sometimes used to facilitate the handling of the dough, to increase the longevity of the bread, and to improve volume and textural attributes such as moistness and tenderness.[13,19,20]

dough conditioners Chemicals used in commercial baking that improve the finished bread product, such as providing better loaf volume and a softer crumb.

crumb The dry particles in the bread crust.

Sugar

Sugar is not an essential ingredient in bread, because sucrose (and eventually glucose) is produced from the hydrolysis of flour starch by enzymes. Added sugar provides food for the yeast, increasing fermentation; however, high sugar levels may repress yeast activity. Flavor, texture, and browning are also affected by the use of added sugar.[13,19,20]

Dough Conditioners

In commercial baking, **dough conditioners** are used to improve the finished bread product, yielding better volume and softer crumb. **Crumb** refers to dry particles in the crust. Conditioners are classified by their functions on the dough:[13,19–24]

- *Oxidizing agents* adjust the acidity of dough and thereby affect the number of disulfide bonds in the gluten and gluten-forming molecules.
- *Reducing agents*, such as L-cysteine, interact with gluten to reduce elasticity.
- *Emulsifiers*, such as mono- and diglycerides, reduce the degree or rate at which bread goes stale.
- *Enzymes*, most commonly fungal amylases, are used for varying purposes, including extending product shelf life, reducing the required mix time, and improving the texture of the finished product.

Making Yeast Breads

The process of making yeast bread comprises mixing, kneading, fermenting/rising, shaping, and baking (see **Figure 12.3**).

Mixing

The most important stage of the bread making process is mixing. Mixing allows all the ingredients to be incorporated uniformly into the mixture. This promotes the development of gluten structures that trap air bubbles from the yeast, allowing the dough to rise. A number of different options are available for mixing:[13,19,20,25,26]

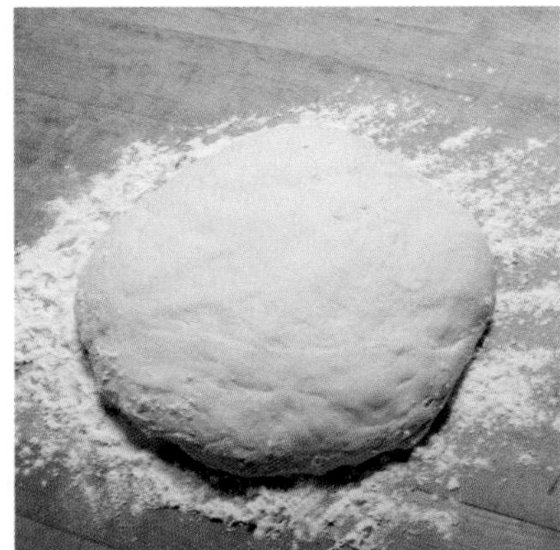
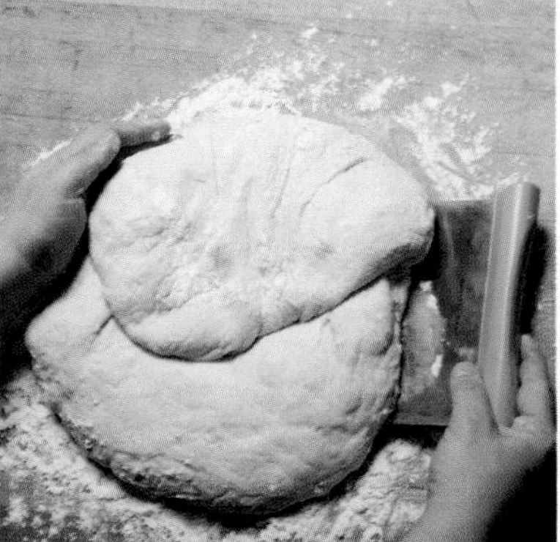
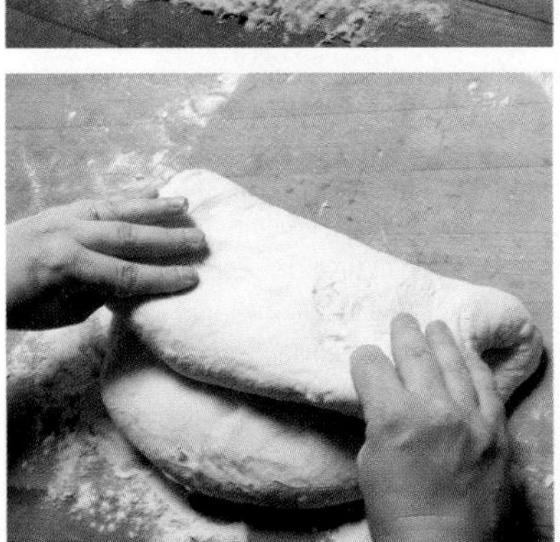
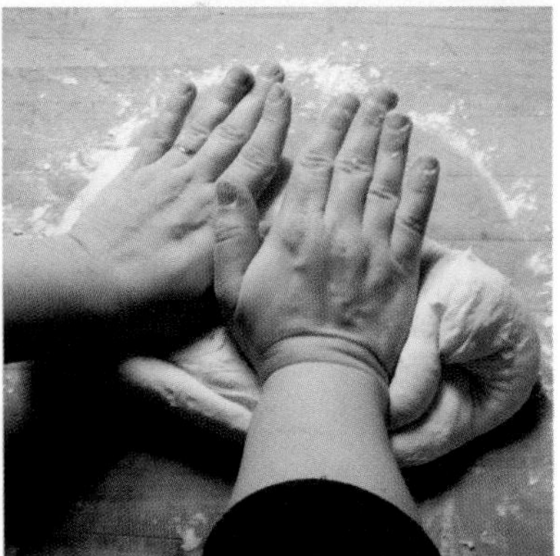
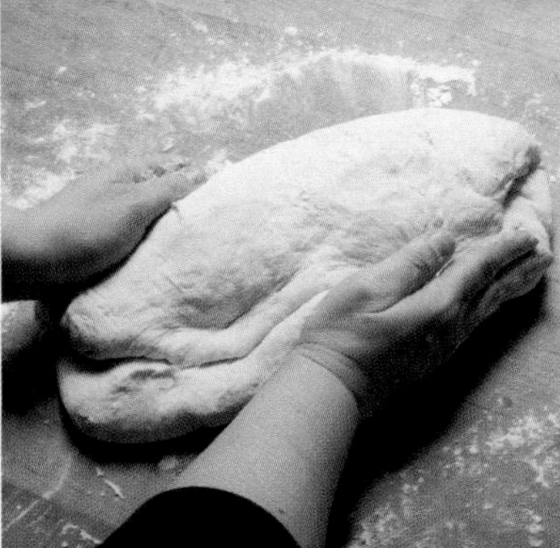
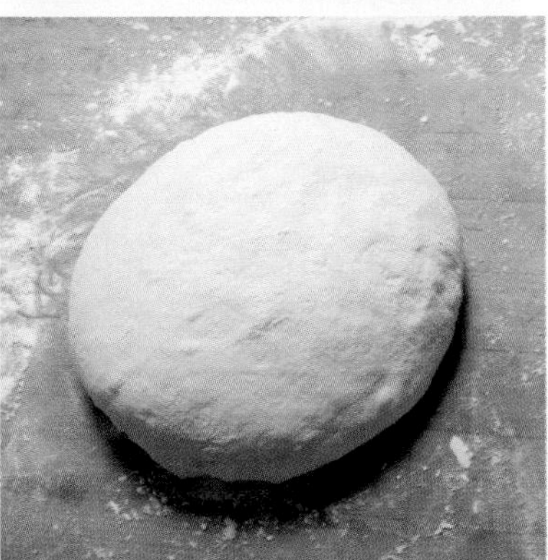

FIGURE 12.3 Making yeast bread consists of a number of steps: mixing, kneading, fermenting/rising, shaping, and baking.

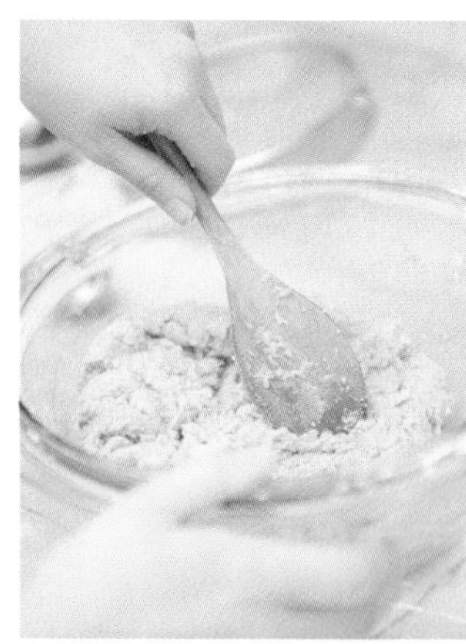

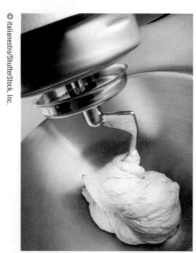

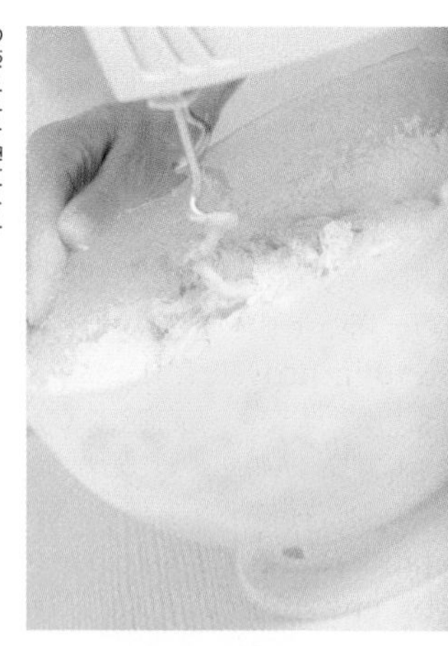

FIGURE 12.4 With straight mixing, all of the ingredients are added at the same time and mixed by hand or a machine. This usually results in a good quality bread product, but there is the possibility that the yeast might not become evenly distributed throughout the dough.

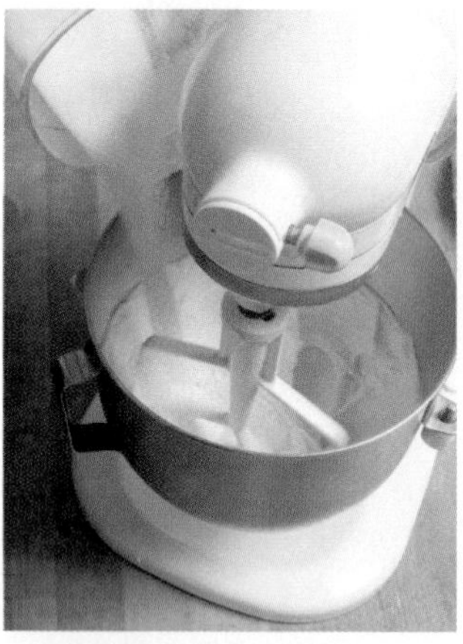

FIGURE 12.5 Batter mixing is a modification of the straight-dough method that eliminates kneading. In this case, stirring develops the gluten. It is the quickest mixing method.

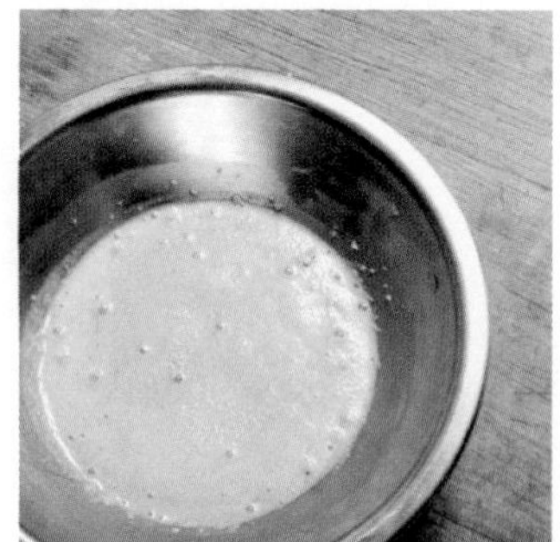

FIGURE 12.6 Sponge mixing is a two-step bread making process. First, a sponge is made and allowed to ferment for a period of time. The sponge is then added to the rest of the ingredients to make the final dough.

- With *straight mixing* (see **Figure 12.4**), activated yeast and the liquid mixture are added to the flour and mixed.
- With *batter mixing* (see **Figure 12.5**), a modified straight mixing method is used that eliminates kneading. This method requires less flour and the yeast mixture is thin. Stirring advances gluten development.
- *Sponge mixing* (see **Figure 12.6**) is a two-step process where the yeast, liquid, and part of the flour are combined and fermented, creating a spongelike texture (in fact, bakers call this thin batter the **sponge**). The remaining ingredients are added to the sponge to make dough.

Kneading

Kneading strengthens the gluten strands that give dough its elasticity and helps to disperse the yeast cells throughout the dough that will form the gas cells that will later be inflated. Kneading is done by hand or machine (see **Figure 12.7**). This process continues until the dough is elastic and smooth (see **Figure 12.8**). If the bread dough is not kneaded enough, it will not be able to hold the tiny pockets of carbon dioxide gas created by the leavening agent (such as yeast or baking powder) and will collapse, leaving a heavy and dense loaf. If the dough is overworked it will become very sticky.[13,19,20]

FIGURE 12.7 Kneading the dough is one of the most important steps in bread baking. This step more than any other will determine the outcome of the bread. Kneading can be performed with a bread machine, a mixer equipped with a dough hook, or by hand.

(a)

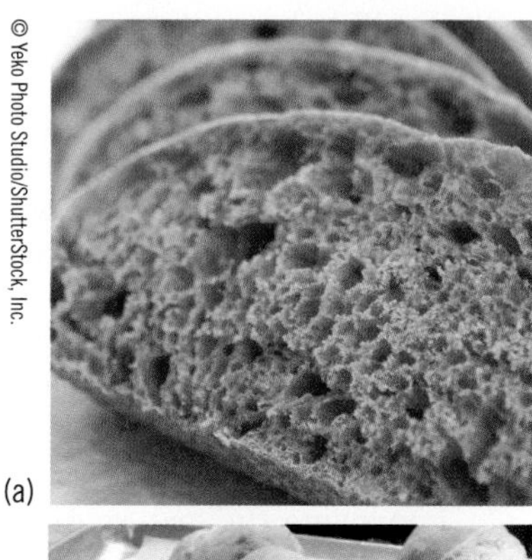

(b)

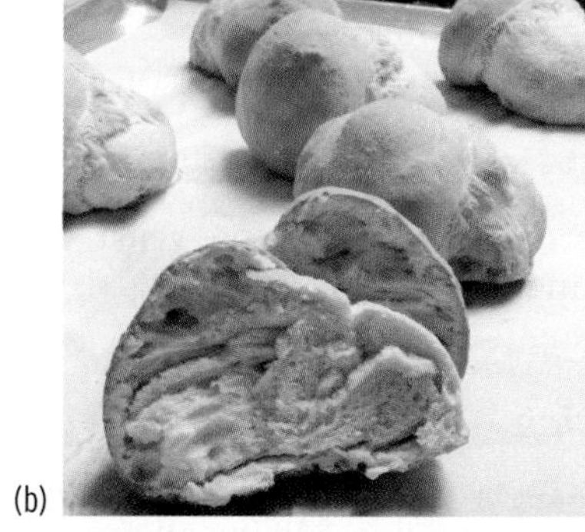

FIGURE 12.8 (a) The dough should be kneaded until it is smooth and moderately elastic. The presence of one or two bubbles beneath the surface of the dough is a sign that the dough is sufficiently well kneaded. (b) Over-kneading may result in a sticky dough, but this is rarely a problem except with powerful commercial mixers.

sponge The use of a mixture of liquid, yeast, sugar, and flour to make a thin batter to allow yeast activity. This mixture is then added to the remaining ingredients to form dough.

Fermenting/Rising

Fermentation caused by the enzyme action of yeast increases acidity, changes the quality of the gluten, and produces carbon dioxide.[13,16,19,20] The fermentation process may take a couple hours or more, depending on the amount of yeast and/or starter and temperature. After the dough is fermented and is molded into the desired shape and placed in a baking pan, it is allowed to rise for a little bit longer, a process known as **proofing**.[13,16,19,20,27]

The temperature and time can affect yeast activity and the degree of fermentation in the baking process. The ideal fermentation temperature is 80–90°F (26–32°C). Yeast cells accelerate their gas production and develop stronger flavors in warmer temperatures; cooler temperatures cause the dough to rise more slowly. The more yeast that is used, the less time that is required to ferment.[13,16,19,20,24]

Problems in the final product are sometimes attributed to effects of fermentation on **oven spring**, which is the sharp rising in volume of bread during the first 10 to 12 minutes of baking (when amylase enzymes are more active). During this time, the dough's water-holding capacity is reduced and the production of carbon dioxide is accelerated, causing gases to expand within the cells.[13,19,20,22]

If the dough ferments for too long, the final product may have a flat or sunken top, a coarse grain, and a thick texture. If the dough is not fermented long enough, the final product may by overly dense and have a thick texture.

Shaping and Decorative Finishes

Shaping the dough not only serves a decorative function but also identifies the bread type and minimizes loss of gases. Decorative finishes include slashing, braiding, and/or the use of a wash or glaze. The type of wash used influences the color, texture, and shine of the crust (see **Figure 12.9**).[2,23,24]

Baking

The final step in making bread is baking. During baking, the dough undergoes different chemical processes. As the temperature of the bread increases, oven spring occurs, enzymes are deactivated, protein denaturation occurs, moisture content is reduced, starch **gelatinization** happens, and the bread browns due to Maillard reactions.[13,19,20]

proofing Stage in bread making where the bread dough is left to rise for the last time after it is molded into a loaf and placed into the baking pan. During this stage, starch is converted into sugars, producing carbon dioxide and alcohol. The result is dough expansion and flavor development.

oven spring The rapid increase in volume in a loaf of bread during the first few minutes of baking.

gelatinization Process that involves heating starch granules in a moist environment; the granules swell as water is absorbed and disrupt the organization of the starch granules.

quick breads Bread products that require no rising or proofing time. Quick breads vary widely in the consistency of their dough or batter.

Quick Breads and Cakes

Bread products that do not require rising or proofing are called **quick breads**. Cakes also fall in this category. Both quick breads and cakes are leavened with chemical leavening agents rather than biological leavening agents such as yeast. One of the more common chemical leavening agents is baking soda (sodium bicarbonate) plus an acid, usually cream of tartar, lemon juice, or cultured buttermilk. This combination elicits an acid–base reaction that releases carbon dioxide. Baking powder has sodium bicarbonate and may be used in place of baking soda, but it already includes an acid acidifying agent (cream of tartar) as well as a drying agent (usually starch), so no additional acid is needed.[13,19,20,24,28]

The quick bread or cake rises when it is heated in the oven. Upon heating, the carbon dioxide gas made by the chemical leavening agent is released, leaving behind small empty pockets of air in the product, which causes the dough or batter to rise. Physical leavening also contributes to making a successful quick bread or cake. Physical leavening is achieved by mixing the dough or batter in a certain way to trap air within the product.

Batters and Doughs

Quick breads and cakes contain the same basic ingredients: flour, a leavening agent, eggs, fat (butter, margarine, shortening, or oil), and a liquid, such as milk. However, they vary widely in the consistency of their dough or batter. There are four main types of quick bread batters and doughs (see **Figure 12.10**):[13,19,20,24,28]

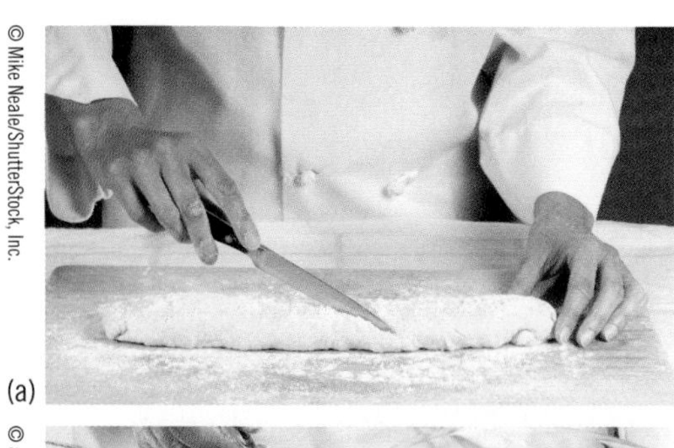
(a) © Mike Neale/ShutterStock, Inc.

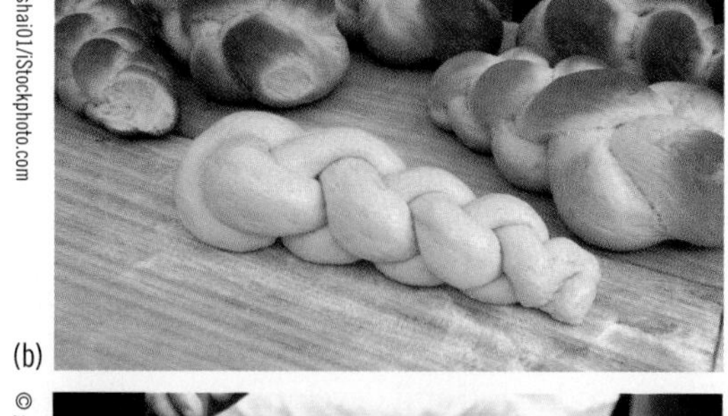
(b) © ishai01/iStockphoto.com

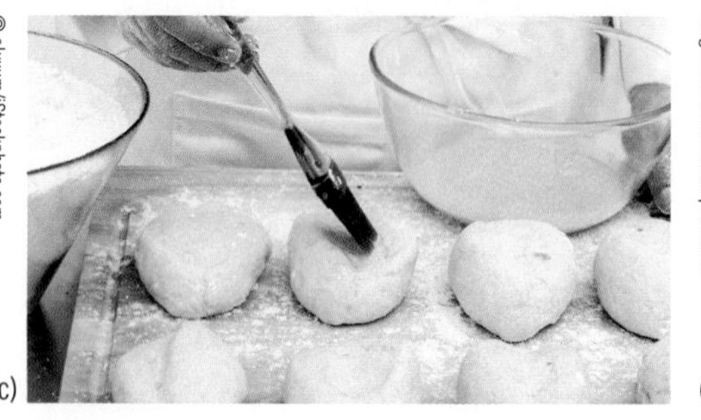
(c) © aluxum/iStockphoto.com

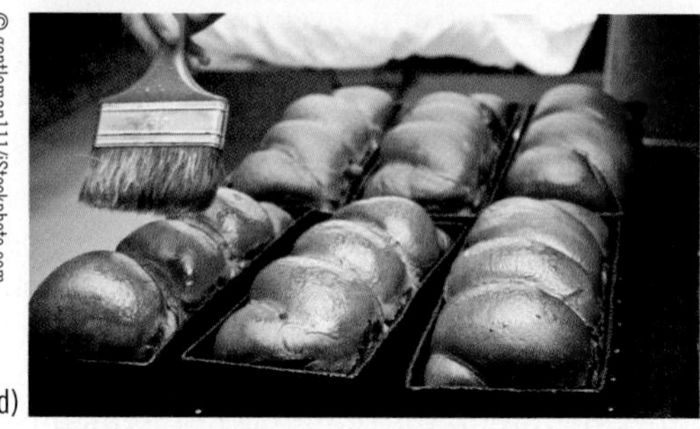
(d) © gentleman111/iStockphoto.com

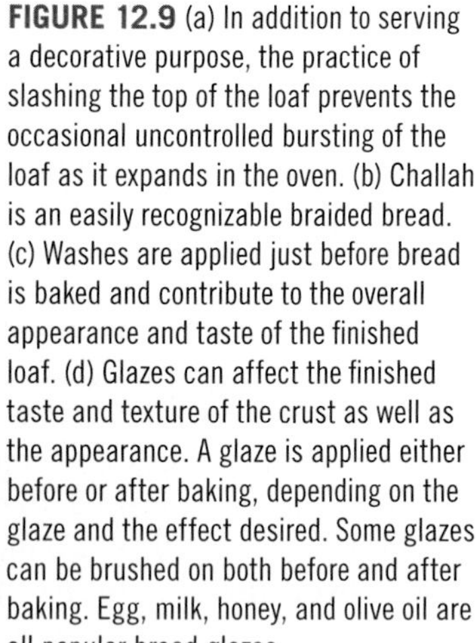
FIGURE 12.9 (a) In addition to serving a decorative purpose, the practice of slashing the top of the loaf prevents the occasional uncontrolled bursting of the loaf as it expands in the oven. (b) Challah is an easily recognizable braided bread. (c) Washes are applied just before bread is baked and contribute to the overall appearance and taste of the finished loaf. (d) Glazes can affect the finished taste and texture of the crust as well as the appearance. A glaze is applied either before or after baking, depending on the glaze and the effect desired. Some glazes can be brushed on both before and after baking. Egg, milk, honey, and olive oil are all popular bread glazes.

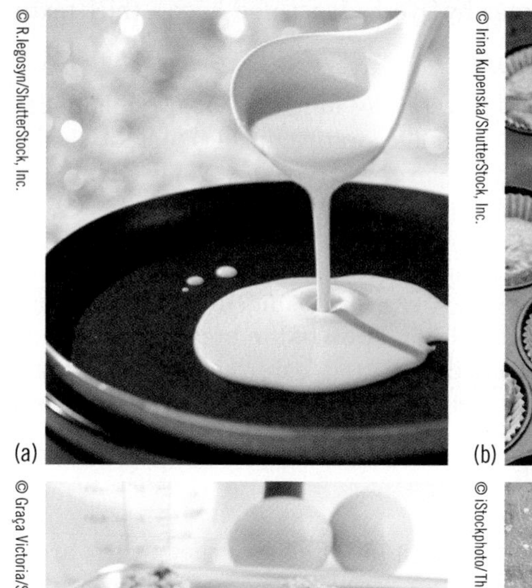
(a) © R.legosyn/ShutterStock, Inc.

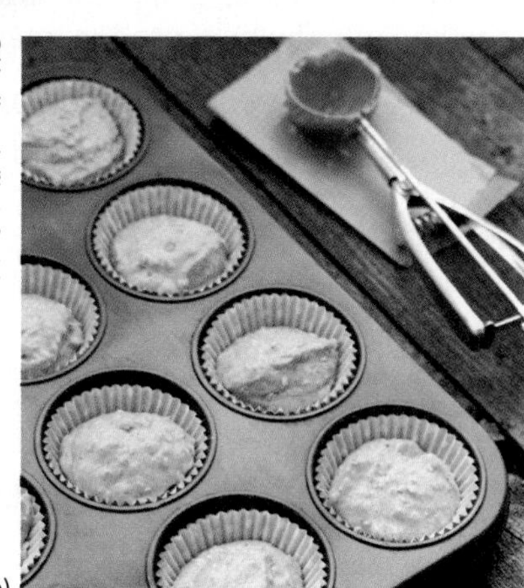
(b) © Irina Kupenska/ShutterStock, Inc.

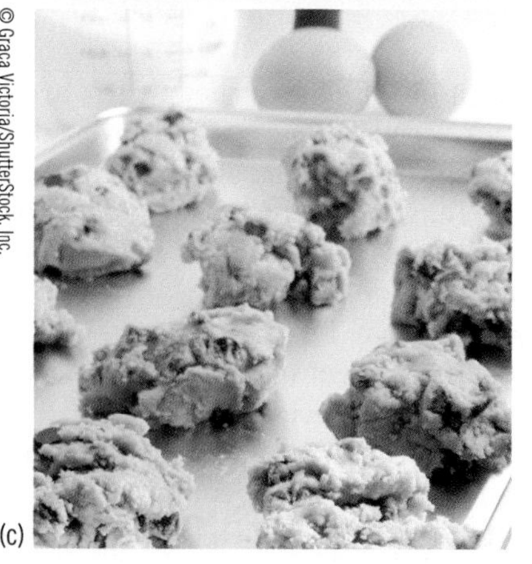
(c) © Graça Victoria/ShutterStock, Inc.

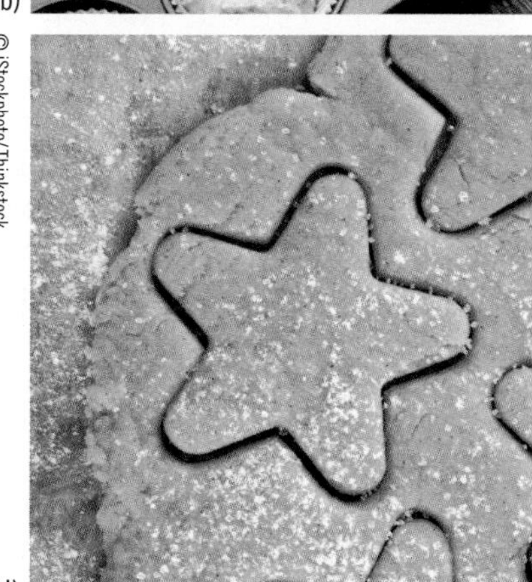
(d) © iStockphoto/Thinkstock

FIGURE 12.10 (a) Pour batters have a liquid consistency because they are equal parts liquid and dry ingredients. Pancake batter is a pour batter. (b) Drop batters, such as cornbread and muffin batters, have a liquid-to-dry ratio of about 1:2. (c) Soft doughs, such as chocolate chip cookies, have a liquid-to-dry ratio of about 1:3. Soft doughs stick significantly to work surfaces. (d) Stiff doughs, such as pie crust dough and sugar cookie dough, are easy to work in that they will only minimally stick to work surfaces, including hands. Stiff doughs are produced with a ratio of approximately 1:8 liquid-to-dry ingredients.

pour batters Call for a liquid-to-dry ratio of about 1:1; pour in a steady stream (for example, pancake batter).

drop batters Call for a liquid-to-dry ratio of about 1:2; example include cornbread and muffin batters.

soft doughs Call for a liquid-to-dry ratio of about 1:3; examples include chocolate chip cookie dough.

- **Pour batters** call for a liquid-to-dry ingredient ratio of about 1:1 and pour in a steady stream (for example, pancake batter).
- **Drop batters** call for a liquid-to-dry ingredient ratio of about 1:2 (for example, cornbread and muffin batters).
- **Soft doughs** call for a liquid-to-dry ingredient ratio of about 1:3 (for example, chocolate chip cookie dough).

- **Stiff doughs** call for a liquid-to-dry ingredient ratio of about 1:8 (for example, sugar cookie dough).

Mixing Methods for Quick Breads and Cakes

The following are the three most common methods for mixing quick bread and cake batters:

- *Blending and stirring:* Also known as the *quick-bread method*, the dry and wet ingredients are measured separately, then quickly mixed together. Wet ingredients often use beaten eggs, which incorporate trapped air so the product will rise. Examples include pancake and muffin batters (see **Figure 12.11**).
- *Wide-sweep stirring:* The dough or batter is repeatedly and rapidly folded over on itself to trap air (this can also be done with beaten eggs or egg white foam). Upon baking, the air escapes the product walls, leaving open air cells, causing the product to rise. Examples include pound cake and sponge cake batters (see **Figure 12.12**).
- *Creaming:* Creaming is the typical method for cake batters. With this method, the butter or hydrogenated fat and sugar are creamed (beaten together). Eggs and liquid flavoring are mixed in with the dry and wet ingredients last (see **Figure 12.13**). This method achieves rise from the initial creaming of the fat and chemical leaveners. A variation of creaming, known as the *shortening method*, is typically used for biscuits and scones. This technique combines chilled fat with the dry ingredients to give the product rise and flakiness.

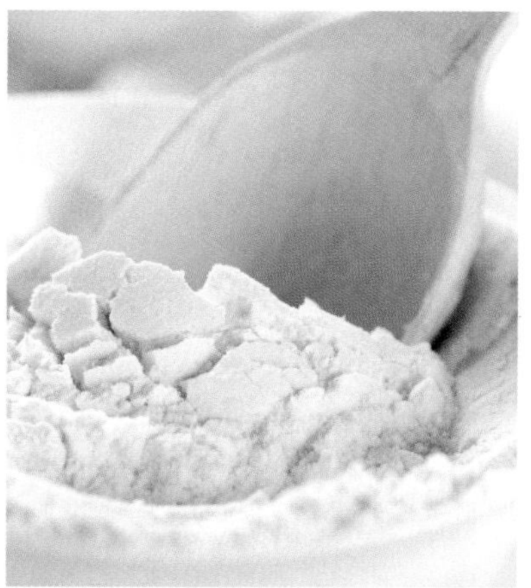

© Sea Wave/ShutterStock, Inc.

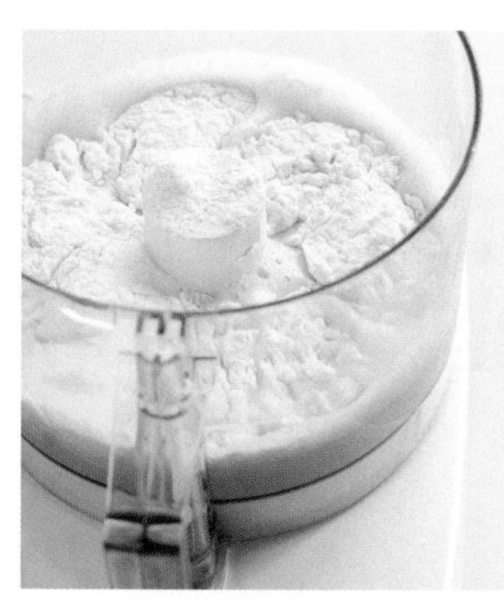

© jreika/ShutterStock, Inc.

FIGURE 12.11 The blending and stirring method is used for pancakes, muffins, corn bread, and dumplings. The dry and wet ingredients are measured separately and then quickly mixed together. Mixing is usually with a tool with a wide head such as a spoon or spatula to avoid overbeating the dough.

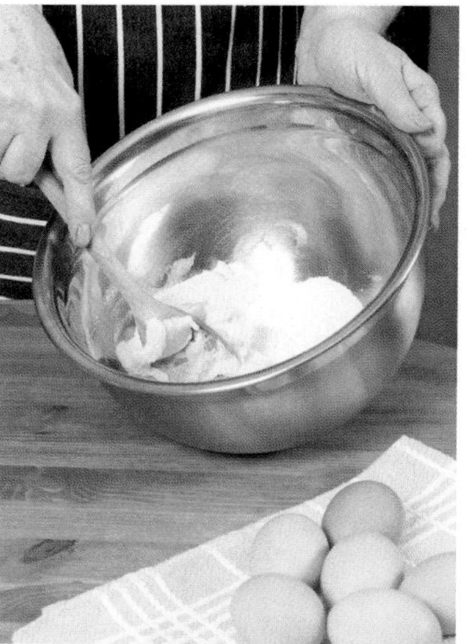

© iStockphoto/Thinkstock

FIGURE 12.12 With the wide-sweep method, the dough or batter is repeatedly and rapidly folded over on itself to trap air. Examples include pound cake and sponge cake batters.

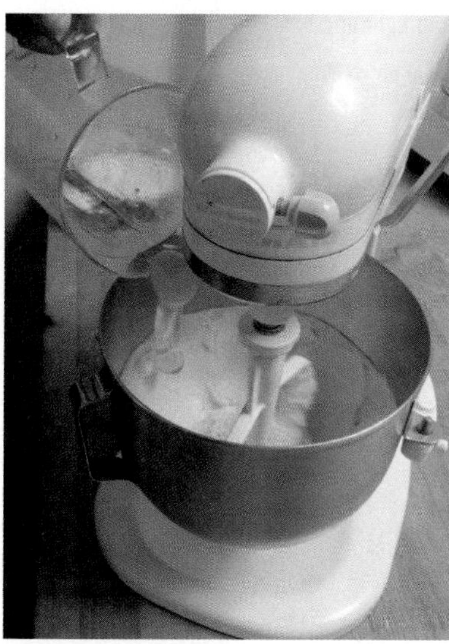

FIGURE 12.13 The creaming method is frequently used for cake batters. The butter and sugar are beaten together until smooth and fluffy. Eggs and liquid flavoring are mixed in, and finally dry and liquid ingredients are added in.

Types of Quick Breads and Cakes

Quick breads include a great variety of breakfast, snack, and dessert foods, such as muffins, pancakes, waffles, nut breads, doughnuts, coffeecakes, biscuits, scones, popovers, cream puffs, and éclairs. Cake types include sponge, angel food, and shortened.[13,19,20,22]

Pancakes and Waffles

Pancakes and waffles are leavened by carbon dioxide gas production, resulting from baking powder or from a sour milk and soda combination (see **Figure 12.14**). Their consistency and texture depends on the proportions of ingredients used—flour, liquid, baking powder or soda, salt, and egg. Waffles are similar to pancakes with the exception that they contain more egg and more fat.

stiff doughs Call for a liquid-to-dry ratio of about 1:8; sugar cookie dough is considered stiff dough.

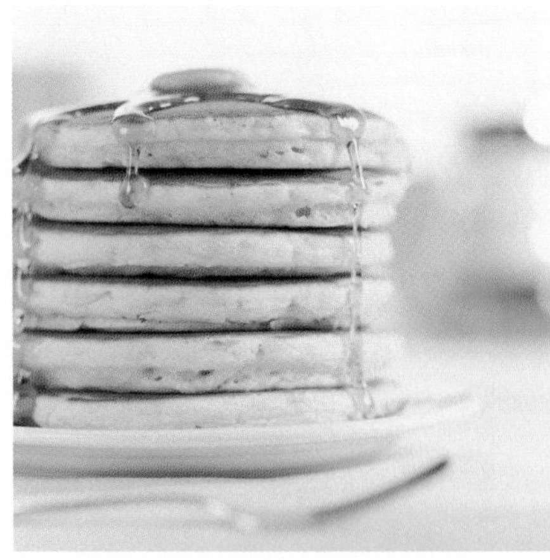

FIGURE 12.14 Pancakes are the result of an acid–base reaction and the proper addition of heat. The chemical reaction results in the formation of gas bubbles. Cooking the pancake at the right temperature traps the air bubbles, resulting in a light and fluffy texture.

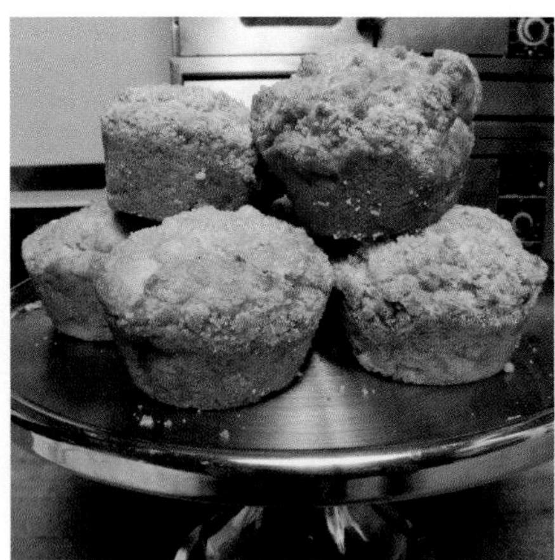

FIGURE 12.15 Most muffin recipes rely on baking soda and an acid or baking powder. The sodium bicarbonate in the baking soda or baking powder reacts with an acid to produce carbon dioxide bubbles during the baking process, resulting in a light and fluffy muffin.

Muffins

Muffins are quick breads that are typically uniform in texture, lightly browned, and have pebbly appearance (see **Figure 12.15**).

Nut Breads and Coffeecakes

Nut breads and coffeecakes are similar to muffins. Nut breads are baked in loaf pans at a lower temperature and for a longer time (see **Figure 12.16**). Coffeecakes are baked in cake or pie pans. Other products in this category include cake doughnuts, hush puppies, and fritters, which are cooked by deep fat frying.

Biscuits and Scones

Biscuits are usually uniform in shape, have an evenly browned and tender crust, and have a flaky texture as a result of their rolled dough. Scones are similar to biscuits but are richer due to the use of eggs and half-and-half or cream in the batter (see **Figure 12.17**).

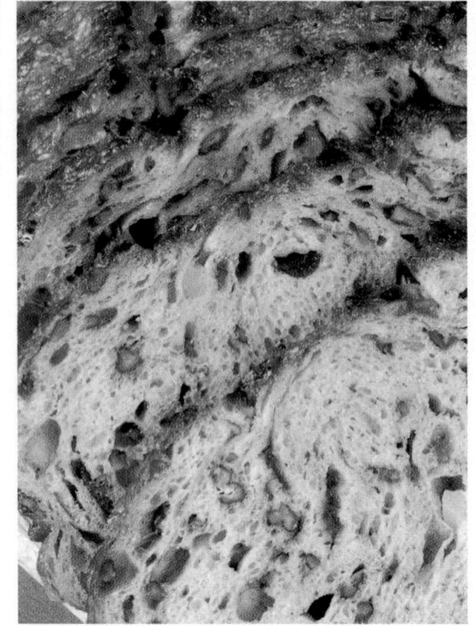

FIGURE 12.16 Nut breads can be made with a variety of different fruits. For examples, bananas, zucchinis, dates, and cranberries are just some of the fruits that are commonly incorporated into nut breads.

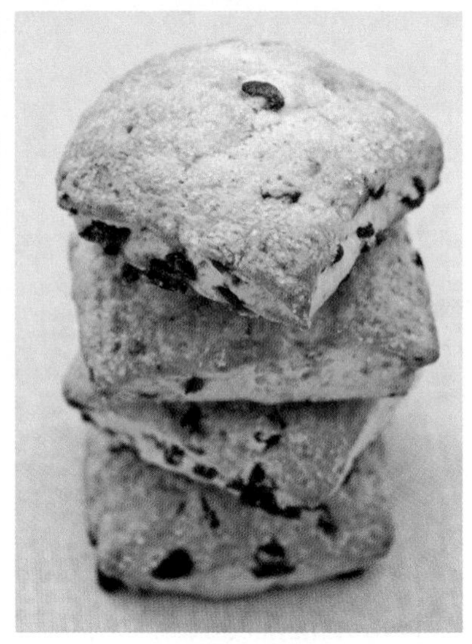

FIGURE 12.17 Scones are usually made of wheat flour, but some recipes call for barley or oatmeal. Baking powder is usually used as the leavening agent. In many countries, scones are usually an accompaniment to sweetened tea.

Popovers

Popover dough is very moist. When cooked, the water in the dough produces steam, which acts as the leavening agent. Popovers are usually baked at a much higher temperature than other baked goods because of the need to convert the water to steam very rapidly. Popovers are typically mixed by the muffin method and have a hollow center and hard crusts (see **Figure 12.18**).

Cream Puffs and Éclairs

Cream puffs and éclairs are similar to popovers in that they are also leavened primarily by steam, but they are made with more fat. Similar to popovers, cream puffs and éclairs have a brown exterior with a large hollow center (see **Figure 12.19**).

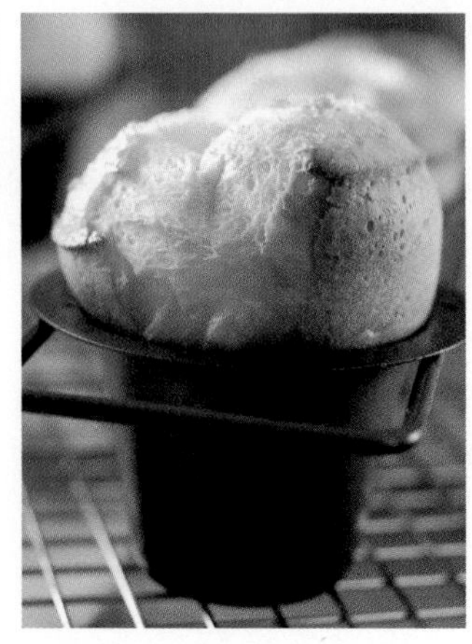

FIGURE 12.18 Popovers are light hollow rolls that are typically baked in muffin tins. The name *popover* comes from the fact that the batter "pops" over the top of the muffin tin while baking.

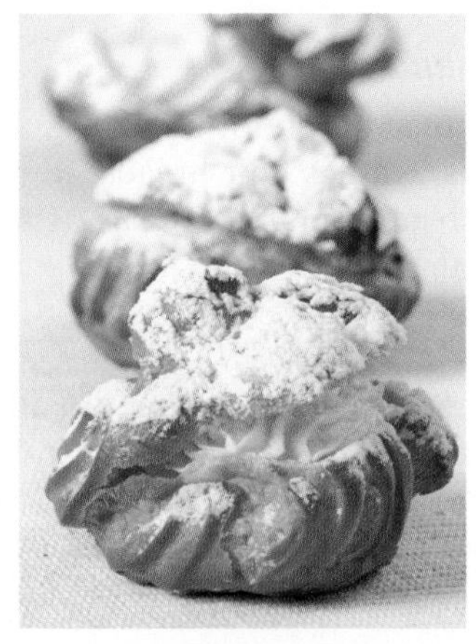

FIGURE 12.19 A popular pastry, cream puffs can be filled with whipped cream, pastry cream, or ice cream.

Sponge Cakes

Sponge cakes are light, porous cakes that are made using self-rising flour, sugar, beaten eggs, and flavorings (see **Figure 12.20**). They have a higher proportion of eggs to flour than other cakes, with very little fat (from the eggs). Although butter or oils may be added to some batters, most sponge cakes do not include shortenings.

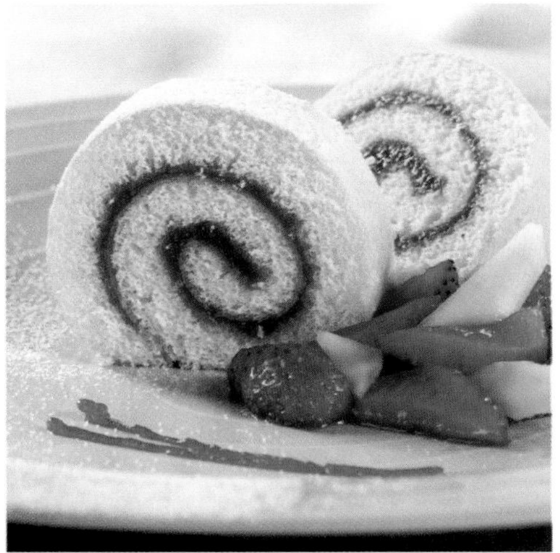

© iStockphoto/Thinkstock

FIGURE 12.20 Sponge cakes are European-style cakes that are used in layer cakes, jelly rolls, and tiramisu. They include very little fat other than that provided by the egg yolks.

Angel Food Cake

Angel food cake is a very light, airy cake made with stiffly beaten egg whites—called a meringue—and no egg yolks or fats (see **Figure 12.21**). Leavening is via the air in the meringue and steam production. Egg white proteins and the starch and flour protein are incorporated into the watery film around air cells, contributing to stability. Sugar is added for flavoring, its stabilizing effect on egg white proteins, and also to counterbalance the effects of the egg protein and flour. Cream of tartar is typically added to lower the pH, stabilize and whiten the foam, and yield a finer-grained product. **Table 12.2** summarizes the roles of quick bread and cake ingredients in the final baked product.

Shortened Cakes

Shortened cakes are made from flour, nonfat dry milk solids, egg, fat, sugar, salt, and baking powder (see **Figure 12.22**). They are leavened mostly by carbon dioxide gas from baking powder (or from soda and buttermilk). Air incorporated into the fat or into the beaten eggs or egg whites also aids in leavening of the mixture.

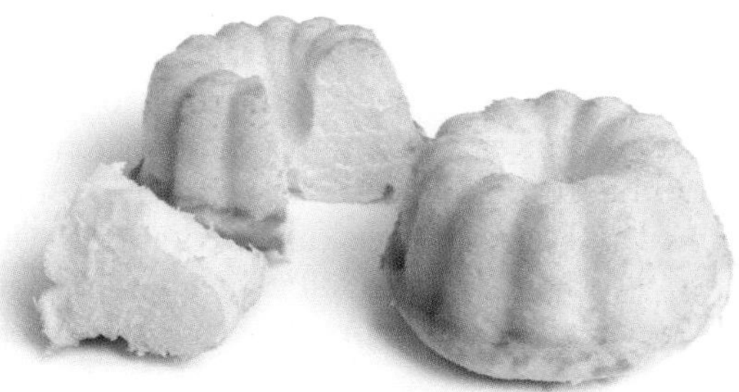

© iStockphoto/Thinkstock

FIGURE 12.21 Angel food cake is a type of sponge cake. It first became popular in the United States in the late 19th century. The name is derived from the cake's airy lightness, which people said was to be the "food of the angels."

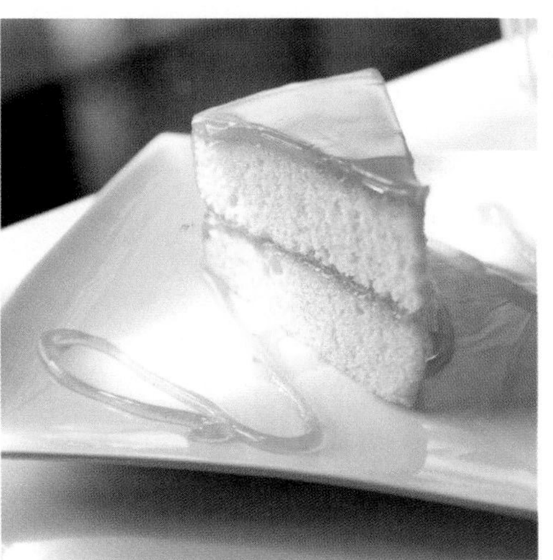

© jomphong/ShutterStock, Inc.

FIGURE 12.22 Shortened cakes, one of the most commonly prepared cakes, are typically served at birthday parties and wedding receptions. Also known as butter, conventional, or creamed cakes, shortened cakes can be made from scratch or from a cake mix.

Bread Selection Criteria

Consumers select breads that have the qualities of freshly baked bread—an appealing aroma, a crispy crust, and a moist, soft crumb.

Staling and Spoiling

Staling refers to the changes that occur in bread after baking as water migrates from the crust to the crumb, resulting in increasing firmness, loss of moisture and flavor, a crumbly texture, and a leathery crust. These changes happen because the starch molecules retrograde into a more solid structure. This occurs gradually at room temperature and more quickly at refrigerator temperatures. Reheating the bread to redistribute the starch may reverse bread staling.[13,20,23,24,28,29]

Bread spoils by mold growth due to moisture and warm temperatures. Spoilage in wheat bread is known as **rope**; it is caused by heat-resistant strains of *Bacillus*, which can multiply rapidly in bread.[13,20,23,24,28,29]

Sensory Research

Food scientists study consumer preferences for what they want in a bread. Positive attributes of bread freshness are a porous appearance and a floury, malty, sweet, buttery aroma. Freshness is an attribute of a food product that often includes how recently a product was produced or harvested, the extent

staling Stiffening of bread that results from changes that occur after baking possibly due to shifting of water from gluten to starch/amylopectin, thereby changing the nature of the gluten network.

rope Bacterial decomposition of bread whereby protein and starch become discolored and sticky.

TABLE 12.2
Ingredients and Quick Breads

Ingredient	Purpose	Too Much	Too Little
Flour	Dry ingredient with protein content; gluten becomes available with proper hydration.	Low rise; gluten network too tight.	Low rise; not enough protein for gluten development.
Mixing/ kneading	Air incorporation and development of gluten; distribution of ingredients.	Low rise; breaks gluten linkages.	Low rise; less air incorporated, more open gluten; uneven texture.
Liquid	Hydration and aids gelatinization and gluten development.	Low rise; dilutes/tenderizes gluten too much.	Low rise; poor gluten development because flour is not hydrated.
Milk	Hydration; fat, sugar, protein source; sometimes scalded and cooked to destroy enzymes for tender, rich bread.	Low rise; if not scalded, nontender results.	Nontender bread due to lack of liquid, fat, and protein.
Egg	Hydration; fat, protein source; tender (fat), richer bread; protein gives structure.	Low rise, too much protein structure.	Nontender due to lack of fat; sometimes flaky (wanted in a croissant).
Sugar	Attracts and holds water due to action of feeding yeast and browning.	Low rise, overproduction of yeast due to too much of a food source.	Low rise; too tight due to lack of food source for yeast.
Fat	Tenderizes because air gets in between the fat globules.	Low rise; oversoftens gluten network (rubbery), weakens gluten structure.	Low rise; tough, no tenderizing.
Salt	Firming effect.	Low rise; overcontrol of yeast.	Open, coarse texture, effect on yeast.

of preservation, and the appearance of not being stale or spoiled. Scientists have found that the sensory properties of foods contribute significantly to consumer freshness perceptions and that sensory characteristics that are perceived to be fresh in one product type are not necessarily fresh in another.[30]

Bread and cake products can be combined with many other flavoring to add to sensory delight. Spices of all varieties have found their way into bread products and cakes over the course of history, as discussed in **Special Topic 12.1**.

Special Topic 12.1

Phytonutrients and Spices

Andrea Roche

Spices have been used for generations by humans as a food additive and in folk medicine to treat ailments. Scientists have found that many spices do in fact have medicinal properties that alleviate symptoms or prevent disease. A growing body of research has demonstrated that commonly used spices—including cinnamon, garlic, cayenne pepper, and cumin—possess antimicrobial properties that, in some cases, can be used therapeutically. Some spices have even been shown in human or animal studies to fight various diseases. For example, saffron, turmeric, and black and green tea contain potent phytochemicals—including carotenoids, curcumins, catechins, and lignan—that may protect against cancer.[1]

Spices are usually made from seeds, although they can also come from bark, root, fruit, or the flowers of plants. They are generally used as dried products. The majority of spices are commercially grown in the tropics. In general, spices are brown, black, or red in color and have a pungent smell.[2,3]

One study found that 10 grams of spice (about 2 tablespoons) contained as many health-promoting antioxidants as 10 servings of fruits and vegetables. Another study of 27 cooking spices found that most had greater disease-fighting antioxidant power per gram than many fruits and vegetables. Virtually all spices are beneficial, essentially free of calories, and can be substituted for salt.[4]

Cinnamon has been used as a spice and as a traditional herbal medicine for centuries. Originating in Sri Lanka and South India, cinnamon is the inner bark of a tropical evergreen tree. Evidence suggests that this sweet, aromatic spice has potential anti-inflammatory, antimicrobial, antioxidant, antitumor, cardioprotective, cholesterol-lowering, and immune-boosting effects. Other studies have demonstrated that cinnamon may act as an insulin mimetic, meaning that it can potentiate insulin activity or stimulate cellular glucose metabolism. Furthermore, animal studies have demonstrated that cinnamon has strong hypoglycemic properties. One study found that half a teaspoon of cinnamon a day lowered blood-sugar levels in patients with type 2 diabetes and brought down their bad cholesterol.[3] The use of cinnamon as an adjunct to the treatment of type 2 diabetes mellitus is a promising prospect, but further research is needed.[2]

Based on folklore, medicinal use of saffron in treating different diseases, and data obtained from scientific investigations over the years, saffron is a strong potential candidate as an anticancer drug.[3] Primarily found in Iran, saffron is the dried stigmas (the part of the plant that receives pollen during fertilization) of the flowers of the saffron crocus plant. This somewhat rare and expensive spice is used in Western cooking as a colorant and for its delicate, unique flavor.

Garlic is a bulb crop; it grows underground much like root vegetables. Garlic contains the phytochemical allicin, which has been found to be a major antimicrobial agent. The mechanism of allicin's antimicrobial action is not yet fully understood; however, once it is, allicin may be used as a model to design new antibiotics.[3]

Capsaicin, better known as hot or cayenne pepper, is produced from the dried, baked, and ground chili pepper. Researchers are examining its potential benefit as a pain suppressant and for its ability to suppress certain cancer cells.[4]

Tumeric is a member of the ginger family and is a common ingredient in curries. Studies have focused on curcumin, the substance that gives turmeric its vibrant, yellow color. This spice has shown promise for treating Alzheimer's disease. Researchers speculate that it may fight the accumulation of destructive proteins in the brain (a hallmark of Alzheimer's) and also counter the inflammation that can worsen the condition. Curcumin might also have cancer-fighting properties. Research has shown that it decreases the proliferation of cancer cells and can cause malignant tumors to self-destruct.[3]

The health effects of tea—primarily from the leaves of various plants and shrubs—have been investigated. Green tea contains bioactive chemicals such as catechins and polyphenols, which are thought to contribute to the beneficial effects, primarily as antioxidants. In general, all tea has been shown to boost the immune system.[1]

Thymoquinone, a bioactive compound identified in the oil of black cumin, has great therapeutic potential as well as an antimicrobial and anticancer agent.[3]

Exciting as these findings are, most of the research in the area of therapeutic spices has involved larger servings and higher concentrations of spice than one would typically add to foods. Whether smaller amounts of cooking spices can affect human health is not well known. However, the possibility adds weight to another reason to include spices generously in your diet, and the potential for their use in higher "doses" as medicine is a tantalizing possibility. Perhaps most important, from a food science perspective, is that they add flavor to food without adding calories, fat, salt, cholesterol, or sugar.

References

1 Underwood A. The new superfoods. *Newsweek*, 2005 Oct 24;146(17). Available at: http://www.thedailybeast.com/newsweek/2005/10/23/the-new-superfoods.html. Accessed August 3, 2012.

2 Gruenwald J, Freder J, Armbruester N. Cinnamon and health. *Crit Rev Food Sci Nutr.* 2010;50(9):822–834.

3 Lai P, Roy J. Antimicrobial and chemopreventive properties of herbs and spices. *Curr Med Chem.* 2004;11:1451–1460.

4 Spice it up: Disease-fighting flavors. *Consum Rep.* 2006;71(1):49.

Choosing Bread

According to the U.S. Department of Agriculture, breads are classified in the grains food group.[31] Any food made from wheat, rice, oats, cornmeal, barley, or other cereal grain is considered a grain product. Grains are divided into two subgroups: whole grains and refined grains. Whole grains contain the entire grain kernel—the bran, germ, and endosperm. Refined grains have been milled, a process that removes the bran and germ. This is done to give grains a finer texture and to improve their shelf life, but it also removes dietary fiber, iron, and many B vitamins. Because refined grains lack the bran and germ, they often are enriched, a process in which certain B vitamins (thiamin, riboflavin,

Phytonutrient Point

Functional Breads Functional breads enriched with calcium, dietary fiber, prebiotic inulin, beta-glucans, oligosaccharides, omega-3 fatty acids, and even ginseng are available.

Innovation Point

Bread Flour The following is a good general rule of thumb: High-protein bread flour is best for yeast breads; low-protein cake flour is best for cakes.

niacin, and folic acid) and iron are added back after processing. Fiber is not usually added back to enriched grains. The USDA recommends consuming at least 3 ounces of whole grains per day and that half of all grains in the diet should be whole grains.[31,32]

Nutritional Properties and Impact on Health

The flour and yeast in breads makes them a good source of B vitamins as well as the minerals magnesium, phosphorus, potassium, iron, and zinc. Breads are also good sources of protein, fiber, and fat. Whole wheat bread has antioxidants (a type of phytonutrient), lignans, and phenolic acids, which have been shown to reduce the risk of heart disease.[33–39]

Despite all the nutritional attributes that breads offer, research shows that nutrients may wane during processing or over time. Processing tends to decrease levels of bioactive components in grains and also alters their bioavailability.[33,40,41] Milling of the grain, mixing, fermentation, and baking all influence the nutritional quality of bread.[40] Factors such as the mixing process used, pH, temperature, and baking time also influence the vitamin content of the finished product:[40]

- Fermentation has been shown to slightly increase the amount of some B vitamins, including thiamine.[42–44] A portion of the riboflavin in bread is derived from yeast, so bread often contains more riboflavin than the original flour. Whole wheat bread made with yeast results in a 30% enrichment in riboflavin, provided that the fermentation is sufficiently long. Sourdough fermentation does not lead to any enrichment of riboflavin.[44]
- Kneading the dough decreases the amount of pyridoxine (a type of B vitamin) present, as does baking, confirming that pyridoxine is easily destroyed by oxygen and heat. However, longer fermentation times have been shown to increase pyridoxine levels.[44]
- Fermentation time and baking temperature influence folate levels.[45,46]
- A reduction in kneading time and a longer fermentation time may help retain carotenoids and vitamin E levels by limiting oxygen incorporation.[47]
- In grains, antioxidants are concentrated in the bran as phenolic compounds, which are also affected by the bread making process.[48,49]
- After the baking process and the bread is cool, changes in the starch occur that may further affect nutritional quality.[35,50,51] However, aside from minimally affecting the pyridoxine content, limited information is available at this time on the effects of storage on other nutrients in bread.[52]

Bread production is driven by consumer and regulatory demands and is based on demographics, convenience, health, and taste.[53] With consumers aspiring towards a healthy lifestyle, breads containing whole grain, multiple grains, or other functional ingredients are prevalent in the marketplace.[54,55] Based on consumer demand, manufacturers will continue to offer functional properties for bread products.

Consumer trends often influence dietary behavior and consumer attitudes over time.[56] Of late, the food industry has made many changes in the products being offered due to the health concerns of consumers, public health officials, and the medical community. All foods are under scrutiny, from fresh produce to packaged foods as well as breads and cakes.

Scientists have been studying the effects of breads and cakes on everything from heart disease to diabetes to metabolic syndrome, because these products are sometimes made with excessive sugar and fat. **Figure 12.23** shows a label from a baked good containing excessive fats, sugar, and calories.

The main ingredient in bread that has proven health benefits is dietary fiber. Whether it is inherent to the actual product or added to it, high-fiber bread is attractive to health-minded consumers.[57,58] Scientists continue to build evidence that whole grain foods can reduce the risk of coronary heart disease, although the exact mechanism of how this happens is not clear.[36,59–68] In addition, mounting research indicates that whole grains may also reduce the risk of type 2 diabetes and certain cancers (including colon and breast cancer) and help people maintain a healthy weight.[34,64,69–79] Scientists have also noted that those populations that consume more whole grains tend to have healthier lifestyles.[80–82]

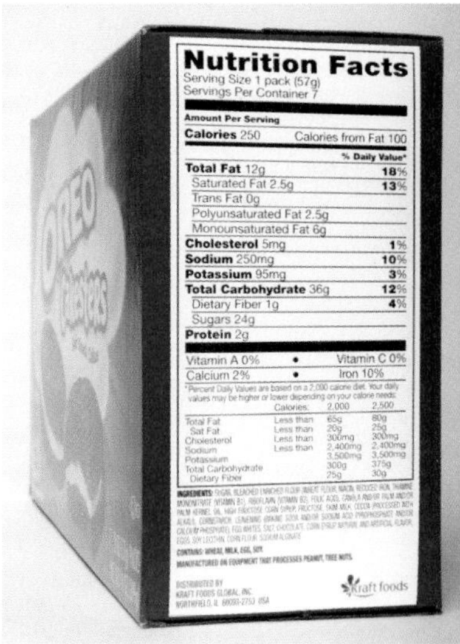
Nutrition Facts
Serving Size 1 pack (57g)
Servings Per Container 7
Amount Per Serving
Calories 250 Calories from Fat 100
% Daily Value*
Total Fat 12g 18%
Saturated Fat 2.5g 13%
Trans Fat 0g
Polyunsaturated Fat 2.5g
Monounsaturated Fat 6g
Cholesterol 5mg 1%
Sodium 250mg 10%
Potassium 95mg 3%
Total Carbohydrate 36g 12%
Dietary Fiber 1g 4%
Sugars 24g
Protein 2g
Vitamin A 0% • Vitamin C 0%
Calcium 2% • Iron 10%
Calories: 2,000 2,500
Total Fat Less than 65g 80g
Sat Fat Less than 20g 25g
Cholesterol Less than 300mg 300mg
Sodium Less than 2,400mg 2,400mg
Potassium 3,500mg 3,500mg
Total Carbohydrate 300g 375g
Dietary Fiber 25g 30g
Kraft foods

FIGURE 12.23 Bread products can be a good source of nutrition unless they have lots of added sugar and fat. Many prepackaged baked goods are high in sugar and fat. Of particular concern are baked goods that contain trans fats, which have been linked to an increased risk of coronary heart disease.

Food Technology

Food scientists, bakers, and food manufacturers all want to create nutritious products that have a relatively long shelf life. With bread, staling is an issue of particular concern. Part of the cause of staling is the shift of water from gluten molecules to starch (amylopectin). This changes the nature of the gluten network in the bread, resulting in less moisture overall as amylopectin undergoes retrogradation. Scientists also have discovered that different types of carbohydrates provide different bread textures and influence the staling process.[83–85]

Recent investigations have focused on the use of hydrocolloids, polysaccharide food substances such as gums, to retain bread freshness. Most of the hydrocolloids that have been tested increase the volume of the loaf and promote moisture retention and water activity. In particular, bread loaves prepared with locust bean gum retained moisture and were softer than those loaves that did not use locust bean gum.[83–85]

As with all food, changes in the bread's texture and flavor will occur over time. Some types of packaging can minimize these changes.[26] Most breads are wrapped in a plastic bag that allows for airflow around the product. Such packaging allows for oxygen to migrate between the product and the packaging in order to maintain product freshness and provide protection; however, depending on how the product is stored, it also may create conditions that accelerate spoilage.[86]

Scientists are currently looking at ways to improve packaging to extend the shelf life of baked goods by using nanotechnology in the form of active packaging. For example, wax paper with cinnamon may offer antimicrobial protection and keep products fresh.[87] Consumers also are seeking sustainable packaging that is environmentally friendly.[88]

Innovation Point

Plant Sterols Scientists are investigating whether adding plant sterols to enhance the nutritional attributes of bread might reduce the risk of cardiovascular disease. Researchers also are seeking ways to reduce sodium without sacrificing quality by substituting potassium salts for sodium chloride.

Going Green with Breads

The advent of the Industrial Age made an enormous impact on the entire food system, including bread production. From mills to mixing machines to vast monocultures of grains, modern technologies have made it possible to produce mass quantities of bread for large populations.[89] However, some of these innovations have had environmental costs. A better understanding between the agriculture and the food system as well as population health will help drive agriculture and the food industry in a greener direction.[89,90]

Wheat

Of all the cereal grains, wheat is by far the most draining on the environment because of its high water demands.[91–93] Several solutions to this problem are being explored:

- Scientists are investigating ways to successfully employ "dry farming" practices for wheat cultivation that require minimal amounts of water and pesticides. Preliminary research shows that alternative farming practices have the potential to reduce agricultural impacts on water quality.[91–93]

- Wheat mills are becoming more energy efficient because of advances in equipment. Mills are being relocated closer to wheat fields to minimize transit time and energy consumption.[91–93]
- The industry is currently exploring compostable packaging that may help the environment. Currently, flour is typically sold in recyclable paper bags.[94] However, demand for environmentally friendly packaging cannot be sacrificed for the safety and quality of the product.[90,95]

Commercial Breads and Cakes

Commercially produced breads and cakes are no doubt convenient, but they do have environmental costs. These costs depend on the types of ingredients, the energy required to produce and ship the product, as well as product and packaging waste. Consumers can affect commercial production practices by demanding products that are environmentally friendly. Consumers can also weigh the options of commercially made bread versus home baked bread. Typically, commercial breads are more energy efficient, because multiple loaves are baked at one time; however, home baking does not require packaging or shipping. Some ideas to consider for greening of breads and cakes is to purchase products that have compostable packaging, that support local bakers, or that are baked at home.

Green Point

Commercial Bread Buying commercial bread is convenient, but home baking offers certain advantages. For example, fewer additives are needed because the shelf life of the product does not need to cover the duration of time that spans production at a commercial facility to reaching a consumer's home.

Food Safety and Foodborne Illness

Packaging requirements for fresh bakery goods are sometimes minimal because the products are meant for immediate consumption. However, like other processed foods, bakery products are subject to physical, chemical, and microbiological spoilage, even with the best-designed packaging.[26,95–98] Any physical and chemical spoilage limits the shelf life of bakery products, but from a health standpoint microbiological spoilage by bacteria, molds, and yeast is of the greatest concern.

Bacteria

Bakery products have been implicated in foodborne illnesses involving *Salmonella* spp., *Listeria monocytogenes*, *Bacillus cereus*, and even the highly toxic *Clostridium botulinum*. Bacteria are most likely to be a problem in high-moisture bakery products packaged under modified atmospheres.[26,95–98] Rope is a more common bacterial contamination resulting from *Bacillus mesentericus*. The contamination originates in the flour. The bread that results has an unpleasant fruity aroma. The crumb deteriorates and the bread becomes soft and sticky due to extracellular slimy polysaccharides.[99–101]

Mold

Fungal mold is a common cause of bread spoilage. Bread is contaminated from the mold spores that are present in the atmosphere during the postproduction phases of bread making—cooling, slicing, packaging, and storage. Rates of mold growth depend on the ingredients used in the bread and the processing method. The most common bread molds are *Penicillium* spp., *Aspergillus* spp., *Cladosporium* spp., *Mucorales* spp., and *Neurospora* spp. Bread molds are a threat to humans because they can produce mycotoxins, which can lead to acute and chronic health effects via ingestion, skin contact, and inhalation and possibly cause death.[102] Researchers found that the addition of sour dough and acid (citric acid, lactic acid, or acetic acid) to commercial white bread delayed the growth of mold, extending the product's shelf-life twofold over that of straight dough bread. Addition of organic acids increased shelf-life up to more than 30 days.[98]

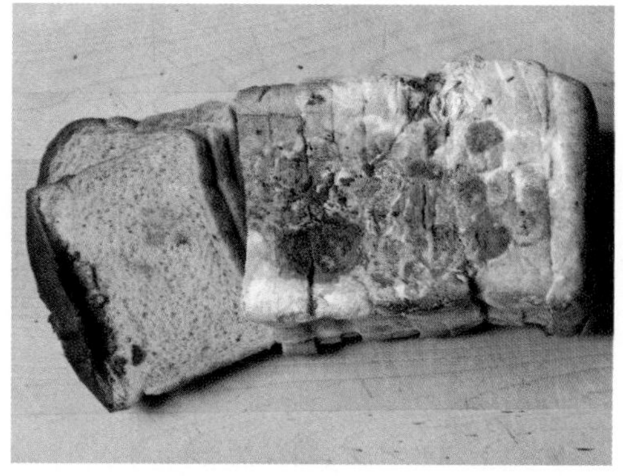

FIGURE 12.24 The most common fermentative yeast is *Saccharomyces cerevisiae*. Although used in the production of bread, if baked bread comes into contact with this yeast the yeast may ferment the sugars in the bread, leading to spoilage. Filamentous yeasts, or chalk molds, create a white growth on the bread's surface.

Yeasts

Yeasts can contaminate baked goods postprocessing through physical contact—for example, by coming into contact with nonsanitized equipment or infected high-sugar foods.[103–105] Two types of yeasts can cause bread spoilage: fermentative yeasts and filamentous yeasts (see **Figure 12.24**).[103] Fermentative yeasts ferment the sugars in the bread; spoilage is signaled by the development of an alcoholic off-aroma. Filamentous yeasts, also known as "chalk molds," create a white growth on the bread surface that is sometimes confused with other types of mold growth. The most common chalk mold is *Pichia burtonii*; it has been shown to be more preservative-resistant than other molds.

Microbial growth is controlled by preservatives and/or refrigeration. However, although refrigeration retards mold growth, it also induces staling. Food-safety techniques such as irradiation and radiation are currently being explored as ways to destroy mold spores.[101]

Fortification and Enrichment

Many of the ready-to-eat cereals and packaged breads are fortified or enriched with nutrients. Nutrients selected for fortification or enrichment are investigated through research rigor to determine the degree of population deficiency as well as establish safety levels. Fortification and enrichment are two different processes:[106]

- *Enrichment:* A process to add back iron, thiamin, riboflavin, niacin, and folic acid at naturally occurring levels
- *Fortification:* A process to add vitamins and minerals in amounts in excess of at least 10% of that normally present in the food

Some examples of each of these processes include enrichment as white flour being enriched with thiamin, riboflavin, niacin and iron, which are lost when wheat is refined. Enriched refined grain products must conform to standards of identity are required by law to be fortified with folic acid as well. **Figure 12.25** shows how the decisions are made for food fortification in the United States.[107]

Chapter Review

Breads have a rich history and are vital to many cultures for both their economic and nutritive value. The cookery behind bread and cake has given humankind a limitless variety of breads; each variety is defined by its unique ingredients and the mixing methods used in its production. The addition of biological (yeast), chemical, or physical leavening agents has allowed for the development of a variety of raised products.

Breads are classified in the grains food group. Any food made from wheat, rice, oats, cornmeal, barley, or other cereal grain is considered a grain product. Grains are divided into two subgroups: whole grains and refined grains. Whole grains contain the entire grain kernel—the bran, germ, and endosperm.

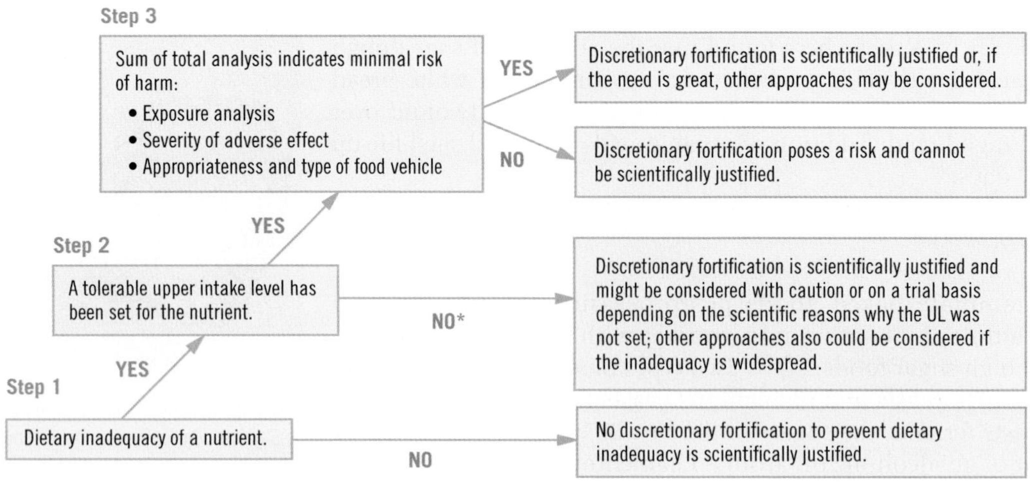

Step 3

Sum of total analysis indicates minimal risk of harm: • Exposure analysis • Severity of adverse effect • Appropriateness and type of food vehicle	YES → Discretionary fortification is scientifically justified or, if the need is great, other approaches may be considered.
	NO → Discretionary fortification poses a risk and cannot be scientifically justified.

Step 2 (YES → Step 3)

A tolerable upper intake level has been set for the nutrient.	NO* → Discretionary fortification is scientifically justified and might be considered with caution or on a trial basis depending on the scientific reasons why the UL was not set; other approaches also could be considered if the inadequacy is widespread.

Step 1 (YES → Step 2)

Dietary inadequacy of a nutrient.	NO → No discretionary fortification to prevent dietary inadequacy is scientifically justified.

FIGURE 12.25 Flow chart for decisions about discretionary food fortification.

*For a number of nutrients, no UL was set because there was insufficient documentation of adverse effects, and the Dietary Reference Intake (DRI) reports language does not include a statement of concern of safety. For example, "There are no reports available of adverse effects from consumption of excess thiamin by ingestion of food and supplements. Because the data are inadequate for a quantitative risk assessment, no Tolerable Upper Intake Level (UL) can be derived." For several other nutrients, the UL was not set because there was insufficient documentation of adverse effects; however, the DRI report language indicated a concern about safety. For example, "No adverse effects have been convincingly associated with excess intake of chromium from food or supplements, but this does not mean that there is no potential for adverse effects resulting from high intakes. Since data on the adverse effects of chromium intake are limited, caution may be warranted."

Source: Reproduced from Institute of Medicine, Food and Nutrition Board. *Dietary Reference Intakes: Guiding Principles for Nutrition Labeling and Fortification.* © 2003 by the National Academy of Sciences, courtesy of the National Academies Press, Washington, DC. Reprinted with permission.

Refined grains have been milled, a process that removes the bran and germ. This is done to give grains a finer texture and to improve their shelf life, but it also removes dietary fiber, iron, and many B vitamins. Because refined grains lack the bran and germ, they are often enriched, a process in which certain B vitamins (thiamin, riboflavin, niacin, and folic acid) and iron are added back after processing. Fiber is not usually added back to enriched grains. Bread remains to be the staff of life.

Learning Portfolio

© ImageState

Study Points

1. Wheat is one of the most important food crops in the world.
2. The essential ingredients for yeast-leavened dough are flour, liquid, yeast, and salt.
3. Yeast is a microscopic one-celled organism. Various factors affect yeast activity in baking, especially fermentation time and temperature.
4. Flour provides protein for bread in the form of glutenin and gliadin, which combine with water to produce gluten. The sheetlike gluten structures trap air and gases made by yeast, causing the bread to rise.
5. Liquid is essential in bread making and may be provided in the form of water, milk, or eggs. It is important for hydration of flour proteins and starch and for dissolving other ingredients.
6. Salt adds flavor, balances the taste of the bread, and retards yeast fermentation. It makes dough less sticky and gluten stretchier, resulting in a lighter product.
7. Quick breads do not require yeast and thus do not require rising or proofing time. Quick breads vary widely in the consistency of their dough or batter.
8. Breads offer many important nutritional attributes; however, research demonstrates that nutrients may decrease during processing or over time. Based on consumer demands, manufacturers will continue to offer functional properties for bread products.
9. Scientists continue to build evidence that whole grain food consumption may reduce risk of coronary heart disease, although the exact mechanism is not clear.
10. Bread stales as a result of changes that occur after baking, including the distribution of water shifting from gluten to starch amylopectin.
11. Consumers can impact the bread industry by demanding that the products are environmentally friendly. A better understanding between the agriculture and food system as well as population health also may help drive of agricultural and industrial change.
12. Bread can become contaminated from mold spores present in the atmosphere during the postproduction phases of bread making. Rates of mold growth depend on the ingredients used and the processing method. Bacterial or yeast contamination of bread products is possible but less likely.

Issues for Class Discussion

1. How does bread production impact the environment? How can the impact of bread production be reduced without affecting the overall supply of bread?
2. Discuss the impact of bread and baked goods on the obesity epidemic. Should bread/cake be named the culprit? Why or why not?

Research Areas for Students

1. Specific grains used in bread that impact health
2. Ways to minimize the environmental impact of bread making
3. Growing grains in diverse climates
4. Incorporation of high-fructose corn syrup into bread and the possible health effects

References

1. Ashton J. *The History of Bread*. Harvard University: The Religious Tract Society; 1904.
2. Assire J, Clavel B. *The Book of Bread*. New York: Flammarion, 1996.
3. Pomeranz Y. *Bread Around the World: Modern Cereal Science and Technology*. New York: VCH Publishers; 1987.
4. Gould JT. Baking around the world. In: Cauvain SP, Young LS (eds.). *Technology of Breadmaking*. 2nd ed. New York: Springer; 2007.
5. Dupaigne B. *History of Bread*. New York: Harry N. Abrams Publishers; 1999.

Key Terms

	page
barm	380
crumb	385
dough conditioners	385
fermentation	380
drop batters	388
gelatinization	387
gluten	384
leavening agent	384
oven spring	387
pour batters	388
proofing	387
quick breads	387
rope	391
soft doughs	388
sponge	386
stiff doughs	389
staling	391
yeasts	380
yeast breads	383

6. Seibel W. Wheat usage in Western Europe In: Faridi H, Faubion JM (eds.). *Wheat End Uses Around the World*. St. Paul, MN: American Association of Food Chemists; 1995.
7. Faridi H, Faubion JM, Qarooni J. Wheat usage in North America. In: Faridi H, Faubion JM (eds.). *Wheat End Uses Around the World*. St. Paul, MN: American Association of Food Chemists; 1995.
8. Kaplan SL. *Good Bread Is Back: A Contemporary History of French Bread, the Way It Is*. Durham, NC: Duke University Press; 2006.
9. McMaster GJ, Gould, JT. Wheat usage in Australia and New Zealand. In: Faridi H, Faubion JM (eds.). *Wheat End Uses Around the World*. St. Paul, MN: American Association of Food Chemists; 1995.
10. Cauvain SP. *Bread Making: Improving Quality*. Boca Raton, FL: Woodhead Publishing; 2003.
11. Cauvain SP, Young LS. *Technology of Breadmaking*. 2nd ed. New York: Springer; 2007.
12. Jacob HE, Reinhart P. *Six Thousand Years of Bread: Its Holy and Unholy History*. New York: Skyhorse Publishing; 2007.
13. Bennion M, Scheule B. *Introductory Foods*. 13th ed. Upper Saddle River, NJ: Prentice Hall; 2009.
14. Dakota Yeast. Available at: http://www.dakotayeast.com/help-fermentation.html. Accessed August 25, 2010.
15. Fleischmann's. Available at: http://www.breadworld.com/FAQ.aspx. Accessed August 15, 2010.
16. Gisslen W. *Professional Baking*. 6th ed. Hoboken, NJ: John Wiley & Sons; 2007.
17. Wing D, Scott A. *The Bread Builders*. White River Junction, VT: Chelsea Green Publishing; 1999.
18. Eliasson AC. *Cereals in Breadmaking: A Molecular Colloidal Approach*. New York: Marcel Dekker; 1993.
19. McGee H. *Keys to Good Cooking: A Guide to Making the Best of Food and Recipes*. New York: The Penguin Press; 2010.
20. Corriher SO. *Cookwise: The Hows & Whys of Successful Cooking with Over 230 Great-Tasting Recipes*. New York: William Morrow and Company; 1997.
21. Seiz K. Dough Conditioner. Baking Management. Available at: http://baking-management.com/rd_applications/bm_imp_9295/. Accessed January 9, 2011.
22. Daem C, Peabody D. Food Study Manual. School of Family and Nutritional Sciences. University of British Columbia. Available at: http://www.library.ubc.ca/ereserve/hunu201/fdmanual/page117.htm. Accessed August 5, 2010.
23. Bloksma AH. Dough structure, dough rheology, and baking quality. *Cereal Food World*. 1990;135(2):237–244.
24. Hui Y-H. *Handbook of food science, technology, and engineering*. Volume 4. Boca Raton, FL: Taylor & Francis; 2006.
25. Department of Foods and Nutrition, Oregon State University. Mixing Methods for Yeast Breads. Available at: http://food.oregonstate.edu/learn/bread.html. Accessed September 17, 2010.
26. Scott Smith J, Hui Y-H (eds.). *Food Processing: Principles and Applications*. Ames, IA: Blackwell Publishing; 2004.
27. Fan J, Mitchell JR, Blanshard JMV. A model for the oven rise of dough during baking. *J Food Engineer*. 1999;41(2):69–77.
28. Hui Y-H (ed.). *Bakery Products: Science and Technology*. Ames, IA: Blackwell Publishing; 2006.
29. Bloksma AH. Rheology of the breadmaking process. *Cereal Food World*. 1990;135(2):228–236.
30. Heenan SP, Dufour JP, Hamid N, et al. Characterization of fresh bread flavor: Relationships between sensory characteristics and volatile composition. *Food Chem*. 2009;116(1):249–257.
31. U.S. Department of Agriculture. Grains Food Group. Available at: http://www.choosemyplate.gov/food-groups/grains.html. Accessed November 3, 2012.
32. U.S. Department of Agriculture. MyPlate. Available at: http://www.choosemyplate.gov. Accessed October 12, 2012.
33. Slavin JL, Jacobs D, Marquart L. Grain processing and nutrition. *Crit Rev Biotech*. 2001;21:49–66.
34. Slavin JL, Martini MC, Jacobs DR Jr, Marquart L. Plausible mechanisms for the protectiveness of whole grains. *Am J Clin Nutr*. 1999;70(3 Suppl):459S–463S.
35. Thompson LU. Antioxidants and hormone-mediated health benefits of whole grains. *Crit Rev Food Sci Nutr*. 1994;34(5–6):473–47.
36. Liu S, Stampfer MJ, Hu FB, et al. Whole-grain consumption and risk of coronary heart disease: Results from the Nurses' Health Study. *Am J Clin Nutr*. 1999;70(3):412–419.
37. Mellena PB, Walsha TF, Herrington DM. Whole grain intake and cardiovascular disease: A meta-analysis. *Nutr Metab Cardiovascular Dis*. 2008;18(4):283–290.
38. Mente A, de Koning L, Shannon HS, Anand SS. Systematic review of the evidence supporting a causal link between dietary factors and coronary heart disease. *Arch Int Med*. 2009;169(7):659–669.
39. Jensen MK, Koh-Banerjee P, Hu FB, et al. Intakes of whole grains, bran, and germ and the risk of coronary heart disease in men. *Am J Clin Nutr*. 2004;80(6):1492–1499.
40. Dewettincka K, Van Bockstaelea F, Kühnec B, et al. Nutritional value of bread: Influence of processing, food interaction and consumer perception. *J Cereal Sci*. 2008;48(2):243–257.
41. Mateo Anson N, Aura AM, Selinheimo E, et al. Bioprocessing of wheat bran in whole wheat bread increases the bioavailability of phenolic acids in men and exerts anti-inflammatory effects ex vivo. J Nutr. 2011;141(1):137–143.
42. Pederson B, Knudsen KEB, Eggum BO. Nutritive value of cereal products with emphasis on the effect of milling. *World Rev Nutr Diet*. 1989;60:1–5.
43. Khetarpaul N, Chauhan BM. Effect of fermentation on protein, fat, minerals and thiamine content of pearl-millet. *Plant Foods Hum Nutr*. 1989;39(2):169–177.
44. Batifoulier F, Verny MA, Chanliaud E, et al. Effect of different breadmaking methods on thiamine, riboflavin and pyridoxine contents of wheat bread. *J Cereal Sci*. 2005;42(1):101–108.
45. Kariluoto S, Aittamaa M, Korhola M, et al. Effects of yeasts and bacteria on the levels of folates in rye sourdoughs. *Int J Food Microbiol*. 2006;106:137–143.
46. Kariluoto S, Vahteristo L, Salovaara H, et al. Effect of baking method and fermentation on folate content of rye and wheat breads. *Cereal Chem*. 2004;81:134–139.
47. Leenhardt F, Lyan B, Rock E, et al. Wheat lipoxygenase activity induces greater loss of carotenoids than vitamin E during breadmaking. *J Agr Food Chem*. 2006;54(5):1710–1715.
48. Hatcher DW, Kruger JE. Simple phenolic acids in flours prepared from Canadian wheat: Relationship to ash content, color, and polyphenol oxidase activity. *Cereal Chem*.1997;74:337–343.
49. Gelinas P, McKinnon CM. Effect of wheat variety, farming site, and bread-baking on total phenolics. *Int J Food Sci Tech*. 2006;41:329–332.

50. Jacobson MR, Obanni M, Bemiller JN. Retrogradation of starches from different botanical sources. *Cereal Chem.*1997;74:511–518.
51. Klucinec JD, Thompson DB. Amylose and amylopectin interact in retrogradation of dispersed high-amylose starches. *Cereal Chem.*1999;76(2):282–291.
52. Perera AD, Leklem JE, Miller LT. Stability of vitamin B_6 during bread making and storage of bread and flour. *Cereal Chem.* 1979;56:577–580.
53. Kohn S. An update of the US baking industry. *Cereal Foods World.* 2000;45(3):94–97.
54. Martin P. Controlling the bread making process: The role of bubbles in bread. *Cereal Foods World.* 2004;49:72–75.
55. Vulicevic IR, Abdel-Aal ESM, Mittal GS, Lu X. Quality and storage life of par-baked frozen breads. *Food Sci Tech.* 2004;37:205–213.
56. Asp E. Consumer trends in consumption. In: Wrigley C (ed.). *Encyclopedia of Grain Science.* Amsterdam; Elsevier; 2004: 322–330.
57. Charalampopoulos D, Wang R, Pandiella SS, Webb C. Application of cereals and cereal components in functional foods: a review. *Inter J Food Micro.* 2002;79 (1-2): 131–141.
58. Kihlberg I, Johansson L, Langsrud O, Risvik E. Effects of information on liking of bread. *Food Quality and Preference.* 2005;16(1):25–35.
59. Keogh GF, Cooper GJ, Mulvey TB, et al. Randomized controlled crossover study of the effect of a highly beta-glucan-enriched barley on cardiovascular disease risk factors in mildly hypercholesterolemic men. *Am J Clin Nutr.* 2003;78(4):711–718.
60. Pins JJ. Do whole-grain oat cereals reduce the need for antihypertensive medications and improve blood pressure control? *J Fam Pract.* 2002;51:353–359.
61. Anderson JW, Hanna TJ, Peng X, Kryscio RJ. Whole grain foods and heart disease risk. *J Am Coll Nutr.* 2000;19(3 Suppl):291S–299S.
62. Butcher JL, Beckstrand RL. Fiber's impact on high-sensitivity C-reactive protein levels in cardiovascular disease. *J Am Acad Nurse Pract.* 2010;22(11):566–572.
63. Jenkins DJ, Kendall CW, Vuksan V, et al. Soluble fiber intake at a dose approved by the US Food and Drug Administration for a claim of health benefits: Serum lipid risk factors for cardiovascular disease assessed in a randomized controlled crossover trial. *Am J Clin Nutr.* 2002;75(5):834–839.
64. Harris KA, Kris-Etherton PM. Effects of whole grains on coronary heart disease risk. *Curr Atherosclerosis Rep.* 2010;12(6):368–376.
65. Coulston AM, Boushey C. *Nutrition in the Prevention and Treatment of Disease.* 2nd ed. Burlingame, CA: Elsevier/Academic Press; 2008.
66. Mann J. Dietary carbohydrate: Relationship to cardiovascular disease and disorders of carbohydrate metabolism. *Eur J Clin Nutr.* 2007;61(Suppl 1):S100–S111.
67. Newby PK, Maras J, Bakun P, et al. Intake of whole grains, refined grains, and cereal fiber measured with 7-d diet records and associations with risk factors for chronic disease. *Am J Clin Nutr.* 2007;86(6):1745–1753.
68. Flight I, Clifton P. Cereal grains and legumes in the prevention of coronary heart disease and stroke: A review of the literature. *Eur J Clin Nutr.* 2006;60(10):1145–1159.
69. Wolfram T, Ismail-Beigi F. Efficacy of high-fiber diets in the management of type 2 diabetes mellitus. *Endocrine Pract.* 2011;17(1):132–142.
70. de Munter JSL, Hu FB, Spiegelman D, et al. Whole grain, bran, and germ intake and risk of type 2 diabetes: A prospective cohort study and systematic. *PLoS Med.* 2007;4(8):e261.
71. Fung TT, Hu FB, Pereira MA, et al. Whole-grain intake and the risk of type 2 diabetes: A prospective study in men. *Am J Clin Nutr.* 2002;76(3):535–540.
72. Montonen J, Knekt P, Järvinen R, et al. Whole-grain and fiber intake and the incidence of type 2 diabetes. *Am J Clin Nutr.* 2003;77(3):622–629.
73. Priebe MG, van Binsbergen JJ, de Vos R, Vonk RJ. Whole grain foods for the prevention of type 2 diabetes mellitus. *Cochrane Systems Rev.* 2008; 23;(1):CD006061.
74. Venn BJ, Mann JI. Cereal grains, legumes and diabetes. *Eur J Clin Nutr.* 2004;58(11):1443–1461.
75. Feldheim W, Wisker E. Studies on the improvement of dietary fibre intake. *Deutsche Lebensmittel-Rundschau.* 2000;96:327–330.
76. Egeberg R, Olsen A, Loft S, et al. Intake of whole grain products and risk of colorectal cancers in the Diet, Cancer and Health cohort study. *British J Cancer.* 2010;24;103(5):730–734.
77. Gråsten SM, Juntunen KS, Poutanen KS, et al. Rye bread improves bowel function and decreases the concentrations of some compounds that are putative colon cancer risk markers in middle-aged women and men. *J Nutr.* 2000;130(9):2215–2221.
78. Dahm CC, Keogh RH, Spencer EA, et al. Dietary fiber and colorectal cancer risk: A nested case-control study using food diaries. *J Nat Cancer Inst.* 2010;102(9):614–626.
79. Hanf V, Gonder U. Nutrition and primary prevention of breast cancer: Foods, nutrients and breast cancer risk. *Eur J Obstet Gynecol Reprod Biol.* 2005;123(2):139–149.
80. Cloetens L, Broekaert WF, Delaedt Y, et al. Tolerance of arabinoxylan-oligosaccharides and their prebiotic activity in healthy subjects: A randomised, placebo-controlled cross-over study. *Br J Nutr.* 2010;103(5):703–713.
81. Liu S, Willett WC, Manson JE, et al. Relation between changes in intakes of dietary fiber and grain products and changes in weight and development of obesity among middle-aged women. *Am J Clin Nutr.* 2003;78(5):920–927.
82. McKeown NM, Yoshida M, Shea MK, et al. Whole-grain intake and cereal fiber are associated with lower abdominal adiposity in older adults. *J Nutr.* 2009;139(10):1950–1955.
83. Rosell CM, Rojas JA, Benedito de Barber C. Influence of hydrocolloids on dough rheology and bread quality. *Food Hydrocolloids.* 2001;15(1):75–81.
84. Sharadanant R, Khan K. Effect of hydrophilic gums on the quality of frozen dough: II. Bread characteristics. *Cereal Chem.* 2003;80(6):773–780.
85. Federation of Bakers. Bread and the Environment: Factsheet 16. Available at: http://www.bakersfederation.org.uk/images/publications/factsheets/fs16-bread-the-environment.pdf. Accessed November 23, 2010.
86. Rodríguez A, Nerín C, Batlle R. New cinnamon-based active paper packaging against Rhizopusstolonifer food spoilage. *J Agri Food Chem.* 2008;56(15):6364–6369.
87. Rogers G. Natural Marketing Institute. Available at: http://www.nhiondemand.com/expertsperspectives/article.aspx?id=68&utm_source=NHI+OnDemand+Newsletter+List&utm_campaign=f2a533f1e5-Experts_Packaging-NMI_Feb01_2011&utm_medium=email. Accessed December 19, 2010.

88. Hazell P, Wood S. Drivers of change in global agriculture. *Philo Trans Royal Soc Lond B Biol Sci*. 2008;363(1491):495–515.
89. Kearney J. Food consumption trends and drivers. *Philo Trans Royal Soc Lond B Biol Sci*. 2010;365(1554):2793–2807.
90. Fernandez U, Vodovotz Y, Courtney P, Pascall MA. Extended shelf life of soy bread using modified atmosphere packaging. *J Food Protection*. 2006;69(3):693–698.
91. Encyclopedia of Oklahoma History and Culture. Dry Farming. Available at: http://digital.library.okstate.edu/encyclopedia/entries/d/dr009.html. Accessed December 5, 2010.
92. Oquista KA, Strock JS, Mullac DJ. Influence of alternative and conventional farming practices on subsurface drainage and water quality. *J Env Qual*. 2006;36(4):1194–1204.
93. Harrington R. Biodegradable and compostable food packaging overview. *Food Production Daily*, August 10, 2010. Available at: http://www.foodproductiondaily.com/Packaging/Biodegradable-and-compostable-food-packaging-overview. Accessed October 22, 2010.
94. Hawkesworth S, Dangour AD, Johnston D, et al. Feeding the world healthily: The challenge of measuring the effects of agriculture on health. *Philo Trans Royal Soc Lond B Biol Sci*. 2010;365(1554):3083–3097.
95. Harter B, Carlson K. Environmental Impacts of Making Bread. Available at: http://www.hellogreentomorrow.com/blog/2010/10/environmental-impacts-of-baking-bread/. Accessed December 2, 2010.
96. Gutiérrez L, Escudero A, Batlle R, Nerín C. Effect of mixed antimicrobial agents and flavors in active packaging films. *J Agri Food Chem*. 2009;57(18):8564–8571.
97. Barber B, Ortolá C, Barber S, Fernández F. Storage of packaged white bread: III. Effects of sour dough and addition of acids on bread characteristics. *Eur Food Res Tech*. 1992;194(5):442–449.
98. Bennett JW, Klich M. Mycotoxins. *Clin Microbiol Rev*. 2003;16(3):497–516.
99. Collins NF, Kirshner LAM, von Holy A. A characterisation of *Bacillus* isolates from ropy bread, bakery equipment and raw materials. *S African J Sci*. 1991;87:62–66.
100. Kirschner LM, von Holy A. Rope spoilage of bread. *S African J Sci*. 1989;85:425–427.
101. Arvanitoyannis IS, Traikou A. A comprehensive review of the implementation of hazard analysis critical control point (HACCP) to the production of flour and flour-based products. *Crit Rev Food Sci Nutr*. 2005;45(5):327–370.
102. Deak T. *Handbook of Spoilage Yeasts*. 2nd ed. Boca Raton, FL; CDC Press; 2008.
103. Fleet GH. Yeasts in foods and beverages: Impact on product quality and safety. *Curr Opin Biotech*. 2007;18(2):170–175.
104. Legan JD, Voysey PA. Yeast spoilage of bakery products and ingredients. *J Applied Microbiol*. 1991;70(5):361–371.
105. Pepe O, Blaiotta G, Moschetti G, et al. Applied and environmental rope-producing strains of *Bacillus* spp. from wheat bread and strategy for their control by lactic acid bacteria. *Microbiology*. 2003;69(4):2321–2329.
106. U.S. Department of Agriculture. Action Guide for Child Care Nutrition and Physical Activity Policies: Glossary. Available at: http://healthymeals.nal.usda.gov/hsmrs/Connecticut/Action_Guide_Child_Care/CCAG_Glossary_BackCover.pdf. Accessed August 8, 2012.
107. U.S. Department of Agriculture. DRI Guiding Principles for Labeling. Available at: http://www.nal.usda.gov/fnic/DRI/DRI_Guiding_Principles_Labeling/124-144.pdf. Accessed August 8, 2012.

CHAPTER 13

Fats and Oils

Mindy Beth Nelkin, MS, RD, MA
Nanna Cross, PhD, RD

Chapter Objectives

THE STUDENT WILL BE EMPOWERED TO:

- Describe how hydrogenated fats made their way into the marketplace and why they were used so pervasively.
- Distinguish among different types of fats, including saturated, monounsaturated, polyunsaturated, trans, and omega fatty acids.
- Discuss the nutritional properties and health impacts of fats.
- Give examples of fatty acids used as functional foods.
- Define two types of rancidity, and explain how to avoid rancidity through proper storage of oils and fats.
- Describe the functions fats play in food preparation and the challenges of replacing trans fats.
- Summarize the technologies involved in developing better fats.
- Compare and contrast the three broad categories of fat substitutes.
- Discuss government regulations affecting the labeling and marketing of products that contain fats.

Historical and Cultural Significance

The history of the current forms of fats and oils that are found in our food supply starts in the late 1800s. In 1897, the French chemist Paul Sabatier discovered the process of hydrogenating oils by using a nickel catalyst to add hydrogen to a fatty acid chain, changing double bonds to single bonds.[1] Shortly after that discovery, Wilhelm Norman, a German chemist, developed a hydrogenation process using hydrogen gas.[2,3] In 1906, the hydrogenation process was patented by Joseph Cormfield and Sons. Proctor & Gamble then obtained the rights to the patent, and Crisco shortening was introduced to consumers in 1911.[2]

One problem with completely hydrogenated vegetable oil is that when all the bonds become saturated the shortening produced has a very hard texture that is unsuitable for baking. Partial hydrogenation, in which just some of the double bonds are saturated with hydrogen and only some are reconfigured from a cis to a trans orientation, solved this problem (see **Figure 13.1**).

Partially hydrogenated margarines and shortening were developed as substitutes for animal fats, butter, and lard in response to public health concerns about the relationship between dietary intakes of saturated animal fats and coronary heart disease.[3] Their use exploded from the 1960s through the 1980s. In fact, by the 1970s margarine had replaced butter as a spread, and margarine sales were two times that of butter.[2] One factor that contributed to the popularity of these products was their low cost, driven by an abundant supply of the soybean, corn, and canola oils used in their production (see **Figure 13.2**).

Nearly all trans fatty acids in the diet come from industrial sources of partially hydrogenated vegetable oil, which is added to processed and ready-to-eat foods, such as margarine and shortening; baked products, such as cakes, muffins, pies, cookies, crackers, and other snack items; and foods fried in fats. The following processed and ready-to-eat foods may contain trans fats:

- Baked foods and dry mixes for baked products such as cookies, crackers, cakes, muffins, pies, sweet breads, and pancakes
- Deep-fried foods such as doughnuts, french fries, onion rings, fried chicken, fried fish, egg rolls, and taco shells
- Sauces and dressings, including cheese sauces and salad dressings
- Snack foods such as microwave popcorn and chips (e.g., potato, corn, tortilla)

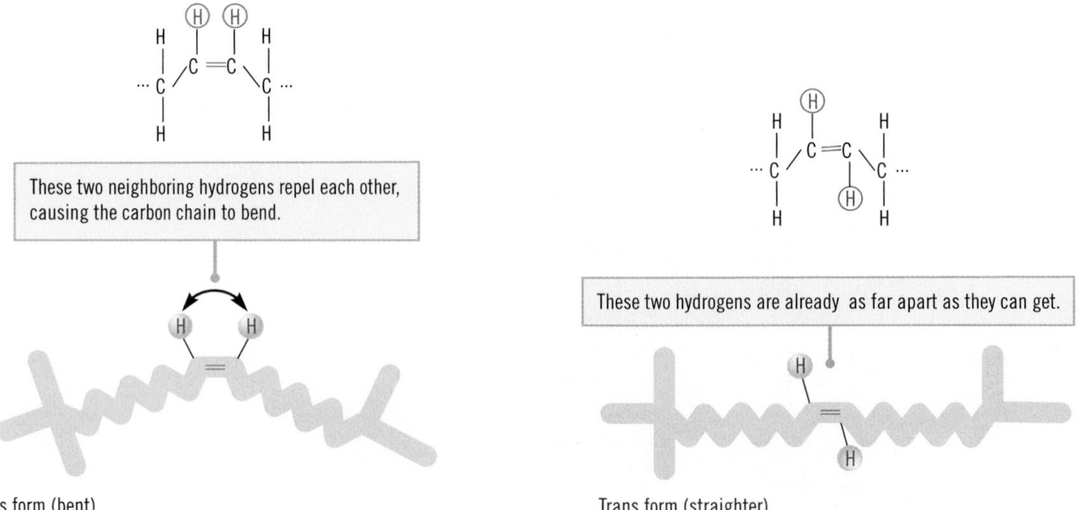
These two neighboring hydrogens repel each other, causing the carbon chain to bend.
These two hydrogens are already as far apart as they can get.
Cis form (bent)
Trans form (straighter)

FIGURE 13.1 In the cis configuration in a naturally unsaturated fatty acid, the hydrogen atoms are on the same side as the carbons, resulting in a kink in the fatty acid chain. When a fatty acid is hydrogenated, the hydrogen atoms are on opposite sides of the carbon, which is called the trans configuration. This makes the hydrocarbon chain relatively straight. The shape of cis and trans fatty acids affects their physical properties.

© iStockphoto/Thinkstock

(a)

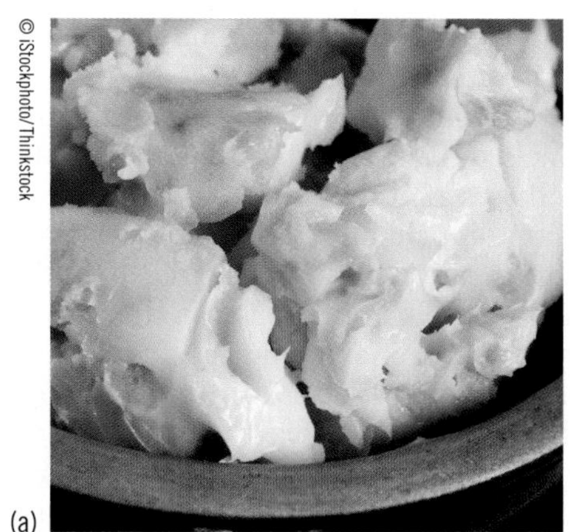

(b)

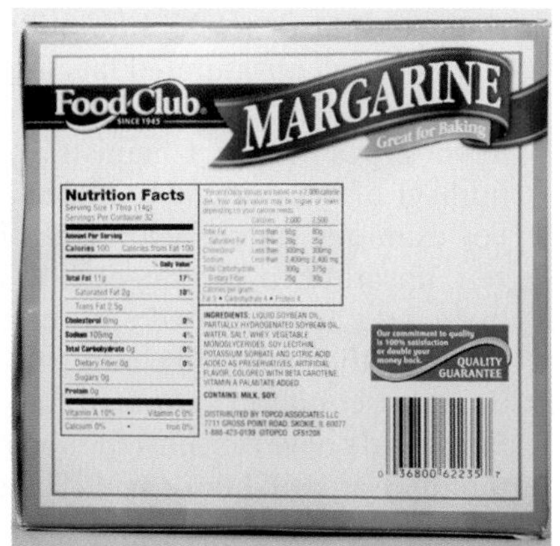

(c)

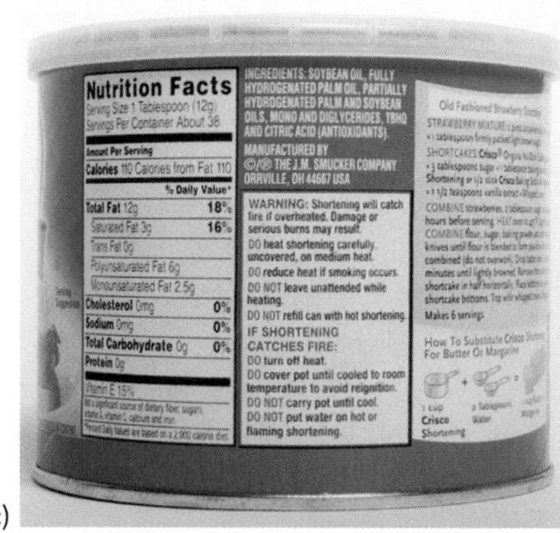

FIGURE 13.2 (a) Lard is derived from pig fat. It was once commonly used in many recipes as a cooking fat or shortening or as a spread similar to butter. It fell into disuse in the mid-20th century due to concerns over its high saturated fat and cholesterol content. (b) Margarine was developed as a replacement for lard and butter. The basic method of making margarine today is emulsifying a blend of hydrogenated vegetable oils with skimmed milk, chilling the mixture to solidify it, and working it to improve the texture. Partially hydrogenated margarine contains trans fats, which have been found to be detrimental to human health. (c) Shortening is hydrogenated vegetable oil. It was developed to replace lard. It is a solid at room temperature and does not require refrigeration. Because it is made from partially hydrogenated vegetable oils, shortening contains trans fats.

- Toppings such as bread crumbs, croutons, icings, nondairy whipped toppings, chocolate chips and syrups, and nondairy creamers

The use of partially hydrogenated fats and trans fats accelerated until the 1980s, when food manufacturers began to respond to consumers' demands to move away from trans fats.[2] In the 1990s, the intake of margarine decreased and the popularity of butter was renewed.[3] Research during this decade began to prove that trans fatty acids are harmful to health. One study showed that a 2% increase in trans fat intake was correlated with a 23% increase in coronary heart disease. Beginning January 1, 2006, the Food and Drug Administration (FDA) mandated that trans fats be included in a food's Nutrition Facts label, prompting food manufacturers to decrease their use of trans fats by finding alternatives. Today, manufacturers are also moving away from solid fats to liquid oils, such as olive oil.

Various technologies are being developed to improve the fats in our diets.[2] These methods will be discussed in more detail in the section on food technology, but some of the more important technologies currently being explored include the following:

- Plant breeding and genetic engineering are being used to produce oil seeds with modified fatty acid composition.
- The hydrogenation process can be modified to reduce or eliminate the formation of trans fatty acids.
- **Fractionation** is the process of physically separating oils into saturated and unsaturated fractions.
- Tropical oils—palm oil, palm kernel oil, and coconut oil—are being used in interesterification processes.[2] **Interestification** is used to produce customized fats by blending highly saturated hard fats (fully hydrogenated vegetable oils) with liquid edible oils to produce fats with intermediate characteristics.[4] Interesterification is able to provide fats with a wide range of melting points, allowing for a variety of food service applications.[5]

fractionation The physical separation of oils into saturated and unsaturated fractions.

interesterification Free fatty acids with the desired degree of saturation and carbon length that can be added to a mixture of triglycerides to develop fats with the desired melting and/or smoke point and stability.

Physical and Chemical Properties

Natural Fatty Acids

Fatty acids in foods exist as triglycerides formed when fatty acids attach to the three carbons of glycerol. Fatty acids differ in the length of their carbon

saturated fatty acids Fatty acids in which all of the hydrogens are saturated and there are no double bonds between the carbon atoms of the fatty acid chain. Stearic acid (18:0) and palmitic acid (16:0) are the most common saturated fatty acids found in food.

monounsaturated fatty acids Fatty acids that have one unsaturated bond. Oleic acid (18:1) is the most common monounsaturated fatty acid. The double bond has a cis configuration.

polyunsaturated fatty acids Fatty acids that have multiple unsaturated bonds. Linoleic acid (18:2) and linolenic acid (18:3) are the most common polyunsaturated fatty acids in vegetable oils used in cooking. The double bonds have a cis configuration.

chain and the degree of saturation. Saturated fats are mostly found in animal fats, whereas unsaturated fats are mostly of plant origin.

Figure 13.3 provides an overview of the chemical structure of the different types of fats. Chemists sometimes designate carbon length and the number of unsaturated bonds in parentheses after the name of the fatty acid. For example, stearic acid (18:0) consists of a chain of 18 carbons and has zero unsaturated carbon–carbon bonds. In **saturated fatty acids**, all of the hydrogens are saturated and there are no double bonds between the carbon atoms of the fatty acid chain. Stearic acid (18:0) and palmitic acid (16:0) are the most common saturated fatty acids found in food. **Monounsaturated fatty acids** have one unsaturated bond. Oleic acid (18:1) is the most common monounsaturated fatty acid. The double bond has a cis configuration. Olive oil contains more oleic acid than any other natural food. **Polyunsaturated fatty acids** have multiple unsaturated bonds. Linoleic acid (18:2) and linolenic acid (18:3) are the most common polyunsaturated fatty acids in vegetable oils used in cooking. The double bonds have a cis configuration.

Partially Hydrogenated (Trans) Fatty Acids

Compared to vegetable oils, the partially hydrogenated (trans) fats developed in the last century offered physical and chemical properties that were advantageous to consumers:[6]

- *Longer shelf life:* Partially hydrogenated fats are less susceptible to oxidation and rancidity, or spoilage, which occurs when the double bonds become saturated with the addition of hydrogen ions. In contrast, vegetable oils have a high concentration of polyunsaturated fatty acids, including linoleic and linolenic acid, and are prone to oxidation or spoilage.[2]
- *Plasticity*: Shortening allows for easier creaming of sugar when used in cake batter and cookie dough, giving the dough or batter

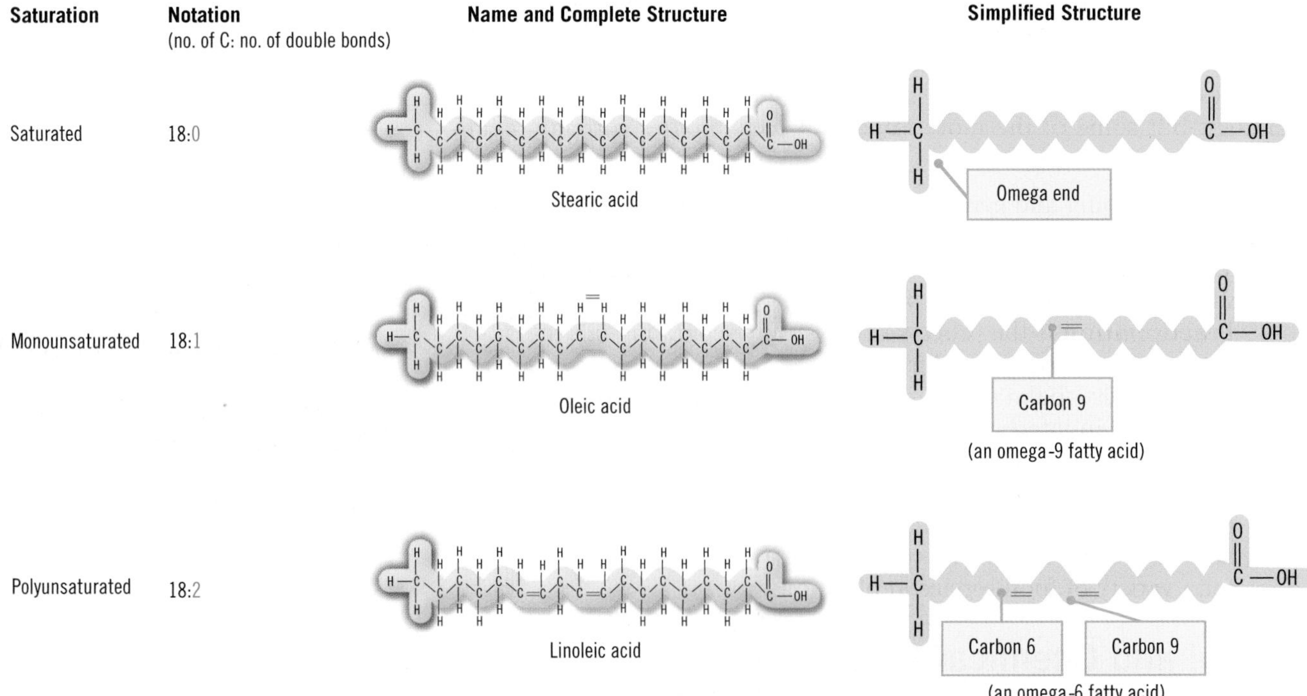

FIGURE 13.3 In a saturated fatty acid, all of the hydrogen atoms are saturated. Unsaturated fatty acids are missing some hydrogens and have one (monounsaturated) or multiple (polyunsaturated) double bonds.

plasticity; that is, suppleness and workability. Using solid fat in baking shortens gluten strands, resulting in flakiness in pie crusts, biscuits, and scones.

- *Higher smoke point:* Partially hydrogenated fats are more stable during cooking and have a higher smoke point than vegetable oils, making them ideal for deep-fat frying.[2]
- *Tactile and other sensory properties:* Partially hydrogenated fats improve mouthfeel, increase food density, and enhance odor.

Natural Sources of Trans Fats

Trans fats are not always the result of industrial hydrogenation processes. They also occur naturally in meat and dairy products as a result of microbial hydrogenation of cis-unsaturated fatty acids in the stomach of ruminant animals (i.e., cattle, bison, sheep, goats).[3,7,8] The concentration of trans fat in ruminant sources of meat and dairy products is 5–8%, compared to 10–60% in partially hydrogenated vegetable oils and 3% in refined vegetable oils.[7–13]

Nutritional Properties

Fats and oils are an important part of the diet. They are calorically dense, with 1 gram of fat providing 9 kcal of energy. They also allow for the digestion of the fat-soluble vitamins, vitamins A, E, D, and K. A diet with too little fat will result in not enough absorption of these important vitamins. Fats also play key roles in our bodies, especially as the building blocks of cell membranes.[14] The *Dietary Guidelines for Americans, 2010* recommends that 20–35% of an adult's daily calories should come from fats, 30–35% of daily calories in children 2 to 3 years of age, and 25–35% of daily calories in children and adolescents 4 to 18 years of age. **Table 13.1** provides information on the fat content of various foods.

Gastronomy Point

Fats and Satiation Fats contribute to our sense of satiation, the feeling of fullness after a meal has ended and the signal that we should stop eating.

plasticity Describes the suppleness or workability of batter or dough.

Green Point

Tropical Oils Tropical oils such as palm oil are gaining in popularity as replacements for trans fats because they have a high smoke point and are good for frying and have similar qualities. Even though they are saturated, they have been found to be less harmful to health than trans fats. Palm oils are a sustainable farming product, and countries such as Malaysia are dependent on them economically. The plantations are examples of renewable agriculture; they rehabilitate farmland, do not degrade forests, do not displace other crops, and require small plots of land to produce a large quantity of crop. Palm oils contain high amounts of vitamin A and can be used to treat deficiencies.

TABLE 13.1
Total Fat, Saturated Fat, Trans Fat, and Cholesterol Content Per Serving*

Product	Common Serving Size	Total Fat (g)	Saturated Fat (g)	%Daily Value for Saturated Fat	Trans Fat (g)	Combined Saturated and Trans Fat (g)	Cholesterol (mg)	%Daily Value for Cholesterol
French fried potatoes± (fast food)	Medium (147 g)	27	7	35%	8	15	0	0%
Butter†	1 tbsp	11	7	35%	0	7	30	10%
Margarine, stick**	1 tbsp	11	2	10%	3	5	0	0%
Margarine, tub**	1 tbsp	7	1	5%	0.5	1.5	0	0%
Mayonnaise†† (soybean oil)	1 tbsp	11	1.5	8%	0	1.5	5	2%
Shortening±	1 tbsp	13	3.5	18%	4	7.5	0	0%
Potato chips±	Small bag (42.5 g)	11	2	10%	3	5	0	0%
Milk, whole±	1 cup	7	4.5	23%	0	4.5	35	12%
Milk, skim**	1 cup	0	0	0%	0	0	5	2%
Doughnut±	1	18	4.5	23%	5	9.5	25	8%
Cookies± (cream filled)	3 (30 g)	6	1	5%	2	3	0	0%
Candy bar±	1 (40 g)	10	4	20%	3	7	< 5	1%
Cake, pound±	1 slice (80 g)	16	3.5	18%	4.5	8	0	0%

* Nutrient values rounded based on FDA's nutrition labeling regulations.
† Butter values from FDA Table of Trans Values, 1/30/95.
** Values derived from 2002 USDA National Nutrient Database for Standard Reference, Release 15.
†† Prerelease values derived from 2003 USDA National Nutrient Database for Standard Reference, Release 16.
± 1995 USDA Composition Data.
Source: Reproduced from U.S. Food and Drug Administration. Revealing trans fats. *FDA Consumer*. Sept–Oct 2003:37(5). Pub No. FDA05-1329C.

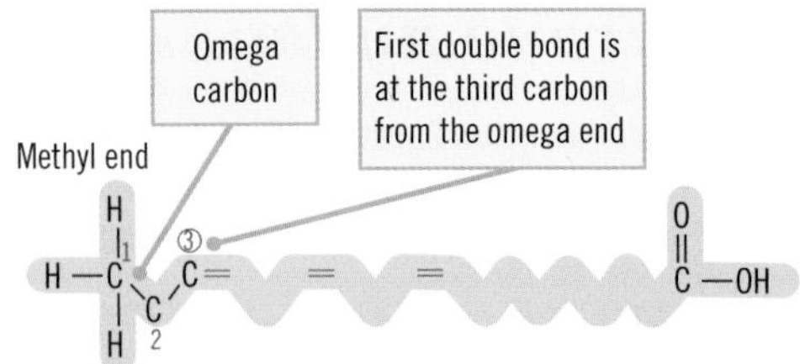

Alpha-linolenic, an omega-3 fatty acid

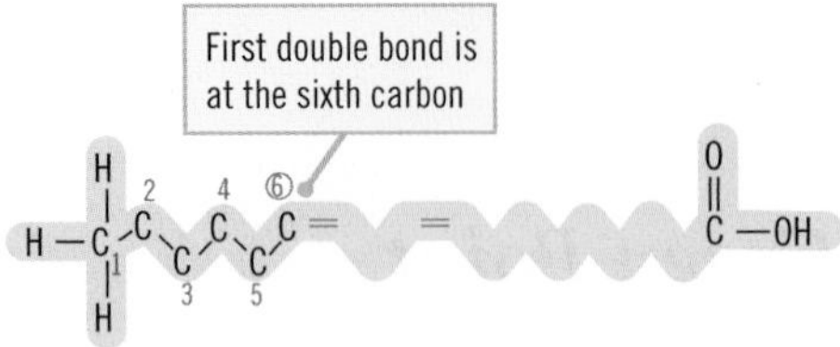

Linoleic, an omega-6 fatty acid

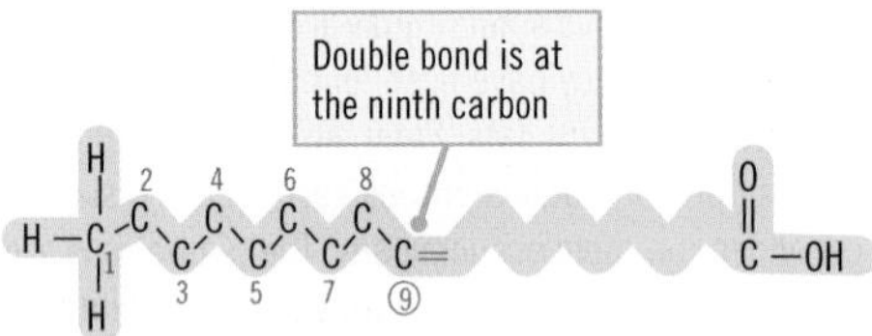

Oleic, an omega-9 fatty acid

FIGURE 13.4 In fatty acids, the carbon atom of the methyl group at the end of the hydrocarbon chain is called the omega carbon. Omega fatty acids are classified by counting from the omega carbon to the position of the first carbon double bond.

TABLE 13.2
Good Sources of Monounsaturated, Omega-3, and Omega-6 Fatty Acids

Monounsaturated Fatty Acids	Omega-3 Fatty Acids	Omega-6 Fatty Acids
Nuts Vegetable oils: • Canola • Olive • High oleic • Safflower • Sunflower	Certain fish: • Salmon • Trout • Herring Vegetable oils: • Soybean • Canola • Walnuts • Flaxseed	Vegetable oils: • Soybean • Corn • Safflower

Source: Courtesy of the U.S. Department of Health and Human Services.

Omega Fatty Acids

Of special note are the omega fatty acids, which play an important role in health (see **Figure 13.4**). Notable omega-3 fatty acids are alpha-linolenic acid (ALA), **eicosapentaenoic acid (EPA)**, and **docosahexaenoic acid (DHA)**. Vegetable oils, including olive and canola oils, and especially flaxseed oil, are high in ALA. Fish, particularly fatty fish such as salmon, are high in EPA and DHA. Foods high in the omega-6 fatty acids (such as linolenic acid) include corn oil, cottonseed oil, sunflower oil, and soybean oil.

Omega-3 and omega-6 fatty acids are considered essential fatty acids because humans do not manufacture these fatty acids in their bodies and they must be consumed in the diet (see **Figure 13.5**). Omega-9, although an important fatty acid, can be made from omega-3 and omega-6 fatty acids, and thus is not considered essential. The ratio of omega-3 to omega-6 fatty acids in the diet has important health implications. By current estimates, the typical Western diet contains too many omega-6 fatty acids in relationship to intake of omega-3 fatty acids. To address this imbalance, food manufacturers are beginning to fortify bread, eggs, and even pet foods with omega-3 fatty acids. Omega-3 fatty acids can also be taken in capsule form as a food supplement. **Table 13.2** lists foods containing healthy fatty acid.

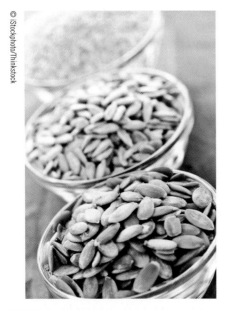

FIGURE 13.5 Sunflower seeds are a good source of omega-6 fatty acids. They also contain omega-3 fatty acids, which can help decrease the risk of coronary artery disease and lower blood pressure.

Impact of Fats on Health

Fats are very energy dense. Only small amounts of intake are required to meet our energy needs. Too much fat in the diet can contribute to weight gain. Overconsumption of fat in general, and certain types of fats in particular, contributes to a host of health issues, including obesity, diabetes, cardiovascular disease, and orthopedic problems.

Dietary fats have an effect on blood lipid and cholesterol profiles. Saturated, monounsaturated, and polyunsaturated fats have been shown to increase high-density lipoprotein (HDL) cholesterol levels (see **Figure 13.6** and **Figure 13.7**). HDL cholesterol is the "good" cholesterol. Saturated fats increase low-density lipoprotein (LDL) cholesterol levels. LDL is considered the "bad" cholesterol. Trans fats have been shown to reduce HDL levels and increase LDL levels. In a healthy diet, less than 7% of daily energy needs come from saturated fats. Cholesterol intake should be limited to no more than 200 mg per day.

Fatty Acids as Functional Foods

Certain fats are beneficial to health. Some may even been considered a functional food or a neutraceutical, depending on their form and whether they are an ingredient in food or taken as a supplement. A **functional food** is any modified food or food ingredient that may provide a health benefit beyond that

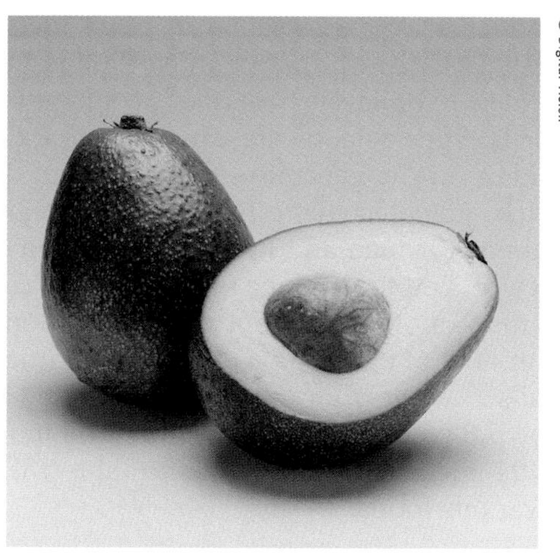

© Digital Vision

FIGURE 13.6 Avocados are rich in monounsaturated fatty acids and other nutrients and have been found to offer protection against coronary heart disease.

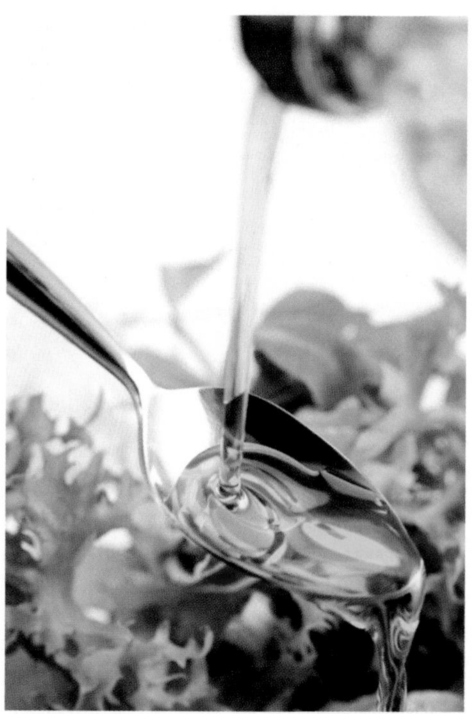

© Laurent Renault/ShutterStock, Inc.

FIGURE 13.7 The main type of fat found in olive oil is monounsaturated fatty acids. Monounsaturated fats may help lower the risk of heart disease by decreasing total cholesterol and low-density lipoprotein cholesterol levels.

of the traditional nutrient it contains, whereas a nutraceutical (the combination of the words *nutrition* and *pharmaceutical*) refers to isolated food dietary components, supplements, ingredients, or the food itself.[15] Food scientists are learning to isolate certain fatty acids and are developing ways to incorporate them into other foods. For example, conjugated linoleic acid (CLA) is currently being promoted as a dietary supplement due to its purported health benefits.[16] Omega-3 fatty acids are being used to fortify foods and animal feed. Docosahexaenoic acid (DHA) and vegetable oils high in n3 fatty acids are being used to help meet the dietary guidelines for fatty acid intake (n3 refers to a double bond found in the third bond from the methyl end of a fatty acid molecule).[17,18]

In a study comparing algae oil to cooked salmon, it was determined that the algal components (DHA plus glycerol) were as good a source of DHA as that found in salmon. These components can be isolated from algae and used as a supplement for vegans and people who do not normally consume fish.[19] DHA also is commonly used in infant formulas as a supplement.

eicosapentaenoic acid (EPA) A type of omega-3 fatty acid that is found in fish oil.

docosahexaenoic (DHA) A type of omega-3 fatty acid that is found in fish oil.

functional food Foods or food components that may offer health benefits beyond basic nutrition.

Health Risks of Trans Fats

Nutrition research has demonstrated a positive linear relationship between dietary intake of trans fatty acids and increased LDL cholesterol and total cholesterol levels.[20–22] However, it was not until the 1990s, 40 years after margarine was introduced into the American diet, that this relationship was established.[21–23] A meta-analysis of studies on the dietary intake of trans fatty acids demonstrated a 23% increase in the incidence of coronary heart disease (CHD) with a 2% increase in energy intake from trans fatty acids.[22] Gram-for-gram replacement of saturated fat with trans fat in the diet was associated with an approximately 15 times greater risk of CHD.[24] Unlike saturated fatty acids, which raise serum levels of HDL cholesterol, trans fatty acids decrease HDL cholesterol levels but increase the ratio of total cholesterol to HDL, thus increasing the risk of CHD and cardiovascular disease (CVD).[25] Other metabolic effects of trans fatty acids are an increase in lipoprotein a, which increases the risk for CVD and cerebrovascular disease,[26] and elevated levels of markers for inflammation, including C-reactive protein and tumor necrosis factor, which also are risk factors for CVD.[27–29]

In 1995, the USDA published a table entitled "Fatty Acid Content of Selected Foods Containing Trans Fatty Acids," using fatty acid values from

Gastronomy Point

Nuts as Snacks The high amount of fiber, protein, and healthy fats make nuts a perfect, satisfying snack. Pair a handful of nuts with a piece of fruit or make a portable trail mix using dried fruit, popcorn, cereals, and/or chocolate chips.

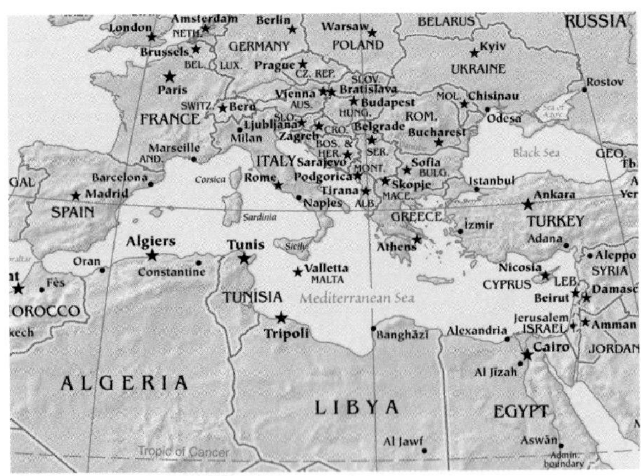

FIGURE 13.8 The traditional diet of people who live in the Mediterranean region is based on legumes, unrefined cereals, fruits, vegetables, and olive oil. It also features moderate consumption of dairy products (mostly as cheese and yogurt), moderate to high consumption of fish, low consumption of meat and meat products, and moderate wine consumption.

Source: Courtesy of the U.S. Central Intelligence Agency/University of Texas Libraries.

selected foods that were sampled and chemically analyzed between 1989 and 1993.[30–32] The primary source of trans fatty acids from this survey was baked goods, such as cakes, cookies, crackers, pies, and breads. Based on this data, two research groups estimated daily trans fatty acid intake in the general population from dietary intake surveys. Harnack and colleagues estimated daily mean trans fat intakes to be 8.4 grams for men and 5.4 grams for women.[30] Allison and colleagues calculated the average trans fatty acid content of foods to be 2.6% of total calories and approximately 5.3 grams of trans fats per day, with 80% of trans fats coming from partially hydrogenated vegetable oils.[31] Meanwhile, the FDA estimated average trans fat intakes to be 5.8 grams per day based on food intake data collected between 1994 and 1996.[19,33,34] Refer to Table 13.1 for the trans fat content of various foods.

Lessons from the Mediterranean Diet

Some oils are healthier than others. For example, results of the Lyon Heart Study determined that people who follow the Mediterranean Diet reap the benefits of a heart healthy regimen.[12] They have a lower incidence of heart disease, largely due to the kinds of fats they consume.[13] The Mediterranean region includes the 16 countries that border the Mediterranean Sea (see **Figure 13.8**). Although languages and culture vary widely in this region, what the people have in common is a diet high in fruits, vegetables, grains, nuts, and fish, with more than half of the fat calories coming from olive oil, which is high in monounsaturated fat. Compared to the typical American diet, a higher percentage of the calories in the Mediterranean diet come from fats; however, the fat is mostly unsaturated. Benefits of unsaturated fatty acids, particularly those found in nuts, are explored further in **Special Topic 13.1**.

Special Topic 13.1

Nuts and Nut Allergies

Allison Stevens, MS, RD, LD

Nuts as a Source of Healthy Fats

Dietary fatty acids and cholesterol are major determinants of two major causes of morbidity and mortality in Americans: cardiovascular disease (CVD) and type 2 diabetes.[1] However, as stated in the *Dietary Guidelines for American, 2010*, unsaturated fats—monounsaturated fatty acids and polyunsaturated fatty acids—have significant metabolic benefits and are actually health promoting.

Several lines of evidence indicate that the type of fat is more important in decreasing metabolic and CVD risk than the total amount of fat in the diet. For example, metabolic studies have established that it is the type of fat, rather than total fat intake, that affects common intermediate risk factors, such as cholesterol levels.[2] Additionally, results from controlled clinical trials and epidemiological studies have shown that replacing saturated fatty acids in the diet with unsaturated fats is more effective in decreasing CVD risk than is reducing total fat intake overall.[3]

Tree nuts, including almonds, Brazils, cashews, hazelnuts, macadamias, pecans, pine nuts, pistachios, and walnuts, are nutrient-dense foods that are particularly high in monounsaturated and polyunsaturated fatty acids (see **Figure A** and **Table A**). (Note that tree nuts are distinct from peanuts, which are considered legumes.) Tree nuts are energy dense, with 45–75% of their calories coming from fats.[4] The fats in nuts are primarily composed of monounsaturated and polyunsaturated fatty acids. Monounsaturated and polyunsaturated fatty acids comprise greater than 75% of the total lipids in nuts.[5] Walnuts have a distinctive fatty acid profile and contain more linoleic acid and alpha-linolenic acid than other tree nuts.[6] The following table provides the energy content and lipid composition for eight common tree nuts and peanuts (a legume).

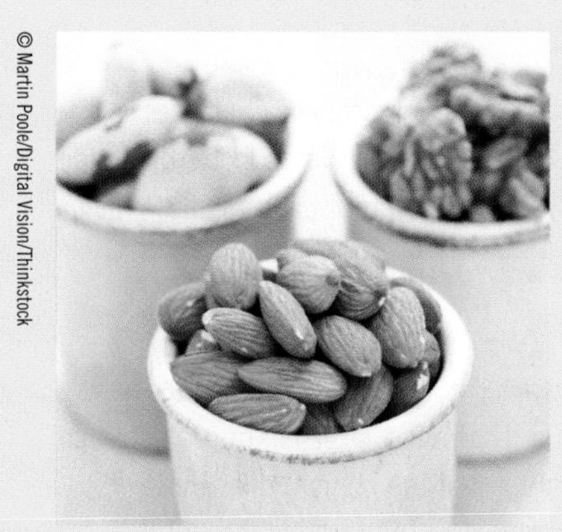

FIGURE A Nuts are a great source of heart-healthy monounsaturated and polyunsaturated fats. Nuts are a great source of heart-healthy monounsaturated and polyunsaturated fats, which may contribute to their cardioprotective benefits.

Nuts as a Source of Phytonutrients

Tree nuts are a source of valuable micronutrients, including folic acid, niacin, and vitamins B_6 and E, and are an important source of the minerals calcium, magnesium, copper, zinc, and phosphorus.[7] Tree nuts also contain phytochemicals, such as phytosterols and flavonoids, which have been associated with a variety of bioactivities, including antioxidant, hypocholesterolemic, and anti-inflammatory actions. These bioactivities may affect the initiation and progression of several processes that can lead to chronic disease such as CVD.[8] Phytosterols, which are sterols found in plants, are poorly absorbed by humans and reduce the intestinal absorption of cholesterol. They have been used as a cholesterol-lowering food ingredient.[9] Flavonoids are polyphenolic compounds present in plant foods. They include flavonols, flavones, catechins, flavanones, anthocyanidins, and isoflavonoids. They may have beneficial health effects because of their antioxidant properties and their inhibitory role in various stages of tumor development in animal studies.[10]

The protein content of most nuts makes up about 10–25% of the total calories, making them a good source of plant protein.[11] However, the biological value of nut protein is not as high as that of animal protein because nuts are missing some essential amino acids.[7] Additionally, tree nuts are a good source of dietary fiber, providing 5–10% of daily fiber requirements.[12] After cereals, nuts are the plant food highest in fiber, followed by legumes, whole grain bread, fruits, and vegetables.[13,14]

Nuts and Disease Prevention

The USDA has approved a qualified health claim for tree nuts, stating, "Scientific evidence suggests but does not prove that eating 1.5 ounces per day of most nuts, as part of a diet low in saturated fat and cholesterol, may reduce the risk of heart disease." The protective effect of nuts on CVD is due to their lipid profile and their vitamin and mineral content. Their high fiber content and wide range of phytonutrients also may play a role.

Additionally, the *Dietary Guidelines for Americans, 2010* concluded that, "consumption of nuts collectively and walnuts, almonds, and pistachio nuts individually, in the context of a healthy diet and when calorie intake is constant, has a favorable impact on CVD risk factors, particularly serum lipid levels." Emerging research also suggests that nut consumption may have a significant impact on diabetes.

TABLE A
Nutrient Composition of Nuts per 1.5 Ounces (43 g)

Type	Energy (kcal)	Total Fat (g)	Saturated Fatty Acids (g)	Monounsaturated Fatty Acids (g)	Polyunsaturated Fatty Acids (g)	Protein (g)
Almonds	254	22.5	1.7	14.3	5.4	9.4
Brazil nuts	279	28.2	6.4	10.4	8.8	6.1
Cashews	244	19.7	3.9	11.6	3.3	6.5
Hazelnuts	275	26.5	1.9	19.	8 3	6.4
Macadamias	305	32.4	5.1	25.2	0.6	3.3
Peanuts	249	21.1	2.9	10.5	6.7	10.1
Pecans	302	31.6	2.7	18.7	8.7	4.0
Pistachios	243	19.6	2.4	10.3	5.9	9.1
Walnuts, English	278	27.7	2.6	3.8	20.1	6.5

Source: Reproduced from the USDA Center for Nutrition Policy and Promotion, Report of the Dietary Guidelines Advisory Committee on the *Dietary Guidelines for Americans, 2010.* Data from USDA, Agricultural Research Service, USDA Nutrient Data Laboratory. 2009. USDA National Nutrient Database for Standard Reference, Release 22. Available at: http://www.ars.usda.gov/ba/bhnrc/ndl.

The Nurse's Health Study indicated that frequent nut consumption (five or more times per week) was associated with a 27% reduction in relative risk of developing diabetes, compared to those who rarely or never ate nuts.[15]

Although nuts are high in fat, epidemiological and clinical studies have shown that nut consumption is not associated with higher body weight. In fact, epidemiological data have been consistent in indicating that those who eat nuts have a lower body mass index (BMI) than those who do not.[16] Additional research indicates that appetite suppression may result from the satiating effects of the high fiber, protein, and energy content of nuts.[12]

Nut Allergies

A food allergy is an abnormal response to a food that is triggered by the body's immune system. In an allergic reaction to tree nuts, the body produces a specific type of antibody called immunoglobulin E (IgE). The majority of nut allergens are seed storage proteins.[11] The presence of specific IgE antibodies to several nuts is a common clinical finding, but the clinical relevance of this cross-reactivity is usually limited. However, allergic reactions to nuts can be severe and even life threatening; fatal reactions following their ingestion have been documented. Food allergy is diagnosed by identifying an underlying immunological mechanism by allergy testing and establishing a causal relationship between food ingestion and symptoms (by giving oral challenges).[17]

More than 160 foods can cause allergic reactions in people with food allergies. The FDA has identified the eight most common allergenic foods: milk, eggs, fish, crustacean shellfish, tree nuts, peanuts, wheat, and soybeans. These eight foods, and any ingredient that contains protein derived from one or more of them, are designated "major food allergens" by the Food Allergen Labeling and Consumer Protection Act.[18] People with nut allergies must read all labels carefully to determine the presence of nuts, nut-derived ingredients, and whether the food was processed in a facility that also processes nuts.

References

1 U.S. Department of Agriculture, Center for Nutrition Policy and Promotion. Report of the Dietary Guidelines Advisory Committee on the *Dietary Guidelines for Americans, 2010.* Available at: http://www.cnpp.usda.gov/Publications/DietaryGuidelines/2010/DGAC/Report/D-3-FattyAcidsCholesterol.pdf. Accessed September 10, 2011.

2 Hu FB, van Dam RM, Liu S. Diet and risk of type II diabetes: The role of types of fat and carbohydrate. *Diabetologia.* 2001;44(7):805–817.

3 Smit LA, Mozaffarian D, Willett W. Review of fat and fatty acid requirements and criteria for developing dietary guidelines. *Ann Nutr Metab.* 2009;55(1–3):44–55.

4 Alasalvar C, Shahidi F. *Tree Nuts: Composition, Phytochemicals, and Health Effects.* Boca Raton, FL: CRC Press; 2009.

5 Venkatachalam M, Sathe SK. Chemical composition of selected edible nut seeds. *J Agric Food Chem.* 2006;54:4705–4714.

6 Ros E, Mataix J. Fatty acid composition of nuts: Implications for cardiovascular health. *Br J Nutr.* 2006;96(Suppl. 2):29S–35S.

7 Brufau G, Boatella J, Rafecas M. Nuts: Source of energy and macronutrients. *Br J Nutr.* 2006;96(Suppl. 2):24S–28S.

8 King JC, Blumberg J, Ingwersen L, et al. Tree nuts and peanuts as components of a healthy diet. *J Nutr.* 2008;138(9):1736S–1740S.

9 Insel P, Ross D, McMahon K, Bernstein M. *Nutrition.* 4th ed. Burlington, MA: Jones & Bartlett Learning; 2011.

10 Hollman PCH, Katan MB. Health effects and bioavailability of dietary flavonols. *Free Rad Res.* 1999;31(Suppl. Dec):S75–S80.

11 Sathe SK, Kshirsagar HH, Roux KH. Advances in seed protein research: A perspective on seed allergens. *J Food Sci.* 2005;70(6):93–120.

12 Coates AM, Howe PR. Edible nuts and metabolic health. *Curr Opin Lipidol.* 2007;18(1):25–30.

13 Salas-Salvadó J, Bulló M, Pérez-Heras A, Ros E. Dietary fibre, nuts and cardiovascular diseases. *Br J Nutr.* 2006;96(Suppl. 2):45S–51S.

14 Pimentel D, Pimentel M. Sustainability of meat-based and plant-based diets and the environment. *Am J Clin Nutr.* 2003;78(3):661S–662S.

15 Hu FB, Stampfer MJ, Manson JE, et al. Frequent nut consumption and risk of coronary heart disease in women: Prospective cohort study. *BMJ.* 1998;317(7169):1341–1345.

16 Mattes RD, Kris-Etherton PM, Foster GD. Impact of peanuts and tree nuts on body weight and healthy weight loss in adults. *J Nutr.* 2008;138:1741S–1745S.

17 Crespo JF, James JM, Fernandez-Rodriguez C, Rodriguez J. Food allergy: Nuts and tree nuts. *Br J Nutr.* 2006;96(Suppl. 2):S95–S102.

18 U.S. Food and Drug Administration. Food Allergies: What You Need to Know. June 2010. Available at: http://www.fda.gov/food/resourcesforyou/Consumers/ucm079311.htm. Accessed September 10, 2011.

Food Preparation and Storage Principles

The uses of fats in cooking are many—they give foods the right combination of texture, aroma, flavor, and mouthfeel. The chef picks oils or solid fats according to their uses in baking, frying, and sautéing and as salad dressings and drizzles.

Gastronomy Point

Nuts as Toppings Use nuts to add crunch to salads or vegetable dishes, or blend nuts with breadcrumbs for a crunchy topping for meats or seafood.

The Most Popular Plant Oils for Cooking

The most popular and healthful oils to cook with are canola oil and olive oil because of their high unsaturated fat content, subtle flavors, and multiple uses in cooking.

Canola Oil

Canola oil is heat stable when cooking and frying. It is usually used as part of a blend in frying oils. Its bland taste makes it a good base for dressings. It can be topped off with a stronger tasting oil to gain the desired flavor or finished with such an oil or essence in drizzles. Olive oil is one such finishing oil, but there are many more, including walnut, shallot, and rosemary oils. Some of the more popular finishing plant oils are almond oil, rice oil, peanut oil, and clove oil. Canola oil is also a good base for mayonnaises, spreads, and margarines (see **Figure 13.9**).

Olive Oil

Olive oil and extra virgin oil, which comes from the first **pressing** of the olive and is known for its intense flavor, are used in dressings and drizzles (see **Figure 13.10**). Olive oils are also used in cooking when a slight olive flavor is desired. Olive oils come in different colors, ranging from green to yellow. The darker green colors are due to chlorophyll. The color of "straw-colored" olive oil is due to the oil's carotenoid content.[25,26]

pressing The process of breaking the cell wall by grinding, flaking, rolling, or pressing under high pressure to liberate oil.

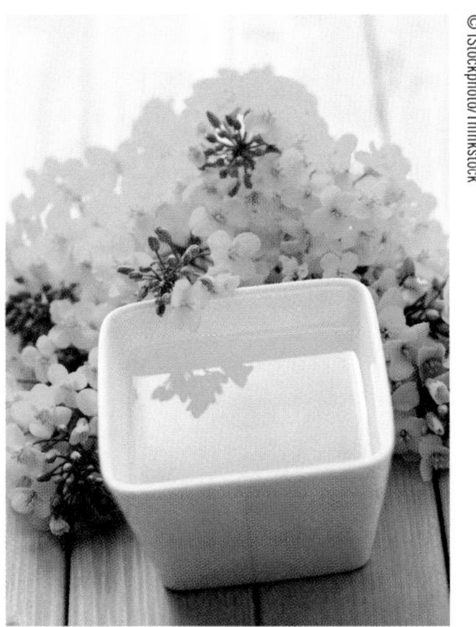

FIGURE 13.9 Canola is made by heating and then pressing the seeds of either rapeseed or field mustard plants. The name *canola* was derived from "Canadian oil, low acid" in 1978 because the oil was first developed in Canada and has low amounts of erucic acid. Canola oil is low in saturated fat and contains both omega-6 and omega-3 fatty acids.

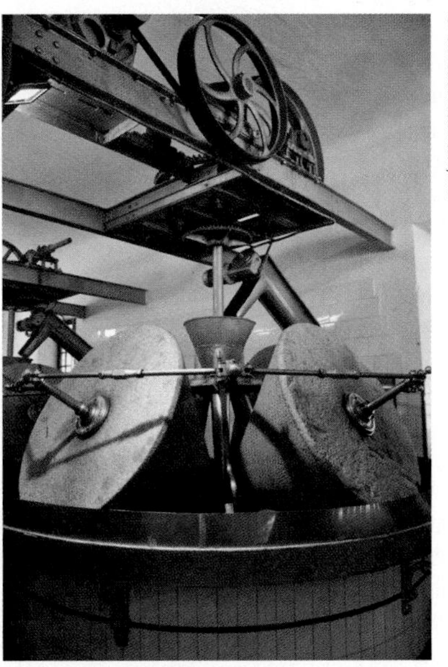

FIGURE 13.10 Traditional methods of making olive oil use a millstone to grind fresh olives into a paste. The paste is then placed in the olive press. An olive press works by applying pressure to the olive paste to separate the liquid oil and water from the solid plant material. The oil and water then are separated by standard decantation.

Other Plant Oils

Many other plant-derived oils are used for specific cooking purposes (see **Figure 13.11**):

- Because of its full flavor and fragrance, hazelnut oil is best used as a finishing oil and in vinaigrettes.
- Walnut oil has a strong, full flavor and is also used in vinaigrettes.

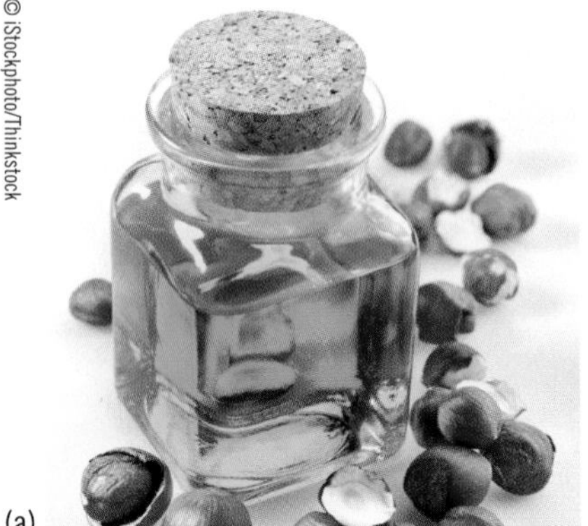

(a)

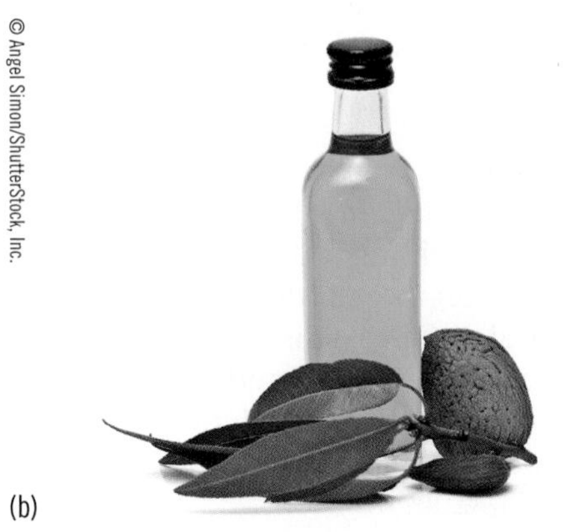

(b)

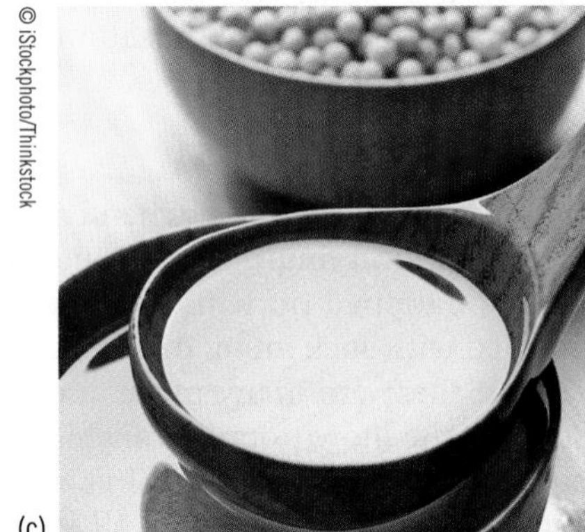

(c)

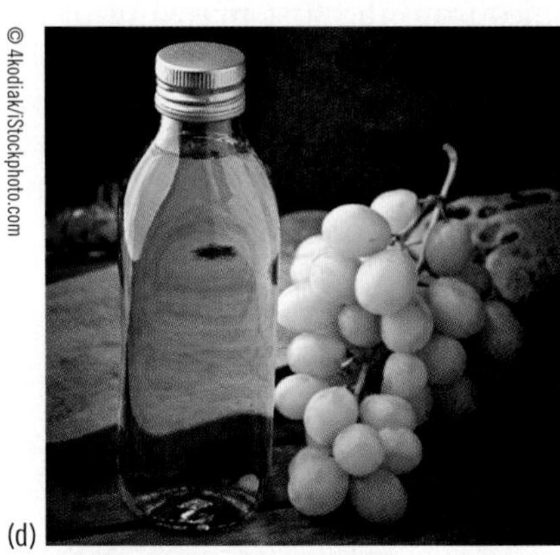

(d)

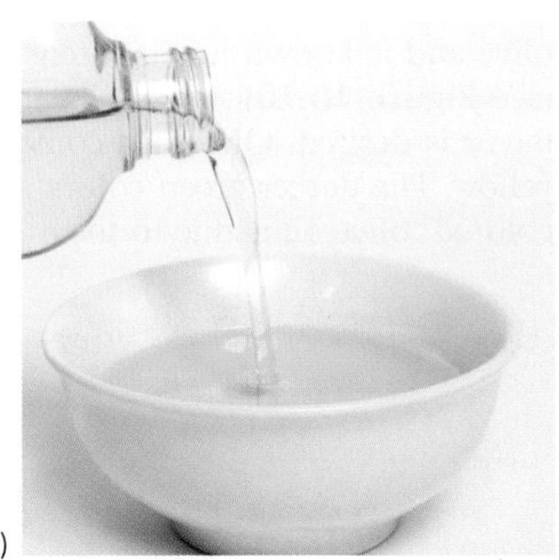

(e)

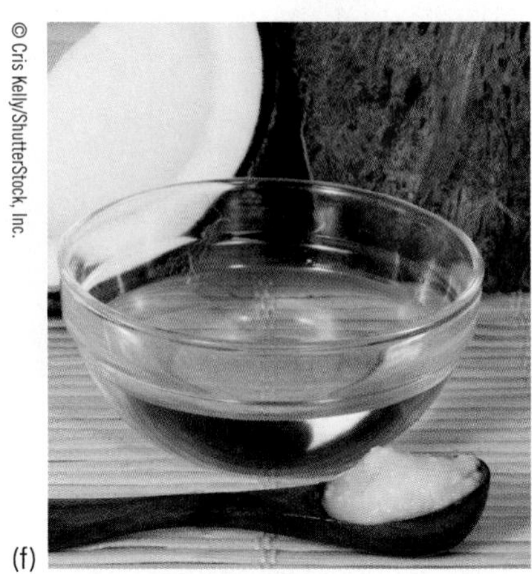

(f)

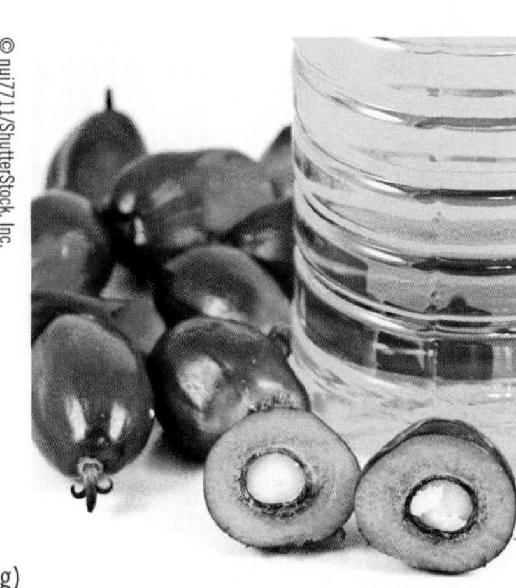

(g)

FIGURE 13.11 A variety of different plant-based oils are used in cooking. The oils have different physical and chemical properties, which are reflected in their uses in cooking. Some oils are used primarily as salad oils and garnishes; others are used for frying and sautéing. (a) Hazelnut oil is produced from pressed hazelnuts. It has a strong flavor and is used as a cooking oil. It has a similar composition to extra virgin olive oil, with high amounts of omega-9 and omega-6 fatty acids. (b) Walnut oil is produced from pressed walnuts. It is about 50% linoleic acid, an essential omega-6 fatty acid. It is also a good source of omega-3 fatty acids. Because of its high price, it is generally used less than other cooking oils. (c) Soybean oil is one of the most widely consumed cooking oils. It is extracted from the seeds of the soybean. The major unsaturated fatty acids in soybean oil are alpha-linolenic acid (7–10%), linoleic acid (51%), and oleic acid (23%). Soybean oil also contains saturated fatty acids: stearic acid (4%) and palmitic acid (10%). (d) Grapeseed oil is made from pressed grapes. It is a good source of linoleic acid and oleic acid. It has a high smoke point, which makes it a good oil for frying and sautéing. (e) Cottonseed oil is made from pressed cotton seeds. Its fatty acid profile generally consists of 70% unsaturated fatty acids, 26% saturated fatty acids and 4% glycerol. Some nutritionists caution against using cottonseed oil in cooking because of its high saturated fat content. (f) Coconut oil is extracted from the kernel or meat of mature coconuts. It is very heat-stable, which makes it well suited to cooking at high temperatures. However, many organizations and groups recommend against the consumption of significant amounts of hydrogenated coconut oil because of its high levels of saturated fats. (g) Palm oil is derived from the fruit of the oil palm. Many processed foods contain palm oil. It is high in saturated fatty acids.

- The light "grapey" flavor of grapeseed oil makes it good for vinaigrettes. It also is a good oil for sautéing because it has a relatively high smoke point.
- Soybean oil is a good frying oil with a high smoke point. It is low in saturated fat and high in the monounsaturated and polyunsaturated fatty acids. A new form of soybean seed is being developed, using traditional plant breeding methods, that has high levels of oleic acid and is being used to replace trans fats and saturated fats. Use of soybean oil is one of the most efficient ways to replace trans fats in foods. It also has a long shelf life and is heat stable due to its high monounsaturated fatty acid content. Furthermore, it is cost-effective and has health benefits. This is a boon for vegetable-based shortenings and baking.[28]
- Cottonseed oil is useful in deep fat frying. It is a more healthful option than hydrogenated soybean oil because it is not hydrogenated. Cottonseed oil has high concentrations of linoleic acid. When blended with canola oil, it also works well for deep fat frying. It is a good replacement for trans fats, and its use significantly decreases the percentage of saturated fatty acids in foods.[27]
- Sunflower oil is rich in tocopherol (vitamin E) and protects against oxidation and rancidity. This trait has been perpetuated in genetically engineered plant lines. Sunflower oil also is being used in new zero-trans fat acid products and trans fat-free Crisco shortenings.
- Tropical oils—palm, palm kernel, and coconut—all have saturated fatty acids and high melting points. These oils are used to replace partially hydrogenated solid fats, especially in baking and confectionary goods.[35–41]

Deep-Fat Frying

Deep-fat frying can be defined as the process of cooking foods by immersing them in an edible oil at a temperature above the boiling point of water.[42–45] It also is referred to as *fat-immersion frying*. The act of immersing a food in an edible oil at high temperatures changes the structure of the food product. On contact, the heat and oil are simultaneously transferred to the food, with the food absorbing the oil. The result is a fried product, with desired changes to the original food's flavor, color, texture, and overall palatability.[46,47] The amount of oil uptake is directly proportional to the amount of moisture lost, thus deep-fat frying is considered a dehydration process (see **Figure 13.12**).[44]

Interestingly, most of the oil uptake or absorption takes place in the cooling off period.[46,47] In efforts to decrease oil absorption by fried foods due to health concerns, pre- and postfrying techniques have been optimized to lower the final oil uptake while maintaining the desired culinary results.[44,47] Prefrying treatments mainly affect the microstructure of the food's crust, with the goal of reducing surface permeability. Postfrying treatments seek to remove surface oil before the postcooling absorption begins.[44]

The following prefrying techniques can be used to decrease oil uptake:[47]

- Blanching
- Air drying
- Steam baking

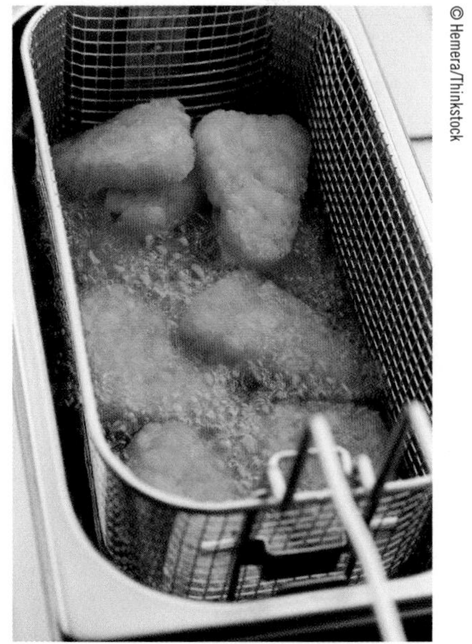

FIGURE 13.12 Deep-fat frying is a popular cooking method. Most deep fryers have a basket that is lowered into a well containing heated oil. The oil and the heat are transferred to the food item, resulting in a slightly crispy cooked food item.

- Osmotic dehydration
- Surface treatments (application of coatings)

Posttreatment techniques used to decrease oil uptake include the following:[47]

- Removing the food item from the fryer while temperatures are still increasing
- Vigorously shaking the basket of fried food items after its removal from the oil
- Postfry drying by means of convection air drying techniques or super heating

Other cooking techniques that can decrease the amount of oil absorption are:[47]

- Cooking for a shorter time and at higher temperatures
- Not putting cold items in hot oil, which increases frying time
- Creating thicker food products because the surface area-to-volume ratio affects total oil absorption (i.e., thinner food items, such as potato chips, absorb more oil)

Most of the oils used in deep frying are high in saturated and trans fats. The American Heart Association recommends limiting trans fat to less than 1% of daily intake, or 2 grams, based on a 2,000 kcal diet.[10,48] The most recent recommendations from the *Dietary Guidelines for Americans, 2010*, recommend avoiding trans fatty acids from industrial sources and limiting those from natural sources to less than 0.5% of calories.[49] Reducing the consumption of deep-fried foods can help people meet this goal.[50–57]

Baking with Fats

Solid fats are most commonly used as spreads and shortenings. In baked goods, fats provide crispness, flakiness, and softness. In addition, fats and oils in baked goods serve multiple functions that are integral to the product, such as tenderizing, ensuring sufficient shelf life, providing flavoring, and adding to the product structure.[3] Points to consider when selecting a fat include the fat's melting point and creaming ability.

The Role of Shortening

Shortenings used in baking may include regular hydrogenated oils, hard fats, emulsified shortenings, fluid shortenings, and traditional butter and margarines.[9] Shortening plays the following roles in baking:

- Shortening incorporates and traps air, which increases the volume of baked goods.[35–36]
- In breads and other yeast-raised products, shortening contributes to the softness of the product and the crumb structure.[37]
- In cakes and cookies, shortening prevents the cohesion of gluten strands present in flour during the mixing process.[37]
- In pastries, shortening adds to the development of a flakey crust by separating the thin layers of dough.[37]

Crystalline Structure

The structure, composition, and polymorphic forms of fat crystals are the most important criteria for the functional properties of shortening and other forms of fats.[36] Fats are a network of crystals with oil trapped inside.[38] This network of fat crystals directly affects the texture of candy, with smaller crystals leading to firmer products (chocolate) and larger crystals producing a crunchy mouth feel.[39–41]

Fats have large alpha crystals, which are formed rapidly if fats are chilled, and beta crystals, which are small. Beta crystals are good for shortening because they can be creamed easily and give a smooth texture. Beta crystals also have a high melting point.

Challenges in Replacing Trans Fats

Some processed baked goods have trans fats. Due to the negative health effects of trans fats, food technologists have been replacing trans fats with other fats. However, baked goods made with trans fat substitutes often differ from those made with trans fats:[3]

- Baked goods without trans fats may suffer in volume and appearance and have the wrong texture.
- The batter of baked goods made without trans fats may not be as soluble and have an altered texture.
- The specific gravity of batter and cream fillings made without trans fats may affect the distribution of the dough.
- Products that do not have trans fats have a shorter shelf life.

The benefits of trans fats in baking have been difficult to duplicate with other fats and oils. The challenge continues to replace trans fat in food products, while maintaining the qualities to which consumers have grown accustomed.

Avoiding Rancidity

Rancidity is the most common cause of "off flavor" in oil.[58] **Hydrolytic rancidity**, the first type of spoilage in fats, is associated with the presence of water.[59] The triglycerides in fats react with water, freeing their fatty acids from glycerol and breaking down into volatile secondary products with an off flavor.[58] **Oxidative rancidity**, the second type of spoilage in oil, is also referred to as auto-oxidation. This occurs when the lipid is catalyzed in the presence of heat or light.

Vegetable oils have higher concentrations of polyunsaturated fatty acids, specifically linoleic acids, and are more susceptible to oxidation.[60] Oxidative rancidity in oils occurs when heat, metals, or other catalysts cause unsaturated oil molecules to convert to free radicals. These free radicals are easily oxidized, yielding hyperperoxide and organic compounds such as aldehydes, ketones, and organic compounds, which cause the undesirable odors and taste.[61]

Lipids can undergo oxidation during exposure to high temperature, during handling, and/or during storage. To prevent oxidation, fats and oils should be kept in a cool, dry place. Oils should be stored in tightly sealed dark bottles or containers to avoid reactions with light, heat, and air. The use of antioxidants in oils can help to protect against rancidity. Storing oils away from metals and avoiding cooking utensils containing copper or iron can also help prevent oxidation reactions.[59]

rancidity Condition produced by oxidation of unsaturated fats present in foods and other products. An unpleasant odor or flavor is generated when the fatty substance is exposed to air.

hydrolytic rancidity Spoilage in fats associated with the presence of water. The triglycerides react with water, freeing their fatty acids from glycerol and breaking down into volatile secondary products with an off flavor.

oxidative rancidity Spoilage in oil that also is referred to as auto-oxidation. Occurs when the lipids are catalyzed in the presence of heat or light.

Gastronomy Point

Storage of Oils Oils should be stored in a cool place (65°F [18°C]) to maintain their integrity and used within 1½ to 3 months. As a general rule, purchase oil as needed and according to the menu. In a commercial kitchen, little inventory remains on the shelves for more than a week.

Improving Fat Intake

As you have learned, not all fats are bad. Many have important health-promotion functions. The key is to eat good fats (monounsaturated and polyunsaturated fatty acids) in moderation and to try and skip the less desirable fats (saturated and trans fats). Savvy menu planning, purchasing, and meal preparation can help to limit the consumption of saturated fats and trans fats while increasing consumption of monounsaturated and polyunsaturated fatty acids.

Menu Planning

The following menu planning tips* can be used to decrease the consumption of saturated and trans fats:

- Increase servings of legumes, fruits, vegetables, and whole grains.
- Serve low-fat (1%) or nonfat milk.
- Limit servings of luncheon meats, hot dogs, and sausage.
- Limit servings of battered or breaded foods that are fried in fat during processing.
- Limit or control the amount of full-fat cheese served. Serve low-fat cheese instead.
- Use broth-based soups rather than cream-based or prepared bases.
- Eliminate or limit the number of desserts served or modify recipe ingredients to lower the fat content.
- Eliminate or limit the service of high-fat snack items, such as cookies, cake, doughnuts, brownies, and chips.
- Offer fresh fruit as an alternative to dessert at each meal.
- Offer mustard, ketchup, and low-fat mayonnaise as alternatives to high-fat spreads.

Gastronomy Point

Storing Butter To store butter, wrap it in an airtight cover. Refrigerate regular butter for up to 1 month and unsalted butter for up to 2 weeks. Both can be frozen for up to 6 months.

Grocery Shopping

Making simple changes when grocery shopping* is an easy way to decrease consumption of saturated and trans fats. One easy way to decrease dietary fat is to make smart selections when purchasing meat:

- Purchase ground chicken or turkey (without skin) to mix with or substitute for lean ground beef.
- Purchase leaner meats, such as ground beef with no more than 15% fat.
- Purchase reduced-fat processed meats, such as frankfurters and deli meats.
- Substitute lean ham for bacon or sausage.

Baked goods are often a source of "hidden" fats. Manufacturers often add fats to baked goods to increase their shelf life and mouthfeel. The following tips can help minimize the amount of hidden fats that make it into your cupboard:

- Purchase lower-fat breads, such as bagels, pita bread, corn tortillas, and English muffins. Avoid higher-fat products, such as croissants, doughnuts, Danish pastries, and sweet rolls. Choose whole-grain breads most often.
- Read the labels. Avoid products with animal fat (lard) or saturated vegetable oils, such as coconut oil, palm oil, or palm kernel oil, and hydrogenated shortening or stick-type margarine.
- For cakes, use angel food cakes or sponge cakes that contain little fat. Regular cake recipes are difficult to modify for reduced fat.
- If commercial baking mixes are used, such as those for muffins and pancakes, purchase only those to which fat must be added so the amount of fat can be controlled. Compare brands because a comparable product may be lower in saturated fat.

---

* This section is reproduced from the Bureau of Health/Nutrition, Family Services and Adult Education, Connecticut State Department of Education. Nutrition Policies and Guidance for the Child and Adult Care Food Program (CACFP)—Planning Healthy Meals, September 2011. Available at: http://www.sde.ct.gov/sde/LIB/sde/pdf/deps/nutrition/CACFP/Healthy_Meals.pdf.

When shopping the dairy aisle, purchase low-fat cheeses and products made with these cheeses. For example, purchase part-skim mozzarella cheese instead of regular mozzarella. Instead of ice cream, purchase low-fat alternatives such as ice milk, frozen yogurt, sherbet, and frozen juice pops.

Purchase low-fat mayonnaise and salad dressings and avoid commercial barbecue sauces and canned sauces. Many of these products are loaded with added fats to improve their shelf life and mouthfeel.

As a general rule, limit use of convenience and prepared items that are higher in fat. Read food labels to compare and evaluate nutrition information for processed food items such as pizza and hot dogs. A different brand of the product may contain less fat. When purchasing from vendors, write specifications for the fat content of products (i.e., specify the percentage of fat contained in meat items and make sure products received are the same as those specified).

Meal Preparation

The way in which a food is prepared* has a huge impact on the final fat content of the finished food item. For example, making just a few changes when cooking meat and poultry can minimize the fat content in the final product:

- Start with the leanest cuts of meat and then trim away any fat.
- When cooking poultry, remove all the fat and skin.
- Meat, poultry, and fish can be roasted on a rack so the fat will drain off.
- Fat can also be drained from cooked ground meats by draining the meat in a colander or using a turkey baster to remove fat that has cooked out of product.
- Meats should be browned by broiling or cooked in a nonstick pan with little or no oil.
- Soups, stews, sauces, broths, and boiled meat should be made ahead of time and then refrigerated and the congealed fat removed prior to serving.
- Use lean ham or a small amount of ham base (omit salt) for seasonings.
- Instead of basting with drippings, keep meat moist with fruit juices or an acceptable oil-based marinade (i.e., one low in monounsaturated or polyunsaturated fats).

Gravies should be made after the fat has hardened and been removed from the liquid. To thicken gravies and sauces without adding fat, mix cornstarch with a small amount of cold water to make a slurry. Slowly stir this mixture into the liquid to be thickened and bring it back to a boil. Cornstarch can be used to replace a roux (a butter-flour mixture used for thickening). Use an amount of cornstarch equal to one-half the amount of flour indicated.

When cooking with fats, remember that a little goes a long way and that a number of nonfat options are available:

- Use only enough salad dressing to lightly coat salad.
- Use nonstick cooking spray in place of oil or shortening for pan-frying and sautéing.

---

* This section is reproduced from the Bureau of Health/Nutrition, Family Services and Adult Education, Connecticut State Department of Education. Nutrition Policies and Guidance for the Child and Adult Care Food Program (CACFP)—Planning Healthy Meals, September 2011. Available at: http://www.sde.ct.gov/sde/LIB/sde/pdf/deps/nutrition/CACFP/Healthy_Meals.pdf.

- For baked goods or other foods, use pan liners and nonstick cooking spray instead of greasing sheet pans.
- Substitute low-fat cheese, such as ricotta, farmer, cottage, or mozzarella, for part of the cheese in recipes.
- Do not add butter, margarine, or oil to cooked vegetables.

Food Technology

Plant Breeding and Genetic Engineering

Vegetable seed oils have been developed by traditional plant breeding, mutations, and gene modification for decades to improve yield as well as functional and nutritional qualities.[32] *Trait-enhanced oilseeds* is the term used to describe oilseeds that have been genetically modified to change their fatty acid composition. The focus of trait-enhanced oilseeds has been to develop new breeds that (1) meet requirements for health, (2) have the functional qualities needed for frying and/or baking, and (3) have a neutral impact on the flavor of food. An example of plant breeding to change fatty acid composition was the elimination of the undesirable erucic acid from rapeseed, which resulted in the development of canola oil.[62,63]

Innovation Point

Technologies to Minimize Trans Fats

New technologies are being developed to decrease or eliminate trans fats through the production of blends. Blends are mixtures of oils with reduced percentages of trans fatty acids and saturated fatty acids. In some instances, hydrogenated oils are used, but in smaller percentages, along with a tropical oil or nonhydrogenated oil.

Improving Stability and Frying Ability

Traditional canola, soybean, and sunflower oilseeds are low in saturated fat and high in linoleic and linolenic acids, which are both polyunsaturated fatty acids. They are suitable for salad dressings, but unsuitable for deep fat frying and for most baked products. Polyunsaturated fatty acids are susceptible to rancidity and lack the plasticity required for baking. However, with the help of modern technology, varieties of these oilseeds have been developed that are low in polyunsaturated fatty acids so heir stability in food processing is improved. These oilseeds are also low in saturated fatty acids and medium to high in monounsaturated fatty acids.[64–72] Fats high in the monounsaturated fatty acid oleic acid are desirable because of its positive effect on serum lipids and because monounsaturated fats are less susceptible to oxidation and rancidity compared to polyunsaturated fatty acids, and therefore are acceptable for deep-fat frying. Two varieties of sunflower and canola seeds have been developed with lower polyunsaturated fatty acids and higher oleic acid content. These changes have made them more stable and more suitable for deep-fat frying.[73]

Improving on Traditional Margarine

Oilseeds have also been developed for use in preparing semi-solid fats for margarine-like spreads and for baking. These fats contain saturated fats, are solid at room temperature, and have the plasticity needed for baking. Soybeans have been developed to increase the amount of saturated fatty acids (stearic and palmitic) for use in preparing semi-solid fats without hydrogenation or the addition of trans fats.[72] Even though saturated fatty acids generally increase LDL cholesterol levels, stearic acid has a neutral effect on serum lipids and cardiovascular risk. Therefore, stearic acid can be added to oil mixtures to raise the melting point for semi-solid fats without adding health risks.

Weighing the Advantages and Disadvantages

An advantage of using trait-enhanced oilseeds to reduce trans fatty acids in the food supply is that no additional chemical processing is required by oilseed processors or food manufacturing plants. Another advantage is that these oils have a longer "fry life," in that they can be used for a longer period of time than other oils or partially hydrogenated fats for deep-fat frying. Although some modified oils are more expensive, the cost of labor for food service operations is less because oil replacement for frying operations is less frequent.

One caveat in using trait-enhanced oilseeds is that formulas for baked products may need to be modified when these fats are used in preparing baked products such as cookies, cakes, and crackers. Also, one of the limitations of trait-enhanced oilseeds is that shortages of seed supplies for planting can impact commercial availability.[73]

Modified Hydrogenation

Traditional hydrogenation of vegetable oils adds hydrogen gas to unsaturated fatty acids under high heat in the presence of a metal catalyst, nickel, to fill unsaturated double bonds.[9] Modifications in the hydrogenation process in the past decade have been successful in lowering trans fatty acid isomers in partially hydrogenated fats to less than 10%.[5] Advantages of the modified hydrogenation process is that readily available traditional soybean, cottonseed, and canola oils can be used and it results in a semi-hard shortening that is appropriate for baking and frostings. However, the disadvantages are that this method does not completely eliminate trans fats and that it requires sophisticated technology.[58–61,74–79]

Fractionation of Fats

Fractionation is a method of hardening liquid oils by adding saturated fatty acids with a higher melting point to transform an oil mixture to a solid fat. It is used in a variety of food processing applications. Fractionation physically separates saturated fatty acids from monounsaturated and polyunsaturated fatty acids. Palm oil, palm kernel oil, and coconut oil contain approximately 50% saturated fatty acids and are good oils for this process. For example, palm oil is fractionated into saturated stearic and monounsaturated oleic acid. Stearic acid is a hard fat that is acceptable for fractionation and isolation because it has a neutral effect on serum lipids.[80]

An advantage to fractionation is that solid fats can be prepared without hydrogenation or the addition of trans fats. A controlled amount of saturated fatty acids can be added to produce fats with (1) varying amounts of saturated fatty acids (45–75%), (2) a range of melting points (61–113°F [16–45°C]), and (3) different degrees of plasticity. The resulting fats can be used in various applications, such as baking and deep-fat frying.[81] A disadvantage of this method is the sophisticated technology it requires.

Interesterification

Interesterification is a method used to change the fatty acid composition of fats and oils by hydrolysis of fatty acids from the glycerol backbone, followed by re-esterification. To achieve interesterification, excess amounts of glycerol are added to a mixture of vegetable oils in the presence of a catalyst. High heat is then applied, resulting in a redistribution of fatty acids on the glycerol molecule. Both chemical and enzymatic methods are used in interesterification. Specific microbial lipases are used for enzymatic interesterification. Enzymes are preferred when triglycerides with a specific fatty acid pattern are desired.

Advantages of interesterification are that free fatty acids with the desired degree of saturation and carbon length can be added to a mixture of triglycerides to develop fats with the desired melting and/or smoke point and stability. For example, highly saturated hard fats from palm, palm kernel, and coconut oil can be combined with liquid oils to yield margarines and shortening with the desired characteristics and with zero trans fats.

Disadvantages of enzymatic interesterification are that it is relatively expensive and that the reaction time is much longer than chemical interesterification.[82,83] The disadvantage of chemical interesterification is that approximately 30% of the fat is lost in the formation of soap and fatty acid methyl esters.[82] A disadvantage to interesterification by either method is that some of these products have saturated fatty acid levels as high as 32%.[84,85]

Reformulating Food Products to Remove Trans Fats

Those in the food manufacturing and food service industries must consider several factors when changing operations to eliminate trans fats. The selection of a modified fat product is based the characteristics of the fat and the qualities needed for the specific food product. For example, the best choice of fat for deep-fat frying may not be suitable for baking. The following factors must also be considered:

- The capacity of the commercial operation to adapt without purchasing new equipment.
- The availability of the chosen modified fat.
- The cost and sensory qualities of the reformulated food product.

Food manufacturers considering a reformulation should keep the following in mind:[54,55]

- Become familiar with the kinds and cost of ingredients on the market from suppliers of fats and/or oils.
- Consider the availability of ingredients and possible fluctuations in price related to supply and demand.
- Evaluate products made with different ingredients, including a test of consumer acceptance through sensory evaluation. Expect to adjust the formula to obtain desirable taste and texture.

Resources for restaurants, schools, and other food service operations changing to trans fat free operations are available from the Cambridge Public Health Department[62,63] and the New York City Department of Public Health and Mental Hygiene.[56,57] The American Heart Association has compiled a list of manufacturers of commercial oil and shortening manufacturers, with detailed information on their products and contact information.[52,53,62,63]

Greening Fats and Oils

Recent technology has allowed green uses for fat and oils, as well as disposal. In this section, two positive trends concerning dietary fat are discussed. The first is the use of fat as biodiesel, which is an alternative fuel produced from domestic resources. Biodiesel is safe for the environment, can be used in any diesel engine, and is more sustainable and less polluting than conventional petroleum diesel.[86] The use of biodiesel fuel has been found to significantly reduce greenhouse gases, carbon dioxide, and sulfur dioxide in air emissions. In addition, biodiesel is biodegradable and non-toxic. Biodiesel is produced from renewable resources, being cooking oil waste. The "fat to fuel" process recycles waste oils that are set to be dumped in landfills or flushed down drains.[86] A secondary positive outcome of using biodiesel is it reduces dependence on limited energy resources and foreign oil.

The second "greening" potential of fat and oil is within its potential method of disposal. The Environmental Protection Agency (EPA) provides a list of problematic fat types that fills our landfills and clogged pipes. These are:[87]

- Yellow grease: deep fryer grease and oil
- Brown grease: found in restaurant grease traps
- Black grease: congealed grease in sewer pipes
- Trap waste: other trap waste

The potential for fat lies in being considered green lies in making it more able to become immiscible. This bioavailability would be achieved by treating the waste fat and oil with anaerobic microorganisms. The EPA claims this would solve the landfill problem, along with save electricity and water from the past usage of fat disposal. In addition, the process is less expensive and less pollutant to our air.[87]

Fat Substitutes

The American Heart Association defines **fat substitutes**, also called *fat mimetics*, as ingredients that mimic one or more of the roles of fat in food, such as providing moisture, mouthfeel, and other characteristics of fat by holding water. **Fat extenders** differ from fat substitutes; they optimize the functionality of fat, allowing for a decrease in the usual amount of fat required by a product.[5]

Fat substitutes are classified into three categories based on their nutrient source: carbohydrate-based, protein-based, and fat-based substitutes. The carbohydrate-based fat substitutes use plant polysaccharides in place of fat. They resemble conventional fats, are stable at cooking and frying temperatures, and provide all the functions of fat while yielding less than 9 calories per gram. Protein-based fat substitutes may be microparticulated, which means that they can be processed into a powder form. Fat-based substitutes are used as barriers to block fat absorption; they also are called *fat analogs*.[88]

Why are fat substitutes used? Some believe that they are needed to decrease the quantity of fat in foods, and in so doing help people lower their total fat intake.[88] The substitutes can be used to provide some or all of the functions of fat, yet yield fewer calories.[5] In order to be used successfully they need to be able to replicate all or some of the functional properties of fat in fat-modified foods, including its sensory qualities. Replicating the taste and mouthfeel provided by fat can be a challenge.[88]

fat substitutes Also called *fat mimetics*, ingredients that mimic one or more of the roles of fat in food, such as providing moisture, mouthfeel, and other characteristics of fat by holding water.

fat extenders Ingredients that optimize the functionality of fat, allowing for a decrease in the usual amount of fat required by a product.

Carbohydrate-Based Substitutes

Carbohydrate-based fat substitutes are made of celluloses, dextrins, gums, and fibers. They are basic components of emulsions and hydrocolloids. Mixed with water, they make gels. They are used in many food products because of their stabilizing and thickening qualities. Carbohydrate-based fat substitutes are used in dairy products such as cheeses and yogurts, frozen desserts, sauces, salad dressings, processed meats, baked goods, spreads, chewing gums, snack products, and fruit purees.

Hydrocolloids

Hydrocolloids are mostly gums and fibers, such as guar gum, xanthan gum, and carboxymethlycellulose. They replace starches and can enhance a food's texture without affecting taste.[11] They can be used to produce thicker sauces. For example, they are a viable option for improving the stability of white sauces during freezing and thawing by reducing structural changes after thawing. White (béchamel) sauces are more stable with gums because the gums interact with amylase in the sauces, decreasing the amount of interaction between amylase molecules.[89–91] Hydrocolloids give manufacturers more options than modified starches to address texture loss and water exudation.

Pectins

Pectin gels are being used more and more often to replace fats while maintaining a product's texture, taste, and stability. Pectin, a water-soluble fiber, is being used in baked goods, as a gelling agent in confectionary items and bakery fillings, and as a stabilizer in yogurts and milk drinks. The primary source of pectin comes from citrus peel and apple pomace.[92] It is a good **emulsifier** because it reduces the surface tension between two immiscible interfaces, allowing them to mix.[14] Pectins are becoming common in low-fat vegetable-based mayonnaises (see **Figure 13.13**).[89]

The use of pectins and fruit purees as fat replacers decreases the amount of saturated fat and total fat in a food. Consumers of foods containing these substances decrease their total fat consumption and increase their fiber intake. The use of fruit purees in particular can also increase the amount of antioxidants in a food. However, pectins and fruit purees may not reduce consumers' overall energy intake and may decrease the intake of certain nutrients.[5]

corn syrup, wheat starch, degerminated yellow
corn flour, honey, palm kernel oil, modified corn
starch, nonfat milk, glycerin, apple puree, fruit
juice concentrate (kiwi, strawberry, red raspberry,
blueberry), canola oil, natural and artificial flavor,
fructooligosaccharides, corn cereal, strawberries,
blueberries, whey, monoglycerides, soy lecithin,
corn starch, nonfat yogurt powder (heat treated
after culturing), soybean oil, invert sugar,
cinnamon, guar gum, caramel color, citric acid,
BHT for freshness, beta carotene for color, red
40, blue 2, cellulose gum, green 3, blue 1, red 40
lake, blue 2 lake.
Vitamins and Minerals: Vitamin A palmitate,

FIGURE 13.13 Fat substitutes are becoming an increasingly common ingredient in processed foods. Food manufacturers use fat substitutes to maintain the original food's characteristics while decreasing the amount of fat.

emulsifier A mixture that requires the suspension of one liquid in another; for example, a mixture of water in margarine, shortening, or ice cream.

Protein-Based Substitutes

The protein-based mimetics are whey (milk protein) and egg protein. Because they provide a creamy mouthfeel, they are good when used in dairy products, such as ice cream and creamy soups. However, they are not useful for frying.

Protein blends combine animal or vegetable protein and gum. These blends are used in frozen and baked goods. It is suggested that the combination of protein and starch hydrocolloid gives a synergistic effect for lowering fat while retaining the texture and character of the product and creating an improved creaminess and mouthfeel. One gram of protein blend or protein-based mimetic replaces 3 grams of fat.[5]

Fat-Based Substitutes

Fat-based substitutes may include alterations of fatty acids and provide fewer calories than regular fats or even no calories. However, emulsifiers and fat-based substitutes may provide up to 9 calories per gram.[5]

Olestra

Olestra (sold as Olean) is a fat analog that has zero calories. It has properties of fat but it cannot be hydrolyzed by gastrointestinal or pancreatic lipases, and it is too large a molecule to be absorbed in the gastrointestinal tract.[5] **Figure 13.14** shows the structure of olestra.

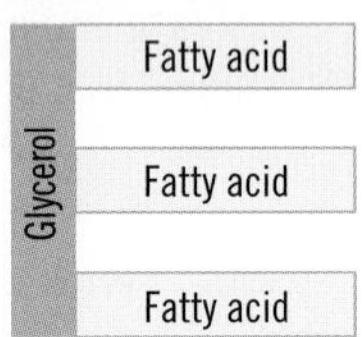

A triglyceride has three fatty acids attached to a glycerol backbone.

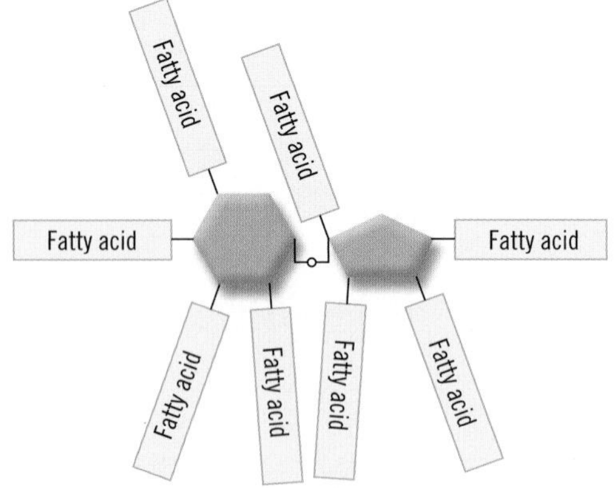

Olestra has six to eight fatty acids attached to a sucrose backbone.

FIGURE 13.14 Olestra is derived from sucrose. Because of this, it can bond with six, seven, or eight fatty acids. The resulting structure of olestra is too large to be absorbed by the intestines and passes through the gastrointestinal tract without being digested.

Fantesk

Fantesk is a branded fat analog that is a mixture of starch, water, and one or more oily substances. It is used in baking and for frostings. It has a smooth texture and easy spreadability and can be used in ice creams and cheeses. It can be used to make foods much lower in fat than their conventional counterparts. The finished product is low in fat and yet has improved texture and volume. The two scientists who developed Fantesk were able to produce the unusual gel by processing starch and oil (such as soy oil) in pressurized superheated steam. Regardless of subsequent processing—be it melting, freezing or drum-drying—the fry oil droplets were found to remain dispersed in the starch.[93]

The Dilemma of Using Fat Substitutes

Fats and oils are a dense form of energy. They offer both health benefits and health risks. The dilemma is that we are developing new fats for snack foods, not making better food choices. While we look to decrease dietary fats for caloric reasons, we are asking industry to develop low- and zero-calorie fat substitutes that have all the other attributes of fat. Consumers eat these fat substitutes in snacks, cookies, and chips rather than getting high-quality fats directly from plant-based and fish sources. Because these substitutes lack the essential nutrients we need, and may even reduce their absorption, food manufacturers then fortify these foods with vitamins and minerals. Many processed foods also have increased amounts of fat and salt.

At a time when Americans are trying to improve their diets by increasing consumption of healthier fats by using olive oil and other unsaturated and monounsaturated oils, food manufacturers are constantly developing new and better ways to fry foods and package high-fat foods. Deep fried foods are as popular as ever. Trans fats carry a health risk, but are foods deep fried in a polyunsaturated oil really a healthier product? Americans seem to consider the perfect dietary fat as one that has zero calories but that allows us to continue eating french fries.

Hydrogenation of vegetable oils unintentionally added trans fat to foods during processing. Beginning in the 1990s, research demonstrated a positive relationship between dietary intake of trans fats and coronary heart disease. Since then, there has been a worldwide effort to reduce or eliminate trans fats from processed foods.[38] Changing the trans fat content of a food without increasing the amount of saturated fat while maintaining functional qualities and consumer acceptance is a complex task—one that requires the expertise and collaboration of members of the nutrition and food science community, the food processing and food service industry, and government regulatory and public health agencies.[3,84]

Food Regulations

Trans Fats Labeling

The FDA published a final rule on July 11, 2003, that requires that the trans fat content be listed on a food item's nutrition label (see **Figure 13.15**). The FDA instituted this requirement based on research that demonstrated a positive relationship between dietary trans fat intake and coronary heart disease and in response to a petition from the Center for Science in the Public Interest.[33] The ruling went into effect on January 1, 2006.

Innovation Point

Margarine Spreads Margarine spreads formulated with plant sterols/stanols have been developed by McNeil Nutritionals (Benecol Spreads) and Unilever (Promise Activ Light Spread). Plant sterols/stanols inhibit the absorption of dietary cholesterol and are recommended as part of a cholesterol-lowering diet.

Nutrition Facts

Serving Size 1/2 cup (56g)
Servings per container: 8

Amount Per Serving			
Calories 200		Calories from Fat 10	
		% Daily Value*	
Total Fat 1g			2%
Saturated Fat 0g			0%
Trans Fat 0g			23%
Cholesterol 0mg			3%
Sodium 0mg			0%
Total Carbohydrate 41g			48%
Dietary Fiber 2g			8%
Sugars 1g			
Protein 7g			
Vitamin A 0%	·	Vitamin C 0%	
Calcium 0%	·	Iron 10%	
Thiamin 35%	·	Riboflavin 15%	
Niacin 20%	·	Folic acid 30%	

*Percent Daily Values are based on a 2,000-calorie diet. Your daily values may be higher or lower depending on your calorie needs.

	Calories:	2000	2,500
Total Fat	Less Than	65g	80g
Sat Fat	Less Than	20g	25g
Cholesterol	Less Than	300mg	300mg
Sodium	Less Than	2,400mg	2,400mg
Total Carbohydrate		300g	375g
Dietary Fiber		25g	30g

Calories per gram:
Fat 9 Carbohydrate 4 Protein 4

FIGURE 13.15 All packaged foods must list the trans fat content on their Nutrition Facts labels. Any food that contains less than 0.5 grams of trans fat per serving can say it contains 0 grams of trans fat.

Butter Products

Federal law mandates that butter must be 80% milk fat. The remaining 20% is milk solids and water. Butter consists of cream, salt, and annatto. The USDA grades butter quality based on its flavor, body, texture, salt, and color. Butter may have a yellow color due to fat-soluble animal pigments. Butter is labeled with Grade AA, indicating superior quality, or Grade A, indicating very good quality. The following labels on butter are regulated by law:

- *Unsalted butter*: No salt has been added.
- *Sweet butter:* Made with sweet cream, instead of sour cream. Usually contains salt.
- *Whipped butter*: Has the same ingredients as butter, but, because air has been incorporated, it has 60–70% fewer calories, fat, cholesterol, and sodium. The inclusion of air also increases volume, which creates a softer, more spreadable consistency when cold.
- *Creamed butter:* Creamed butter has the high fat component separated from whole milk as a result of the creaming process. According to federal standards, it must contain 80% milk fat or more.[2]
- *Light or reduced calorie butter*: Has half the fat of regular butter, through the addition of skim milk, water, and gelatin. This and other spreads are not good for baking.

Fat Substitutes

Fat substitutes can be categorized as food additives or as supplements and must meet the approval of the FDA. Those Generally Recognized as Safe (GRAS) include cellulose gel, dextrins, guar gum, and gum arabic. Labels on foods made with fat substitutes must comply with the Nutritional Labeling and Education Act of 1990, which states that the label must list the usual name and the energy or nutrient contributions.[5]

Chapter Review

Partially hydrogenated fats and trans fats was in full use until the 1980s, when the case against trans fats—for health reasons—reached its peak. One study showed that a 2% increase in trans fat intake correlated with a 23% increase in coronary heart disease. Beginning on January 1, 2006, the Food and Drug Administration (FDA) mandated that trans fats be included on the Nutrition Facts label.

Thereafter, the use of omega fatty acids, which play an important role in health, was encouraged, especially sources of omega-3 fatty acids like alpha-linolenic acid (ALA), eicosapentaenoic acid (EPA), and docosahexaenoic acid (DHA). Vegetable oils, including olive and canola oils, and especially flaxseed oil, are high in ALA. Fish, particularly fatty fish such as salmon, are high in EPA and DHA. Foods high in the omega-6 fatty acids (such as linolenic acid) include corn oil, cottonseed oil, sunflower oil, and soybean oil.

Prior to this, most of the oils used in deep frying are high in saturated and trans fats. The American Heart Association recommends limiting trans fat to less than 1% of daily intake, or 2 grams based on a 2,000 kcal diet. The most recent recommendations from the *Dietary Guidelines for Americans, 2010* recommend avoiding trans fatty acids from industrial sources and limiting those from natural sources to less than 0.5% of calories.[4] Reducing the consumption of deep-fried foods can help people meet this goal.

Baking and cooking with fats provide crispness, flakiness, and softness. In addition, fats and oils in baked goods serve multiple functions that are integral to the product, such as tenderizing, ensuring sufficient shelf life, providing flavoring, and adding to the product structure. Points to consider when selecting a fat include the fat's melting point and creaming ability.

The crystalline structure, composition, and polymorphic forms of fat crystals are the most important criteria for the functional properties of fats in the cooking process. Fats are a network of crystals with oil trapped inside. This network of fat crystals directly affects the texture of candy, with smaller crystals leading to firmer products (chocolate) and larger crystals producing a crunchy mouth feel. Fats have large alpha crystals, which are formed rapidly if fats are chilled, and small beta crystals. Beta crystals are good for shortening because they can be creamed easily and give a smooth texture. Beta crystals also have a high melting point.

Rancidity is the most common cause of "off flavor" in oil. Hydrolytic rancidity, the first type of spoilage in fats, is associated with the presence of water. The triglycerides in fats react with water, freeing their fatty acids from glycerol and breaking down into volatile secondary products with an off flavor. Oxidative rancidity, the second type of spoilage in oil, also is referred to as auto-oxidation. This occurs when the lipid is catalyzed in the presence of heat or light.

Fat substitutes are classified into three categories based on their nutrient source: carbohydrate-based, protein-based, and fat-based substitutes. The carbohydrate-based fat substitutes use plant polysaccharides in place of fat. They resemble conventional fats, are stable at cooking and frying temperatures, and provide all the functions of fat while yielding less than 9 calories per gram. Protein-based fat substitutes may be microparticulated, which means that they can be processed into a powder form. Fat-based substitutes are used as barriers to block fat absorption; they also are called *fat analogs*. Fat substitutes or replacements have been developed but have been met with their own challenges.

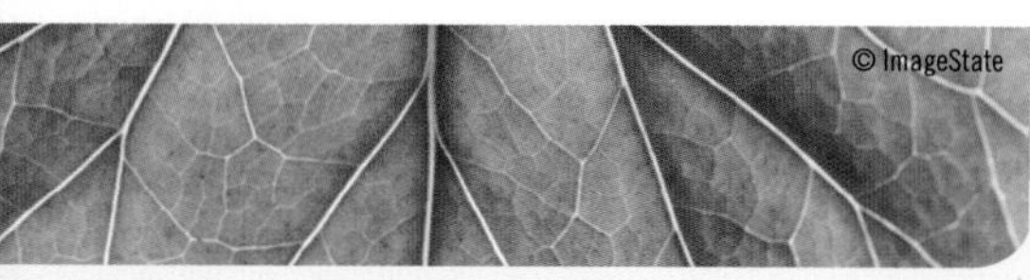

Learning Portfolio

Key Terms

	page
docosahexaenoic acid (DHA)	409
eicosapentaenoic acid (EPA)	409
emulsifier	424
fat extenders	423
fat substitutes	423
fractionation	405
functional food	409
hydrolytic rancidity	417
interesterification	405
monounsaturated fatty acids	406
oxidative rancidity	417
plasticity	407
polyunsaturated fatty acids	406
pressing	413
rancidity	417
saturated fatty acids	406

Study Points

1. Compared to vegetable oils, hydrogenated fats have a longer shelf life, greater plasticity, and a higher smoke point. Hydrogenated fats also are less susceptible to oxidation and spoilage.
2. Nearly all trans fatty acids in the diet come from industrial sources. Partially hydrogenated vegetable oil is added to processed and ready-to-eat foods, such as margarine and shortening; baked products, such as cakes, muffins, pies, cookies, crackers, and other snack items; and deep-fat fried foods.
3. Natural sources of trans fats are found in meat and dairy products as a result of microbial hydrogenation of cis-unsaturated fatty acids in the stomachs of ruminant animals.
4. Fats have a number of important biological functions. They are the building blocks of cell membranes. They are a dense form of energy, with 1 gram of fat supplying 9 kcal of energy. Only small amounts of intake are required to meet our energy needs. Fats aid the absorption of the fat-soluble vitamins A, E, D, and K. A diet with too little fat will result in not enough absorption of these important vitamins. Too much fat in the diet can contribute to weight gain and possibly certain chronic diseases.
5. Dietary fats affect blood lipid profiles and cholesterol levels. A normal lipid profile has a total cholesterol level of under 200 mg, with healthy HDL levels and controlled LDL values. Saturated fats have a negative effect on this lipid profile.
6. Research in the 1990s proved that trans fatty acids are harmful to health. Studies have shown that a 2% increase in trans fat intake results in a 23% increase in coronary heart disease.
7. Food manufacturers have started replacing hydrogenated vegetable oils in their food products in response to research on the negative health effects of these fats and the FDA's mandate that the amount of trans fats be listed on all food labels.
8. The Lyon Heart Study determined that people who follow the Mediterranean Diet reap the benefits of a heart healthy regimen.
9. Vegetable seed oils have been developed by traditional plant breeding, mutations, and gene modification for decades to improve yield as well as the functional and nutritional qualities of seed oils.
10. Fat substitutes are ingredients that mimic one or more of the roles of fat in food, including the sensory and physical functions of fat. They are classified into three categories based on their nutrient source: carbohydrate-based, protein-based, and fat-based substitutes.

Issues for Class Discussion

1. Why are tropical oils important? What are their health implications? Can they replace trans fats in restaurant cooking and processed foods?
2. What are the ethical dilemmas facing farmers who produce tropical oils? Can they serve the local population or must they grow the crop for export? What about deforestation?
3. How safe are genetically enhanced oilseeds? Will such foods help meet the food needs of a growing global population? Can genetically enhanced seeds improve the health of populations?

Research Areas for Students

1. Enhancements in genetically modified oilseeds and traditionally bred oilseeds
2. The prominence of tropical oils in the global market
3. Safety of enhanced oilseeds and tropical oils on health
4. Fortification of animal feeds and processed foods with fatty acids and phytochemicals

References

1. Britannica Online Encyclopedia. Encyclopedia Britannica. 2010. Available at: http://www.britannica.com.
2. Tarrago-Trani MT, Phillips KM, Lemar MS, Holden JM. New and existing oils and fats used in products with reduced trans fatty acid content. *J Am Diet Assoc.* 2006;106(6):867–880.
3. Eckel RH, Borra S, Lichtenstein AH, Yin-Piazza SY. Understanding the complexity of trans fatty acid reduction in the American diet: American Heart Association Trans Fat Conference 2006: Report of the Trans Fat Conference Planning Group. *Circulation.* 2007;115(16):2231–2246.
4. Cunningham ER. What are interesterified fats? *J Am Diet Assoc.* 2007;107(4):704.
5. Position of the American Dietetic Association: Fat replacers. *J Am Diet Assoc.* 2005;105(2):266–275.
6. American Heart Association. Prepared Foods and Mixes Without Trans Fat. Face the Fats Restaurant Resources. 2010. Available at: http://www.heart.org/HEARTORG/GettingHealthy/FatsAndOils/FacetheFatsRestaurantResources/Prepared-Foods-Mixes-without-Trans Fat_UCM_304092_Article.jsp. Accessed September 10, 2011.
7. Byrne J. UK Saturated Fat Proposals Have EU-Wide Implications, Caobisco. March 2010. Available at: http://www.bakeryandsnacks.com/Formulation/UK-saturated-fat-proposals-have-EU-wide-implications–Caobisco. Accessed March 30, 2010.
8. Stender S, Astrup A, Dyerberg J. Ruminant and industrially produced trans fatty acids: Health aspects. *Food Nutr Res.* 2008. DOI: 10.3402/fnr.v52i0.1651.
9. Ackman RG, Mag TK. Trans fatty acids and the potential for less in technical products. In: Sebedio JL, Christie WW (eds.). *Trans Fatty Acids in Human Nutrition.* Dundee, UK: The Oily Press; 1998:35–58.
10. Wolff RL, Precht D, Molkentin J. Occurrence and distribution profiles of trans 18:1 acids in edible fats of natural origin. In: Sebedio JL, Christie WW (eds.). *Trans Fatty Acids in Human Nutrition.* Dundee, UK: The Oily Press; 1998:1–33.
11. U.S. Department of Agriculture. National Nutrient Database for Standard Reference, Release 21. Available at: http://www.ars.usda.gov/nutrientdata. Accessed September 10, 2011.
12. American Heart Association. Lyon Diet Heart Study. 2010. Available at: http://www.americanheart.org/presenter.jhtml?identifier=4655. Accessed October 10, 2010.
13. American Heart Association. Mediterranean Diet. 2010. Available at: http://www.americanheart.org/presenter.jhtml?indentifier=4644. Accessed October 10, 2010.
14. U.S. Department of Health and Human Services, U.S. Department of Agriculture. Fats. In: *Dietary Guidelines for Americans, 2005.* Available at: http://www.health.gov/dietaryguidelines/dga2005/document/html/chapter6.htm?debugMode=false. Accessed September 10, 2011.
15. Ferguson LR. Nutrigenomics approaches to functional foods. *J Am Diet Assoc.* 2009;109(3):452–458.
16. Position of the American Dietetic Association: Fortification and nutritional supplements. *J Am Diet Assoc.* 2005;105(8):1300–1311.
17. Nettleton JA. Striving to increase compliance with dietary guidelines for fatty acid intake: A call for a multifaceted dietary approach. *J Am Diet Assoc.* Oct 2007;107(10):1723–1725.
18. Fiber One. General Mills. Available at: http://www.fiberone.com/Product/Default.aspx. Accessed September 10, 2011.
19. U.S. Department of Agriculture. 1989–91 Continuing Survey of Food Intakes by Individuals and 1989–91 Diet and Health Knowledge Survey on CD-ROM. NTIS accession number: PB96-501747 1996.
20. Mensink RP, Katan MB. Effect of dietary trans fatty acids on high-density and low-density lipoprotein cholesterol levels in healthy subjects. *N Engl J Med.* 1990;323:439–445.
21. Lichtenstein AH, Ausman LM, Jalbert SM, Schaefer EJ. Effects of different forms of dietary hydrogenated fats on serum lipoprotein cholesterol levels. *N Engl J Med.* 1999;340:1933–1940.
22. Mozaffarian D, Katan MB, Ascherio A, et al. Trans fatty acids and cardiovascular disease. *N Engl J Med.* 2006;354:1601–1613.
23. Valenzuela A, Morgado N. Trans fatty acid isomers in human health and in the food industry. *Biol Res.* 1999;32:273–287.
24. Ascherio A, Katan MB, Zock PL, et al. Trans fatty acids and coronary heart disease. *N Engl J Med.* 1999;340:1994–1998.
25. Executive Summary of the Third Report of the National Cholesterol Education Program (NCEP) Expert Panel on Detection, Evaluation, and Treatment of High Blood Cholesterol in Adults (Adult Treatment Panel III). *JAMA.* 2001;285:2486–2497.
26. Almendingen K, Jordal O, Kierulf P, et al. Effects of partially hydrogenated fish oil, partially hydrogenated soybean oil, and butter on serum lipoproteins and Lp[a] in men. *J Lipid Res.* 1995;36:1370–1384.
27. Mozaffarian D, Pischon T, Hankinson SE, et al. Dietary intake of trans fatty acids and systemic inflammation in women. *Am Soc Clin Nutr.* 2004;79:606–612.
28. Lopez-Garcia E, Schulze MB, Meigs JB, et al. Consumption of trans fatty acids is related to plasma biomarkers of inflammation and endothelial dysfunction. *J Nutr.* 2005;135:562–566.
29. Mensink RP. Metabolic and health effects of isomeric fatty acids. *Curr Opin Lipidol.* 2005;16:27–30.
30. Harnack LA, Lee S, Schakel SF, et al. Trends in the trans fatty acid composition of the diet in a metropolitan area: The Minnesota Heart Survey. *J Am Diet Assoc.* 2003;103:1160–1166.
31. Allison DB, Egan SK, Barraj LM, et al. Estimated intakes of trans fatty and other fatty acids in the US population. *J Am Diet Assoc.* 1999;99:166–174.
32. Exler J, Lemar L, Smith J. Fat and Fatty Acid Content of Selected Foods Containing Trans Fatty Acids. (Special purpose table no. 1.) Beltsville, MD: Beltsville Human Nutrition Research Center, Nutrient Data Laboratory; 1995; Computer file released by U.S. Department of Agriculture.
33. U.S. Food and Drug Administration. Guidance for Industry: Trans Fatty Acids in Nutrition Labeling, Nutrient Content Claims, Health Claims; Small Entity Compliance Guide. 2003. Available at: http://www.fda.gov/Food/GuidanceComplianceRegulatoryInformation/GuidanceDocuments/FoodLabelingNutrition/ucm053479.htm. Accessed September 10, 2011.
34. U.S. Department of Agriculture, Agricultural Research Service. Data Tables: Results from USDA's 1994–96 Continuing Survey of Food Intakes by Individuals and 1994–96 Diet and Health Knowledge Survey, Table Set 10. Washington, DC: USDA, Agricultural Research Service; 1997.
35. Omar MN, Nor-Nazuha MN, Nor-Dalilah MN, Sahri MM. Frying performance of palm-based solid frying shortening. *Pak J Biol Sci.* 2010;13(6):298–302.

36. Mayamol PN, Balachandran C, Samuel T, et al. Zero trans shortening using rice bran oil, palm oil and palm stearin through interesterification at pilot scale. *Int J Food Sci Tech*. 2009;44(1):18–28.
37. Daniels RL. Ultra Blends Enzymatic Solutions: Simplified. Sustainable. Reliable. 2011. Available at: http://cms.bnpmedia.com/uploaded/SFWB%5CUltraBlends%20Enzymatic%20Solutions%20Brochure.pdf. Accessed August 14, 2012.
38. Dibildox-Alvarado E, Rodrigues JN, Gioielli LA, et al. Effects of crystalline microstructure on oil migration in a semisolid fat matrix. *Crystal Growth Design*. 2004;4(4):731–736.
39. Vuillequez A, Koza L, Youssef B, et al. Thermal and structural behavior of palm oil: Influence of cooling rate on fat crystallization. *Macromolecular Symposia*. 2010;290(1):137–145.
40. Meng Z, Liu Y, Shan L, Jin Q, Wang X. Reduction of graininess formation in beef tallow-based plastic fats by chemical interesterification of beef tallow and canola oil. *J Am Oil Chem Soc*. 2010;87(12):1435–1442.
41. Rousseau D, Ghosh S, Park H. Comparison of the dispersed phase coalescence mechanisms in different tablespreads. *J Food Sci*. 2009;74(1):E1–E7.
42. Daniel DR, Thompson LD, Shriver BJ, et al. Nonhydrogenated cottonseed oil can be used as a deep fat frying medium to reduce trans fatty acid content in french fries. *J Am Diet Assoc*. 2005;105(12):1927–1932.
43. Scott-Thomas C. Researchers Breed Non-GM Soybeans for Trans Free Oil. FoodNavigator-USA.com. September 17, 2010. Available at: http://www.foodnavigator-usa.com/Science/Researchers-breed-non-GM-soybeans-for-trans-free-oil. Accessed August 13, 2010.
44. Bouchon P. Understanding oil absorption during deep-fat frying. *Adv Food Nutr Res*. 2009;57:209–234.
45. Bouchon P, Aguilera JM, Pyle DL. Structure oil-absorption relationships during deep-fat frying. *J Food Sci*. 2003;68(9):2711–2716.
46. Choe E, Min DB. Chemistry of deep-fat frying oils. *J Food Sci*. 2007;72(5):R77–R86.
47. Ziaiifar AM, Achir N, Courtois F, et al. Review of mechanisms, conditions, and factors involved in the oil uptake phenomenon during the deep-fat frying process. *Int J Food Sci Tech*. 2008;43(8):1410–1423.
48. Lichtenstein AH, Appel LJ, Brands M, et al. Diet and lifestyle recommendations revision 2006: A scientific statement from the American Heart Association Nutrition Committee. *Circulation*. 2006;114:82–96.
49. Dietary Guidelines Advisory Committee. Report of the DGAC on the *Dietary Guidelines for Americans, 2010*. Part D. The Science Base. Section 3: Fatty Acids and Cholesterol. USDA. CNPP. Available at: http://www.cnpp.usda.gov/DGAs2010-DGACReport.htm. Accessed on September 10, 2011.
50. Hillyer CD. Regulating trans fats: Worldwide trends. *INFORM*. 2007;18(5):356–357.
51. Stender S, Dyerberg J, Astrup A. Consumer protection through a legislative ban on industrially produced trans fatty acids in foods in Denmark. *Scand J Food Nutr*. 2006;50:155–160.
52. Canadian Nutrition Labeling and Claims Regulations. Appendix 4. Current Regulatory Context. Food and Nutrition. Health Canada. 2006. Available at: http://www.hc-sc.gc.ca/fn-an/nutrition/gras-trans-fats/tf-ge/tf-gt_rep-rap-eng.php. Accessed September 10, 2011.
53. Aase S. Taking trans fat off the menu: What you can learn from trans fat bans at Sheikh Khalifa Medical City and the Cleveland Clinic. *J Am Diet Assoc*. 2009;109:1148–1151.
54. Remig V, Franklin B, Margolis S, et al. Trans fats in America: A review of their use, consumption, health implications, and regulation. *J Am Diet Assoc*. 2010;110:585–592.
55. Dunford N. FAPC-134. Formulating food products with low trans fats. *Food Technology Fact Sheet*. Robert M. Kerr Food & Agricultural Products Center. Oklahoma Cooperative Extension Service. Oklahoma State University.
56. Dunford NT. FAPC-164. Low trans fat and trans free fat update. *Food Technology Fact Sheet*. Robert M. Kerr Food & Agricultural Products Center. Oklahoma Cooperative Extension Service. Oklahoma State University.
57. New York City Department of Health and Mental Hygiene. The Regulation to Phase Out Artificial Trans Fat in New York City Food Service Establishments (Section 81.08 of the New York City Health Code). Available at: http://www.nyc.gov/html/doh/html/transfat/english/faqs.html. Accessed September 10, 2011.
58. Nollet LML, Pegg RB, Shahidi F. Off flavors and rancidity in foods. In: Nollet LML (ed.). *Handbook of Meat, Poultry, and Seafood Quality*. Hoboken, NJ: Wiley-Blackwell; 2007.
59. Vaclavik V, Christian EW. *Essentials of Food Science*. 3rd ed. New York: Springer; 2008.
60. Angulo O, López Aguilar JR, Valerio Alfaro G, et al. Evaluation of a simple and sensitive sensory method for measuring rancidity in soybean oils. *Grasas y Aceites*. 2006;57(2).
61. Purcaro G, Moret S, Conte LS. HS–SPME–GC applied to rancidity assessment in bakery foods. *Eur Food Res Tech*. 2007;227(1):1–6.
62. Cambridge Public Health Department. Phasing Out Trans Fat in Cambridge Food Service Establishments. How to Comply: What Restaurants, Caterers, Mobile Food Vendors, and Others Need to Know. Available at: http://www.cambridgepublichealth.org. Accessed September 10, 2011.
63. Canola Council of Canada. Canola Oil—The Myths Debunked. Available at: http://www.canolacouncil.org/canola_oil_the_truth.aspx. Accessed September 10, 2011.
64. Hammond EG, Fehr WR. Improving the fatty acid composition of soybean oil. *J Am Oil Chemist Soc*. 1984;11:1713–1716.
65. Nutrition Regulation Map. 2009. FitFrying.com. Available at: http://fitfrying.com/map/nutrition-regulation-map.php. Accessed September 10, 2011.
66. Beizaie SS. What California Restaurant Operators Need to Know About the State's Trans Fats and Menu Labeling Requirements: New Restrictions Take Effect on January 1, 2011. Holland & Knight LLP. Available at: http://www.hklaw.com/publications/What-California-Restaurant-Operators-Need-to-Know-About-the-State-rsquos-Trans-Fats-and-Menu-Labeling-Requirements-nbspNew-Restrictions-Take-Effect-on-January-1-2011-12-15-2010/. Accessed November 15, 2012.
67. Mount TL, Warner K, List GR, et al. Low-linolenic acid soybean oils-alternatives to frying oils. *J Am Oil Chemist Soc*. 1994;71:495–499.
68. Liu K. Soy oil modification: Products and applications. *INFORM*. 1999;10:868–878.
69. Kleingartner LW. NuSun sunflower oil: Redirection of an industry. In: Janick J, Whipkey A. (eds.). *Trends in New Crops and New Uses*. Alexandria, VA: ASHS Press; 2002:135–138.

70. Gupta MK. Sunflower oil. In: Gunstone FD (ed.). *Vegetable Oils in Food Technology*. Boca Raton, FL: CRC Press; 2002:128–156.
71. Przybylski R, Mag T. Canola/rapeseed oil. In: Gunstone FD (ed.). *Vegetable Oils in Food Technology*. Boca Raton, FL: CRC Press; 2002:98–127.
72. Wang T. Soybean oil. In: Gunstone FD (ed.). *Vegetable Oils in Food Technology*. Boca Raton, FL: CRC Press; 2002:18–58.
73. NuSun Sunflower Oil. Today's Healthy Oil Choice. National Sunflower Association. Mandan, ND. Available at: http://www.sunflowernsa.com/uploads/resources/12/nusun_healthyoil_brochure2010.pdf. Accessed September 10, 2011.
74. Purcaro G, Moret S, Conte LS. HS–SPME–GC applied to rancidity assessment in bakery foods. *Eur Food Res Tech*. 2007;227(1):1–6.
75. Higgins NW. Low Trans Stereoisomer Shortening Systems. US Patent Application No. 20040146626.
76. King JW, Holliday RL, List GR, Snyder JM. Hydrogenation of vegetable oils using mixtures of supercritical carbon dioxide and hydrogen. *J Am Oil Chemist Soc*. 2001;78:107–113.
77. Wright AJ, Wong A, Diosady LL. Ni catalyst promotion of a cis-selective Pd catalyst for canola oil hydrogenation. *Food Res Int*. 2003;36:1069–1072.
78. Mondal K, Lalvani, SB. A second order model for the catalytic-transfer hydrogenation of edible oils. *J Am Oil Chemist Soc*. 2000;77:1–8.
79. Lalvani SB, Mondal K. Electrochemical hydrogenation of vegetable oils. US Patent Application No. 20030213700.
80. Deffense E. Fractionation of palm oils. *J Am Oil Chemist Soc*. 1985;62:376–385.
81. North American Product Groups. The Choice for Palm. Loders Croklaan. Available at: http://northamerica.croklaan.com/ProductGroups/OurProductGroups. Accessed September 10, 2011.
82. Kellens M. Oil modification processes. In: Hamm W, Hamilton RJ (eds.). *Edible Oil Processing*. Boca Raton, FL: CRC Press; 2000:129–173.
83. Birschbach P, Fish N, Henderson W, Willrett D. Enzymes: Tools for creating healthier and safer foods. *Food Technol*. 2004;58:20–26.
84. List GR, Pelloso T, Orthoefer F, et al. Preparation of zero trans soybean oil margarines. *J Am Oil Chemist Soc*. 1995;72:383–384.
85. Satchithanandam S, Oles CJ, Spease CJ, et al. Trans, saturated, and unsaturated fat in foods in the United States prior to mandatory trans fat labeling. *Lipids*. 2004;39:11–18.
86. American Heart Association. Zero Grams Trans Fat Product Contact List. Face the Fats Restaurant Resources. Available at: http://www.heart.org/HEARTORG/GettingHealthy/FatsAndOils/FacetheFatsRestaurantResources/0-Grams-TransFat-Prduct-Contact-List_UCM_305092_Article.jsp. Accessed September 10, 2011.
87. Environmental Protection Agency. Biodiesel: Fat to Fuel. Available at: http://www.epa.gov/region9/waste/biodiesel. Accessed August 17, 2012.
88. York D. Increasing CHP Productivity While Reducing Biosolids Volume and Climate Changing Gases. Available at: http://www.epa.gov/region9/waterinfrastructure/training/energy-workshop/docs/2010/020110FinalFecHawaiiPresentationHiMauiOahuKuai.pdf. Accessed August 17, 2012.
89. American Heart Association. Fat Substitutes. 2010. Available at: http://www.americanheart.org/presenter.jhtml?identifier=4633&debugMode=false. Accessed September 10, 2011.
90. Daniells S. Options Abound for Low-Fat, Vegetable-Based Mayonnaise. March 2, 2010. Available at: http://www.foodnavigator.com/Science-Nutrition/Options-abound-for-low-fat-vegetable-based-mayonnaise. Accessed August 13, 2012.
91. Daniells S. Hydrocolloids May Enhance White Sauces in Ready Meals. March 26, 2010. Available at: http://www.foodnavigator.com/Science-Nutrition/Hydrocolloids-may-enhance-white-sauces-in-ready-meals. Accessed August 13, 2012.
92. Daniells S. White Sauce Stability Boosted by Gums. August 19, 2009. Available at: http://www.foodnavigator.com/Science-Nutrition/White-sauce-stability-boosted-by-gums. Accessed August 13, 2012.
93. Daniells S. Pectin-Stabilized Oil Bodies to Offer Pre-emulsified Oil. February 19, 2008. Available at: http://www.foodnavigator.com/Science-Nutrition/Pectin-stabilised-oil-bodies-to-offer-pre-emulsified-oil. Accessed August 13, 2012.

CHAPTER 14

Sugar and Sugar Substitutes

SeAnne Safaii, PhD, RD, LD

Chapter Objectives

THE STUDENT WILL BE EMPOWERED TO:

- Summarize the history, processes, and products of the cane and beet sugar industries.
- Review the chemistry of the different types of sugar molecules.
- Compare and contrast the many types of sweeteners, both nutritive and non-nutritive.
- Identify food label ingredients that reveal the presence of added sugars.
- Explain how sugar's properties apply to food preparation.
- Discuss the basics of candy making.
- Review information on the impact of sugar on Americans' health.
- Review the food safety history of non-nutritive sweeteners.

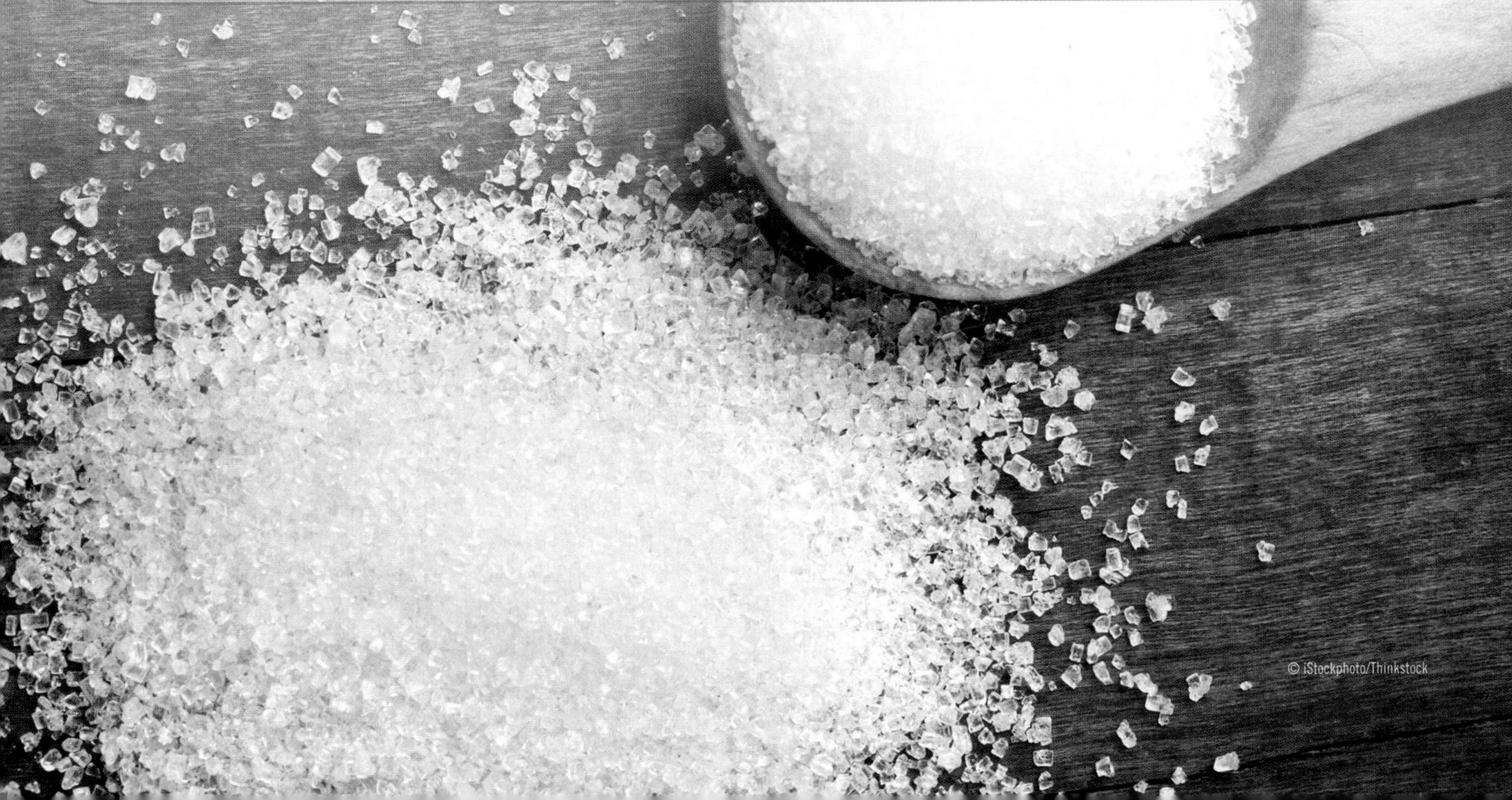

Historical, Cultural, and Ecological Significance

The history of sugar is a tale of global exploration, slavery, and capitalism. Today's modern sugar industry also is affected by global politics. The first recorded use of sugarcane leads is from New Guinea in 8000 B.C.; the earliest evidence of the use of crystalline sugar is from approximately 500 A.D. in India. Today, global consumption of sugar is approximately 120 million tons a year, and its use is expanding at a rate of about 2 million tons per year. The European Union, Brazil, and India are the top three producers of sugar, accounting for some 40% of annual worldwide production.[1–3]

Products of the Sugar Industry

Although numerous types of sugars and syrups are available in the marketplace, originally sugar came from two sources: sugarcane or sugar beet. Sugar, or sucrose, which is a disaccharide comprised of glucose and fructose, is found in the following forms:

- *Raw sugar* is granulated, solid, or coarse and is brown in color. It forms when the moisture from the juice of the sugarcane evaporates.
- *Granulated sugar* is the familiar white table sugar.
- *Brown sugar* is made from the sugar crystals from molasses syrup.
- *Confectioner's sugar*, also known as powdered sugar, is finely ground sugar.
- *Turbinado sugar* is unrefined sugar made from sugarcane juice.

Other commonly used sugars include fructose, which is the naturally occurring sugar in fruit. It also is called *levulose* or *fruit sugar*. Honey, which is produced by honeybees, is a combination of fructose, glucose, and water.

Sugarcane

Sugarcane (*Saccharum* spp.) is a type of grass that grows in tropical regions. It requires a lot of sunlight and water. The plants take 6 to 12 months to reach maturity. Sugarcane is harvested by chopping the stems from the plant. The roots are left in the ground to grow new stems, and a new crop. To extract sugar, the cane is crushed by large rollers, similar to how wheat is milled into flour.[1] The sweet juice that emerges from the crushed stems is filtered and then thickened by heating and evaporation. Eventually, crystals form, which are the starting material for the refining process.[3] The final raw sugar looks like the soft brown sugar found in most grocery stores. Additional refining is necessary to get the white crystal sugar that we use in food preparation. The juice that remains is sweet and is used to make molasses, which is usually turned into cattle food or sent to an alcohol distillery.[3]

The fiber left over after crushing the sugarcane stalks is called *bagasse*. Burning bagasse at the factory produces both electricity and steam, which are used to further process sugar. The heat produced from large furnaces can be used to boil water and make low-pressure steam for the sugar-making process. Bagasse also is a renewable, carbon-neutral fuel. Technically, the carbon dioxide produced is removed from the atmosphere by the new crop of growing canes (resulting in net zero carbon dioxide emissions). Thus, a well-run sugarcane refinery is environmentally friendly.[1] In contrast, when a large power station produces electricity, it burns fossil fuels that cannot be replaced and that contribute to global warming.

Bagasse is used in construction materials, such as insulation, and in biodegradable tableware. It also is used as a biofuel.[4] In Brazil, sugarcane produces one of the best raw materials for ethanol because it is easy to extract sugar for the fermentation process. Sugarcane grows well in Brazil's tropical climate, and Brazil produces more of it than any other country. Brazilian ethanol factories burn the bagasse efficiently and cleanly, providing enough electricity to power sugarcane refineries and to sell as surplus. In 2006, Brazil achieved energy independence through its sugarcane crop and oil resources.[5]

Beet Sugar

Sugar beets (*Beta vulgaris*) are also a source of sugar. The sugar beets are grown in the ground and harvested in autumn. Sugar beets require nearly four times the land area of the equivalent sugarcane crop, but they can be grown a variety of different climates.[1]

After the beets are harvested they are washed and then sliced into thin chips. This increases the surface area, making it easier for sugar extraction. The beets are mixed with hot water, and the sugary juice is diffused. The flesh of the sugar beet is pressed to remove any remaining juice. The remaining pulp is sent to a drying plant and turned into animal feed. The juice is then cleaned, boiled, steamed, and evaporated in a process similar to that used for cane sugar. The remaining sweet liquid is a byproduct called beet molasses, which is usually turned into cattle food or sent to an alcohol distillery.[1]

Beet sugar factories, like cane sugar factories, use steam and electricity and have cogeneration stations where high-pressure steam is used to produce electrical power. However, the leftover pulp from the beet cannot be used to fuel the boilers in the same way that bagasse can. Beet pulp is, however, a source of animal feed,[1] and it is an excellent food for lactating dairy cows. Beet pulp feed can be fed fresh to cows from October to February, and pulp that is stored in silos can be provided as feed throughout the year.[6] Growers of sugar beets in the United States and Canada often use genetically modified varieties of sugar beets for weed control. This technology significantly reduces dependency on chemical applications and cultivation, resulting in reduced consumption of fossil fuels.[3]

> ***Green Point***
>
> **Organic Sugar** Sugar sold in the United States that is labeled organic must meet specific USDA requirements that specify that the sugarcane has been cultivated without the use of chemical pesticides or herbicides. Organic sugar will perform identically to refined sugar. The demand for organic sugar has increased because the major organic food producers require organic sugar for their beverages, dairy products, cereals, chocolate products, confectionaries, and preserves.

Physical and Chemical Properties

Recall that sugars are simple carbohydrates consisting of either one basic sugar unit or a few small units linked together. Carbohydrates are composed of carbon (C), hydrogen (H), and oxygen (O). Carbohydrates are linked together by condensation reactions and broken apart by hydrolysis reactions. Each condensation reaction links two monosaccharides together, producing a water molecule. Each hydrolysis reaction uses a water molecule to break the linkage between the two monosaccharide units of a larger molecule.[7]

Carbohydrates are classified according to the number of basic sugar units that are linked together. They are classified as monosaccharides, disaccharides, oligosaccharides, and polysaccharides (see **Figure 14.1**):

- **Monosaccharides** are simple sugars composed of one basic unit. Glucose, fructose, and galactose are monosaccharides. Honey and corn syrup are made of monosaccharides.
- **Disaccharides** are sugars composed of two monosaccharides that have joined together as a result of a dehydration synthesis reaction

> **monosaccharides** Simples sugar composed of one basic unit. Examples include: glucose, fructose, and galactose.
>
> **disaccharides** Sugars composed of two monosaccharides that have joined together as a result of a dehydration synthesis reaction that results in a glycosidic bond. Disaccharides are present in cane and beet sugar (sucrose), milk sugar (lactose) and malt sugar (maltose).

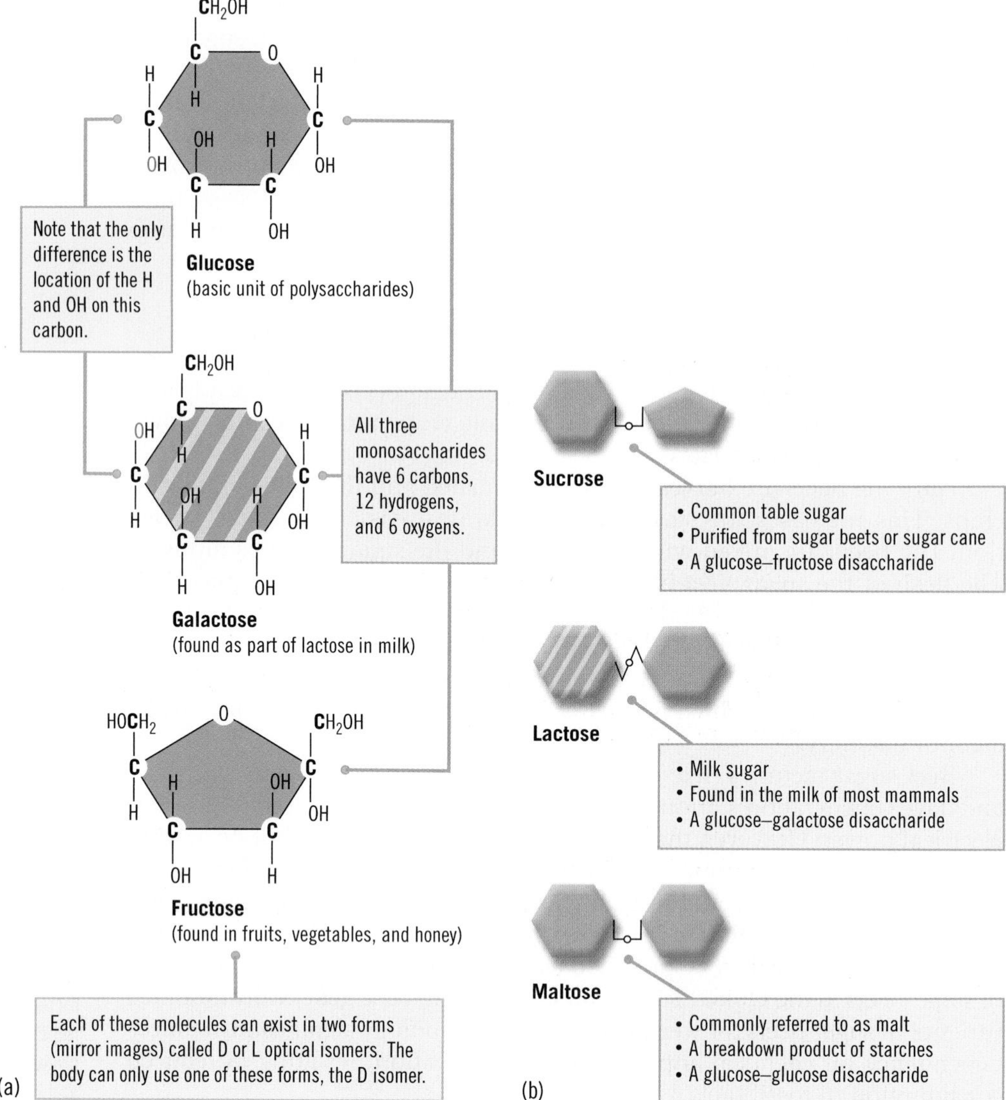

Note that the only difference is the location of the H and OH on this carbon.
Glucose
(basic unit of polysaccharides)
All three monosaccharides have 6 carbons, 12 hydrogens, and 6 oxygens.
Galactose
(found as part of lactose in milk)
Fructose
(found in fruits, vegetables, and honey)
Each of these molecules can exist in two forms (mirror images) called D or L optical isomers. The body can only use one of these forms, the D isomer.
(a)
Sucrose
• Common table sugar
• Purified from sugar beets or sugar cane
• A glucose–fructose disaccharide
Lactose
• Milk sugar
• Found in the milk of most mammals
• A glucose–galactose disaccharide
Maltose
• Commonly referred to as malt
• A breakdown product of starches
• A glucose–glucose disaccharide
(b)

FIGURE 14.1 (a) Monosaccharides are the simplest form of carbohydrate. They cannot be broken down into simpler sugars by hydrolysis. They are the building blocks of more complex sugars such as oligosaccharides and polysaccharides. (b) Disaccharides consist of two monosaccharides connected by a glycosidic bond. The most common disaccharides are sucrose, lactose, and maltose.

that results in a glycosidic bond. Disaccharides are present in cane and beet sugar (sucrose), milk sugar (lactose) and malt sugar (maltose).

- **Oligosaccharides** are typically composed of 3 to 10 monosaccharide units. They are found in small amounts in foods. Fructo-oligosaccharides are found in many vegetables and consist of short chains of fructose molecules. The most common of the oligosaccharides—raffinose and stachyose—are found in dried beans, peas, and lentils. These carbohydrates are broken down by intestinal bacteria.
- **Polysaccharides** are composed of long chains of monosaccharide units bound together by glycosidic bonds. They usually have more than 10 monosaccharide units. The basic units are linked as straight chains or branched chains, long and short. The various linkages are what give different polysaccharides their unique properties and behaviors in water and with heating. Amylopectin (see **Figure 14.2**) and glycogen (see **Figure 14.3**) are two important polysaccharides.

oligosaccharides Typically composed of 3 to 10 monosaccharide units. They are found in small amounts in foods.

polysaccharides Composed of long chains of monosaccharide units bound together by glycosidic bonds. They usually have more than 10 monosaccharide units. The basic units are linked as straight chains or branched chains, long and short. Amylopectin and glycogen are two important polysaccharides.

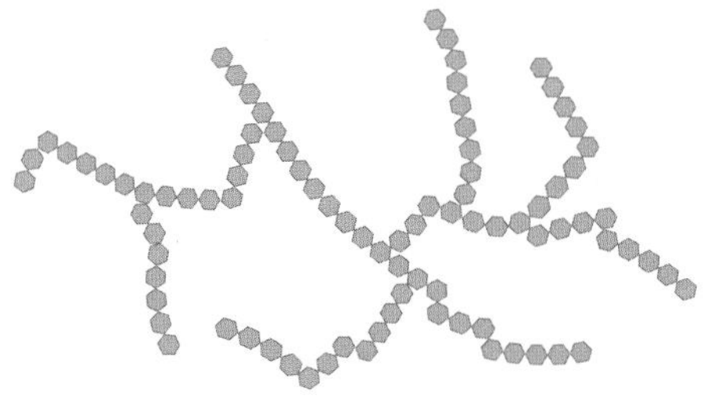

FIGURE 14.2 Amylopectin is a highly branched polysaccharide that is the primary component of starch. Plants store energy as starch. When the plant cells require energy, the plant hydrolyzes the starch, releasing glucose subunits.

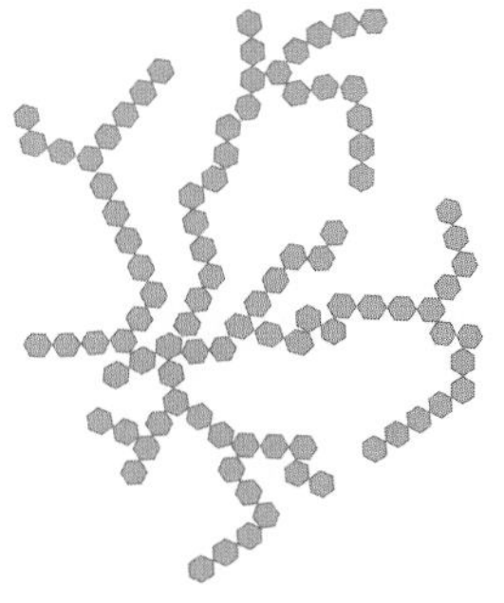

FIGURE 14.3 Glycogen is a highly branched polysaccharide. It is used as a form of energy storage in animals. Because it is so similar to amylopectin, it is sometimes referred to as animal starch.

Gastronomy Point

Prebiotics and Probiotics Oligosaccharides have become popular additives to foods recently because they act as prebiotics. Prebiotics are the nondigestible food ingredients—mostly oligosaccharides—that probiotic bacteria thrive on. Together prebiotics and probiotics can help to maintain a healthy digestive system. Similar to fiber, prebiotics are processed through the digestive system and fermented in the colon through bacterial activity. The fermentation process helps the growth of "healthy" gut bacteria.

Types of Sugars and Sweeteners

Foods and food products contain many different types of sugars. Some are naturally occurring, whereas others are added. In addition, many types of sugar substitutes, or sweeteners, are used in food products. Sugar substitutes can be helpful for those trying to lower their sugar intake, but not all sugar substitutes are lower in energy. Some sweeteners are still pending approval. They have not yet been recognized as **Generally Recognized as Safe (GRAS)** by the Food and Drug Administration (FDA).

The three basic classifications of compounds that add sweetness to foods are caloric sweeteners (of which table sugar is one), artificial sweeteners (those not found in nature), and sugar alcohols.[3,7,8] Food manufacturers supply products using a combination of many different natural and artificial sweeteners, which leads to some differences in use and preference.[1,3] **Table 14.1** lists the content and attributes of many sweeteners.

Generally Recognized as Safe (GRAS) A designation given to a food or drug by the Food and Drug Administration (FDA) when it is approved for public use.

caloric sweetener Substance that gives a pleasant sensation of sweetness to foods and that can be absorbed and yield energy in the body. Includes simple sugars, sugar alcohols, and high-fructose corn syrup.

Caloric or Nutritive Sweeteners

Digestible carbohydrates that provide energy are called **caloric sweeteners**, or nutritive sweeteners.[8]

Table Sugar

Table sugar, also known as refined granulated sugar, is produced from sugarcane (see **Figure 14.4**) by the multistep process described earlier. The sugarcane is harvested and then sent to a sugar mill (see **Figure 14.5**). The stalk of the plant is ground to release the sugar. The sugar is then boiled in water until it thickens into a syrup from which the sugar crystallizes. The crystals are then spun in a centrifuge. A portion of the molasses that is produced is removed to produce raw sugar, which is then crystallized, dried and packaged.

Beet sugar is processed in a similar process. The natural sugar stored in the beet root is separated from the rest of the plant material and boiled for extraction. It is filtered and then allowed to crystallize.

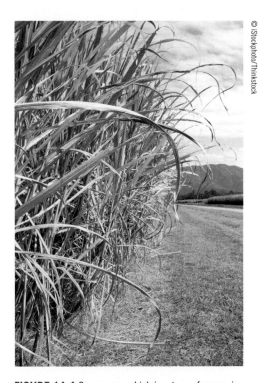

FIGURE 14.4 Sugarcane, which is a type of grass, is the world's largest crop. The main product of sugarcane is sucrose, which accumulates in the stalk. The sucrose is extracted and purified in specialized mill factories.

Molasses

Molasses is the filtrate that remains after sucrose crystals have been removed from the sugarcane juice. After the first crystallization process, the molasses remaining is sweet and light colored (see **Figure 14.6**). After each cycle of crystallization, the molasses becomes darker and bitterer and increases in mineral content. The darkest molasses is called *blackstrap molasses*.

TABLE 14.1
Comprehensive Sweetener Chart

Sweetener	Sweetness Relative to Sugar (Sucrose = 1.0)	Energy (kcal/g)	Attributes	Functionality in Food Products	Effect on Blood Sugar and Metabolism
Nutritive Sweeteners					
Sucrose (white table sugar)	1.0	4.0	Bulking agent Texture enhancer Substrate for yeast Control of crystallization Good humectant Inhibition of starch gelatinization and protein denaturation	Extends shelf life of baked goods through moisture retention. Achieves moist, fine crumb in cakes. Lowers freezing point in frozen dairy products. Enhances and balances flavor. Enhances mouth feel in beverages.	Increases blood sugar. Too much in diet may be linked to obesity.
Fructose	1.1–1.7	4.0	Low glycemic index Reducing sugar Good humectant	Controls surface cracking in cookies.	Increases blood sugar.
Lactose	0.2–0.6	4.0	Bulking agent Reducing sugar Flow agent	Induces Maillard browning in baked goods.	Increases blood sugar.
Polyol (Sugar Alcohols)					
Xylitol	1.0	2.4	Good humectant High negative heat of solution Does not promote tooth decay	Enhances cooling effect. Provides moisture to baked goods. Promotes glossiness of frostings.	Increases blood sugar. Partially absorbed in small intestine; unabsorbed sugar alcohols may be metabolized by bacteria in the gastrointestinal tract.
Maltitol	0.9	2.1	Similar solubility, melting point, and sweetness as sucrose Low hygroscopicity	Maintains plasticity of gum. Base ingredient for hard candy.	Increases blood sugar. Partially absorbed in small intestine; unabsorbed sugar alcohols may be metabolized by bacteria in the gastrointestinal tract.
Erythritol	0.7	0.2	Noncaloric (0.2 kcal/g) High digestive tolerance Zero glycemic index Does not promote tooth decay Good heat and acid stability High negative heat of solution	Improves baking stability and shelf life. Adds bulk and body to dairy products. Freezing point depression in dairy products. Produces characteristic glass, texture, snap, and melt in calorie-reduced chocolate.	Increases blood sugar. Partially absorbed in small intestine; unabsorbed sugar alcohols may be metabolized by bacteria in the gastrointestinal tract.
Mannitol	0.7	1.6	Low hygroscopicity Chelates iron and copper ions	Dusting agent on gum. Prevents stickiness on hard candy.	Increases blood sugar. Partially absorbed in small intestine; unabsorbed sugar alcohols may be metabolized by bacteria in the gastrointestinal tract.
Sorbitol	0.5	2.6	Good humectant Chelates iron and copper ions	Aids in compressibility of tablets. Helps control water activity in food systems. Crystal inhibitor in frozen desserts.	Increases blood sugar. Partially absorbed in small intestine; unabsorbed sugar alcohols may be metabolized by bacteria in the gastrointestinal tract.

Sweetener	Sweetness Relative to Sugar (Sucrose = 1.0)	Energy (kcal/g)	Attributes	Functionality in Food Products	Effect on Blood Sugar and Metabolism
Isomalt	0.5	2.1	Low hygroscopicity Inhibits moisture absorption Low cooling effect	Achieves crisp texture in baked goods. Used to create cake decorations and dessert garnishes.	Increases blood sugar. Partially absorbed in small intestine; unabsorbed sugar alcohols may be metabolized by bacteria in the gastrointestinal tract.
Lactitol	0.4	2	Similar properties to sugar Low cooling effect Low hygroscopicity	Highly versatile sweetener. Improves shelf life and stability of confections.	Increases blood sugar. Partially absorbed in small intestine; unabsorbed sugar alcohols may be metabolized by bacteria in the gastrointestinal tract.
Non-nutritive Sweeteners					
Saccharin	300–600	0	Heat stable Good solubility and stability Bitter, metallic aftertaste	Used in diet beverages, jelly, baked goods, chewing gum.	No effect. Not digested or absorbed.
Aspartame	160–220	0	Can leave a lingering sweet aftertaste Enhances fruit flavors Unstable to prolonged heat, although available in encapsulated form May hydrolyze at pH > 5 Most stable at pH 3–5 Subject to Maillard browning	Used in carbonated beverages, dry beverage mixes, frozen desserts, and fillings. Enhances fruity and citrus beverage flavors.	No effect. Digested and absorbed. Must have warning for those with PKU.
Neotame	7,000–13,000	0	Good stability Slow onset Slight lingering taste Flavor masking/ enhancing properties	Sweetener in carbonated and still beverages, dairy products, and bakery products. Flavor enhancing effects in chewing gum.	No effect. Not digested or absorbed.
Acesulfame K	200	0	Stable over a wide range of temperatures and pH Readily soluble	Excellent heat stability in baked goods. Used in dry beverage mixes, confections, carbonated soft drinks, chewing gum, dry dessert mixes, and baked goods.	No effect. Not digested or absorbed.
Sucralose	400–800	0	Heat and pH stability Similar onset and duration as sucrose Long shelf-life	Used in baked goods, extruded products, and beverages. Stable during ultra high temperature (UHT) processing and pasteurization.	No effect. Not digested or absorbed.
Stevia (Rebaudioside A or Reb-A)	300	0	Heat and pH stability Non yeast-fermentable substrate Low hygroscopicity No Maillard reaction	Used in dry beverage mixes, confections, carbonated soft drinks.	No effect. Digested and absorbed.

Sources: Data from Bennion M, Scheule B. *Introductory foods.* 13th ed. Columbus, OH: Prentice Hall; 2010; Higashiyama T. Novel functions and applications of trehalose. *Pure Appl Chem.* 2002;74(7):1263–1269; American Heart Association. Sugars 101. 2010. Available at: http://www.americanheart.org. Accessed December 28, 2010; U.S. Food and Drug Administration. Artificial sweeteners: No calories … Sweet! *FDA Consumer Magazine.* July–August 2006. Available at: http://www.fda.gov/fdac/features/2006/406_sweetners.html. Accessed February 21, 2011; Calorie Control Council. Information About Aspartame. 2005. Available at: http://www.aspartame.org. Accessed February 11, 2010; McNeil Nutritionals. Splenda No Calorie Sweetener Fact Sheet. 2011. Available at: http://www.splenda.com. Accessed February 11, 2011; and American Academy of Family Physicians. Stevia Sweeteners: What You Need to Know. 2010. Available at: http://familydoctor.org/online/famdocen/home/healthy/food/general-nutrition/1006/1010.html. Accessed March 11, 2010.

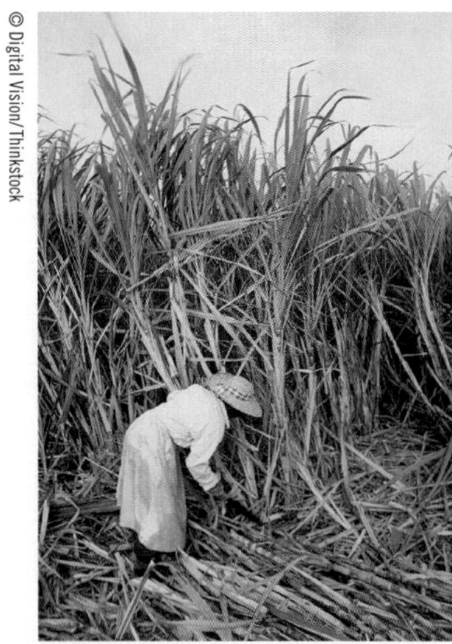

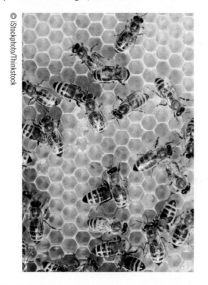
© Digital Vision/Thinkstock

FIGURE 14.5 Mills extract the raw sugar from freshly harvested canes. The raw sugar is then further refined to produce white sugar, which is 99% sucrose.

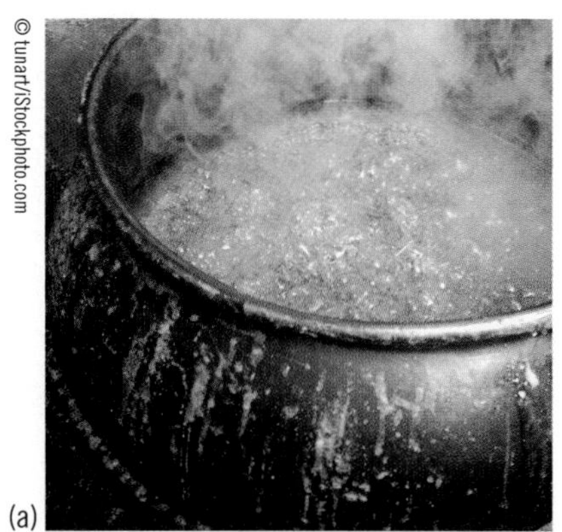
© tunart/iStockphoto.com

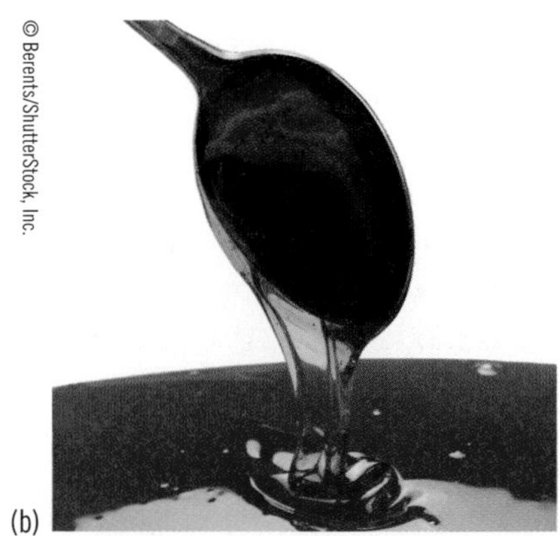
© Berents/ShutterStock, Inc.

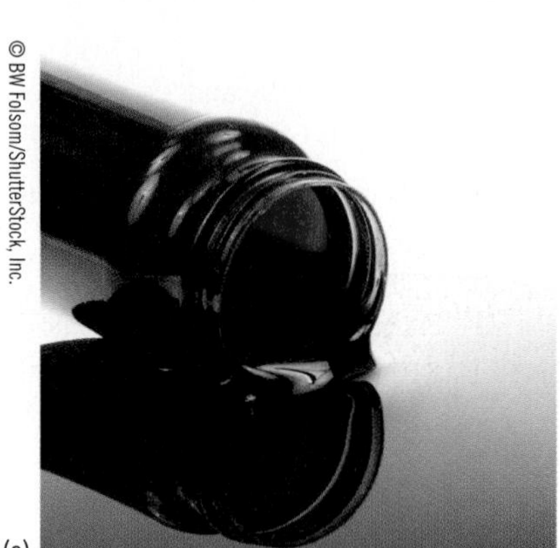
© BW Folsom/ShutterStock, Inc.

FIGURE 14.6 (a) The crystallization process. (b) The result of the first crystallization and boiling of sugar crystals is a light-colored, viscous molasses. It has a high sugar content because it is from the first processing of the canes. (c) Blackstrap molasses is produced after the third boiling of the sugar syrup. By this point, the majority of the sucrose from the original juice has been removed. Blackstrap molasses contains trace amounts of vitamins and is a significant source of several minerals, such as calcium, magnesium, potassium, and iron. Because of its vitamin and mineral content, blackstrap molasses is sold as a health supplement and often is added to animal feed.

© iStockphoto/Thinkstock

FIGURE 14.7 Honeybees produce honey from flower nectar. The bees transform the nectar into honey through a process of regurgitation and then store it in wax honeycombs inside the beehive. Beekeepers encourage overproduction of honey so the excess can be taken from the colony. Honey has approximately the same relative sweetness as that of granulated sugar.

Honey

Honey starts out as flower nectar, which is then harvested by honeybees, modified in their bodies, regurgitated into the wax cells of the honeycomb in the beehive, and concentrated by evaporation (see **Figure 14.7**). Honey is about 17% water; however, when stored, it tends to crystallize out of its liquid solution. This process is easily reversed by heating. Honey has a variety of carbohydrates, including fructose, glucose, maltose, and sucrose. According to the FDA, honey that contains more than 8% sucrose is considered adulterated. The USDA has set various grades for honey based on the product's moisture content, minimum total solids, flavor, aroma, and clarity. In recent years, crop pollinators and honey manufacturers have been concerned about the effects of colony collapse disorder, which is discussed in **Special Topic 14.1**.

Special Topic 14.1

Honeybees in Trouble

Debra Silverman, MS, RD

The honeybee population (see **Figure A**) in the United States has experienced escalating losses since 2006.[1,2] The losses have been blamed on colony collapse disorder (CCD), although scientists are still unclear on exactly what causes it. Pollination of crops by honeybees contributes $14 billion annually to U.S. agriculture.[2] Significant declines could cause traumatic economic consequences for the agricultural industry, affecting the U.S. food supply and creating food shortages.

Colony collapse is characterized by the disappearance of most adult bees from their hives. Some researchers think that infection, compounded by nutritional stress due to habitat loss, may be responsible for CCD. This hypothesis suggests that bees infected with the protozoan *Nosema ceranae* are metabolically stressed. The bees become very hungry and leave their colony to forage but fail to find enough food (a problem that is exacerbated by habitat loss) and lack the energy to return to their colony. Foraging behavior in honeybees is mainly determined by the individual's nutritional status rather than the hive's honey stores. The loss of agricultural land and native vegetation—largely due to real estate development—may be reducing the bees' ability to forage.[1]

Other researchers have found evidence of multiple pathogens in CCD honeybees, indicating compromised immune systems. Neonicotinoid pesticides have also been suspected of contributing to CCD. Some believe that the long-term use of in-hive pesticides used to control honeybee parasites also may be involved. Another study found unusual ribosomal RNA fragments in the guts of CCD bees. These ribosomal fragments indicate viral infection and may serve as biomarkers for CCD colonies.[2]

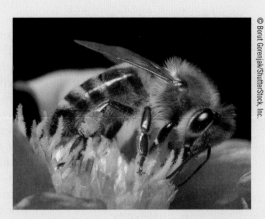

FIGURE A The honeybees that make the type of honey collected by beekeepers are of the genus *Apis*. Honeybees pollinate dozens of important agriculture crops, including rapeseed, broccoli, cucumbers, melons, cotton, and apples, to name just a few. The collapse of honeybee colonies will have a huge economic impact.

CCD losses were estimated at 23% for the winter of 2006–2007 and 36% for 2007–2008.[2] These catastrophic losses highlight the need to increase funding for CCD research. Understanding the causes for colony collapse may prevent devastation of the U.S. agricultural industry and consequential food shortages in future years.

References

1 Naug D. Nutritional stress due to habitat loss may explain recent honeybee colony collapses. *J Bio Con.* 2009;4(7):2369–2372.

2 Johnson RM, Evans JD, Robinson GE, Berenbaum MR. Changes in transcript abundance relating to colony collapse disorder in honeybees (*Apis melliflora*). *PNAS.* 2009;106(35):14790–14795.

Maple Syrup

Maple syrup comes from sap collected from sugar maple trees (see **Figure 14.8**). To produce syrup, water from the sap is evaporated by boiling, yielding a concentration of no more than 35% water. It takes about 40 gallons of sap to yield 1 gallon of maple syrup.

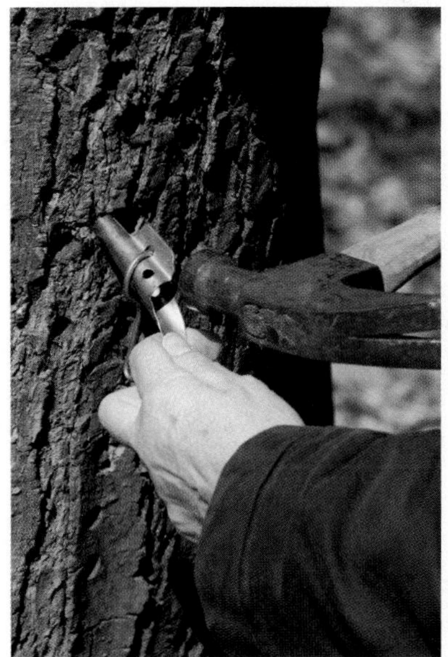

FIGURE 14.8 Maple syrup is made from the sap of sugar maple, red maple, or black maple trees. In cold climates, maple trees store starch in their trunks and roots before winter. In the spring, the starch is converted to sugar, which rises up in sap. The sweet sap can be collected from the trees by drilling holes in the trunks and collecting the sap that is exuded. The sap is then heated, leaving behind a concentrated sugar syrup.

Crystalline Fructose

Crystalline fructose is usually made from corn. Corn is milled to produce cornstarch and then further processed to make corn syrup, which is primarily glucose. Enzymes are added so the glucose is converted into fructose. The fructose crystallizes out of the solution and is then dried and milled.

Crystalline fructose is used primarily by food processors. When it is used in combination with sucrose, it yields a sweeter product than if either sugar were used alone, allowing manufacturers to use less of both sugars. Food scientists and technologists favor pure crystalline fructose because of its functional properties.

Corn Syrup

Corn syrup is produced by adding an enzyme to corn starch and water. The resulting corn syrup consists primarily of glucose, but it also contains D-glucose (dextrose) and maltose. Corn syrup is used as a nonsweet thickener in foods.

High-Fructose Corn Syrup

High-fructose corn syrup (HFCS) starts out as cornstarch and is then chemically or enzymatically converted to glucose and some short polymers of glucose.

stevia A non-nutritive sweetener obtained from the leaves of a South American plant that is 300 times sweeter than sucrose.

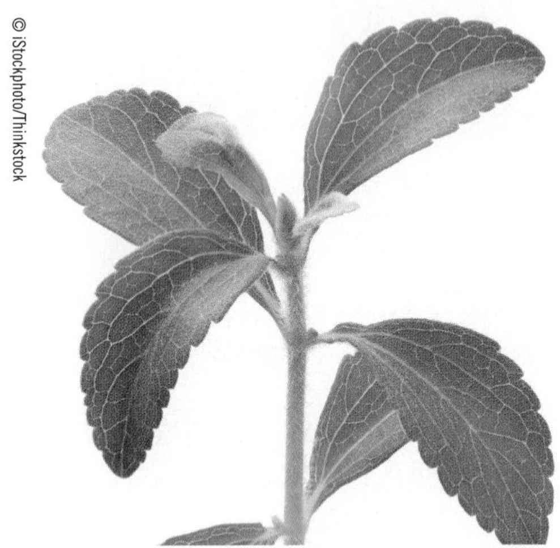

FIGURE 14.9 Stevia is a popular sugar substitute. Because stevia is 300 times sweeter than sugar and has a negligible effect on blood sugar levels, it has gained increased attention as a possible sweetener in low-sugar, low-carbohydrate foods.

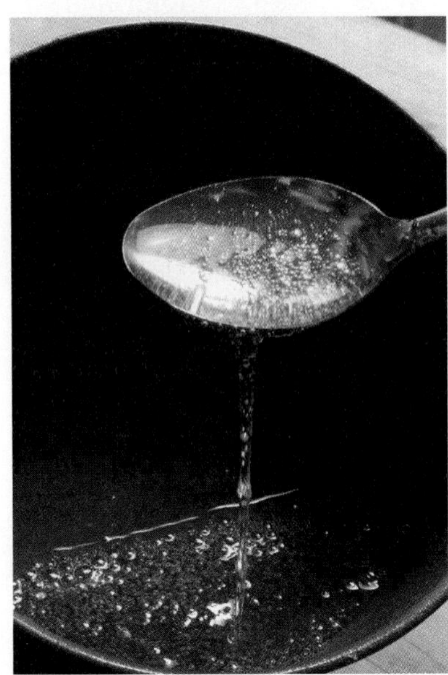

FIGURE 14.10 Invert sugar is a syrup that is a mixture of glucose and fructose. Bakers and candy makers use invert sugar because it is less prone to crystallization.

Another enzyme, glucose isomerase, is then used to convert some of the glucose into fructose, in order to make the syrup sweeter. The final product is about 55% fructose. Its primary use is as a sweetener in sodas and fruit-flavored drinks. HFCS is the most common added sweetener in processed foods and beverages.

HFCS has been linked to obesity due to the fact that it is used in so many products, especially processed foods and soft drinks.[3,4,8] Consumption of large amounts of HFCS, along with other types of sugar, has also been linked to dental caries, poor nutrition, and increased triglyceride levels. However, the evidence is insufficient to state that HFCS is less healthy than are other types of added sweeteners. According to the Academy of Nutrition and Dietetics, studies comparing HFCS and sucrose have found no significant differences in a person's fasting blood glucose, insulin, leptin, and ghrelin levels. These studies further suggest that the type of added sugar (sucrose, HFCS, honey, or fruit juice concentrate) is not of concern but rather the amount of total calories that these sweeteners contribute to the overall diet. Both the American Medical Association and the Academy of Nutrition and Dietetics made statements in 2008 that HFCS does not appear to contribute to obesity any more than other caloric sweeteners.[9] More research is underway to assess the caloric contribution of HFCS in the diet.[10]

Trehalose

Trehalose is a disaccharide of two glucose molecules. In nature, it can be synthesized by bacteria, fungi, plants, and invertebrates. Extracting trehalose used to be difficult and costly, but an inexpensive extraction technology has been developed so it can be extracted from starch.

The enzyme that digests trehalose is only found in the small intestine. Consequently, trehalose is not digested for 2 to 3 hours after eaten, leading to lower rises in blood glucose levels, which make it a good alternative sweetener for those with diabetes. The stability of this disaccharide makes it attractive for use in the food industry.[11–13]

Tagatose

Tagatose is a useful molecule that has the same bulk as sugar and that is almost as sweet. It is a natural sweetener that is present in only small amounts in fruits and dairy products, but it can be made commercially from galactose through an enzymatic process. It has only 1.5 calories per gram because less than 20% of ingested tagatose is absorbed in the small intestine. Although tagatose is digested in the same way that fructose is, its limited absorption means that it is metabolized mainly in the large intestine. The short chain fatty acids in tagatose promote the growth of bacteria that have been shown to improve colon health. Consequently, the prebiotic potential of tagatose is often stressed for the foods that use this sugar replacer.[11,12]

Stevia

Stevia is an herbal sweetener extracted from a South American shrub of the Sunflower family (see **Figure 14.9**). Stevia glycosides are 250–300 times sweeter than sugar. Stevia was recently granted the status as GRAS.[8]

Invert Sugar

Invert sugar is a clear, liquid form of sugar that is sweeter than granulated sugar (see **Figure 14.10**). It is made commercially by dissolving sucrose in water, heating the solution, and then adding an acid, such as cream of tartar, to yield two equal portions of glucose (dextrose) and fructose (levulose). Because this type of sugar resists crystallization, it often is used by professional confectioners who require a sugar that yields a smooth texture.

Identifying Added Sugars in Foods

Sugar from natural sources is found in the American diet from sources such as fruit (fructose) and milk (lactose) or as table sugar added during the processing or preparation of a food product.[14] It often is difficult for consumers to tell by looking at the Nutrition Facts label if a food contains added sugar because the line for "sugars" includes both those that are found naturally in the food and those that have been added during processing. However, even though the amounts of added sugars are not identified on the label, savvy consumers can spot added sugars on the ingredients list by looking for the following ingredients:

- Brown sugar
- Corn sweetener
- Corn syrup
- Fruit juice concentrates
- High-fructose corn syrup
- Honey
- Invert sugar
- Malt sugar
- Molasses
- Raw sugar
- Sugar
- Sugar molecules ending in "ose" (dextrose, fructose, glucose, lactose, maltose, sucrose)
- Syrup

non-nutritive sweeteners Substances that give a pleasant sensation of sweetness to foods, but that supply limited or no energy to the body; also called artificial or alternative sweeteners.

saccharin A non-nutritive sweetener that is about 300 to 700 times sweeter than sucrose.

aspartame A non-nutritive sweetener that is 200 times sweeter than sucrose.

phenylketonuria (PKU) A rare genetic disease caused by a lack or deficiency of the enzyme phenylalanine hydroxylase that breaks down the essential amino acid phenylalanine.

Artificial Sweeteners

Artificial sweeteners also are called low-calorie sweeteners or **non-nutritive sweeteners** because they provide virtually no energy. They are used in foods to control weight and blood glucose levels and to prevent dental caries.[14,15]

Saccharin

The oldest artificial sweetener on the market is **saccharin**. Discovered in 1879 by an American chemist, it is approximately 300 to 400 times sweeter than sugar. The safety of saccharin has been under investigation for 50 years. Its safety and that of other sugar substitutes are discussed in **Special Topic 14.2**. It does not affect blood sugar. It is marketed as tabletop sweeteners Sweet 'N Low, Sugar Twin, and Necta Sweet.[16]

Aspartame

The sweetener **aspartame** was discovered by accident in 1965. Made of two amino acids, phenylalanine and aspartic acid, it is approximately 200 times sweeter than sugar. The FDA requires that foods containing aspartame have the following label: "Phenylketonurics: Contains Phenylalanine" (see **Figure 14.11**). Individuals with **phenylketonuria (PKU)** cannot metabolize phenylalanine; it can build up in the body and cause harm.

Due to its sweetness, only small amounts are necessary to sweeten foods. It is found in 6,000 products in the United States. The majority of aspartame consumption, 70%, is from soft drinks. It has been the most studied sweetener, with over 200 studies indicating that the long-term consumption of aspartame does not cause health problems. It does not affect blood sugar.

Aspartame is not stable at high temperatures. Consequently, it has limited use in baking unless it is added at the end of the cooking cycle. It is marketed as the tabletop sweeteners NutraSweet and Equal.[16,17]

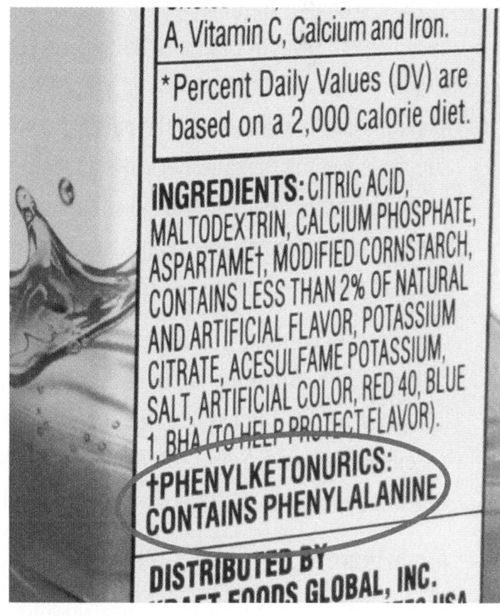

FIGURE 14.11 People with phenylketonuria do not have the enzyme needed to metabolize the amino acid phenylalanine. In the absence of this enzyme, phenylalanine levels can build up in the body, resulting in damage to the central nervous system and ultimately brain damage. People with phenylketonuria must read food and beverage levels to ensure they do not consume foods that contain phenylalanine, which includes foods sweetened with aspartame.

Special Topic 14.2

Safety of Non-nutritive Sweeteners: A History

SeAnne Safaii, PhD, RD, LD

Non-nutritive sweeteners can help consumers reduce calorie intake, control weight, manage chronic diseases, and prevent cavities. Because of the improved quality of non-nutritive sweeteners, the food industry has seen a marked rise in their use.

Much controversy surrounds the safety and consumption of non-nutritive sweeteners. They have been around since the 1950s, but between 1999 and 2004 more than 6,000 new products containing non-nutritive sweeteners were launched. They are in so many products that most people consume them without even knowing it. The following are the six FDA-approved non-nutritive sweeteners:

- Saccharin (approved for use prior to the Delaney Clause, which was passed in 1958 to give the FDA control over the use of non-nutritive sweeteners)
- Aspartame (approved for use in 1981)
- Acesulfame potassium, or "ace-K" (approved for use in 1988)
- Sucralose (approved for use in 1998)
- Neotame (approved for use in 2002)
- Rebaudioside A (Reb-A), a highly purified form of stevia (approved for use in 2008)

An *acceptable daily intake (ADI)* has been established for each additive. The ADI is the amount of each additive that can be consumed on a daily basis over a lifetime without risk to health.[1–3] Non-nutritive sweeteners are classified as additives and are often combined with nutritive sweeteners and/or sugar alcohols for volume or desired flavor.

Saccharin

In 1977, research showed that ingestion of saccharin in male rats caused bladder tumors. Because of this, the FDA proposed a ban on saccharin based on the Delaney Clause of the Federal Food, Drug, and Cosmetic Act, which was enacted in 1958. The Delaney Clause prohibits the addition of any chemical to the human food supply that causes cancer in humans or animals. At the time, saccharin was the only artificial sweetener available on the market, and the public did not want diet products removed. Congress intervened and allowed saccharin to remain in the food supply as long as the label carried the following warning: "Use of this product may be hazardous to your health. This product contains saccharin which has been determined to cause cancer in laboratory animals."[4] Since then, more than 30 human studies have been completed; the results found in rats have not been replicated in humans. The result has been that saccharin is now deemed safe for human consumption.[4] The ADI for saccharin is 5 mg/kg body weight, and products cannot exceed 12 mg per fluid ounce in beverages and 30 mg per serving in processed foods.

One problem with the original study on rats is that it used amounts of saccharin that were hundreds of times higher than would normally be ingested by humans. In 2000, the National Toxicology Program (NTP) of the National Institutes of Health recommended that saccharin be removed from the list of potential carcinogens. A warning no longer appears on saccharin-containing products.[2] However, one danger of saccharin remains. Saccharin belongs to a class of compounds known as sulfonamides, which can cause allergic reactions in individuals who cannot tolerate sulfa drugs. Reactions can include headaches, breathing difficulties, skin eruptions, and diarrhea.

Aspartame

Aspartame, or L-α-aspartyl-L-phenylalanine methyl ester, was approved for use as a sweetener by the FDA in 1981 and expanded for use in carbonated beverages in 1983. It has been approved for use in over 100 countries. An ADI of 50 mg/kg of body weight has been established for aspartame. This would be equivalent to consuming 20 diet soft drinks per day. Aspartame is hydrolyzed in the gut into aspartic acid, methanol, and phenylalanine. Because aspartame breaks down into phenylalanine, the FDA requires that foods containing it carry a warning label for people with phenylketonuria (PKU), a rare condition in which a person is born without the ability to properly break down the amino acid phenylalanine. Phenylalanine is also found in commonly consumed foods. For example, a serving of nonfat milk contains 6 times more phenylalanine and 13 times more aspartic acid than a beverage sweetened 100% with aspartame.[2,5]

Aspartame is one of the most controversial artificial sweeteners. Numerous websites, books, and articles state various reasons why aspartame should not be consumed. A comprehensive review of its safety was recently published by the Scientific Committee on Food.[5,6] The authors concluded that current intakes of aspartame are well below the ADI and that aspartame is not a carcinogen, nor is it associated with neurobehavioral disorders.

Acesulfame K

Acesulfame K, or 5,6-dimethyl-1,2,3-oxathiazind-4(3H)-one-2,2-dioxide, has been an approved sweetener since 1988 and yet most people are not even aware of its existence in their foods and beverages. On ingredient labels, it is listed as acesulfame K, acesulfame potassium, Ace-K, or Sunette. Pharmacokinetic studies have demonstrated that 95% of the sweetener consumed is excreted unchanged in the urine. More than 90 studies have been conducted on the safety of Acesulfame K and have shown it to be safe when consumed in moderation.[2] The ADI has been established at 17 mg/kg of body weight.

Sucrolose

Sucralose, or trichlorogalactosucrose, was approved for limited use in 1998. In 1999, it was given approval for use as a general-purpose sweetener. Because sucralose is one of the newer artificial sweeteners to hit the market, fewer long-term studies of its safety have been conducted (compared to saccharin and aspartame). Sucralose is poorly absorbed, and most of it is excreted unchanged in the feces. The FDA reviewed research studies in humans and animals and concluded that sucralose does not present a carcinogenic, reproductive, or neurological risk to humans.[3] An ADI of 5 mg/kg of body weight has been established.

Neotame

In 2002, the FDA approved a new sweetener called Neotame (N-[N-3,3-dimethylbutyl)-L-α-aspartyl]-L-phenylalanine-1-methyl ester). Neotame is chemically related to aspartame, but it does not pose a danger to individuals with PKU because such a small amount is needed for sweetness. It is much sweeter than aspartame, having a sweetness approximately 7,000 to 13,000 times that of sucrose. Although researchers have looked at possible links to cancer as well as reproductive and developmental toxicity, human and animal studies have failed to find evidence of these effects.[3] An ADI of 2 mg/kg of body weight has been established.

Stevia

Stevia, or rebaudioside A or Reb-A, was approved for use in 2008. Only its highly purified form, rebaudioside A (Reb-A), has received FDA approval. (Stevia has been sold as a dietary supplement for many years. Dietary supplements do not have to go through the FDA approval process.) Reb-A-based sweeteners are considered safe for consumption as tabletop sweeteners and as ingredients in foods and beverages. The studies on which the FDA based its approval were specific to Reb-A; therefore, its approval is only for this form and does not extend to other stevia-derived sweeteners.

Stevia has not been shown to affect blood pressure or blood glucose levels; however, health risks could develop in people with diabetes or high blood pressure if stevia is combined with diabetes or blood pressure–lowering drugs.[1,6] Additionally, limited research is available on the effects of stevia on pregnant or breastfeeding women; thus, it is recommended that these women avoid using stevia sweeteners of any kind.[1]

References

1 Mayo Clinic. Diabetes Nutrition: Including Sweets in Your Meal Plan. 2008. Available at: http://mayoclinic.com/health/diabetes-nutrition/DA00130/NSECTIONGROUP=2. Accessed February 24, 2011.

2 Kroger M, Meister K, Kava R. Low-calorie sweeteners and other sugar substitutes: A review of the safety issues. *Comp Rev Food Sci Food Safety.* 2006;5:35–47.

3 International Programme on Chemical Safety. WHO Food Additives Series S: 52 Neotame. 2004. Available at: http://www.inchem.org/documents/jecfa/jecmono/v52je08.htm. Accessed April 27, 2010.

4 Sugar Substitutes: Americans Opt for Sweetness and Lite. 2006. Available at: http://www.sc.edu/healthycarolina/pdf/facstaffstu/nutrition/SugarSubstitutes.pdf. Accessed February 11, 2011.

5 Sugar alcohols fact sheet. Food Insight. 2008. Available at: http://www.foodinsight.org/Resources/Detail.aspx?topic=Sugar_Alcohols_Fact_Sheet. Accessed February 20, 2011.

6 American Academy of Family Physicians. Stevia Sweeteners: What You Need to Know. 2010. Available at: http://familydoctor.org/online/famdocen/home/healthy/food/general-nutrition/1006/1010.html. Accessed March 11, 2010.

acesulfame-K A non-nutritive artificial sweetener that is 150 to 200 times sweeter than sugar that enhances and sustains the sweet taste of foods and beverages. It is heat stable, so it can be used in baked products.

sucralose A non-nutritive sweetener made from sucrose that is 600 times sweeter than sugar.

neotame A sweetener that is 8,000 times sweeter than sugar. It is heat stable and can be used in baking.

sugar alcohols Also called polyols, compounds formed from monosaccharides by replacing a hydrogen atom with a hydroxyl group. Used as nutritive sweeteners.

Acesulfame-K

Acesulfame potassium, or **acesulfame-K**, was discovered in Germany in 1967. It is 200 times sweeter than sugar. Because it is not digested, it is non-caloric and does not affect blood sugar. Due to its stability in heat, it can be used in cooking and baking. It is marketed as Sunnette in food products and as Sweet One or Swiss Sweet as a tabletop sweetener.[16,18]

Sucralose

Sucralose is derived from sugar but has had chlorine atoms added. It is 600 times sweeter than sugar. It is stable under extreme pH conditions and at high temperatures, so it can be used in baking. (It is the most heat stable of all the non-nutritive sweeteners.) Because the absorption of sucralose is limited, it adds no caloric value to foods and does not affect blood sugar. It is currently used in over 4,500 products, including soft drinks. It is sold under the brand name Splenda.[16,19]

Neotame

The most recently approved non-nutritive sweetener is **neotame**. It is 8,000 times sweeter than sugar. Although similar to aspartame, products containing neotame do not have to carry the warning label for PKU because the amount of phenylalanine in it is negligible. Neotame is heat stable and can be used in baking.[16,20,21]

Sugar Alcohols

Sugar alcohols, also called *polyols*, are a group of lower-calorie, carbohydrate-based sweeteners. These compounds are formed commercially from monosaccharides by replacing a hydrogen atom with a hydroxyl group. They also occur naturally in fruits and vegetables. Polyols are considered nutritive sweeteners, but they provide only about half as many calories as sugar.

The body absorbs polyols slower than other sugars, which is important for diabetics. They are used as a food ingredient, often to replace sugar, in many sugar-free and reduced-calorie foods because they improve bulk, mouth feel, and texture compared to low-calorie sweeteners. The substitution of polyols for sugar is in equal amounts; that is, 1 cup for 1 cup.

Foods sweetened with polyols or sugar alcohols may be labeled as "sugar free." The FDA has approved the use of the health claim "does not promote tooth decay" for sugar-free products that contain polyols, which includes many gums.[10,15,22–24] The caloric values of polyols range from 0.2 to 3.0 calories per gram. The following polyols are commonly used in processed foods:

- Sorbitol
- Mannitol
- Xylitol
- Erythritol, Erythritol
- Isomalt (Palatinat)
- Lacititol
- Maltitol
- HSH (hydrogenated starch hydrolysates)

Future Artificial Sweeteners

A number of new non-nutritive sweeteners are currently under review by the FDA:

- *Alitame* is a peptide that is about 2,000 times sweeter than sugar. It has minimal caloric value because of the miniscule amounts necessary to achieve sweetness.

- *Cyclamates* are 30 times sweeter than sugar, but they were banned from use in the United States due to a study implicating sodium cyclamate to bladder cancer in rats. Cyclamates are still used as sweeteners in other countries.
- *Neohesperdine dihydrochalcone*, which is derived from grapefruit rinds, is 1,500 times sweeter than sugar. It is currently approved in the United States as a flavor modifier, not as a sweetener.
- *Thaumatin* is a small protein extracted from an African berry that is 2,000 times sweeter than sugar. It is approved by the FDA as a flavor modifier but not as a sweetener.
- *Glycyrrhizin*, derived from licorice extract, is 30 times sweeter as sugar. It is not yet approved as a sweetener, but it is approved as a flavor enhancer.[4,8]

Roles of Sugar in Food Preparation

Sugar serves many important functions in food preparation by interacting with molecules of protein or starch during baking and cooking processes:[4]

- It tenderizes food by absorbing water, inhibiting gluten development in flour, and delaying starch gelatinization.
- It helps delay coagulation in egg custards and other baked protein dishes.
- It incorporates air into shortening in the creaming process.
- It caramelizes and undergoes Maillard reactions under heat, imparting cooked and baked foods with a pleasing color and aroma.
- It speeds the growth of yeast by acting as a food source.
- It helps regulate the gelling of fruit jellies and preserves.
- It prevents spoilage.
- It recrystallizes to varying degrees, allowing for a wide variety of candies and the smoothness and flavor of ice cream.

Sugar easily changes form in food preparation. With the application of heat, sugar melts, changing into the liquid state. Sugar can undergo severe chemical breakdown, as seen in carmelization, or it can be subject to milder changes, such as hydrolysis. Hydrolysis of sucrose results in the formation of equal amounts of glucose and fructose, or *invert sugar*. The specific term for this hydrolysis is called *inversion*. A mixture of sucrose and invert sugar will crystallize less easily than will sucrose by itself. Therefore, when making crystalline candies, cream of tartar is often added to ensure that a moderate amount of invert sugar will be formed, which helps achieve a smooth texture. A slow rate of cooking also results in inversion, whereas fast boiling will allow less time for inversion. Another method of causing hydrolysis is by adding the enzyme invertase. This enzyme is used commercially to catalyze sucrose inversion.[3,8]

Baking

Sugar plays a number of important roles in the baking process.

Egg Foams

Sugar serves as a whipping aid to help stabilize beaten egg foams in cakes. As sugar crystals disperse among the proteins, they help delay protein coagulation. This causes protein bonds to form at a higher temperature, which helps the cakes set and form their solid structure.[4]

Innovation Point

New (Old) Natural Sweetener: Agave Nectar Once used by the Aztecs to flavor food and drinks, agave nectar comes from the blue agave plant that thrives in the volcanic soils of southern Mexico. In recent years, it has gained in popularity as a natural sweetener. Agaves are large, spiny succulents. It takes 7 to 10 years for the agave to grow large enough for sap to be extracted from its core. The sap is filtered and heated to a low temperature to break it down into sugars. Because of its high fructose content (70–80%), it is sweeter than table sugar. The taste of agave nectar is similar to honey, yet it has the same functions as sugar in browning, moisture retention, softening, and food preservation.

Innovation Point

Fiber Fiber can be used as a texturizing agent and may serve as a major sugar replacement in baked goods in the future.

Creaming

The creaming process causes sugar crystals to become intermingled with shortening molecules. The sugar's irregular crystals trap very small air cells into the shortening. During baking, the air cells expand when filled with carbon dioxide and other gases, promoting lightness.[4]

Leavening

Sugar provides a source of nourishment for yeast growth. Moisture and warmth cause yeast cells to break down sugar so carbon dioxide gas is released at a faster rate than if only flour were present. Thus, the leavening process is accelerated in the presence of sugar, and the dough rises at a faster and more consistent rate.[4] **Figure 14.12** shows a cake baked without adequate sugar; note the lack of leavening.

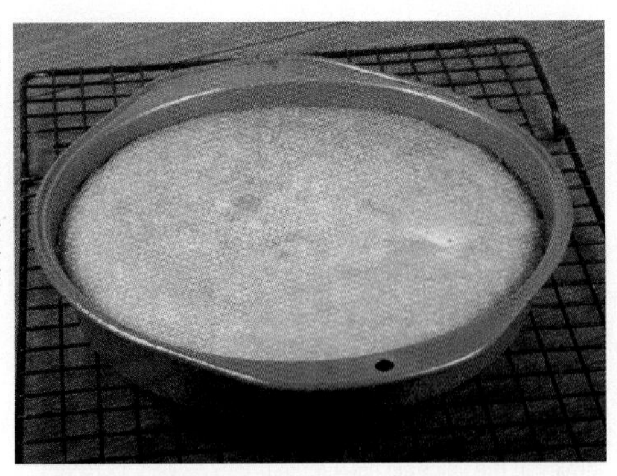

FIGURE 14.12 If enough sugar is not present during the baking process, the resulting cake will be flat and brown because of a lack of leavening.

Gluten Formation

When batters or doughs are mixed, the sugar acts as a tenderizer by absorbing water, which slows gluten development. It does this by competing with gluten-forming proteins for water. The full hydration of proteins is prevented, leaving the batter or dough less rigid. This gives the final baked product a tender crumb and good volume.[4]

Gelatinization

During baking, heat causes starch in flour to absorb liquid and swell. (Recall that this is called *gelatinization*.) As the liquid is absorbed, the batter changes form, entering into a solid state, thus "setting" the cake. Sugar acts to slow gelatinization by competing with the starch for liquid. This raises the temperature required for the cake to set. The leavening agents and sugar produce a fine, uniformly grained cake with a soft, smooth crumb texture.[4]

Caramelization

When sugar is heated above its melting point, it changes from a colorless liquid to a golden brown liquid and develops an appealing flavor and aroma. Sugar contributes to the golden-brown, crisp surface of breads, cakes, and cookies; this surface browning improves moisture retention in baked products, prolonging freshness.[3,8]

Maillard Reactions

When cooked at high oven temperatures, sugar chemically reacts with proteins in the baking product, contributing to the food's browned surface. Recall that the nonenzymatic browning of breads, cakes, and cookies is due to Maillard reactions, which is also called Maillard browning. The more golden brown the surface appears, the higher the sugar content of the baked good.[4]

Candy Making

When sugar and water are combined, at a certain point no more sugar will dissolve unless more water is added or the temperature is raised. This is the basic principle of candy making. As the temperature is raised, more sugar can be added until the new saturation point is reached. As the temperature is then lowered, the solution now has more sugar in it than would have been possible without heating. Because the product has an artificially induced saturation point, it is chemically unstable and will try to correct itself by crystallizing the sugar back into a solid state. Undisturbed cooling will produce large crystals (rock candy), and rapid cooling with agitation will produce small crystals. Crystal formation also can be reduced by adding an acid (e.g., cream of tartar, lemon juice), a fat (e.g., butter, milk, chocolate), or a protein (e.g., egg white, gelatin).

Candies produced from this process of manipulating boiled sugar solutions are classified as crystalline or amorphous. **Crystalline candies** are soft, smooth, and creamy, and the sugar crystals are so tiny that they cannot be felt by the tongue. Fudge, panache, divinity, and creams are all types of crystalline candies (see **Figure 14.13**).[3,8] In contrast, **noncrystalline (amorphous) candies** are, as their name implies, without form. Amorphous candies have a higher concentration of sugar than crystalline candies. Their syrups are so viscous that sugar crystals cannot form. They come in a variety of forms, including chewy caramels and hard brittles (see **Figure 14.14**).[8] Both crystalline and amorphous candies require careful cooking to ensure that the correct final temperature is achieved.

crystalline candy Candy that contains crystals in its final form, such as fudge and fondant.

noncrystalline (amorphous) candy Candy that does not contain crystals, such as taffy and caramels.

bound water The portion of the total water content of a product that is bound to chemicals in food.

Crystalline Candies

The concentration of sugar in crystalline candies is lower than that in amorphous candies; consequently, they are not boiled as long or at as high a temperature. When making crystalline candy, the water is boiled out, creating a concentrated sugar solution. Water often is defined as *bound* or *free*, meaning that a portion of the total water content of a product is either bound to chemicals in food or free to evaporate (become vapor). One of the processes used to reduce the amount of free water in candy is concentration through adding sugar and heating. **Bound water** is less able to take part in chemical reactions, thus increasing the stability of the final food product. Hard candies are stable in dry climates but will rapidly cake under humid conditions.

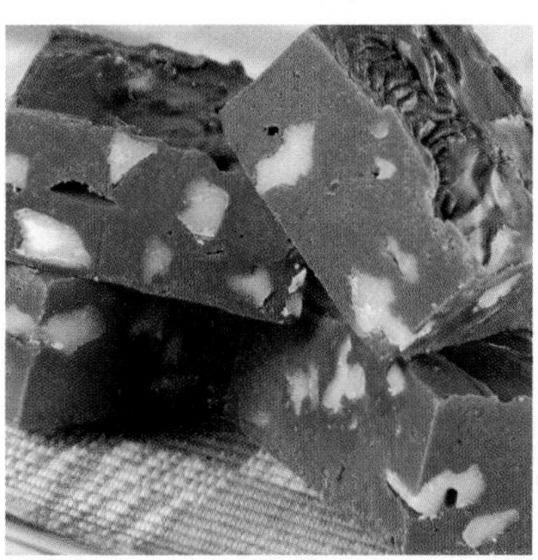

© iStockphoto/Thinkstock

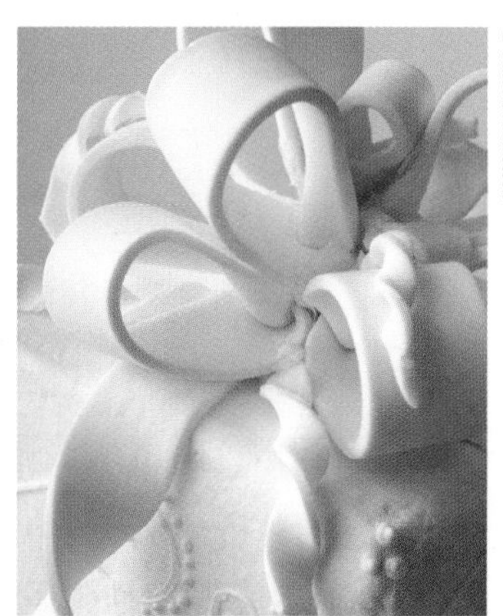

© VStock/Thinkstock

FIGURE 14.13 Crystalline candies have an organized sugar structure that is formed through the process of crystallization. Crystalline candies, such fudge or fondant, are smooth, creamy, and easily chewed.

It is important to use a pan with even heating characteristics to ensure accurate, even temperature readings. A small error of 1 or 2 degrees below the correct temperature will cause the candy to be too soft; conversely, cooking at 1 or 2 degrees above the required temperature will create a crumbly or hard product. Another factor that affects the firmness of crystalline candy is the rate of heating. If a candy is heated too slowly, too much of the sugar will become inverted, and the candy may remain too soft and not set properly.[8] If an acidic ingredient, such as cream of tartar, is present, the rate of heating is extremely important because sugar inversion will occur. A small amount of cream of tartar can have the same effect in a solution heated slowly to the final boiling point as a large amount of cream of tartar in a rapidly heated solution to the same boiling point.

Weather also can influence the outcome of crystalline candy making. If candy is made on a rainy day, the end product may be too soft. This is due to the hygroscopic nature of sugar—it attracts water readily.[4] In extremely humid environments, moisture will be removed from the air and absorbed by the cooling candy. The moisture level in crystalline candy is so critical to the firmness that just small variations in moisture and temperature can affect the end product. To compensate for high humidity, crystalline candies should be cooked to 1 degree higher than the recipe indicates.

The crystalline candy solution should be left undisturbed during cooling. If disturbed, premature crystallization may occur, resulting in a grainy product. If the solution is cooled to room temperature and then beaten, crystallization will occur more slowly, and the product will have a smoother texture.

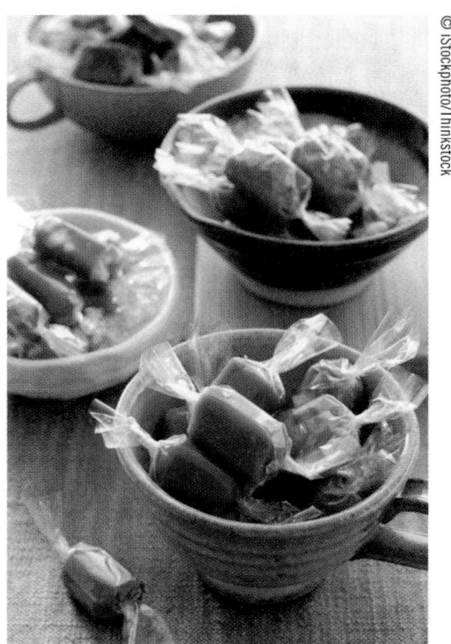

© iStockphoto/Thinkstock

FIGURE 14.14 Amorphous candies usually have higher sugar concentrations than crystalline candies and do not have an organized sugar crystal structure. They may be chewy, hard, or brittle. Caramels, nut brittles, and toffees are examples of amorphous candies.

Noncrystalline Candies

In noncrystalline candies, the sugar does not crystallize. The crystallization process is prevented by (1) cooking to very high temperatures so the finished product hardens quickly, before the crystals have a chance to develop, (2) adding interfering substances (such as butter or corn syrup) that impede crystals from forming, or (3) a combination of these two methods. Noncrystalline candies include brittles, caramels, and taffy.

Impact on Health

Sugar adds pleasure to meals—a taste preference for sweets appears to be inborn.[7] The position of the Academy of Nutrition and Dietetics, based on research evidence, is that dietary sugars are not an independent risk factor for any particular disease, nor do they appear responsible for behavioral changes. Sugars can, however, contribute to acid production in the mouth, which promotes dental caries, and they supply energy (kilocalories) with few nutrients.[22] The connection of sugar to dental caries is explored further in **Special Topic 14.3**.

Special Topic 14.3

Role of Sugar in Dental Caries

Carole Palmer, EdD, RD, LDN

Dental caries is a multifactorial disease that is initiated when acids in the mouth demineralize tooth enamel. Dental plaque, the film that is constantly forming on the chewing surfaces and along the gum line of the teeth, harbors bacteria that feed on dietary carbohydrates. The bacteria metabolize the carbohydrates to acids, which are then excreted onto tooth enamel surfaces. The acids destroy the tooth enamel, and the bacteria then invade the inner tooth, resulting in dental caries.[1]

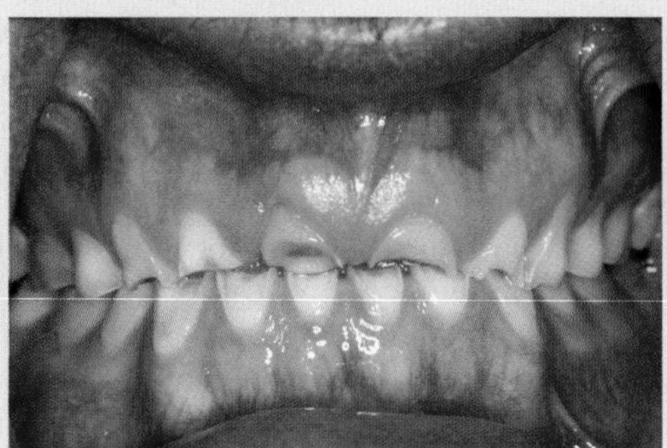

© E.H.Gill/Custom Medical Stock Photo

FIGURE A Acid erosion of the teeth is the loss of tooth structure by acids. Consumption of foods and beverages with a pH below 5.0 may start the process of dental erosion. Of particular concern, are acidic beverages such as carbonated soft drinks, fruit juices, and some wines.

Demineralization of the tooth enamel occurs over time either from this bacteria-moderated mechanism or from direct contact of the tooth enamel with acid-containing foods and beverages or stomach acid. Acid erosion is a slow process (see **Figure A**); any habit that involves prolonged contact between acids and tooth enamel over time is a risk factor for enamel demineralization.

A number of misconceptions exist about the dietary factors responsible for dental caries. One misconception is that any food left on the teeth causes caries. In fact, only foods containing carbohydrates—not fats, proteins, or food fibers—can serve as food sources for acid-producing bacteria. Another common misconception is that sucrose is the primary causative factor of caries and that avoiding "sweets" will prevent dental caries. In fact, all of the simple sugars—fructose, glucose, galactose, maltose, and lactose as well as sucrose—can be cariogenic (caries promoting). Today, the most common sweetener added to food is high fructose corn syrup, which is cariogenic as well. Starch alone is considered less cariogenic than sugar because it must be hydrolyzed in the mouth by salivary amylase into shorter chain sugars before it can be metabolized by caries-causing bacteria and thus may be swallowed before this reaction occurs to any extent.[2,3]

Factors Determining the Cariogenic Potential of Foods

The cariogenic potential of foods is determined by more than merely the types of sugars consumed, however. The *physical form* of the carbohydrate-containing foods may also play a role in cariogenic potential. Because cariogenic bacteria can feed on sugars as long as they are in direct contact with teeth, foods that are less rapidly cleansed from the mouth, such as dried fruits or starch/sugar combinations, are potentially more cariogenic than foods or beverages that are cleared more rapidly, such as fresh fruits, sugared beverages consumed normally (not sipped slowly), and high-fiber foods.[4,5] Starch/sugar combinations may be more cariogenic than sugars alone because their physical form leads to the distribution of small particles throughout the mouth, which may contribute to their retention in the oral cavity.[6]

The most important risk factor for dental caries development, however, is the *overall pattern of eating* rather than the types or amounts of cariogenic foods consumed.[7] This is because the total overall time that the teeth are exposed to acids from any source is the greatest risk factor for caries development.[8,9] Therefore, an eating plan of three meals a day and no snacking would be less cariogenic than an eating plan that includes many meals and snacks throughout the day, even if the food composition of the two plans were the same.[10,11] Sipping on a sugar-containing beverage over time is more harmful to the teeth than consuming it all at once at one sitting.[5] For this reason, in young children juice provided in baby bottles or "sippy cups" is often a major contributor to severe early childhood caries.

Minimizing the Cariogenic Potential of the Diet

The primary dietary carbohydrate recommendation to reduce caries risk is to minimize the frequency of contact between simple sugars and dental plaque on a daily basis.[7] This may involve reducing the overall frequency of consumption of foods and drinks containing cariogenic carbohydrates, limiting these carbohydrates to mealtimes rather than between meals, and/or changing the physical form of snacks and drinks consumed between meals to reduce oral contact time.

References

1 Loesche WJ. Role of *Streptococcus mutans* in human dental decay. *Microbiol Rev.* 1986;50(4):353–380.
2 Bowen BH. Food components and caries. *Adv Dent Res.* 1994;8:215–220.
3 Woodward M, Walker ARP. Sugar consumption and dental caries: Evidence from 90 countries. *Brit Dent J.* 1994;176:297–302.
4 Rugg-Gunn AJ. *Nutrition and Dental Health.* Oxford: Oxford University Press; 1994.
5 Ismail AI, Burt BA, Eklund SA. The cariogenicity of soft drinks in the United States. *J Am Dent Assoc.* 1984;109:241–245.
6 Garcia-Closas R, Garcia-Closas M, Serra-Majem L. A cross-sectional study of dental caries, intake of confectionery and foods rich in starch and sugars, and salivary counts of *Streptococcus mutans* in children in Spain. *Am J Clin Nutr.* 1997;66:1257–1263.
7 Kandelman D. Sugar, alternative sweeteners and meal frequency in relation to caries prevention: New perspectives. *Brit J Nutr.* 1997;77:S121–S128.
8 van Palenstein Helderman WH, Matee MIN, van der Hoeven JS, Mikx FHM. Cariogenicity depends more on diet than the prevailing mutans streptococcal species. *J Dent Res.* 1996;75:535–545.
9 Stephan RM. Changes in hydrogen ion concentrations on tooth surfaces and in carious lesions. *J Am Dent Assn.* 1940;27:718–723.
10 Palmer CA, Kent R Jr, Loo CY, et al. Diet and caries-associated bacteria in early childhood caries. *J Dent Res.* 2010;89(11):1224–1229.
11 Gustafsson BE, Quensel CE, Lanke SL, et al. The Vipeholm dental caries study. *Acta Odont Scand.* 1954;11:232–364.

Current Sugar Consumption Versus Recommendations

Most Americans consume too much sugar. Added sugars displace vital nutrients and fiber, and they may contribute to obesity when energy intake exceeds the body's needs.[25] According to NHANES, the average person in the United States consumes about 105 pounds of added sugar per year, or about 30 teaspoons of added sugar a day.[26] Because of this, the *Dietary Guidelines for Americans* has recommended that consumers "choose and prepare food and beverages with little added sugars."[27] See **Special Topic 14.4** for more on sugar and the U.S. obesity crisis.

The Dietary Reference Intakes (DRI) suggest that total sugars (sugars intrinsic to foods, such as fruit and milk, *plus* added sugars) account for no more than 25% of a person's daily total calories (equivalent to 125 grams of sugar, or 31 teaspoons). This recommendation is higher than that

Special Topic 14.4

The U.S. Obesity Crisis

Sung Eun Choi, PhD, RD

Obesity is the most common nutrition-related problem in the United States and is considered a major risk factor for cardiovascular disease, certain types of cancer, and type 2 diabetes. Obesity is defined as a body mass index (BMI) of 30 or greater, which is calculated from a person's height and weight.

During the past 20 years there has been a dramatic increase in obesity in the United States.[1] **Figure A** shows the extent of the obesity crisis across each of the states. In 2010, no state had a prevalence of obesity of less than 20%. Thirty-six states had a prevalence equal to or greater than 25%, and twelve of these states—Alabama, Arkansas, Kentucky, Louisiana, Mississippi, Missouri, Oklahoma, Tennessee, West Virginia, Michigan, South Carolina, and Texas—had a prevalence of obesity equal to or greater than 30%.

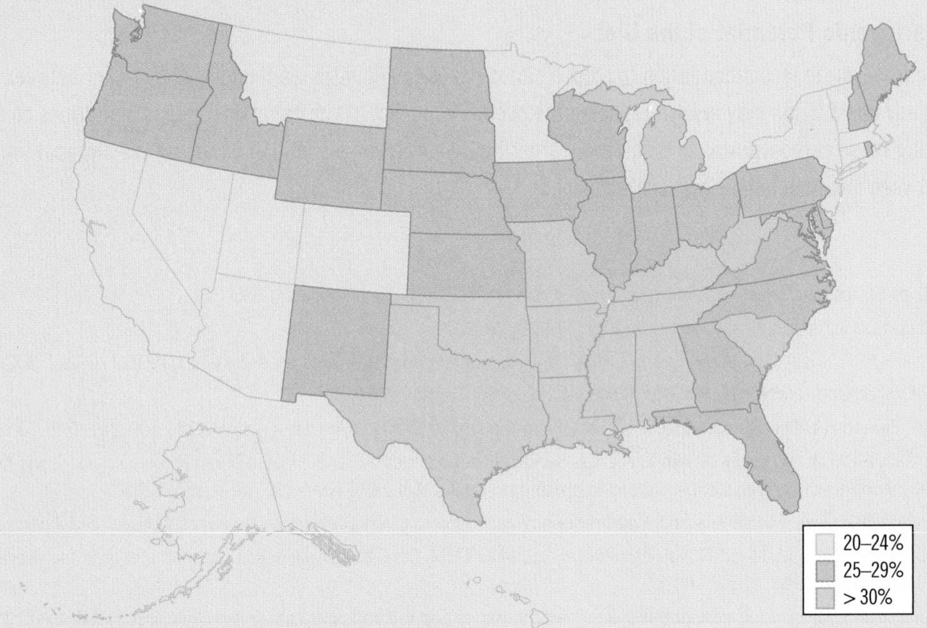

FIGURE A Percentage of the adult population with obesity (BMI ≥ 30), 2010.

Source: Reproduced from the Center for Disease Control and Prevention. U.S. Obesity Trends: Trends by State 1985–2010. Available at: http://www.cdc.gov/obesity/data/trends.html.

References

1 Centers for Disease Control and Prevention. U.S. Obesity Trends: Trends by State 1985–2010. Available at: http://www.cdc.gov/obesity/downloads/obesity_trends_2010.pdf. Accessed December 30, 2010.

recommended by the World Health Organization (WHO) and the Food and Agriculture Organization (FAO), which suggest that sugars account for no more than 10% of total energy intake.[28,26] Based on a 2,000-calorie diet, this would equal only about 12 teaspoons of a sugar a day, which is far less than what most Americans eat now. Consider the following sobering fact: According to the *Dietary Guidelines for Americans, 2010*, no more than 5–15% of calories from solid fats and added sugars combined can be reasonably accommodated in the recommended USDA Food Patterns that have been designed to meet nutrient needs and optimal health.[27]

Sweeteners and Weight Gain

The relationship between sweeteners and artificial sweeteners to weight gain may be linked to the effect our perceptions of sweetness have on our feelings of satiety, or how much we need to eat to feel satisfied.[15,26] It is well documented that repeated exposure to a flavor trains a person's flavor preferences. Most people don't like the bitter taste of coffee at first, but after multiple exposures their taste buds get used to it. Similarly, when people cut back on their intake of salt or fat, there will eventually be a preference for lower levels of these in their diets after several weeks. People who switch to skim milk will tell you that whole milk tastes too strong for them. The same is true for salty foods. In contrast, when cutting back on sugar, artificial sweeteners are often substituted; therefore, people's taste buds do not get a chance to get used to consuming less of a sweet taste.[29]

Artificial sweeteners are hundreds to thousands of times sweeter than sugar. Artificial sweeteners, particularly because they are very sweet, have been shown to promote sugar cravings and sugar dependence. This is due to repeated exposure to artificial sweeteners, most commonly and extensively through the consumption of diet beverages. Repeated exposure trains flavor preference, correlating a person's habitual intake of a flavor and his or her preferred passion for that flavor. Therefore, with repeated intake of artificial sweeteners, one may experience sugar cravings and end up with a greater dependence on sugar.[29]

Going Green

During the nineteenth century, people relied on a range of natural materials (wool, wood, etc.) to provide the essentials of life. This changed significantly during the twentieth century with the Industrial Revolution, which caused humans to become almost totally dependent on fossil fuels to produce the fuels, polymers, and chemicals required for modern-day life. Today, in an effort to become less reliant on nonrenewable resources and more green, researchers are working on the development of a biodegradable plastic called polyactide, or PLA. Derived completely from the sugars in corn, sugar beets, sugarcane, and other plants, a plastic part made from PLA can biodegrade after its life cycle in 90 to 120 days in a landfill. Contrast this with petroleum-based plastics, which take approximately 1,000 years to decompose.[30–32] Another green effort is the use of bagasse, which is produced as a byproduct of sugarcane refining, as an alternative to conventional tree-based paper products. Bagasse "disposable" paper products are 100% compostable within 180 days.[32]

Chapter Review

Sugar is an important energy source and an element in food that provides a pleasing taste. Nutritionally, it provides energy, but very few nutrients. Table sugar is crystalline sucrose produced commercially from sugar beets or sugarcane. Monosaccharides are the building blocks of sugars and complex carbohydrates. Sweeteners can be classified as nutritive or non-nutritive depending on if they yield calories. Non-nutritive sweeteners have increased in popularity, and there are now six FDA-approved varieties available. Each of these has a different level of sweetness when compared to sucrose. Sugar plays a variety of important roles in cooking. Sugar serves many important functions in food preparation by interacting with molecules of protein or starch during baking and cooking processes:[4]

- It tenderizes food by absorbing water, inhibiting gluten development in flour, and delaying starch gelatinization.
- It helps delay coagulation in egg custards and other baked protein dishes.
- It incorporates air into shortening in the creaming process.
- It caramelizes and undergoes Maillard reactions under heat, imparting cooked and baked foods with a pleasing color and aroma.
- It speeds the growth of yeast by acting as a food source.
- It helps regulate the gelling of fruit jellies and preserves.
- It prevents spoilage.
- It recrystallizes to varying degrees, allowing for a wide variety of candies and the smoothness and flavor of ice cream.

Learning Portfolio

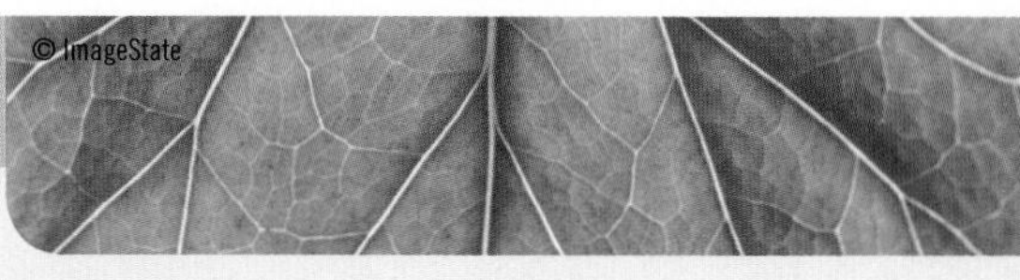

Study Points

1. Processed sugar has been used by humans for thousands of years.
2. Table sugar is crystalline sucrose produced from sugar beets or sugarcane.
3. Monosaccharides are the building blocks of carbohydrates. Glucose, fructose, and galactose are important monosaccharides.
4. Sugar alcohols (polyols) may be used with low-calorie sweeteners to improve the bulk, mouth feel, and texture of certain foods.
5. The six non-nutritive sweeteners approved for use in the United States are saccharin, aspartame, acesulfame-K, sucralose, neotame, and rebaudioside A (stevia).
6. Sugar provides an important source of energy in the diet, but little nutrition. Foods that contain relatively large amounts of sugar have low nutrient density.
7. In the preparation of candy, sugar is boiled. Candies are classified as crystalline or noncrystalline (amorphous) depending upon their internal organization.

Issues for Class Discussion

1. Does excessive sugar consumption necessarily lead to obesity?
2. What is the link between sugar and dental caries?
3. Does sugar cause hyperactivity in children?

Research Areas for Students

1. Safety of artificial sweeteners
2. Effects of sugar cash crops on sustainable development in developing countries
3. Health problems attributed to sugar consumption

References

1. Sugar Technology International. Available at: http://www.sucrose.com/home.html. Accessed February 4, 2011.
2. Meditz SW, Hanratty DM (eds.). *Caribbean Islands: A Country Study*. Washington, DC: GPO for the Library of Congress; 1987.
3. McWilliams M. *Food Fundamentals*. 8th ed. Upper Saddle River, NJ: Pearson–Prentice Hall; 2006.
4. The Sugar Association, Inc. Available at: http://www.sugar.org. Accessed February 1, 2011.
5. Szwarc F. Use of Bio-fuels in Brazil. 2004. Available at: http://unfccc.int/files/meetings/cop_10/in_session_workshops/mitigation/application/pdf/041209 szwarc-usebiofuels_in_brazil.pdf. Accessed January 20, 2011.
6. Norel R, Chahine M, Beard P. Ensiling pressed beet pulp. University of Idaho Department of Agricultural and Life Sciences, University of Idaho Extension; January 2007. Available at: http://www.srcoop.com/articles/beetpulp_bulletin.pdf. Accessed January 12, 2011.
7. Whitney E, Rolfes SR. *Understanding Nutrition*. 12th ed. Belmont, CA: Wadsworth.
8. Bennion M, Scheule B. *Introductory Foods*. 13th ed. Columbus, OH: Prentice Hall; 2010.
9. Corn Refiners Association. High Fructose Corn Syrup Facts. Available at: http://www.corn.org/products/sweeteners/high-fructose-corn-syrup. Accessed July 5, 2011.
10. American Academy of Family Physicians. Stevia Sweeteners: What You Need to Know. 2010. Available at: http://familydoctor.org/online/famdocen/home/healthy/food/general-nutrition/1006/1010.html. Accessed March 11, 2010.
11. Murphy, MM, Douglass JS, Birkett A. Resistant starch intake in the United States. *J Am Diet Assoc.* 2008;108:67–78.
12. Insel P, Ross D, McMahon K, Bernstein M. *Nutrition*. 4th ed. Burlington, MA: Jones & Bartlett Learning; 2011.
13. Higashiyama T. Novel functions and applications of trehalose. *Pure Appl Chem.* 2002;74(7):1263–1269.

Key Terms

	page
acesulfame-K	446
aspartame	443
bound water	449
caloric sweetener	437
crystalline candy	449
disaccharides	435
Generally Recognized as Safe (GRAS)	437
monosaccharides	435
neotame	446
noncrystalline (amorphous) candy	449
non-nutritive sweeteners	443
oligosaccharides	436
phenylketonuria (PKU)	443
polysaccharides	436
saccharin	443
stevia	442
sucralose	446
sugar alcohols	446

14. American Heart Association. Sugars 101. 2010. Available at: http://www.americanheart.org. Accessed December 28, 2010.
15. U.S. Food and Drug Administration. Artificial sweeteners: No calories ... Sweet! *FDA Consumer.* 2006;40:(4):27–28. Available at: http://permanent.access.gpo.gov/lps1609/www.fda.gov/fdac/features/2006/406_sweeteners.html. Accessed November 17, 2012.
16. Calorie Control Council. Saccharine Facts. 2010. Available at: http://www.saccharin.org. Accessed February 11, 2011.
17. Calorie Control Council. Information About Aspartame. 2005. Available at: http://www.aspartame.org. Accessed February 11, 2010.
18. American Academy of Family Physicians. Acesulfame K: What You Need to Know. 2010. Available at: http://familydoctor.org/online/famdocen/home/healthy/food/general-nutrition/1006/1008.html. Accessed February 11, 2011.
19. McNeil Nutritionals. Splenda: No Calorie Sweetener Fact Sheet. 2011. Available at: http://www.splenda.com. Accessed February 11, 2011.
20. Prakash I, Corliss G, Ponakala R, Ishikawa G. Neotame: The next-generation sweetener. *Food Technology*. 2002;56(7): 28–45.
21. Sweeteners Holdings. Neotame Fact Sheet. 2002. Available at: http://www.neotame.com. Accessed February 11, 2011.
22. Academy of Nutrition and Dietetics. Position of the American Dietetic Association: Use of nutritive and non-nutritive sweeteners. *J Am Diet Assoc.* 2004;104:255–275.
23. International Food Information Council Foundation. Nutrition Fact Sheet: Polyols. 2008. Available at: http://www.foodinsight.org/Resources/Detail.aspx?topic=Sugar_Alcohols_Fact_Sheet. Accessed February 20, 2011.
24. International Food Information Council Foundation. Facts About Low-Calorie Sweeteners. 2006. Available at: http://www.ifc.org. Accessed February 11, 2011.
25. International Food Information Council Foundation. Questions and Answers About Low-Calorie Sweeteners, Appetite, and Weight Management. 2009. Available at: http://www.foodinsight.org/Resources/Detail.aspx?topic=Questions_and_Answers_About_Low_Calorie_Sweeteners_Appetite_and_Weight_Management. Accessed February 11, 2011.
26. U.S. Department of Agriculture, Agricultural Research Service. What We Eat in America: NHANES, 2005–2006. 2009. Available at: http://www.ars.usda.gov/Services/docs.htm?docid=13793. Accessed February 11, 2011.
27. U.S. Department of Agriculture, U.S. Department of Health and Human Services. *Dietary Guidelines for Americans, 2010.* 7th ed. Washington, DC: U.S. Government Printing Office; December 2010.
28. Bhargava A, Amialchuk A. Added sugars displaced the use of vital nutrients in the National Food Stamp Program Survey. *J Nutr*. 2007;137:453–460.
29. Yang Q. Gain weight by "going diet?" Artificial sweeteners and the neurobiology of sugar cravings. *Yale J Biol Med*. 2010;83: 101–108.
30. The sustainability of NatureWorks polylactide polymers and Ingeo polylactide fibersa: An update of the future. Initiated by the 1st International Conference on Bio-based Polymers (ICBP 2003), November 12–14, 2003, Saitama, Japan.
31. Burk MJ. Sustainable production of industrial chemicals from sugars. *Int Sugar J*. 2010;112:30–35.
32. Eco Products. Our Materials. 2010. Available at: http://www.ecoproducts.com/our_materials.html. Accessed February 12, 2011.

CHAPTER 15

Beverages

Renee Reynolds, MS, RD, LDN
Carole Palmer, EdD, RD, LDN

Chapter Objectives

THE STUDENT WILL BE EMPOWERED TO:

- Understand the origins and ecology of coffee and tea and discuss the cultural underpinnings of coffee and tea consumption and the role each plays in everyday life.
- Know how coffee and tea are grown and processed.
- Discuss the aesthetic properties, including aroma, flavor, and texture, of coffee and tea.
- Identify the phytonutrients in coffee, tea, and sports beverages and possible beneficial health effects of consumption.
- Evaluate food safety issues with regard to beverages and current regulations that are in place to protect human health and safety.
- Identify the ecological impact of coffee, tea, and sports beverages and environmentally friendly options available to consumers.

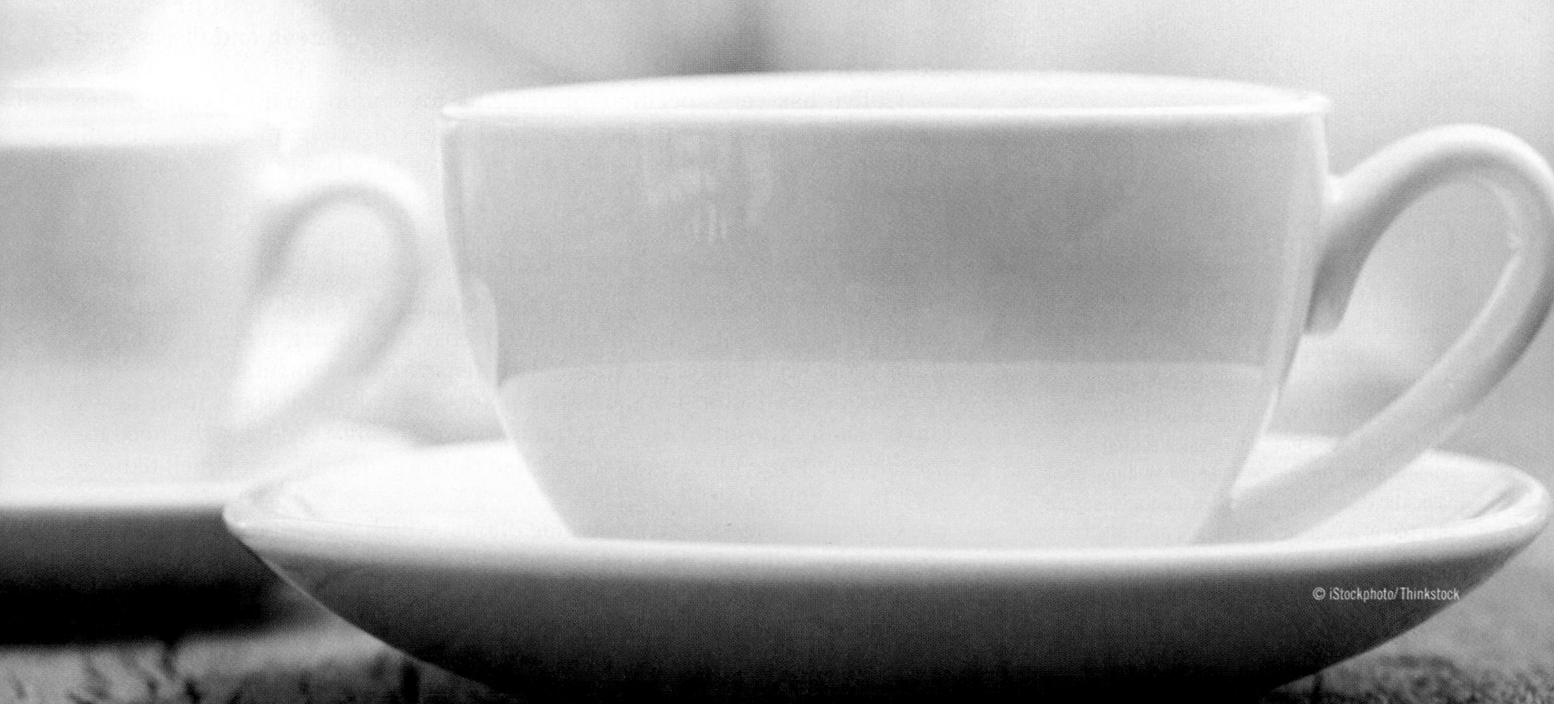

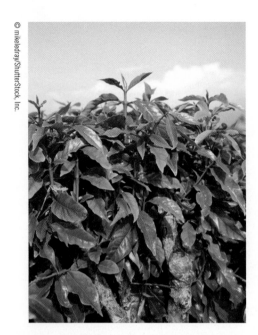

FIGURE 15.1 *Coffea* plants are shrubs or small trees that grow well in dry, tropical climates. The most commonly cultivated species grow best in the cool temperatures found at high elevations. Trees will grow fruits after 3 to 5 years and remain productive for approximately 50 to 60 years.

Coffee

Historical, Cultural, and Ecological Significance

The origins of coffee as a beverage are unclear. Several legends attribute the discovery of coffee to different people; however, the most popular is the story of Kaldi. According to this legend, in the 9th century Kaldi, an Ethiopian goat herder, noticed that after his herd grazed on the fruit of the coffee plant, which grew wild on the plateaus of central Ethiopia, they began to prance and dance excitedly.[1–3] Coffee made its way to Arabia in the 1200s, where it was most likely used for medicinal purposes.[2,3] Arabs closely guarded coffee beans and their cultivation, refusing to allow foreigners to see their plantations or to transport fertile beans outside of the region.[4] Soon coffeehouses opened in Mecca and other parts of the Arab world.

By the 1600s, the Dutch began growing coffee in India and Java (now called Indonesia).[4,5] The Dutch colonies were the major suppliers of coffee to Europe.[4] Venetian traders brought coffee to Europe in 1615, and Venice was home to the first European coffeehouse, which was established in 1645.[4] Coffeehouses opened in Austria, France, Germany, Holland, and England, where they were sites of social interaction and political discussion.[6] In the late 1600s, coffee finally made its way to North America, making its debut in Virginia.[2] The cultivation of the plant soon spread to Central and South America.[4]

Ecology

Coffee is a member of the botanical family Rubiaceae, which comprises 500 genera and over 6,000 species.[7] Coffee's genus is *Coffea*, and the two species that are used for global coffee production are *Coffea arabica* (arabica coffee) and *Coffea canephora* (robusta coffee).[2,7] Two other species, *Coffea liberica* (Liberica coffee) and *Coffea dewevrei* (excelsa coffee), are grown on a much smaller scale.

Arabica coffee continues to grow naturally on the plateaus of Central Ethiopia (see **Figure 15.1**).[2] The plant self-pollinates, and subsequently it is less likely to undergo mutations. Differences in the taste of the final coffee product are based on variations in the soil, moisture, and climate in which the plant is grown.[3] However, coffee has been selectively bred to improve certain characteristics, such as cup quality, caffeine content, and disease and drought resistance.[7]

Coffee has very specific requirements for commercial cultivation (see **Figure 15.2**).[7] Important factors include the correct temperature, rainfall, sunlight, wind, and type of soil. Requirements vary based on the variety of coffee grown.[5]

Shade- Versus Sun-Grown Coffee

Coffee has traditionally been grown under a canopy of shade trees because the coffee plant does not generally tolerate extensive exposure to direct sunlight.[8] Shade-grown cultivation practices have extensive environmental value.[9] Shade trees act as protection for the coffee plants, safeguarding them from heavy rain and sun exposure, helping to maintain soil quality, reducing the need for weeding, and providing natural mulch in the form of leaf litter, which reduces need for chemical fertilizers.[10]

Conversion to sun-grown coffee plants, which are sun tolerant and can grow without the shade canopy, intensified in the 1970s.[8] It was initially

Green Point

Coffee Farms A large number of studies conducted in Central and South America, as well as Indonesia, over the past 15 years have shown that shade-grown coffee farms are correlated with an increased number and species of birds, improved bird habitat, soil protection/erosion control, carbon sequestration, natural pest control, and improved pollination. Shade-grown coffee plantations serve as a sort of refuge for the types of habitats that are generally under threat worldwide.

thought that increased sun exposure would protect the plants against coffee leaf rust (*Hemililaia vastatrix*), a coffee pathogen that dates back to the 1860s and is spread via wind and rain from spores and lesions on the underside of the leaves.[11] With less shade exposure, it was expected that moisture would dry more readily, inhibiting the fungus. Even though the coffee leaf rust was not as devastating as expected, the use of sun-grown coffee was eventually associated with higher yields and touted to farmers as being more profitable.

Unfortunately, despite the higher output, sun-grown coffee is associated with greater soil erosion, acidification, and greater amounts of toxic runoff from pesticides.[12] Additionally, new sun-grown varieties require extensive management and more inputs, such as the use of chemical fertilizers, insecticides, fungicides, and water (see **Figure 15.3**).[10] In fact, farmers who cultivate shade-grown coffee devote only 2% of their expenses to chemical inputs, whereas those growing semi-modern or modern sun-grown varieties devote 19–25%.[8] When incorporating the cost of inputs, as well as the negative environmental externalities, sun-grown coffee production is actually substantially more costly than shade-grown coffee in the long term.

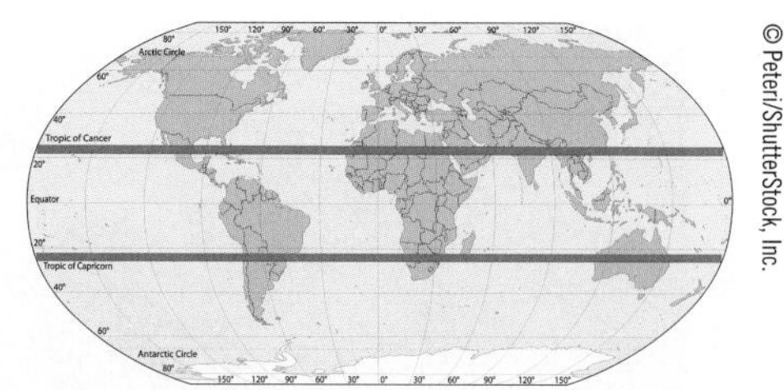

FIGURE 15.2 Cultivation of coffee is limited to tropical regions located between 25 degrees North and 25 degrees South latitude.

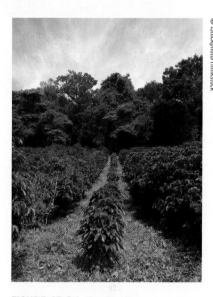

FIGURE 15.3 In the short term, sun grown coffee results in higher yields, but at a steep price. Plantations of sun-grown coffee require large inputs of pesticides, herbicides, and fertilizers. This means that these hazardous chemicals then leach into local water supplies and ecosystems.

Coffee Production

The coffee plant produces berries (see **Figure 15.4**). Typically, one coffee berry contains two seeds (the coffee beans).[2] Prior to the roasting and grinding of the coffee, the berries (which also are called *cherries*) must first undergo processing, which includes removal of the coffee bean from the fruit and subsequent drying.[3] Processing plays a crucial role in coffee production because careful and correct processing will help ensure a clean-tasting coffee without any off-tastes.

The two main methods of processing are wet and dry. The dry method is the older of the two methods and is very simple: The berries are picked and placed in the sun to dry. They are usually spread in a thin layer and raked

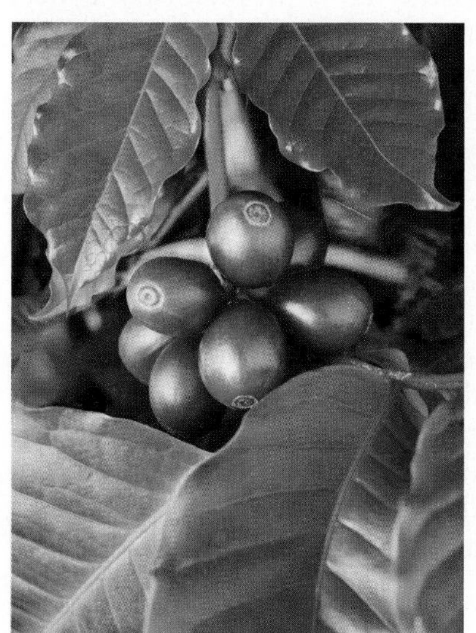

FIGURE 15.4 The coffee beans are contained in coffee berries. Once ripe, coffee berries are picked, processed, and dried. The seeds are then roasted to varying degrees, depending on the desired flavor.

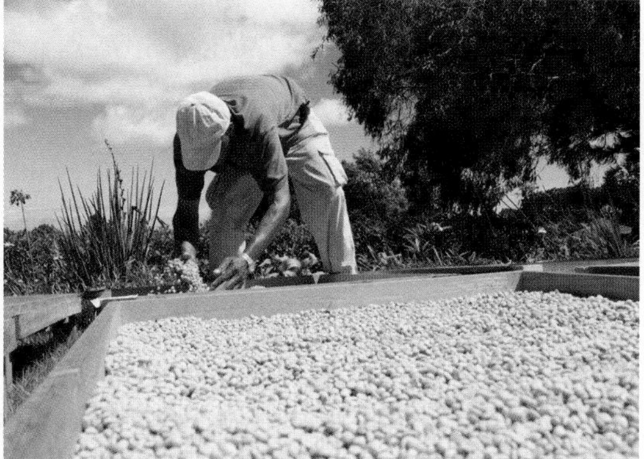

FIGURE 15.5 The dry process is the oldest method of processing coffee. With this method, the berries are cleaned, usually by hand, using a sieve. The cherries are then spread out in the sun on concrete or brick patios and raked periodically to ensure drying and prevent mildew. The drying process is extremely important because it affects the final quality of the coffee. If dried too long, the beans will be brittle and will break. If the beans are too moist, they are vulnerable to fungi and bacteria.

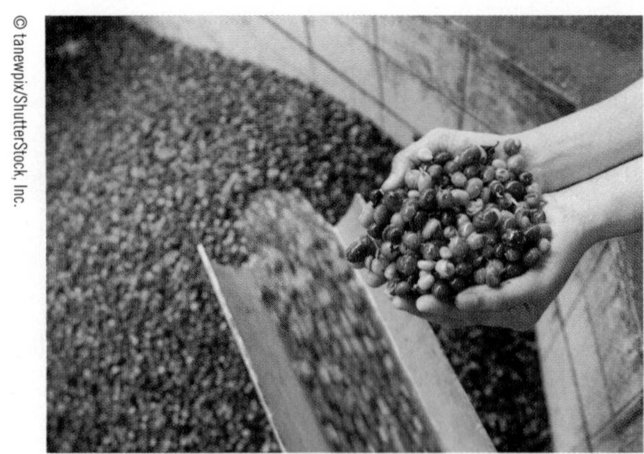

FIGURE 15.6 With wet processing, the fruit is removed from the seeds before drying. The skin of the cherry and some of the pulp is removed by pressing the fruit through a screen while submerged in water. The remaining pulp is removed by the ferment-and-wash method, whereby the remainder of the pulp is removed by breaking down the cellulose by fermenting the beans with bacteria and then washing them with large amounts of water.

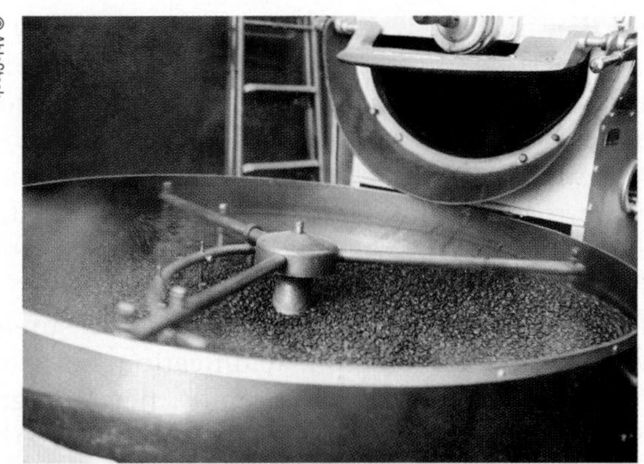

FIGURE 15.7 Roasting of the green coffee beans results in chemical changes that produce the characteristic flavor of coffee by causing the green coffee beans to expand and to change in color, taste, smell, and density. Drum roasters are one of the most common types of roasters. They have a rotating drum that tumbles the beans in a heated environment.

every so often to ensure that all of the seeds receive the same amount of sun exposure (see **Figure 15.5**).[1,3] The dry processing method can take anywhere from 10 days to 3 weeks. After the drying is complete, the husk of the fruit will be removed by a machine, revealing the prized beans.

In the wet method, the outer skin and the pulp of the berries are removed by a machine immediately following harvest (see **Figure 15.6**). This removal of the outer skin is called *pulping*.[2] However, the beans are still covered by a thin parchment-like skin.[2,3] After processing in fermenting and washing tanks, the beans are dried for several weeks, after which milling machines remove the skin.[2]

The type of processing used can affect the flavor profile of the coffee. The dry process produces a coffee that is heavy in body, sweet, smooth, and complex, whereas the wet process produces a cleaner, brighter, and fruitier coffee.[3]

Roasting

Roasting of the coffee bean is thought to be the single most important factor influencing the coffee's final flavor.[3] The beans are roasted at up to 900°F (482°C) for a period of up to 16 or 17 minutes (see **Figure 15.7**).[2] During roasting, a volatile oil called caffeol is released, sugars within the bean caramelize, and the bean develops a slightly burned flavor. The longer the coffee bean roasts, or the higher the roasting temperature, the darker the bean. The two main types of roasts are medium and dark; however, four types of roasts are officially recognized: light/pale, medium, dark/full roast, and darkest roast.[1] Medium roasts have a delicate flavor and aroma, whereas darker roasts have a more bitter taste.

Preservation and Storage

Once the coffee beans have been roasted, they start to lose their aroma, as well as the volatile caffeol. The best way to preserve the flavor and aroma of coffee beans is to place the roasted beans in an airtight container and then freeze them if they will not be used within 2 weeks. Coffee beans will keep in the freezer for up to 3 months and can be ground frozen, as they are needed. Once coffee is ground, its aroma and flavor diminish quickly. Ground coffee sold in stores is usually packaged in vacuum-packed tins, foil-lined packets, or plastic bags to prevent exposure to oxygen. Keeping coffee away from excessive air, moisture, heat, and light will help guarantee optimal flavor.[1]

Grading

A standardized, generalized system for grading coffee beans does not exist, and coffee grading terminology varies by country. However, most coffees tend to be graded on the same characteristics, including appearance (bean size, uniformity, and color), the number of defective beans per sample, and cup quality, which takes into account the flavor and body of the brewed coffee. One consistent reference across countries is the use of standardized screens to measure the size of the beans. The lack of uniform coffee grading can make it difficult to interpret the quality of the beans unless one is familiar with each country's grading criteria.[13]

Additives

The world's very first coffee drinkers experimented with the addition of different ingredients, such as spices, to help enhance the coffee's flavor. Two well-known additives include chicory and fig. The famous New Orleans coffee features chicory, which complements dark roast beans by adding a peppery flavor.[1] In Great Britain, fig is added to impart body and a slight sweetness and fruitiness.

Flavored coffee is also very popular. A wide range of flavors are available, including hazelnut, vanilla, chocolate, cinnamon, and Irish crème. Because the flavor is added to the whole beans prior to grinding and brewing, the flavor must be quite strong. Many of today's flavorings are artificial and are accompanied by substances such as propylene glycol (a solvent) that help to dissolve the flavors, preserve them, and aid in carrying the flavoring into the pores of the bean.[3] In addition to flavoring agents, the most popular additive throughout the world is milk.[14]

Green Point

Coffee Farming It is estimated that 37 gallons of water are needed to grow the coffee beans needed for a single cup of coffee when using industrial farming practices.

Innovation Point

Coffee Taste Variations in the soil, moisture, and climate contribute to differences in the taste of coffee. Coffee has been selectively bred in order to improve certain characteristics such as cup quality, caffeine content, disease, and drought resistance.

Brewing

There is no single best way to make coffee, and there are a wide variety of brewing methods (see **Figure 15.8**).[14] One of the most common brewing methods is the filter method, whereby finely ground coffee is placed into a paper or reusable cone-shaped filter and water is poured over the top. The brew filters through the unit into a pot and is ready to drink; the coffee grounds remain in the upper unit.[14] The standardized recipe for a cup of filtered coffee is two level tablespoons of coffee grounds per cup.[2]

Other notable coffee brewing techniques include Turkish coffee, the French press, and espresso:

- *Turkish coffee*, which is popular in the Middle East, North Africa, the Caucasus, and the Balkans, is made with finely ground coffee beans that are boiled in a small copper pot. The coffee then is served in a cup and the grounds are allowed to settle. Sugar is added to taste.[14]
- The *French press method* uses a plunger to extract the most flavor from the ground beans. Coarse ground coffee is placed in the press and then hot water is added. The brew steeps for 3 to 5 minutes and then the plunger is pushed down, which separates the coffee grounds from the brew.[14]

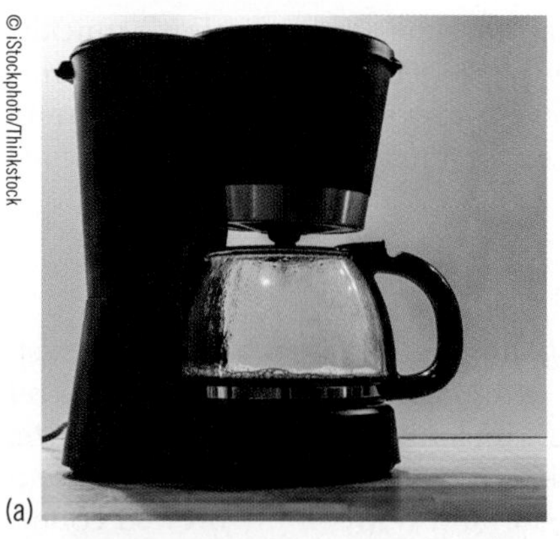

© iStockphoto/Thinkstock

(a)

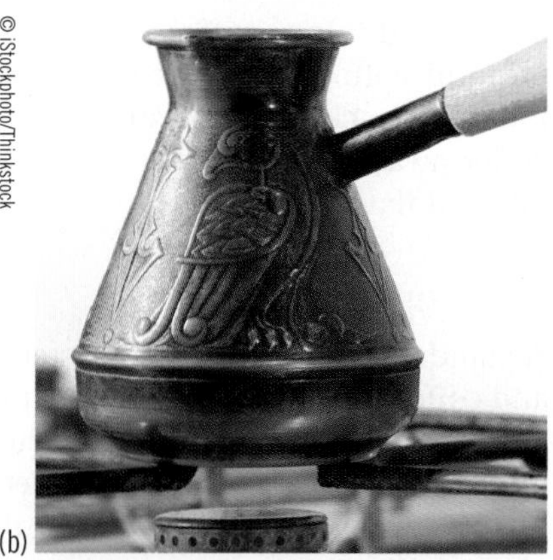

© iStockphoto/Thinkstock

(b)

© George Doyle/Stockbyte/Thinkstock

(c)

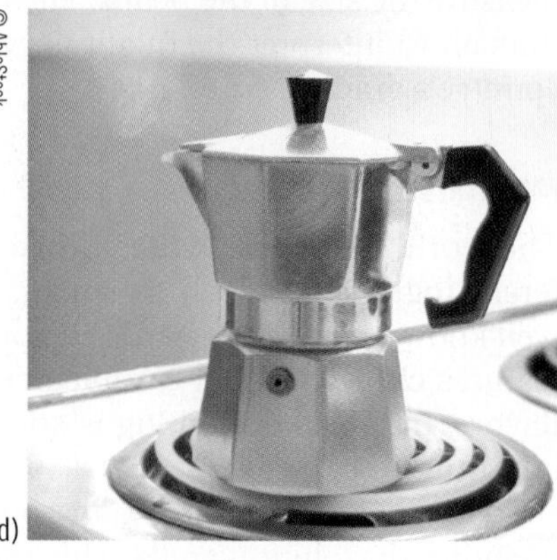

© AbleStock

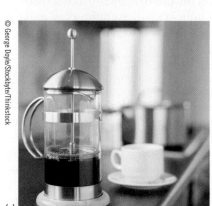

(d)

FIGURE 15.8 (a) In the United States, most homes have a coffee pot. With this method of brewing, hot water is dripped through a filter containing ground coffee. The hot coffee brew then drips into the pot below. (b) The Turkish brewing method dates back to the 16th century. Roasted and then finely ground coffee beans are boiled in a copper pot called a cezve. The resulting brew, which is quite strong and flavorful, is then served in a cup and the grounds are allowed to settle. (c) With the French press, hot water is added to the glass pot and the brew is allowed to form. After 4 to 5 minutes, the hot water is then forced through the coffee grounds by a plunger, resulting in a full-bodied brew. (d) Stove-top espresso makers produce coffee by passing hot water pressurized by steam through ground coffee beans.

- *Espresso*, the quintessential Italian drink, has been enjoyed by Italians for decades and is now adored by Americans as well. The stove-top espresso maker, originally known as the moka pot, uses pressure to force very finely ground, dark-roasted coffee to produce the espresso brew.[13]

Gastronomy Point

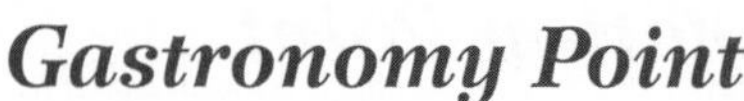

Espresso A "shot" of espresso is quantified as 1 ounce and is typically served in an espresso cup, which holds up to 2½ ounces.

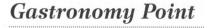

Desired Aesthetic Properties

When selecting coffee, personal preference determines whether it is shade-grown or sun-grown, ground or whole bean, medium or dark roast, flavored, or decaffeinated. Important considerations include budget, methods of production, and the effects of production on the environment.

Several specific properties of coffee can also contribute personal preference:

- *Acidity* is defined as a pleasant tartness, snap, or twist with an underlying sweetness; acidity adds sharpness and "life" to coffee.[1,3] Coffee with low acidity exhibits a soft, smooth, mellow taste.
- The *mouth feel* or *body* of the coffee takes into account the feelings of heaviness, tactile richness, and thickness when the coffee is swished in the mouth. It also describes the coffee's texture, such as oily, buttery, or thin.[3]
- **Aroma**, in the context of coffee, is attributed to the gases and products of the aromatic oils that are released by roasting.[3]
- The *finish* refers to the "resonant silence" at the end of a sip—the immediate sensation after the coffee is swallowed. Some coffees possess a chocolate finish, whereas others exhibit berry tones.[3]

aroma Fragrance/smell of coffee or tea.

- The *flavor* takes into account sweetness, which results from caramelization after roasting, and bitterness, which is naturally present in some beans and results from the decomposition products formed during roasting.[1]

Menu Planning

The consumption of coffee is widespread throughout the world inside and outside of the home.[15] Coffee can be enjoyed at any time of day. In the United States and other European countries, it is part of the morning ritual, consumed with breakfast or on the go. The "coffee break" is an essential component of American business culture and plays an important role in maintaining social contact in a work environment.[6] Coffee still remains a drink over which people can discuss, develop, and exchange ideas; it accompanies academic conferences and business meetings to facilitate exchanges and communication.[15] In some countries, including France, Italy, Austria, Hungary, and Switzerland, coffee follows the midday meal.[6]

Over the last decade, a niche for specialty coffees has been created by environmentally conscious consumers. Coffee producers and distributors have begun to take advantage of this opportunity to promote coffees that are produced sustainably.

Nutritional Properties

Coffee contains more than a thousand different chemicals. It is composed of carbohydrates, lipids, nitrogenous compounds, vitamins, minerals, alkaloids, and phenolic compounds.[16] The USDA Nutrient Database reveals that an 8-ounce cup of brewed coffee can provide 1–5% of the Recommended Daily Allowance (RDA) of magnesium in adult men and 6–18% of the RDA of niacin in adult men. There has been some speculation as to whether these micronutrients contribute to some of the proposed health benefits of coffee consumption; however, the current literature does not provide studies to support or negate this hypothesis.

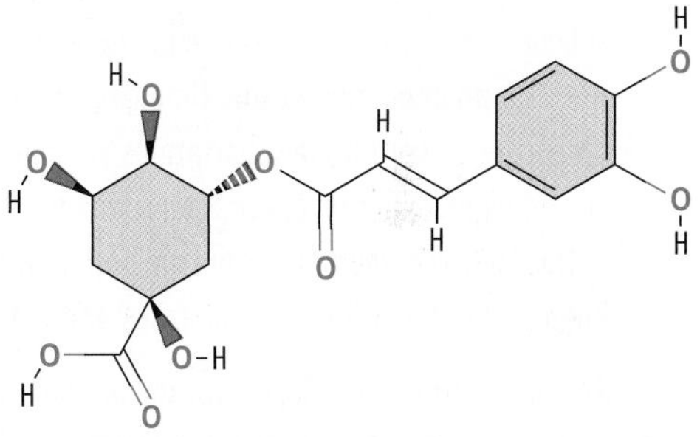

Bioactive Compounds

Bioactive compounds in coffee include chlorogenic acid, caffeine, and diterpenes.[17]

Chlorogenic Acids

Chlorogenic acids are a family of esters that form between quinic acid and trans-cinnamic acids (both of which are dietary phenols).[18] The most abundant chlorogenic acid in coffee is 5-O-caffeoylquinic acid (see **Figure 15.9**).[17] Coffee is the richest dietary source of chlorogenic acids, with 7 ounces of brewed coffee supplying 70–350 mg. The same amount of coffee supplies 30–350 mg of caffeic acid.

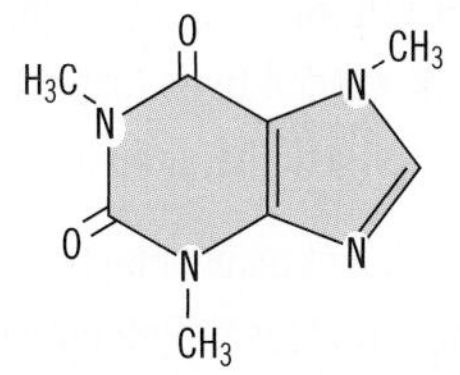

Caffeine

Caffeine is an alkaloid that occurs naturally in coffee beans (see **Figure 15.10**). At the levels of intake associated with coffee consumption, caffeine's biological effects are exerted on the adenosine receptor. Adenosine is an endogenous compound and has inhibitory effects on the central nervous system.[17] Through antagonism of adenosine (that is, the blocking of adenosine receptors), caffeine acts as a stimulant. The amount of caffeine in coffee varies. A recent study analyzed 14 different specialty coffees at coffee shops in the United States and

Phytonutrient Point

Chlorogenic and Caffeic Acid Both chlorogenic and caffeic acid have antioxidant activity in the lab; however, their activity in the human body is unclear; both acids are extensively metabolized, and the metabolites have less antioxidant activity than the parent compounds.

chlorogenic acid A dietary phenol that has been found have antioxidant effects.

caffeine Alkaloid compound that occurs naturally in coffee beans and tea leaves; a stimulant that acts on the adenosine receptors as cinnamic acids.

FIGURE 15.9 5-O-caffeoylquinic acid is an important phenol found in coffee. Coffee represents one of the richest dietary sources of chlorogenic acid.

FIGURE 15.10 Caffeine is a plant alkaloid that acts as a central nervous system stimulant. Found in beverages such as coffee, tea, and soft drinks, it is the world's most widely consumed psychoactive drug. Although toxic at very high doses, everyday consumption has low health risks.

found that the amount of caffeine in 8 ounces of coffee ranged from 72–130 mg.[19] The USDA Nutrient Database estimates that one 8-ounce cup of brewed coffee provides 95 mg of caffeine.

People often drink caffeinated beverages for their stimulating effects. Other beverages, such as alcoholic beverages, have the opposite effect, acting as central nervous system depressants. For information on one type of alcoholic beverage, see **Special Topic 15.1** on distilled liquors.

Special Topic 15.1

Distilled Liquors

Bekah Angoff

History of Distilled Liquors

The process of distillation goes back to 3500 B.C. when Arab chemists used the technique to create perfumes and scents for medicinal use. In the fourth century B.C. Aristotle recorded the benefits of distilling seawater to make it drinkable. As far back as 2,000 years ago, concentrated alcohols were used in China by alchemists and consumed by the privileged class. By the thirteenth century in China, distilled liquor was produced commercially.[1]

The origin of the word *distill* comes from the Latin word *destillare*, meaning "to drip."[1,2] The first publication devoted solely to the process and nature of distilling is from Italy in 1500; it was called *Liber de arte distillandi.* The publication highlighted the act of purifying substances, which is where the name *spirit* originated, as the product took on a "pure and ethereal" reputation.[2]

The first crafted sprits and waters of life (*eau de vie* or *aqua vitae*) were produced in Salerno, Italy, around 1100 at the local medical school. They were thought to be of "pure essence" and were considered to be a fundamental element, along with water, air, earth, and fire. The apothecaries at this time gave customers these spirits as cordials to stimulate the circulatory system. As belief in the medicinal properties of spirits grew, variations were developed. In the fifteenth century, brandy was created and named after the German term for "burnt wine." In France, armagnac was made from leftover wine that was in danger of spoiling. In the 1600s, more sprits were crafted. In Holland, gin was made from rye and juniper, and in France brandy making was perfected in the Cognac region. In the West Indies, the English distilled rum from molasses and cane sugar.[2]

As more cultures developed spirits, production became more streamlined. The distilling process became more intricate, with most spirits going through a double-distillation process. The purified substances were consumed not only for spiritual or medicinal means but also for pleasure. With distilleries growing in size and number, addiction became a problem. Government agencies in Europe started to regulate alcohol production, which lessened the issue of addiction and abuse, but it did not eliminate it.

In America around this time, the production of alcohol was even greater than in England. In the early 1700s, rye was distilled in the northern colonies, and corn was distilled into whisky in Kentucky. At the end of the Revolutionary War, moonshine distilleries popped up, usually in distressed or poor areas of the South. Poor farmers made "hooch" from their corn crops in order to generate an additional source of revenue. In fact, distilled spirits were more lucrative than fresh corn! Government entities became aware of the sales and thought it was profit that needed to be taxed. In 1862, the Office of Internal Revenue was formed to gather proper taxation from all profits made on this crop, as well as other industrious activity.

Consumption of alcohol increased in the United States over the next 60 years. By 1920, many of the country's problems were thought to be caused by alcohol. Prohibition became law with the Eighteenth Amendment to the U.S. Constitution, which made it illegal to produce or consume alcohol. However, people found many ways to circumvent the law. Speakeasies popped up, providing libations in cloaked locations, and doctors prescribed cordials to patients, much like the apothecaries did in the fifteenth century. Home-crafted alcohol was imbibed, usually in the form of moonshine or "bathtub gin." Around this time, the first cocktails were developed, from the gin and tonic (England) to the martini. The first well-known American cocktail, the Sazerac (brandy and bitters), was created in New Orleans. When the Eighteenth Amendment was repealed in 1933, the floodgates opened to the cocktail boom, which continues today as the craft of mixology.[2]

The Process of Distillation

The purpose of distillation is to purify a liquid. The process starts with a liquid, which in the case of making distilled liquor, is a fermented mash of grapes, wheat, barley, corn, potato, or another grain, fruit, or vegetable. The first distilled alcohols were made from fruits, such as grapes and plums. Grains also were used, with fermented rice being used in China and barley in Europe.[1]

The liquid mixture is prefermented by yeast. The distillation process ends any residual yeast activity because the mixture reaches a temperature that is too high for the yeast to live. The first liquors were put through a simple process; for example, wine or beer was put into a container with a tube attached at the top. The liquid was boiled and the resulting steam traveled through the tube, where it condensed along the way and was collected in a container at the end of the tube. Today, the process is basically the same, but an alternate tube is placed in the center of the main line, which eliminates impurities and water (see **Figure A**). With two areas for the alcohol vapors to cool, the distillate is at its purest form and strongest alcohol content (potency) because the process concentrates the original proof of the starting fermented product.[1,2]

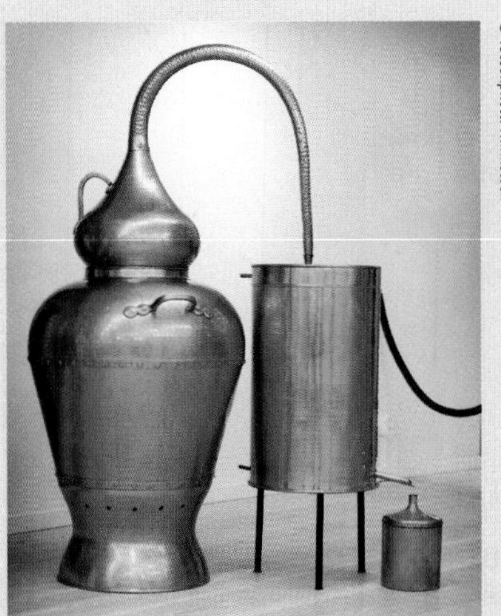

FIGURE A A distilled beverage, spirit, or liquor is an alcoholic beverage that is produced by distilling (i.e., concentrating by distillation) ethanol produced by means of fermenting grain, fruit, or vegetables.

The distillate is then aged, filtered, and adjusted in order to make it palatable. Often, pure distillate is too strong to ingest, having an alcohol content of 90–95%. The aging process lessens the alcohol concentration to a palatable percentage of around 30–40%. (Moonshine often is consumed at distilled potency, making it hazardous to ingest.[2])

Impact on Health

Alcohol consumption has varied through history, but today alcohol plays a large role in most cultures. Intoxication, which means "poisoning," is the result of excessive alcohol consumption; indeed, alcohol is toxic to the human body. Symptoms of intoxication, or drunkenness, include impaired vision and motor and cognitive functions.

Alcohol consumption has been shown to influence the development of certain health problems, such as hypertension and gout, as well as being the subject of dangerous addiction. Over time, chronic alcohol use can damage the liver because it is responsible for metabolizing the alcohol. The kidneys also are affected because they are the organs responsible for filtering waste, so the passage of toxic alcohol damages them. As body systems weaken over time due to alcohol abuse, more health risks present themselves. Alcohol should be consumed in moderation.

References

1 CU Boulder Organic Chemistry Undergraduate Courses. Distillation. 2011. Available at: http://orgchem.colorado.edu/hndbksupport/dist/dist.html. Accessed November 26, 2011.

2 McGee H. *On Food and Cooking*. New York: Simon & Schuster; 2004.

Diterpenes

Cafestol and kahweol (see **Figure 15.11**) are fat-soluble compounds classified as **diterpenes,** which have been associated with increasing serum total cholesterol and low-density lipoprotein (LDL) cholesterol concentrations in humans.[20] The majority of these compounds is removed by paper filters. Scandinavian boiled coffee, Turkish coffee, and French press coffee contain high levels of cafestol and kahweol, ranging from 6–12 mg/cup, whereas filtered, percolated, and instant coffees contain lower levels, ranging from 0.2–0.6 mg/cup.[17] The mechanism for how these compounds affect lipoprotein metabolism is not clear. A meta-analysis of 14 randomized controlled trials that examined the effect of coffee consumption on serum cholesterol

diterpenes Naturally occurring organic compounds that are found in some essential oils and are thought to have antibacterial, antiviral, antifungal, and expectorant properties.

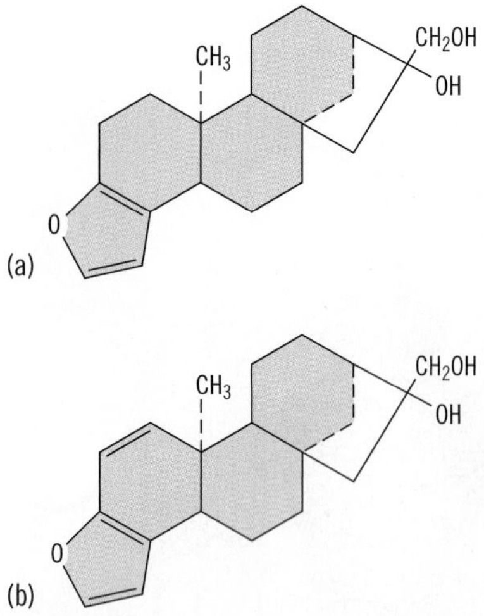

FIGURE 15.11 (a) Cafestol, a diterpene molecule present in coffee beans, may have beneficial effects on serum cholesterol levels. A typical bean of Coffea arabica contains about 0.6% cafestol by weight. (b) Kahweol is a diterpene molecule found in coffee beans of Coffea arabica. It is structurally related to cafestol.

concentrations did find that consumption of boiled coffee dose-dependently increased serum total and LDL cholesterol concentrations but that filtered coffee had little effect on the increase on serum cholesterol.[21]

Impact on Health

Coffee's effects on human health have been disputed over the past few decades. Initial studies found that heavy coffee consumption (five to six cups per day) was correlated with increased risk of cardiovascular disease.[22] These initial studies, however, were epidemiological, and they did not control adequately for unhealthy factors, such as cigarette smoking and physical inactivity.[23] Indeed, recent prospective cohort studies have *not* found a significant association between coffee consumption and the risk of coronary heart disease (CHD). Two separate meta-analyses conducted in 1992 and 1994 that combined 10 different prospective cohort studies, also did not support an association between coffee consumption and CHD risk.[24] Since those meta-analyses, further studies, including large cohort groups in the United States, Scotland, and Finland, have not found a significant association.[25,26]

The health benefits of coffee are currently being investigated, most notably the link between coffee consumption and type 2 diabetes mellitus. Epidemiological research—as well as large, prospective cohort studies in the Netherlands, the United States, Finland, and Scotland—have shown that coffee consumption is associated with a significant dose-dependent reduction in the risk of developing type 2 diabetes mellitus. Two of the largest prospective cohort studies were the Health Professionals Follow-up Study (41,934 men) and the Nurses' Health Study (84,276 women), both of which were conducted in the United States.[27] Results indicated that men who drank at least six cups of coffee per day had a 54% lower risk of developing type 2 diabetes mellitus than men who did not consume coffee, whereas women who drank at least six cups of coffee per day had a 29% lower risk than women who did not drink coffee.[22]

Additionally, the higher the caffeine consumption in the cohorts, the higher the risk reduction. One meta-analysis from 2009 that considered data from over 500,000 individuals in prospective cohort studies showed that drinking three to four cups of coffee daily may reduce the risk of developing type 2 diabetes mellitus by 25%.[22]

The biological mechanisms by which coffee has this antidiabetic effect are still being investigated. Researchers continue to explore coffee's effects on glucose tolerance, as well as insulin sensitivity. A 2010 study showed that the potential antidiabetic compound might be caffeine. Although studies have yet to be conducted in humans, scientists from Nagoya University stated that their results in lab mice indicated that caffeine is one of the most effective antidiabetic components in coffee, although the potential mechanism is unknown.[28]

Epidemiological research also supports claims that coffee consumption may prevent Parkinson's disease and liver disease (cirrhosis and hepatocellular carcinoma).[22] The potential mechanisms for both of these effects are still being explored; at present, it is premature to begin recommending coffee consumption as a means to prevent either disease. The links between coffee and suicide risk, cancer, osteoporosis/hip fracture risk, and mineral deficiencies also are being investigated; research is preliminary, at best, in these areas.

In conclusion, coffee consumption is associated with a significantly decreased risk of type 2 diabetes mellitus in both epidemiological and prospective cohort studies. Additionally, case-control and prospective cohort studies suggest that coffee consumption is associated with decreased risk of hepatic injury, cirrhosis, and hepatocellular carcinoma.[29–32] Overall, coffee does not appear to pose significant health risks; instead, moderate amounts (three to four cups/day) may actually result in health benefits.

Food Safety and Foodborne Illness

The primary food safety concerns with coffee include the presence of chemical residues, such as pesticides; improper processing; inadequate storage conditions; and contamination.[33] Because coffee is not eaten raw and is subject to soaking, fermentation, drying, roasting, and brewing, there is little, if any, residue from pesticides.[34] The results of a National Coffee Association study released in 2010 that evaluated the pesticide residue in 50 different commercial coffee brews found that brewed coffee has a negligible pesticide residues.[35]

One of the most well-known contaminants in coffee is a type of mycotoxin. **Aflatoxins** are a large group of closely related compounds that are metabolic products of the fungus *Aspergillus*. Aflatoxins are highly carcinogenic.[35]

Ochratoxin A (OTA) is another mycotoxin produced by two genera of fungi: *Penicillium* and *Aspergillus*. OTA contamination tends to occur most commonly in cereals, fresh grapes, dried vine fruit, wine, beer, coffee, and cocoa. OTA contamination in coffee has been shown to be a postharvest problem. One of the best ways to avoid contamination is to control the amount of water available in the coffee beans to prevent mold growth.[36]

aflatoxin Mycotoxin (fungus) in coffee.

ochratoxin A (OTA) A mycotoxin produced by *Penicillium* and *Aspergillus* fungi.

In the late 1990s, the Food and Agriculture Organization (FAO) of the United Nations, the International Coffee Organization (ICO), and the European coffee industry collaborated to create a project to address OTA contamination in coffee. The main objectives of this project are to support the development of best practices to help minimize levels of OTA contamination throughout the production, processing, handling, and transportation of coffee. The project has a two-step approach: (1) to build up local expertise in coffee producing countries and (2) to develop ongoing national training programs. In 2002, the European coffee industry released a Code of Practice that outlines best practices for operators along the coffee production chain to follow to minimize the risk of OTA contamination.[36]

Green Point

Pesticide Residue A study conducted by the National Coffee Association that evaluated the pesticide residue in 50 different commercial coffee brews found that brewed coffee has a negligible amount of pesticide residue.

Going Green with Coffee

As more value is placed on environmental sustainability, more green coffee options will become available. Several initiatives are already underway:

- The American Birding Association, the Smithsonian Migratory Bird Center, the National Arbor Day Foundation, and the Rainforest Alliance have led a campaign for shade-grown and organic coffees that use sustainable farming practices.
- The International Coffee Organization outlines some of the main sustainability programs; these guidelines can help environmentally conscious consumers choose coffee products that align with their values.
- Organic certification for coffee products ensures that there is no use of agrochemicals (see **Figure 15.12**). Organic standards also include nature conservation through prohibition of clearing primary ecosystems, biodiversity preservation, and soil and water conservation.[37]
- The Smithsonian Migratory Bird Center has stringent standards for bird-friendly certification; these standards promote shade-grown coffee production, which is economically, environmentally, and socioculturally responsible. If the growing conditions of the

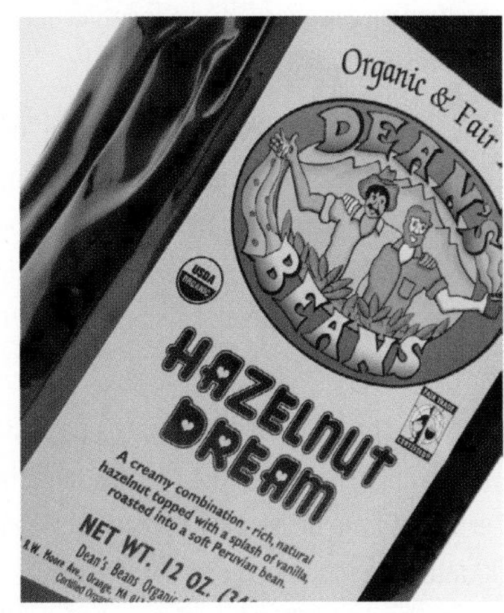

FIGURE 15.12 In the United States, the certification of organic coffee crops is overseen by the United States Department of Agriculture (USDA). U.S. organic certification discourages the use of chemicals within 3 years preceding the harvest of the crop. In addition, any fertilizers used must be 100% organic.

fair trade Movement that seeks to empower farmers and farm workers, protect the environment, and help farmers develop appropriate business skills to compete in a global market.

coffee meet organic standards and if certain shade-grown criteria are met, then the coffee is given a bird-friendly label.[9] The market for organic, shade grown coffee, based upon the Smithsonian Migratory Bird Center's stringent criteria, reached $3.5 million dollars in 2008, averaging to a 145% annual increase between 2000 and 2008.[9]

- **Fair trade**, which is discussed in detail in **Special Topic 15.2**, aims to empower farmers and farm workers, to protect the environment, and to give farmers appropriate business skills to compete in a global market.[37] Fair Trade coffee is held to high social standards and high environmental standards that ensure that natural ecosystems are not degraded and that cultivation of the land is done sustainably.

Special Topic 15.2

Fair Trade Coffee

Veronica Salsberg, BS

According to the Fair Trade Federation, *fair trade* is "an economic partnership based on dialogue, transparency, and respect." The fair trade movement includes a global network of producers, traders, marketers, advocates, and consumers whose mission is to focus on building equitable trading relationships between consumers and economically disadvantaged farmers and artisans throughout the world. The Fair Trade Federation (FTF) is a trade federation established in 1994 and based in Washington, DC. It encompasses fair trade producers, importers, wholesalers, retailers, nongovernmental organizations, and individuals committed to providing fair wages and good employment opportunities to economically disadvantaged farmers and artisans in developing and developed countries. The FTF also serves as a clearinghouse of information on fair trade, organizes conferences, and provides marketing resources and networking opportunities for its members.[1]

The FTF has adopted several key principles to help guide its members. These principles are based on the creation of opportunities for the economically disadvantaged through the sustainable development of management skills and financial and technical expertise, equity in gender, payment of fair prices, promotion of safe and healthy work environments, encouragement of environmentally sustainable production practices, and education of the public on the importance of purchasing fair trade goods and the need for change in the practices of conventional trade.[1]

The idea of fair trade has been around for some time, but the relatively recent fair trade movement arose to address important social and ethical issues in international trade. A key example of this is the international coffee market. Agricultural products such as coffee are sensitive to growing conditions and temperature fluctuations, so coffee beans are therefore subject to exaggerated boom-bust cycles and chronic price fluctuations. Booms cause coffee prices to go up when farm output is low; busts cause prices to drop dramatically when there are bumper crops. Fair Trade seeks to stabilize these price fluctuations and provide farmers with access to international markets and fair wages for their labor.[2]

Coffee is produced by some of the poorest countries in the world, but it is consumed by the wealthiest nations. The United States is the largest coffee-consuming country, importing more than 22% of the global coffee crop.[2] Coffee is one of the most valuable commodities exported from developing countries, second only to petroleum. For many of the world's least developed countries, such as Ethiopia and Guatemala, coffee exports comprise 50% or more of their export earnings. However, many of the individual coffee growers are small-scale operations and their businesses financially marginal. Fair trade can help these growers make a decent living.

The notion of fair trade is catching on, with most supermarkets carrying at least some fair trade products. Although fair trade products may cost a little more than conventional or noncertified products, consumers are willing to pay for them. In 2008, Fair Trade certified coffee sales increased by 14%. This may be greatly due to fair trade organizations working to promote awareness in order to create market demand. According to Stacy Wagner, the public relations manager at Fair Trade USA, a nonprofit organization based in California, 50% of American households are aware of fair trade coffee, up from only 9% in 2005.[3]

Representatives from businesses, including Starbucks, Peet's, and Green Mountain Roasters, all report a consumer push for socially responsible business practices, and the majority of these business strive to meet consumer demands. Starbucks offers fair trade coffee among its other coffee options and has socially responsible business guidelines for its coffee buyers.[3] Grocer Shaw's Supermarket started carrying Equal Exchange Fair Trade Coffee in 1996 and has greatly expanded its program based on growing sales. A spokeswoman for Shaw's explained that carrying fair trade coffee makes sense because the prices are reasonable, the products are of good quality, and the consumers who purchase them appreciate helping small farmers.[2]

Rodney North, spokesman for Equal Exchange, explains how the fair trade movement is not unfamiliar to the food industry and actually closely resembles the first stages of the push toward marketing organically certified foods. North explains that organic foods first started out in consumer cooperatives that represented a small niche of the American supermarket industry; from there, the certified organic industry found its first audience and later expanded into more mainstream channels. North states, "[the Fair Trade Label] is kind of like the [USDA] organic seal. It's something that enough people are looking for that it's helpful to have."[2] For the socially responsible coffee drinker, there are more options today than ever before, and future trends reports indicate that consumer education, awareness, and fair trade investment will continue to grow.

References

1 The Fair Trade Federation. 2005 Report: Fair Trade Trends in North American and the Pacific Rim. 2005. Available at: http://www.fairtradefederation.org/ht/a/GetDocumentAction/i/278. Accessed November 1, 2011.

2 Fagnani S. Fair share: Socially responsible coffee and food are gaining acceptance in supermarkets, delivering a nice ROI for participating retailers. *Supermarket News*, April 12, 2004: 35.

3 Haight C. The problem with fair trade coffee. *Stanford Soc Innov Rev.* 2011:9(3);74–79.

Tea

Historical, Cultural, and Ecological Significance

Tea is one of the most popular beverages worldwide; it is the second most widely consumed beverage after water.[38] Tea's origins trace back to China. The Chinese Emperor Shen-Nung, known as the father of Chinese agriculture and medicine, is credited with the discovery of tea in 2700 B.C. when tea leaves accidentally blew into his pot of boiling water.[39]

By the fourth century, tea was an integral part of Chinese life, used mainly for medicinal purposes. Leaves were applied topically to soothe wounds, and people would crush and mix the bitter leaves with shallots, ginger, salt, and orange in attempts to make it more palatable.[15] Tea also was used by Buddhist monks to help with meditation practices because it helped to boost concentration and banish fatigue (see **Figure 15.13**).[38]

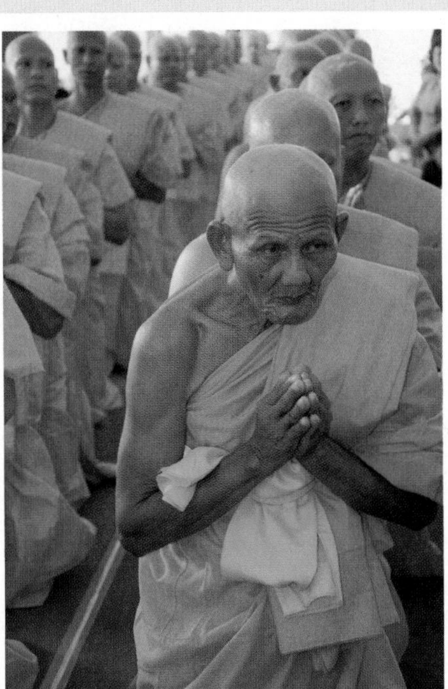

FIGURE 15.13 Buddhists were some of the first to harness the mysticism surrounding tea. In the highly symbolic Buddhist tea ceremony, followers enter an almost barren tea room and ritualistically consume tea offered by a tea master, all the while focusing on peace and simplicity.

Buddhist monks were the first to bring tea to Japan in the sixth century and helped spread tea throughout Southeast Asia.[15] In the sixteenth century, Portuguese, Dutch, and other European traders and missionaries visited Asia and were introduced to the beverage.[40] The Dutch East India Company fueled the mania for tea in Great Britain, bringing the first consignment of Chinese tea to Europe in 1610.[41] The drink became an integral part of British life, appealing to lords and ladies, as well as men and women of the working class.[38] Tea continued to spread throughout Europe, and then to North America in the 1700s (making its debut in Manhattan) and to South America and Australia in the nineteenth and twentieth centuries.[41]

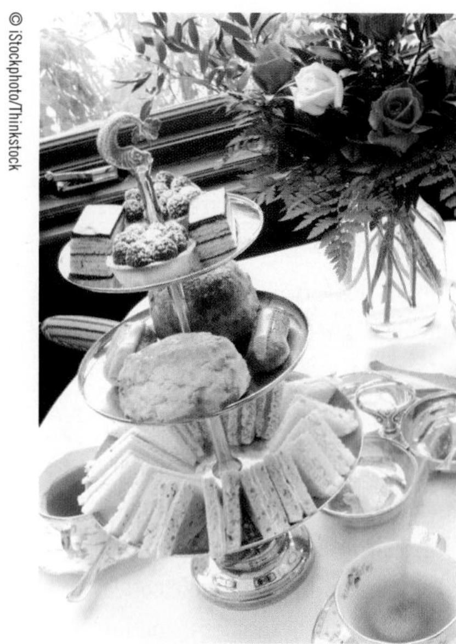

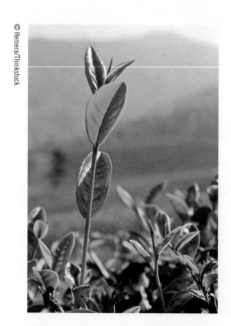

FIGURE 15.14 Afternoon tea is a small snack typically eaten between 3 and 5 P.M. The custom of afternoon tea originated in England in the 1840s.

Use by Specific Cultures

Tea is a beverage that transcends cultures, but specific customs pertaining to it are an integral component of the Chinese, Japanese, British, Indian, Russian, and American cultures:

- Tea originated in China, and it continues to permeate Chinese life. Green tea is consumed throughout the day and with meals. It also is a means by which the Chinese welcome guests.[40]
- The Japanese tea ceremony developed slowly over time and is reflective of Japanese cultural history. The Japanese consider the ceremony a means by which the spirit, man, and nature come together.[40] The ceremony consists of making and drinking green tea in an established tea room. The careful art of making the tea and special rules of etiquette distinguish the Japanese ceremony.[42]
- Late afternoon tea became a custom in the British culture in the nineteenth century; Anna Maria Stanhope, Duchess of Bedford, is attributed with making afternoon tea a social event and using it as a means to boost her energy and mood (see **Figure 15.14**).[38]
- Tea also is popular in Russia, where dark, strong tea sweetened with jam, sugar, or honey is preferred.[38]

Ecology

The tea plant, *Camellia sinensis*, is an evergreen that grows in tropical and subtropical regions (see **Figure 15.15**).[41] The two main varieties are Chinese tea, *Camellia sinensis sinensis*, which has small leaves, and Assam tea, *Camellia sinensis assamica*, which has larger leaves.[43] The finest teas are grown at 3,000 to 7,000 feet above sea level.[44] The cooler temperatures and harsher conditions encourage the leaves to mature more slowly and develop complexity, which optimizes the flavor of tea.[40,41] Cultivated tea is mainly grown on plantations, large estates, or in gardens.[40]

The tea plant is indigenous to Southwestern China and the Assam region of India, but it is now grown in approximately 35 different tropical and subtropical countries.[45] Although tea production is widespread, 75% of global tea production takes place in China, India, Sri Lanka, and Kenya.[45] Wild tea plants can grow up to 30 feet tall; however, when cultivated for commercial use, the plant is pruned to waist height (3 to 4 feet).[41,46]

FIGURE 15.15 Tea is produced from the leaves of *Camellia sinensis*. Common names include tea plant, tea tree, and tea shrub. The most common forms of tea, including white tea, green tea, and black tea, are all produced from the leaves of this species.

Tea plants cross-breed readily, which has resulted in a number of different hybrids with subtle differences in flavor.[39] The plant's small, white flowers produce one to three seeds, which resemble hazelnuts.[41] Traditionally these seeds were used to cultivate new tea plants. Today, however, cultivation methods include the propagation of new plants from cuttings taken from tea plants with desirable qualities, such as high yield or a special flavor.[41] To harvest tea, the leaves are plucked from the mature plant. At lower elevations and in warmer climates, tea is harvested once the plants reach 2½ years of age; tea plants at higher elevations and in cooler climates tend to be harvested at 5 years of age. The first leaves harvested are termed the "first flush" and are usually the best quality.[38] Tea plants adjust to the local soil and climate, which has a large impact on the flavor of the tea.[39] Specific types of tea varieties thrive in different climates; for example, oolong variety tea plants prefer cold, frozen climates, whereas other varieties grow optimally with little water and less fertile soil in warmer climates.[39]

Tea Production

The differences among the various types of tea result from different forms of processing and the associated oxidation.[44] The four stages of tea processing result in four different varieties: black, green, oolong, and white. Processing includes withering, rolling, fermentation, and drying (see **Figure 15.16**).[41] The withering stage removes excess moisture from the leaves. Withering can be done traditionally, whereby the leaves are spread across trays or sections called *tats*. However, today mechanized systems, which reduce the withering time, are preferred.[43] As the leaves lose moisture, a chemical withering also occurs, wherein the proteins and carbohydrates break down into amino acids and simple sugars and the concentrations of caffeine and polyphenols increase.[43] (See **Table 15.1** for the caffeine levels in tea.) In the rolling stage, the leaves are crushed and broken into small pieces. The traditional method of rolling is done by hand. Different varieties of rolling machines are now used; however, the traditional method produces tea with a smoother flavor.[41] The next stage, fermentation, is actually a misnomer because biological fermentation does not occur; rather, a series of chemical reactions take place in which the polyphenols in the tea leaves are oxidized.[43] During this stage, the broken leaves are spread on tables and spend a matter of hours in a controlled environment with steady temperature, humidity, and aeration.[43] The enzyme polyphenol oxidase initiates oxidation, which causes the leaves to turn a copper color.[41] The last process is drying, which uses heat to inactivate the polyphenol enzymes, dry the leaves, and caramelize the sugars.[43]

Gastronomy Point

Herbal Teas Herbal teas, known as *tisane*, are not made from the leaves of the tea plant; they are infusions of leaves, roots, bark, seeds, or flowers of other plants.

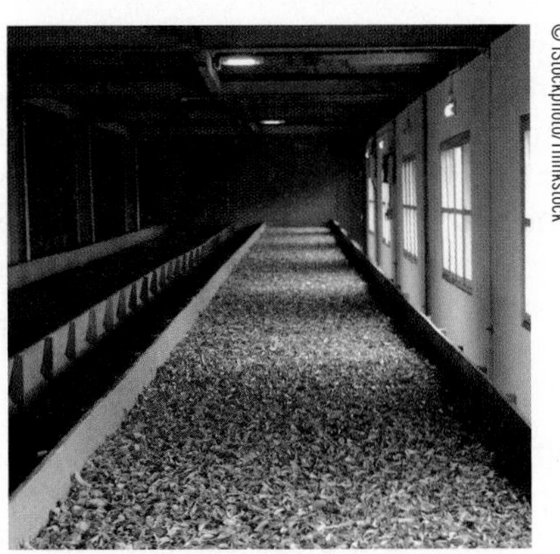

(a)

© iStockphoto/Thinkstock

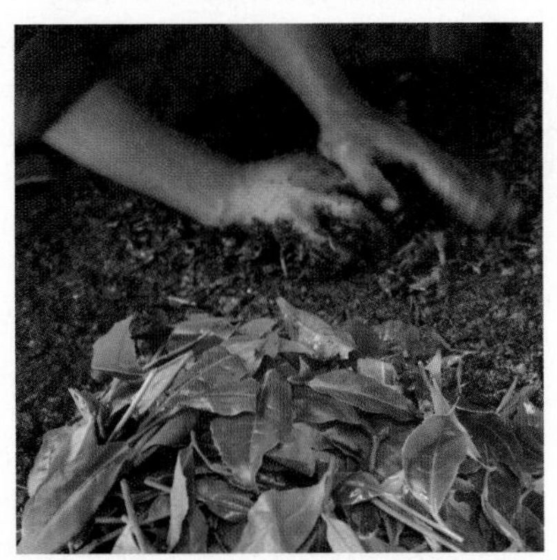

(b)

© YinYang/iStockphoto.com

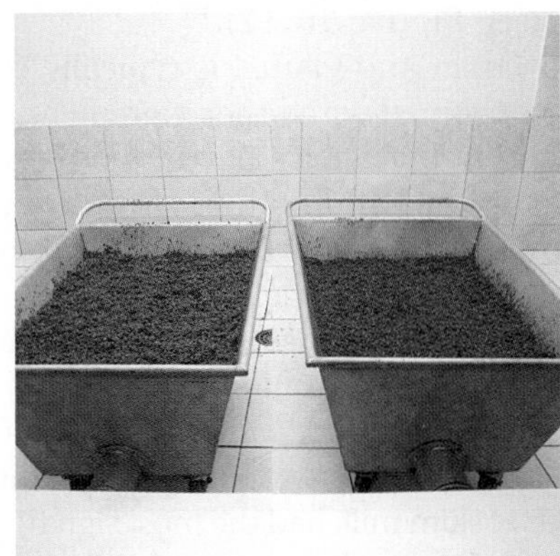

(c)

© iStockphoto/Thinkstock

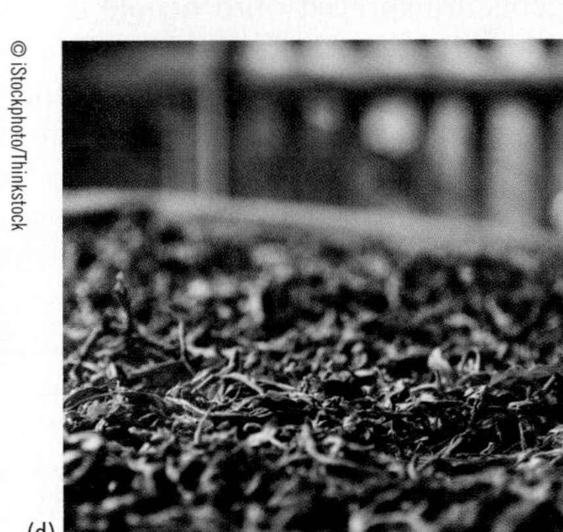

(d)

© onecleanvision/iStockphoto.com

FIGURE 15.16 (a) Withering is the process of removes excess water from the leaves. The leaves are left in the sun or cooled with fans to remove moisture. This process also promotes the breakdown of leaf proteins and increases the amount of caffeine present. (b) With rolling, the tea leaves are torn and bruised in order to speed oxidation. Some of the leaf's juices may also be released, further aiding in oxidation. (c) During fermentation, the leaves are left in a climate-controlled room where they turn progressively darker as the chlorophyll in the leaves is broken down and tannins are released. (d) During drying, additional moisture is removed from the tea. Baking is the most common way to dry tea.

TABLE 15.1
Caffeine Content of Tea

Type of Tea	Caffeine in One 6-ounce Cup*
Green tea	8–36 mg
Oolong	12–55 mg
Black	25–110 mg

*As a comparison, coffee generally contains 60–180 mg of caffeine per cup.

Source: Data from U.S. Department of Agriculture. National Agricultural Library. Nutrient Data Library. Available at: http://ndb.nal.usda.gov/ndb/foods/show/4320. Accessed September 7, 2012.

© iStockphoto/Thinkstock

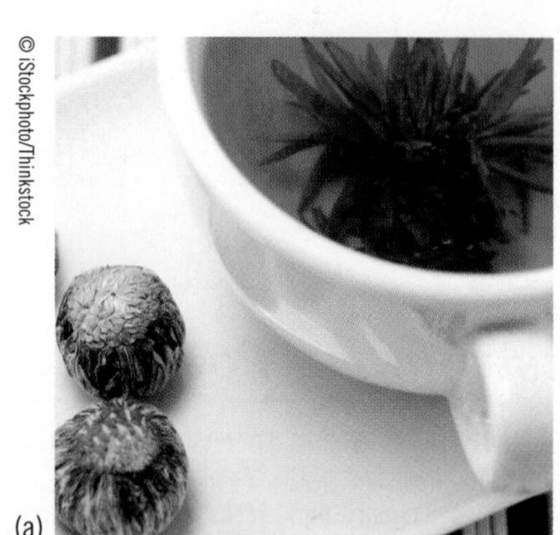

(a)

© Wollertz/ShutterStock, Inc.

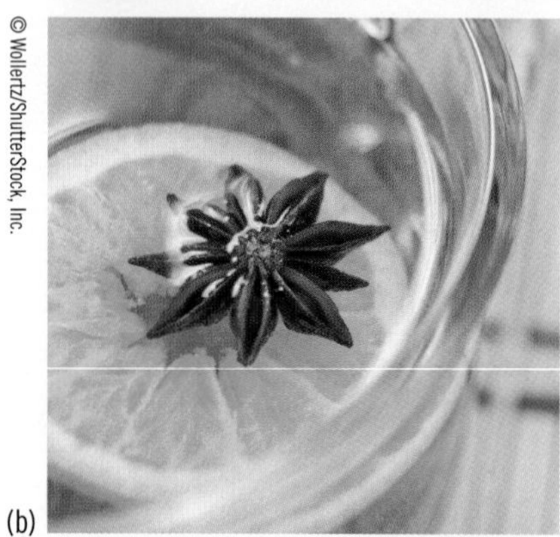

(b)

© Hemera/Thinkstock

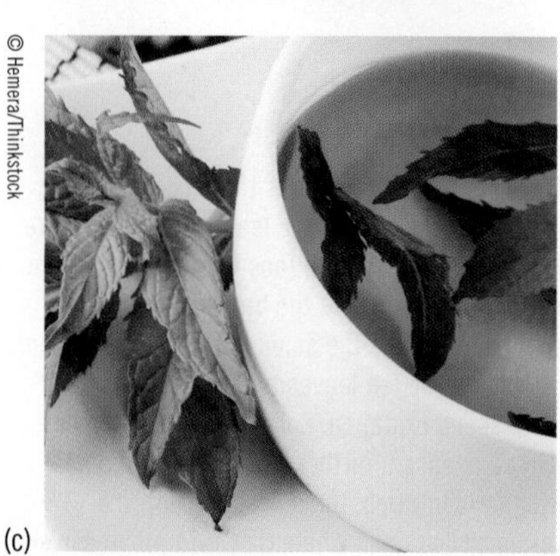

(c)

FIGURE 15.17 A variety of flowers, fruits, and flavorings are added to tea. Spiced teas have spices and fruit rinds mixed in with the tea leaves. Common additives include mint, chamomile, orange, vanilla, and jasmine.

Grading

When grading black tea, two main factors are taken into account: size of the tea leaves and the method of production.[44,47] Whole, large tea leaves will result in a higher grade. The method of production can either be traditional, whereby most of the processing is done by hand with limited use of machinery, or mechanized, which is known as the Crush, Tear, and Curl (CTC) process.[47] Mechanical processing damages the leaves, resulting in a lower grade.

Although there are distinct grading criteria for black tea, there is no standardized method for grading green or oolong teas. Methods of grading green and oolong teas change from country to country and from region to region. Although the grading system is not universal, similar considerations are taken into account, including the variety of the tea plant, the region where the tea is grown, and the stage at which the leaves are picked.[47]

Preservation and Storage

Tea leaves are very dry and will readily absorb water and any chemicals or odors from the air.[39] Tea should be stored in an airtight aluminum container in a cool, dark place. It is important to protect tea from odors, moisture, light, and air in order to optimize its flavor. It is recommended that any tea be used within 6 months to a year after purchasing.[40] Conventional tea bags tend to have greater surface area than loose leaf tea and become stale sooner.[40] When buying tea bags, it is best to buy small numbers in individual packages.

Additives

Tea additives have been used for centuries. The most popular flowers added to tea include jasmine, chrysanthemum, gardenia, and magnolia. Examples of flavored tea include orange, peach, vanilla, and black currant. Flavoring agents are sprayed onto heated tea leaves, whereas spiced teas have spices and fruit rinds mixed into the tea leaves (see **Figure 15.17**).[40]

Green tea, which is most popular in Japan and China, is typically consumed plain. However, black tea often is consumed with other ingredients. In Russia, a slice of lemon is added to "brighten" black tea's flavor; a dollop of raspberry jam, sugar, or honey also is a traditional addition. In Great Britain, black tea is customarily consumed with milk. Casein, a protein in milk, binds with polyphenols, giving the tea a smoother, less astringent taste.[40]

The formation of polyphenol–milk protein complexes has lead some researchers to investigate how added milk might reduce the total antioxidant capacity of black tea. A 2010 study published in the *Nutrition Research Journal* analyzed and compared five different brands of black tea after different amounts of whole milk, low-fat milk, and skim milk were added. Adding skim milk had the most significant effect on decreasing the available antioxidants. One explanation of this finding is that whole milk contains more fat-soluble antioxidants, and when the amount of fat in the milk is reduced, these antioxidants are eliminated.[48] Overall, a review of the literature shows inconsistencies regarding milk's effect on tea. However, it is difficult to interpret the studies because they consider different polyphenolic tea components and use different antioxidant assay systems.[49]

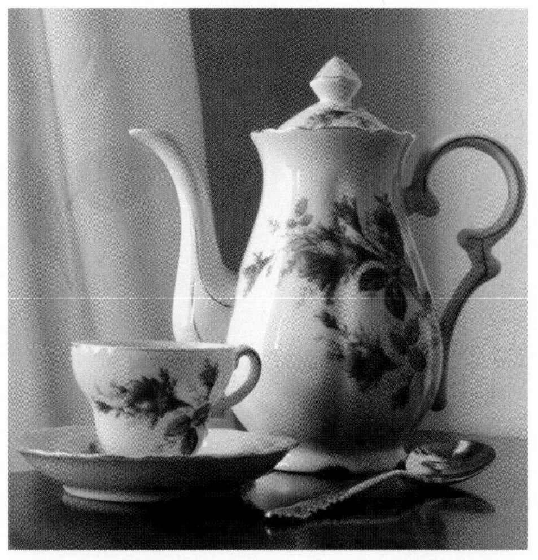

FIGURE 15.18 Due to the long popularity of tea and its role in many cultures, teapots have long been a form of decorative art. For example, when afternoon tea became popular in Britain, beautifully designed china and porcelain teapots and tea cups became widely popular and were produced by such companies as Wedgewood and Royal Worcester.

Brewing

For thousands of years, it was customary to add compressed or powdered tea leaves to a kettle or cup.[40] The Ming dynasty popularized the teapot and shaped the tea brewing methods practiced today. The traditional tea brewing method involves a tea kettle, a tea pot, and a tea strainer.

The kettle is typically made of metal; higher quality kettles have a chromium-plated copper body.[40] The kettle is used to boil the water, which is then added to the teapot. The teapot holds the tea as it brews, or steeps (see **Figure 15.18**). The tea leaves are suspended in the hot water, expanding and flavoring the brew. Once the tea has steeped for the appropriate amount of time, the strainer is used to catch the loose leaves when the tea is poured from the teapot. Teapots with built in strainers are very easy to find, and automatic, electric tea kettles are now available and becoming increasingly popular. A tea infuser may also be employed in tea brewing. It is a perforated metal receptacle in which a measured amount of loose tea leaves are placed (see **Figure 15.19**).[40] The infuser is then placed in either the teapot or tea cup before boiling water is added.

Brewing methods vary and are essentially based on personal preference. Both loose teas and tea bags are available for brewing (see **Figure 15.20**). Loose leaf tea has longer tea leaf pieces, and, because of this, it has a better flavor compared to tea bags, which have shorter, crushed tea leaves. Advances are being made, however, with Lipton now selling long-leaf teas in bags.[38]

When preparing loose leaf tea, use 1 teaspoon of loose leaf tea for every 6 ounces of water.[40] Water is another consideration because it can have a direct effect on the tea's flavor. Hard water, which contains minerals and other chemicals, can impair the taste of the tea and also affect its coloring.[39]

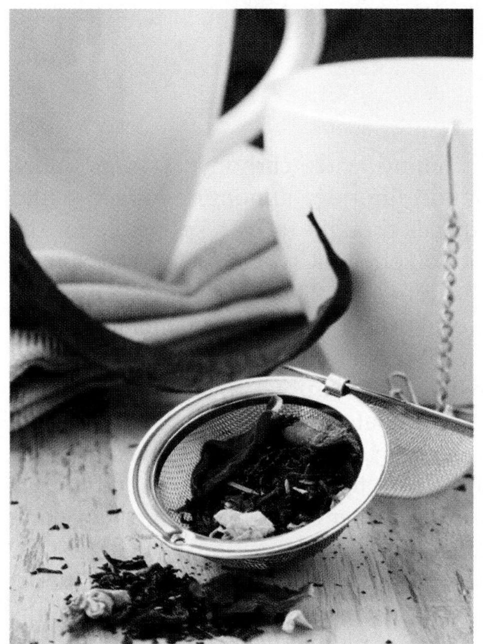

FIGURE 15.19 Loose leaf tea can be placed in a tea infuser for steeping. Tea infusers are sometimes called teaballs or tea makers.

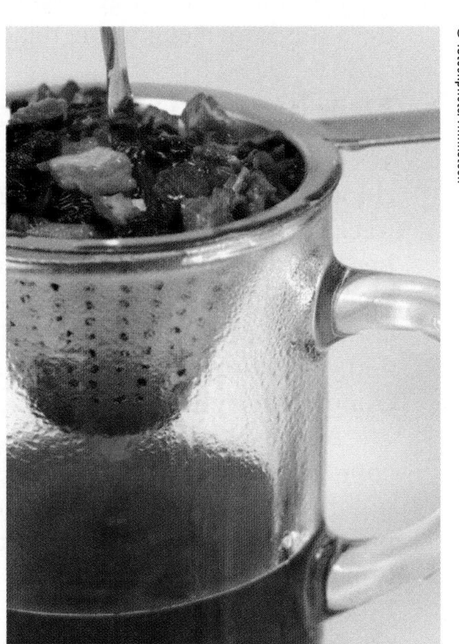

(a)

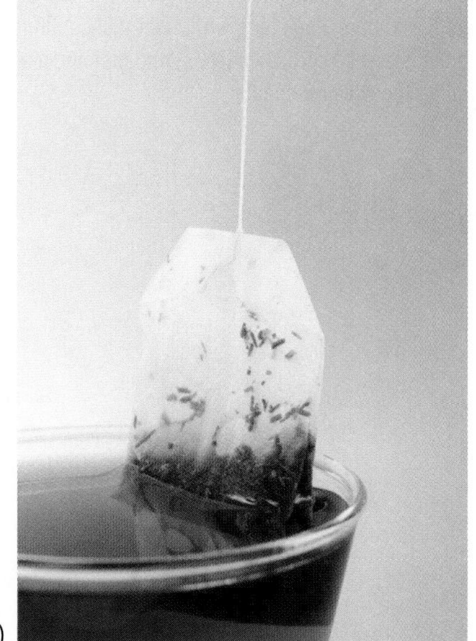

(b)

FIGURE 15.20 (a) Loose leaf tea will produce a better flavor. The loose tea is added directly to the teapot and then strained out after steeping, or a tea ball can be used to contain the tea within the water. (b) A tea bag is a fast, easy way to make a good cup of tea. However, because the tea leaves have been crushed during the production process, the result will not be as good as that made by loose leaf tea.

Natural spring water is best for brewing; however, filtered water will suffice.[38] Water should be heated to the appropriate temperature to guarantee optimal flavor: from 160–175°F (71–79°C) for green tea, 180–190°F (82–88°C) for oolong tea, and a full, rolling boil (212°F [100°C]) for black tea.[40] After the water is added, sufficient time is needed for the brewing process. The appropriate time depends on the leaf size and type of tea. Generally, the smaller the leaf size, the quicker the tea infuses.[40] One to 3 minutes of time to steep is sufficient for loose leaf green tea and 3 to 5 minutes for black tea. When using a tea bag, approximately 3 minutes are needed.[40]

Desired Aesthetic Properties

The taste of a tea beverage depends on a number of different factors, including the soil and weather where the tea was grown; the age of the leaves at harvest; the processing methods used, including how long the leaves are allowed to oxidize and the type of wood used in the drying process; and the use of additives/flavorings.[38] The tea's color, pungency, and body come from polyphenols. The essential/aromatic oils give the tea its fragrance and flavor.[40]

Specific terms are used to describe the cup quality of tea. As with coffee, the *aroma* alludes to the smell, whereas the *body* details how the tea feels on the tongue. Other terms, such as *brisk* (slightly tangy) or *flowery* (hint of floral sweetness), are specific to certain varieties of tea.[38]

Gastronomy Point

Green Tea Tea originated in China, and it continues to permeate Chinese life. Green tea is consumed throughout the day and with meals.

Meal Planning

Tea is often consumed without accompaniment; however, it is also popular to savor baked goods, such as scones, cookies, or biscuits, while sipping a cup of hot tea. The versatility of the tea depends on the particular variety. For example, breakfast blend teas, which consist of a blend of black teas, can accompany a morning meal, whereas green tea makes a great beverage to sip on its own throughout the morning and afternoon. Teas can also be paired with certain meals. A general guideline is to match the type of tea with food from the same geographic region.[38]

Gastronomy Point

Pairing Tea Laura C. Martin's book, *Tea, the Drink that Changed the World*, lists the following tea/food pairing suggestions: Japanese green tea with seafood, fish, and rice; black teas with meat dishes; Chinese black tea with hot, spicy foods; and jasmine tea with delicately flavored meals.

Nutritional Properties

Tea includes polyphenols, alkaloids, amino acids, carbohydrates, proteins, chlorophyll, volatile organic compounds, fluoride, aluminum, minerals, and trace elements.[50] One group of chemicals thought to be responsible for the beneficial health effects of tea are the polyphenols, which include a group of plant chemicals called *catechins* (see **Figure 15.21**).[51] White and green tea contain epicatechin (EC), epigallocatechin (EGC), epicatechin gallate (ECG), and epigallocatechin gallate (EGCG), whereas oolong and black teas contain complex polyphenols called theaflavins and thearubigins.[52]

As the tea plant grows, fluoride accumulates in the leaves.[53] The fluoride content of tea varies, depending on the type of tea. Fluoride levels in green, oolong, and black teas are lower and closer to those recommended for the prevention of dental caries.[53] Caffeine is another component of tea; preparation methods, such as brewing time, the amount of tea and water used for brewing, and whether the tea is loose or in tea bags, will have a direct impact on the amount of caffeine.[53] Generally speaking, 8 ounces of tea contains approximately half the amount of caffeine as coffee.[54] Black teas contain the most caffeine: 64–112 mg per 8 ounces. Oolong tea contains 29–53 mg per 8 ounces. Green and white teas contain the least: 24–39 mg per 8 ounces and 32–37 mg per 8 ounces, respectively.[51]

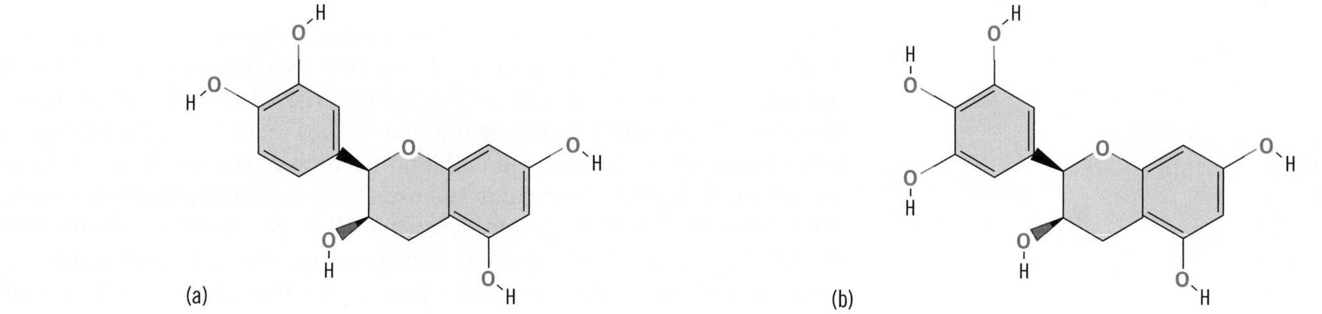

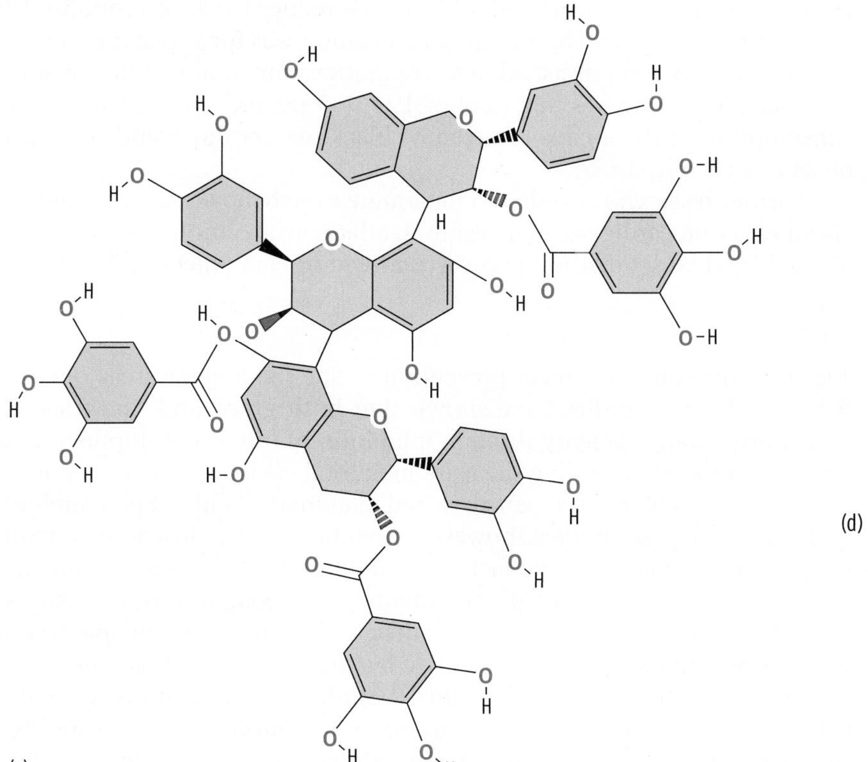

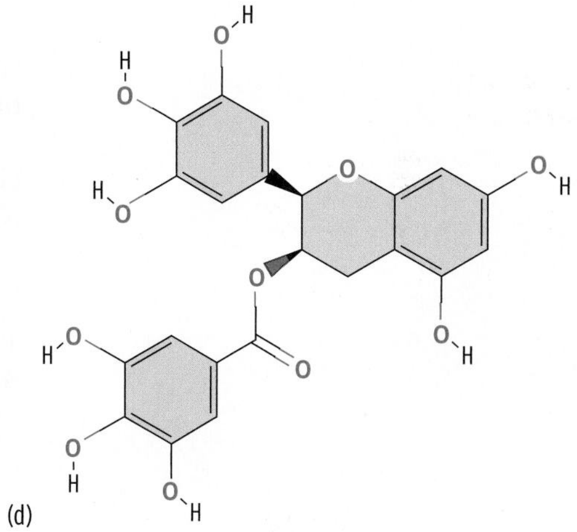

FIGURE 15.21 Teas contain catechins that have been found to have antioxidant properties. White and green tea have been shown to have high concentrations of (a) epicatechin, (b) epigallocatechin, (c) epicatechin gallate, and (d) epigallocatechin gallate.

Tea contains 14–27 μg/L of aluminum; variations are due to different soil conditions, different harvesting periods, and water quality. Aluminum is neurotoxic and is eliminated from the body through the kidneys. At present, it is unclear how much aluminum in tea is bioavailable. Overall, tea consumption does not appear to carry a high risk of aluminum toxicity.[55]

Flavonoids in tea can inhibit the bioavailability of dietary sources of nonheme iron, which is found in plant foods, dairy products, and iron supplements, by inhibiting intestinal absorption.[53] When drinking tea with a meal, it is recommended to consume foods that enhance iron absorption, such as foods rich in vitamin C or animal foods with heme iron (i.e., red meat). Tea consumed between meals does not seem to affect iron absorption.[55]

Impact on Health

Much research today is devoted to studying the association between tea consumption and disease prevention, most notably cancer and cardiovascular disease but also dental caries and periodontal disease, among others. Most studies have focused on the effects of green tea in particular.

Cardiovascular Disease

A meta-analysis conducted in 2001 examined 10 prospective cohort studies and 7 case-control studies and concluded that tea consumption of 24 ounces per day is associated with an 11% decreased risk of myocardial infarction.[46] Scientists emphasized, however, that the studies included in the analysis may have shown a bias due to preferential publication of studies showing a protective effect. Since this meta-analysis, prospective cohort studies have shown mixed results.[53] A more recent, relatively large prospective cohort study in 40,530 Japanese adults reported that green tea consumption is associated with reduced mortality due to all causes and cardiovascular-related mortality specifically.[56] The study showed that daily consumption of five or more cups of green tea is associated with a 26% reduced risk of mortality from cardiovascular disease. The strongest association was for stroke prevention. A recent meta-analysis published in 2009 that examined nine different studies (involving 4,379 strokes in a pool of 194,965 people) concluded that daily consumption of three cups of green or black tea per day could prevent the onset of ischemic stroke.[56]

Further research is needed to determine exactly how tea has such a beneficial effect on cardiovascular health. Under consideration are the effects of tea on blood vessel dilation and vascular endothelial function.[53]

Cancer

Tea consumption and cancer prevention is one the biggest areas of current research. Animal studies have shown that both green and black tea have cancer-preventative activity through inhibition of tumor development at different organ sites, including the skin, lung, oral cavity, esophagus, stomach, small intestine, colon, liver, pancreas, and mammary gland.[57] Epidemiological and clinical human studies, however, have been inconclusive. Inconsistent results may be due to several factors, including the types of teas studied, the methods of production, the bioavailability of tea compounds, differences in tea preparation and consumption, genetic variation in how people respond to tea consumption, and other lifestyle factors, such as tobacco and alcohol use, physical activity, or weight status.[51] Studies continue, however, and scientists are now focusing more attention on the effects of tea flavonoids on cell-signaling pathways; tea may help modulate the pathway that transforms healthy cells to cancerous cells.[53] Further studies are needed to evaluate the relationship between tea consumption and cancer risk.

Oral Disease

Tea also has been linked to reduced risk of dental caries and periodontal disease. Studies have shown that green, black, and oolong teas have extracts that inhibit the growth and acid production of cavity-producing bacteria in a test tube.[53] More studies involving human subjects are needed; however, results from a study involving 6,000 14-year old children in the United Kingdom are promising. The results indicated that those with higher tea consumption had significantly fewer dental caries relative to nondrinkers.[58]

A 2009 study concluded that there was a modest association between intake of green tea and periodontal disease prevention. The scientists evaluated the relationship between the intake of green tea and periodontal parameters. Every cup of green tea per day was associated with a 0.023 decrease in the mean periodontal disease after adjusting for confounding variables.[59] In vitro studies have indicated that the polyphenols in green tea inhibit the growth and adherence of periodontal pathogens, as well as their production of virulence factors. Further research in this arena is indicated and may soon result in recommendations.

Other Diseases

Tea's effects on other diseases, including osteoporosis and kidney disease, also are being studied. In terms of osteoporosis, results of studies are mixed; more studies are needed to determine whether tea consumption helps to prevent development of osteoporosis or reduce the risk of osteoporotic fractures.[53] With respect to kidney stones, more investigation is also needed, as studies and recommendation remain unclear. Coffee and tea are two of the more popular beverages consumed. Both have antioxidant properties and have been shown to be beneficial to health. Another beverage, wine, has also been shown to contain antioxidants that may be beneficial to health. See **Special Topic 15.3** for more on wine.

Special Topic 15.3

Wine and Winemaking

Jordan Tillery

History of Winemaking

According to an ancient fable, a Persian princess discovered wine. The princess had lost favor with the king and was planning to commit suicide. When she found a jar of grapes that had spoiled, she considered them to be poisonous and decided to consume them. Instead of the negative effects she had been hoping for, she became very happy and all of her anxieties lifted. The king adored her once more, and she rejoined her ranks in the court. Thus began grape fermentation and wine production.[1]

Wine has been a part of human history for many centuries. Over the years it has served many purposes—medicinal, religious, economic and social. Exact locations and dates when wine was first discovered are still unknown; however, more and more artifacts are being revealed. Based on the available evidence, it is thought that wine was produced and consumed as early as 6000 to 4000 B.C. around the areas of Mesopotamia and the Caspian Sea.[1] The first written reference to wine goes back to the ancient Egyptians. Only the privileged had access to this fermented beverage; some pharaohs and others of high status were buried with wine in order to ease their way into the underworld.[1]

The ancient Greeks also made wine. In Greece, wine was accessible to everyone, and it was used for everything from medicinal purposes to social rituals. When the Romans came through Greece around 1000 B.C., they took with them a knowledge of and taste for wine.[2] Upon arriving back in Italy, the Romans perfected the art of wine production. By considering the a region's particular soil and climate, they created different types and flavors of wine. The Romans may have been the first people to store wine in glass because glass blowing became popular around this time as well. In addition to perfecting the art of winemaking, the Greeks and Romans even had Gods of wine, known as Dionysus and Bacchus, respectively.[3]

Wine became a huge export from Italy once other countries heard about its benefits and wonderful taste. England, Spain, France, and Germany received the Italian imports and began production themselves. France started experimenting with different winemaking methods and soon became one of the largest wine producers in the world—it remains so today. Spain, Italy, and France accounted for 51% of the world wine production in 2004.[4]

The popularity of wine continued to spread through Europe and eventually over to Mexico. By the 1770s, California was already a growing power in wine manufacturing and distribution. Today, vineyards make up a relatively large portion of California, and this single state produces about 90% of American wines.[4]

The Winemaking Process

Winemaking is more complicated than just letting grapes spoil and extracting their juices (see **Figure A**). Harvesting the grapes is one of the most important steps in the winemaking process. The grapes are picked when they are at their ripest. The grapes are then put into a machine that crushes them and removes the stems. At this point, the grapes can either be pressed to extract the juices or left to drain (referred to as "free run"). Instead of being crushed or pressed, some red grapes are introduced whole into a closed vat in order to extract their juices.[5]

After the extraction processes are complete, the juice is allowed to ferment.[6] The yeast feeds on sugars from the grape juice, starting the fermentation process. Fermentation works best at the ideal temperature of 77°F (25°C).[5]

Next is the filtration process. The extracted grape juice is forced through a variety of screens. Once the juice is filtered of impurities and solids, it is refrigerated to prevent further yeast growth and also to allow carbon dioxide to keep the yeast cells suspended in the liquid. Once the wine has been filtered and clarified, it is allowed to age either in storage barrels or in bottles. Either screw caps or corks can be used during the bottling process; however, wines aged in bottles typically already have a cork closure.[5]

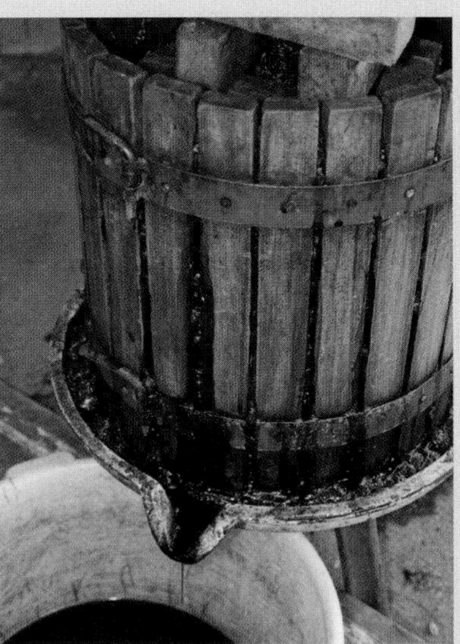

FIGURE A Winemaking involves a number of different steps, all of which are critical in producing a wine of optimal taste.

Defining and Choosing Wines

The three different colors of wine—white, red, and pink—have slightly different properties. White wine is made by removing the skin of the grapes before pressing, whereas red wine is pressed from whole grapes, including the skin and the seeds inside. Pink wine is just a mixture of the other two. Multiple factors come into play when selecting a wine. As with many products, the taste, smell, texture, and mouth feel are very important when choosing a wine.[5]

Impact on Health

The skin and seeds of the pressed grapes are what give red wine its redeeming qualities. Reservatrol is one of the polyphenolic compounds found in wine, especially red wine, which has been shown to have healthful benefits.[7] Other compounds found in wine are flavonols and anthocyanins. Flavonols reduce the level of LDL cholesterol (the "bad cholesterol") in the blood, and they raise the level of HDL cholesterol (the "good cholesterol").[8] Anthocyanins, which contribute to the red, purple, and blue colors of many fruits, including grapes, have been shown to lower rates of coronary heart disease.[7,8] Light-to-moderate consumption of wine may improve cardiovascular health by increasing the amount of HDL cholesterol, decreasing the risk of clot formation, reducing inflammation, and increasing antioxidant activity.[8]

Even though wine has many admirable qualities, it must be consumed in moderation. Overconsumption of wine, or any alcohol for that matter, can have detrimental effects on the body. How much wine should be consumed for maximum benefits? Most medical authorities state that men should limit their consumptions to one to two 4-ounce servings a day and women to one serving a day to receive the maximum health benefits.[9]

References

1 Professional Friends of Wine. Wine History. 2011. Available at: http://www.winepros.org/wine101/history.htm. Accessed November 4, 2011.

2 Cornell University. Songs of the Vine. 2008. Available at: http://rmc.library.cornell.edu/ewga/exhibition/introduction/index.html. Accessed November 9, 2011.

3 Encyclopedia Mythica Online. Dionysus. Available at: http://www.pantheon.org/articles/d/dionysus.html. Accessed November 4, 2011.

4 Goodhue R, Green R, Heien D, Martin P. California wine industry evolving to compete in 21st century. *California Agr.* January 2008;62(1):12–18.

5 Encyclopædia Britannica. Wine. 2011. Available at: http://www.britannica.com/EBchecked/topic/645269/wine. Accessed November 3, 2011.

6 McGovern PE, Fleming SJ, Katz SH. *The Origins and Ancient History of Wine.* Amsterdam: Gordon and Breach Publishers; 1996.

7 Wrolstad RE. The Possible Health Benefits of Anthocyanin Pigments and Polyphenolics. The Linus Pauling Institute; Oregon State University. Available at: http://lpi.oregonstate.edu/ss01/anthocyanin.html. Accessed December 3, 2011.

8 PubMed Health. Health and wine. *A.D.A.M. Medical Encyclopedia.* Available at: http://www.ncbi.nlm.nih.gov/pubmedhealth/PMH0002684. Accessed December 2, 2011.

9 Yale-New Haven Hospital. A Glass of Red Wine a Day Keeps the Doctor Away. Available at: http://www.ynhh.org/about-us/red_wine.aspx. Accessed December 3, 2011.

Food Safety

One of the main food safety concerns regarding tea involves pesticide residues. Because tea is the second most popular beverage worldwide, it is monitored to ensure that pesticide residues are below the Maximum Residue Limits (MRLs).[59] FAO has a panel that reviews residues, analytical aspects, metabolism, environmental fate, and use patterns of pesticides. Meanwhile, the World Health Organization (WHO) reviews toxicological and related data and estimates acceptable daily intakes (ADIs) of pesticides. International agencies including the FAO, WHO, and the European Economic Commission (EEC/EC) have created MRL levels for tea-growing countries; when tea contains residues that exceed the MRLs, a country's exports will decline, negatively affecting trade revenues.[59]

Another area of tea safety concern involves sun-brewed tea; when tea is prepared in this manner, the water does not reach a high-enough temperature to kill pathogens or bacteria that may be present (see **Figure 15.22**). In 1996, the Centers for Disease Control and Prevention released guidelines and recommendations for brewing iced tea in order to reduce the potential for bacterial contamination, which include (1) brewing iced tea at 195°F (90°C) for 3 to 5 minutes; (2) storing iced tea for no longer than 8 hours; (3) and cleaning the tea brewer/storage dispenser/faucet daily.[60]

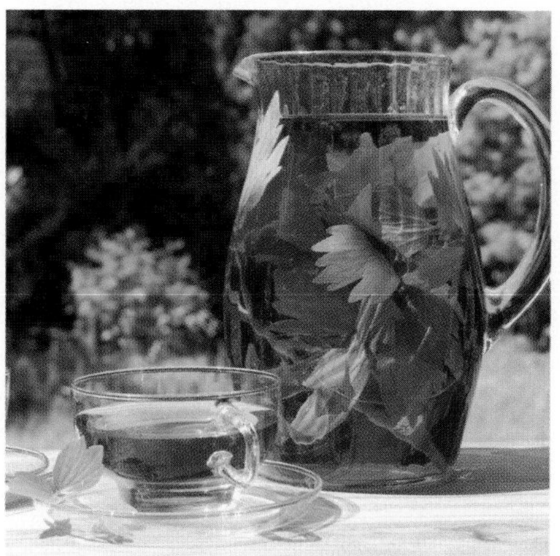

FIGURE 15.22 With sun-brewed tea, the tea is left to brew in a pitcher outside, with the heat coming from the sun. Although a summer favorite, it is best to use caution with sun-brewed tea to avoid foodborne illness.

The issue of fluorosis has received considerable attention from the scientific community. Different teas contain varying amounts of fluoride, and with moderate consumption (a liter or less per day) there seems to be no risk of excess fluoride intake. Fluoride levels in brick tea, however, may pose a problem. Brick tea is tea made from blocks of whole or finely ground black tea, green tea, or postfermented tea leaves that have been packed into molds and pressed into a block. Brick tea contains a range of 0.5–1.7 mg fluoride per 8-ounce serving. Tibetan children and adults who consume large amounts of brick tea have shown symptoms of **fluorosis** (fluoride excess), including axial skeletal pain and spinal rigidity.[53]

fluorosis A condition caused by exposure to excessive amounts of fluoride that is characterized by skeletal changes and by mottled tooth enamel.

Studies have shown that consumption of large volumes of instant tea over prolonged periods also can increase the risk of fluorosis. A 2005 study used two independent testing laboratories to evaluate the mean fluoride concentrations per liter in tea solutions. The results ranged from 1.0–6.5 parts per million (ppm). Notably, some teas exceeded the Environmental Protection Agency's safety limit of 4.0 ppm for drinking water and the Food FDA's limit of 1.4–2.4 ppm for bottled beverages. The typical American diet supplies less than 0.5 mg of fluoride a day. When combined with fluoridated water intake, consumption may be as high as approximately 1.0 mg of fluoride/day. Intake of 10 mg/day for prolonged periods of time can result in preclinical skeletal fluorosis.[61]

Food Technology

Tea has come a long way in terms of cultivation, production, packaging, and preparation. Many of the innovations in tea technology in the twentieth century have taken root in America.

In 1904, New Yorker Thomas Sullivan began placing single servings of loose leaf tea in hand-sewn silk bags instead of small canisters.[38] In 1952, the Lipton Tea Company developed a four-sided bag known as the "Flo-thru," which guaranteed adequate space for the tea leaves to expand and release optimal flavor.[38] Over time, the quality of tea bags has improved substantially, as has the grade of tea placed inside the bag. Consumer demand for higher quality tea bags has led to the introduction of a pyramid-shaped tea bag, which is made of a silken nylon material that allows room for longer leaf tea.[62]

Gastronomy Point

Tea Bags Tea bags are extremely popular today. More than 50% of the tea consumed in the United States is made from tea bags.

Phytonutrient Point

Ready-to-Drink Tea The polyphenol concentration of ready-to-drink teas is substantially lower relative to other teas. The highest polyphenol concentrations are found in brewed hot tea.

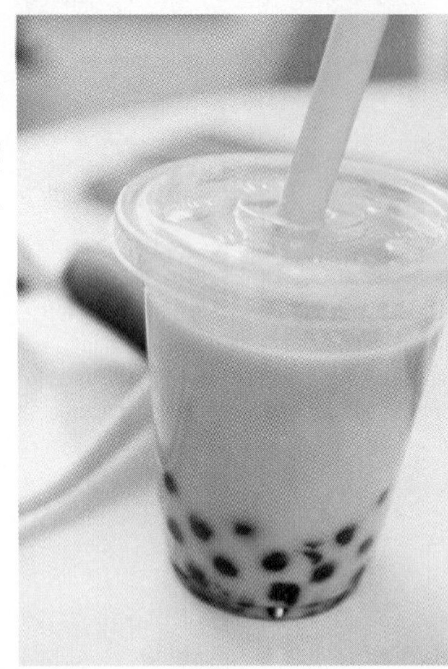

FIGURE 15.23 Bubble tea, which originated in Taiwan, is usually made with tea blended with fruit, milk, or syrup and small, chewy tapioca balls.

An Englishman, Richard Blechynden, is credited with inventing sweetened iced tea at the St. Louis World Fair in 1904, and its popularity soon spread across America.[39] Instant tea and iced tea mixes were formulated in the 1940s and 1950s.[44] Ready-to-drink iced tea is one of the fastest-growing sectors of the American tea market, largely due to its convenience. The tea is ready-to-drink in easy-to-carry bottles, cans, and plastic containers.[38]

Bubble tea, also known as "pearl tea drink" or "boba," has become increasingly popular in the United States (see **Figure 15.23**). Bubble tea, a concoction of cold, infused tea with black tapioca "pearls" and sweet flavoring, originated in Taiwan in the 1980s.[38]

Going Green with Tea

In 2008, the Center for Research on Multinational Corporations released a report outlining the social, economic, and ecological conditions of six of the most important tea-producing countries: India, Sri Lanka, Vietnam, Indonesia, Kenya, and Malawi. Tea production raises several environmental issues, including habitat conversion, energy use, and agrochemical use.[45] Converting forests and natural animal habitats into tea plantations may qualify as the most environmentally damaging effect of tea production because it not only leads to species reduction but also causes considerable soil erosion.[63] Deforestation also is a problem because the drying process commonly involves burning firewood from natural forests. The multiple steps of tea production also require an enormous amount of energy.[45] Lastly, because tea is mainly grown on plantations and in a monoculture, tea producers rely heavily on large quantities of pesticides, which have detrimental impacts on the environment, including:[59]

- Reduction in soil biodiversity
- Water pollution
- Development of pesticide-resistant crops
- Resurgence of pests or outbreak of secondary pests
- Toxic pesticide residues

Alternative methods of pest management are exist, including integrated pest management (IPM). IPM uses an effective and environmentally sensitive approach to pest management that relies on commonsense practices, such as mechanical trapping devices, natural predators (insects that eat other insects), insect growth regulators, mating disruption substances, and the use of biological pesticides.[64]

In terms of social and economic aspects of tea production, the following issues were highlighted in the 2008 report:[45]

- Poor working conditions with low wages
- Low job and income security
- Discrimination along ethnic and gender lines
- Lack of protective gear
- Inadequate basic facilities, such as housing, drinking water, and food

More environmentally and socially conscious options are available for consumers, including fair trade teas and teas from producers that belong to the Ethical Tea Partnership (ETP) monitoring and improvement program (see **Figure 15.24**). The ETP is a not-for-profit membership organization of tea companies that share a vision of a thriving tea industry that is socially just and environmentally sustainable. The ETP has local staff in Kenya, Malawi, India, Indonesia, Sri Lanka and China, and a London-based team. Together with a set of partner organizations, the ETP runs a range of assurance, producer support, and strategic programs to improve the sustainability of the tea sector, the lives of tea workers, and the environment in which tea is produced. The ETP was established in 1997 and currently has more than 25 international members.[65]

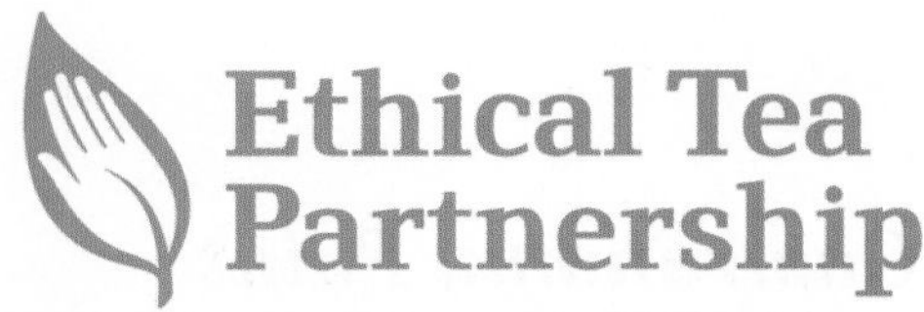

FIGURE 15.24 Producers who adhere to Ethical Tea Partnership criteria for the environment and workers rights can use the ETP logo as marketing tool.

Source: Courtesy of the Ethical Tea Partnership.

Sports Beverages

Historical, Cultural, and Ecological Significance

Sports beverages made their debut in the mid-1960s, and their effectiveness was showcased by way of the Florida Gators football team. In the summer of 1965, University of Florida football coaches noticed that their players were adversely affected by heat and heat-related illnesses and that their performance on the field suffered as a consequence.[66] University physicians and researchers eventually realized that both fluid and electrolyte losses, which occurred on the football field during practice and games, were not being replenished. A beverage containing a precise combination of carbohydrates and **electrolytes**—ions in body fluids that are integral to metabolic and energetic processes—was soon concocted and called "Gatorade."

As the Florida Gators improved their performance and began to win more games, other college and university football coaches across the country took note and began demanding the beverage, which increased sales nationwide.[66] Gatorade soon became the official sports drink of the National Football League (NFL). Sports beverage consumption is widespread among professional and recreational athletes alike. Sports drinks also appeal to those who do not engage in particular sports or physical activity on a daily basis.

A **sports drink** is a beverage designed to quench thirst faster than water and replenish the sugar and minerals lost from the body during physical exercise.[67] Although plain water is a good thirst quencher, it is a poor rehydrator because it takes approximately 30 to 60 minutes for it to be absorbed and distributed throughout the body.[68] When exercise lasts longer than an hour, muscle and liver glycogen stores become depleted, and a sports drink is indicated. A sports drink is superior to water in that it helps to maintain the physiological drive to drink.[69] During exercise, thirst is not a reliable guide because hot weather and/or strenuous exercise can cause large fluid losses before a person feels thirsty.[68] A wide variety of sports drinks are on the market; some replace carbohydrates and electrolytes; others contain protein, specific amino acids, and fat; and some provide herbs, vitamins, and caffeine (see **Figure 15.25**).[70]

electrolytes Ions in bodily fluids that are integral to metabolic and energetic processes; include chloride, sodium, and potassium.

sports drink Beverage designed to quench thirst faster than water and replenish the sugar and minerals lost from the body during physical exercise.

osmolality/osmolar solution Concentration of a solution expressed as osmoles of solute per liter of solution or as milliosmols per kilogram (mOsm/kg) of water.

hyponatremia Condition when blood serum sodium falls below normal levels.

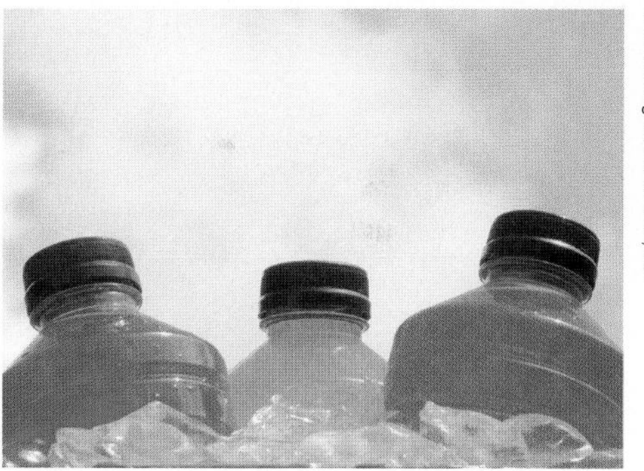

FIGURE 15.25 Since their introduction in the 1960s, the number of sports drinks on the market has exploded. Sports drinks to satisfy every need have been developed. In addition to electrolytes, many are now infused with vitamins, proteins, amino acids, herbs, and caffeine.

Physical and Chemical Properties

The desirable composition of a sports beverage includes a carbohydrate fuel source, such as glucose, sucrose, or glucose polymers, and electrolytes, such as sodium, potassium, and chloride, which are the main electrolytes lost in sweat when exercise exceeds 1 hour.[68]

Several different studies have suggested that the optimal amount of carbohydrate replacement during exercise ranges from 6–8%, which allows carbohydrates to be absorbed rapidly while maximizing gastric emptying rates. The carbohydrates provided in the beverage will help to fuel both the muscles and the brain, maintaining blood glucose levels and promoting the uptake of carbs into the muscle cells.[69]

The **osmolality** (i.e., the concentration of the **osmolar solution**) for a sports drink should be close to that of human body fluids.[70] The amount of optimal electrolyte ranges from 70–165 mg/240 mL for sodium and 30–75 mg/240 mL for potassium. The electrolytes not only replenish those which are lost during exercise, but they also help to enhance palatability of the beverage.[68] The provision of electrolytes is also helpful in preventing muscle cramps. Sodium replacement is particularly critical in preventing **hyponatremia**, a

Gastronomy Point

Sports Beverages For a sports beverage to be marketed successfully, the beverage must be highly palatable as well as appealing in appearance and texture. The electrolytes help to enhance flavor; interestingly, carbonation may actually decrease palatability.

condition characterized by dangerously low blood sodium levels. Hyponatremia is caused by prolonged heavy sweating with failure to replace sodium or by excessive plain water intake.[71] **Table 15.2** lists the desirable content of sports beverages.

Other sports beverage additives include protein and caffeine. Carbohydrate is the preferred fuel for both short- and longer-duration endurance exercise, whereas protein is not a major contributor to energy supply. Protein's main purpose in the body is structural. When added to sports beverages, protein may be in the form of casein, whey, soy, or individual amino acids. The most commonly used amino acids include branched-chain amino acids (BCAAs), such as leucine, isoleucine, and valine.[70]

gluconeogenesis Production of new glucose by metabolic pathways within the cell.

It is thought that when glycogen and blood glucose levels fall due to prolonged exercise, BCAAs will be used to produce energy via **gluconeogenesis**—the production of glucose by metabolic pathways within the cells. Thus, supplementation may delay the onset of fatigue.[70] Additionally, BCAAs can decrease synthesis of serotonin, a neurotransmitter in the brain, which is associated with early fatigue.[72] However, to date, no studies have confirmed the effectiveness of BCAAs in blunting the effects of fatigue.

An overwhelming amount of literature over the past 30 years has evaluated the effect of caffeine on endurance exercise performance. Low doses of 5–6 mg/kg body weight have shown performance-enhancing effects.[70] Studies have shown that moderate caffeine ingestion from supplements, coffee, or tea (3–6 mg/kg body weight) prior to and/or during exercise sessions lasting more than an hour can increase time to exhaustion, decrease the rate of perceived exertion, and increase glycogen sparing (forgoing the use of body glucose reserves for energy).[70] Caffeine's mechanism of action is still not clearly understood. Caffeine has a broad range of effects on a metabolisms, hormones, and physiology.[73] However, caffeine that has been *added to* a sports beverage has not been clearly shown to have a performance-enhancing effect. **Table 15.3** lists the amount of caffeine in a variety of beverages and foods. One popular beverage that is a common source of caffeine is carbonated soft drinks, which are discussed in **Special Topic 15.4**.

TABLE 15.2
Composition of Sports Beverages

Component	Comment
Fuel source	Contains carbohydrate: glucose, sucrose, and glucose polymers (maltodextrin). Goal intake is 60–70 g/hr (approximately 1 liter of a 6–8% carbohydrate drink).
Electrolytes	Contains sodium (70–165 mg per 240 mL) and potassium (30–75 mg per 240 mL) to replace electrolytes lost in sweat when exercise is longer than 3 to 4 hours in duration. Electrolytes also enhance palatability.
Rapid absorption	Contains 6–8% carbohydrates. A high carbohydrate concentration slows gastric emptying and intestinal absorption.
Palatability	Flavored beverages enhance consumption. Electrolytes enhance flavor. Carbonation may decrease the amount of fluid consumed.

Source: Reproduced from Fink HH, Burgoon LA, Mikesky AE. *Practical Applications in Sports Nutrition.* 2nd ed. Sudbury, MA: Jones and Bartlett Publishers; 2009.

TABLE 15.3
Caffeine Content in Different Beverages and Foods

Beverage/Food	Size	Caffeine/mg
Coffee, decaf	150 mL (5 oz)	2–5
Tea	150 mL (5 oz)	40–80
Hot cocoa	150 mL (5 oz)	1–8
Chocolate milk	225 mL	2–7
Jolt Cola	12 oz	100
Josta	12 oz	58
Mountain Dew	12 oz	55
Surge	12 oz	51
Diet Coca-Cola	12 oz	45
Coca-Cola	12 oz	64
Coca-Cola Classic	12 oz	23
Dr. Pepper	12 oz	61
Mello Yellow	12 oz	35
Mr. Pibb	12 oz	27
Pepsi Cola	12 oz	43
7-Up	12 oz	0
Mug Root Beer	12 oz	0
Sprite	12 oz	0
Ben & Jerry's no-fat coffee fudge frozen yogurt	1 cup	85
Starbucks coffee ice cream	1 cup	40–60
Dannon coffee yogurt	8 oz	45
100 Grand bar	1 bar (43 g)	11.2
Krackel bar	1 bar (47 g)	8.5
Reese's Peanut Butter Cup	1 pack (51 g)	5.6
Kit Kat bar	1 bar (46 g)	5
Raisinets	10 pieces (10 g)	2.5
Butterfinger bar	1 bar (61 g)	2.4
Baby Ruth bar	1 bar (60 g)	2.4
Special Dark chocolate bar	1 bar (41 g)	31
Chocolate brownie	1.25 oz	8
Chocolate chip cookie	30 g	3–5
Chocolate ice cream	50 g	2–5
Milk chocolate	1 oz	1–15
Bittersweet chocolate	1 oz	5–35

Source: Reproduced from the U.S. Food and Drug Administration. Medicines in My Home: Caffeine and Your Body. 2007. Available at: http://www.fda.gov/Drugs/ResourcesForYou/Consumers/BuyingUsingMedicineSafely/UnderstandingOver-the-CounterMedicines/ucm093517.htm

Special Topic 15.4

Carbonated Beverages and Soft Drinks

Christina Ypsilantis

Carbonated waters were first used for medicinal purposes in Europe's natural hot spas. These waters contain strong tastes and odors from dissolved chemicals and minerals produced by volcanic action below the earth's surface. Europeans bathed and drank from these tonic waters for medical cures. The spas claimed that the waters cured rheumatism, gout, nephritis, and dyspepsia, among many other things. Scientists eventually discovered that when carbonated waters are trapped under the earth, the carbon dioxide begins to dissolve in the water. The waters only begin to fizz when the carbon dioxide reaches the water's surface. (This is similar to when soda is unopened in the can. Soda does not begin to fizz until the cap is snapped off.)[1]

Bottling "Medicinal Waters"

At first, interest in bottling carbonated water was driven by a desire to provide the public easier access to its medicinal attributes. In the late 1700s, the British scientist Joseph Priestly mixed carbon dioxide and water to create carbonated water. He collected carbon dioxide to use in his experiments by trapping the vapors given off by fermenting beer. The taste of the carbonated water was quite tangy and bitter, similar to the early spa waters (or to a modern-day club soda). Priestly found that the carbonated waters neutralized the acidity in the stomach.[1]

The scientist responsible for bringing these artificially created carbonated waters to the United States was a Yale University chemistry professor named Benjamin Silliman. He spent a great deal of time figuring out how to bottle carbonated water without the contents exploding out of the bottle; this is how soda "pop" received its name.[1]

Adding Flavorings

Until 1850, carbonated beverages were bland and bitter; it wasn't until flavorings were added that they started to be consumed based on taste (although initially soda flavorings were added to carbonated water only for medicinal purposes). In the mid-1800s sugar and flavorings began to be added to carbonated water. Pharmacists would add roots, herbs, and leaves to improve the taste of the carbonated water as well as to provide additional curatives. For example, raspberry leaves, ribwort, nettles, birch bark, currant leaves, dandelion, sassafras, and strawberry leaves were all added to carbonated water.[1]

Pharmacists created new soda flavors and began to create artificial colors in laboratories. One artificial color, caramel, which is created by burning sugar, is still used to color cola beverages today. Prior to the passage of the Pure Food and Drug Act, pharmacists were allowed to experiment with any dye or flavoring they wanted.[1]

The Advent of Soft Drinks

Flavored carbonated beverages gained popularity as tasty beverages consumed just for pleasure instead of for potential medicinal benefit (see **Figure A**). These beverages were termed *soft drinks* to differentiate them from alcoholic (*hard*) alternatives.

The production of soft drinks starts with finely purified water. Soft drink manufacturers filter tap water through fine, clean sand and gravel to remove any impurities from the water before further processing. Flavorings—sugars, syrups, and/or sugar substitutes—then are added to the purified solution. After the base of the soft drink has been made, it goes through a carbonator or a carbo-cooler, which carbonates the syrup–water mixture.[2]

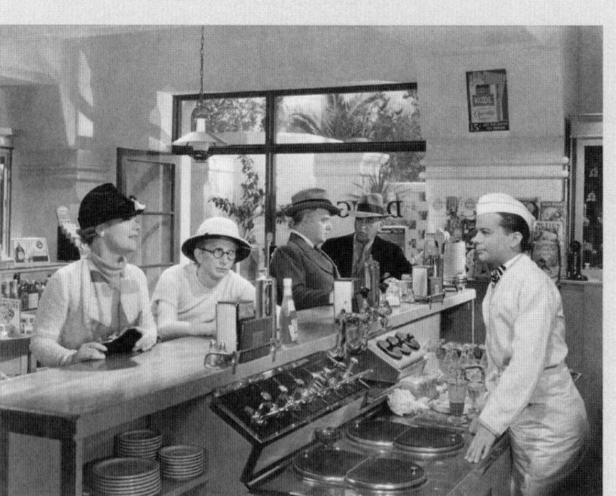

FIGURE A Prohibition, which outlawed the sale and consumption of alcohol in the 1920s, also might have helped to make carbonated sodas more popular. In the 1920s, most drugstores had soda fountains. People who once congregated in bars were now congregating at the soda fountains.

The most common sweetener used in soft drinks is high-fructose corn syrup. Most diet soft drinks contain non-nutritive chemical sweeteners. Some of these non-nutritive sweeteners have been approved by the FDA, whereas others have not. Aspartame is a popular chemical sweetener that is found in Diet Coke.

Health Concerns

A number of heath issues have been associated with soft drink consumption. The consumption of soda has increased about 300% over the past 20 years, and sodas are the leading source of added dietary sugars in the United States. One study found that adolescents understood that sugared and artificially sweetened sodas were unhealthy, but yet they still consumed them.[3] Typically, one regular 12-ounce soda supplies 140 calories and about 9 teaspoons of sugar—an alarming amount of sugar for just one beverage.[4] The country's high rate of soda consumption has been linked to the rising rate of obesity and type 2 diabetes.

Children are becoming obese and are beginning to develop type 2 diabetes because they are not consuming healthful foods and beverages but are instead opting for sugary foods and beverages. This has sparked debate in many school districts about banning the sale of soft drinks in schools. Regular soda consumption is associated with metabolic syndrome, osteoporosis, kidney problems, dental caries, and negative caffeine reactions.[4] It is important to educate all generations, but especially youth, to curb their consumption of these unhealthy and non-nutritious beverages.

Overall, the history of soda has evolved immensely—beverages that started out as medical cures with natural flavorings have become sodas with artificial flavorings that are a detriment to health. The evolution of soda is still ongoing; it could perhaps take a turn in a positive and nutritious direction, or it could plateau. The most important point is to consume everything in moderation. A diet based on whole and natural foods and beverages rather than artificial ones is the more healthful option.

References

1 Tchudi SN. *Soda Poppery: The History of Soft Drinks in America.* New York: Charles Scribner's Sons; 1986.

2 Australian Refreshment Beverage. How Soft Drinks Are Made. 2004. Available at: http://www.australianbeverages.org/scripts/cgiip.exe/WService=ASP0002/ccms.r?PageID=10055.

3 Stop drinking soda? How this beverage could affect your health. *Mayo Clinic Women's Healthsource.* 2010;14;1–2.

4 Frank-White N, Frank E. Diet vs. sugar-sweetened soda preferences and attitudes in a sample of adolescents. Open Pediatr Med J. 2010;4:23–25.

Impact on Health and Athletic Performance

Adequate fluid intake is the number one nutrition intervention for all athletes because hydration status is a critical determinant of the athlete's physiological capacity to train, compete, and recover successfully (see **Table 15.4**). Even the slightest levels of dehydration (~2% of body water levels) can adversely affect exercise performance.[69]

TABLE 15.4
Adverse Effects of Dehydration on Exercise and Performance

Body Weight Loss	Adverse Effects on Performance
1%	The thirst threshold. Leads to decrease in physical work capacity.
2%	Stronger thirst, vague discomfort, loss of appetite.
3%	Dry mouth, increasing hemoconcentration, reduction in urine output.
4%	Decrease of 20–30% in physical work capacity.
5%	Difficulty concentrating, headache, sleepiness.
6%	Severe impairment in ability to regulate body temperature during exercise; increased respiratory rate, leading to tingling and numbness of extremities.
7%	Collapse is likely if combined with heat and exercise.

Individual fluid and electrolyte needs are variable during physical exercise because people differ in their metabolic rate and body mass and the environmental conditions in which they exercise.[74] Hydration goals, therefore, must be highly individualized. Fluid should be consumed at rates that closely match the athlete's sweating rates.[68] As noted earlier, plain water is only sufficient for exercise lasting less than an hour. One of the most effective ways to prevent dehydration is the consumption of sports beverages because they encourage voluntary intake, stimulate fast absorption of sugar and electrolytes, promote rapid and complete rehydration, and improve performance.[69]

The literature strongly highlights the importance of adequate hydration and its beneficial effects on performance. (However, an important caveat is that the majority of sports nutrition research has been conducted on young, highly trained male athletes, so the results cannot be generalized to the entire population.[70]) In 2005, a panel of international experts convened for the American College of Sports Medicine Roundtable on Hydration and Physical Activity. The experts combed through a wide array of sports nutrition research and formulated several consensus statements. Additionally, they conducted an evidence-based analysis of hydration and determined the best recommendations for fluid, electrolyte, and carbohydrate intake before, during, and after exercise.[74]

In terms of sports performance, substantial fluid deficits greater than 2% of baseline body weight can induce loss of performance capacity via degradation of physical and mental performance, increased cardiovascular strain, changes in metabolism, and decreased heat tolerance. Additionally, dehydration negatively affects short-term memory, working memory, psychomotor and visual motor skills, arithmetic ability, and mood. A consensus statement recognized that drinking carbohydrate–electrolyte sports beverages enhances performance in comparison to plain water during prolonged (45 to 50 minutes) exercise, as well as during high-intensity, intermittent exercise. In recent years, the sports drink industry has started to promote beverages containing **ergogenic aids**, which are substances or practices believed to improve athletic performance that are taken before, during, or after physical activity. See **Special Topic 15.5** for more on the addition of ergogenic aids to sports drinks. Other sports drinks tout that they contain valuable phytonutrients. See **Special Topic 15.6** for more about sports drinks and phytonutrients.

ergogenic aids Substances or practices believed to improve athletic performance that are taken before, during, or after physical activity.

Special Topic 15.5

Ergogenic Aids in Sport Drinks

Michelle Palladino

Now more than ever within the world of sports and nutrition, the supplement industry has erupted, with specific emphasis on fitness and athletics. Within the past 5 to 10 years, the use of performance enhancers, or ergogenic aids, has taken off. Ergogenic aids are substances or practices believed to improve one's athletic performance that are taken before, during, or after physical activity. Ergogenic aids can be grouped into five major categories: mechanical (weight training), psychological (meditation), physiological (HGH, blood doping), pharmacological (anabolic steroids), and nutritional (sports drinks).[1]

Although most of these classifications of ergogenic aids are directed at athletes, nutritional ergogenic aids, specifically sports drinks, affect the everyday consumer because of their widespread availability.[2] The wide variety of commercial sports drinks, including Gatorade and PowerAde, provide at least 50–80 calories and contain 14–17 grams of carbohydrate (sucrose, glucose, and fructose) per 8 ounces of water. The carbohydrates act as ergogenic aids by enhancing stomach emptying, improving fluid absorption, and increasing the body's energy supply. The electrolytes in sports drinks—especially calcium, magnesium, sodium, potassium, and chloride—act as ergogenic aids by conserving fluid in the muscle cells and replacing those lost through sweat.[2,3]

Aside from water, carbohydrates, and electrolytes, other ergogenic aids are being added to commercial sports drinks, including folic acid, amino acids, zinc, and vitamins A, E, B_1, B_2, B_6, and B_{12}.[1] These ergogenic aids are believed to optimize muscle growth, repair, and contractility, as well as enhance glycogen metabolism, energy production, and aerobic activity.[3]

Although some studies have shown ergogenic benefits from sports drinks, the research findings are usually specific to athletes performing more than 1 hour of strenuous endurance exercise, such as long-distance running or repetitive exercises in summer heat. In these circumstances, the carbohydrates within these beverages are immediately used by muscles, promoting a rapid increase in energy. The results do not necessarily apply to the typical (often sedentary) American. The ease of availability of sports drinks concerns many dietitians, who argue that if vigorous exercise is not being preformed then the carbohydrates in sports drinks are simply stored as fat within adipose tissue. The combination of a sedentary lifestyle with an overconsumption of these beverages may lead to obesity as well as an increased risk of developing type 2 diabetes.[1,3]

According to the Academy of Nutrition and Dietetics, it is unnecessary for most athletes, and especially the average American consumer, to consume the additional ergogenic aids provided in sports drinks if they are eating a nutritious and wholesome diet.[1] Nutritional ergogenic aids should be used with caution and only after evaluation of the product for safety, value, and potency.

References

1 Academy of Nuritition and Dietetics. Position of the American Dietetic Association, Dietitians of Canada, and the American College of Sports Medicine: Nutrition and athletic performance. *J Am Diet Assoc.* 2010;100(12):1543–1546.

2 Tokish J, Kocher M, Hawkins R. Ergogenic aids: A review of basic science, performance, side effects, and status in sport. *Am J Sports Med.* 2004;32(6):1543–1553.

3 Ahrendt D. Ergogenic aids: Counseling the athlete. *Am FamPhysician.* 2001;63(5):913–23.

Special Topic 15.6

Phytonutrients in Sports Beverages

Rene Reynolds, MS, RD, LDN

Phytonutrients, or phytochemicals, are chemicals produced by plants that may have beneficial effects on health. Phytonutrients are not essential, and there is limited evidence of the health effects of each specific chemical. Examples of phytonutrients include carotenoids, chlorophyll, chlorophyllin, curcumin, fiber, flavonoids, phytosterols, and resveratrol. Beverages with naturally occurring phytochemicals include orange juice, cranberry juice, tea, and red wine.[1]

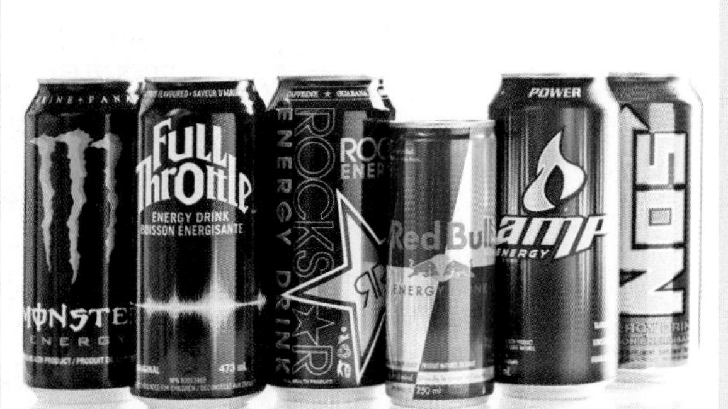

A wide variety of sports energy drinks are available in the marketplace. They are marketed primarily toward young men and sports enthusiasts.

Phytochemicals reached mainstream status in 2008. Initially, sports beverages did not contain any phytonutrients, and solely consisted of carbohydrates, electrolytes, and water. However, today some sports beverages incorporate phytonutrients to distinguish themselves in the marketplace. Phytonutrient-added sports beverages are relatively new and are not very widespread. Currently, no convincing evidence indicates that they enhance sports performance.[2]

One example of a sports drink with added phytonutrients is one that has microencapsulated citrus phytochemicals. The encapsulation conceals the bitter taste of these compounds while supposedly conveying the benefits of citrus fruits.

Sports energy drinks are common on grocery store and health food store shelves today. These drinks are formulated to contain stimulants and additives to boost energy and mental concentration. The first and most well-known energy beverage is Red Bull, which was first introduced in 1997 and accounts for the majority of energy drinks sold in the United States.[3] The target market for sports drinks includes men 15 to 30 years of age and sport enthusiasts.[3] Based on Red Bull's success, hundreds of other energy drinks are now available.

The most common ingredient in energy beverages is caffeine, which is commonly combined with taurine, glucuronolactone, guarana, and B vitamins to create an appealing "energy blend."[3] Guarana is one of the most commonly used ingredients; it contains an array of phytochemicals, including theophylline, theobromine, tannins, saponins, and caffeine. Guarana can enhance the effects of caffeine.[4]

Acai and green tea are also being added to energy drinks because of the phytochemicals they contain. Again, the effects of phytochemicals—alone or within sports or energy beverages—on exercise and sports performance have not been well researched.

References

1 Oregon State Info Center. Phytochemicals. Available at: http://lpi.oregonstate.edu/infocenter/phytochemicals. Accessed May 2011.
2 Sloan E. Getting Ahead of the Curve: Phytochemicals. Available at: http://beta.rodpub.com/uploads/trendsense-0110.pdf. Accessed May 2011.
3 Higgins JP, Tuttle TD, Higgins CL. Energy beverages: Content and safety. *Mayo Clin Proc.* 2010;85(11):1033–1041.
4 Ask the Experts: Are Energy Drinks Safe to Consume? Available at: http://chnr.ucdavis.edu. Accessed May 2011.

Food Safety and Regulations

Consumption of sports drinks is well warranted in athletes during and after vigorous physical activity and poses little if any health risks. Energy drinks, however, can pose significant dangers to health when they overused or misused. The debate continues over the safety of energy drinks; some people feel that regulations are too lax. Regulation of energy beverages globally is not standardized, and the United States does not have strict regulations—energy beverage companies are free to make energy and performance-enhancement claims at their own discretion. Due to the absence of strong oversight, the industry exhibits very aggressive marketing.[73]

The caffeine content of energy drinks ranges from 70–150 mg/serving, and one bottle may contain up to three servings.[75] Although healthy adults can consume up to 400 mg of caffeine daily, drinking several bottles of an energy drink can result in excessive caffeine intake, characterized by nervousness, irritability, sleeplessness, abnormal heart rhythms, and upset stomach.[75] To minimize risk from energy beverages, it is recommended to:

- Limit consumption to 500 mL, or two cans per day.
- Rehydrate with water or appropriately formulated sports beverages after/during intense physical exercise.[76]
- Avoid mixing alcohol with energy beverages. Mixing with alcohol before consuming an energy drink during exercise is very dangerous.

Making Sports Drinks Green

The biggest sustainability issue in terms of sports beverages is the use of plastic bottle packaging. The production of these bottles uses an immense amount of water as well as energy derived from fossil fuels.[77] Additionally, most clear plastic bottles are made from polyethylene terephthalate (PET), which may yield leach harmful chemicals, including endocrine disruptors.[70]

As customer concern shifts to the environment, many beverage companies are beginning to put sustainability measures in place. For example, Coca-Cola launched a new annual sustainability report in early 2011 outlining different initiatives, including the use and delivery of 2.5 billion "PlantBottle" packaging bottles in nine major markets.[78] These bottles consist of 30% plant-based material and are 100% recyclable. Many companies are trying to incorporate the use of bioplastics, which are derived from cornstarch and natural polymers. Nestle, for example, has pledged to develop bottles produced entirely from recycled or renewable material by 2020.[79] Companies also are looking into redesigning the shape of bottles to reduce the amount of plastic used.

Another green option for consumers is to create their own sports beverages at home and drink them from a reusable 1-liter container. A recipe can be as simple as 4 teaspoons sugar/honey, 1 teaspoon salt, and 4 ounces orange juice. Another way to avoid plastic bottles is to mix sports drink powders with tap water and transport the beverage in a metal canteen or a reusable water bottle.

Chapter Review

The two main types of coffee bean roasts are medium and dark. Medium roasts have a delicate flavor, and darker roasts have a more bitter taste. Keeping coffee away from excessive air, moisture, heat, and light will guarantee optimal flavor. The most common brewing method for coffee today is the filter method. The standardized recipe for a cup of filtered coffee is 2 level tablespoons of coffee grounds for each cup.

Coffee contains more than a thousand different chemicals and is composed of carbohydrates, lipids, nitrogenous compounds, vitamins, minerals, alkaloids, and phenolic compounds. Current research indicates that coffee consumption is associated with a significant dose-dependent reduction in the risk of developing type 2 diabetes mellitus. In addition, coffee does not appear to pose significant health risks. Main areas of coffee safety concern include chemical residues, such as pesticides; proper processing; storage conditions; and contamination. One of the most well-known contaminants in coffee is a mycotoxin called aflatoxin. Coffee can be designated as fair trade, organic, or bird friendly, which can help customers select coffee that is produced in an environmentally and socially responsible manner.

The four different stages of tea processing result in four different varieties of tea: black, green, oolong, and white. The taste of the tea beverage depends on the processing method, the region where the tea is grown, the weather, the use of additives/flavorings, the type of soil in the tea garden, age of the leaves when they are plucked, how long the leaves are allowed to oxidize, and the type of wood used in the drying process. Many different tea additives are used; flavoring agents are sprayed onto heated tea leaves; spices and fruit rinds can be mixed into the tea leaves; and honey or milk can also be added to the brewed tea. Tea is composed of a wide variety of ingredients, and the chemicals thought to be responsible for the beneficial health effects of tea include polyphenols. However, flavonoids in tea can inhibit the bioavailability of dietary sources of nonheme iron. Because tea is the second most popular beverage worldwide, it is monitored carefully to ensure that pesticide residues are below the Maximum Residue Limits (MRLs).

Tea consumption is correlated with beneficial cardiovascular effects; researchers are investigating the potential mechanisms, which include the impact of tea on blood vessel dilation and vascular endothelial function. Investigations continue to look at tea's ability to reduce cardiovascular disease risk, prevent cancer, osteoporosis, kidney stones, and assist in weight loss. Ready-to-drink tea is one of the fastest growing sectors of the American tea market. The polyphenol concentration of ready-to-drink teas is substantially lower relative to other (hot, brewed) teas. Environmental issues concerning tea production include habitat conversion, energy use, and agrochemical use. There are options for consumers who are environmentally and socially conscious, including fair trade teas and tea certified by the Ethical Tea Partnership (ETP).

Sports beverages made their debut in 1965 and were used by the University of Florida football team to replenish fluids and electrolytes lost and boost performance. When exercise lasts more than an hour, a sports drink is indicated because muscle and liver glycogen stores start to deplete. During exercise, thirst is not a reliable guide as large fluid losses can occur prior to feeling thirsty.

A sports beverage includes a carbohydrate fuel source (such as glucose or sucrose) and electrolytes (potassium, chloride, and sodium). The carbohydrate helps to fuel both the muscles and brain, maintaining blood glucose levels and promoting the uptake of carbs into the muscle cells. Low doses of caffeine (5–6 mg/kilogram body weight) have shown performance-enhancing effects in athletes. Adequate fluid intake is the number one nutrition intervention for all athletes because hydration status is a critical determinant of the athlete's physiological capacity to train, compete, and recover successfully. The goal for minimum fluid replacement during most activities should be to limit fluid deficits to less than 2% of baseline body weight. Drinking carbohydrate–electrolyte sports beverages enhances performance in comparison to plain water during prolonged (45 to 50 minutes) exercise, as well as during high-intensity, intermittent exercise.

Learning Portfolio

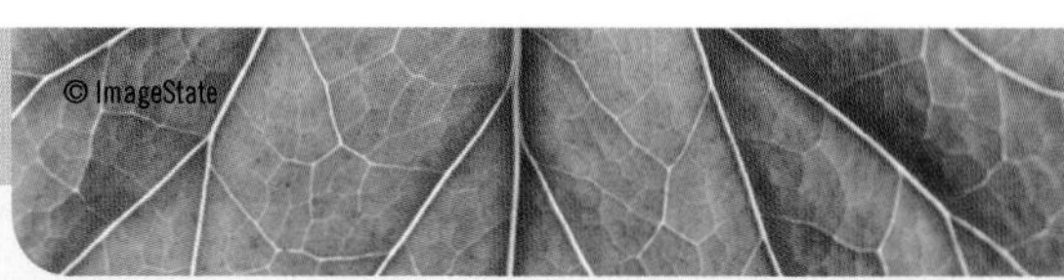

Coffee

Study Points

1. Although the origins of coffee are unclear, it made its way to Arabia in the 1200s. By the 1600s, coffee was introduced to Europe and coffeehouses quickly spread, providing a venue for social interaction and political discussion.
2. Coffee has specific requirements for commercial cultivation. Temperature, rainfall, sunlight, wind, and type of soil must all be taken into account. Shade-grown coffee practices have extensive environmental value. Variances in the soil, moisture, and climate where the coffee beans are grown contribute to the differences in the taste of coffee.
3. The two main types of coffee bean roasts are medium and dark. Medium roasts have a delicate flavor, and darker roasts have a more bitter taste.
4. Keeping coffee away from excessive air, moisture, heat, and light will guarantee optimal flavor.
5. There is no standardized, generalized system for grading coffee beans.
6. The most common brewing method today is the filter method. The standardized recipe for a cup of filtered coffee is 2 level tablespoons of coffee grounds for each cup.
7. Coffee contains more than a thousand different chemicals and is composed of carbohydrates, lipids, nitrogenous compounds, vitamins, minerals, alkaloids, and phenolic compounds.
8. Current research indicates that coffee consumption is associated with a significant dose-dependent reduction in the risk of developing type 2 diabetes mellitus. In addition, coffee does not appear to pose significant health risks.
9. Main areas of coffee safety concern include chemical residues, such as pesticides; proper processing; storage conditions; and contamination. One of the most well-known contaminants in coffee is a mycotoxin called aflatoxin.
10. Coffee can be designated as fair trade, organic, or bird friendly, which can help customers select coffee that is produced in an environmentally and socially responsible manner.

Issues for Class Discussion

1. What is the role/responsibility of Starbucks and other large coffee chains in increasing demand for sustainably produced coffee?
2. What are some potential strategies and incentives to shift coffee production back to shade-grown methods?
3. What is the role of coffee in American culture?
4. What are some of the effects of globalization on coffee and the spread of American coffee chains internationally?

Research Areas for Students

1. Substances in coffee that may offer health benefits
2. Effects of "green" food labels on consumer buying behavior
3. New sustainable coffee practices
4. Depth of consumer knowledge/awareness regarding coffee production methods

Key Terms

	page
aflatoxin	467
aroma	462
caffeine	463
chlorogenic acid	463
diterpenes	465
electrolytes	481
ergogenic aids	486
fair trade	468
fluorosis	479
gluconeogenesis	482
hyponatremia	481
ochratoxin A (OTA)	467
osmolality/osmolar solution	481
sports drink	481

Tea

Study Points

1. Tea originated in China and became an integral part of Chinese life. Different cultures have developed their own tea customs and ceremonies, and one of the most well known is the Japanese tea ceremony.
2. China, India, Sri Lanka, and Kenya are responsible for 75 percent of global tea production.
3. The first leaves harvested are the best quality and are called the "first flush." The finest teas are grown at 3,000–7,000 feet above sea level.
4. The four different stages of tea processing result in four different varieties of tea: black, green, oolong, and white. The taste of the tea beverage depends on the processing method, the region where the tea is grown, the weather, the use of additives/flavorings, the type of soil in the tea garden, age of the leaves when they are plucked, how long the leaves are allowed to oxidize, and the type of wood used in the drying process.
5. Many different tea additives are used; flavoring agents are sprayed onto heated tea leaves; spices and fruit rinds can be mixed into the tea leaves; and honey or milk can also be added to the brewed tea.
6. Tea is composed of a wide variety of ingredients, and the chemicals thought to be responsible for the beneficial health effects of tea include polyphenols. However, flavonoids in tea can inhibit the bioavailability of dietary sources of nonheme iron.
7. Because tea is the second most popular beverage worldwide, it is monitored carefully to ensure that pesticide residues are below the Maximum Residue Limits (MRLs).
8. Tea consumption is correlated with beneficial cardiovascular effects; researchers are investigating the potential mechanisms, which include the impact of tea on blood vessel dilation and vascular endothelial function. Investigations continue to look at tea's ability to reduce cardiovascular disease risk, prevent cancer, osteoporosis, kidney stones, and assist in weight loss.
9. Ready-to-drink tea is one of the fastest growing sectors of the American tea market. The polyphenol concentration of ready-to-drink teas is substantially lower relative to other (hot, brewed) teas.
10. Environmental issues concerning tea production include habitat conversion, energy use, and agrochemical use. There are options for consumers who are environmentally and socially conscious, including fair trade teas and tea certified by the Ethical Tea Partnership (ETP).

Issues for Class Discussion

1. How popular is tea in America compared to other parts of the world?
2. How can tea production be made more environmentally friendly? Is the fair trade movement and ETP certifications helpful in promoting environmentally-friendly cultivation practices?

Research Areas for Students

1. Tea and weight loss.
2. Impact of adding milk, sugar, and other additives on tea's antioxidant properties.
3. Tea consumption and oral health.
4. Tea consumption and bone health.
5. Effects of tea on stress levels/blood pressure.

Sports Beverages

Study Points

1. Sports beverages made their debut in 1965 and were used by the University of Florida football team to replenish fluids and electrolytes lost and boost performance.
2. When exercise lasts more than an hour, a sports drink is indicated because muscle and liver glycogen stores start to deplete. During exercise, thirst is not a reliable guide as large fluid losses can occur prior to feeling thirsty.
3. A sports beverage includes a carbohydrate fuel source (such as glucose or sucrose) and electrolytes (potassium, chloride, and sodium). The carbohydrate helps to fuel both the muscles and brain, maintaining blood glucose levels and promoting the uptake of carbs into the muscle cells.
4. Low doses of caffeine (5–6 mg/kilogram body weight) have shown performance-enhancing effects in athletes.
5. Adequate fluid intake is the number one nutrition intervention for all athletes because hydration status is a critical determinant of the athlete's physiological capacity to train, compete, and recover successfully. The goal for minimum fluid replacement during most activities should be to limit fluid deficits to less than 2% of baseline body weight.
6. Drinking carbohydrate–electrolyte sports beverages enhances performance in comparison to plain water during prolonged (45 to 50 minutes) exercise, as well as during high-intensity, intermittent exercise.
7. Regulation of sports beverages is not standardized, and the United States does not have strict regulations on energy drinks. Therefore, energy beverage companies are free to make energy and performance enhancement claims at their own discretion.
8. The biggest environmental issue in terms of sports beverages is the use of plastic bottles. The production of these bottles uses an immense amount of water as well as energy derived from fossil fuels.

Issues for Class Discussion

1. Should sports energy drinks be regulated?
2. Is it ethical for marketers to target sports drinks to nonathletes? Should sports beverages be sold in schools?

Research Areas for Students

1. Caffeine's mechanisms of action in enhancing athletic performance
2. Effect of branched-chain amino acids in sports beverages
3. Effect and role of phytonutrients during and after athletic activities
4. Effect of energy drinks on athletic performance
5. Preventive measures for hyponatremia

References

1. Roden C. *Coffee: A Connoisseur's Companion.* New York: Random House; 1994.
2. Coffee. In: *World Book Encyclopedia.* Chicago: World Book Inc.; 2006.
3. Davids K. *Coffee: A Guide to Buying, Brewing, and Enjoying.* 5th ed. New York: St. Martin's Press; 2001.
4. Coffee Science Information Centre. The History of Coffee. 2010. Available at: http://coffeeforums.wordpress.com. Accessed September 6, 2012.
5. International Coffee Organization. Ecology and Physical Properties of Coffee. 2010. Available at: http://www.ico.org/ecology.asp. Accessed September 6, 2012.
6. Heise U. *Coffee and Coffeehouses.* Atglen, PA: Schiffer; 1987.
7. International Coffee Organization. Botanical Aspects. Available at: http://www.ico.org/botanical.asp. Accessed September 6, 2012.
8. Perfecto I, Rice RA, Greenberg R, et al. Shade coffee: A disappearing refuge for biodiversity. *Bioscience.* 1996;46(8):598.
9. Rice R, Bedoya M. The Ecological Benefits of Shade-Grown Coffee. 2010. Available at: http://nationalzoo.si.edu/scbi/migratorybirds/coffee/bird_friendly/ecological-benefits-of-shade-grown-coffee.cfm. Accessed September 6, 2012.
10. Commission for Environmental Cooperation. Shade-Grown Coffee. Available at: http://www.cec.org/Page.asp?PageID=1180&SiteNodeID=419. Accessed December 16, 2010.
11. Coffee Research Organization. Coffee Diseases and Pests: Coffee Rust. Available at: http://www.coffeeresearch.org/agriculture/rust.htm. Accessed January 8, 2011.
12. Watson K, Achinelli ML. Context and contingency: The coffee crisis for conventional small-scale coffee farmers in Brazil. *Geographic J.* 2008;174(5):223–234.
13. Banks MM, McFadden C, Atkinson C. *The World Encyclopedia of Coffee.* Leicester, UK: Lorenz Books; 2006.
14. International Coffee Organization. Roasting and Making Coffee. Available at: http://www.ico.org/making_coffee.asp. Accessed January 8, 2011.
15. Standage T. *A History of the World in 6 Glasses.* New York: Walker & Company; 2006.
16. Higdon J. *An Evidence-Based Approach to Dietary Phytochemicals.* New York: Thieme Medical Publishers; 2007.
17. Linus Pauling Institute. Coffee. 2005. Available at: http://lpi.oregonstate.edu/infocenter/foods/coffee. Accessed September 6, 2012.
18. Clifford M. Chlorogenic acids and other cinnamates: Nature occurrence and dietary burden. *J Sci Food Agric.* 1999;79:362–372.
19. McCusker R, Goldberger B, Cone E. Caffeine content of specialty coffees. *J Analytic Toxicol.* 2003;27(7):520–522.
20. Urgert R, Van der Weg G, Kosmeijer-Schull T, et al. Levels of cholesterol-elevating diterpenes cafestol and kahweol in various coffee brews. *J Agric Food Chem.* 1995;43(8):2167–2172.
21. Jee S, He J, Appell L, et al. Coffee consumption and serum lipids: A meta-analysis of randomized controlled clinical trials. *Am J Epidemiol.* 2001;153(4):353–362.
22. Higdon JV, Frei B. Coffee and health: A review of recent human research. *Crit Rev Food Sci Nutr.* 2006;46(2):101–123.
23. Willett WC, Stampfer MJ, Manson JE, et al. Coffee consumption and coronary heart disease in women: A ten-year follow-up. *JAMA.* 1996;275(6):458–462.
24. Kawachi I, Colditz GA, Stone CB. Does coffee drinking increase the risk of coronary heart disease? Results from a meta-analysis. *Br Heart J.* 1994;72(3):269–275.
25. Woodward M, Tunstall-Pedoe H. Coffee and tea consumption in the Scottish Heart Health study follow-up: Conflicting relations with coronary risk factors, coronary disease, and all cause mortality. *J Epidemiol Community Health.* 1999;53(8):481–487.
26. Kleemola P, Jousilahti P, Pietinen P, et al. Coffee consumption and the risk of coronary heart disease and death. *Arch Intern Med.* 2000;160(22):3393–3400.
27. Salazar-Martinez E, Willett WC, Ascherio A, et al. Coffee consumption and risk for type 2 diabetes mellitus. *Ann Intern Med.* 2004;140(1):1–8.
28. Yamauchi R, Kobayashi M, Matsuda Y, et al. Coffee and caffeine ameliorate hyperglycemia, fatty liver, and inflammatory adipocytokine expression in spontaneously diabetic KK-ay mice. *J Agric Food Chem.* 2010;58(9):5597–5603.
29. Gallus S, Tavani A, Negri E, LaVecchia C. Does coffee protect against liver cirrhosis? *Ann Epidemiol.* 2002;12(3):202–205.
30. Gelatti U, Covolo L, Franceschini M, et al. Coffee consumption reduces the risk of hepatocellular carcinoma independently of its aetiology: A case control study. *J Hepatol.* 200542:528–534.
31. Inoue M, Yoshimi I, Sobue T, Tsugane S, JPHC Study Group. Influence of coffee drinking on subsequent risk of hepatocellular carcinoma: A prospective study in Japan. *J Natl Cancer Inst.* 2005;97(4):293–300.
32. Shimazu T, Tsubono Y, Kuriyama S, et al. Coffee consumption and the risk of primary liver cancer: Pooled analysis of two prospective studies in Japan. *Int J Cancer.* 2005;116(1):150–154.
33. Nelson G, Waugh T. Food Safety in the Coffee Industry. 2002. Available at: http://www.slideserve.com/oakley/food-safety-in-the-coffee-industry. Accessed September 5, 2012.
34. Coffee Review. Coffee and Health: Pesticides and Chemicals. 2001. Available at: http://www.coffeereview.com/reference.cfm?ID=121. Accessed January 8, 2011.
35. McCarthy JP, Adinolfi J, McMullin WC, et al. National Coffee Association Survey of Pesticide Residues in Brewed Coffees. 2010.
36. Food and Agriculture Organization of the United Nations. Reducing Ochratoxin A in Coffee. Available at: http://www.coffee-ota.org/mycotoxins_what.asp. Accessed December 15, 2010.
37. Fair Trade USA. Fair Trade Overview. Available at: http://www.transfairusa.org/content/about/overview.php. Accessed December 16, 2010.
38. Martin LC. *Tea: The Drink That Changed the World.* Rutland, VT: Tuttle Publishing; 2007.
39. Chuen LK, Sin LK, Yu LT. *The Way of Tea.* Singapore: Barron's Educational Series; 2001.

40. Perry S. *The New Tea Book.* San Francisco: Chronicle Books; 2001.
41. Tea. In: *World Book Encyclopedia.* Chicago: World Book Inc.; 2006.
42. Tanaka S, Tanaka S. *The Tea Ceremony.* 3rd ed. Tokyo: Kodansha America; 1998.
43. Encyclopedia Britannica. Tea Production. Available at: http://www.britannica.com/EBchecked/topic/585098/tea-production. Accessed December 15, 2010.
44. Tea Association of the USA. About Tea. Available at: http://www.teausa.com/general/501g.cfm. Accessed December 15, 2010.
45. Van Der Wal S. *Sustainability Issues in the Tea Sector.* Amsterdam: Center for Research on Multinational Corporations; 2008.
46. Peters U, Poole C, Arab L. Does tea affect cardiovascular disease? A meta-analysis. *Am J Epidemiol.* 2001;154(6):495–503.
47. Wissotzky Tea. The grading of tea. Available at: http://www.wtea.com/about-tea_grading.aspx. Accessed February 2, 2011.
48. Ryan L, Petit S. Addition of whole, semi-skimmed, and skimmed bovine milk reduces the total antioxidant capacity of black tea. *Nutr Res.* 2010;30(1):14–20.
49. Kyle JA, Morrice PC, McNeill G, Duthie GG. Effects of infusion time and addition of milk on content and absorption of polyphenols from black tea. *J Agric Food Chem.* 2007;55(12):4889–4894.
50. Cabrera C, Gimenez R, Lopez MC. Determination of tea components with antioxidant activity. *J Agric Food Chem.* 2003;51(15):4427–4435.
51. National Cancer Institute. Tea and cancer prevention: Strengths and limitations of the evidence. 2010. Available at: http://www.cancer.gov/cancertopics/factsheet/prevention/tea. Accessed February 5, 2011.
52. Balentine DA, Paetau-Robinson I. Tea as a source of dietary antioxidants with a potential role in prevention of chronic diseases. In: *Herbs, Botanicals, and Teas.* Lancaster, PA: Technomic Publishing; 2000: 265–287.
53. Higdon J. Tea catechins and polyphenols: Health effects, metabolism, and antioxidant functions. *Crit Rev Food Sci Nutr.* 2003;43(1):89–143.
54. Lakenbrink C, Lapczynski S, Maiwald B, Engelhardt UH. Flavonoids and other polyphenols in consumer brews of tea and other caffeinated beverages. *J Agric Food Chem.* 2000;48(7):2848–2852.
55. Cabrera C, Artacho R, Gimenez R. Beneficial effects of green tea: A review. *J Am Coll Nutr.* 2006;25(2):79–99.
56. Kuriyama S, Shimazu T, Ohmori K, et al. Green tea consumption and mortality due to cardiovascular disease, cancer, and all causes in Japan: The Ohsaki study. *JAMA.* 2006;296(10):1255–1265.
57. Yang CS, Maliakal P, Meng X. Inhibition of carcinogenesis by tea. *Ann Rev Pharmacol Toxicol.* 2002;42:25–54.
58. Jones C, Woods K, Whittle G, et al. Sugar, drinks, deprivation and dental caries in 14-year-old children in the northwest of England in 1995. *Community Dent Health.* 1999;16(2):68–71.
59. Gurusubramanian G, Rahman A, Sarmah M, et al. Pesticide usage pattern in tea ecosystem, their retrospects and alternative measures. *J Environ Biol.* 2008;29(6):813–826.
60. Schreck S. Did You Know? Iced Tea Safety. 2010. Available at: http://www.foodsafetynews.com/2010/06/did-you-know-iced-tea-safety. Accessed February 2, 2011.
61. Whyte MP, Essmyer K, Gannon FH, Reinus WR. Skeletal fluorosis and instant tea. *Am J Med.* 2005;118(1):78–82.
62. Tea and Coffee. Available at: http://www.teaandcoffee.net. Accessed February 2, 2011.
63. Clay JW. *World Agriculture and the Environment.* Washington, DC: Island Press; 2004.
64. Environmental Protection Agency. Integrated Pest Management Principles. 2012. Available at: http://www.epa.gov/opp00001/factsheets/ipm.htm. Accessed February 2, 2011.
65. Ethical Tea Partnership. Enabling Change Across the Tea Sector. 2011. Available at: http://www.ethicalteapartnership.org. Accessed February 5, 2011.
66. Gatorade. History. Available at: http://www.gatorade.com/history. Accessed May 2011.
67. Sports Drink. Available at: http://encarta.msn.com/dictionary. Accessed May 2011.
68. Insel P, Ross D, McMahon K, Bernstein M. *Nutrition: MyPlate Update.* Burlington, MA: Jones & Bartlett Learning; 2012.
69. Murray B. Preventing Dehydration: Sports Drinks or Water? Available at: http://gssiweb.com. Accessed May 2011.
70. Maurer J. Sports Beverages. 2005. Available at: http://www.dswfitness.com/docs/SportsBeverages.pdf. Accessed September 5, 2012.
71. Sax L. Polyethylene terephthalate may yield endocrine disruptors. *Env Health Perspectives.* 2010;118:445–448.
72. Bonci L. Energy drinks: Help, harm, or hype? *Sports Sci Exchange.* 2002:1.
73. Higgins JP, Tuttle T, Higgins C. Energy beverages: Content and safety. *Mayo Clin Proc.* 2010;85(11):1033–1041.
74. Casa DJ, Clarkson PM, Roberts WO. American College of Sports Medicine roundtable on hydration and physical activity: Consensus statements. *Curr Sports Med Rep.* 2005;4:115–127.
75. Ask the Experts: Are Energy Drinks Safe to Consume? Available at: http://chnr.ucdavis.edu. Accessed May 2011.
76. Pollard J. Energy and sports drinks. *Health Hints.* 2006;10.
77. Bartels E. Green dilemma: Gatorade versus vitamin water. *Portland Tribune.* 2009.
78. Coca-Cola launches new annual sustainability report. Available at: http://processtechnology.drinks-business-review.com/news/coca-cola-launches-new-annual-sustainability-report-070211. Accessed May 2011.
79. Epstein J. Sustainable Beverage Packaging: Time to Lighten Up. 2010. Available at: http://www.aeb.com/news_events/blog/bid/11483/Sustainable-Beverage-Packaging-Time-to-Lighten-Up. Accessed October 3, 2012.

CHAPTER 16

Food Preservation and Packaging

Jennifer Lerman, RD, LDN

Chapter Objectives

THE STUDENTS WILL BE EMPOWERED TO:

- Identify the basic principles behind food spoilage and the techniques used to overcome and prevent it.
- List the methods and types of packaging food processors use to preserve and extend the shelf life of foods.
- Discuss unique challenges food processors face relating to the development of safe, usable, and environmentally friendly preservation and packaging techniques.
- Explain how government agencies encourage, regulate, and protect the food supply in relation to pesticides, irradiation, and packaging materials.
- Identify strategies for making food processing and packaging more environmentally friendly.

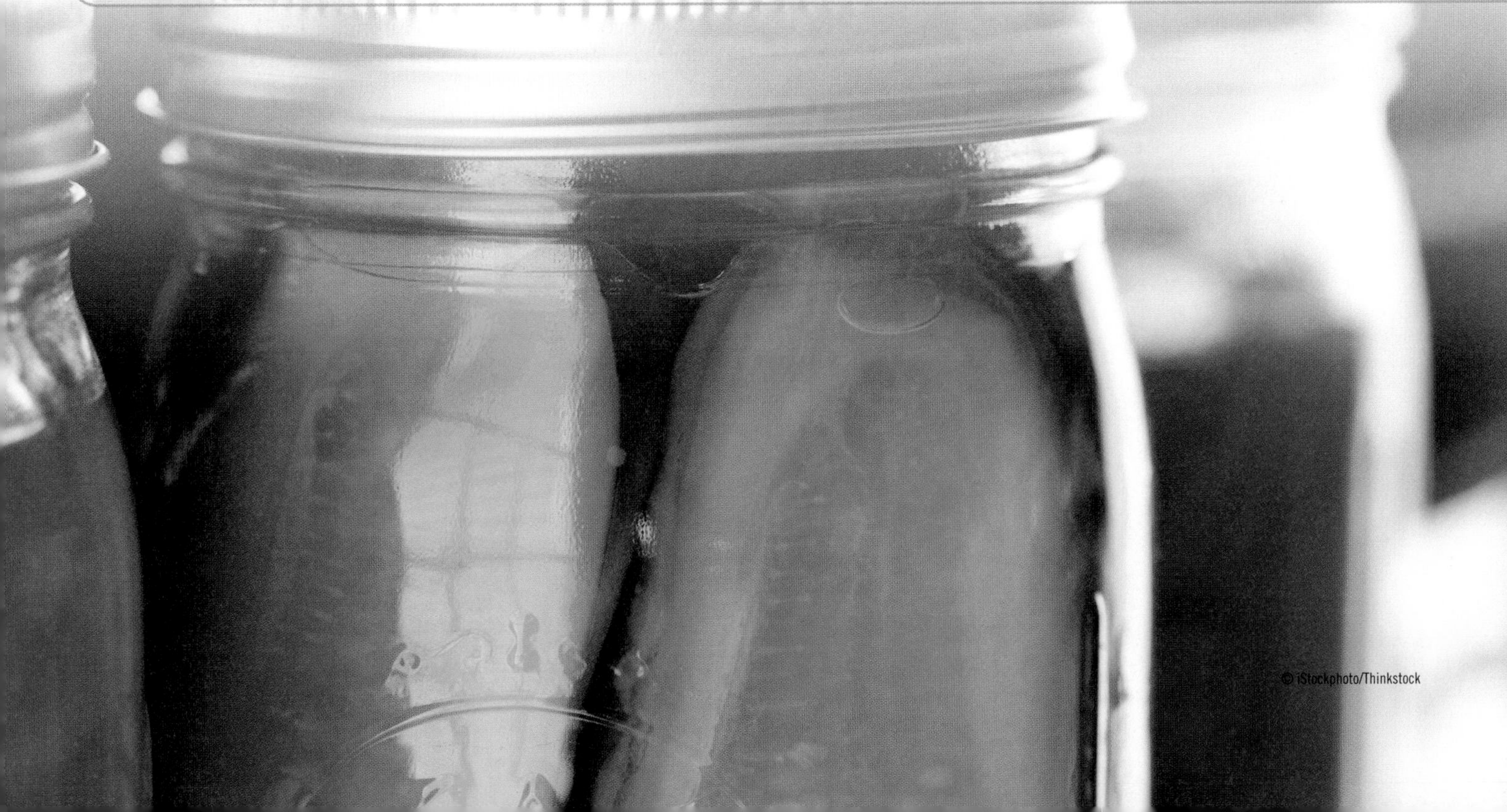

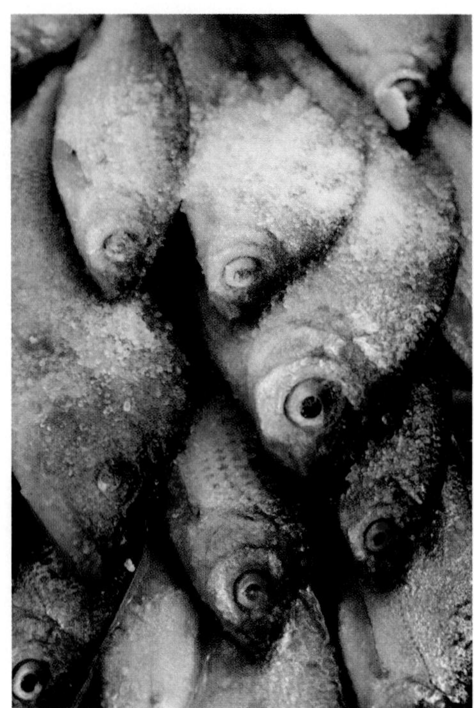

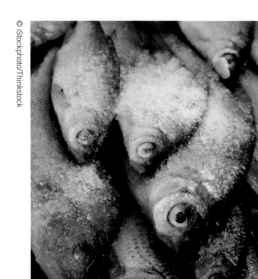

FIGURE 16.1 Salting is commonly used to preserve foods such as bacon, ham, fish, and beef. It also is used to make pastrami and corned beef. Foods that have been heavily salted can be stored for years without turning rancid.

Food Preservation

The advent of food preservation techniques enabled humans to survive harsh environments and take long journeys. Most importantly, it allowed societies to move away from the "hunter-gatherer" method of survival. For thousands of years, people relied on a number of techniques to preserve food, including combinations of drying, smoking, salting, pickling, and fermenting. These methods of food preservation are still used today, as well as newer techniques, such as canning, freezing, freeze-drying, irradiation, and pasteurization.[1] Scientific advances now allow us to have a more complete knowledge of how these techniques work.

Water Activity and Osmotic Stress

Salt, or sodium chloride, has been used as a food preservative for thousands of years.[1] Salt and other preservatives, such as sodium benzoate and potassium sorbate, work to preserve food by reducing the water activity (a_w) in fresh food. Water activity is a measure of the relative vapor pressure of a food as compared with the vapor pressure of pure water.[2,3] Many unprocessed foods have a water activity greater than 0.95, which is high enough for microorganisms to thrive.[2] Specific bacteria have varying limits of a_w with different preservation solutes. For example, bacterial growth may occur at an a_w of 0.95 if sodium chloride is used for preservation, versus 0.92 if sugar is used. An a_w of less than 0.8 is thought to be the lowest that can support bacterial growth; fungi are able to grow on a_w of greater than 0.6 (see **Table 16.1**).[4]

Salt preserves food by essentially drying it out, thereby lowering the water activity (see **Figure 16.1**). The mechanism by which salt reduces a_w is **osmosis**, the process of water molecules moving from a less concentrated solution to a more concentrated solution to achieve equilibrium. Salt added to food creates a more concentrated solution on the outside versus the inside of the food's cells. Osmosis draws water out of the food into the more concentrated surroundings. If a drying mechanism also is added—for example, smoke or warm air—the water drawn out of the food evaporates, and the process of osmosis toward equilibrium begins again, further drying and preserving the food.[1] Salt is an effective preservative; however, its overuse in American food products raises significant health concerns, as discussed in **Special Topic 16.1**.

osmosis Movement of water molecules across a membrane toward a more concentrated solution to achieve concentration equilibrium.

TABLE 16.1
Water Activity (a_w) of Some Common Foods

Food Item	a_w
Liverwurst	0.96
Cheese spread	0.95
Red bean paste	0.93
Caviar	0.92
Fudge sauce	0.83
Soft moist pet food	0.83
Salami	0.82
Soy sauce	0.80
Peanut butter, 15% total moisture	0.70
Dry milk, 8% total moisture	0.70

Source: Reproduced from U.S. Food and Drug Administration, Inspections, Compliance, Enforcement, and Criminal Investigations, Water Activity (a_w) in Foods. Available at: http://www.fda.gov/ICECI/Inspections/InspectionGuides/InspectionTechnicalGuides/ucm072916.htm. Accessed December 16, 2010.

Special Topic 16.1

Sodium Intake and Food Processing

Jennifer Lerman, RD, LDN

Current understanding of the relationship between health and diet indicates that a diet high in sodium increases blood pressure. High blood pressure is a risk factor for many conditions, including stroke, heart disease, heart failure, and kidney disease.[1] Because of these associations, the 2005 *Dietary Guidelines for Americans* recommended that people at high risk (those who already have hypertension, are African American, or are middle-aged or older) limit their intake of sodium to 1,500 mg of sodium per day. Other people were advised to consume less than 2,300 mg per day, which is roughly the equivalent of 1 teaspoon of salt, although it depends on the brand and variety of salt used. The more recent *Dietary Guideline for Americans, 2010* advises that because 70% of the U.S. population now falls into one of the high-risk categories, the recommendation is that *all* people consume less than 1,500 mg of sodium per day, and that this reduction should be achieved gradually over time to allow for taste perceptions to change.[2] A recent Centers for Disease Control and Prevention (CDC) report based on data from the National Health and Nutrition Examination Survey (NHANES) indicates that less than 10% of adults achieve the sodium limits recommended.[3] It is estimated that the average American consumes more than 3,400 mg of sodium daily.[4]

The major source of sodium in the American diet is processed and restaurant foods. Estimates are that more than 75% of sodium intake comes from these foods, with only 10% coming from salt added at the table and during cooking.[3] One result of the excessive addition of sodium to processed and packaged foods is a growing public concern about the sodium content of the food supply (see **Figure A**). Congress recently asked the Institute of Medicine (IOM) to offer strategies on how to reduce sodium intake to recommended limits. In its report *Strategies to Reduce Sodium Intake in the United States*, the IOM recommends that the Food and Drug Administration (FDA) change the GRAS ("generally recognized as safe") status of sodium. This will then allow the FDA to regulate sodium content in food further and slowly require food manufacturers to reduce the sodium content of their products. Despite these recommendations, no definitive federal regulatory action regarding sodium has been implemented to date.[5]

For their part, members of the food manufacturing industry have been taking steps to begin reducing sodium levels in packaged foods. Low- and reduced-sodium alternatives to many foods are currently available in the marketplace. Methods for reducing sodium already being used include salt substitutes, which often contain potassium salts (however, these can be dangerous for people with kidney disease). Some companies also have started using sea salt, which can be manufactured to be slightly lower in sodium because it contains other minerals, such as calcium and magnesium, and has larger crystals, thereby reducing the amount of sodium per volume.[6,7] Other substitutes, such as powdered plant extracts, have been developed that may be used in the future to achieve sodium reduction in processed foods.[8] Mechanical changes have also been studied based on targeting the way people perceive salty tastes. One approach is to "layer" salt in foods, providing high- and low-sodium parts and essentially tricking the tongue into tasting a saltier product.[9] Other researchers have found that only 20% of salt dissolves on the tongue to be tasted; by restructuring the shape of the salt crystal, a 25% sodium reduction can be achieved in a food product with no change in taste.[10]

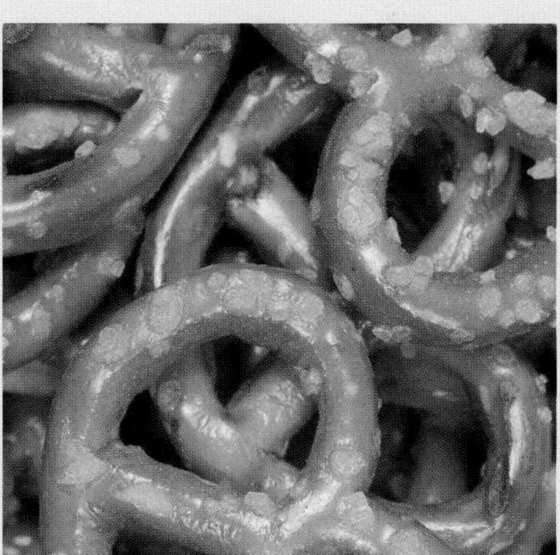

FIGURE A Sodium is added to a large percentage of processed foods, and it is not always as noticeable an ingredient like the topping on these pretzels.

A number of large food manufacturers have announced plans to further reduce sodium in their products. Companies such as Kraft, ConAgra, Unilever, and General Mills have pledged to reduce sodium in some or all of their products by 10% to 20% by 2015.[8] Some companies are also participating in the National Salt Reduction Initiative (NSRI), which is a collaboration between cities, national health groups, and companies that is designed to reduce sodium intake by the public in participating cities. Studies are being carried out to determine whether this initiative will be successful.[11]

In considering sodium reduction, it must be remembered that the goal of reducing dietary intake of sodium must be balanced with the reason sodium is being used in processed food—the food needs to remain free from pathogenic microbial growth and have an appealing taste and texture.[12] Companies now are putting considerable effort into achieving this goal without sacrificing quality or safety.

References

1 Institute of Medicine. *Dietary Reference Intakes for Water, Potassium, Sodium, Chloride, and Sulfate.* Washington, DC: National Academies Press; 2004.

2 U.S. Department of Agriculture, Center for Nutrition Policy and Promotion. *Report of the Dietary Guidelines Advisory Committee on the Dietary Guidelines for Americans, 2010.* Available at: http://www.cnpp.usda.gov/DGAs2010-DGACReport.htm. Accessed December 12, 2010.

3 Centers for Disease Control and Prevention. Sodium intake among adults—United States, 2005–2006. *MMRW.* 2010;59(24):746–749.

4 Kuhn ME. Strategies for reducing sodium in the US. *Food Technol.* 2010;64(5):34–36.

5 Mitka M. IOM recommends federal regulation over the salt content of certain foods. *JAMA.* 2010;303(22):2238–2240.

6 Heller L. Campbell Soups to Be Made with Lower Sodium Sea Salt. February 24, 2006. Available at: http://www.foodnavigator-usa.com/Financial-Industry/Campbell-soups-to-be-made-with-lower-sodium-sea-salt. Accessed January 1, 2011.

7 Zeratsky K. Nutrition and Healthy Eating: Is Sea Salt Better for Your Health Than Table Salt? Mayo Clinic. Available at: http://www.mayoclinic.com/health/sea-salt/AN01142. Accessed January 1, 2011.

8 Lee GH. A salt substitute with low sodium content from plant aqueous extracts. *Food Res Int.* Available at: http://www.sciencedirect.com/science/article/pii/S0963996910004515. Accessed June 13, 2012.

9 Daniells S. Smart Salt Distribution Can Cut Salt Without Extra Additives. Food Navigator Online. November 6, 2009. Available at: http://www.foodnavigator.com/Science-Nutrition/Smart-salt-distribution-can-cut-salt-without-extra-additives. Accessed January 1, 2011.

10 FoodProcessing.com. PepsiCo Reduces Sodium by Restructuring Salt. March 3, 2010. Available at: http://www.foodprocessing.com/industrynews/2010/050.html. Accessed January 1 2011.

11 Scott-Thomas C. Low-Sodium Products Decline in Popularity, Says NPD. Food Navigator Online. April 26, 2010. Available at: http://www.foodnavigator-usa.com/Financial-Industry/Low-sodium-products-decline-in-popularity-says-NPD. Accessed December 12, 2010.

12 Scott-Thomas C. The Next Steps in Evaluating Sodium Reduction. Food Navigator Online. November 17, 2010. Available at: http://www.foodnavigator-usa.com/Financial-Industry/The-next-steps-in-evaluating-sodium-reduction. Accessed December 12, 2010.

Innovation Point

Liquids Originally, liquid foods were pasteurized in their containers; now, through a continuous-flow process, liquids can be pasteurized continuously and poured into sterile containers, improving the efficiency of the process.

Other preservatives, such as sugar (used to preserve fruit as in jam, for example), salts other than sodium chloride, protein, and humectants (which promote moisture retention), also are added to food to reduce water activity. By lowering the water activity and increasing osmotic stress on microbes, the food environment becomes unfavorable to microbial growth and reproduction.

Different strains of bacteria and fungi have different minimum water activities as well as other varying requirements for growth. For these reasons, different foods require different treatments with preservatives in order to prevent the growth of microorganisms.[5]

Acidity

Another method of food preservation is to adjust the pH of a food product's environment. Frequently, this is accomplished by adding a weak acid preservative, such as benzoic, sorbic, citric, propionic, acetic, or lactic acid, or by lowering the pH with a stronger acid. Similar to salting and refrigeration, the addition of an acid has a detrimental effect on microorganism growth. Weak acids may be more effective than strong acids at preventing microbial growth because they do not dissociate in the pH range of typical foods. The nondissociated weak acids are able to permeate the microorganism's cell membrane. Once inside the microbe, they either bind to enzymes, inactivating them, or they dissociate, lowering the internal pH of the microorganism.

Acidification of the microbe's internal environment disrupts the organism's ability to function and grow. The microbe reacts by pumping protons outside its membrane to restore normal pH, which reduces the energy available for growth and reproduction.[4]

Stronger acids also can be added to food for preservation. The flavor and texture of the food may be more negatively influenced with strong acids than with weak acids because more of the acid may be needed to prevent microbe growth. Strong acids do dissociate in most foods and thus cannot pass through microbial cell membranes. However, strong acids can inhibit microorganisms by denaturing enzyme proteins embedded in the cell membrane and by creating a high proton gradient that can cause migration of protons across the membrane, which can affect ion transport molecules on the membrane surface. In some instances, strong acids denature enough of the microbe's membrane to destroy it, and the microbe dies.[4]

A review of food labels will often reveal the use of preservatives (see **Figure 16.2**). Note that microorganisms can adapt to various mechanisms of preservation and become resistant to them over time. For example, in one laboratory experiment the dangerous bacteria *E. coli* O157 became resistant to acid in 17 minutes. The adaptation of microorganisms to preservation techniques represents a significant area of future monitoring and research to ensure the continued safety of the food supply.[4]

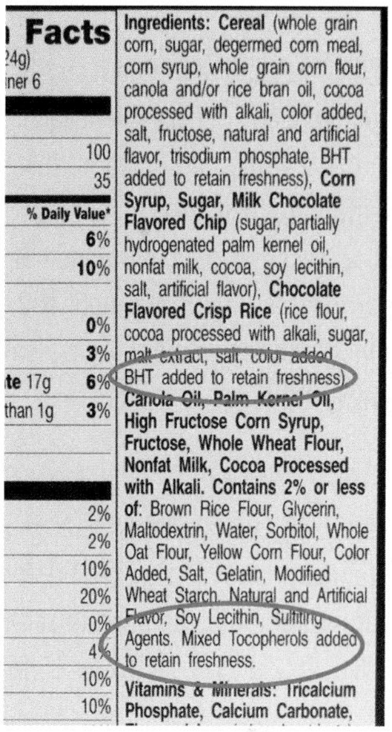

Ingredients: Cereal (whole grain corn, sugar, degermed corn meal, corn syrup, whole grain corn flour, canola and/or rice bran oil, cocoa processed with alkali, color added, salt, fructose, natural and artificial flavor, trisodium phosphate, BHT added to retain freshness), Corn Syrup, Sugar, Milk Chocolate Flavored Chip (sugar, partially hydrogenated palm kernel oil, nonfat milk, cocoa, soy lecithin, salt, artificial flavor), Chocolate Flavored Crisp Rice (rice flour, cocoa processed with alkali, sugar, malt extract, salt, color added, BHT added to retain freshness), Canola Oil, Palm Kernel Oil, High Fructose Corn Syrup, Fructose, Whole Wheat Flour, Nonfat Milk, Cocoa Processed with Alkali. Contains 2% or less of: Brown Rice Flour, Glycerin, Maltodextrin, Water, Sorbitol, Whole Oat Flour, Yellow Corn Flour, Color Added, Salt, Gelatin, Modified Wheat Starch, Natural and Artificial Flavor, Soy Lecithin, Sulfiting Agents. Mixed Tocopherols added to retain freshness. Vitamins & Minerals: Tricalcium Phosphate, Calcium Carbonate,

FIGURE 16.2 Chemical preservatives must be included in the ingredient list if present in a food. The FDA requires that the preservative's common name and function (e.g., mold inhibition, flavor protection) must be included in the ingredient list.

Thermal Processing

Early on, it was recognized that applying heat through cooking helped make food safer to eat. Heating food was also found to extend an item's shelf life. The process of heating food to preserve it is known as *thermal processing*, and it is discussed further in **Special Topic 16.2**. Thermal processing inactivates and kills microbes and denatures enzymes and other proteins. The application of heat is particularly important to inhibiting microbial growth in nonacidic foods. However, thermal processing has some negative effects, including the loss of heat-sensitive (and, depending on the heating medium, sometimes water-soluble) nutrients as well as the inadvertent destruction of nonpathogenic bacteria.[3]

Special Topic 16.2

Thermal Food Processing

Aisling Whelan

During the past 25 years, consumer demand for convenient and varied food products has grown. Consumers have become accustomed to an enormous choice of foods at the grocery store, regardless of the season. This demand has created a need for faster production, improved quality, and longer shelf life. Thermal food processing is one of many techniques developed to address this need. *Thermal processing* is the term used to describe the combination of temperature and time aimed at eliminating a desired number of microorganisms from a food product. Thermal processing methods include boiling, pasteurization, and ohmic heating.[1]

Boiling

Sterilization by boiling is the simplest method of heat preservation. Just 10 minutes of boiling of any food product renders it free of microorganisms. However, in order to stay free of microorganisms the sterilized food must not come into contact with any unsterile objects or be exposed to the air.[2] In the food industry, this can be achieved through "in-container sterilization."

Just like the boiling method, sterilization refers to the addition of heat to a product to remove all traces of microorganisms (or remove them to commercially acceptable levels). The major methods of sterilization are in-container and UHT (ultra-high-temperature) sterilization. With in-container sterilization, the product is packed into the container and then both the container and the product are sterilized using a heating method such as boiling. Sterilization is completed following a heat treatment of 239–248°F (115–120°C) for 10 to 20 minutes. This process is typical of canned and some bottled products. With UHT, or aseptic processing, the product and the package are sterilized separately. The heat treatment is 275–284°F (135–140°C) for 3 to 5 seconds. The package, once sterilized, is filled with the sterile product, and the whole thing is sealed under sterile conditions. This process is typical of "long-life" milk as well as some packaged fruit juices and soups.

Pasteurization

Pasteurization is a method used to preserve foods and beverages and extend their shelf life through heat. Invented by Louis Pasteur, pasteurization revolutionized the food industry by establishing a simple process to extend the shelf life of milk (fruit juices and other beverages can also be pasteurized). Pasteurization destroys non-spore–forming pathogenic microorganisms. The heat treatment is 161.6–165.2°F (72–74°C) for 15 to 30 seconds. Pasteurization does not seek to kill all the microorganisms in food, only the harmful ones.

Ohmic Heating

The newest heat preservation technique is *ohmic heating*. Ohmic heating—also referred to as resistance hating, joule heating, or electroheating—preserves foods that are in a semi-suspended state, such as a sauce. Ohmic heating does not require as much heat as the other processes discussed, and thus it results in a higher-quality food. Examples of foods treated with ohmic heating are liquid eggs, orange juice, and other fruit juices.[2]

Advantages and Disadvantages

The major benefit of thermal food processing is the inactivation of foodborne pathogens. Foodborne illnesses can be life threatening, and the use of thermal processing techniques can virtually eliminate the risk of becoming ill from certain foods. Other lesser known benefits of thermal food processing are improved digestibility and improved palatability. Thermal processing can also enhance the functional properties of antioxidants.

The negative effects associated with thermal food processing are the loss of certain nutrients as well as the formation of compounds that negatively affect flavor, perception, texture, and color. One example of this is the Maillard reaction between proteins and sugars that occurs when milk is exposed to higher heats, causing browning and discoloration of the milk.[3]

Impact on Food Supply

The invention of the thermal food processing techniques continues to have a major impact on the food supply. The average consumer is presented with hundreds of food options on a daily basis, ranging widely in cost, nutritional content, and taste. Without thermal food processing, this variety of products would simply not be possible.

Although thermal processing has expanded our food supply, decreased the cost of food, and helped make food more accessible to the entire population, it has also become associated with the high-calorie, sugar- and fat-laden items that contribute to our nation's obesity epidemic. The problem does not lie in the science of thermal food processing; after all, heat preservation techniques do not add calories, as they simply increase the shelf life of foods. Thermal food processing is a major contributor to modern day food science innovation. With its continued use, thermal food processing will continue to ensure that an abundance of food is both accessible and affordable to the growing population.

References

1 Pereira RN. Environmental impact of novel thermal and non-thermal technologies in food processing. *Food Res Int.* 2010 Aug;43(7):1936–1943.

2 Brown A. *Understanding Food: Principles and Preparation.* 4th ed. New York: Wadsworth; 2011.

3 Van Boekel M. A review of the beneficial aspects of food processing. *Mol Nutri Food Res.* 2010 Sept;54(9):1215–1247.

Blanching

Blanching is another form of heat treatment (see **Figure 16.3**). With blanching, the food is held at a temperature of less than 212°F (100°C) for 2 to 3 minutes. This can be accomplished by placing the food in boiling water or exposing it to steam. The goal is to inactivate enzymes naturally found in the food tissue while maintaining the food's appealing taste, appearance, and texture. In addition, blanching forces air out of the food, decreasing the rate of oxidative degradation. Blanching is typically a first step in processing, followed by freezing, canning, or drying the food.[3]

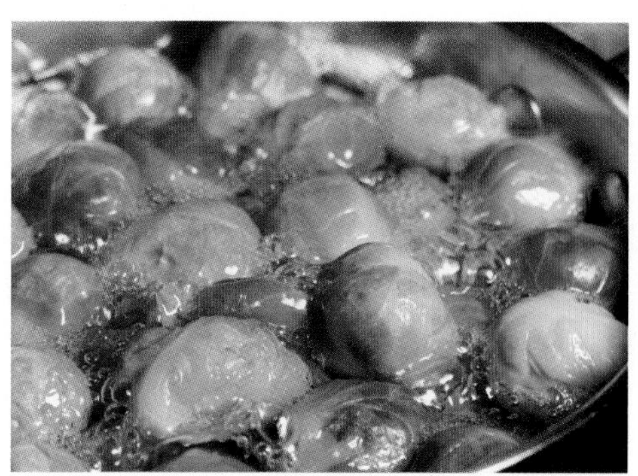

FIGURE 16.3 Vegetables often are blanched before they are frozen and packaged. Blanching cleans the surface of the vegetables and softens them, making them easier to pack. Blanching also preserves the vitamin and mineral content of the food and brightens its color.

Pasteurization

Another method of thermal processing is pasteurization (see **Figure 16.4**). This method is named after Louis Pasteur, a microbiologist and chemist who established that microorganisms caused food spoilage. With pasteurization, the food or beverage is heated to between 140–212°F (60–100°C) for a certain amount of time, depending on the particular food or beverage, to kill a large number of pathogenic microorganisms (see **Table 16.2**).[3] Because not all microbes are destroyed, pasteurized foods are often refrigerated to keep them from spoiling.[6]

Foods that are frequently pasteurized include milk, ice cream mix, and liquid eggs.[6] A variety of different types of pasteurization can be used, including high-temperature, short-time (HTST); higher-heat, shorter-time (HHST); and ultra-high-temperature (UHT). The higher the heat, the shorter the time needed to pasteurize a food. For example, the FDA recommends holding milk for 30 minutes if pasteurizing it at 145°F (63°C), compared to 0.01 seconds if pasteurizing at 212°F (100°C).[7] Shorter times can be advantageous to manufacturers. In addition, when very high temperature processing is used, all viable microorganisms in a product are killed so when placed in a sterile container a product that may normally need refrigeration, such as milk or cream, can be stored at room temperature. However, the benefit of treatment at a lower temperature (or for very short time) is the elimination of disease-causing microbes without the unwanted denaturing and coagulation of proteins that might occur in these foods if they were treated with higher temperatures.

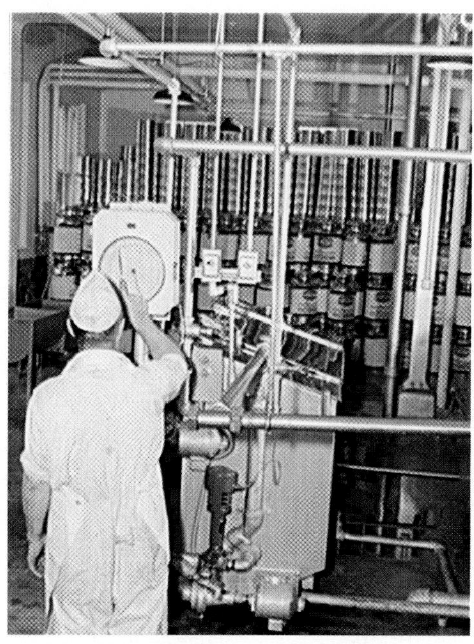

FIGURE 16.4 Pasteurization was developed by Louis Pasteur in 1864. The practice became commercialized around the late 1800s and early 1900s. In addition to improving consumer safety, pasteurization can improve the quality and shelf life of foods.

Courtesy of Library of Congress, Prints & Photographs Division, FSA/OWI Collection, [LC-USF34-063463-D].

TABLE 16.2
Pasteurization Temperature Versus Time Required

Temperature	Time
145°F (63°C)	30 minutes
161°F (72°C)	15 seconds
191°F (89°C)	1.0 second
194°F (90°C)	0.5 seconds
201°F (94°C)	0.1 seconds
204°F (96°C)	0.05 seconds
212°F (100°C)	0.01 seconds

Source: Reproduced from U.S. Department of Agriculture. Pasteurized Milk Ordinance (PMO) 2007: Standards for Grade "A" Pasteurized, Ultra-Pasteurized and Aseptically Processed Milk & Milk Products, Grade "A" Pasteurized Milk Ordinance (2007 Revision). Available at: http://www.fda.gov/Food/FoodSafety/Product-SpecificInformation/MilkSafety/NationalConferenceonInterstateMilkShipmentsNCIMSModel-Documents/PasteurizedMilkOrdinance2007/UCM063945. Accessed December 26, 2010.

Gastronomy Point

Raw Milk Proponents of raw milk believe that raw milk tastes better and confers health benefits. However, according to the CDC, FDA, and a number of other organizations, consumption of raw milk is unadvisable because of the risk of foodborne illness.

According to the FDA, foodborne illness associated with milk and dairy products has been greatly reduced by milk sanitation ordinances, including pasteurization.[8] Today, fewer than 1% of foodborne outbreaks are associated with milk, compared to an estimated 25% of outbreaks in 1938.[8] Because dairy was seen as an essential food group to promote health and adequate nutrition in the United States, the United States Public Health Service (USPHS) initiated research into enhancing safety of these foods in the early 1900s. The USPHS and FDA continue to update the ordinance describing safe handling and processing of milk in the form of the Pasteurized Milk Ordinance (PMO).[8]

It is important to note that the FDA and CDC strongly encourage the pasteurization of milk, although it is not currently mandated by federal law.[9] Although milk sold interstate must be pasteurized, individual states regulate the sale of "raw," or unpasteurized, milk to consumers.[9,10] Raw milk may not cause illness in the majority of the population, but it can be harmful for children, people with compromised immune systems, and pregnant women.

Canning

aseptic packaging Process whereby food can be batch heated in a sterile fashion and then placed in a sterilized container.

Clostridium botulinum A pathogenic bacterium that produces a neurotoxin and grows in anaerobic conditions, making it one of the major safety concerns to food processors.

Another well-known method of heat processing for preservation is canning (see **Figure 16.5**). During this type of processing, food is held for a number of minutes at a temperature greater than 230°F (110°C).[3] With traditional canning, the food is heated and held at a high temperature once it is already inside the packaging material. Alternatively, in a newer process, food can be batch heated in a sterile fashion and then placed in a sterilized container. This is known as **aseptic packaging**. Canned foods are not considered sterile, although they are devoid of pathogenic bacteria or other microbes that can grow at room temperature.[6] During the canning process, the pathogen of most concern is ***Clostridium botulinum***, a bacteria that produces a deadly neurotoxin. It can grow in anaerobic (oxygen-free) conditions and produce spores, and it is resistant to high temperatures. Because of this, it can survive in canned goods. Of particular concern are low-acid canned foods because *C. botulinum* can reproduce quickly in low-acid environments.

Canning also is a popular method of home food preservation. In fact, it is becoming increasingly popular, with sales of canning supplies increasing by 50% in recent years.[11] The home canning method involves using either a pressure canner or a boiling water canner, filling the jars with the food to be canned, putting lids on the jars, and then placing the cans in boiling water or pressurized containers at specific temperatures or pressures for a set amount of time based on the particular food (see **Figure 16.6**).[12] The canning equipment is designed to allow the lids to seal onto the jars to prevent spoilage even if the food is stored at room temperature. The National Center for Home Food Preservation recommends using home-canned foods within a year.[13] It also is important to protect home-canned foods from anaerobic bacteria, such as *C. botulinum*, by the inclusion of natural or added acids, salt, or sugar.[14] For more information on safety considerations and home canning, see **Table 16.3**.

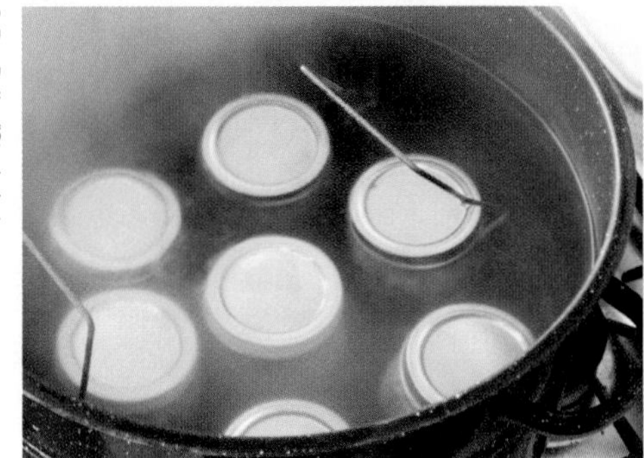

FIGURE 16.5 With canning, food is heated and sealed in an airtight container. Canned foods have a long shelf life, ranging from 1 to 5 years. Canning was developed in the early 1800s in response to a contest sponsored by the French military to develop a new food preservation method. Nicolas Appert developed canning and won the prize of 12,000 francs.

Considerations for Food Processors

When food processors are planning how to can and package foods, they make a number of economic and technical decisions. For example, they must evaluate the maximum cooking time and temperature a food can sustain without changes in taste, flavor, or texture. They also must consider the cost of packaging materials and the heating and sealing equipment. All decisions must ensure the destruction of dangerous microbes and preservation of the food. One difficulty that must be overcome is fully heating all of the contents within a package to the proper temperature. This is affected by whether the food is solid, liquid, or both. The phase of the ingredients in the package will

TABLE 16.3
Safety Considerations in Home Canning

- Make sure you use the latest canning methods and recommendations.
- Do not use outdated publications or cookbooks, even if they were handed down from trusted family cooks.
- Use the right equipment for the kind of foods that you are canning.
- Follow these recommendations to ensure that home-canned fruits and vegetables are safe:
  - Use a pressure canner.
  - Be sure the gauge of the pressure canner is accurate.
  - Use up-to-date process times and pressures for the kind of food, the size of jar, and the method of packing food in the jar.
- Before eating home-canned fruits and vegetables, check to make sure that:
  - The jar lid is firmly sealed and concave.
  - No liquid is leaking from the jar.
  - No liquid spurts out when you open the jar.
  - No unnatural or "off" odors can be detected.

Source: Reproduced from Van D. Home-Canned Vegetables: Delicious and Safe. August 9, 2010. FoodSafety.gov. Available at: http://www.foodsafety.gov/blog/home_canning.html. Accessed June 8, 2012.

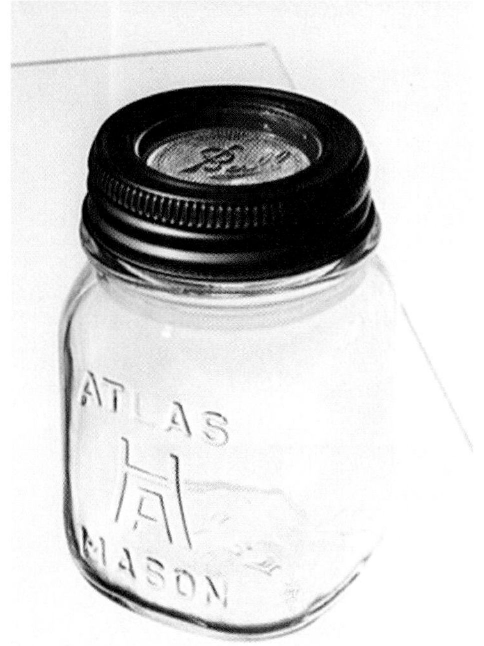

FIGURE 16.6 Home canning usually uses Mason jars. The food is added to the jars and then the filled jars are processed in a type of pressure cooker called a canner. The canners often have specialized racks to hold multiple jars. The jars are cooked in the canner at a high enough temperature to kill *C. botulinum* throughout the entire food product.

Courtesy of Library of Congress, Prints & Photographs Division, FSA/OWI Collection, [LC-USW3-019342-C].

determine if conduction heats the interior or whether convection currents can help to transfer heat. In addition, some of the equipment can cause the contents of the package to move. All of these aspects will change the time and temperature needed to effectively heat the package contents to destroy pathogenic microorganisms.

If canning techniques are not completed properly, problems will result. If a canned good is not heated to a high enough temperature or held there for a long enough time or if it becomes contaminated during or after processing and sealing, it can spoil. Some signs of damaged cans include leakage from seams, rust, and bulging ends, which indicates that gas-producing microorganisms are multiplying inside.[6]

Regardless of which method of thermal processing is used, processors must be careful to quickly cool products to proper temperatures. Particularly when a food is heated in large batches, complete cooling to storage temperatures within a short time frame is needed to prevent microorganism overgrowth. The appropriate temperature is specific for the particular food item. For example, pasteurized milk must be brought to below 40°F (4.4°C) so microbes that grow well between 45°F (7.2°C) and 161°F (72°C) do not spoil the milk while it is cooling. Other foods, such as canned goods, may need to be cooled quickly to room temperature so microorganisms that grow at high temperatures, known as **thermophiles**, do not reproduce and damage the food while the cans are cooling.[6] Standards of good manufacturing practice and hazard analysis and critical control point (HACCP) plans are commonly used by companies to ensure that these safety measures are being met.

thermophiles Organisms that can live in high temperatures.

Refrigeration and Freezing

Storing food at cold temperatures is another method of food preservation. Microbes have specific temperature ranges in which they grow and reproduce well. The majority of microorganisms that affect food cannot reproduce well below 40°F (4.4°C), which is the proper upper limit refrigeration temperature for most foods.[15] However, retardation of microbial growth does not mean that the pathogens are gone or that they are not multiplying at all. In fact, some pathogens can still grow at cold temperatures; thus, other methods of preservation are sometimes used in conjunction with refrigeration for preservation.[16] Note that once food products are removed from refrigerator temperatures, conditions again become favorable for bacterial growth and multiplication.[4]

Cold temperatures inhibit microbial growth by slowing the microbes' enzymatic activity and growth rate and inhibiting protein synthesis. Cold temperatures also affect the microbes' nutrient requirements, density, and the liquidity of their cell membranes. The solubility of particles inside and outside the microbes also is affected. Not only does food remain safer at these lower temperatures due to decreased microbial growth, its quality is preserved longer as the food's own enzymes are inactivated, slowing deterioration.[3,4,16]

Nonprocessed fresh produce often has low levels of bacteria after harvest because the outside of most produce does not provide a favorable environment for microbial growth. However, once produce is cut, peeled, or shredded, its nutrients become accessible for pathogen growth. In this situation, produce must be held at temperatures that are low enough to inhibit microbial growth. Prior to slicing and packaging, some produce is first washed in an antimicrobial solution to remove pathogens.[16]

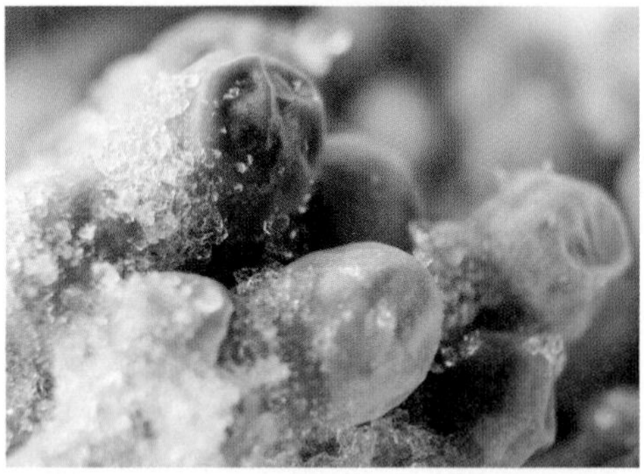

FIGURE 16.7 Freezer burn does not affect the safety of the food, but it can negatively affect its taste and color.

Freezing foods (–0.4°F to –14°F [–17.5°C to –10°C]), in contrast to refrigeration at warmer temperatures, causes liquid water within the food to become solid ice. At freezer temperatures, microbial growth ceases almost completely, as does enzyme activity that would usually degrade the quality of a food product. Nutrients are also generally preserved during freezing. The major factor affecting food quality at freezer temperatures is the formation of ice crystals. When the crystals form, they damage cell walls within the food product, and once the food is thawed it can be mushy or degraded in other ways (see **Figure 16.7**). Careful control of the freezing process can minimize this problem by keeping crystals small and uniform. However, crystal formation is also dependent on the size and type of food, not just the freezing process. Additionally, once a food is frozen, it must be maintained at a low temperature throughout processing and distribution in order to maintain quality. This is both difficult and costly to accomplish.[3]

Drying, Smoking, and Freeze-Drying

Similar to many other preservation methods, drying, smoking, and freeze-drying are all methods that slow the growth of microorganisms by removing water from the food. An added benefit of these methods is that the removal of water reduces the weight and volume of the food being dehydrated.[3] This benefits food processors by reducing shipping costs and allowing for the transportation of larger amounts of food in less space. Many groups of people benefit from the dehydration of food, from NASA astronauts, to military personnel, to mountaineers and hikers.

Most dehydration methods require large amounts of energy and typically rely on evaporation, vaporization, or sublimation.[3] Other processes besides water loss occur during dehydration that can change the food product, including Maillard browning and loss of volatile compounds, which can affect both the look and taste of the food.[3] Various machines and tools can be used to accomplish dehydration, including spray dryers, vacuums, conveyors, and drying cabinets, in addition to new technologies such as microwaves and infrared freeze-dryers (see **Figure 16.8**).[3,17]

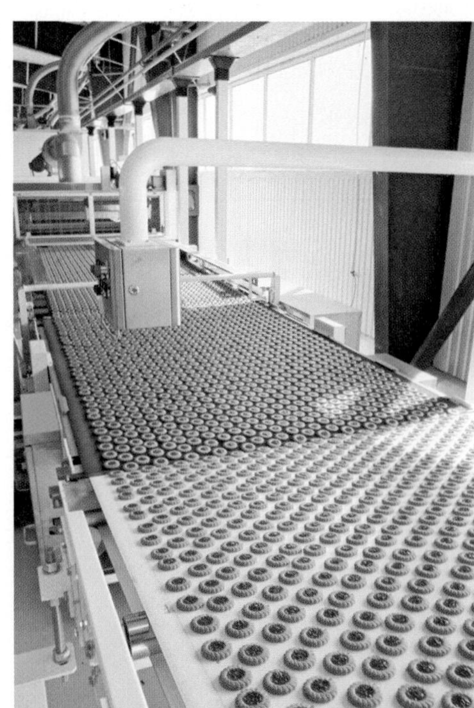

FIGURE 16.8 Although an ancient technology, dehydration is still a popular food preservation method. Today, food manufacturers use heaters and fans to speed the dehydration process.

Dehydration often is combined with other methods to kill microorganisms, preserve food, and enhance flavor. In particular, smoking was an early method found to both preserve and enhance the quality of certain foods. The application of smoke to food, most often meat, often is combined with drying to both dehydrate and smoke the product. The heat also may kill microbes, and the dehydration hinders microbial growth. The acid and alcohol products in smoke that are generated when wood burns damage the microorganisms on the food's surface. Additionally, smoke contains phenols that act as antioxidants, inhibiting rancidity. Smoking does have its faults, including the deposition of polycyclic hydrocarbons on the surface of the food, which have been found to have adverse health effects. Liquid smoke can be used as an alternative to enhance a food's flavor.[3]

Freeze-drying, also known as **lyophilization**, is another method of food preservation involving removal of water. Freeze-drying is perhaps best known to the public in the form of "astronaut food" sold in museums or in the form of freeze-dried instant coffee sold in grocery stores. Freeze-drying is also used to add fresh fruits and vegetables to processed foods. For example, freeze-dried strawberries can be added to packaged cereal. The basic process involves freezing the food and then placing it in a vacuum to create pressure to cause the solid ice in the food to turn directly into vapor, a process called **sublimation**.[18] The majority of the water in the food is thereby removed, preserving the food and greatly reducing its weight. The food then is placed into air-tight packaging or vacuum sealed so the food cannot reabsorb moisture from the air (see **Figure 16.9**). Food preserved in this way is often rehydrated with water or another liquid before consumption. This process is used for pharmaceutical products as well.

Innovation Point

Dehydrated Food A new technology that can be used to create fruits and vegetables comparable to freeze-dried versions uses microwaves and a vacuum. This method is currently used to dehydrate food and live cultures.

lyophilization Freeze-drying.

sublimation The phase change whereby a material goes directly from solid to gas, bypassing the liquid phase.

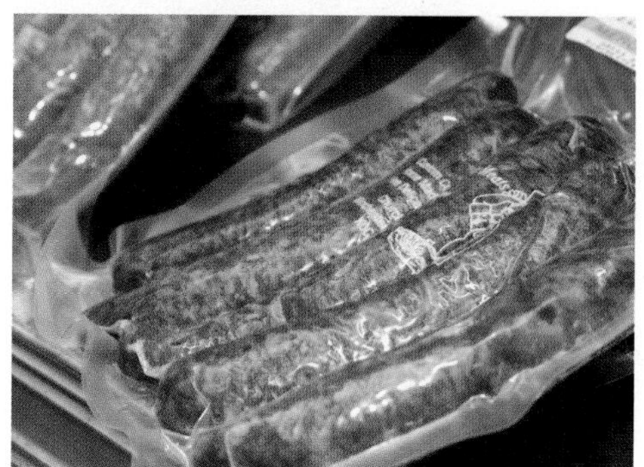

© Jupiterimages/Photos.com/Thinkstock

FIGURE 16.9 With vacuum packaging, air is removed from the package prior to sealing. The goal is usually to remove oxygen and moisture from the container in order to extend the shelf life of food. Vacuum packaging also reduces the volume of the contents and package.

Fermentation

Fermentation is a food preservation technique that cultures around the world have used for centuries. The concept behind fermentation is to encourage the growth of "friendly" bacteria that inhibit the growth of pathogenic bacteria.[3] Different cultures traditionally produced fermented foods that were unique to the particular region or climate. For example, kimchi is a fermented cabbage from Korea (see **Figure 16.10**), and crème fraîche is a fermented cream originally developed in France. Fermentation was a particularly useful method of preserving foods in damp climates where drying foods was difficult, especially before the advent of airtight packaging materials.[1] Other familiar fermented foods are yogurt, prosciutto, bread, cheese, wine, and even chocolate, which is made from fermented cacao beans.[1]

Flavors in fermented foods are stronger, in part because the bacteria or yeast involved in the fermentation process produce acids.[1] These acids help to preserve the food and add flavor.[3] By breaking down sugars, fermented foods can be easier for some people to digest.[1] This is seen with foods such as yogurt, which can sometimes be eaten comfortably by people with lactose intolerance. Pickling and fermentation overlap as preservation techniques because pickled foods, those to which vinegar has been added, also can begin to ferment by creating their own acids.

Fermentation of some foods produces carbon dioxide that contributes to leavening and rising, as in yeast breads. Oftentimes, the fermentation process is induced by the addition of starter cultures. Once the cultures are added, the food is placed in an appropriate environment to encourage growth of the friendly yeast or bacteria. In recipes, this often is noted by instructions to place yeast bread in a warm location to rise.[1]

In addition to providing preservation, fermented foods have traditionally been a dietary source of probiotics. Probiotics are thought to encourage gastrointestinal tract health by promoting friendly bacteria in the gut and thereby inhibiting pathogenic bacteria.[4] Research is ongoing regarding other possible health benefits of probiotics. Note that studies done on probiotic bacteria typically examine a specific genus, species, or strain of bacteria, thus the results may not apply to all probiotics or to all fermented foods.[19,20] Varying "doses" of probiotics have been studied, which may not translate easily to food servings. Finally, labeling and health claims for probiotics may not be regulated or standardized, depending on whether the items are marketed as supplements or as foods. These factors complicate our understanding of the health benefits of fermented foods.

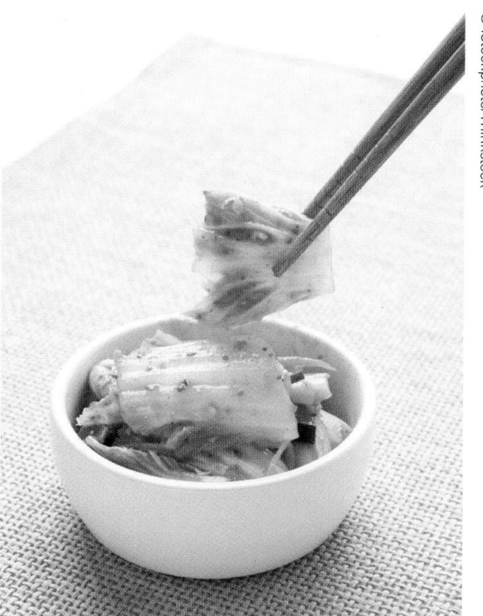

© iStockphoto/Thinkstock

FIGURE 16.10 Kimchi is a traditional fermented Korean dish made with vegetables, most often cabbage, radishes, and cucumbers, and seasonings. Hundreds of varieties of kimchi are available.

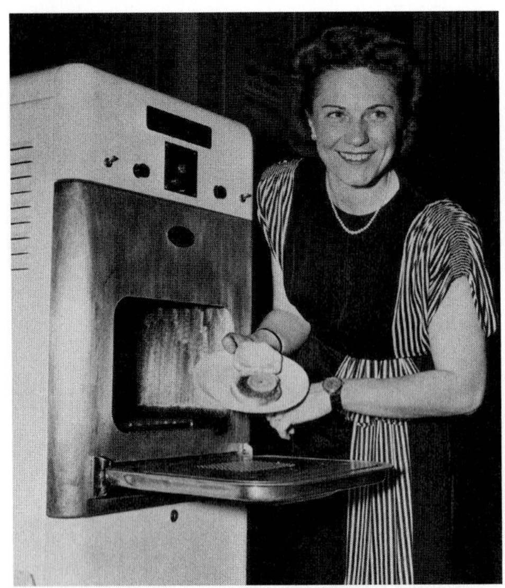

FIGURE 16.11 The first commercial microwave oven was sold in 1947, but these early microwave ovens were large and expensive. It was not until 1967 that the first countertop microwave was available for home use. Today, microwave ovens are found in most kitchens.

irradiation The exposure of food products to ionizing radiation in the form of gamma rays, X-rays, or electron beams to kill microbes.

Microwaves and Irradiation

Energy can also be used to heat and preserve foods. Common methods include microwave ovens and irradiation. During World War II it was discovered that radar generated heat; this finding was then applied to the development of microwave ovens (see **Figure 16.11**).[21] Microwaves create heat through the movement of high-frequency radio waves (moving at 2 billion cycles per second) that energize some molecules within food.[22] As the molecules become energized, they begin to move and become hot. The heat from these molecules is then transferred to other molecules, thus heating the food. Microwave ovens now are found in many homes and are used to cook, reheat, and defrost foods. Commercially, microwave ovens also are used to temper, precook, and dry foods, such as pasta.[21]

Irradiation is the exposure of food products to ionizing radiation in the form of gamma rays, X-rays, or electron beams.[3] Testing of radiation for preservation of food began in the 1920s and was continued by the military in the 1950s as a way to protect rations from pathogens.[23] Irradiation involves the formation of free electrons, ions, and free radicals within a food. Free electrons and free radicals damage DNA by breaking its bonds, thereby impairing growth and reproduction of both the tissue in the food and any microorganisms within it.[3,24]

In the United States, irradiation is considered an "additive" and is thus regulated by the FDA. The radiation dose is measured in kilograys (kGy). Exposure to radiation is classified as low, medium, or strong; the various strengths accomplish different types of preservation:

- *Low-dose radiation* is used to eradicate insects and to inhibit sprouting, maturation, and growth. It extends the shelf life of foods such as ripe fruits and vegetables.[3]
- *Medium-dose radiation* is also known as *pasteurizing radiation*; it is used to reduce microbial populations in a food product. Food is exposed to a dose of radiation (1–10 kGy) which reduces, but does not completely destroy, pathogens.[25]
- *High-dose radiation* is not typically allowed under FDA regulations except for the sterilization of dry spices and seasonings and frozen packaged meat used by NASA astronauts.[26] Doses in the range of 42–77 kGy, which are considered high, can sterilize a product. High doses will even destroy the highly resistant spores of *C. botulinum*.[25]

The FDA only allows certain foods to be irradiated. FDA guidelines specify the type of food, the purpose of the irradiation, and the maximum dose of radiation allowed for that food and purpose. For example, shell eggs are allowed to be irradiated at a maximum of 3 kGy to control the growth of *Salmonella* spp. A complete, updated list can be found on the FDA's website.[26]

The FDA also requires that foods that have been irradiated be labeled both with the irradiation symbol and the words "treated with radiation" or "treated by irradiation" (see **Figure 16.12**). If a food product that was irradiated does not have a label, the FDA requires a sign or some other notification that is conspicuous to the end consumer. The FDA does not require that a food product that contains an *ingredient* that was irradiated be labeled as irradiated.[27]

It is important to note that food often is irradiated when it is already in its packaging material. In these cases, the packaging is also irradiated. The FDA has an extensive list of packaging materials, additives, and coatings that are allowed for use in a product being irradiated.[27] When polymers, which are often found in packaging, are exposed to radiation, they create both cross-linkages and chain scission. Cross-linking connects chains of polymers, whereas chain scission breaks them apart. Cross-linkages are stable, but chain scissions can migrate out of the packaging material and into food. Thus,

Gastronomy Point

Fermented Foods Fermented foods are widely found in many cultures and often are prized for the added layer of flavor added by the fermentation process.

packaging material must be tested if it is intended for use with irradiated foods.[23]

With irradiation, as with many techniques applied to food processing, there also is the question of whether the food remains safe to consume. Various consumer groups are concerned about food treated by irradiation because of the negative connotations of radiation.[23] Numerous agencies worldwide, including the Centers for Disease Control and Prevention (CDC), the World Health Organization (WHO), the International Atomic Energy Agency (IAEA), and the Food and Agricultural Organization of the United Nations, support the use of irradiation.[3,23] Critics of food irradiation raise concern about radiolytic products (found in very small amounts in irradiated foods) and the loss of some nutrients. Radiolytic products are volatile compounds that some think are carcinogenic, but they are thought to be safe for humans in the amounts found in irradiated foods.[24] Nutrient losses—particularly thiamine, as well as vitamins A, C, and E—have been found but are comparable to losses found with other types of processing methods.[24] On the whole, the risks of food irradiation are thought to be less dangerous to the majority of the population than the risk of pathogenic growth.

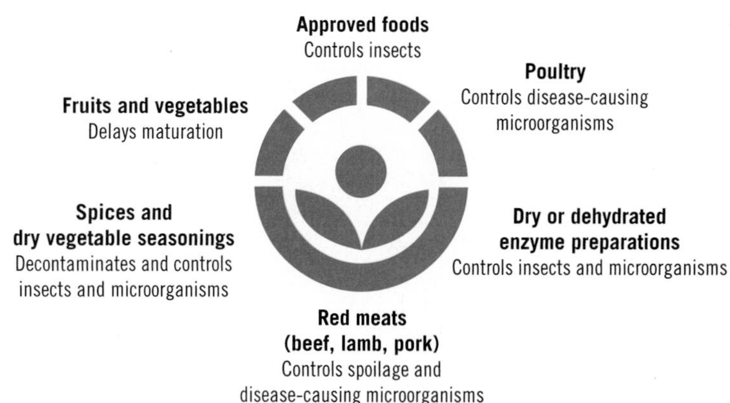

FIGURE 16.12 The Radura is the international symbol that indicates that a food has been irradiated. The FDA requires that irradiated foods have a label with either the statement "treated with radiation" or "treated by irradiation," along with the Radura.

In addition to concerns about consumer safety, another obstacle to implementing irradiation as a major preservation technique is the initial cost associated with starting a new method of preservation. In the United States, for example, most food manufacturers have already invested considerable time and money in techniques such as freezing, canning, or other methods. At this point, manufacturers have little incentive to invest money into a new system of preservation. In countries that have less developed manufacturing and preservation systems, the capital needed to begin irradiating food may be prohibitive.[3]

Effects of Preservation on Nutrient Composition

As may be expected, nutrient composition can be affected by the preservation method used. In particular, vitamin composition and (to a lesser extent) mineral retention can be affected by heat, pH, light, oxidation, water solubility, and other applications.[28] Numerous studies have examined differences in vitamin and mineral composition of foods processed by various methods, though the results are somewhat confounded by natural variations in foods.[29] For example, vitamin and mineral content are affected by the maturity of the fruit or vegetable, where it was grown, and the length of time it was transported or stored before processing.[28,29]

Vitamin C (ascorbic acid) is one of the most often studied vitamins because it is highly susceptible to damage from heat, drying, oxidation, and simple tissue damage (e.g., slicing).[28,29] Thiamine also is the subject of much research because it is destroyed by high heat and nonacidic conditions.[28] USDA data on spinach, for example, shows that the amount of thiamine present in spinach that was frozen or canned is less than that in cooked fresh spinich.[29] Compared to fresh spinach, frozen and canned spinach also has less riboflavin, niacin, vitamin B_6, and folate.[29] These differences are expected because the introduction of heat, water, acid, and other treatments applied during preservation can detrimentally affect numerous vitamins, as shown in **Table 16.4**. Macronutrients also can be affected by preservation. For example, fats can undergo oxidation when exposed to light, and proteins and amino acids can be denatured by acid and heat.[28]

TABLE 16.4
Vitamin Content of Fresh, Frozen, and Canned Vegetables (1 Cup per Serving)

Food	Thiamin (mg)	Riboflavin (mg)	Niacin (mg)	B_6 (mg)	Folate (μg)
Green Beans					
Fresh, boiled	0.093	0.121	0.768	0.070	41
Frozen, boiled	0.047	0.122	0.517	0.081	31
Canned	0.022	0.061	0.277	0.041	43
Green Peas					
Fresh, boiled	0.205	0.122	0.862	0.230	46
Frozen, boiled	0.102	0.160	2.368	0.181	94
Canned	0.182	0.090	1.664	0.095	53
Peaches					
Fresh	0.041	0.053	1.370	0.043	7
Frozen	0.033	0.088	1.633	0.045	8
Canned*	0.029	0.063	1.609	0.050	8
Spinach					
Fresh, raw	0.023	0.217	0.217	0.059	58
Frozen, boiled	0.148	0.334	0.834	0.258	230
Canned	0.034	0.295	0.830	0.214	210
Tomatoes					
Fresh, raw	0.067	0.034	1.069	0.144	27
Canned	0.117	0.089	1.821	0.043	13

* Canned in heavy syrup and drained.
Sources: Data from U.S. Department of Agriculture, Agricultural Research Service. 2011. USDA National Nutrient Database for Standard Reference, Release 24. Available at: http://www.ars.usda.gov/Services/docs.htm?docid=22114. Accessed December 18, 2012.

Despite the seeming nutritional advantage of fresh foods over processed ones, recent reviews and studies have cautioned that some of these data may be misleading. Many vitamins naturally degrade in fresh foods once the food is harvested, especially in fruits and vegetables that are transported long distances before reaching the store shelf. Therefore, nutrient composition of foods picked at peak maturity and immediately blanched and frozen or canned may actually be better than that of the "fresh" produce typically available at the grocery store.[29]

Newer Technologies in Food Preservation

New food preservation technologies are being researched and developed by the food industry to improve the quality, efficiency, safety, and shelf life of food and to meet consumers' demands for high-quality foods. Mechanical food processing methods to extend shelf life are constantly being developed. The FDA mandates how much of a food product's microorganism population must be reduced for a food processing method to be considered successful. For example, in juice pathogenic microbes have to be reduced by 100,000. Developers study new methods to determine if the treatment adequately reduces the size and growth rate of the microorganism population. Because thermal treatment of food may affect a food's flavor, texture, and other quality indicators, nonthermal processing is emerging as an important area of development.

High Pressure

One area of interest is the use of pressure to inactivate microorganisms (see **Figure 16.13**). This process is known as high hydrostatic pressure processing or **ultra-high-pressure (UHP) processing.**[3] UHP is preferred for some foods because it can reduce microbial populations without subjecting the food to high temperatures, which can result in a higher-quality product.[3] Foods processed in this way are placed under uniform pressure of up to 100,000 pounds per square inch; living microbes are destroyed by anything greater than 60,000 pounds per square inch.[3,30] (The reason food does not explode from this pressure is that the pressure is applied evenly across the entire surface and interior of the food.) The pressure is applied for a few minutes, usually after the food has been placed in a package. Following UHP, the food, if it is nonacidic, must then be refrigerated to inhibit spores from growing. Some companies have touted the added safety, freshness (because it is not thermally processed), and freedom from preservatives this method confers to their commercial products.[31]

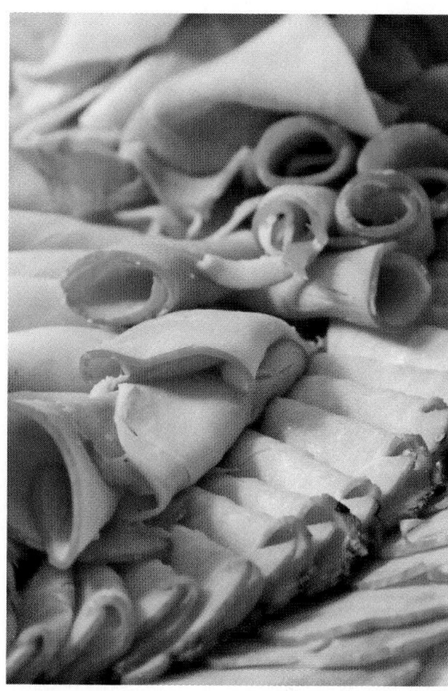

FIGURE 16.13 UHP can be applied to a variety of foods, including fruits and vegetables, meats, and seafood. Some deli meats are treated with UHP, including sliced ham, turkey, and chicken.

High Pressure and High Temperature

When combined with high temperatures, high pressure processing can result in sterile food products.[31] This process is called **pressure-assisted thermal sterilization (PATS)**. It often is used with low-acid canned products.[32] PATS can inactivate *C. botulinum* spores at lower temperatures (250°F; 121°C) and a shorter holding time (3 minutes) than more traditional processing methods.[32]

Nonthermal Processing Methods

Other new technologies being proposed include using ultraviolet (UV) irradiation, low-energy X-ray irradiation, pulsed light, and ultrasound to reduce microbial activity in food. Researchers are also combining some of these methods with high pressure, increased temperatures, or other methods to create both high-quality and safe preserved food products.[32]

ultra-high-pressure (UHP) processing Use of pressure to inactivate microorganisms; also known as high hydrostatic pressure processing.

pressure-assisted thermal sterilization (PATS) A process used in low-acid canned products that can inactivate *Clostridium botulinum* spores with lower temperatures (49°F; 121°C) and lower holding time (3 minutes) than traditional methods of processing.

Refined Thermal Techniques

Thermal methods continue to be refined. Recent advances include the use of microwaves and electricity to heat food and reduce microbial populations. A new method of microwave heating called *continuous microwave processing* was recently designed for aseptic sterilization of sweet potato puree. In this process, the puree is passed through a tube and the microwave energy is directed at the center of the product in order to heat it from the inside out. Because the heating is quick, the temperature is consistent throughout the product, and cooling occurs at the end of the process, continuous microwave processing is quite efficient and has been found to retain higher amounts of beta-carotene than when the food is processed using more traditional methods.[33]

Another newer thermal method of processing food is ohmic heating (also known as electrical resistance heating or electroheating).[3] With this method, electrodes that are in direct contact with the food run electricity through the product, heating it evenly and inactivating microorganisms. It preserves quality because the heating is quick and uniform. A similar method, but one that is not considered a thermal method, is pulsed electric fields (PEF), whereby a liquid is subjected to very fast pulses of electricity. It is thought that the electrical pulses destroy microbial cell membranes, thus inactivating pathogens and spoilage organisms.[34]

Antimicrobial Chemicals

A number of antimicrobials have shown promise as potential food preservatives. These chemicals can be sprayed onto raw or finished foods or mixed in as an ingredient. The foods can also be dipped into an antimicrobial solution.[34] Consumer demand has recently encouraged food processors to look at natural antimicrobials that will safely preserve products, enabling the manufacturer to use the label "natural." Another product used in the food production process that is of concern to consumers is pesticides. See **Special Topic 16.3** for more information on pesticides.

A number of natural chemicals have been found that have the potential to inhibit microorganisms. These include essential oils, lysozyme, lactoferrin, lactoperoxidase system (LPS), fatty acids, chitosan, and nisin, among other compounds. A few of these, including fatty acids and essential oils, which include plant oils such as mint and citrus essential oil, are hydrophobic and thus interact better with microorganisms that have lipophilic cell membranes. The disadvantage of this property is that it sometimes causes the chemicals to be sequestered in fatty portions of a food. Lactoferrin is a protein that binds to iron. It is found in human and animal fluids. Lactoferrin keeps iron from microbes, preventing them from growing and reproducing properly. It also is thought to remove lipopolysaccharides from the microbes' cell membranes, forming pores on the cell surface. LPS is also found in human and animal fluids, such as milk and colostrum. It consists of an enzyme, lactoperoxidase, which catalyzes a reaction to create cyanosulphurous acid and cyanosulphuric acid. Both chemicals cause detrimental effects to bacteria, fungi, and viruses. Although these chemicals have been studied, many are not yet in wide use as antimicrobials in the United States.[34]

Special Topic 16.3

Pesticides in Our Food

Jennifer Lerman, RD, LDN

Pesticides are used in food production to kill, repel, or reduce any kind of pest that may be present. According to the Environmental Protection Agency (EPA), the government body that regulates these chemicals, pesticides include insecticides, fungicides, rodenticides, insect repellents, weed killers, antimicrobials, and swimming pool chemicals. Before any pesticide can be sold or used in the United States, the EPA must review and register it.[1] When pesticides are to be used on food, the EPA requires manufacturers to submit data indicating the amount of pesticide residue remaining on the food, including both raw and processed varieties of the agricultural product. The agency also requires studies to be submitted showing both short- and long-term toxicity of the pesticide. These studies often are performed on animals using amounts of the pesticide that are greater than the levels expected to be found as residue on food.

The EPA pays particular attention to pesticide exposure in children and infants when evaluating pesticides. Infants and children are progressing through stages of growth and development that are sensitive to chemicals, and they may consume a more limited variety of foods than adults and eat more calories per kilogram of body weight. Thus, pesticides may pose a greater risk to this subset of the population.[2]

The Food Quality Protection Act

In 1996, Congress passed the Food Quality Protection Act (FQPA), which mandated the EPA to review all previously registered pesticides within 10 years to ensure continued safety. As a result of continued reassessment and monitoring, some pesticides have been removed from the market.[3] For example, the pesticide aldicarb, an *n*-methyl carbamate insecticide used on products such as cotton, potatoes, and citrus fruits, is no longer an approved pesticide because of its neurotoxic effects. Despite its termination, aldicarb will not disappear immediately. Although the pesticide's registration with the EPA was terminated in October 2010, the chemical will not be phased out of production until 2014, and it may still be used until 2018.[4]

Persistent Organic Pollutants

Perhaps the greatest concern regarding pesticides in our food supply comes from persistent organic pollutants (POPs), which do not break down in nature and have been found to have toxic properties. An example is the organochlorine pesticides, including diphenyltrichoroethane, otherwise known as DDT. The danger in these POPs is that even when they are banned from use or phased out voluntarily, they remain in the environment and can continue to contaminate the food supply for many years.

A limited number of studies have looked at the chemical contamination of food to estimate total dietary intake of these chemicals. One recent study of chemical contamination of the U.S. food supply revealed that multiple pesticide chemicals were found in detectable amounts in 31 commonly consumed foods. Nearly every food studied contained chemical residues, and most contained more than one type of chemical. The authors of the study estimated a daily intake of a number of pesticides. Although none of these values exceeded the EPA or European Union reference doses, it is not known at this time how multiple chemical residues may act cumulatively within humans.[5] Another recent review of prenatal and childhood exposure to pesticides indicates that there may be an association between increased exposure and impaired neurodevelopment.[6] If accurate, it would imply that limiting exposure to pesticides in the food supply may be an important public health objective.

A related concern is the contamination of food products with other POPs, such as industrial chemicals not designed for use as pesticides but that enter the food chain via environmental contamination. Examples of these types of chemicals are mercury, perfluorinated compounds (PFCs), polychlorinated biphenyls (PCBs), and polybrominated diphenyl ethers (PBDEs). Oftentimes, it is difficult to pinpoint where exposure to these chemicals is coming from because the contaminants are found in water, dust, and other generalized places. Studies have shown, however, that even after these chemicals are banned, they are still found in human tissues.[7] For example, PBDEs, which were used as flame retardants, have been found in human breast milk, fetal liver tissue, and in fish and bird tissues. This chemical is found to have detrimental effects on the liver, thyroid, and brain. PBDEs are not currently banned in the United States, although major U.S. manufacturers have been voluntarily phasing out versions of the chemical in recent years.[8]

Research related to the dangers of pesticide and other chemical exposure is complicated by the fact that it is difficult to prove that pesticide exposure causes a certain outcome, such as cancer, as well as the fact that pesticide exposure comes from both food and nonfood products and can vary by location and by dietary pattern. Thus, more research is needed to direct agencies such as the EPA toward regulations that create not only a safer environment but also a safer food supply.

References

1 Environmental Protection Agency. Setting Tolerances for Pesticide Residues in Foods. Available at: http://www.epa.gov/pesticides/factsheets/stprf.htm. Accessed November 20, 2010.

2 Environmental Protection Agency. Protecting the Public from Pesticide Residues in Food. Available at: http://www.epa.gov/pesticides/factsheets/protect.htm. Accessed November 20, 2010.

3 Environmental Protection Agency. Accomplishments Under the Food Quality Protection Act. Available at: http://www.epa.gov/pesticides/regulating/laws/fqpa/fqpa_accomplishments.htm. Accessed November 20, 2010.

4 Environmental Protection Agency. Agreement to Terminate All Uses of Aldicarb. Available at: http://www.epa.gov/oppsrrd1/REDs/factsheets/aldicarb_fs.html. Accessed November 20, 2010.

5 Schecter A, Colacino J, Haffner D, et al. Perfluorinated compounds, polychlorinated biphenyls, and organochlorine pesticide contamination in composite food samples from Dallas, Texas, USA. *Environ Health Persp.* 2010;118(6):796–802.

6 Jurewicz J, Hanke W. Prenatal and childhood exposure to pesticides and neurobehavioral development: Review of epidemiological studies. *Int J Occ Med Env Health.* 2008;21(2):121–132.

7 Doucet J, Tague B, Arnold DL, et al. Persistent organic pollutant residues in human fetal liver and placenta from Greater Montreal, Quebec: A longitudinal study for 1998 through 2006. *Environ Health Persp.* 2009;117(4):605–610.

8 Environmental Protection Agency. Polybrominated Diphenylethers (PBDEs). Available at: http://www.epa.gov/oppt/pbde. Accessed December 16, 2010.

Scientists are hard at work trying to determine which methods and chemicals work best and how combining multiple methods can improve food safety. Research is currently focused on whether using multiple methods works synergistically or additively. Clearly, as advances in technology arise, food processors are looking to apply new methods for improvements in quality, cost, and efficiency. It must be determined which methods are most effective, for both food safety and cost of processing, for the greatest number of foods. It is worth watching for new trends—advances in processing and preservation are important for both the safety and nutritional quality of the food we eat.[34]

Food Packaging

Food packaging advances have improved food processing and extended the shelf life of food items (see **Figure 16.14**). Packaging advances have made it possible to ship food safely over long distances and provide the means to provide consumers with detailed information about their food. In some cases, packaging also can be used to trace the path that foods take from field to table. New materials can even communicate information to processors and consumers to further improve food quality and safety.[35]

FIGURE 16.14 Many types of packaging are used to protect food from the outside environment, ensuring that it is transported safely from the manufacturing plant to the consumer's table.

Common Packaging Materials

Packaging is designed to protect the food from microbes, air, water, and physical damage and is based on the type of food being contained. Manufacturers also consider how the packaging material itself interacts with the food. For example, some foods may brown in the presence of a certain material, and carbonated or acidic beverages may degrade some types of packaging. Manufacturers also assess the stability of the material structure during shipping, stacking, and storage. For many products, tamper resistance also is a concern. Many packages use more than one type of material in the final product.[35]

The main types of materials used in food packaging are paper, plastic, metal, and glass. As technology has advanced, some of these materials have become more popular than others.

Glass

Made from heated silica, sodium carbonate, and stabilizers, glass is believed to be the original food packaging, first used in 3000 B.C. It is still used primarily because of its ability to contain foods without reacting with them, to withstand processing temperatures, to keep out air and water, and to allow for product visibility. It also is reusable and thus environmentally friendly. Unfortunately, glass is heavy and breakable, and therefore not as well suited to transportation as some other materials.[35]

Paper and Paperboard

These lightweight packaging alternatives have also been used for centuries. Paper, which is made from pulped cellulose fibers derived from wood, can be treated for direct food contact or turned into thicker paperboard that can either have direct contact with food or be used for outer packaging or shipping. Paper and paperboard can be waxed or laminated with a plastic polymer such as polyethylene to improve resistance to water and oils. Kraft paper, a heavy-duty processed paper, is used for flour and sugar bags; parchment paper, a thin acid-treated paper, is used for butter. Solid board, a form of paperboard with numerous layers that is then laminated, is used for milk and juice cartons. Paper also can be laminated with aluminum for added moisture resistance to package foods such as dried soups.[35]

Green Point

Transportation Costs Because of transportation costs, including the high costs of fossil fuels, the weight and volume of a particular packaging material are vitally important to the manufacturer in keeping costs down and maintaining a small carbon footprint.

Green Point

Thermoplastics Thermoplastics are easy to remold and are thus good candidates for recycling programs.

Metals

Aluminum and other metals, such as steel, are also used for food packaging. Lightweight, flexible aluminum can be used to make cans for beverages. It blocks light, air, and moisture extremely well. It cannot be welded, so it can only be used in seamless containers. In addition to laminating paperboard, aluminum is also rolled into thin sheets of foil that are used as a food wrap or, when thicker, for food trays. Aluminum also is used in metalized films, a combination of plastic and metal that is very flexible and is well known for its use as snack packaging.

Aluminum is expensive compared to other metals, which is one reason tin and steel are used for food packaging as well. Steel must be coated in tin, chrome, and often a lacquer to prevent corrosion upon contact with food. The combination of tin and steel is called tinplate; tin-free steel is also known as chrome oxide or electrolytic chromium coated steel. Tinplate can be hermetically sealed, allowing it to be used in aseptic packaging. Both tinplate and tin-free steel are strong and can be easily decorated. They are used for canned goods, metal ends of packages, processed foods, and bottle caps as well as other types of packages (see **Figure 16.15**).[35]

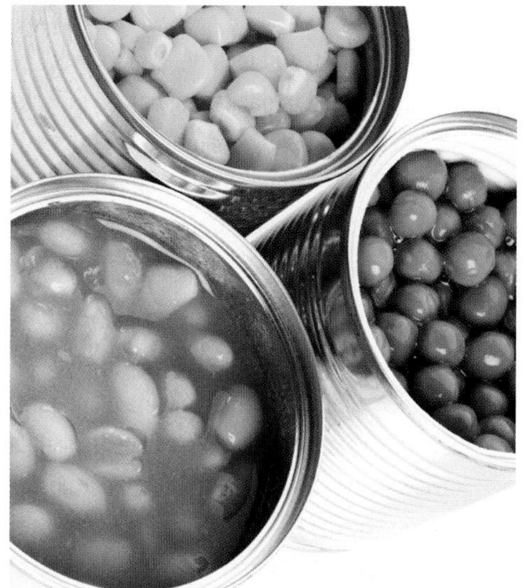

FIGURE 16.15 Metal cans are a versatile packaging material and can be used with a diverse array of foods and beverages. Most cans are made of tinplate or aluminum.

Plastics

Another common packaging material used for many types of food is plastic. The EPA describes *plastic* as polymers made from chains of molecules consisting of hydrogen, carbon, oxygen, and/or silicon.[36] The molecules originate from heating petroleum or other substances. **Thermoplastics** are the category of plastics commonly used for food packaging; they soften every time they are heated and thus can be reshaped, molded, and, more importantly, recycled.[35] The most commonly used plastics in food packaging are polyvinyl chloride (PVC), polystyrene, polyamide, polyolefins, and polyesters. The latter two are the most common and include polyethylene, polypropylene, and polyethylene terephthalate (PETE).[1] Polyethylene is the most inexpensive plastic. It can be high density, which is stiff, or low density, which is flexible, as used in bread bags and squeeze bottles.[35] PETE is widely used in items such as carbonated drink bottles because it is clear and virtually impermeable to the carbonation gases.

thermoplastics Category of plastics used for food packaging because they soften when heated and can be reshaped, molded, and recycled.

The particular type of plastic used in a food package is based on the specific qualities that it provides and its intended use (see **Figure 16.16**). For example, if a food is meant to be both microwaved and served in its plastic tray, a rigid plastic that can withstand a microwave with no migration of chemicals and without melting, such as polypropylene, will be used.[35] Additional information on the safety of packaging materials, particularly plastics, is discussed in **Special Topic 16.4**.

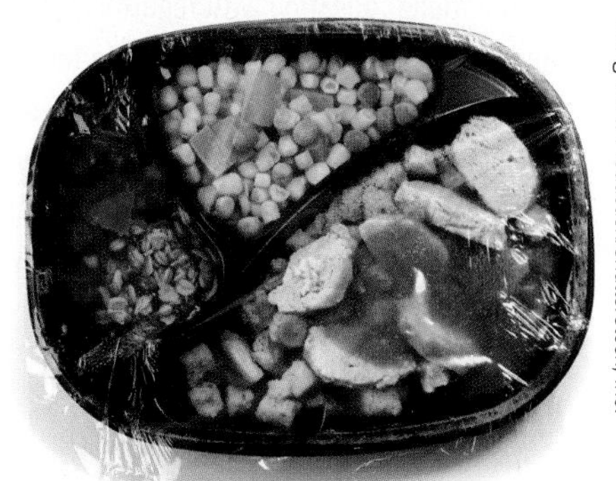

FIGURE 16.16 The packaging for a particular food must meet several objectives. It must provide physical protection, it must protect the food from the outside environment, it must deter tampering, and it must be convenient.

Special Topic 16.4

Safety of Packaging Material

Jennifer Lerman, RD, LDN

Before a material can be used in food packaging in the United States, the FDA must be notified of its use. This requirement stems from the Federal Food, Drug, and Cosmetic Act (FD&C), which describes a food additive as "any substance the intended use of which results or may reasonably be expected to result, directly or indirectly, in its becoming a component or otherwise affecting the characteristics of any food (including any substance intended for use in producing, manufacturing, packing, processing, preparing, treating, packaging, transporting, or holding food; and including any source of radiation intended for any such use)."[1] This definition indicates that because materials and chemicals used in packaging can be expected to migrate to some extent into a food, their safety must be ascertained before use. The FD&C Act, passed in 1958, exempted substances that are GRAS and that were in common use in food prior to the act becoming law. More recently, in the 1997 Food and Drug Administration Modernization Act (FDAMA), the process for obtaining approval for packaging material was streamlined. Now, manufacturers and suppliers are allowed to submit Food Contact Notifications to the FDA for new materials being used in food packaging. The FDA has 120 days to review the notification and object if concerns arise with regard to the packaging material.[2]

Determining whether a food-contact substance is safe is the main goal of notification and FDA review. The Code of Federal Regulations [21 CFR 170.3(i)] defines safe as a "reasonable certainty in the minds of competent scientists that a substance is not harmful under the intended conditions of use."[3] The number of tests and studies the FDA requires to make determinations about the safety of food-contact substances depends on the end consumer's estimated daily intake of that chemical. In one review, 85% of substances submitted for review between 2000 and 2006 had exposure levels of less than 150 μg per day. At this level, only short-term genetic toxicity tests are required by the FDA to assess the safety of the substance. If dietary exposure is greater than this amount, additional studies and tests are done to verify the safety of the food-contact substance.[4]

Despite the effort that goes into assuring the safety of food-contact chemicals, safety concerns surround some of these substances. A well-known recent example of a food-contact chemical with safety concerns is bisphenol A (BPA). Used in cans as a lining and in polycarbonate plastics, BPA has come under scrutiny after some studies showed disruption of sexual maturation in rodents and an association with heart disease in adult humans, among other findings.[5] A report from the National Toxicology Program notes "some concern for effects on the brain, behavior, and prostate gland in fetuses, infants, and children at current human exposures to bisphenol A."[6] The amount of BPA that is safe for human consumption is not known definitively, although the EPA and the European Food Safety Authority (EFSA) consider a tolerable dose to be 50 micrograms per kilogram per day. However, the European Commission Scientific Committee on Food Safety has proposed a limit of 10 micrograms per kilogram per day.

An additional question with regards to BPA is how much BPA migrates into food from packaging material. A recent study of canned, fresh, and plastic-wrapped foods in the United States showed a range of BPA levels in foods that varied based on the brand, type of food, and pH.[5] Because a variety of factors clearly play a role in how much BPA is consistently being consumed, and it is not yet known what levels of consumption are safe, some manufacturers have removed BPA from their packaging materials.[7] The FDA is currently continuing research into BPA. It also is in support of reasonable steps to reduce human exposure to BPA and supports industry efforts to remove BPA from infant bottles, cups, and formula can linings.[6]

References

1 Food, Drug, and Cosmetic Act, 21 U.S.C. 321 §201(s). Available at: http://www.fda.gov/RegulatoryInformation/Legislation/FederalFoodDrugandCosmeticActFDCAct/FDCActChaptersIandIIShortTitleandDefinitions/ucm086297.htm. Accessed June 8, 2012.

2 U.S. Food and Drug Administration. Regulatory Report: FDA's Food Contact Substance Notification Program. Available at: http://www.fda.gov/Food/FoodIngredientsPackaging/FoodContactSubstancesFCS/UCM064161. Accessed November 29, 2010.

3 21 CFR 170.3(i). Available at: http://cfr.vlex.com/vid/170-3-definitions-19706720. Accessed November 29, 2010.

4 U.S. Food and Drug Administration. Regulatory Report: Assessing the Safety of Food Contact Substances. Available at: http://www.fda.gov/Food/FoodIngredientsPackaging/FoodContactSubstancesFCS/UCM064166. Accessed November 29, 2010.

5 Schecter A, Malik N, Haffner D, et al. Bisphenol A (BPA) in U.S. food. *Environ Sci Technol.* 2010;44(24):9425–9430.

6 U.S. Food and Drug Administration. Update on Bisphenol A for Use in Food Contact Applications. January 2010. Available at: http://www.fda.gov/NewsEvents/PublicHealthFocus/ucm197739.htm#current. Accessed November 29, 2010.

7 Hickman M. Major producers to ditch BPA from packaging. *Independent.* November 1, 2010. Available at: http://www.independent.co.uk/life-style/health-and-families/health-news/major-producers-to-ditch-bpa-from-packaging-2121837.html. Accessed November 29, 2010.

Advances in Food Packaging Technologies

The food packaging industry is constantly researching new packaging techniques and materials to increase the shelf life of foods and to make foods easier to transport.

Modified Atmosphere Packaging

Fresh produce spoils, in part, due to respiration of the living cells. Living cells degrade large molecules of starch, sugar, and organic acids to produce energy, carbon dioxide, and water. Respiration rates increase when cells are injured, such as when a food is cut. High rates of respiration are known to decrease the shelf life of fresh foods.[37]

Food processors have found that modifying the air within a package is a useful method to reduce respiration rates. This process, called **modified atmosphere packaging (MAP)**, was first used in 1927 with apples, which were stored in a lower oxygen, higher carbon dioxide environment to extend their shelf life. MAP began being used commercially in the late 1970s for meat; it was later used for fresh produce, pasta, coffee, and baked goods, among other products. A number of different packaging techniques can be considered MAP. They include vacuum packaging because air is removed (this is a type of modification of atmosphere), and packaging material that is impermeable to outside air (thus keeping the food product in a modified atmosphere during distribution and storage).[38]

modified atmosphere packaging (MAP) The deliberate manipulation of the gases or the diffusion of gases within a food package to enhance shelf life and reduce spoilage.

Depending on the food, different combinations of gases—including oxygen, nitrogen, and carbon dioxide—are used to create the right environment to extend shelf life. Lowering oxygen and increasing carbon dioxide concentrations also inhibits the growth of aerobic microorganisms in produce and other foods.[38] Because oxygen also causes fats to go rancid and antioxidants to degrade, decreasing oxygen concentrations also can reduce these undesirable changes.[37,38] In packages of meat, high oxygen is usually used to achieve the correct red color that consumers expect. Nitrogen, an inert gas, also is typically used because it does not interact with foods and does not dissolve into the foods; it can thus be used to fill a package to keep it from collapsing. It can replace oxygen or help maintain package integrity when carbon dioxide dissolves into some types of foods.[38]

Polymers Used in MAP

A variety of polymers are used to seal foods in MAP, including PVC, polyethylene terephthalate (PET), polyethylene, and polypropylene. The material is chosen based on the food being packaged and what qualities are needed. For example, some foods are packaged in a semipermeable polymer with a modified atmosphere of gases that changes over time (due to the selective permeability of the material). The final mixture of gas concentrations is designed to extend shelf life. This is known as *equilibrium modified atmosphere packaging*. Other polymers are selected for their sealing capabilities, antifogging capabilities, and mechanical properties (i.e., how well the packaging works mechanically with the structure of the food and the equipment being used).[38]

Disadvantages

MAP has both advantages and disadvantages. If not properly designed, MAP can make food more dangerous by allowing for the growth of anaerobic microbes; of particular concern is the dangerous, toxin-producing *C. botulinum*. MAP can also affect the volatility and flavor profile of the packaged food, adversely affecting taste.[37] Another major disadvantage is that MAP is ineffective once a package is opened because the atmosphere then becomes the same as the outside environment. MAP also can be costly for manufacturers and may increase package volume size.[38] It can increase discoloration of some foods, such as lettuce, although it inhibits enzymatic browning of some foods (e.g., peach, kiwi, mango).[37]

Green Point

Extending Shelf Life MAP, edible films, and other technologies reduce waste by extending shelf life, thereby reducing the amount of food that enters landfills.

edible films Materials applied to foods that provide a benefit to the food and can be consumed by the end user; they typically allow for selective gas exchange to preserve quality, while retaining moisture or preventing microbial growth.

intelligent packaging Technology built into a package that lets a food processor, distributor, seller, or consumer know something about the internal or external environment of the package.

Advantages

Advantages of MAP include retention of antioxidants, such as vitamin C and carotene, because there is less oxygen available to degrade them.[37] Another significant advantage is the preservation of a food for a longer time without the use of chemical preservative ingredients.[38] In summary, MAP, although effective at extending shelf life, may be more useful when combined with other methods, such as antimicrobials and edible films.[37]

Edible Films

Another important innovation in food packaging has been the advent of edible films. **Edible films** are materials applied to foods that provide a benefit to the food and can be consumed by the end user; they typically allow for selective gas exchange to preserve quality, while retaining moisture or preventing microbial growth.[38] Waxes applied to fruit and vegetables were the earliest edible films. They aid in retaining moisture to extend shelf life.

Advances have allowed processors to combine antimicrobial chemicals with edible films to inhibit microbial growth and spoilage and further extend shelf life.[37] The types of antimicrobials added to edible films include essential oils, fatty acid esters, organic acids, nitrites, and sulfites. One natural edible coating with inherent antimicrobial properties is chitosan, a polymer derived from crab and shrimp shells.[34] This material has been used extensively in food products, both as a functional ingredient and as an edible coating. Any material used as an edible film is intended to be consumed; thus, it must either be approved as a food additive or considered a GRAS ingredient.[39]

Edible films have been proposed as a promising technique for extending shelf life when combined with MAP. Benefits of edible films include reduction in packaging materials and enhanced biodegradability; they are also useful as vehicles for delivering antimicrobial chemicals (see **Figure 16.17**). Like other food packaging technologies, future advances may result in a more widespread application of edible films.[37]

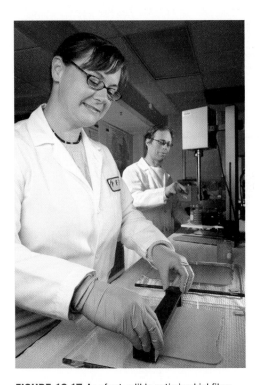

FIGURE 16.17 As of yet, edible antimicrobial films have not yet hit products on grocery store shelves. However, these materials have huge potential commercial applications for preventing microbial growth on foods.

Courtesy of the USDA Agricultural Research Service. Photo by Peggy Greb.

Intelligent and Active Packaging

Recent technological advances have brought about new "smart" packaging that interacts with the package's external or internal environment. Smart packaging is currently divided into two main categories: active and intelligent.

Intelligent Packaging

Packaging containing sensors and indicators that let a food processor, distributor, seller, or consumer know something about the package's environment is called **intelligent packaging**.[40] For example, an intelligent package may have a freshness indicator, which changes color when it measures a critical concentration of ethylene or another ripening chemical. The color change communicates a message about what has happened inside the package.

Intelligent packaging devices are available that can indicate whether a minimum or maximum temperature has been reached. For example, food processors can use such devices to learn whether the temperature inside the package has reached that needed for sterilization. Similarly, a consumer can determine when a beverage has been cooled to an ideal drinking temperature for consumption.[40] Other devices can measure moisture, gas, or microbial concentration or growth. Some technologies, such as the radio frequency identification (RFID), can wirelessly transmit signals for tracking and other purposes, such as information about spoilage.[41] RFID also can be used for stock rotation. Active RFIDs typically contain a sensor and a paper battery to power the transmission, whereas passive RFIDs are powered by the reading device, which is usually a type of scanner.[40,42]

Green Point

Edible Films Edible films can help reduce waste by reducing the amount of packaging a food needs to stay safe and fresh.

Another group of complex sensory devices are *time temperature integrators* (TTIs). These devices sense temperature changes in a product over time, representing the change with a color change on the exterior package. The technology used includes sensing enzymes, biochemical reactions, and mechanical changes within the product. Various techniques have been employed; for example, the devices can use polymeric changes or diffusion in the sensor based on pH or temperature changes. Newer models use photosensitive crystals and rely on changes in the polar molecule concentration caused by temperature changes to trigger a color change on the indicator.[40]

A number of obstacles have emerged that are preventing the widespread use of TTI technology. Some are concerned whether the sensory information on the surface of a package accurately represents temperature changes deeper inside of it. In addition, at present the technology is relatively costly—$0.05 to $0.20 per package.[40]

Active Packaging

In contrast to intelligent packaging, **active packaging** not only senses changes within a product, but performs some function to actually correct the change.[40] In active packaging, spoilage reactions or chemicals, such as excess water, oxygen, or ethylene, are counteracted with scavenging chemicals.[41] For example, if excess oxygen, which would normally create oxidation and rancidity, is detected, oxygen scavengers added to the package would absorb the oxygen. Other compounds used in active packaging can release carbon dioxide, which works as an antimicrobial and extends shelf life. Moisture can be controlled with humidity controllers that can either prevent the loss of moisture that would dry out foods or, alternatively, absorb moisture that seeps into packages of dry or powdered goods to prevent clumping of ingredients. In addition to food processors, the U.S. military is keenly interested in the use of technology to extend the shelf life and portability of foods. Read more about the military's interest in processed foods in **Special Topic 16.5**.

active packaging Packaging that releases scavenging chemicals in response to spoilage reactions or the presence of chemicals or compounds, such as excess water, oxygen, or ethylene.

Innovation Point

Smart Packaging Smart packaging represents an advance in technology that will aid in food safety, traceability, and quality. It is hoped that in the future the technology will become more precise, less expensive, and more widespread.

Special Topic 16.5

Military Packaging: Technology in Action[1]

Jennifer Lerman, RD, LDN

The U.S. military uses many of the packaging advances discussed in this chapter. The military is unique because the food, or rations, that it serves must withstand extreme environments and abuses while remaining safe and edible for extended periods of time. Because of these requirements and because it operates on a very large scale, food packaging and preservation are essential concerns for the military; it participates in significant amounts of research and testing of new technologies.

Not only must military ration packaging protect and preserve food, it must also be designed with consideration of weight, disposability, and functionality of the packaging material. Rations may need to be dropped from the air, stored on a damp ship, or carried through sweltering deserts or frigid arctic environments. The packaging cannot add too much extra weight to the food, and it cannot create excessive waste that will need to be disposed of in the field. It also must be easy to open and may need to double as a serving container. Additionally, the packaging may also need to help heat or insulate the food and beverages for consumption. These physical conditions are considered and accommodated by packaging researchers and testers in the military.

Meals, Ready to Eat

A main item of concern for these testers is the well-known military rations known as Meals, Ready to Eat, or MREs. MREs need to be shelf stable for 3 years at 80°F (26°C) or for 6 months at 100°F (38°C). They must remain of acceptable quality and free from microorganism growth. They must be tested to ensure they meet these standards and put through other physical tests, such as vibrations and drops from 21 inches after being held at 100°F (38°C) and –20°F (–29°C) for 2 days.

Packaging material must protect the food from oxygen and moisture. The MRE entrée packaging is made of a quad-laminate—four materials layered on top of each other—each with various beneficial properties needed to protect the food. The layers currently include polyolefin, aluminum foil, polyamide, and pigmented polyester. Layering these various materials protects the food from off-odors from the packaging material, moisture, oxygen, and changes encountered in the physical environment (such as high temperatures during sealing or low temperatures in cold weather).

Packages That Heat Themselves

The U.S. military uses a number of innovative packaging technologies. For example, since 1993 MREs have included a flameless ration heater, or FRH. This electrochemical heater contains mostly iron and magnesium within a package made of polyester scrim and high-density polyethylene. The packaging must have strong moisture-barrier properties because with the addition of less than 2 ounces of water in the field this component undergoes an exothermic reaction that is hot enough to heat the MRE entrée to a temperature of 100°F (38°C) in less than 12 minutes. The FRH also has the ability to insulate the ration and keep it warm for up to 1 hour. In an extension of this technology, the military also created a larger heating package for the unitized group ration (UGR). This box contains a full meal (entrée, vegetable, starch, and dessert) for 18 people in four family-style trays stacked on top of one another. A single pull-tab must be pulled to activate the heating component around each tray. Within 45 minutes of pulling the tab, the meal is heated and ready to serve. The components within the FRH and UGR packaging are actually used to cook the food.

Ultrasonic Sealing

One packaging innovation the military is currently working on is ultrasonic sealing. This technology is being studied to overcome the issue of contamination of the seal of packaged foods due to the food material getting stuck in the seal area. Currently, food pouches are formed, filled, and then sealed. For foods containing liquids—such as soups, entrées with a sauce, and beverages—the food can get on the package material and inhibit the ability of the packaging material to form a good seal. Ultrasound technology can seal the package properly even if food material is in the way. An additional benefit is that heat is targeted to the two layers being joined, while maintaining lower heat on the outside of the package. This technology has the potential to reduce waste and spoilage caused by contamination due to faulty seals.

Other Innovations

The military is working to develop a number of innovative food processing technologies. Currently, to preserve many MRE components, the military uses retort processing, whereby food held within its pouch or tray is sealed, heated, and held for a predetermined number of minutes at 240–250°F (115–121°C). However, this can result in lower quality food secondary to the high heat and holding time. It also is thought that some nutrients are lost during this process. Recently, the military has been working toward approval of microwave sterilization to replace some of the retort processing. The benefit of microwave processing is reduced time, which preserves freshness and nutrients. The military has also spent nearly 20 years working on high-pressure processing (HPP). By processing foods at a pressure of 87,000 pounds per square inch, bacteria are killed without compromising the quality of the food. This type of processing is particularly useful for foods that do not react well to the high heat sterilization temperatures of retort or microwave processing.

Military packaging and processing, as well as new research in these areas, holds promise for innovations in civilian food technology in the future. As the military pushes research into food processing to improve the quality and safety of rations for its soldiers, the benefits are sure to extend to commercial food processing.

References

1 U.S. Army Natick Soldier Research, Development and Engineering Center, NSRDEC Packaging Integration Team. Overview of Military Packaging. Public Affairs Office Release U11-068. Natick, MA; 2011.

Quality Control

Controlling the quality of preserved or fresh foods is an essential component of food packaging. One major detriment of packaged foods is flavor changes that occur over time. A main reason that packaged foods develop off flavors are chemical changes within the food, such as oxidative reactions causing rancidity in lipid portions of the product. Methods used to prevent these changes have been discussed in previous sections. However, another major issue food processors must deal with is the interaction of food products with packaging materials. Two issues can occur: the first is **flavor scalping**, which is the absorption of volatile food flavors by packaging materials, the second is the migration of packaging materials into food.[43]

flavor scalping The absorption of volatile food flavors by packaging materials.

Polyethylene, one of the most common materials in food packaging, is a major contributor to flavor scalping because it is lipophilic and thus easily absorbs nonpolar molecules, which include aroma molecules. Also, because many flavor and aroma molecules are volatile, transfer of these molecules can happen across airspace inside the package. A variety of factors, including surface area of the packaging, concentration and composition of aromatic chemicals, pH, and temperature, among other factors, affect the rate and degree of volatile chemical migration and flavor scalping.[43]

To reduce the migration of packaging chemicals into foods, flavor and odor absorbers are added to packaging materials. The absorbers are designed to remove volatile packaging chemicals that escape into the food package. In addition, barrier materials are used to keep packaging and food from interacting. These barriers are useful both for limiting flavor scalping and migration of packaging materials into food, and they include laminating of packaging material with polymers or metal. Some newer technologies include coating packaging materials with a combination of chemicals, such as silica oxide, PET, or nanoparticles. The migration of chemicals from packaging into food products is an important consideration with regard to food safety. The chemicals in packaging materials are considered food additives; they must not be harmful when consumed.[41] See **Table 16.5** for more on common food additives.

Green Point

Flavor Scalping Flavor scalping can be an issue when recycled plastics are used in packaging because not all absorbed flavors can be removed. Studies have shown less than 50% of absorbed terpenes are removed with chemical washing. These chemicals can affect the flavor new product packaged in the recycled container.

TABLE 16.5
Types of Food Additives
As you have learned in this chapter, many types of chemicals and additives are added to food products. The following table offers a summary of types of common food ingredients, why they are used, and some examples of the names that can be found on product labels. Some additives are used for more than one purpose.

Type of Additive	Functions	Examples of Uses	Names Found on Product Labels
Preservatives	Prevent food spoilage from bacteria, molds, fungi, or yeast (antimicrobials); slow or prevent changes in color, flavor, or texture; delay rancidity (antioxidants); maintain freshness	Fruit sauces and jellies, beverages, baked goods, cured meats, oils and margarines, cereals, dressings, snack foods, fruits and vegetables	Ascorbic acid, citric acid, sodium benzoate, calcium propionate, sodium erythorbate, sodium nitrite, calcium sorbate, potassium sorbate, BHA, BHT, EDTA, tocopherols (vitamin E)
Sweeteners	Add sweetness with or without the extra calories	Beverages, baked goods, confections, table-top sugar, substitutes, many processed foods	Sucrose (sugar), glucose, fructose, sorbitol, mannitol, corn syrup, high fructose corn syrup, saccharin, aspartame, sucralose, acesulfame potassium (acesulfame-K), neotame

(*continues*)

TABLE 16.5
Types of Food Additives (*continued*)

Type of Additive	Functions	Examples of Uses	Names Found on Product Labels
Color additives	Offset color loss due to exposure to light, air, temperature extremes, moisture, and storage conditions; correct natural variations in color; enhance colors that occur naturally; provide color to colorless and "fun" foods	Many processed foods, such as candies and snack foods, margarine, cheese, soft drinks, jams/jellies, gelatins, pudding and pie fillings	FD&C Blue Nos. 1 and 2, FD&C Green No. 3, FD&C Red Nos. 3 and 40, FD&C Yellow Nos. 5 and 6, Orange B, Citrus Red No. 2, annatto extract, beta-carotene, grape skin extract, cochineal extract or carmine, paprika oleoresin, caramel color, fruit and vegetable juices, saffron (Note: Exempt color additives are not required to be declared by name on labels but may be declared simply as colorings or color added)
Flavors and spices	Add specific flavors (natural and synthetic)	Pudding and pie fillings, gelatin dessert mixes, cake mixes, salad dressings, candies, soft drinks, ice cream, BBQ sauce	Natural flavoring, artificial flavor, and spices
Flavor enhancers	Enhance flavors already present in foods (without providing their own separate flavor)	Many processed foods	Monosodium glutamate (MSG), hydrolyzed soy protein, autolyzed yeast extract, disodium guanylate or inosinate
Fat replacers (and components of formulations used to replace fats)	Provide expected texture and a creamy "mouth-feel" in reduced-fat foods	Baked goods, dressings, frozen desserts, confections, cake and dessert mixes, dairy products	Olestra, cellulose gel, carrageenan, polydextrose, modified food starch, microparticulated egg white protein, guar gum, xanthan gum, whey protein concentrate
Nutrients	Replace vitamins and minerals lost in processing (enrichment), add nutrients that may be lacking in the diet (fortification)	Flour, breads, cereals, rice, macaroni, margarine, salt, milk, fruit beverages, energy bars, instant breakfast drinks	Thiamine hydrochloride, riboflavin (vitamin B_2), niacin, niacinamide, folate or folic acid, beta-carotene, potassium iodide, iron or ferrous sulfate, alpha tocopherols, ascorbic acid, vitamin D, amino acids (L-tryptophan, L-lysine, L-leucine, L-methionine)
Emulsifiers	Allow smooth mixing of ingredients, prevent separation Keep emulsified products stable, reduce stickiness, control crystallization, keep ingredients dispersed, and help products dissolve more easily	Salad dressings, peanut butter, chocolate, margarine, frozen desserts	Soy lecithin, mono- and diglycerides, egg yolks, polysorbates, sorbitan monostearate
Stabilizers, thickeners, binders, texturizers	Produce uniform texture, improve "mouth-feel"	Frozen desserts, dairy products, cakes, pudding and gelatin mixes, dressings, jams and jellies, sauces	Gelatin, pectin, guar gum, carrageenan, xanthan gum, whey
pH control agents and acidulants	Control acidity and alkalinity, prevent spoilage	Beverages, frozen desserts, chocolate, low-acid canned foods, baking powder	Lactic acid, citric acid, ammonium hydroxide, sodium carbonate
Leavening agents	Promote rising of baked goods	Breads and other baked goods	Baking soda, monocalcium phosphate, calcium carbonate
Anticaking agents	Keep powdered foods free-flowing, prevent moisture absorption	Salt, baking powder, confectioner's sugar	Calcium silicate, iron ammonium citrate, silicon dioxide
Humectants	Retain moisture	Shredded coconut, marshmallows, soft candies, confections	Glycerin, sorbitol

Type of Additive	Functions	Examples of Uses	Names Found on Product Labels
Yeast nutrients	Promote growth of yeast	Breads and other baked goods	Calcium sulfate, ammonium phosphate
Dough strengtheners and conditioners	Produce more stable dough	Breads and other baked goods	Ammonium sulfate, azodicarbonamide, L-cysteine
Firming agents	Maintain crispness and firmness	Processed fruits and vegetables	Calcium chloride, calcium lactate
Enzyme preparations	Modify proteins, polysaccharides and fats	Cheese, dairy products, meat	Enzymes, lactase, papain, rennet, chymosin
Gases	Serve as propellant, aerate, or create carbonation	Oil cooking spray, whipped cream, carbonated beverages	Carbon dioxide, nitrous oxide

Source: Reproduced from U.S. Food and Drug Administration and the International Food Information Council. Food Ingredients and Colors. April 2010. Available at: http://www.fda.gov/Food/FoodIngredientsPackaging/ucm094211.htm#types. Accessed April 27, 2011.

Going Green with Food Processing and Packaging

Food packaging is a significant source of **municipal solid waste (MSW)** in the United States. Containers and packaging, both for food and nonfood products, comprised 30.8% of MSW generated in 2008 (as shown in **Figure 16.18**).[44] Packaging for food represents 50% of sales of packaging material; furthermore, food packaging contributes to MSW at a greater rate than other products because people consume food multiple times per day.[35]

municipal solid waste (MSW) Solid material that must be disposed of; food packaging contributes significantly to MSW.

Source Reduction

One of the major methods of reducing the amount of MSW produced by food packaging is source reduction, which is the practice of using less material to package and ship items (see Figure 16.18). Today, aluminum cans, tinplate cans, and plastic beverage bottles all use much less material to create the same volume package than those used in 1970s.[35] This clearly reduces MSW because less material is thrown away if the product was originally packaged using less material. For food processors, it is both environmentally and economically friendly to develop effective methods of source reduction.

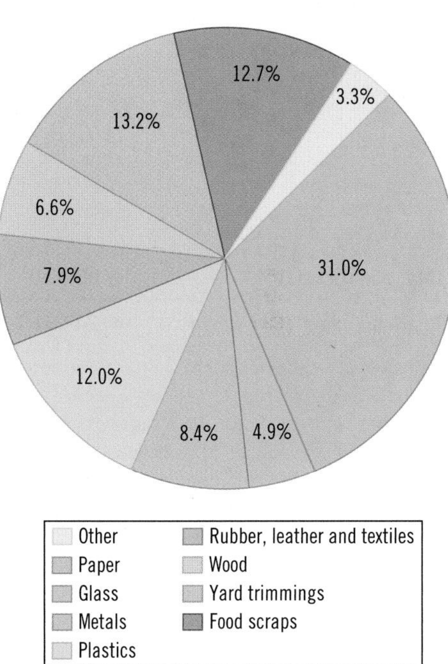

FIGURE 16.18 Food packaging is a major component of municipal solid waste. Efforts are ongoing to reduce the amount of material used in packages and to make the material that is used easier to reuse or recycle.

Source: Reproduced from Municipal Solid Waste Generation, Recycling, and Disposal in the United States: Facts and Figures for 2008. Available at: http://www.epa.gov/osw/nonhaz/municipal/pubs/msw2008rpt.pdf. Accessed January 2, 2011.

Composting

In the commercial sector, composting, or the breakdown of organic material, applies mostly to food scraps created during processing. By composting these materials to create natural fertilizer, food processors aid in the reduction of MSW.[35] This is an important goal because recent statistics indicate that food scraps comprised 12.7% of MSW generated in 2008.[44]

Biodegradable Packaging

Biodegradable packaging—created from cellulose, starch, chitosan and other ingredients—can be broken down in the environment into soil, water, and other organic components. One technique for creating it is to ferment starches with microbial action to produce moisture-resistant biodegradable packaging.[35]

Recycling

Recycling is a well-known method of reusing material. Many materials used in food packaging can be recycled, including paper, aluminum, steel, and most types of plastic.[35] The most recent report by the EPA on MSW indicates that Americans recycle approximately 33.2% of MSW generated yearly (see **Table 16.6**).[44] Many food and beverage packages are recycled at a high rate, including 48.2% of aluminum beer and soda cans.[35]

Green Point

Steel Cans Steel cans are at least 40% lighter now than they were in 1970.[35]

TABLE 16.6
Generation and Recovery of Materials in MSW—2008* (in millions of tons and percent of generation of each material)

Material	Weight Generated	Weight Recovered	Recovery as Percent of Generation
Paper and paperboard	77.42	42.94	55.5%
Glass	12.15	2.81	23.1%
Metals			
Steel	15.68	5.29	33.7%
Aluminum	3.41	0.72	21.1%
Other nonferrous metals†	1.76	1.21	68.8%
Total metals	**20.85**	**7.22**	**34.6%**
Plastics	30.05	2.12	7.1%
Rubber and leather	7.41	1.06	14.3%
Textiles	12.37	1.89	15.3%
Wood	16.39	1.58	9.6%
Other materials	4.50	1.15	25.6%
Total materials in products	**181.14**	**60.77**	**33.5%**
Other wastes			
Food, other**	31.79	0.80	2.5%
Yard trimmings	32.90	21.30	64.7%
Miscellaneous inorganic wastes	3.78	Negligible	Negligible
Total other wastes	**68.47**	**22.10**	**32.3%**
Total municipal solid waste	**249.61**	**82.87**	**33.2%**

* Includes waste from residential, commercial, and institutional sources.
† Includes lead from lead-acid batteries.
** Includes recovery of other MSW organics for composting.
Note: Details might not add to totals due to rounding. Negligible = Less than 5,000 tons or 0.05 percent.
Source: Reproduced from Environmental Protection Agency. Municipal Solid Waste Generation, Recycling, and Disposal in the United States: Facts and Figures for 2008. Available at: http://www.epa.gov/osw/nonhaz/municipal/pubs/msw2008rpt.pdf. Accessed January 2, 2011.

Challenges

Food processors may experience difficulty achieving reductions in packaging because of added research and development costs and finding balance between this goal and consumer demand. For example, consumer demand may tend toward more packaging material because it is convenient for consumers to have individually wrapped servings and to be able to prepare food directly in the containers in which it is sold.[35]

Chapter Review

Food preservation and food packaging technologies have advanced significantly throughout the years. This chapter has explained the scientific and technical innovations that have allowed manufacturers to reduce microbial growth leading to spoilage, ship food longer distances, and increase the amount of time food stays fresh on store shelves and in home pantries. These innovations have changed the way we work, shop, cook, and store foods;

therefore, the importance of preservation and packaging on society should not be overlooked. As advances continue in these fields, the food industry is tackling new problems, such as pesticide contamination, waste disposal, chemical contamination, and sodium content in processed foods. It is imperative that these health and environmental issues remain in the forefront to ensure a sustainable and safe food supply.

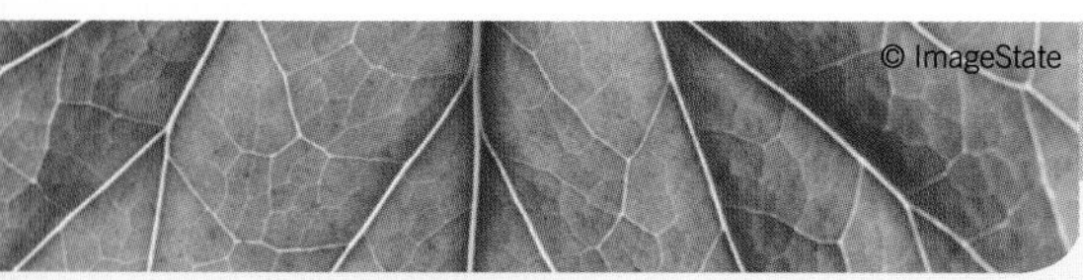

Learning Portfolio

Key Terms

	page
active packaging	517
aseptic packaging	502
Clostridium botulinum	502
edible films	516
flavor scalping	519
intelligent packaging	516
irradiation	506
lyophilization	505
modified atmosphere packaging (MAP)	515
municipal solid waste (MSW)	521
osmosis	496
pressure-assisted thermal sterilization (PATS)	509
sublimation	505
thermophiles	503
thermoplastics	513
ultra-high-pressure (UHP) processing	509

Study Points

1. High water activity (a_w) in food allows for microbial growth; many methods of preservation work by reducing a food's water activity.
2. Heat is an important food preservation method because it inactivates and kills microbes and denatures enzymes and proteins.
3. *C. botulinum* is a dangerous anaerobic bacterium that must be safeguarded against in preservation methods such as canning and MAP.
4. Canning, freezing, drying, fermenting, and pasteurizing are methods used to preserve food by inhibiting microbial growth and enzymatic activity.
5. Irradiation damages DNA and thus inhibits microbial reproduction. Irradiated foods must be labeled as such; however, food products containing irradiated ingredients do not have to be labeled.
6. New methods of preservation, particularly nonthermal ones, are constantly being developed and tested with the intention of improving quality, taste, and shelf life of preserved foods.
7. Food packaging extends shelf life, creates a barrier to the external environment, allows for transport, and provides a method of communication with the consumer.
8. Food packaging materials are selected based on the specific properties they provide in combination with the use for which they are intended.
9. MAP, edible films, and intelligent/active packaging are newer packaging technologies that extend shelf life and reduce food and solid waste.
10. Food packaging materials interact with food and can affect the flavor and safety of that food.
11. Manufacturers must consider source reduction, disposability, and recycling potential of packaging materials because food packaging contributes greatly to manufacturing costs and landfill waste.

Issues for Discussion

1. Discuss the advantages and disadvantages of current preservation techniques and how they affect the safety of the U.S. food supply.
2. Raw and unpasteurized foods, such as raw milk, are sometimes lauded for their health benefits. Discuss the pros and cons of unpasteurized foods as well as the dilemmas surrounding regulation of these products.
3. Discuss the pros and cons of irradiation. Do you think the public's fears are justified? Do the potential dangers of irradiation outweigh its benefits?
4. A delicate balance must be achieved between innovation and safety when it comes to government regulation of food packaging materials. Based on the description of the FDA process for reviewing safety of food packaging materials presented in Special Topic 16.4, is the United States too lenient or too stringent with manufacturers with regard to allowing new packaging materials?
5. Discuss the pros and cons of pesticides use on food crops. How does the rising cost of food in general and the high cost of organic food affect this discussion?

Research Ideas for Student

1. Techniques used to protect foods from *E. coli* O157
2. Home food preservation methods and safety concerns
3. The health benefits of probiotics
4. Shared responsibility of municipalities, consumers, and manufacturers in reducing food packaging's contributions to municipal solid waste
5. Susceptibility of local food supplies to a terrorist attack

References

1. Shephard S. *Pickled, Potted, and Canned: How the Art and Science of Food Preserving Changed the World*. 2nd ed. New York: Simon and Schuster; 2006.
2. U.S. Food and Drug Administration. Inspections, Compliance, Enforcement, and Criminal Investigations, Water Activity (a_w) in Foods. Available at: http://www.fda.gov/ICECI/Inspections/InspectionGuides/InspectionTechnicalGuides/ucm072916.htm. Accessed December 16, 2010.
3. Floros JD. Feeding the world today and tomorrow: The importance of food science and technology. *Comp Rev Food Sci Food Safety.* 2010;9(1):572–599.
4. Beales N. Adaptation of microorganisms to cold temperatures, weak acid preservatives, low pH, and osmotic stress: A review. *Comp Rev Food Sci Food Safety.* 2004;3(1):1–20.
5. Doyle ME, Glass KA. Sodium reduction and its effect on food safety, food quality and human health. *Comp Rev Food Sci Food Safety.* 2010;9(1):44–56.
6. Adams MR, Moss MO. *Food Microbiology*. 3rd ed. Cambridge, UK: RSC Publishing; 2008.
7. U.S. Food and Drug Administration. PMO 2007: Grade "A" Pasteurized Milk Ordinance (2007 Revision). Available at: http://www.fda.gov/Food/FoodSafety/Product-Specific Information/MilkSafety/NationalConferenceonInterstate MilkShipmentsNCIMSModelDocuments/Pasteurized MilkOrdinance2007/ucm063836.htm. Accessed December 26, 2010.
8. Moskin J. Preserving time in a bottle (or a jar). *New York Times Online*. May 26, 2009. Available at: http://www.nytimes.com/2009/05/27/dining/27cann.html. Accessed January 2, 2011.
9. U.S. Food and Drug Administration. Raw Milk—Associated Public Health Risks. January 24, 2007. Available at: http://www.fda.gov/Food/FoodSafety/Product-SpecificInformation/MilkSafety/ConsumerInformationAboutMilkSafety/ucm181965.htm#slide. Accessed December 26, 2010.
10. U.S. Food and Drug Administration. FDA and CDC Remind Consumers of the Dangers of Drinking Raw Milk. March 1, 2007. Available at: http://www.fda.gov/NewsEvents/Newsroom/PressAnnouncements/2007/ucm108856.htm. Accessed January 16, 2011.
11. U.S. Food and Drug Administration. PMO 2007: Standards for Grade "A" Pasteurized, Ultra-Pasteurized and Aseptically Processed Milk & Milk Products, Grade "A" Pasteurized Milk Ordinance (2007 Revision). Available at: http://www.fda.gov/Food/FoodSafety/Product-SpecificInformation/Milk Safety/NationalConferenceonInterstateMilkShipments NCIMSModelDocuments/PasteurizedMilkOrdinance2007/UCM063945. Accessed December 26, 2010.
12. National Center for Home Food Preservation. General Canning Information: Recommended Canners. Available at: http://www.uga.edu/nchfp/how/general/recomm_canners.html. Accessed January 2, 2011.
13. National Center for Home Food Preservation. Storing: Home Canned Foods. Available at: http://www.uga.edu/nchfp/how/store/store_home_canned.html. Accessed January 2, 2011.
14. Moskin J. Some canning dos and don'ts. *New York Times Online*. May 26, 2009. Available at: http://www.nytimes.com/2009/05/27/dining/27cbox.html?_r=1%26ref=dining. Accessed January 2, 2011.
15. *ServSafe Coursebook*. 5th ed. Chicago, IL: National Restaurant Association Educational Foundation; 2008.
16. Harris, LJ, Farber JN, Beuchat LR, et al. Outbreaks associated with fresh produce: Incidence, growth, and survival of pathogens on fresh and fresh-cut produce. *Comp Rev Food Sci Food Safety.* 2003;2(suppl 1):78–141.
17. Clark PJ. Processing innovations. *Food Technol.* 2009; 63(8):100–102.
18. Institut National de la Recherche Agronomique (INRA). Improving the Freeze-Drying Process. Available at: http://www.international.inra.fr/research/some_examples/improving_the_freeze_drying_process. Accessed December 28, 2010.
19. Food and Agriculture Organization/World Health Organization Joint Working Group. *Guidelines for the Evaluation of Probiotics in Food.* London, Ontario, Canada. April 30 and May 1.
20. National Institutes of Health, National Center for Complementary and Alternative Health. An Introduction to Probiotics. Available at: http://nccam.nih.gov/health/probiotics. Accessed December 21, 2010.
21. Tang J, Hao F, Lau M. Microwave heating in food processing. In: Yang XH, Tang J (eds.). *Advances in Bioprocessing Engineering.* Singapore: World Scientific Publishing; 2002.
22. U.S. Food and Drug Administration. How Do Microwaves Work? FDA/CFSAN Food Safety A to Z Reference Guide, 2007. Available at: http://www.fda.gov/Food/Resources ForYou/StudentsTeachers/ucm110552.htm. Accessed June 26, 2011.
23. Morehouse K, Komolprasert V. Irradiation of food and packaging: An overview. *ACS Symposium Series* 2004;875:1–11. Available at: http://www.fda.gov/Food/FoodIngredients Packaging/IrradiatedFoodPackaging/ucm081050.htm. Accessed December 21, 2010.
24. Irradiation and food safety: Scientific status summary. *Food Technol.* 2004;58(11):48–55.
25. Effect of preservation technologies on microbial inactivation in foods. *Comp Rev Food Sci Food Safety.* 2003;2 (suppl 1):42–45.
26. U.S. Food and Drug Administration. Foods Permitted to Be Irradiated Under FDA Regulations (21 CFR 179.26). Available at: http://www.fda.gov/Food/FoodIngredients Packaging/IrradiatedFoodPackaging/ucm074734.htm. Accessed December 21, 2010.
27. Code of Federal Regulations. Title 21: Food and Drugs. Part 179—Irradiation in the Production, Processing and

Handling of Food. Available at: http://ecfr.gpoaccess.gov/cgi/t/text/text-idx?c=ecfr%26sid=911a36a52aad0759b094cf95b467782e%26rgn=div5%26view=text%26node=21:3.0.1.1.10%26idno=21. Accessed December 21, 2010.

28. Morris A, Barnett A, Burrows O. Effect of Processing on Nutrient Content of Foods. *CAJANUS*. 2004;37(3):160–164. Available at: http://www.ops-oms.org/English/CFNI/cfni-caj37No304-art-3.pdf. Accessed June 26, 2011.
29. Rickman, JC, Barrett DM, Bruhn CM. Nutritional comparison of fresh, frozen, and canned fruits and vegetables. Part 1. Vitamins C and B and phenolic compounds. *J Sci Food Agric.* 2007;87:930–944.
30. Ramaswamy R, Balasubramaniam VM, Kaletunc G. High Pressure Processing. Ohio State University Extension Fact Sheet. Available at: http://ohioline.osu.edu/fse-fact/0001.html. Accessed December 29, 2010.
31. Swientek B. High pressure treats luncheon meats, deli salads. *Food Technol.* 2010;64(7):114.
32. Clark PJ. Nonthermal processing on the front burner. *Food Technol.* 2010;64(7):113.
33. Parrott D. Microwave technology sterilizes sweet potato puree. *Food Technol.* 2010;64(7):66.
34. Corbo MR, Bevilacqua A, Campaniello D, et al. Prolonging microbial shelf life of foods through the use of natural and non-thermal approaches. *Int J Food Sci Tech.* 2009;44:223–241.
35. Marsh K, Bugusu B. Food packaging: Roles, materials, and environmental issues. *J Food Sci.* 2007;72(3):R39–R55.
36. Environmental Protection Agency. Plastics: Common Wastes and Materials. Available at: http://www.epa.gov/osw/conserve/materials/plastics.htm. Accessed December 31, 2010.
37. Rojas-Graü MA, Oms-Oliu G, Soliva-Fortuny R, Martín-Belloso O. The use of packaging techniques to maintain freshness in fresh-cut fruits and vegetables [review]. *Int J Food Sci Tech.* 2009;44:875–889.
38. Phillips C. Modified atmosphere packaging and its effects on the microbiological quality and safety of produce [review]. *Int J Food Sci Tech.* 1996;31:463–479.
39. Pavlath AE, Orts W. Edible films and coatings: why, what and how? In: Embuscado ME, Huber KC (eds.). *Edible Film Coatings and Food Applications*. New York: Springer. 2009:1–23.
40. Brody AL. Intelligent packaging: A power tool for food. *Food Technol.* 2010;64(5):79–81.
41. Tarver T. Novel ideas in food packaging. *Food Technol.* 2008;62(10):54–59.
42. Yam KL, Takhistov PT, Miltz J. Intelligent packaging: Concepts and applications. *J Food Sci.* 2007;70(1):R1–R10.
43. Sajilata MG, Savitha K, Singhal RS, Kanetkar VR. Scalping of flavors in packaged foods. *Comp Rev Food Sci Food Safety.* 2007;6(1):17–35.
44. Environmental Protection Agency. Municipal Solid Waste Generation, Recycling, and Disposal in the United States: Facts and Figures for 2008. Available at: http://www.epa.gov/osw/nonhaz/municipal/pubs/msw2008rpt.pdf. Accessed January 2, 2011.

Appendix A *Herbs and Health*

Kimberly Owen

An *herb*, by definition, is "a seed-producing annual, biennial, or perennial that does not develop persistent woody tissue but dies down at the end of a growing season; a plant or plant part valued for its medicinal, savory, or aromatic qualities."[1] Herbs are used for everything from promoting health and healing to improving memory; increasing energy; and enhancing love, fertility, and creativity.

Herbs are a concentrated food, consisting of vitamins, minerals, and trace elements as well as various other chemicals. Seeds, leaves, stems, bark, roots, flowers, and extracts of herbs are traditionally ground into a paste and consumed fresh or briefly cooked as part of a recipe. Introducing herbs into cooking can boost flavor without adding excess sodium, sugar, or fats to one's diet. Fresh herbs have a stronger flavor than dried herbs; therefore less is needed to enhance the flavor of a dish.[2] Fresh herbs should be added last in the cooking process to preserve their flavor.[1]

Herbs are considered to be a functional food. Functional foods are "foods that provide benefit beyond basic nutrition."[2] A budding subfield of nutrition is studying foods that do not provide macronutrients, vitamins, or minerals, but that do "interact with the body to support health and prevent abnormality and disease."[2] Researching the potential of herbs as functional foods is a tiresome task given that there are more than 20,000 varieties of edible herbs in existence.[3] For each herb, research is conducted on the herb itself, a meal based on the food, and the role of the food in the diet. The goal of this research is to identify the single bioactive compound(s) that generate the known health benefit.

Globalization and the Internet now allow us to access a wider variety of herbs grown all over the world. We are able to get herbs that are native to a certain region and climate that we are not able to grown in our own. Free trade and commerce make it even more important for consumers to make sure they are buying from a reputable supplier.

In the United States, the largest market for herbs is as supplements.[3] In 1994, the Dietary Supplement Health and Education Act (DSHEA) was passed. According to the DSHEA, a *dietary supplement* is:

> A product, other than tobacco, that is intended to supplement the diet and contains one of the following dietary ingredients: a vitamin, mineral, herb or other botanical, an amino acid, dietary substance to supplement the diet by increasing the total daily intake, or a concentrate, metabolite, constituent, extract, or a combination of these ingredients.[4]

Accurate labeling is the responsibility of the company producing the supplement. The supplement label must contain the following phrase: "This statement has not been evaluated by the food and drug administration. This product is not intended to diagnose, treat, cure or prevent any diseases."[4] In addition, the label must make known the name and quantity of each active and inactive ingredient.[4] For botanical ingredients such as herbs, the part of the plant form which the ingredient was derived also is required. For example, coriander seeds and cilantro come from the same plant, yet they have distinctly different taste, texture, and nutritional benefits.[5]

The United States Pharmacopeia (USP) is a nonprofit health organization that independently tests over-the-counter herbal supplements to verify product integrity, purity, and potency. The USP's job is to make sure that what it states on the label matches the actual product contents. Products that meet the USP's standards for quality control are awarded a USP certified symbol on their packaging. Participation in the USP is voluntary and, as a result, many herbal supplement companies do not participate. The USP differs from the FDA in that the FDA tests effectiveness and safety, whereas the USP tests that the product content matches the product labeling.[4] The FDA reserves the right to remove a product form the market only *after* it has been shown to be unsafe or harmful.

In conclusion, it is best to consume fresh or dried herbs as flavor enhancers for whole foods. If you choose to consume herbs in supplemental form, it is best to educate yourself on the contents of the supplement and the company from which the supplement is produced and to choose wisely.

Table A.1 provides information on herbs that have been studied by the National Toxicity Program. **Table A.2** presents additional research areas and health concerns with regard to the use of herbs.

TABLE A.1
Herbals and Herbal Components that Have Been Examined by the National Toxicity Program (NTP)

Herb/Herbal Component	Uses and/or Precautions
Aloe vera gel	Widely used as both a dietary supplement and as a component of cosmetics. Ninth most popular supplement based on U.S. sales (2002). The gel has been used for centuries as a treatment for minor burns and is increasingly being used in products for internal consumption.
Black cohosh	Used to treat symptoms of premenstrual syndrome, dysmenorrhea, and menopause. Ranked 11th in sales in 2002.
Bladderwrack	A source of iodide used in treatment of thyroid diseases. Also used as an ingredient in weight-loss preparations.
Comfrey	Consumed in teas and in salads. However, it contains pyrrolizidine alkaloids (e.g., symphatine), which are known to be toxic. Used externally as an anti-inflammatory agent in the treatment of bruises, sprains, and other external wounds. Based in part on NTP studies on the alkaloid components of comfrey, the FDA has recommended that manufacturers of dietary supplements containing this herb remove them from the market.
Echinacea purpurea	Extract from this plant is the most commonly used medicinal herb in the United States (2002). It is used as an immunostimulant to treat colds, sore throats, and the flu.
Ephedra	Also known as Ma Huang, this herb was 21st in sales in 2002. Traditionally used as a treatment for symptoms of asthma and upper respiratory infections. Often found in weight loss and "energy" preparations, which also usually contain caffeine. Use has been associated with side effects such as heart palpitations; psychiatric and upper gastrointestinal effects; and symptoms of autonomic hyperactivity, such as tremor and insomnia, especially when take with other stimulants.
Ginkgo biloba	Fourth highest in sales (2002). Ginkgo fruit and seeds have been used medicinally for thousands of years. The extract of green-picked leaves has been increasing in popularity in the United States. *Ginkgo biloba* extract promotes vasodilatation and improves blood flow. It also appears beneficial for short-term memory loss, headache, and depression.
Ginseng and ginsenosides	Ginseng ranked 13th in sales of medicinal herbs in 2002, down from 4th in 1996. Ginsenosides are thought to be the active ingredients in ginseng. Ginseng has been used as a treatment for a variety of conditions, including hypertension, diabetes, and depression. However, it has also been associated with various adverse health effects.
Goldenseal	Traditionally used to treat wounds, digestive problems, and infections. Goldenseal was 17th in sales in 2002. It is currently used as a laxative, tonic, and diuretic. Mistakenly thought to disguise the presence of other drugs in drug tests.
Green tea	Extract of green tea is used for its antioxidative properties. Green tea was 15th in sales in 2002.
Kava kava	The 25th most widely used medicinal herb (2002), this herb has psychoactive properties and is sold as a calmative and as an antidepressant. A recent report of severe liver toxicity has led to restrictions of its sale in Europe and has apparently affected sales in the United States. Some components may alter efficacy/toxicity of therapeutic agents.

Herb/Herbal Component	Uses and/or Precautions
Milk thistle	Milk thistle extract ranked 8th in sales in 2002. It is used to treat depression and several liver conditions, including cirrhosis and hepatitis. It also has been used to increase breast milk production.
Pulegone	A major terpenoid constituent of the herb pennyroyal. It is found in lesser concentrations in other mints. Pennyroyal has been used as a carminative insect repellent, emmenagogue (an herb that stimulates blood flow in the pelvic area and uterus), and as an abortifacient. Pulegone has well-recognized toxicity to the liver, kidney, and central nervous system.
Senna	Senna acts as a laxative. Its use has increased due to the removal of one of the most widely used chemical-stimulant type laxatives from the market.
Thujone	A terpenoid found in a variety of herbs, including sage and tansy, and in high concentrations in wormwood. Suspected as the causative toxic agent associated with drinking absinthe, a liqueur flavored with wormwood extract.

Source: Adapted from National Toxicology Program Fact Sheet. Updated 2011. Available at: http://ntp.niehs.nih.gov/ntp/htdocs/liason/factsheets/HerbMedFacts.pdf. Accessed April 27, 2011.

TABLE A.2
Research Areas and Health Concerns for the Use of Herbs

Herb	Other Common Names	Research Areas	Health Concerns
Arnica	Mountain tobacco, leopard's bane, wunderkraut	Muscle pain, stiffness, osteoarthritis	May increase effects of anticoagulants.
Astragalus	Huang chi, huang qi, milk vetch	Weak immune system, fatigue	May interact with immunosupressants.
Cayenne	Capsicum, red pepper, African chilies	Musculoskeletal pain, osteoarthritis, digestive problems	May cause digestive disorders, skin irritation.
Cordyceps	Caterpillar fungus, dong chon xai cao, semitake	Weak immune system, poor endurance	May reduce blood sugar levels.
Devil's claw	Grapple plant, harpagophytum, wood spider	Muscle pain, digestive problems, fever	May interfere with antidiabetes drugs.
Echinacea	Purple coneflower, black Sampson, Indian head	Weak immune system, colds, infections	May interfere with immunosuppressants.
Elderberry	Elderberry syrup, American elder	Colds, flu, fever, weak immune system, excess body water	May interact with diuretics or laxatives.
Ginger	*Zingiberis rhizoma*, ginger root, Jamaica ginger	Nausea, vomiting, motion sickness, osteoarthritis	May interact with anticoagulants and diabetes drugs.
Ginseng	Chinese ginseng, ciwuija, Russian root	Poor endurance, low energy, weak immune system	May interfere with anticoagulants.
Gotu kola	Indian pennywort, hydrocotyle, kaki kuda	Varicose veins, edema	May interfere with hypoglycemic medications.
Guarana	Guarana gum, zoom cocoa, Brazilian cocoa	Excess body fat, lethargy	Contains caffeine.
Rhodiola	Golden root, Arctic root	Lethargy, fatigue, poor endurance	May interact with other herbs.
Valerian	Mexican valerian, garden heliotrope, tagara	Insomnia, anxiety, depression	May interact with other sedatives.
Willow bark	White willow, purple osier, bay willow	Fever, muscle pain, osteoarthritis	May interact with anticoagulants

References

1. Herb. (n.d.). Dictionary and Thesaurus—Merriam-Webster Online. Available at: http://www.merriam-webster.com/dictionary/herb. Accessed February 14, 2011.
2. Tapsell LC, Hemphill I, Cobiac L, et al. Health benefits of herbs and spices: The past, the present, the future. *Med J Aust.* 2006;185(4):S4–S24.
3. Klein M, Obermeyer W. U.S. Spending Millions to See if Herbs Truly Work: Medline Plus. National Library of Medicine, National Institutes of Health. 2010. Available at: http://www.nlm.nih.gov/medlineplus/news/fullstory_106729.html. Accessed January 10, 2011.
4. Cassileth BR, Heitzer M, Wesa K. The public health impact of herbs and nutritional supplements. *Pharmceutical Biol.* 2009;47(8):761–767.
5. Frey C, Rouseff RL. *Natural Flavors and Fragrances: Chemistry, Analysis, and Production*. Washington, DC: American Chemical Society; 2005.

Appendix B *Spices and Health*

Abby Calcutt

Background

Turmeric is a **spice** that is being researched for its potential health benefits. The spice is derived from *Curcuma longa*, which is in the Ginger family.[1] Turmeric is responsible for giving curries their yellow hue and sharp, earthy flavor. It is a common spice in Southeast Asian and Indian cuisines.

The active constituent in turmeric is curcumin (diferuloylmethane). Curcumin is classified as a **phytochemical** and also as a lipophilic polyphenol. Typically, curcumin comprises between 2–5% of turmeric. Research indicates that the majority of the therapeutic effects of turmeric can be attributed to curcumin.[2]

Curcumin has had many different uses over the centuries. In addition to its use in Asian and Indian cuisines, today it is being used as coloring and flavoring agent in foods.[3] It can be found in some mustards, cheeses, yogurts, and dry mixes. In various cultures, curcumin has been used as an herbal remedy to treat a broad spectrum of illnesses and autoimmune diseases.[3] It also has many uses in Ayurvedic medicine, which is the traditional medicine of India, where it is considered as having antioxidant, antiseptic, analgesic, anti-inflammatory, and antimalarial properties.[4]

Curcumin's antioxidant properties have been attributed to its chemical structure. Researchers have found that curcumin prevents the abduction of electrons by promoting the oxidation of the polyunsaturated fatty acid linoleate.[1] Thus, curcumin inhibits lipid peroxidation.

spice A flavorful component of a plant other than the leaves used in cooking. Examples include turmeric and ginger (rhizome); celery, cumin, and poppy (seed); allspice (fruit); and cinnamon (bark).

phytochemical Any biologically active compound found in plants. Many are considered beneficial in the prevention of chronic diseases.

Currently, researchers are investigating curcumin as a therapy for multiple illnesses. Its anti-inflammatory properties, ability to alleviate joint pain, and the chemopreventative properties are just a few of the areas being explored.

Curcumin has also been studied with regard to its effects on melanomas and head and neck, breast, colon, pancreatic, prostate, and ovarian cancers.[1] Some of the most in-depth examinations of curcumin's influence on cancer have been on the spice's anti-inflammatory properties. More than 60 clinical trials on curcumin's anti-inflammatory effects have been conducted or are currently underway.[5,6] Researchers have found that curcumin may reduce injury to cells through the attenuation of oxidative stress and suppression of inflammation.[7,8] Studies have also found that curcumin inhibits cell proliferation, promotes apoptosis, and acts as a COX-2 inhibitor.[7]

Although the number of clinical trials is growing, at present no standard has been set for an appropriate curcumin supplement dosage. Studies in which animals or participants were given varying amounts of curcumin have found few adverse symptoms at high consumption amounts.[7] The studies reviewed administered 450 mg to 12,000 mg of curcumin. Some individuals experienced mild nausea and diarrhea when given doses greater that 8,000 mg daily.[7]

One review article from 2010 discussed that multiple studies have indicated that curcumin is ineffective or that it produces adverse effects. One example that was specified related to enzymes in the lung, lymph, and skin. A chemical study found that a higher amount of DNA fragmentation and base damage in the presence of copper and isozymes of cytochrome p450 were associated with higher amounts of curcumin exposure.[6]

Discussion and Conclusion

The body of research is growing, but currently both the number of completed clinical trials and the size of existing clinical trials have been small, typically having fewer than 25 individuals with cancer. Positive results have been reported with respect to curcumin's effect on inhibiting cancer cell proliferation or promoting apoptosis in various settings in vivo and in vitro. However, not enough data is available to formulate recommendations or to generalize to all types of cancer.

Curcumin has been found to influence various cancer cells that other treatments have had little impact upon, such as pancreatic cancer cells. This, along with investigating other health benefits linked to the phytochemical may prompt further research. The highly variable dosages of curcumin given to participants and its bioavailabity must be kept in mind by researchers and professionals reviewing the literature. Also, the greatest improvements with some curcumin treatments were seen in the most damaged cells. As a result, curcumin might not serve a great purpose in the prevention of cancer.

Another point to consider is that, as with any supplemental nutrition study, individuals may have consumed turmeric or curcumin independent of the study, which could skew the results. Also, curcumin may not be a suitable treatment for everyone. Multiple sources warn that individuals with gallstones or susceptibility to gallstones should avoid turmeric. More research may elucidate the intricacies of the relationship between curcumin and cancer, and eventually its potential as a therapeutic treatment will be better understood.

References

1. Wilken R, Veena MS, Wang MB, Srivatsan ES. Curcumin: A review of anti-cancer properties and therapeutic activity in head a neck squamous cell carcinoma. *Mol Cancer.* 2011;10:12.
2. Chattopadhyay I, Biswas K, Bandyopadhyay U, Banerjee RK. Turmeric and curcumin: Biological actions and medicinal applications. *Curr Sci.* 2004;87:44–50.
3. Ammon HP, Wahl MA. Pharmacology of *Curcuma longa*. *Planta Med.* 1991;57:1–7.
4. Aggarwal BB, Sundaram C, Malani N, Ichikawa H. Curcumin: The Indian solid gold. *Adv Exp Med Biol.* 2007;595:1–75.
5. Kelland K. Scientists say curry compound kills cancer cells. *Reuters.* October 8, 2009. Available at: http://uk.reuters.com/article/2009/10/28/us-cancer-curry-idUKTRE59R1E020091028.
6. Bar-Sela G, Epelbaum R, Schaffer M. Curcumin as an anti-cancer agent: Review of the gap between basic and clinical applications. *Curr Med Chem.* 2010;17:190–197.
7. Patel VB, Misra S, Patel BB, Majunder AP. Colorectal cancer: Chemopreventative role of curcumin and resveratrol. *Nutri Cancer.* 2010;62:958–967.
8. Heng MC. Curcumin targeted signaling pathways: Basis for anti-photoaging and anti-carcinogenic therapy. *Int J Dermatol.* 2010;49:608–622.

Appendix C *Measurement Conversions and Equivalents*

Weight Conversions	
1 gram	1,000,000 micrograms
1 gram	1,000 milligrams
1 kilogram	1,000 grams
1 kilogram	2.2 pounds
1 microgram	0.001 milligrams
1 milligram	1,000 micrograms
1 ounce	28.35 grams
1 pound	16 ounces
1 pound	454 grams

Volume Conversions	
1 cup	0.5 pint
1 cup	16 tablespoons
1 cup	236.59 milliliters
1 cup	8 fluid ounces
1 fluid ounce	0.125 cup
1 fluid ounce	2 tablespoons
1 fluid ounce	29.6 milliliter
1 gallon	128 fluid ounces
1 gallon	16 cups
1 gallon	3.79 liters
1 gallon	4 quarts
1 gallon	8 pints
1 jigger	3 tablespoons
1 liter	0.85 Imperial gallon
1 liter	1.06 quart
1 liter	1,000 milliliters
1 milliliter	0.03 fluid ounce
1 pint	16 fluid ounces
1 pint	2 cups
1 quart	2 pints
1 quart	32 fluid ounces
1 quart	4 cups
1 quart	946.36 milliliters
1 tablespoon	0.0625 cup
1 tablespoon	0.5 fluid ounce
1 tablespoon	14.79 milliliters
1 tablespoon	3 teaspoons
1 teaspoon	0.33333 tablespoon
1 teaspoon	4.93 milliliter
1 teaspoon	60 drops
1 teaspoon	Approximately 5 grams dry weight
1/3 cup	16 teaspoons
1/3 cup	5 tablespoon + 1 teaspoons

Length Conversions	
1 centimeter	0.01 meter
1 centimeter	0.394 inches
1 foot	12 inches
1 inch	2.54 centimeters
1 meter	39.37 inches

Can Equivalents		
Can Size	**Ounces**	**Cups**
2	19–20 ounces	2½ cups
2.5	29 ounces	3½ cups
3	48 ounces	5¾ cups
10	98–108 ounces	3 quarts
211	12 ounces	1½ cups
303	14.5–16 ounces	2 cups
Buffet	8 ounces	1 cup

Scoop Equivalents*	
Scoop Size	**Amount**
6	⅔ cup
8	½ cup
10	⅖ cup
12	⅓ cup
16	¼ cup
20	3 ⅕ tablespoons
24	2 ⅔ tablespoons
30	2 ⅕ tablespoons
40	⅔ cup

* The scoop number indicates the number of scoops it takes to make 1 quart.

Source: Reproduced from U.S. Department of Agriculture. Nutritive Value of Foods. *Home and Garden Bulletin*, 72, p. 9. Available at: http://www.nal.usda.gov/fnic/foodcomp/Data/HG72/hg72_2002.pdf. Accessed August 6, 2012.

Glossary

acesulfame-K A non-nutritive artificial sweetener that is 150 to 200 times sweeter than sugar that enhances and sustains the sweet taste of foods and beverages. It is heat stable, so it can be used in baked products.

acidification When carbon dioxide is absorbed by oceans, it changes the chemistry of the seawater, which can impair marine life and adversely affect the oceanic food web.

actin Thin filament in muscle fibrils that binds with myosin in muscle contraction and relaxation.

active packaging Packaging that releases scavenging chemicals in response to spoilage reactions or the presence of chemicals or compounds, such as excess water, oxygen, or ethylene.

adaptation The gradual decrease in the ability to distinguish between odors over time.

affective tests Sensory tests used to determine differences in acceptability or preference between products.

aflatoxin Mycotoxin (fungus) in coffee.

agribusiness A complex system of businesses involved in the production and packaging of food. It includes farmers, both large and small operations, and the companies that provide the inputs, such as seeds, chemicals, and lines of credit, needed to produce agricultural products. This system also includes businesses involved in the processing, packaging, transportation, and marketing of food.

agroecosystem An agricultural system that includes cropland, pasture, land for livestock, and uncultivated land adjacent to a farm that supports vegetation and wildlife and the corresponding atmosphere, soil, groundwater, and drainage. A sustainable agroecosystem maintains natural resources and does not rely on artificial inputs to manage pests and disease outbreaks among the crops.

air cell The pocket of air usually found at the large end of an egg between the outer and inner shell membranes.

al dente Italian phrase meaning "to the tooth" used to describe cooked pasta that is tender yet firm enough to be resistant when bitten.

albumen The clear substance consisting of water-soluble protein that surrounds the yolk of an egg.

aleurone The layer between the bran and endosperm in cereal kernels.

amino acids Organic molecules containing carbon, hydrogen, oxygen, and nitrogen. Twenty-two amino acids are found in nature. The basic structure of amino acids involves an alpha-carbon atom linked to an amino (NH2) group, a carboxylic group (COOH), a hydrogen atom, and a side group denoted by the letter R.

amyloplast An organelle in some plant cells that stores starch; commonly found in starchy plants such as tubers and fruits.

analytical tests Sensory tests used to detect discernible differences.

anthropogenic effect That which is created by or caused by human activity.

aquaculture The farming of fish and other aquatic species.

aroma Fragrance/smell of coffee or tea.

aseptic packaging Process whereby food can be batch heated in a sterile fashion and then placed in a sterilized container.

aspartame A non-nutritive sweetener that is 200 times sweeter than sucrose.

barm Foam at of the top of fermenting beer that was used as yeast for bread.

biobased product A commercial or industrial product or package made of at least 25% biological products, renewable agricultural materials (including plant, animal, and marine materials), or forestry materials.

biocapacity The regenerative capacity and the availability of the natural resources of the planet.

biodiversity The variety of life forms that make up a community, including plants, animals, fungi, and microorganisms. In recent years, the term has come to stand for the concepts and principles of conservation.

biofilm A collection of microorganisms that form a surface-like lining.

bivalve Mollusk characterized by having two shells attached by a hinge.

blanch To cook produce for 1 to 2 minutes to destroy plant enzymes that can affect color and flavor.

bound water The portion of the total water content of a product that is bound to chemicals in food.

bran The high-fiber outer layers of cereal kernels that protect the endosperm and germ.

brown rice Hulled, unprocessed whole grain rice.

bulgur Cracked wheat produced from steamed and dried or roasted wheat berries.

butter A milk product made by churning cream until it reaches a semisolid state.

buttermilk A cultured dairy product made by adding a harmless bacterial culture to fresh, pasteurized low-fat or nonfat milk. Once heated, lactic acid is produced, resulting in a liquid with a thick texture and tangy flavor.

caffeine Alkaloid compound that occurs naturally in coffee beans and tea leaves; a stimulant that acts on the adenosine receptors as cinnamic acids.

caloric sweetener Substance that gives a pleasant sensation of sweetness to foods and that can be absorbed and yield energy in the body. Includes simple sugars, sugar alcohols, and high-fructose corn syrup.

candling A process that uses light to help determine the quality of an egg.

carbohydrates One of the four major classes of nutrients. With an energy value of 4 calories per gram, these compounds are one of the most basic nutrients in foods.

carmelization A series of reactions involving dehydration, isomerization, and polymerization, resulting in the formation of polymeric caramels (caramel colloids). Caramels are responsible for the dark brown colors of certain foods.

carotenoids Plant compounds known for their yellow-orange color and antioxidant properties.

case control study A case series on individuals who have the disease of interest and a group of similar individuals who do not have the disease. Exposure comparisons can be made.

case report Detailed reports of a condition or disease in a single individual. Case reports can be suggestive, but it is often difficult to exclude alternative explanations for a condition/disease. These studies are usually used to study rare diseases.

case series Compiled from multiple case reports describing the same conditions. Routine surveillance programs can often be used to compile a case series.

casein The main protein found in milk. Under certain conditions it coagulates, forming clumps; this is a key step in making cheese.

cellulose A homo-polysaccharide of glucose that is indigestible by human enzymes. Cellulose is the predominant component of plant cell walls and, being indigestible, has no caloric contribution.

cephalopod Mollusk with a small internal shell.

cereals Edible kernels from plants of the grass family.

chalazae The twisted cordlike strands of egg white that anchor the yolk in the center of the white.

chlorogenic acid A dietary phenol that has been found have antioxidant effects.

chloroplast Organelle in plant cells where photosynthesis takes place; contains the green pigment chlorophyll.

choline A micronutrient essential for breaking down fats to produce energy and maintain cell membranes.

chromoplast A plant cell organelle that contains colored compounds other than chlorophyll.

climacteric fruits Fruits that continue to ripen once picked.

Clostridium botulinum A pathogenic bacterium that produces a neurotoxin and grows in anaerobic conditions, making it one of the major safety concerns to food processors.

cohort study Participants are classified based on the presence or absence of exposure and then followed over time to assess disease development. In a retrospective cohort study, the disease of interest has already occurred at the time the study begins; in a prospective cohort study, the disease has not yet occurred.

collagen Connective tissue found in meats that will break down and form gelatin under moist heat.

comminution The process of finely dicing meat during industrial food processing.

complete protein Proteins containing all essential amino acids. Examples include meat and dairy proteins, soybeans.

consumer panel A panel selected from the public according to the demographics necessary to taste test a product.

conventional agriculture Industrialized agricultural system characterized by mechanization, crop monocultures, and the use of chemical fertilizers and pesticides. Its emphasis is on productivity and profitability.

converted rice Long-grain rice that is parboiled before milling.

couscous A semolina grain rolled into small, round pellets.

cracked wheat Wheat berries that are crushed or cut into small pieces.

cream A rich, liquid form of milk that contains at least 18% milk fat. It is more viscous than milk and is an off-white or yellowish color.

creaming The process by which milk fat begins to rise and form a layer at the top when fresh milk stands for a while.

crème fraîche A thin sour cream made from unpasteurized cream and bacteria that is popular in French cuisine.

crop yield Also called agricultural output; the amount of a crop harvested per unit over a given period of time; can refer to the crop as a whole as well as to an individual plant.

cross-sectional survey Examines individuals with respect to both exposure and disease at a specific point in time. Because exposure and disease are assessed at the same time, it can be difficult to determine whether the exposure predated the disease.

crumb The dry particles in the bread crust.

crustacean Invertebrate with a jointed external skeleton.

cryoprotectant A molecule that protects biological tissue against structural damage (due to ice formation) during freezing and thawing.

crystalline candy Candy that contains crystals in its final form, such as fudge and fondant.

curd The semisolid portion created when milk coagulates.

curdling The process by which milk separates into its solid and liquid components, typically caused by overcooking, high heat, or the presence of acids or salt.

curing Preservation technique used in making meat products such as sausage and frankfurters.

cytoplasm Fluid inside a plant or animal cell that contains the organelles.

degermed cornmeal Cornmeal produced with the bran and germ removed prior to milling the corn endosperm.

descriptive panel A panel commonly used to determine differences between food samples. The descriptive panelist is experienced in the type of food being tested and receives extensive training prior to the testing.

descriptive tests Sensory tests designed to provide information on the specific sensory characteristics of food samples and to quantify the sensory differences.

dietary fiber Carbohydrates and lignin that are intrinsic to a plant's structure but that are indigestible by human digestive enzymes.

Dietary Guidelines for Americans Nutrition, dietary, and food safety recommendations that are designed to promote health and reduce the risk of chronic disease for healthy Americans ages 2 years and older. The *Dietary Guidelines for Americans* are the foundation of federal nutrition policies, nutrition education programs, and information activities.

difference tests Sensory tests designed to detect discernible differences.

disaccharides Sugars composed of two monosaccharides that have joined together as a result of a dehydration synthesis reaction that results in a glycosidic bond. Disaccharides are present in cane and beet sugar (sucrose), milk sugar (lactose) and malt sugar (maltose).

dispersion Formed when substances called colloids are too large to dissolve in a solvent. Instead, they remain in the solvent as an unstable dispersion. Dispersions are further classified as suspensions or emulsions.

diterpenes Naturally occurring organic compounds that are found in some essential oils and are thought to have antibacterial, antiviral, antifungal, and expectorant properties.

docosahexaenoic acid (DHA) A type of omega-3 fatty acid that is found in fish oil.

double-blind placebo-controlled design A design whereby neither the participants nor the investigator knows who has been assigned to a treatment or a placebo group. This study design is usually considered to provide the most compelling evidence of a cause-and-effect relationship.

dough conditioner Chemicals used in commercial baking that improve the finished bread product, such as providing better loaf volume and a softer crumb.

drop batter Calls for a liquid-to-dry ratio of about 1:2; examples include cornbread and muffin batters.

dry heat cooking methods Meat preparation methods that do not include the addition of liquid, such as broiling, grilling, frying, and roasting.

duo-trio test A difference test in which three samples are presented at the same time. A reference is designated, and the judge is asked to select the one most similar to the reference.

durum A type of hard wheat that is higher in protein than other wheat types; it is used for pasta.

ecological literacy An understanding of the interconnected systems and associated relationships that sustain the web of life.

ecosystem A dynamic complex of plant, animal, and microorganism communities, as well as the nonliving environment, that interact and function as a unit.

ecosystem services Benefits society obtains from ecosystems, including food and water; the regulation of floods, drought, land degradation, and disease; soil formation and nutrient cycling; and cultural, recreational, spiritual, religious, and other nonmaterial benefits.

edible films Materials applied to foods that provide a benefit to the food and can be consumed by the end user; they typically allow for selective gas exchange to preserve quality, while retaining moisture or preventing microbial growth.

egg foam Created when the albumen (egg white) is whipped; when heated, the air expands and the protein in the egg foam solidifies, creating a light texture for soufflés, cakes, and meringues.

egg product The result of removing eggs from their shells and processing them into liquid, frozen, and dried forms.

egg white Common name used for the albumen that surrounds the yolk of an egg.

eicosapentaenoic acid (EPA) A type of omega-3 fatty acid that is found in fish oil.

elastin Connective tissue found in meats that must be physically removed or trimmed prior to consumption of the meat product.

electrolytes Ions in bodily fluids that are integral to metabolic and energetic processes; include chloride, sodium, and potassium.

emulsifier A mixture that requires the suspension of one liquid in another; for example, a mixture of water in margarine, shortening, or ice cream.

emulsion A type of dispersion where the colloidal particles disperse completely within the medium (the second phase). Milk, mayonnaise, and gravies are examples of emulsions.

endosperm The large inner portion of cereal kernels that contains large amounts of starch in a protein matrix.

enrichment Adding back of nutrients after processing of a food. The Flour Enrichment Act of 1972 mandated the addition of thiamin, riboflavin, niacin, and iron to flour.

enzymatic browning Process whereby the enzyme polyphenol oxidase (PPO) catalyzes the oxidation of phenols into brown-colored melanins.

enzyme Biocatalysts that speed up the rate of biochemical reactions, without getting destroyed themselves. Not all proteins are enzymes, but all enzymes are proteins. Each enzyme catalyzes a specific type of reaction.

ergogenic aids Substances or practices believed to improve athletic performance that are taken before, during, or after physical activity.

fair trade Movement that seeks to empower farmers and farm workers, protect the environment, and help farmers develop appropriate business skills to compete in a global market.

farina Coarsely ground wheat endosperm.

fat extenders Ingredients that optimize the functionality of fat, allowing for a decrease in the usual amount of fat required by a product.

fat substitutes Also called fat mimetics, ingredients that mimic one or more of the roles of fat in food, such as providing moisture, mouthfeel, and other characteristics of fat by holding water.

fatty acid Aliphatic chains with a carboxylic acid (–COOH) functional group.

fermentation The general transformation of organic substances, such as simple sugars, into smaller molecules by the action of microorganisms.

finfish Aquatic vertebrate with gills, fins, and an internal skeleton.

finishing diet The diet fed to livestock animals immediately prior to slaughter.

flavor The combined sense of taste, odor, and mouthfeel.

flavor scalping The absorption of volatile food flavors by packaging materials.

flexitarian diet A primarily vegetarian eating plan, but its adopters occasionally eat meat.

fluorosis A condition caused by exposure to excessive amounts of fluoride that is characterized by skeletal changes and by mottled tooth enamel.

food foam Two-phase system where air is dispersed in a continuous liquid or solid phase.

food insecurity When households have difficulty providing enough food for all their members due to lack of resources.

food science Encompasses the investigation of better ways to select, preserve, process, package, and distribute food products.

fortification Addition of certain nutrients to a food as a means to prevent specific nutrient deficiencies in the population.

fractionation The physical separation of oils into saturated and unsaturated fractions.

freezer burn Shriveled cells on food that have lost too much moisture due to sublimation.

fruitarian diet Diet characterized by consumption of fruits, nuts, seeds, and, in some cases, legumes.

functional fiber Indigestible carbohydrates that have been isolated, extracted, or manufactured and that have been clinically proven to have a physiological benefit.

functional food Foods or food components that offer health benefits beyond basic nutrition.

gelatinization Process that involves heating starch granules in a moist environment; the granules swell as water is absorbed and disrupt the organization of the starch granules.

Generally Recognized as Safe (GRAS) A designation given to a food or drug by the Food and Drug Administration (FDA) when it is approved for public use.

genetically modified organisms (GMOs) Organisms that have been transformed by the insertion of one or more transgenes (genes not naturally found in the organism). Organisms in which the genetic material (DNA) has been altered in a way that does not occur naturally.

germ The smallest part of the cereal kernel; it produces a sprout for a new plant.

gluconeogenesis Production of new glucose by metabolic pathways within the cell.

gluten The protein complex formed from the fractions gliadin and glutenin when flour is mixed with water.

glutinous rice Short-grain rice that produces sticky clumps desired for sushi and rice cakes, also called sticky or waxy rice.

glycemic index (GI) A ranking system that quantifies the effect that food carbohydrates have on blood glucose levels.

glycemic load Calculated by taking the glycemic index of a food, multiplying it by the grams of carbohydrates in the serving, and dividing by 100. Takes into account the quality as well as the quantity of carbohydrates by considering serving sizes of carbohydrate-containing foods.

glycerol A three-carbon compound with three alcohol (hydroxyl) groups, each of which is esterified with a fatty acid.

glycogen The primary carbohydrate in animal muscle; it is converted to lactic acid after slaughter.

grading A voluntary process in which meat products are rated for their quality.

grain General term for all cereals and cereal plants.

greenhouse effect A naturally occurring process whereby gasses trap heat in the atmosphere. Human activities have generated more of these gases, particularly carbon dioxide, resulting in the warming of earth's atmosphere.

groats Whole cereal kernels, such as oat groats.

gustatory Relating to the sense of taste.

half and half A combination of cream and whole milk with more than 18%, but less than 30%, milk fat.

health claim Claim on a food label that state that there is a relationship between a substance or nutrient in the food product and a disease or health-related condition. Such claims must be reviewed and approved by the FDA.

hedonic scale A test that uses pictures applicable to questions of sensory intensities.

heirloom Plants from seed of older times.

herbicide A type of pesticide used to kill unwanted plants. Herbicides target a specific type of plant while leaving others intact. Plants can produce natural herbicides in reaction to an encounter with an undesirable species or substance.

holding time The minimum and maximum time after preparation that a product can be used for a sensory test.

hominy Corn endosperm.

hominy grits Coarsely milled hominy.

homocysteine An amino acid produced in the body and a potential contributor to heart disease and certain age-related diseases when blood levels are elevated.

homogenization A process whereby the fat globules in milk are reduced in size and evenly distributed throughout the liquid.

hormonal growth promotants (HGPs) Hormones administered to livestock to promote weight gain prior to slaughter.

humectants Food components used to retain moisture in the matrix.

hydrogenation The addition of hydrogen atoms to an unsaturated fatty acid, causing the double bonds (unsaturated) to become single bonds (saturated).

hydrolysis Chemical reaction where a water molecule is used to split a compound into simpler molecules.

hydrolytic rancidity Spoilage in fats associated with the presence of water. The triglycerides react with water, freeing their fatty acids from glycerol and breaking down into volatile secondary products with an off flavor.

hyponatremia Condition when blood serum sodium falls below normal levels.

imitation cheese A product similar to processed cheese, but the butterfat is replaced by vegetable oil, nonfat milk, or whey solids mixed with water.

incomplete protein Proteins that lack one or more essential amino acid. Most plant proteins are incomplete proteins.

inspection A federally mandated process whereby trained officials inspect meat processing plants to ensure food safety.

instant or quick-cooking cereal Precooked cereal that only requires rehydration.

intelligent packaging Technology built into a package that lets a food processor, distributor, seller, or consumer know something about the internal or external environment of the package.

interesterification Free fatty acids with the desired degree of saturation and carbon length that can be added to a mixture of triglycerides to develop fats with the desired melting and/or smoke point and stability.

intervention study A type of prospective cohort study where the exposure is controlled by the investigator. These studies can be considered therapeutic (secondary prevention) or preventative. Dietary Approaches to Stop Hypertension (DASH) was an intervention study.

irradiation The exposure of food products to ionizing radiation in the form of gamma rays, X-rays, or electron beams to kill microbes.

kasha Roasted buckwheat groats.

lactic acid Biological compound that builds up in animal carcasses after slaughter, reducing the pH of the meat.

lacto vegetarian diet Diet characterized by the consumption of plant-based foods and the addition of dairy products.

lacto-ovo vegetarian diet Diet characterized by the consumption of plant-based foods and the addition of dairy products and eggs.

lactose Milk sugar composed of glucose and galactose.

laying hens Domesticated chickens raised solely for the purpose of egg production.

leavening agent An ingredient in leavened bread that incorporates gas bubbles into the dough, causing it to rise.

lecithin A phospholipid found in the cell membrane of egg yolks; used as an emulsifier in cooking.

legumes A class of vegetables that have edible seed pods, including beans, peas, lentils, and peanuts. Sometimes referred to as pulses.

light cream Cream containing more than 18%, but less than 30%, milk fat; also called table cream or coffee cream.

lipids Organic compounds that are soluble in organic solvents. Like carbohydrates, lipids are composed of carbon, hydrogen, and oxygen; however, lipids have higher proportions of hydrogen and less of oxygen.

living systems The animate, interconnected components and processes of ecosystems (no matter how small or large).

low-fat milk Milk in which some of the fat has been removed; contains 1% milk fat.

lutein A carotenoid found in eggs and green leafy vegetables that may act as an antioxidant, protecting the eyes from cataracts and age-related macular degeneration.

lycopene Bright red compound found in tomatoes and some other red fruits and vegetables.

lyophilization Freeze-drying.

macaroni General term for all dried pasta products made with wheat flour and water.

macrobiotic diet An eating regimen first popularized in Japan; a predominantly vegetarian diet that is based on grains and supplemented with local vegetables. People following this diet avoid highly processed or refined foods and most animal products.

Maillard reaction Nonenzymatic chemical reaction that occurs between reducing sugars and amino groups of amino acids and proteins; results in a brown color and change in flavor.

malt Sprouted, dried barley.

marbling Fat interspersed throughout muscle tissue.

meal Coarsely ground cereal milled finer than grits but not as fine as flour.

meat extenders Protein substances added to meat; sometimes used synonymously with "meat fillers," which are usually carbohydrate substances.

metabolic diet study Randomized control trial conducted in a clinical research center where study participants are randomized into test or control groups and fed an experimental diet or a "regular" diet, respectively.

methane Greenhouse gas produced by livestock.

metmyoglobin Compound formed when myoglobin is exposed excessively to oxygen and the iron converts to the ferric state, causing the meat to become brownish-red.

milling The process of grinding grain in a mill.

mineral Elements other than carbon, hydrogen, oxygen, and nitrogen that are present in foods. Minerals are heat stable and are classified as major or trace, depending on their concentrations in plants and animals.

modified atmosphere packaging (MAP) The deliberate manipulation of the gases or the diffusion of gases within a food package to enhance shelf life and reduce spoilage.

moist heat cooking methods Meat preparation methods that include the addition of a liquid (e.g., water), such as braising, stewing, simmering, and steaming.

molecular gastronomy Form of modern gourmet cooking that seeks to identify all the physical and chemical changes that occur during food production and cooking to create the best flavor and texture.

mollusk Invertebrate with a hardened shell.

monoculture The cultivation of a single crop year-to-year on the same land.

monosaccharides Simple sugar composed of one basic unit. Examples include: glucose, fructose, and galactose.

monounsaturated fatty acids Fatty acids that have one unsaturated bond. Oleic acid (18:1) is the most common monounsaturated fatty acid. The double bond has a cis configuration.

mouthfeel The way that a particular type of food feels in the mouth.

municipal solid waste (MSW) Solid material that must be disposed of; food packaging contributes significantly to MSW.

myoglobin Primary pigment found in meats.

myosin Thick filament in muscle fibrils that binds with actin in muscle contraction and relaxation.

natural eggs Eggs that do not have artificial ingredients or added color. The term natural is not regulated by the USDA. The term does not limit the use of antibiotics, type of feed, or define the laying hen housing system. Use of the term on a product requires an explanation of the use of the word "natural"; e.g., "no added colorings or artificial ingredients."

neotame A sweetener that is 8,000 times sweeter than sugar. It is heat stable and can be used in baking.

nitric oxide myoglobin Pigment found in cured meats that causes the meat to turn pink.

nonclimacteric fruits Fruits that only ripen when left on the plant.

noncrystalline (amorphous) candy Candy that does not contain crystals, such as taffy and caramels.

nonenzymatic browning The most common type of browning in processed foods. These reactions occur at elevated temperatures and include the caramelization of sugars and Maillard reactions between amino acids and sugars.

nonfat milk Also referred to as skim milk and fat-free milk, this milk has as much of the milk fat removed as possible. In order to be labeled as nonfat, it must contain less than 0.5% milk fat.

non-nutritive sweeteners Substances that give a pleasant sensation of sweetness to foods, but that supply limited or no energy to the body; also called artificial or alternative sweeteners.

nutrient content claim Statement that a food company can place on a product label that reflects the product's nutrient content. For example, a package label may state that the product "Contains 100 calories." Companies can also state that a particular food is a "good source" of a nutrient or that a food is a "high" source of a nutrient.

nutrigenomics Study of how food affects our genes and the way our bodies respond to nutrients.

nutrition ecology An interdisciplinary science that encompasses all aspects of the food chain and the entire nutrition system and their effects on health, the natural environment, society, and the economy.

nutrition transition The major shift in the types of foods consumed by human populations and the resultant effect upon body composition and health.

ochratoxin A (OTA) A mycotoxin produced by *Penicillium* and *Aspergillus* fungi.

olfactory Relating to the sense of smell.

oligosaccharides Typically composed of 3 to 10 monosaccharide units. They are found in small amounts in foods.

omega-3 fatty acids Polyunsaturated fatty acids that have their first double bond on the third carbon from the methyl end of the fatty acid chain. They are essential to the human diet and include docosahexaenoic acid (DHA), eicosapentaenoic acid (EPA), and alpha-linolenic acid (ALA).

omega-6 fatty acids Polyunsaturated fatty acids that have the first double bond on the sixth carbon atom from the methyl end. These essential PUFAs, when consumed in moderate amounts, help regulate metabolism, stimulate growth of skin and hair, and maintain bone health. Dietary sources include palm, soybean, rapeseed, and sunflower oils.

omnivore diet Diet characterized by the consumption of both plant-based foods and animal products.

osmolality/osmolar solution Concentration of a solution expressed as osmoles of solute per liter of solution or as milliosmols per kilogram (mOsm/kg) of water.

osmosis Movement of water molecules across a membrane toward a more concentrated solution to achieve concentration equilibrium.

ovalbumin The main protein found in the albumen or egg white; it makes up 60–65% of the total protein in an egg.

oven spring The rapid increase in volume in a loaf of bread during the first few minutes of baking.

ovo vegetarian diet Diets characterized by the consumption of plant-based foods and the addition of eggs.

oxidative rancidity Spoilage in oil that is also referred to as auto-oxidation. Occurs when the lipids are catalyzed in the presence of heat or light.

oxymyoglobin Compound formed when the myoglobin pigment comes into contact with oxygen, causing the meat to become bright red.

paired comparison test A difference test in which two samples are presented, and the judge is asked to select the one that has more of a particular characteristic.

papillae Rough bulges or protuberances in the surface of the tongue, some of which contain taste buds.

parboiling The partial cooking of food as the first step in the cooking process.

pasta General term for any macaroni or noodle product.

pasteurization The process of heating a food or beverage to a high enough temperature to destroy harmful pathogenic bacteria.

pasteurized processed cheese Products created by combining shredded or ground pasteurized cheeses with emulsifiers and flavors; they are less expensive than natural cheeses and have a longer shelf life, because they do not ripen with age.

peptide bond (or amide bond) Covalent bond between the nitrogen of one amino acid with the carbon of the carboxylic group of the adjacent amino acid.

pescatarian (pesco vegetarian diet) Diet characterized by the exclusion of all meat except from fish and may include eggs or dairy products.

phenolic compound Substances that affect the taste, aroma, mouthfeel and nutrient content of fruits and vegetables that contain them.

phenylketonuria (PKU) A rare genetic disease caused by a lack or deficiency of the enzyme phenylalanine hydroxylase that breaks down the essential amino acid phenylalanine.

phospholipid The resulting diglyceride when one of the fatty acids in a triglyceride is replaced by a phosphate group.

photosynthesis Process whereby plants use sunlight, water, and carbon dioxide to create oxygen and glucose.

phytochemical Any biologically active compound found in plants. Many are considered beneficial in the prevention of chronic diseases.

phytonutrients (or phytochemicals) Non-nutritive chemicals derived from plants that may play a role in disease prevention and human health.

plant-based diet A diet that is primarily made up from plant food sources but may include some animal products.

plasticity Describes the suppleness or workability of batter or dough.

polished white rice Milled brown rice with a smooth surface due to the rubbing away of the bran and germ from the rice kernels during milling.

polysaccharides Composed of long chains of monosaccharide units bound together by glycosidic bonds. They usually have more than 10 monosaccharide units. The basic units are linked as straight chains or branched chains, long and short. Amylopectin and glycogen are two important polysaccharides.

polyunsaturated fatty acid Fatty acids that have multiple unsaturated bonds. Linoleic acid (18:2) and linolenic acid (18:3) are the most common polyunsaturated fatty acids in vegetable oils used in cooking. The double bonds have a cis configuration.

pome A fleshy fruit with a middle core and seeds; examples include apples and pears.

population or correlational study Study that uses data from entire populations to compare event (such as disease) frequencies with an exposure in different groups during the same time period or in the same group at different times. Because these studies look at whole populations rather than individuals, it is impossible to link an individual exposure with the occurrence of disease in that individual—a major limitation of this type of study.

pour batter Calls for a liquid-to-dry ratio of about 1:1; pours in a steady stream (for example, pancake batter).

pressing The process of breaking the cell wall by grinding, flaking, rolling, or pressing under high pressure to liberate oil.

pressure-assisted thermal sterilization (PATS) A process used in low-acid canned products that can inactivate *Clostridium botulinum* spores with lower temperatures (49°F; 121°C) and lower holding time (3 minutes) than traditional methods of processing.

primary structure Linear arrangement of amino acids in a protein chain.

processed cheese food A product containing less real cheese than processed cheese; it typically has added water, milk solids, and/or vegetable oil to make it softer and more spreadable. It must have a minimum fat content of 23% and a maximum of 44%.

profiling A group of highly trained panelists work together to develop the vocabulary needed to provide specific descriptions of food samples; used to detail the specific flavors (flavor profiling) or textures (texture profiling) of a food or beverage.

proofing Stage in bread making where the bread dough is left to rise for the last time after it is molded into a loaf and placed into the baking pan. During this stage, starch is converted into sugars, producing carbon dioxide and alcohol. The result is dough expansion and flavor development.

protein coagulation Congealing and separating out of denatured proteins.

protein complementation Combining two or more different protein sources to have a better amino acid balance than when consuming either protein alone.

protein denaturation The disruption of bonds that make up the tertiary and secondary structure of proteins. Can occur through the addition of heat, alcohol, acids, salts, enzymes, and mechanical shear.

proteins Complex polymers of amino acids.

pullets An alternate term for laying hens.

quaternary structure How multiple peptide chains are aggregated together by hydrogen bonds, disulfide linkages, and salt bridges into a final specific protein shape.

quick bread Bread products that require no rising or proofing time. Quick breads vary widely in the consistency of their dough or batter.

rancidity Condition produced by oxidation of unsaturated fats present in foods and other products. An unpleasant odor or flavor is generated when the fatty substance is exposed to air.

randomized design A study design whereby individuals are randomly assigned to a treatment or control group.

ranking test A difference or preference test in which more than two samples are presented and all samples are compared by ranking them from lowest to highest for the intensity of a specific characteristic.

rating difference test Test to differentiate among multiple samples that uses a rating scale. Products are ranked using a rating scale to assess for differences between samples.

ratite Flightless bird such as ostrich and emu.

raw food diet Diet that may or may not consist entirely of vegetarian foods; comprises mostly uncooked or unprocessed foods.

raw milk Milk in its natural form that has not undergone processing such as pasteurization and homogenization.

reduced-fat milk Milk in which some of the fat has been removed; contains 2% milk fat.

refined flour Wheat flour that has the germ and bran removed and usually has been whitened as well.

rennin An enzyme derived from calves' stomachs that is used to coagulate the milk protein casein.

resistant starch (RS) Starch that cannot be enzymatically digested by humans.

resveratrol A strong antioxidant and anti-inflammatory compound found in red wine, grape juice, and peanuts.

retort pouch A flexible container that is aseptic or void of microorganisms.

rope Bacterial decomposition of bread whereby protein and starch become discolored and sticky.

saccharin A non-nutritive sweetener that is about 300 to 700 times sweeter than sucrose.

Salmonella Rod-shaped bacteria responsible for many foodborne illnesses.

saturated fatty acids Fatty acids in which all of the hydrogens are saturated and there are no double bonds between the carbon atoms of the fatty acid chain. Stearic acid (18:0) and palmitic acid (16:0) are the most common saturated fatty acids found in food.

saturated solution Solution that has the maximum amount of solute that can be dissolved in the solvent.

scorching Burning of milk that occurs when casein micelles and whey protein drop to the bottom of the pan, stick, and burn.

secondary structure Foldings or coilings within a protein structure that are stabilized by hydrogen bonding.

semolina Durum flour used for production of pasta and couscous.

sensory evaluation The scientific measurement method of food quality based on sensory characteristics as perceived by the five senses.

shell Outer covering of egg, composed mainly of calcium carbonate; may be white or brown depending on the breed of chicken.

shell membranes Two membranes, outer and inner, that surround the albumen (white) of an egg; they provide a protective barrier against bacterial penetration.

shellfish Freshwater or saltwater invertebrate with a hard external skeleton or shell.

slurry A starch mixed in a cool or cold liquid.

soft dough Calls for a liquid-to-dry ratio of about 1:3; an example includes chocolate chip cookie dough.

solution When solute molecules completely dissolve in a solvent without precipitating out.

sour cream A cultured dairy product made by adding a harmless bacterial culture to pasteurized, homogenized light cream. Sour cream has a milk fat content no less than 18%.

spice A flavorful component of a plant other than the leaves used in cooking. Examples include turmeric and ginger (rhizome); celery, cumin, and poppy (seed); allspice (fruit); and cinnamon (bark).

sponge The use of a mixture of liquid, yeast, sugar, and flour to make a thin batter to allow yeast activity. This mixture is then added to the remaining ingredients to form dough.

sports drink Beverage designed to quench thirst faster than water and replenish the sugar and minerals lost from the body during physical exercise.

staling Stiffening of bread that results from changes that occur after baking possibly due to shifting of water from gluten to starch/amylopectin, thereby changing the nature of the gluten network.

starch gelatinization The loss of molecular organization within starch granules characterized by irreversible swelling and loss of birefringence.

starch gelation Process whereby amylose molecules leach out of the starch granules and form intermolecular hydrogen bonds. The result is a three-dimensional network of amylose molecules with entrapped water and starch granules. Responsible for the texture of many sauces and puddings.

stevia A non-nutritive sweetener obtained from the leaves of a South American plant that is 300 times sweeter than sucrose.

stiff dough Calls for a liquid-to-dry ratio of about 1:8; sugar cookie dough is considered stiff dough.

stone The pit of a fruit; found in fruits such as cherries, plums, and peaches.

structure/function claim Claim on a food package that describes the role of a substance in the food in maintaining a structure in or function of the human body. Such claims do not require preapproval by FDA.

sublimation The phase change whereby a material goes directly from solid to gas, bypassing the liquid phase.

sucralose A non-nutritive sweetener made from sucrose that is 600 times sweeter than sugar.

sugar alcohols Also called polyols, compounds formed from monosaccharides by replacing a hydrogen atom with a hydroxyl group. Used as nutritive sweeteners.

suspension A type of dispersion where the large colloidal molecules remain suspended in the media and are visibly distinct, such as when starch is suspended in cold water.

sustainable agriculture An agricultural system that is founded in the principles of ecology; sustainable agriculture is economically viable, socially conscious, and capable of maintaining high productivity.

syneresis "Weeping" of a starch gel due to rapid heating or cooling.

taste bud One of the small parts of gustatory and supportive cells; usually found on the upper surface of the tongue.

tertiary structure Final three dimensional structure of protein that involves numerous noncovalent interactions between amino acids.

texture The sensory manifestation of the structure or inner makeup of products in terms of their feel as measured by tactile nerves on the surface of the skin of the hands, lips, or tongue.

textured soy protein (TSP) A protein-rich meat alternative made from defatted soy flour or soybeans.

thermophiles Organisms that can live in high temperatures.

thermoplastics Category of plastics used for food packaging because they soften when heated and can be reshaped, molded, and recycled.

triangle test A difference test in which three samples are presented simultaneously (two of which are the same), and the judge is asked to identify the odd sample.

ultra-high-pressure (UHP) processing Use of pressure to inactivate microorganisms; also known as high hydrostatic pressure processing.

ultra-high-temperature (UHT) processing A high-heat pasteurization method where milk is heated to 280–300°F (138–150°C) for 2 to 6 seconds.

ultra-pasteurization A high-heat pasteurization method where milk is heated to 275°F (135°C) for 2 to 4 seconds.

umami Taste category based on glutamate compounds, which are commonly found in meats, mushrooms, soy sauce, fish sauce, and cheese.

vacuole The largest structure in the plant cell; it holds a mixture of sugars, enzymes, pigments, and other compounds that contribute to a food's flavor.

vegan Diet characterized by the consumption of exclusively plant-based foods and lifestyle habits that strive to exclude any animal derived products.

vegetarian diet Diet characterized by the consumption of plant-based foods with some (eggs and/or dairy) or no animal products.

vermicomposting The use of earthworms to convert organic waste into a nutrient-rich paste that can be used to replenish the soil.

vitamins Organic, nutritionally essential compounds that are mostly heat labile. They are classified as water soluble or fat soluble.

vitelline membrane A colorless membrane that surrounds the yolk.

water activity (a_w) The ratio of the vapor pressure of a food sample (p) to the vapor pressure of pure water (p_0) at the same temperature. In thermodynamic terms, it is a measure of the energy status of water in a system.

wheat berry A raw, unprocessed wheat kernel.

whey The liquid portion of coagulated (curdled) milk.

whipping cream Cream with enough fat content to be whipped into a foam; it comes in two varieties: light whipping cream, which contains between 30% to 36% milk fat and is used in ice cream and as a thickener in soups and sauces, and heavy cream, which is better for whipping and contains at least 36% milk fat.

whole milk Milk as it comes from the cow; composed of water (88%), milk fat (3.5%), and other milk solids (8.5%), such as protein, lactose, and minerals.

yeast A microscopic one-celled fungus used as a leavening agent. Saccharomyces cerevisiae is the species most commonly used in baking.

yeast bread Bread that is leavened by the action of yeast, which converts the fermentable sugars present in dough into the gas carbon dioxide. This causes the dough to expand or rise as the gas forms pockets or bubbles. When the dough is baked, the yeast dies and the air pockets "set," giving the baked product a soft and spongy texture.

yogurt A cultured dairy product made by combining bacterial cultures to milk; it is creamy and has a slightly tart aftertaste.

yolk The yellow, usually spherical, portion of an egg surrounded by the albumen that serves as nutrition for the developing chick in a fertilized egg; the yolk is a major source of vitamins and minerals. It contains almost half the egg's protein and all of the fat and cholesterol.

zeaxanthin A carotenoid found in eggs and green leafy vegetables that may act as an antioxidant, protecting eyes from cataracts and age-related macular degeneration.

Index

C

D

E

F

G

H

I

K

L

M

N

O

P

Q

R

S

T

U

V

W

Y

Z